BARRON'S

MCAT®

Medical College Admission Test®

3RD EDITION

Jay Cutts, M.A.
Director
Cutts Graduate Reviews
Albuquerque, New Mexico

Mariel Campbell, M.A.
Biology Instructor
Department of Biology and Biotechnology
Central New Mexico Community College
Albuquerque, New Mexico

Louis Gotlib, M.A.T.
Chemistry Teacher
Wissahickon High School
Ambler, Pennsylvania

Nicholas Christopher Hostetter, M.A.
Child Protective Services Worker
West Virginia Department of Health
and Human Resources
Hamlin, West Virginia

Beth Jakubanis, L.C.S.W.
Adjunct Professor
California State University, Northridge
California State University, Los Angeles
Los Angeles, California

Daniel Milton Oman, Ph.D.
Founder
PhysicsandCalculus.com
(Private tutoring and online learning)
Singapore

Robert Oman, Sc.M., Ph.D.
President
Oman Consulting, Inc.
St. Petersburg, Florida
Singapore

John R. Smolley, M.D.
Health Sciences Instructor
Albuquerque, New Mexico

J. Shield Wallace, Ph.D.
Professor of Chemistry
Central New Mexico Community College
Albuquerque, New Mexico

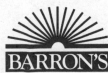

BARRON'S

All inquiries should be addressed to:
Barron's Educational Series, Inc.
250 Wireless Boulevard
Hauppauge, New York 11788
www.barronseduc.com

ISBN: 978-1-4380-7792-5

ISSN #: 2163-3347

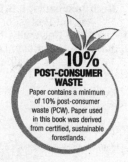

10%
POST-CONSUMER
WASTE
Paper contains a minimum
of 10% post-consumer
waste (PCW). Paper used
in this book was derived
from certified, sustainable
forestlands.

PRINTED IN THE UNITED STATES OF AMERICA
9 8 7 6 5 4 3 2 1

About the Authors

JAY CUTTS is director of the Cutts Graduate Reviews. He has taught the MCAT and other graduate exams since 1990 and specializes in individualized instruction on advanced cognitive skills for problem solving, critical analysis, and control of time. He has personally helped more than 1000 students worldwide get accepted to medical, graduate, and law school. In his spare time he plays Eastern European music on the accordion and is the author of *Death by Haggis*.

MARIEL CAMPBELL has conducted research in mammalian parasitology and disease epidemiology in the United States and South America. She also has more than 15 years experience teaching biology at the community college and university levels, including biology for health sciences, comparative anatomy, and human anatomy and physiology.

LOUIS GOTLIB is a Phi Beta Kappa graduate of The Johns Hopkins University and the University of North Carolina. He has taught many levels of chemistry over the past 30 years, and has coauthored Barron's GED and CLEP review books. His hobbies are playing chess and collecting slide rules.

NICHOLAS CHRISTOPHER HOSTETTER has a B.A. in sociology from Mary Washington College and an M.A. in sociology from Marshall University. He has nearly 10 years of experience working with the developmentally disabled, the homeless, and seniors. He has taught sociology at Bluegrass Community and Technical College and at Mountwest Community and Technical College. He is currently a child protective services worker with the West Virginia Department of Health and Human Resources.

BETH JAKUBANIS is a lecturer at California State University Northridge and California State University, Los Angeles, where she teaches Social Welfare and Clinical Practices to undergraduate and graduate students. She also provides continuing education to therapists in practice. Her psychotherapy private practice is located in Tarzana, California. Beth graduated from the University of California, Los Angeles, in 2008 with her masters in social welfare.

DANIEL MILTON OMAN received his M.S. in physics and his Ph.D. in electrical engineering from the University of South Florida in Tampa, Florida. After some time researching solar energy and teaching undergraduate physics students, he joined AT&T Bell Laboratories and Lucent Technologies in the semiconductor industry, where he worked on technology improvement and product engineering management. Since 2010, he has been running his own tutoring business in Singapore, specializing in physics, chemistry, and biology. He is also the founder of the online science learning website *www.physicsandcalculus.com*.

ROBERT OMAN received his Ph.D. in Physics from Brown University in Providence, Rhode Island. He was president of Oman Consulting, Inc., and the developer of the MCAT Physics Tutor website. He taught mathematics and physics at several colleges and universities and did research for Litton Industries, United Technologies, and NASA, where he developed the theoretical model for the first pressure gauge sent to the moon.

JOHN R. SMOLLEY earned his M.D. from the University of Utah and was a Ph.D. candidate in physiology. He practiced medicine full time for 15 years (psychiatry) and did a post-doctoral fellowship in membrane electrophysiology. Currently he is an MCAT instructor in Albuquerque and teaches health sciences to a variety of aspiring practitioners. John loves flying amateur rockets, growing culinary mushrooms, stargazing, and jazz.

J. SHIELD WALLACE holds a Ph.D. degree in bioorganic chemistry. He currently teaches courses in general and organic chemistry primarily to preprofessional students. Before his tenure at CNM, Professor Wallace held research and development positions with Sanofi-Aventis Pharmaceuticals, Sandia National Laboratories, and the United States Air Force. For the past several years, he has been preparing students for the chemistry-related aspects of the MCAT exam through review and strategy workshops.

Contents

Preface ix

Introduction 1

Orientation to the MCAT 1

Your Plan of Attack 7

Timing Strategy 9

Testing Strategy 15

Three-Month Study Plan 33

Practice, Practice, Practice: Online Resources 33

PART 1: BIOLOGICAL AND PHYSICAL SCIENCES

1 General Chemistry 37

Atomic Structure and the Periodic Table 37

Ionic and Covalent Bonding 57

States of Matter 71

Stoichiometry 93

Thermochemistry and Thermodynamics 107

Kinetics and Equilibrium 122

Solution Chemistry 137

Acid–Base Chemistry 149

Electrochemistry 165

Summary 173

General Chemistry Practice Exercises 174

Answer Key 181

Answers Explained 181

2 Physics 183

Math and Units of Measurement 183

Motion, Falling Bodies, and Projectiles 188

Forces (Including Friction) 198

Mass and Weight 207

Work, Energy, and Power 212

Torque and Equilibrium 223

Fluids 234

Mechanical Waves and Sound 245

Simple Harmonic Motion 258

Electrostatics...262
DC Circuits..270
Capacitance..278
Electromagnetism..281
Reflection, Refraction, Polarization, and Diffraction.......................................285
Mirrors and Lenses..293
Atoms and Nuclei..300
Summary...307
Physics Practice Exercises...308
Answer Key..316
Answers Explained...316

3   Biology..319
Cell Biology..319
Cell Metabolism and Enzymes..338
Microbiology...359
DNA and Protein Synthesis...368
Eukaryotic Cell Replication...398
Meiosis and Genetic Variability..404
Genetics...412
Population Genetics and Hardy–Weinberg..420
Evolution..421
Human Anatomy and Physiology...429
Developmental Biology..511
Summary...517
Biology Practice Exercises...518
Answer Key..527
Answers Explained...527

4   Organic Chemistry..531
Organic Compound Functional Groups...531
The Covalent Bond..533
Molecular Structure and Spectra..552
Separation and Purification Techniques...575
Hydrocarbon Compounds...588
Oxygen Functional Group Compounds...610
Amines...636
Answers to Practice Questions..644
Summary...649
Organic Chemistry Practice Exercises...650
Answer Key..657
Answers Explained...657

5 Biochemistry..659

   Amino Acids and Proteins...659

   Carbohydrates 669

   Lipids...677

   Principles of Bioenergetics...681

   Metabolism 683

   Summary 702

   Biochemistry Practice Exercises 703

   Answer Key 706

   Answers Explained...706

PART 2: SOCIAL SCIENCES

6 Psychology..711

   Sensory Processing...711

   Cognition and Language 716

   Psycho-Bio Constructs of Behavior..734

   Social Constructs of Behavior...763

   Learning, Attitude, and Behavior..766

   The Notion of Self and Identity Formation...773

   Attitudes and Beliefs That Affect Social Interactions......................................784

   Actions and Processes Underlying Social Interactions 790

   Summary 796

   Psychology Practice Exercises 797

   Answer Key 802

   Answers Explained...802

7 Sociology...805

   Theoretical Approaches...806

   Culture..807

   Socialization...810

   Social Institutions..814

   Elements of Social Interaction 815

   Demographic Characteristics of Society 817

   Social Class..821

   Prejudice and Discrimination..824

   Spatial Inequality 824

   Health Disparities..825

   Healthcare Disparities...826

   Summary 826

   Sociology Practice Exercises 827

   Answer Key 830

   Answers Explained...830

PART 3: CRITICAL REASONING

8 Critical Analysis and Reasoning Skills.................................835

An Overview..835

Tackling the Passage.....................................837

Understanding the Questions.............................846

Getting the Answer.......................................852

Sample Passage...857

Summary..868

Critical Analysis Practice Exercises....................869

Answer Key...885

Answers Explained..885

PART 4: PRACTICE TESTS

Practice Test 1.......................................893

Answer Key...974

Answers Explained..976

Practice Test 2......................................1003

Answer Key..1081

Answers Explained.......................................1083

Index...1107

Preface

This book is a fresh, up-to-date approach to the current MCAT. It is designed to help you, today's premed student, master the MCAT and get accepted to medical school. I'd like to share with you some of the elements that make this book uniquely effective.

First, Barron's *MCAT* contains more than just a direct and comprehensive review of science. It also teaches critical strategies, including those for test taking, problem solving, and the Critical Analysis and Reasoning section.

Second, an amazing team of MCAT prep specialists, educators, and scientists, as well as premed students, have given generously of their time and expertise to create this resource for you. These contributors were specifically chosen for their depth of practical experience in working with MCAT students as well as for their expertise in their fields. Together we represent nearly 100 years of hands-on teaching and test prep experience!

Third, the Barron's staff and the authors share the conviction that this book can best serve the premed community through your input. Most of the authors work with students on a daily basis and find their input invaluable. We also asked a team of over 60 current premed students to review the book before publication. Their feedback has helped us make sure that this book meets your needs.

I personally stand by the quality of this book. If you don't feel you're getting everything you need out of it, contact me through my website: *http://www.cuttsreviews.com/premed/*. At that site you can also access our other fine materials to support your prep, including our free MCAT Solution of the Week and our premed forum. Check the forum for discussions, updates, and corrections. The MCAT is still evolving, so be sure to come to my website for up-to-the-minute information. Sign in now so we can help you get started mastering the MCAT!

On behalf of all of us involved with this book, I wish you success in your pursuits.

Jay B. Cutts, MA
Director, Cutts Graduate Reviews

ACKNOWLEDGMENTS

I would like to thank the following people: Wayne Barr, Bob O'Sullivan, and Linda Turner at Barron's for their kind and wise guidance; the primary authors Mariel Campbell, Louis Gotlib, Chris Hostetter, Beth Jakubanis, Daniel and Robert Oman, John Smolley, and Shield Wallace for their extremely conscientious work; the additional authors Fahd Anzaar, Cynthia Arias, Michael Bisogno, Charles Buxbaum, Darrin Doran, Ashley Outlaw Frank, Jeff Grell, Steven Patrick Morrissey Jerrems, Sarah Jin, Sankar Kaliappan, Gary Montry, Ege Ozdemir, Katelyn Robillard, Hannah Rose, Pratik Shah, and Paige Souder for contributing according to their areas of expertise. We also thank the *123HelpMe.com* website for allowing us to adapt some of their essays.

I also want to thank the premed student review panel for their generous feedback: Avneesh Aggarwa, Sana Ahmad, Anton Alder, Terry Archer-Liefde, Jaishri Atri, Dylan Bailey, Lauren Barr, Husain Bawany, Nicole Beers, Jessica Chen, Cheng Cheng, Ify Chinedozi, Hannah Cunningham, John Cusimano, Donald DeSanto, Maleesa Dunsworth, Jennifer E. McBride, Maria Esposito, Amir Essani, Scott Fligor, Maria Galvez, Meera Gebrae, Chris Genovese, Jennifer Ginsberg, Reem Hamade, Rabia Hamidani, Taylor Harms, Guy Helman, Mitch Izower, Pauline Jackson, Cindy Jovin, Daniel Reid, Hajra Khan, Christine Khong, Stuart Kyllo, Ngan Lam, Zi-Qi Liew, David Livermore, Samaa Lutfi, Gina M. Labellarte, Erin M. Visalli, Reehan Malhance, Christopher Manzella, Bianca Martinez, Christine Mesa, Grant Riesberg, Momtaz Nahar, Anh Nguyen, Jackline Odhiambo, Drumil Pate, Janki Pate, Marylul Poupart, Gabriel Quinones-Medina, Nate Rhodes, Ajleeta Sangtani, Chris Schiller, Cole Seifers, Lance Slatton, Lanre Udu, Huong Vu, Austin Wetmore, Jessica Wheeley, Ariel White, Jessica Wickes, Chris Wright, Shaleena Young, and Arthurine Zakama.

Finally, I want to thank the premed advisors who helped us prepare revisions for the post-2015 MCAT—Ann Caplea, Walsh University; Carrie Christensen, St. Catherine College; and Khalilah Reddie, University of Massachusetts at Lowell—and also the premed and medical school students who provided valuable feedback: Amal Algahmi, Carolina Chiou, Michael Flowers, Mark Hoffman, Alex Karel, and Tyler Rhoades.

Jay Cutts

Introduction

→ **ORIENTATION TO THE MCAT**
→ **YOUR PLAN OF ATTACK**
→ **TIMING STRATEGY**
→ **TESTING STRATEGY**
→ **THREE-MONTH STUDY PLAN**

The introduction will help you master how to prepare for and take the MCAT. You should reread this section regularly to review these important strategies for doing your best on all parts of the MCAT. If you have not already read the preface to this book, do so now. It directs you to online resources to support your test preparation.

ORIENTATION TO THE MCAT

The Medical College Admission Test (MCAT) is a computer-based test given multiple times a year. The Association of American Medical Colleges (AAMC), which manages the MCAT, provides extensive information about the MCAT on their website at *www.aamc.org*. Be sure to visit this site and thoroughly review the available information.

The MCAT

The MCAT measures both your factual knowledge and problem-solving ability in the areas of biochemistry, biology, physics, general chemistry, organic chemistry, psychology, and sociology. In addition, many MCAT questions test your ability to read graphs, charts, and diagrams and to apply analytical reading and logic skills. The Critical Analysis and Reasoning Skills section of the test measures your ability to read and to analyze written material. All questions are multiple-choice, with four answer choices. No points are deducted for wrong answers on the MCAT. For this reason, be sure to fill in an answer for each question, even if you have not worked on the question.

TIP

Free MCAT Solution of the Week and Prep Planner.

Sign up now!

MCAT MATH STRATEGIES

MCAT questions typically require only basic math calculations. You cannot use a calculator. Don't worry, though. You shouldn't need one.
The most important math strategy is accuracy!
Estimate to make sure you are in the right range.
Write out each step of your calculations.

The four sections of the MCAT are the following:

Chemical and Physical Foundations of Biological Systems ("Chem/Phys")
Biological and Biochemical Foundations of Living Systems ("Biological")
Psychological, Social, and Biological Foundations of Behavior ("Psych/Soc")
Critical Analysis and Reasoning Skills ("CARS")

The first two sections above test biological and physical sciences and are covered in Part 1 of this book (Chapters 1 through 5). Part 2 reviews psychology and sociology (Chapters 6 and 7). Part 3 reviews the critical analysis section (Chapter 8).

CHEMICAL AND PHYSICAL FOUNDATIONS OF BIOLOGICAL SYSTEMS

The Chem/Phys section includes questions that draw on the following topics:

General Chemistry (33%)
Physics (25%)
Biochemistry (25%)
Organic Chemistry (15%)
Biology (2%)

THE CHEM/PHYS SECTION

59 questions
95 minutes
8–9 passages with 4–8 questions each
About 12–15 independent questions

Passages typically give background information, describe experiments, or set up a situation to be analyzed. Physics passages can be either purely physics or presented in a medical or biological context. The independent questions are not based on a passage and are not related to each other. They are placed in clusters of three to five questions, and the clusters appear in three to four places throughout the test, with one cluster typically at the end.

BIOLOGICAL AND BIOCHEMICAL FOUNDATIONS OF LIVING SYSTEMS

The Biological section includes questions that draw on the following topics:

Biology (65%)
Biochemistry (25%)
Organic Chemistry (6%)
General Chemistry (4%)

THE BIOLOGICAL SECTION

59 questions
95 minutes
8–9 passages with 4–8 questions each
About 12–15 independent questions

Passages typically give background information, describe experiments, or set up a situation to be analyzed. The independent questions are not based on a passage and are not related to each other. They are placed in clusters of three to five questions, and the clusters appear in three to four places throughout the test, with one cluster typically at the end.

Note that of the five science areas—biochemistry, biology, general chemistry, organic chemistry, and physics—all except physics can appear in either of the two science sections. Biochemistry is equally represented in both sections. Organic chemistry occurs more frequently in Chem/Phys (15%) but also accounts for 6% of Biological. General chemistry occurs in about 4% of Biological questions and Biology occurs in about 2% of Chem/Phys. Even the Psych/Soc test sections can include physical and biological science concepts.

PSYCHOLOGICAL, SOCIAL, AND BIOLOGICAL FOUNDATIONS OF BEHAVIOR

The Psych/Soc section includes questions that draw on the following topics:

Psychology (60%)
Sociology (30%)
Biology (10%)

THE PSYCH/SOC SECTION

59 questions

95 minutes

8–9 passages with 4–8 questions each

About 12–15 independent questions

Psych/Soc passages can be either purely psychology or sociology or can be presented in a medical or biological context.

CRITICAL ANALYSIS AND REASONING SKILLS

The CARS section presents long passages drawn on topics from the Humanities and Social Sciences.

THE CRITICAL ANALYSIS SECTION

53 questions

90 minutes

About 8 passages with 5–7 questions each

No independent questions

MCAT Scores

All sections are scored on a 15 point scale of 118 to 132. For each section, your score is derived from the total number of questions you get right (raw score). You are not penalized for wrong answers, and all correct answers are worth the same amount. The raw score is converted to the 15 point scale (scaled score) according to a curve based on the scores of recent test takers. The following table shows approximately how raw scores compare with scaled scores. Notice that a few more correct answers often results in a higher scaled score.

Score requirements for admissions to medical schools vary widely from school to school. In general, scores of 124 or below are not competitive. Scores in the 125 to 126 range may be competitive at some schools but will not be competitive at many others. Scores of 127 on each section will most likely be considered strong by many schools. Students applying to the most competitive schools, however, may need scores above 129. Schools often look at the combined score for all three numerically scored sections. As a result, a high score in one section can compensate for a slightly lower score in another section.

To convert a score on the pre-2015 MCAT to the new scale, add 117. For example, an old score of 10 is equal to 127 on the new scale.

Table 1. Converting Raw Scores to Scaled Scores

Chem/Phys, Biological, Psych/Soc		Critical Analysis	
Raw Score	Scaled Score*	Raw Score	Scaled Score*
0–3	118	1–2	118
4–7	119	3–6	119
8–12	120	7–11	120
13–17	121	12–15	121
18–21	122	16–19	122
22–25	123	20–24	123
26–29	124	25–29	124
30–34	125	30–34	125
35–40	126	35–39	126
41–46	127	40–43	127
47–50	128	44–45	128
51–53	129	46–47	129
54–55	130	48–49	130
56–57	131	50–51	131
58–59	132	52–53	132

*These scaled scores are an approximation. They vary from exam to exam.

Test Day Schedule

Table 2 shows you what your test day schedule may look like.

Table 2. MCAT Test Day Schedule

Examinee agreement and optional tutorial	15 minutes
Chemical and Physical Foundations	95 minutes (59 questions)
Break (optional)	10 minutes
Critical Analysis and Reasoning	90 minutes (53 questions)
Break (optional)	30 minutes
Biological and Biochemical Foundations	95 minutes (59 questions)
Break (optional)	10 minutes
Psychological, Social, and Biological Foundations	95 minutes (59 questions)
Chance to void test and survey	10 minutes
Total content time (not including breaks)	6 hours, 15 minutes

Be sure to consult the AAMC website for other details and changes about the test day.

Importance of the MCAT

Medical school admissions committees typically make their decisions based on MCAT scores, undergraduate GPA, your personal statement, your interview, letters of recommendation, and your experience, including the types of courses you have taken, your volunteer experiences, and internships you have done. Think of the MCAT and GPA as the first hurdles. If you have a low MCAT score and GPA, the committee may not look at the rest of your application. Because the GPA is difficult to increase in your last semester or two, a strong MCAT score may be your best chance to be seriously considered by the admissions committee.

WHAT ADMISSIONS COMMITTEES CONSIDER

MCAT

GPA

Personal statement

Interview

Letters of recommendation

Experience: Types of courses, volunteer work, internships

Features of the Computer MCAT

A number of features available on the computer MCAT will help you organize your test taking. You can practice these strategies by taking the MCAT practice exams provided online by AAMC. You need to learn and master these features. Some of the features are available only on the practice tests and are not available on the actual MCAT. These include search, notes, pause, solutions, self-diagnosis, and item numbering.

AAMC offers at least three practice tests on their website. Additional tests will be added over time. The online test allows you to practice the features of the computer exam.

When you begin the test, you can choose whether the test will be timed or not, which type of questions you want to do, whether you want to see the solutions, and so on. These are very helpful features of which you should take advantage. However, these features are for practicing only. They are **not** available on the actual MCAT.

Once the test begins, some features will be available that are also on the actual MCAT. The session will begin with introductory screens that provide a tutorial on using the testing features. Be sure to go through this thoroughly now. On your actual test day, you should not need to review the tutorial. The tutorial covers:

- Use of the mouse
- Marking and unmarking
- Strikeout
- Reviewing
- Scroll bar
- Highlighting on the sciences and Verbal Reasoning sections
- Exhibits

A few of these features may be confusing at first. Strikeout allows you to cross off an answer choice that you believe is wrong. You can undo a strikeout at any time. Marking a question does not mean marking an answer. It is a feature that allows you to mark a question that you would like to come back to later. The test instructions suggest that when you do come back to the question later and select an answer, you should unmark it. However, this is not necessary. You will still get credit for the answer even if you leave the question marked.

The Review feature allows you to see a list of all of the questions on the section and a breakdown of which ones are marked, which ones are answered, and which ones are unanswered. You can then click on a question you want to look at again. This feature can be helpful, especially toward the end of the test, to make sure you have answered everything. While on the Review screen, be careful not to click Exit. Exit does not take you out of Review mode; it ends the section. To get out of Review mode, you must select a question to review.

Once the tutorial ends (both on the practice and actual MCAT), you will be taken to the Chemistry/Physics section. Here, as is true on the Biological and Critical Analysis sections, you will see a split screen. The left panel contains the passage, and the right panel contains all of the questions for that passage. You will usually need to scroll to see the lower parts of the screen.

Below the split screens, in the lower right-hand corner are the buttons for Previous, Next, Mark, and Review. Slightly above these, in the left panel, is the button for Exhibit. Clicking this brings up a new, small screen with an additional display, usually the Periodic Table. This appears even on the Critical Analysis section. At the left end of the bottom bar is a display showing which question you are on and the time remaining. Note that the clock counts down and that it displays seconds as well as hours and minutes. When you have finished all the questions for a passage, simply click Next to go to the next passage.

To record an answer for a question, you have to click in the circle next to the answer choice. Clicking on any other part of the answer results in striking out that answer choice. Note that striking out a choice has no effect on receiving credit for an answer. If you strike out three answer choices, you will not get credit for the remaining answer unless you click its circle. If you click an answer that you previously struck out, the strikeout will automatically be removed.

The Review button gives you an overview of all the questions for the section. From the Review screen, you can double click on a question to be taken to the passage that the question is associated with, along with the other questions for that passage. When you finish reviewing that question, you can use the Previous or Next buttons to go on to other passages. Instead, you can click the Review button to choose any question.

At the bottom of the Review page are three or four buttons. Review All starts you back at the beginning of the test. Review Incomplete takes you in order only to passages for which there is a question that you have not yet answered. Review Marked appears only if you have marked any questions. It takes you in order only to passages where you marked an item. Finally, the End button ends the current section, preventing you from doing any further work on it.

You can navigate through a section in several ways. The default method is to simply go in order. When you have finished answering all the questions on a screen, click Next. A second method is to skip around, choosing which passages to work on. To do this, use the Next or Previous button to view other passages quickly. The final method of navigating through the section is to use Review. Depending on which review option you choose, you will be taken to passages where there are questions that you either have not answered or have marked. You can also choose a particular question to review. In all cases, Review will take you back to the section. At that point, you can use the Previous or Next buttons again, or you can go back to Review.

Practice navigating the MCAT with Barron's online MCAT: *http://barronsbooks. com/tp/mcat*

YOUR PLAN OF ATTACK

You must accomplish two tasks to get a top score on the MCAT.

1. Review as much content as possible.
2. Master the critical testing, timing, and problem-solving strategies that can boost your score.

> **THE TWO KEYS TO MCAT SUCCESS**
>
> 1. Review content
> 2. Master test-taking strategies

Most people need to do both of these to earn a top score. Many people assume that reviewing content is the only way to improve on the MCAT. In reality, using the right strategies often turns out to be the fastest and most reliable way to gain points. Comprehensive content review gives you the knowledge needed on the MCAT. Using strategies gives you the tools for using that knowledge to gain points.

Science Review Plan

The AAMC publishes an MCAT Topic Outline that lists all possible categories and topics that might appear on the MCAT. If you can master that list, you will be familiar with any topic that shows up on the test. Barron's *MCAT* covers all of the topics on the MCAT Topic Outline.

The biggest obstacle to effective studying is simply that you have to review a vast amount of material. We have organized your review for you by focusing on the concepts that you will need on the test. Calculate the number of weeks that are left until your test. Then divide up the contents of this book evenly so that you have a weekly assignment. At the end of this introduction is a three-month plan for organizing your study time.

If you have a hard time organizing yourself, find a person whom you trust and respect, who is well organized, and who is willing to help you organize your study time. The person does not need to be familiar with the MCAT. Make an informal agreement with this person that if he or she is willing to be your mentor during your study period, you will promise to give 100 percent. Your mentor should be willing to be brutally direct with you about your study efforts and progress.

Three or four months of study time is enough to make progress. Six to eight months, or even longer, is better. In fact, many students start during the summer of the year before they will take their MCAT. Students usually have more free time in the summer. A plan to study during the school year often falls flat. Start early!

Some people sabotage their study efforts by taking on too many other obligations. If, during the months you are studying for the MCAT, you are also planning to take a few classes, work a couple of jobs, do an internship, and get in a vacation to an exotic resort, you have shortchanged yourself. Ideally, during the summer leading up to your MCAT, you should take on no more than 20 hours a week of work or school obligations and keep all other activities to a minimum.

> **ARE THESE OBLIGATIONS SABOTAGING YOUR EFFORTS?**
>
> Work, school, travel plans, family obligations, extracurricular activities, and volunteer positions all take time.
> Cut back for success.

Keep a Realistic Eye on Your Progress

Start with a diagnostic test, using a test in this book or a test published by AAMC. At least once a month, take another test to see how you are scoring. If your scores are not steadily increasing, redo your study plan. Evaluate what you are getting wrong. Is it content knowledge or is it strategy? Remember that almost always, a careful look at your test-taking strategies will show how you could have gained more points even without knowing more content.

Other Aspects of the Admissions Process

During the summer at the end of which you will take your MCAT, you also need to be preparing other parts of the admissions process. These include writing a personal statement and gathering letters of recommendation. Check with your premed advisor immediately to make sure you will have met the prerequisites for medical school admissions. Ask your advisor about the requirements for completing volunteer opportunities, internships, and research experience.

MASTERING STRATEGIES

Whenever you work on a practice question in this book, you should also work on test-taking strategies. Almost all questions have some element of strategy. Remember that the MCAT is testing your problem-solving ability as well as your science, pyschology, and sociology knowledge. Many questions on the sciences are actually testing your ability to analyze graphs; interpret written material; and break down, synthesize, and problem solve with new information.

Timing strategy is also critical on the test. We will take a close look at the art and science of timing strategy. The difference between getting accepted to medical school and not getting accepted can often be a matter of readjusting timing on the test.

TEST ANXIETY AND LEARNING DISABILITIES

If you find that test anxiety often gets in the way of performing your best on a test, you will probably find that mastering the timing strategies and testing strategies will eliminate much of the anxiety. For many people, anxiety is centered around the conflict between wanting to speed up to get to more questions and needing to slow down to be more accurate. A good timing strategy tells you how much time to spend on a question and when to move on. You can work this out and perfect it before going into your actual MCAT.

Another common aspect of test anxiety is that you, the test taker, do not think the same way as the test writers. You have your own reasons for choosing your answer over theirs.

Testing strategy helps you understand the underlying reasons why one answer must be correct and the other answer that you were considering actually has a fatal flaw. With some practice, you can learn what the test writers are looking for.

If you have a learning disability, or believe you may have one, that affects your ability to complete the test at the same speed and with the same accuracy as other people do, you can inquire about taking the test under special conditions.

DISABILITIES

Test takers with disabilities may be entitled to take the test under special conditions.

TIMING STRATEGY

What does *timing strategy* mean, and why is it important? You may say, "I need to learn how to get to all the questions. That's the only way I can get more points." Let's examine that idea and see if it is true.

We have all developed certain strategies for taking tests over the years. These strategies operate on a subconscious level. You are, in fact, making certain decisions about how to use your time continually throughout a test, without being conscious of many of these decisions.

For example, when a test section begins, what do you do first? Most people simply go to the first question and start reading it at the beginning. However, that is only one of many possible things you could do when the section starts. It is an assumption that you may have developed from your past test-taking experiences. We will examine this and other assumptions to determine what is actually the best thing to do in each situation.

How many questions do you hope to work on? Should you be pushing yourself to work faster or letting yourself relax and work more carefully? When you finish one question, which question should you work on next? If you are having trouble with a question, should you guess and move on now or spend more time on it? How much time is OK to spend on a question? If you get stuck on a question and cannot think of anything else to do with it, should you guess and move on or do something else?

If you were taking the test right now, you would be making the above decisions; however, your decisions would probably not be the best ones for the MCAT. As you study the best way to make these decisions, try to discover what your subconscious assumptions about timing strategy are so you will not be led astray by past test-taking patterns.

A NEW TIMING STRATEGY FOR THE MCAT

The timing strategy that will bring you success on the MCAT is different from the strategy that you use for college tests.

Step 1. Test Layout

The first step is to know the "geography" of each test section. You need to know how many questions the section contains, how many problem sets, how many independent questions, and where the independent questions are. You also need to know how much time is allotted for the section. Review the most recent MCAT information so that you are up to date on this.

TIP

**CONTROL
YOUR TIME**

**Learn to control
the clock so it
doesn't control
you!**

Step 2. Keeping Track of Time

You will need to keep track of time during the test. Some people get anxious when they pay attention to time. However, with practice, most find that keeping track of time is the key to controlling your time. Trying to judge time by feeling alone is very inaccurate and takes up part of your mental processing ability. You are not allowed to bring a watch into the testing center. You will use the clock on the computer to keep track of time.

HOW TO USE THE MCAT CLOCK

You should keep track of time for the whole section. When only a few minutes are left, you will fill in answers for any questions that you have left blank up to this point. The clock on the computer will show you when only a few minutes are left. You should also keep track of time to know how much time you have spent on a particular question. To do this, you need to write down the approximate time when you start a question. If you find yourself wrestling with that question, you will quickly be able to see how much time you have spent.

When you are practicing on paper, even untimed, you should keep track of time. So you will need to use a timepiece for that. Remember that on the actual test, you can use only the timer on the screen.

TIP

**THE SCIENCE OF
TIMING STRATEGY**

**Discover the
absolutely most
efficient way to
use your time on
the MCAT.**

Step 3. Understanding Timing

Let's look at a hypothetical model that can help you understand MCAT timing. During an MCAT, many factors will determine how you will do on each question. These include how well you have learned the science facts, how much practicing you have done, and how well you have learned testing strategies. These also include how well you slept the night before, how alert or tired various systems of your body are, and how many or how few distractions are in your mind about other things in your life. In other words, countless factors, many of which are beyond your control, affect how clearly you may be able to think.

Now imagine that, if you were going to take the MCAT tomorrow, you had an all-knowing perspective, had an omniscient viewpoint, and could actually determine exactly how long it would take you to arrive at the correct answer for each question on the test. For example, you might know that for question 17, you would get the right answer after 4 minutes and 17 seconds and not a second before. (Remember that this is hypothetical. In real life, you obviously cannot know this.)

With this knowledge, see if you could plan out the perfect timing strategy. To keep things simple, suppose a test section had 10 questions and you had 15 minutes to complete it. Also suppose that you could determine the following times (in minutes and seconds) needed to get each question right.

Table 3. Hypothetical Test Section

QUESTION	TIME	QUESTION	TIME
1	4:03	6	0:29
2	0:47	7	2:26
3	7:38	8	1:40
4	1:12	9	2:30
5	3:55	10	3:15

Which question would you answer first? Would you start with question 1, or would you start somewhere else? Which question would you do second? Third?

Answering the quickest question first makes sense. That is question 6, which requires 0 minutes and 29 seconds. Because every question is worth 1 point, regardless of how difficult it is, to get the most points, just choose the quickest questions.

Following this logic, the second question that you would do is question 2 at 0 minutes and 47 seconds, then question 4, and so on. Here is a chart of the best timing strategy.

Table 4. Best Strategy for Taking the Hypothetical Test

QUESTION	TIME USED	TIME LEFT
6	0:29	14:31
2	0:47	13:44
4	1:12	12:32
8	1:40	10:52
7	2:26	8:26
9	2:30	5:56
10	3:15	2:41
~~5~~	3:55 not enough time	

This would give you seven correct answers and you would guess cold on the remaining three questions. Notice that after answering question 10, not enough time is left to answer the next easiest question, question 5.

Now here is the difficulty. Suppose that you need to get eight questions right in order to earn the score you want. The above result is one short of your goal. How could you tweak it? Do you see that there is no way to get more points? If you try to save time on certain questions by going faster, you will get those questions wrong.

Obviously, you will not know how long it will take you to do a question on the real test, but this exercise brings out several important points. This strategy can be simulated in two steps.

1. Choose the best (easiest) question to work on next.
2. Give each question the full time that it needs.

TWO STEPS TO PERFECT TIMING

Choose the next easiest passage to work on.
Give each question the time that it needs.

If you answer questions in order, you will most likely work on some very difficult questions and leave some easy questions undone. Later on, we will discuss a strategy for choosing what to work on. Also, if you regularly quit questions too soon—guessing and moving on to the next question—you will not be giving each question the time it needs. Many people leave a trail of 15 or 20 wrong answers in their wake because they do not give any of the questions enough time.

Another lesson of the omniscient viewpoint model is that you do not need to have a specific goal for how many questions you are going to attempt. If you have a goal, you will inevitably rush to meet it. Let the test tell you how far you can get. You simply need to choose what to work on next and give it the time it needs.

To approximate choosing the next quickest question, scan through a test section before you begin working on it. Identify which passages seem to be the most difficult. These are the passages you will do last if at all. Note that you are choosing whole passages, not individual questions. In our example, you chose one question at a time. In actuality, you will choose passages. Within a passage, some questions will be easy and some will be hard. However, trying to pick only the easy questions from all the passages would be far too difficult and time consuming. You would have to set up the whole passage and then maybe answer only a few questions. In addition, you would be forced to work on even the hardest passages. Choosing passages that are easier and then working on all of the questions in that passage seems to work better for most people.

As you practice the MCAT, you will begin to know what the minimum number of passages is that you can finish on a section even on a bad day. Suppose you can always get through seven passages. When you skim through the section, you will find the four hardest passages. Those are the ones you will cut on your first pass through the section. You will now have five or six passages that you will have plenty of time to work on. Remember that it is not up to you to know how many questions you will get to; the test will tell you that. However, you should adjust your expectations so that they are in line with reality.

You start a test section by skimming through, looking quickly at each passage, and ranking the passages so that you know which ones seem the hardest. You then work on the easiest passages. If you choose the next easiest passage to work on and give each question the time that it needs, you might not get the score you were hoping for; however, you will get the best score that is possible for you that day. Your goal, as you perfect your timing, is to become 100 percent efficient. You must realize that you cannot increase your score by going faster or trying to get to more questions. If you save time on a question but get it wrong, you have wasted all the time you spent on it.

What about giving each question the time that it needs? In our example of the omniscient viewpoint, you knew exactly what that time was. In reality, you do not. Obviously, spending 10 minutes on a question is too long, even if you get it right. Spending only 1 minute is too short. Many questions cannot be answered in 1 minute. How long is OK to spend on a question?

Many people get an internal warning when they have spent more than 1½ minutes on a question. This is probably based on exams in college classes. For the MCAT, a cutoff of 1½ minutes or 2 minutes is too short. The exact amount of time that will optimize the score probably varies among people. However, experience suggests that you should allow at least 3 minutes on hard questions and quite possibly 4 or even 5. Remember that you will have to give this extra time to only a handful of questions, but those are the very questions that will increase your score.

Here is a good model for understanding timing. A particular test section may contain 20 questions that you can get right in 2 minutes or less for each. The remaining questions cannot be gotten right in 2 minutes each, no matter how hard you try. They will require more time. If you limit yourself to 2 minutes per question, you will get your first 20 right but every question after that will be wrong. This may sound unrealistic. In fact, though, it is typical of timed sections for beginning MCAT students—21 questions right, 20 questions wrong, and 9 guesses. Notice that all of the time spent on those 20 incorrect questions, possibly 30 minutes or more, was wasted. In fact, the test taker could have gotten 6 of them right by chance in 1 minute by simply filling in answers.

Once you are willing to spend 3 to 5 minutes on a question, if necessary, how do you know when you have given the question all the time that it needs? If you are getting close to 4 or 5 minutes and still have no inkling, just guess and move on. However, if you guess and move on after only 2 or 3 minutes, you will be cheating yourself out of points. Never plan to come back to a question later. Usually you will not have time. Choose an answer now while you are still on the question. If necessary, rest your eyes for a few seconds, take a breath, and then do whatever you need to be certain of your answer.

Step 4. Evaluating Your Timing

Let's take a look at how typical students might use their time before they study test-taking strategies and then see how much they can improve.

Typical Performance and Possible Improvement

In the table below, the test taker's first attempt at a timed section resulted in working on 50 of the 59 questions and not working on the other 9. Of the questions that the student actually worked on, 20 were correct and 30 were wrong. Of the 30 wrong answers, 20 of them were the result of strategy errors. The other ten were questions for which the student did not know the needed science facts. The student did not take time to put down cold guesses for the questions that were not worked. The student got a total of 20 questions right for a score of 122.

TIP

THE POWER OF TIMING STRATEGY

Theoretically, you can increase your score from 122 to 127 just with better timing strategy!

Table 5. First Attempt at Timing

59 Total Questions			SCORE	
ATTEMPTED 50		LEFT 9		
20 right	30 wrong	0 right	Total right = 20	Score = 122
	20 poor strategy	10 science lacking		

In this next attempt, the student simply took the time to put guesses down for the 10 questions he or she did not work on. By chance, the student would get 2 to 3 more points. Notice that this is enough to move the score to 123.

Table 6. Results with Guesses for Unworked Questions

59 Total Questions			SCORE	
ATTEMPTED 50		LEFT 9		
20 right	30 wrong	2 right	Total right = 22	Score = 123
	20 poor strategy / 10 science lacking			

Below, the student chose which passages to work on instead of just doing the first ones. The 10 questions for which this person did not know enough science will now become the 10 cold guesses. The student can find 10 easier questions to work on and get right. In other words, the student is now getting 30 of the 50 right by choosing easier questions. The student still answered 20 questions wrong because of strategy. The total is now 32, for a scaled score of 125.

Table 7. Results with Choosing Which Passages to Work On

59 Total Questions				SCORE	
ATTEMPTED 50			LEFT 9		
20 right	20 wrong	10 right	2 right	Total right = 32	Score = 125
	20 poor strategy				

By adding these two strategies, the student went from a 122 to a 125. That is a very big improvement and is due to timing strategy alone. Then the student added in the strategy of taking more time on 5 of the 20 questions that were strategy errors. This means that the student did not answer as many questions, 34 instead of 42, and actually left more questions not worked on, 24 instead of 9. The student still answered the original 20 correctly plus the 10 more from picking passages with easier science. Next the student worked on the 5 remaining questions. Because the student attempted 5 questions instead of 20, the student had enough time to get the questions correct.

Table 8. Results When Some Questions Are Sacrificed to Work Longer on Others

59 Total Questions				SCORE	
ATTEMPTED 35			LEFT 24		
20 right	5 right	10 right	6 right	Total right = 41	Score = 127

When you do a timed section, you can evaluate how effective your timing strategy is by looking at the variables we just considered. Notice that at first, this student missed a lot of the questions that had been worked on. By the end, everything that was worked on was correct, even though fewer were attempted. When you look at the questions you actually worked on, how many of those did you get wrong? If it is more than just a couple, you may get more points by answering fewer questions. If you got more than 5 or 6 wrong, you are quite probably not spending enough time on each question.

You should always write down the amount of time you spend on each question, even when you are working untimed and certainly when you are taking a timed section. Look at the questions you answered wrong. How much time did you spend on each one of them? If you spent only 1 to 3 minutes on a question that you got wrong, you may be stopping too soon. Evaluate to what extent you might have been missing science information on a question and to what extent you knew the facts but were lacking strategy. This will help you focus on your testing strategies as well as on timing.

WRITE DOWN YOUR TIME

Whether practicing timed or untimed, always write down the amount of time you spend on a question. Use the information to evaluate your timing.

Summary of Your Timing Strategy

1. Use the clock on the computer to keep track of time for the whole section and for each question.
2. Scan the whole section, and identify the hardest passages. You will cut the hardest passages your first time through the section. Cut enough passages so that you can easily get through the remaining passages with time to spare.
3. On the science passages, start with the independent questions. Most people find them quicker as there is less setup.
4. Go to the first passage that you had not marked for cutting. Do all of the questions in that passage—even the ones that are difficult—before going on to the next passage. Skip the passages you had agreed to cut.
5. Each time you begin a question, write down the time as displayed on the computer. As you are working on the question, if you start to get the feeling that it is taking a long time, glance at the clock. If you have spent less than 4 minutes, you can still take some time with the question. If you are missing science information and believe you have done everything you can to answer the question, guess and move on even if you have spent less than 3 or 4 minutes. However, if you are in doubt, always err on the side of spending more time. After 5 minutes, if you are not close to an answer, guess and move on.
6. You do not need to keep track of time used for reading or setting up a passage. Keep track of time only while you are working on a specific question.
7. If you have enough time to start a new passage but not enough to finish it, do not read the setup. Skim the questions and look for any that you can answer without reading the setup. Then look for questions that ask for simple facts from the setup.
8. When the time for a section is about halfway over, you may find it effective to go to the harder passages—the ones you agreed to cut at first—and answer the easiest questions. Then return to the easier passages and continue working them thoroughly.
9. When 5 minutes are left for the whole section, go back and put down answers for everything you have not worked on. You will get 1 in 4 right by chance.
10. Use the remaining time to keep working until the end. Remember that even one more right answer could increase your score by 1 point on the 15-point scale.

TESTING STRATEGY
Why Is Strategy Important?

In addition to timing strategy, there are many testing strategies that will help you avoid unnecessary work, avoid careless errors, double-check answers, and solve complex problems by better organizing the information and having more sophisticated problem-solving tools.

Problem-solving strategy is particularly important on the MCAT. In recent years, the MCAT has changed from strictly a test of science facts to a test of problem-solving ability.

THE IMPORTANCE OF TESTING STRATEGY

The MCAT is a test of problem solving at least as much as it is a test of science.

The test gives you complex information that draws from several areas of science in order to see if you can understand the information, organize it, synthesize new information from it, and then solve the problem.

Virtually all MCAT takers report that there are many science questions, including psychology and sociology, that they have gotten wrong even though they knew the science. They could have gotten these questions right if they had used better strategies. When you do practice questions, whether timed or untimed, review the reasons for your wrong answers. If you find that you did not know some science facts, this tells you what you need to review. However, even if you were missing science knowledge, there are often strategies you could have used to get to the right answer.

If you knew the science and still got it wrong, look carefully to see what happened. Did you fail to give the question enough time? Why? Were you trying to do too many questions? Were you not keeping track of time? Did you get into an "anxious" mode? Reviewing your errors is a powerful way to learn about your test-taking patterns and adjust them.

> ## LEARNING TO WORK QUICKLY WITH STRATEGIES
>
> At first, new strategies can seem to take a lot of time. By giving yourself plenty of time to experiment with new strategies now, they will become second nature to you by the time you take your test. Then you will be able to apply them quickly.

Below are the important strategies that can help you boost your score. Remember that in our review of typical performance above, our test taker went from a score of 122 to a score of 125 by using timing strategy and then to a score of 127 by using testing strategy.

Do All the Questions in a Set

When working on a passage, both in physical and social science and in critical analysis, do all of the questions in the set, even if some are difficult. Even though you are choosing the easiest passages, some of the questions will be hard. Do not plan to come back to a question later in the test. Most test takers do not have time to go back. Even if you did have time, you would have to set up the passage from the beginning again. Complete the question the first time, giving it the full amount of time it needs, up to 4 or 5 minutes.

If after 5 minutes you are not close to an answer, put down your best guess. Do not leave it blank. When guessing, be very careful not to choose an answer just because it seems good. You will probably be falling for a distractor.

What is a distractor? The test writers build a wrong answer into the question that may look better than the real answer for various reasons. It may just make sense. It may use wording from the passage that seems familiar. It may contain numbers or patterns that seem related to the passage. It may draw on emotionally charged issues (for example, "C. Everyone should have access to affordable health care.") The distractor is designed in a way that draws you to it if you do not know the real answer.

Unless you have a clear reason to choose one answer over another when you are down to two, it is safer to use this rule of thumb: Choose the answer that is lowest on the computer screen. Then you have a true 50:50 chance of being right. If you grasp at straws for an answer that feels better, you are more likely to pick the distractor.

TIP

TESTING STRATEGY

Do all the questions in a set before going on to the next set!

You should have to guess only very rarely. Guess only if you have used your full 4 to 5 minutes on a question or if you are clearly missing critical science information and have tried to see how far you can get using strategies alone. You should never guess just because the question is hard and you want to save time. You need to give each question the full amount of time that it requires.

If one question in the passage is stumping you, it is fine to go on to other questions in that passage. After you have worked on the other questions, answering the harder one may be easier. Remember that you do not go on to the next passage until you have worked on every question in the current passage.

Use Your Eyes, Not Your Memory

Most test takers have a strong habit of reading the setup and a question and then trying to work out the answer in their head. They try to remember what they read and what the question is asking. Your memory is not accurate enough to do this well. It is overwhelmed by the amount of information it is trying to absorb.

Train yourself to look back at the printed information continually for the facts that you need. This takes a burden off of the processing functions of your memory. Some people complain that they have to go back and forth between the questions and the passage continually, reminding themselves of what they have already read. This is actually the best way to process information on the MCAT. The minute you have finished reading something and have turned your eyes away, the memory of what you read begins to change. Details become blurred or confused. The brain starts interpreting what it remembers. You can notice for yourself that you occasionally get a question wrong because you remembered information from the passage inaccurately.

> **DON'T TRUST YOUR MEMORY**
>
> The MCAT will overwhelm your ability to remember accurately what you have read. Go back and reread as often as necessary to make sure you have the facts correct.

After reading a question and considering the first answer choice, you may no longer accurately remember what the question is asking, especially if it is a complex question. Get in the habit of going back and briefly looking at the question again before going on to the next answer choice.

The habit of relying on memory is a strong one and a difficult one to change. You may have the feeling that answering the question from your memory is faster than going back and reading again. It is faster, but it is also far less accurate.

When reviewing a question you got wrong, look for signs that you remembered things inaccurately or did not bother to go back and look for the facts. Notice if you misconstrued the question or the answer choice. These indicate a reliance on memory instead of real facts.

Reading the Setup for a Passage

In the sciences, the passage will often contain a lot of information that you will not need. Many of the questions can be answered without referring to the passage at all. Glance very briefly at the passage, and then go directly to the questions. Focus on what you need for that question. Doing simpler questions first can be helpful. This will help orient you to the passage. Do not be intimidated by very complex passages.

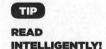
TIP

READ INTELLIGENTLY!

The efficient reader reads less but focuses on the important information.

Use Visual Aids

This strategy is a corollary of "use your eyes, not your memory." Memory is not very effective at keeping distinct categories separate. In contrast, a picture can compare and contrast two categories in columns in a way that is extremely clear. Much MCAT strategy, both on sciences and in critical analysis, depends on keeping two categories distinct, so using visual aids is a critical tool.

EXAMPLE

Consider two different vehicles owned by Maria. Her truck is red. She also has a Subaru. The Toyota has a camper top. Maria could sleep in the back of the Subaru if she sleeps sideways. The four-wheel drive is great for camping in the desert. The silver vehicle is cooler in the desert than the red one, even if it has only all-wheel drive. What Maria likes most about her older vehicle is that when she sleeps in it in the desert, which she does without being sideways, it has an air conditioner in case she needs it.

Answer this question without looking back. Does the four-wheel drive vehicle have air conditioning? Even if you go back and review the words in the above paragraph, you will probably have to do a lot of mental work to keep the two categories—truck and car—straight. Now let's look at how much clearer it is to organize this same information visually and graphically.

Use two columns to compare and contrast the two vehicles. The first sentence says the truck is red, so truck and red go in the same column.

truck	
red	

The next sentence shows that in contrast to truck and red, there is a Subaru. This goes in the contrasting column. Notice that each line so far represents a certain quality. The first line represents body style. The line for Subaru represents make. This helps show what is known about each category. So far, the body style and color of the Subaru are not known.

truck	
red	
	Subaru

The next fact is that "the Toyota has a camper top." Because the Toyota cannot be the Subaru, this information goes in the first column.

truck	
red	
Toyota	Subaru
camper top	

The next fact tells us that it is possible to sleep in the Subaru but only sideways.

truck	
red	
Toyota	Subaru
camper top	
	sleep only sideways

"The-four wheel drive is great for camping in the desert." This information is not related to anything else that is already known so far. Scan the rest of the facts for clues. The next sentence says that the silver vehicle is all-wheel drive. Because silver is not red, all-wheel drive vehicle belongs in the second column. Because all-wheel drive is not four-wheel drive, four-wheel drive goes in the first column.

truck	
red	silver
Toyota	Subaru
camper top	
	sleep only sideways
four-wheel drive	all-wheel drive
great for camping in desert	

Does the last sentence provide anything new? "What Maria likes most about her older vehicle is that when she sleeps in it in the desert, which she does without being sideways, it has an air conditioner in case she needs it." Fill in the blank rows.

truck	
red	silver
Toyota	Subaru
camper top	
	sleep only sideways
four-wheel drive	all-wheel drive
great for camping in desert	cooler in desert

Using a two-column visual organizer allows you to sort the information more reliably than doing it by memory. At the same time, a visual organizer allows you to compare and contrast information quickly and effortlessly.

The visual aid also shows us what is not known. This is particularly helpful because memory tends to fill in blanks based on assumptions. Is the Subaru a sedan? You might have assumed so. You might have assumed it was not. The truth is that this information

TIP

A PICTURE REALLY IS WORTH A THOUSAND WORDS

Pictures are much better at keeping distinctions straight.

is unknown. The space in the second column that represents body type is blank. What else is unknown about the Subaru? What facts are missing for the Toyota?

Whenever information needs to be compared or contrasted, remember to use a visual aid. You will be able to ask for an unlimited amount of scratch paper during the test, although you will be given a limited amount at one time.

Because the test is on computer, any sketches or drawings that appear on the screen have to be redrawn on scratch paper in order to manipulate them. Get used to doing this when practicing, even if you are practicing with a paper test. Making columns is one of the most powerful organizing tools, but you can experiment with other ways of visually organizing information. For example, you can use sketches and make circles to represent sets. If you make an error because you did not have the information organized well enough, do the problem again using visual aids.

Big Picture Thinking vs. Detail Thinking

Big picture thinking and detail thinking are two distinct mental modes of processing information. Detail thinking is linear. It focuses narrowly on the problem and forges straight ahead, using calculations. Big picture thinking is global and holistic. It does not focus on a goal but rather tries to see as much as possible. It steps back from the situation and looks at the situation freshly. For many people, the brain is not able to operate in these two modes at the same time. While one is activated, the other is not accessible.

LEFT BRAIN VS. RIGHT BRAIN

Testing strategy teaches you how to use both sides of your brain for success.

Both of these processing styles are necessary for the MCAT. In fact, part of what the MCAT is testing is your ability to use these two styles at the appropriate times. Problem solving requires the ability to use both. Because the two modes typically cannot be used together, problem solving requires learning when to use each and how to switch between them.

Most people have a preference for one of these styles over the other. Even if you are naturally an intuitive thinker, you may find that because the MCAT involves science, math, time pressure, and psychological pressure, you automatically switch into detail thinking. This may prevent you from using your greatest asset—the ability to see the big picture.

Try to discover which of these modes comes most naturally to you. Start to notice when you are using big picture thinking and when you are using detail thinking. Do you resist switching from one to the other?

ARE YOU STUCK IN DETAIL MODE?

DETAIL THINKING

Good at cranking out details. Bad at remembering why.

One sign that you are stuck in detail mode is that you have failed to see the obvious. Consider this problem. A couple of pizzas are to be divided among seven people, leaving a third of the total pizza for the next day. On the next day, the remainder of the pizza is divided among five people but only after a quarter of the original amount is thrown away. How much is left? Suppose a test taker comes up with the answer of 2.17 pizzas. This person's detail thinking may have followed all of the details and come up with an answer. A big picture perspective, however, indicates that there were only two pizzas to start with. There must have been a calculation error at some stage. Big picture thinking is a reality check on detail thinking.

A person locked into detail thinking often speeds ahead and does not want to slow down, look around, or change directions. If you feel this way, be sure to switch to big picture thinking occasionally to make sure you are on the right track.

ARE YOU STUCK IN BIG PICTURE MODE?

You can also be stuck in big picture mode. One sign of this is not having the focus to deal with details. The person stuck in big picture mode has a general sense of the passage; however, he or she would rather guess on a challenging question and move on than deal with having to crunch numbers, organize information, and problem solve. Many of the testing strategies presented in this introduction are good tools for helping you dig more deeply into the details.

TIP

BIG PICTURE THINKING

Good at planning. Bad at doing the detail work.

THE BIG PICTURE SANDWICH

How can you coordinate these two modes? Do not expect to use them at the same time. Most people find that this is not possible. You can, however, switch between them. One powerful tool for doing this is the big picture sandwich. Start each problem from a big picture perspective. Understand what you are dealing with, and organize your plan of attack. Then switch to detail thinking to analyze the data. Finally, before leaving the problem, switch back to big picture thinking to make sure your answer makes sense and that you have not left anything out. During the process of solving the problem, you may also need to switch back and forth several times within the framework of the big picture sandwich.

Consider this more closely. When orienting to a passage or question, use the big picture to see if you understand the situation, to see where there is some confusion, to consider what the plan of attack should be, and to organize the information. Then switch to detail mode, comparing facts, doing calculations, and reorganizing information. If you get to a dead end or lose track of what you are doing, switch back to big picture mode. When you have solved the problem, switch back to big picture mode to see if your answer makes sense and if you have understood the question correctly. Check whether you have missed anything. Big picture mode also allows you to monitor how confident you are in your answer. If your confidence level is low, you are not yet done.

THE BIG PICTURE SANDWICH

Start with the big picture.
Deal with the details.
Double check using the big picture.
Using the big picture sandwich teaches your left brain and right brain how to work hand in hand.

The Road Map

On more complex problems, as you start off by using the big picture to understand the situation and come up with a plan of attack, you should actually write out a road map of how you are going to solve the problem. If you do not do this, you may easily lose track of your original plan, skip some steps, or forget to do something. By writing the plan down before switching into detail mode, you can quickly check the big picture at a glance as you proceed through the problem.

A road map can look quite simple. Consider the following.

1. Calculate the volume in beaker *A*.
2. Calculate the volume in beaker *B*.
3. Add 1 and 2.
4. Divide step 3 in half.

This road map would give the average volume for the contents of two different beakers. It is fairly simple. However, if the volume calculations are going to be a little complicated or if your mind is tired, you could easily get lost or miss a step if you did not have a written road map in front of you.

If a particular step is complex, break it into subparts. Remember that you do not need a road map on simpler questions. If, while working on a problem, you have lost track of what you are doing and why, go back to big picture mode and set up a road map. Whenever you miss a question, check to see if you got lost or missed something. If you did, your plan should have been written down, not left up to memory.

> **ROAD MAP**
>
> Write down your plan for solving the problem. Don't keep it in your head.
> With a written plan, you can't get confused!

If you find yourself staring at a problem and not knowing exactly how you are going to approach it, take some extra time to work on a plan before analyzing the answer choices. If you still do not have a plan, begin analyzing the answers. That may give you some insight into how to solve the problem. However, once you have the insight, step back for a moment and clarify your plan. Remember that to a large extent, the MCAT is testing your problem-solving abilities. Effective problem solving requires a systematic plan.

The KING Approach—The Secret to Systematic Problem Solving

For many MCAT students, coming up with a systematic plan seems at first to be a matter of luck. They feel as though a plan either presents itself or does not. If it does not, they feel there is nothing they can do about it. In fact, there are ways to develop a systematic plan consciously.

Consider this situation. Kayla comes to her MCAT tutor with a problem on which she has spent more than half an hour and that she could not solve. She has tried everything she could think of. The tutor asks her a question, and Kayla responds. Then the tutor asks another question. She responds again. After the third question, Kayla sees the answer. The process took 3 minutes.

This is a very common scenario. What did the tutor and Kayla do together that Kayla could not do on her own? The tutor did not provide any information or even suggest strategies for solving the problem. The tutor simply asked questions that Kayla had not asked herself. The secret is in which questions to ask.

What are the right questions? We can represent them with the acronym KING.

K—What do I **K**now?
I—What else can be **I**nferred from what I know?
N—What would I **N**eed to know to get the answer?
G—How do I **G**et there?

TIP

THE KING APPROACH

Ask yourself the right questions in order to get the right answers.

These questions help your mind dig into the situation. Start by asking yourself what you already know. This may seem pointless at first because what you already know may seem obvious. However, consciously identifying this information brings it into the active processing part of your memory. Try it. Sometimes people feel they do not know anything. However, there are always some facts that can be identified, no matter how trivial they may seem.

The KING approach is one of the most powerful problem-solving tools. Use it regularly at first, even if it does not seem necessary, in order to learn how to use it. The steps do not always have to be done in order. However, you should usually start with what you know.

The Generic Way to Answer a Question

Use a systematic approach on every question. Many people simply read through a question quickly and then look at the first answer choice. This is not necessarily an effective, systematic way to problem solve. Here is how the process can be broken down and made more systematic.

HOW TO ANSWER A QUESTION

STEP 1 Orient yourself to the question.

STEP 2 Decide on a plan of attack.

STEP 3 Make a first pass through the answers. Quickly eliminate answers that are clearly wrong.

STEP 4 Make a second pass through the remaining answers. Carefully and thoroughly apply strategies.

STEP 1. READ THE QUESTION

Without yet looking at the answer choices, read the question carefully and orient to it. Is anything confusing or ambiguous? Is it clear what the question is looking for? Sometimes you should take a moment to mentally picture the situation that the question deals with. Many people feel that they should get through the question quickly in order to get to the "important" part—the answer choices. In fact, taking the time to be well oriented to the question can help you avoid many errors.

STEP 2. ASK WHAT'S NEXT

Consider how to start working on the question. Do not simply start reading answer choice A. There is often a better way to start. Sometimes you should go back to the setup and clarify concepts and facts. Often you should create a sketch, organize the information graphically, and/or make a road map. Sometimes specific information is stated in the passage that will determine the answer. Find this first before looking at answer choices. This is a common strategy for Critical Analysis.

STEP 3. FIRST PASS THROUGH THE ANSWERS—PROCESS OF ELIMINATION

After completing Step 2, look at the answer choices. Make a first pass through the answers, eliminating only those answers that are clearly out. You are learning strategies that will allow you to evaluate answers in depth. However, do not use those strategies during this pass. In-depth strategies require extra time. You might, for example, spend a lot of time carefully evaluating answers A through C, only to find that answer D is obviously the right one. The time spent on A, B, and C would have been wasted. The first pass gives you a quick overview of the answers. Save in-depth analysis for the second pass.

Be conservative about eliminating answers at this point. Eliminate only those answers that are very clearly incorrect. If you have any uncertainty, leave the answer in until the second pass. Answers can often be categorized as going in the right direction or in the wrong direction. For example, if the correct answer is a substance that will make a solution more acidic, then NaOH would go in the wrong direction. Acetic acid would go in the right direction but still might not be the correct answer because of other factors. Answers that go in the wrong direction are clearly out.

STEP 4. SECOND PASS WITH IN-DEPTH ANALYSIS

Go to the remaining answer choices, and use strategies to determine the correct answer. There may only be two choices left at this point or there may be three or all four.

Especially if there are only two answers left, identifying the difference between the two can help focus more specifically on how to solve the problem. Consider the following:

(A) 3.1754×10^6

~~(B)~~

(C) 18

~~(D)~~

With only A and C remaining, it is clear that the problem does not require precise calculation but rather is an issue of order of magnitude. Estimation alone may give the answer.

The Adversarial Approach—The Secret Weapon

Right now, you are probably getting 5, 10, 15 or more questions wrong that you will be able to get right by using good strategies. These are the questions that will raise your score by 1, 2, 3, or even more points on the 15-point scale. These questions probably all have one thing in common. You can get down to two possible answers on them but are then choosing the wrong one.

The adversarial approach is the most powerful tool for finding which of two answers is correct. Nearly every Critical Analysis passage requires the adversarial approach. It is also the strategy of choice on many science questions. We will look at how the strategy works in both cases.

> **THE ADVERSARIAL APPROACH**
>
> To overcome your own blind spots, defend to the death the answer you don't like and attack to the death the answer that you do like.

In Critical Analysis, when two possible answers are left, most people intuitively feel better about one answer than another and at first they simply pick the answer that feels better to them. When it becomes apparent that this leads to many wrong answers, test takers begin to look more carefully at the two answers, comparing them and trying a little harder to evaluate them. Notice that when you do this, there is still a bias toward the answer that seemed better in the first place. This bias often prevents a test taker from being objective. So despite making the effort, you still get many wrong answers.

Even when you become committed to being more objective, it is difficult to do so. The power of our biases cannot really be overcome simply by wanting to be objective. You need a specific, active strategy to achieve objectivity. We will draw our strategy—the adversarial approach—from the American legal system.

In some legal systems, one attorney argues both sides of a case before the judge. It is that attorney's responsibility to understand both sides, evaluate them, and present a balanced perspective. In America, however, an adversarial system is used. Each side is represented by its own attorney. Each attorney focuses only on his or her perspective, either attacking or defending a position. By eliminating the constraint of being balanced, the system allows each side to pursue one point of view aggressively. The judge then has the responsibility to synthesize both sides. In theory, the adversarial system results in a clearer picture of each side of the issue.

How does this apply to the MCAT sciences and Critical Analysis? Suppose that you have eliminated answers B and C. Answer A seems strong to you. Answer D seems unlikely. You can now apply the four steps of the adversarial approach. They do not have to be applied in a specific order.

(STEP 1) Attack the answer you like.
(STEP 2) Defend the answer you do not like.
(STEP 3) Defend the answer you like.
(STEP 4) Attack the answer you do not like.

Steps 1 and 2 are the most counterintuitive and thus the most powerful. Imagine that you are an attorney and that it is your job to prove that choice A is correct. Once you have done this, you switch positions and become the attorney who must prove that choice A is indisputably wrong.

In Steps 3 and 4, you are justifying your original bias, which may turn out to be correct. However, you are now doing so in more depth. As you try to prove that choice A is correct, you may discover that doing so is difficult. As you try to prove that choice D is incorrect, you may discover some merits to it.

By focusing all your attention on finding the defense for an answer, you see things that you simply would not have seen before when you were impartially reviewing both choices. The same holds true for the attack. By doing all four steps, you will have the best chance of seeing all the points you did not see before. Remember that as you apply this approach, you are not yet in the judge's position of weighing the pros and cons. That will come at the end. The most common error in applying the adversarial approach is falling back into the judge's position too soon and therefore failing to attack from the extreme standpoint and defend from the extreme standpoint. If you continue to get wrong answers, work harder at attacking and defending from the extremes.

The Critical Analysis chapter will discuss what constitutes a defense of an answer and an attack of an answer. On the sciences, you are working not only with formulas and facts but also with logic. When you are down to two answers and you are not able to make any further progress, you can often get a new perspective by trying to attack and defend each answer in turn.

Ambiguity

Sometimes the wording in a question or an answer choice is confusing. The wording may have two different interpretations.

EXAMPLE

You are responsible for collecting research information from three hospitals, two clinics, and five universities. Each institution must have its own unique data collection form.

TIP

CONFUSION IS YOUR FRIEND

If you can notice when you are confused, you will be able to do something about it.

Do you see the ambiguity in this statement? You must identify ambiguity or confusion if it exists. Many people are resistant to feeling confused. They may hope they will catch on later. In fact, it is very helpful to notice confusing wording, identify why it is confusing, and then find a way to resolve the confusion.

In the above example, does creating a unique form for each institution require making ten forms or three forms? The word *institution* may strike some people as ambiguous. A hospital could be one institution and a clinic another. Alternatively, the sentence could mean that Hospital A is one institution and Hospital B is another. How is the test taker supposed to know the correct interpretation?

The MCAT cannot contain a question that is truly ambiguous. It must contain some evidence that will show which interpretation is intended. To deal with an ambiguity, first identify the two interpretations. Then ask which of those interpretations would be defendable based on the information and evidence given in the test. Consider the rest of the passage.

EXAMPLE

You are responsible for collecting research information from three hospitals, two clinics, and five universities. Each institution must have its own unique data collection form. Data must be collected within a week of the time it is compiled and must be delivered directly to the office of the research coordinator. Each of the ten institutions is responsible for double checking the accuracy of its form. You are responsible for getting the signature of the head of staff at each hospital and clinic, but the universities do not need to have their forms signed.

The phrase "each of the ten institutions" defines how the word *institution* is being used.

Working Backward from Answer Choices

TIP

TESTING ANSWER CHOICES

Let the answer choices work for you. Testing answers gives you valuable information.

This is similar to the adversarial approach but not quite as rigorous. Test an answer choice by temporarily assuming it is correct. Would that result in any contradictions? Would the answer fit the data? Testing an answer choice can help you see things about it that you would not see otherwise.

BIGGER OR SMALLER?

On questions that require a calculation, working backward from an answer means that you put the answer into the calculation and see if the result is correct. If the result is too small or too big, you can save time by considering whether you should try a smaller or a larger answer choice.

EXAMPLE

A scientist can add carbon-12 to a reaction only in units of whole numbers of moles (and not in fractions of a mole) but must ensure that there are at least 975 g of carbon so that the carbon will react completely with the oxygen present. What is the smallest number of moles of carbon the scientist must add?

(A) 47

(B) 80

(C) 100

(D) 122

Testing answer choices (multiplying the answer choice times 12 g/mole) is easier and more reliable than dividing 975 by 12. Start with numbers that are easy and foolproof. Choice C is easy and results in 1200 grams. Now apply logic. Choice C cannot be eliminated because if choice B does not give enough, choice C could still be the smallest number of moles to give at least 975 grams. However, choice D is out. What is the plan of attack now?

If choice B is less than 975, then choice C will be the answer. If choice B is more than 975, it is the answer unless choice A is also more than 975. A quick test of choice A shows that because it is less than half of 100, it will yield fewer than 600 grams. Answer A is out.

Now it will be necessary to do the multiplication (80×12). This is still simpler and more foolproof than dividing 975 by 12. The result, 960, is too small. Choice C is the answer.

Estimation

The previous example used estimation. Estimation is a powerful tool. Even though it may not result in an exact answer, it can help eliminate answers, sometimes pinpointing the correct one.

EXAMPLE

To four decimal places, what is the decimal equivalent of $\frac{133}{262}$?

(A) 0.3573

(B) 0.4932

(C) 0.5076

(D) 0.7433

Estimation tells you that the fraction is around half. However, although estimation is an approximation, it does tell you for certain that the fraction is above half (half of 262 would be 131). Any number below half cannot be the correct answer. So choices A and B are out. Because the fraction is only $\frac{2}{262}$ above half, which is a little less than a one-hundredth, choice D is much too big.

Graphs

On problems with one or more graphs, be systematic. First orient yourself to each graph separately. What are the variables? How are the axes labeled? Which elements need to be distinguished and which do not?

For example, consider a graph titled "Solubility of Compound *A* in Carbon Tetrachloride." Determine whether the graph includes compounds other than Compound *A*. If it does not, then Compound *A* is an insignificant fact that can be ignored. The graph might indicate, however, that you would have to distinguish temperatures, pressures, and concentrations. A second graph titled "Solubility of Compound *A* in Water" would indicate that water must be distinguished from carbon tetrachloride.

If more than one graph is shown, the next step is to examine how the graphs are related to each other. Which elements are the same, and which are different? Taking time to do this before answering the questions will help keep the information clear.

> **GRAPHS**
>
> Orient yourself carefully. How are the axes labeled? What do the graphs distinguish? Errors in reading graphs can be completely avoided by careful reading.

Put Down Cold Guess Answers for Any Question You Are Not Going to Work On

There is no penalty for wrong answers. Be sure to put down an answer for each question that you have skipped. Do not spend time trying to eliminate answers. You should either work a question thoroughly or put down a cold guess. On the computer test, simply click on the answer to which the cursor is nearest when the question comes up. It is not necessary to move the cursor into the answer oval. Simply click on any part of the answer. This saves you time from trying to aim. You will get one question in four right by chance!

Alternate Hand Mousing

During the computer test, you will need to both manipulate the mouse and make notes on scratch paper. Some people find it helpful to manipulate the mouse with their nondominant hand so that they do not have to switch hands in order to write notes. Practice this well in advance of the actual test to see if it works for you.

Always Look at All of the Answers

One of the most common causes of errors is choosing an answer that looks good without having considered all of the answers. Even if you are confident in an answer, you are setting yourself up for falling for distractors if you do not at least quickly look at the remaining answers. This is one of the most important strategies for avoiding careless errors. Train yourself to do this on every single question.

EXCEPT, NOT, LEAST, and I, II, III Questions

Questions that use the words EXCEPT, LEAST, or NOT are logically confusing. Consider the question "All of the following are brown EXCEPT . . ." Your attention will focus on the quality of being brown, but the correct answer is the opposite. It is very easy to get confused and choose an answer that is brown. When an MCAT question asks for an exception—for the opposite of what the test taker would normally look for—the word EXCEPT, NOT, or LEAST is capitalized to draw your attention to it.

"DON'T LOOK AT THAT ELEPHANT" QUESTIONS

Questions with EXCEPT, NOT, or LEAST point you away from what you would normally focus on. Be prepared!

Orient to exception questions by reminding yourself that you are looking for three of whatever is expected, such as three brown things, and that these three are the wrong answers. The correct answer will be whatever is remaining when you identify the three brown answers. Holding out three fingers to remind yourself can be helpful. Use this strategy in conjunction with the strategy of going back and skimming the question stem before looking at each answer choice. Keep an eye on your errors in untimed practice to see if you have a tendency to stumble on exception questions.

The I, II, III questions have slightly more complex logic than regular questions, though most people do not have trouble understanding them. You can use a special strategy with these, though.

EXAMPLE

According to the passage, which of the following statements would Sir Isaac Newton have agreed with?

  I.   Petr sa prebudil v kozmickej lodi.
  II. Gravity is a figment of the imagination.
  III. Kapitanka varila mu polievku.

(A) I only
(B) I and II only
(C) II and III only
(D) I, II, and III

The first step in a I, II, III question is to look at the answer choices. Notice which Roman numerals appear in more than one answer. Look for Roman numeral answers that are clearly right or wrong. What answer choices are then eliminated?

Now can you answer the question? If II is wrong, what is left?

Stamina

The MCAT is a very long test. You will get tired. Your brain will not be at its optimum at all times during the test. You can do some simple things to maximize your endurance during the test.

Intense brain activity consumes large amounts of oxygen. Combined with the fact that you are sitting still for hours during the test, your brain will probably become oxygen deprived. When you start feeling tired and your thinking is foggy or unfocused, stretch and flex your arms and legs. Yawn and breathe deeply. During the test, you need to be moderately unobtrusive about this. However, frequent mild stretching and deep breathing will help you think more clearly.

Your eyes will also become overworked in the test. The eyes are involved not only in seeing what is on the screen but in mental processing as well. When you have trouble focusing your attention, try closing your eyes or covering them with the cupped palms of your hand. Shifting your focus to a point in the far distance can also relax the eye muscles. You can do this with your eyes opened by looking out a window or with your eyes closed.

When you are tired, you may be more bothered by distractions. Assume that you will have distractions during your test day, and be prepared for them. Practice for stamina by doing several test sections in a row or by taking a test section with 5 minutes less than the normal time limit. Occasionally working on questions in a noisy or distracting environment may help you practice for distractions.

During the week before your test, you may find it helpful to simulate the schedule of the test day. Keep a note card with approximate times that each section will start and finish, along with break times. During the time that will be devoted to a test section on your actual test day, do not eat, drink, or use the bathroom. If you find that you have trouble following that schedule, such as needing to use the bathroom, getting hungry, or having low blood sugar, adjust your eating and drinking patterns. Identifying any areas of anxiety that you have can also be helpful, such as a fear of not finding the test center, of not waking up on time, or of not getting the score you need. Come up with a backup plan for each concern. Dealing with these concerns in advance may help you get a good night's sleep the night before your test.

Analyzing Your Testing Strategy

After completing a section, either timed or untimed, go over each wrong answer to determine what strategies you could have used to avoid the error. On the following pages is a worksheet you can use to do that, along with a list of possible errors that you can refer to.

> ### THE KEY TO GOOD TIMING
>
> Always analyze your timed test sections carefully to see how you could have improved timing and strategy.

If you answered a question wrong, look at it carefully. Sometimes MCAT students look at a wrong answer and decide it was "just a careless error." In the authors' experience, errors are usually not due to carelessness. They are due to incorrect timing strategy or testing strategy. Every error gives you a chance to learn how to approach the test more effectively. Do not be too quick to dismiss an error as careless. Use the checklist on pages 32–33 to remind yourself of the possible causes of errors.

Analyzing Wrong Answers

Use a worksheet like this to evaluate your wrong answers every time you do a test section. For each question you answered wrong, put down the time you spent on it and the reasons you got it wrong. Choose your reason from the master list of reasons. Then review the strategy for avoiding that error. You do not need to include questions on which you guessed cold.

Note: This page may be photocopied.

ANALYSIS OF ERRORS

Example: Q #15   Time: 3:30   Reason: Did math wrong, time pressure

Test # _____ **Section:** _____

Q # _____   Time: _____   Reason: _____

Q # _____   Time: _____   Reason: _____

Q # _____   Time: _____   Reason: _____

Q # _____   Time: _____   Reason: _____

Q # _____   Time: _____   Reason: _____

Q # _____   Time: _____   Reason: _____

Q # _____   Time: _____   Reason: _____

Q # _____   Time: _____   Reason: _____

Q # _____   Time: _____   Reason: _____

Q # _____   Time: _____   Reason: _____

Q # _____   Time: _____   Reason: _____

Q # _____   Time: _____   Reason: _____

Q # _____   Time: _____   Reason: _____

Q # _____   Time: _____   Reason: _____

Q # _____   Time: _____   Reason: _____

Q # _____   Time: _____   Reason: _____

Q # _____   Time: _____   Reason: _____

Q # _____   Time: _____   Reason: _____

Q # _____   Time: _____   Reason: _____

Q # _____   Time: _____   Reason: _____

Q # _____   Time: _____   Reason: _____

Q # _____   Time: _____   Reason: _____

Q # _____   Time: _____   Reason: _____

Q # _____   Time: _____   Reason: _____

LIST OF REASONS FOR ERRORS

1. **DID NOT USE BIG PICTURE.** Got lost in details. Did not step back to see the big picture. Missed obvious information because focus was too narrow.

2. **TIME PRESSURE.** Not careful enough because of feeling rushed to get on to other questions. Tried to do too many.

3. **COULD NOT ORGANIZE INFO.** Confused by complex details, facts, concepts. Lacked tools to organize the information. Got lost part way through. Did not use visual aids—drawing, charts, columns—when needed. Did not create a systematic roadmap of how to solve the problem.

4. **DID MATH WRONG.** Made a calculation mistake because of failure to double-check or write down each step.

5. **MISREAD QUESTION OR FACTS.** Misinterpreted part of the question or info. Did not apply strategy for ambiguous questions. Did not orient well to the question. Read something into the problem or made an unwarranted assumption.

6. **SPENT LESS THAN 3 MINUTES.** Chose a wrong answer on a question that could have been answered correctly with more time. Did not keep track of time. Felt hesitant to spend 4 or 5 minutes.

7. **REMEMBERED SOMETHING INACCURATELY.** Did not double-check the facts. Used memory instead of eyes. Rushed.

8. **THOUGHT YOU HAD IT RIGHT.** Did not take an extra moment to see if you missed anything. Did not challenge your answer or defend other answers.

9. **DID NOT READ ALL ANSWER CHOICES.** Chose an answer without using the other answers as a double-check. Tried to save time by not reading all answers.

10. **DID NOT CHECK YOUR CONFIDENCE LEVEL.** Did not notice that you were not confident about the answer. Unsure of answer but did not want to take more time. Did not use double checking or big picture to increase confidence. Chose an answer you did not like because all of the others seemed wrong. Did not go back and start from scratch with all answers.

11. **DID NOT KNOW WHAT STRATEGIES TO USE ON QUESTION.** Did not use KING approach. Did not step back to see big picture. Did not use diagram to organize the information. Did not use adversarial approach. Did not work backward from answer choices. Did not use imagination or intuition to get new insights into the problem. Did not check whether some answers were too big or too small.

12. **GOT UNCOMFORTABLE OR ANXIOUS AND QUIT QUESTION TOO SOON.** Let physical/psychological discomfort level dictate your timing strategy instead of controlling time yourself. Did not use the tension between two answers to help you analyze more deeply (adversarial approach).

13. **FELL FOR A DISTRACTOR.** Chose an answer that felt right or that seemed good for a vague reason. Did not use adversarial approach. Did not give the question enough time. When guessing, tried to justify one answer instead of using a random rule of thumb.

14. **PICKED RIGHT ANSWER BUT PUT WRONG LETTER.** Do not yet have perfect strategy for double checking that you have clicked the right answer.

15. **GOT DOWN TO TWO ANSWERS AND PICKED WRONG ONE.** Did not use adversarial approach. Tried adversarial approach but did not argue all the way to the end. Not able to turn energy of frustration into energy for analysis. Did not give the question a full 4 to 5 minutes. Did not use estimation. Did not focus on what the difference was between the two answers.

16. **DID NOT USE PROCESS OF ELIMINATION.** Could have gotten closer to an answer by eliminating wrong answer choices.

17. **BECAME DISCOURAGED BY COMPLEX SETUP.** Did not remember that you do not need to understand everything in the setup. Did not go directly to the questions.

18. **FORGOT TO TAKE TIME TO FILL IN AN ANSWER.**

19. **BECAME CONFUSED BY GRAPHS.** Did not orient to each graph. Did not analyze the relationship between graphs.

20. **COULD NOT RESOLVE AN AMBIGUITY.** Did not identify the two (or more) possible interpretations and ask which interpretation was defendable.

21. **CRITICAL ANALYSIS. DID NOT GET THE MAIN IDEA.** Did not analyze the setup clearly enough for big picture. Did not find the main dichotomies. Got too bogged down in detail. Not enough practice scanning passage for structure. Thrown off by a difficult topic.

22. **CRITICAL ANALYSIS. MISSED AUTHOR'S TONE QUESTION.** Did not see answers in terms of continuum.

THREE-MONTH STUDY PLAN

Here is a plan to organize your studying over three months. The AAMC tests referred to below are the actual MCAT exams published by AAMC.

You do not need to do all sections of an assigned test at the same time except when a full mock test is assigned. After completing a test section, be sure to review both your timing and testing strategies. Also identify science areas that you need to review further.

For a six-month study plan, go through the three-month plan twice. During the first three months, do only the Barron's practice tests and save the AAMC tests for the final three months.

PRACTICE, PRACTICE, PRACTICE: ONLINE RESOURCES

Now that you know the strategies that will help you do well on the MCAT, be sure to use them whenever you do the exercises and practice tests in this book and, of course, when you take your actual MCAT. In addition to all of the tests and practice questions in this book, you can get even more practice with our two additional tests (with complete explanations) online at *http://barronsbooks.com/tp/mcat/.*

Table 9. Three-Month Study Plan

	BARRON'S CHAPTERS	PRACTICE TESTS
FIRST MONTH		
Week 1	Read Table of Contents and Introduction.	Barron's Practice Test 1. All sections, timed.
Week 2	Read Chemistry chapter.	Barron's Chemistry end-of-chapter practice questions.
Week 3	Read Critical Analysis chapter.	Barron's Critical Analysis end-of-chapter practice questions.
Week 4	Read Physics chapter.	Barron's Physics end-of-chapter practice questions.
SECOND MONTH		
Week 5	Read Biology chapter.	Barron's Biology end-of-chapter practice questions.
Week 6	Read Organic Chemistry and Biochemistry chapters.	Barron's Organic Chemistry and Biology end-of-chapter tests.
Week 7	Read Psychology and Sociology chapters.	Barron's Psychology and Sociology end-of-chapter tests.
Week 8	Review Critical Analysis chapter.	AAMC test, timed.
Week 9	Review Chemistry and Physics chapters and the Introduction.	Barron's Practice Test 2, untimed.
THIRD MONTH		
Week 10	Review Biology chapter.	Barron's online Practice Test 1, science sections, timed.
Week 11	Review Organic Chemistry and Biochemistry chapters.	Barron's online Practice Test 1, critical analysis and psych/soc sections, timed.
Week 12	Review Critical Analysis chapter.	Barron's online Practice Test 2 as a full mock test, timed.
Week 13	Review Psychology and Sociology chapters.	Any new AAMC material, timed.

PART 1
Biological and Physical Sciences

Periodic Table of the Elements

1	2	3	4	5	6	7	8	9	10	11	12	13	14	15	16	17	18
1 **H** 1.0																	2 **He** 4.0
3 **Li** 6.9	4 **Be** 9.0											5 **B** 10.8	6 **C** 12.0	7 **N** 14.0	8 **O** 16.0	9 **F** 19.0	10 **Ne** 20.2
11 **Na** 23.0	12 **Mg** 24.3											13 **Al** 27.0	14 **Si** 28.1	15 **P** 31.0	16 **S** 32.1	17 **Cl** 35.5	18 **Ar** 39.9
19 **K** 39.1	20 **Ca** 40.1	21 **Sc** 45.0	22 **Ti** 47.9	23 **V** 50.9	24 **Cr** 52.0	25 **Mn** 54.9	26 **Fe** 55.8	27 **Co** 58.8	28 **Ni** 58.7	29 **Cu** 63.5	30 **Zn** 65.4	31 **Ga** 69.7	32 **Ge** 72.6	33 **As** 74.9	34 **Se** 79.0	35 **Br** 79.9	36 **Kr** 83.8
37 **Rb** 85.5	38 **Sr** 87.6	39 **Y** 88.9	40 **Zr** 91.2	41 **Nb** 92.9	42 **Mo** 95.9	43 **Tc** (98)	44 **Ru** 101.1	45 **Rh** 102.9	46 **Pd** 106.4	47 **Ag** 107.9	48 **Cd** 112.4	49 **In** 114.8	50 **Sn** 118.7	51 **Sb** 121.8	52 **Te** 127.6	53 **I** 126.9	54 **Xe** 131.3
55 **Cs** 132.9	56 **Ba** 137.3	57 **La** 138.9	72 **Hf** 178.5	73 **Ta** 180.9	74 **W** 183.9	75 **Re** 186.2	76 **Os** 190.2	77 **Ir** 192.2	78 **Pt** 195.1	79 **Au** 197.0	80 **Hg** 200.6	81 **Tl** 204.4	82 **Pb** 207.2	83 **Bi** 209.0	84 **Po** (209)	85 **At** (210)	86 **Rn** (222)
87 **Fr** (223)	88 **Ra** (226)	89 **Ac†** (227)	104 **Rf** (261)	105 **Db** (262)	106 **Sg** (266)	107 **Bh** (264)	108 **Hs** (277)	109 **Mt** (268)	110 **Ds** (281)	111 **Rg** (280)	112 **Cn** (285)	113 **Uut** (284)	114 **Fl** (289)	115 **Uup** (288)	116 **Lv** (293)	117 **Uus** (294)	118 **Uuo** (294)

★

58 **Ce** 140.1	59 **Pr** 140.9	60 **Nd** 144.2	61 **Pm** (145)	62 **Sm** 150.4	63 **Eu** 152.0	64 **Gd** 157.3	65 **Tb** 158.9	66 **Dy** 162.5	67 **Ho** 164.9	68 **Er** 167.3	69 **Tm** 168.9	70 **Yb** 173.0	71 **Lu** 175.0
90 **Th** 232.0	91 **Pa** (231)	92 **U** 238.0	93 **Np** (237)	94 **Pu** (244)	95 **Am** (243)	96 **Cm** (247)	97 **Bk** (247)	98 **Cf** (251)	99 **Es** (252)	100 **Fm** (257)	101 **Md** (258)	102 **No** (259)	103 **Lr** (260)

†

General Chemistry

1

- → ATOMIC STRUCTURE AND THE PERIODIC TABLE
- → IONIC AND COVALENT BONDING
- → STATES OF MATTER
- → STOICHIOMETRY
- → THERMOCHEMISTRY AND THERMODYNAMICS
- → KINETICS AND EQUILIBRIUM
- → SOLUTION CHEMISTRY
- → ACID–BASE CHEMISTRY
- → ELECTROCHEMISTRY

The General Chemistry section of the MCAT covers the topics typically taught in two semesters of an introductory inorganic chemistry course. College chemistry courses differ in the content they cover. By reviewing this chapter, however, you will be familiar with the topics that usually appear on the MCAT. The MCAT primarily tests an understanding of general concepts rather than memorization of equations or isolated facts. This chapter reviews and summarizes those facts and concepts that you need to understand. Keep in mind that calculations on the MCAT are kept to a minimum and that calculators of any kind are not allowed on the test.

ATOMIC STRUCTURE AND THE PERIODIC TABLE

All matter is made of atoms. An understanding of the structure of atoms allows us to explain the specific chemical and physical properties of elements and of compounds. The structure of the atom was worked out through a series of experimental and theoretical approaches, and this detailed knowledge of the structure of the atom led to an understanding of the arrangement of the modern periodic table. The logical, predictable organization of the periodic table allows chemists to apply knowledge about atoms in a way that is practical and relevant.

Electronic Structure and Quantum Theory

The current model of the atom is based on quantum mechanics. Quantum mechanics describes (as accurately as nature allows) the location and motion of electrons. It is these electrons that give each element its unique (and highly predictable) properties, which affect the types of bonds an atom forms, the compounds it forms, and the behavior of the element when alone or when combined chemically. These properties allow us to relate atomic structure to location on the periodic table. The periodic nature of chemical and physical properties is of great value in understanding the properties of compounds. It is the basis for predicting the properties of new substances.

BASICS OF ATOMIC STRUCTURE

Atoms are composed of **protons**, **neutrons**, and **electrons**. Even though these basic sub-atomic particles are themselves made of even smaller particles, almost all of the chemistry needed for the MCAT can be explained in terms of protons, neutrons, and electrons. The protons and neutrons are located in the **nucleus** of the atom, which is small and very dense. Electrons are most likely to be located in the spaces outside the nucleus known as orbitals, which are regions with a high probability of electron location. All the atoms of a particular element have the same number of protons.

Protons have a relative charge of +1 and a mass of 1 atomic mass unit (amu). The atomic number (represented by the letter Z) of an element is equal to the number of protons in the nucleus of that element. The identity of the atom is determined by the number of protons in the nucleus.

Neutrons are particles with a relative mass almost identical to that of the proton, but they have no charge. Neutrons are also located in the nucleus of the atom. The neutrons contribute to the mass of the atom but not to the charge.

The electrons are located outside the nucleus. Electrons have a mass equal to about $\frac{1}{1836}$ that of a proton, and their mass is typically not included in the mass of the atom. The charge of the electron is opposite in sign but equal in magnitude to the charge of a proton, namely –1. The masses of the proton and neutron are not exactly equal to each other; however, for all calculations on the MCAT, the two particles can be assumed to have masses equal to 1 amu.

The properties of three main subatomic particles of the atom can be summarized in Table 1.1.

Table 1.1 Subatomic Particles of the Atom

Particle	Relative Mass	Relative Charge	Location
Proton (p⁺)	1 amu*	+1	Nucleus
Neutron (n)	1 amu*	0	Nucleus
Electron (e⁻)	$1/1836 \approx 0$ amu	–1	Outside nucleus

*amu = atomic mass unit

In a neutral atom, the number of protons will equal the number of electrons.

Mass Number

NUCLIDE SYMBOLS

Make sure you know how to quickly determine the number of protons, neutrons, and electrons from a nuclide symbol.

The mass number is the sum of the number of protons and neutrons in an atom's nucleus. It is represented by the letter A. Using the isotope carbon-12 as a standard, 1 amu is defined as exactly $\frac{1}{12}$ the mass of a carbon-12 atom. One amu is equal to 1.66×10^{-24} grams. The use of atomic mass units is for convenience only.

Because the mass number of an atom equals the number of protons plus neutrons and the atomic number equals the number of protons, the number of neutrons can be obtained by subtracting the atomic number from the mass number (or, expressed in symbols, $A - Z$).

An atom of iron-56, $^{56}_{26}$Fe, has an atomic number of 26 and a mass number of 56. This particular atom has 26 protons and 26 electrons and 30 (56 – 26) neutrons. The symbol that shows the element along with its atomic number and mass number is called a **nuclide symbol**.

Isotopes and Average Atomic Mass

Isotopes are atoms of an element with differing numbers of neutrons (the number of protons and electrons does not change). The isotopes of an element have the same atomic number but different mass numbers. An isotope is named for its mass number. Thus, an atom of the isotope of carbon with a mass number of 13 is called carbon-13 (abbreviated C-13, or ^{13}C). The mass number must be specified but the atomic number need not be, because, by definition, all atoms of carbon have an atomic number of 6.

Figure 1.1 shows three isotopes of lithium. All have three protons and three electrons. They would be referred to as lithium-6, lithium-7, and lithium-8. All would exhibit the same chemical properties, which are determined by the electron arrangement of the atom.

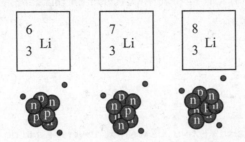

Figure 1.1. Isotopes of lithium

The atomic weights listed on most periodic tables show a weighted average (or average atomic mass) of the isotopes of an element found in nature. This is in contrast to the mass number, which refers to a specific isotope.

The **average atomic mass** of an element is a weighted average based on the fractional abundance of each isotope and the mass of each isotope. The fractional abundance of an isotope is the percentage expressed as a decimal. Thus, an isotope that made up 45% of all the atoms in a sample would have a fractional abundance of 0.45. The sum of all the fractional abundances is equal to 1.00.

> **Average atomic mass:** the weighted average of the masses of the isotopes of an element
>
> **Mass number:** the number of protons and neutrons in a specific isotope of an element

Practice Question

Silicon consists of three isotopes, with masses and abundances as shown in Table 1. Calculate the average atomic mass of a silicon atom.

Table 1 Isotopes of Silicon

Isotope	Mass (amu)	Abundance
Si-28	27.97	0.921
Si-29	28.97	0.045
Si-30	29.96	0.034

Solution: The calculation to determine the average atomic mass would be

$$(27.97 \text{ amu})(0.921) + (28.97 \text{ amu})(0.045) + (29.96 \text{ amu})(0.034) = 28.08 \text{ amu}$$

As a quick check, the average must be within the range of the lightest and heaviest isotopes listed, and will likely be closest to the most abundant isotope. A more general form is:

$$\text{Average Atomic Mass} = \Sigma \text{ (abundance)}_i\text{(mass)}_i$$

TEST QUESTION

A sample of boron was analyzed with a mass spectrometer and found to consist of 80% of boron-11 and 20% of boron-10. Based on this sample, what is the average atomic mass of boron?

(A) 10.20 amu

(B) 10.50 amu

(C) 10.80 amu

(D) 11.20 amu

(C) One way to solve this is to use a weighted average and do the calculation:

$$(0.80)(11) + (0.20)(10) = 10.80$$

Another way, which does not involve a calculation, is to use the fact that the average must be between 10 and 11, because the average cannot be higher than the highest mass nor lower than the lowest one. Because 80% of the atoms analyzed have a mass of 11 amu, the average must be closer to 11. Only choice C meets both criteria.

THE BOHR MODEL OF THE HYDROGEN ATOM: SPECTRA, GROUND, AND EXCITED STATES

TIP

Energy and frequency are directly related.

The nucleus was discovered by Ernest Rutherford in 1911. His "gold foil" experiment showed that the atom had a very small, positively charged center, now known as the nucleus. The volume of an atom is mostly taken up by the electrons. Max Planck hypothesized that the energy emitted by atoms (whether as visible light or other forms of electromagnetic radiation) came in discrete units called **quanta**. The energy of a quantum is directly proportional to the frequency of the radiation emitted. The energy is given by the equation:

$$E = h\nu$$

TIP

The letter ν is the Greek letter "nu" and not a v. Some people prefer to use the letter f as an abbreviation for frequency.

in which E is the energy in joules, h is the constant 6.63×10^{-34} J · s (now known as Planck's constant) and ν (sometimes given as f) is the frequency in Hertz or s^{-1}.

The first modern model of the atom was developed by Niels Bohr around 1913. Bohr developed a model of the hydrogen atom with a single electron traveling around the proton in an orbit, much like the way planets in the solar system orbit the sun. This model, later proven incorrect, was called the **planetary model**. Bohr's model could explain the emission of specific spectral lines from a hydrogen atom when it was energized. Unlike a classical model, in which energy is continuous, Bohr described an atom in which only specific energies were "allowed," a direct result of the quantum nature of the atom predicted by Planck.

TIP

The MCAT does NOT require that you memorize the values of constants, such as h.

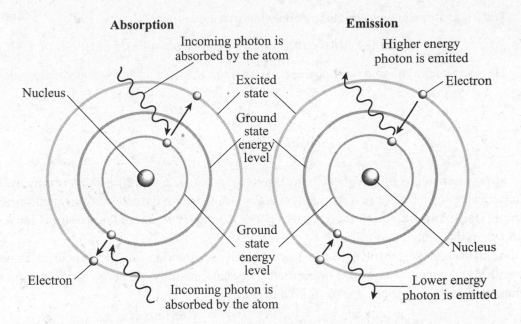

Absorption

Incoming photon is
absorbed by the atom

Excited
state

Nucleus

Ground
state
energy
level

Ground
state
energy
level

Electron

Incoming photon is
absorbed by the atom

Emission

Higher energy
photon is emitted

Electron

Nucleus

Lower energy
photon is emitted

Figure 1.2. Absorption and emission of photons by atoms

Bohr described the energy emitted by an atom using the formula (This does not need to be memorized for the MCAT):

$$\Delta E = R_H \left(\frac{1}{n_i^2} - \frac{1}{n_f^2} \right),$$

where ΔE is the amount of energy emitted or absorbed, R_H is a constant equal to 2.18×10^{-18} J, and n_i and n_f are the initial and final energy states of the electron. This energy can then be related to the wavelength and frequency of the energy by the equations

$$c = \lambda v \text{ and } E = hv,$$

which can be combined to give

$$E = \frac{hc}{\lambda},$$

where c is the speed of light, 3×10^8 m/s, and λ is the wavelength (in meters).

> **ENERGY, FREQUENCY, AND
> WAVELENGTH RELATIONSHIPS**
>
> Energy and wavelength are inversely related.
> Wavelength and frequency are inversely related.

TIP

Patterns such as direct, inverse, and inverse square relationships are common on the MCAT. Be familiar with them.

A typical calculation applying the Rydberg equation is shown below:

Calculate the energy, wavelength, and frequency of light emitted when an electron moves from an energy level of $n = 4$ to an energy level of $n = 2$.

$$\Delta E = R_H \left(\frac{1}{16} - \frac{1}{4} \right) = -4.1 \times 10^{-19} \text{ J}$$

(The negative sign indicates that energy was emitted.)

The frequency can be solved for by applying $E = h\nu$.

$$4.1 \times 10^{-19} \text{ J} = (6.63 \times 10^{-34} \text{ J} \cdot \text{s})(\nu) \text{ and } \nu = 6.0 \times 10^{14} \text{ s}^{-1} \text{ or Hz}$$

The wavelength is found by applying $c = \lambda\nu$ so that

$$\lambda = \frac{c}{\nu} = \frac{3 \times 10^8 \text{ m/s}}{6.0 \times 10^{14} \text{ s}^{-1}} = 5 \times 10^{-7} \text{ m}$$

$$= 500 \text{ nm}$$

Energy transitions from higher energy levels to $n = 2$ are known as the Balmer Series, with initial values of n from 3 to 6 giving light in the visible region of the electromagnetic spectrum. Transitions from $n > 1$ to $n = 1$ give energies in the UV region of the spectrum and are known as the Lyman Series.

In any calculation involving an energy transmission, the sign on the value of ΔE shows whether the energy is absorbed or emitted. The same quantity of energy is involved for a transition from $n = 2$ to $n = 4$ as from $n = 4$ to $n = 2$.

ENERGY IN ELECTRON TRANSITIONS

When an electron moves between two energy levels, the quantity of energy involved is the same whether the electron is going to a higher or lower energy level.

If energy is absorbed, the value is positive. If energy is released, the value is negative.

An **emission spectrum** shows the energies of electromagnetic radiation given off by electrons during the transition from a higher to a lower level, whereas an **absorption spectrum** indicates the energy absorbed by electrons in moving from a lower energy state (often called the ground state) to a higher energy state (the excited state).

Quantum Numbers

Quantum mechanics gives the solution to a wave equation developed by Erwin Schrodinger that describes the most probable location of electrons outside the nucleus of the atom. The fundamental nature of the atom is such that it limits the ability to determine the exact location of the electrons. This limitation is described by the Heisenberg Uncertainty Principle.

Emission spectrum: higher state to lower state
Absorption spectrum: lower state to higher state

The solution of the wave equation yields three quantum numbers. These numbers provide detailed knowledge of the most likely location of electrons that is possible. Each quantum number gives specific information about an electron.

The **principal quantum number (n)** or energy level (the term "shell" is sometimes used, but energy level is the preferred term) can have any integral value from 1 to infinity. In physical terms, this quantum number corresponds to the distance of the electron from the nucleus. The greater the value of n, the greater is the distance from the nucleus. The energy difference from $n = 1$ to $n = 2$ is larger than from $n = 2$ to $n = 3$ and so on.

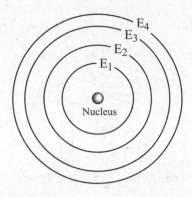

Figure 1.3. Energy levels (principal quantum number n)

Each energy level has a greater size, so that as the energy levels increase, the number of electrons that can occupy that energy level also increases. The number of electrons that can occupy any given energy level is given by the formula $2n^2$. The first energy level can hold two electrons, the second energy level eight electrons, the third eighteen, and so on.

The **azimuthal (angular momentum) quantum number (l)** refers to the shape of the region in space, within a given distance (value of n), where the electrons have a high probability of being located. These regions in space are sometimes called sublevels. For any given value of n, the value of l may range from 0 up to $n-1$. Each value of l is more commonly represented by a letter as shown in Table 1.2. Each sublevel has a specific abbreviation.

Table 1.2 Azimuthal Quantum Numbers

l value	Label
0	s
1	p
2	d
3	f

Other values exist, but for practical purposes only sublevels s, p, d, and f are used.
Each of the sublevels has a specific shape. The s sublevels are spherical, as shown below.

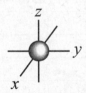

Figure 1.4. The s orbital shape

The p orbitals have a "bi-lobed shape," and there are three of them, each oriented along the x-, y-, or z-axis, as shown in Figure 1.5.

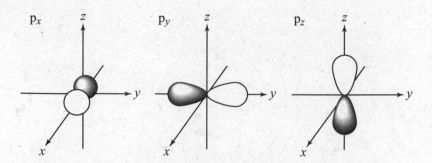

Figure 1.5. The p orbitals shape

The d orbitals are more complex. There are 5 arrangements, each with identical energy (referred to as degenerate). Their shapes are shown in Figure 1.6.

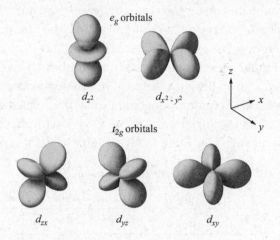

Figure 1.6. The d orbital shapes

The shapes of the seven possible f orbitals are more complex still and it is far more important to know that there are 7 f orbitals (with values of –3 through 0 and up to + 3) for m_l (**magnetic quantum number**—see below) values that are allowed when $l = 3$.

We can also summarize the allowed values of l based on n values as shown in Table 1.3.

Table 1.3 Sublevels in Levels

If n =	l is allowed to have values of	Labels
1	0	1s
2	0	2s
	1	2p
3	0	3s
	1	3p
	2	3d
4	0	4s
	1	4p
	2	4d
	3	4f

This means that each value of n (principal quantum number or energy level) places limits on the possible values of the sublevel.

The **magnetic quantum number (m_l)** describes the orientation of the specific shape (sublevel) where electrons are located. The allowed values of m_l range from $-l$ through 0 and up to $+l$, meaning that there are $2l + 1$ values possible. The set of three quantum numbers (n, l, and m_l) defines an orbital, a region in space in which there is a high probability of an electron being located.

An s sublevel has only one possible m_l value (or orbital): 0.

A p sublevel has an l value of 1 and three possible m_l values: -1, 0, or $+1$.

A d sublevel has an l value of 2 and 5 orbitals (or m_l values): -2, -1, 0, $+1$, and $+2$.

An f sublevel has an l value of 3 and 7 orbitals (or m_l values): -3, -2, -1, 0, $+1$, $+2$, and $+3$.

The **spin quantum number (m_s)**, which describes electrons, is the only quantum number that is independent of the other values of quantum numbers. Electrons have spin values that are designated as either $+\frac{1}{2}$ or $-\frac{1}{2}$. In order for two electrons to occupy a single orbital they must have opposite spins. This is known as the **Pauli Exclusion Principle**. It guarantees that each electron in an atom will have its own unique set of four quantum numbers.

An orbital may be unoccupied (empty), have one electron in it (in which case it could have a spin of either $+\frac{1}{2}$ or $-\frac{1}{2}$), or be full, with two electrons, in which case one electron must have the $+\frac{1}{2}$ spin and the other the $-\frac{1}{2}$ spin. Electrons with opposite spins on the same orbital are said to be paired.

> ## QUANTUM NUMBER SUMMARY
>
> Principal quantum number = energy level
> Azimuthal quantum number = sublevel
> Magnetic quantum number = orientation

Each sublevel has a specific number of orbitals and electrons, as summarized in Tables 1.4 and 1.5.

Table 1.4 Orbitals and Electrons in Different Sublevels

l value	Number of Orbitals ($m_l = 2l + 1$ values)	Maximum Number of Electrons = $2m_l$
0	1	2
1	3	6
2	5	10
3	7	14

Table 1.5 Maximum Number of Electrons in an Energy Level

Energy Level	Maximum Number of Electrons
1	**2** (2 electrons in the 1s)
2	**8** (2 electrons in the 2s and 6 in the 2p)
3	**18** (2 electrons in the 3s, 6 in the 3p, and 10 in the 3d)
4	**32** (2 electrons in the 4s, 6 in the 4p, 10 in the 4d, and 14 in the 4f)

**NUMBER OF ELECTRONS
IN A GIVEN ENERGY LEVEL**

The principal quantum number n will be able to hold a maximum of $2n^2$ electrons.

For $n = 1$, $2n^2 = 2$

For $n = 2$, $2n^2 = 8$

TEST QUESTION

Which set of quantum numbers is not allowed?

(A) $n = 2$, $l = 1$, $m_l = 0$, $m_s = +\frac{1}{2}$

(B) $n = 2$, $l = 1$, $m_l = -1$, $m_s = +\frac{1}{2}$

(C) $n = 2$, $l = 0$, $m_l = 0$, $m_s = -\frac{1}{2}$

(D) $n = 2$, $l = 2$, $m_l = 1$, $m_s = -\frac{1}{2}$

(D) Recall that the principal quantum number, n, sets limits on the allowed values of l

(l can have a value from 0 to $n - 1$) and that m_l can range from –1 through +1, including

0. The allowed spin values are $+\frac{1}{2}$ and $-\frac{1}{2}$. Choice D has a value of l that exceeds $n - 1$.

Orbitals, Configurations, and Filling Diagrams

There are two ways to show the information about the most likely location of the electrons in an atom. An orbital **filling diagram** is a detailed summary of the electrons showing the electrons in each of the energy level and sublevel, as well as the spin of the electrons. A shorthand version is known as an **electron configuration**.

An **Aufbau diagram** shows the specific order in which the energy levels and sublevels are filled. In the ground state of an atom, the energy levels fill from low to high as shown in Figure 1.7.

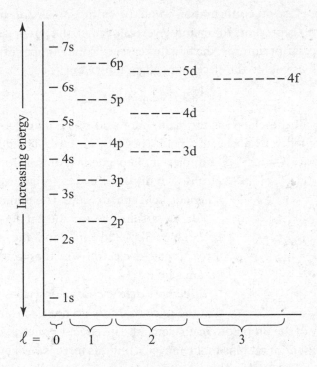

Figure 1.7. Aufbau diagram

The diagram shows that electrons fill in from "low to high," in the order: 1s, 2s, 2p, 3s, 3p, 4s, 3d, and so on. The s sublevels can have up to 2 electrons, the p sublevels, up to 6 electrons, and the d sublevels, up to10, and so on. The electrons "fill in" from low to high energy. This means that the 4s sublevel fills before the 3d sublevel.

One can think of each line in the above diagram as an orbital, with the ability to "hold" up to two electrons.

To show the spins of the electrons in an orbital, arrows are typically used, with an arrow pointing up indicating a + ½ spin and an arrow pointing down indicating a − ½ spin.

Hund's rule addresses one final feature that governs the arrangement of electrons in the atom, namely, that within a specific energy level and sublevel the electrons remain unpaired as much as possible.

Figure 1.8 shows the filling diagram for an atom such as nitrogen, with 7 electrons.

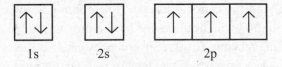

Figure 1.8. Electron filling diagram for nitrogen

Notice how the seven electrons in the nitrogen atom fill in the lowest available sublevels first, and then go on to the next highest levels. Each orbital has a maximum of two electrons, and when the 2p orbitals are reached, the electrons stay "unpaired" as much as possible.

A shorthand version known as a **configuration** describes the number of electrons in each sublevel, but not the spin. The spin can be determined by applying Hund's rule.

For nitrogen, the electron configuration would be written $1s^22s^22p^3$. In an entry such as $2p^3$, the 2 (coefficient) represents the energy level (value of n), the p represents the sublevel (l value), and the superscript number, the 3 in this case, tells the number of electrons.

For an atom such as cobalt, the electron configuration would be:

$$1s^22s^22p^63s^23p^64s^23d^7$$

Atoms in which all the electrons are paired are said to be **diamagnetic**. Diamagnetic atoms are slightly repelled by a magnetic field. They may also weakly repel a magnetic field.

HUND'S RULE

Just as everyone on a bus would like his or her own seat, each electron would like its own orbital.

Examples of diamagnetic atoms include Mg, Zn, and Ar. Atoms with unpaired electrons are weakly attracted to a magnetic field and are said to be **paramagnetic**.

For an arsenic atom, the configuration would be $1s^22s^22p^63s^23p^64s^23d^{10}4p^3$, and the atom would have three unpaired electrons in the 4p sublevel, making it paramagnetic.

Effective nuclear charge describes the attractive pull that the nucleus exerts on the electrons of an atom. This force explains many of the properties of an element. The effective nuclear charge is primarily the result of the number of protons in the nucleus, but this force is weakened by a shielding, or partial blocking effect, caused by all of the electrons except the outermost ones. The outermost electrons are known as valence electrons.

Valence electrons are the outermost energy level electrons in an atom. They are the electrons most directly involved in determining the chemical properties of the elements. The number of valence electrons can be found by locating all the electrons in the outermost energy level, based on the ground state electron configuration. For example, in the example of arsenic above, for which the configuration is $1s^22s^22p^63s^23p^6\mathbf{4s^2}3d^{10}\mathbf{4p^3}$, the highest occupied energy level is 4, and between the 4s and 4p orbitals there are a total of 5 electrons, giving arsenic 5 valence electrons. The older column notation on periodic tables (using Roman numerals, and A and B designations) is helpful for determining the number of valence electrons for elements with columns headed by A. The Roman numeral represents the number of valence electrons. Thus a sulfur atom has six valence electrons (the column heading is VIA). The same answer would be obtained by writing out the configuration $1s^22s^22p^6\mathbf{3s^23p^4}$ and noting that the highest energy level used is 3, with a total of six electrons between the 3s and 3p orbitals.

TIP

VALENCE ELECTRONS AND AN ELEMENT'S LOCATION ON THE PERIODIC TABLE

Be able to quickly tell the ending of an electron configuration and the number of valence electrons for an atom from its location on the periodic table.

A convenient shorthand for configurations is the **noble gas core notation** method, in which the configuration shows all the electrons for the previous noble gas (group VIIIA or 18 on the periodic table) in brackets. This is convenient because it lets one focus on the outer energy level or valence electrons, which can be a time-saver for atoms with many electrons. Two examples follow.

Iodine with 53 electrons would be [Kr] $5s^24d^{10}5p^5$, where the [Kr] indicates $1s^2\ 2s^2\ldots$ up through $4p^6$. The seven valence electrons are still shown.

Iridium with 77 electrons would be [Xe] $6s^24f^{14}5d^7$.

TEST QUESTION

The element with the electron configuration $1s^2 2s^2 2p^6 3s^2 3p^6 4s^2 3d^{10} 4p^6 5s^1 4d^{10}$ is

(A) Silver, which is diamagnetic

(B) Silver, which is paramagnetic

(C) Cadmium, which is diamagnetic

(D) Cadmium, which is paramagnetic

(B) The configuration matches that of silver, element 47. Notice that instead of ending $5s^2 4d^9$, silver has an electron shift from the 5s orbital to the 4d orbital, completing the d sublevel and adding stability to the atom. Because there is at least one unpaired electron, silver is paramagnetic. It is not enough to look only at the ending of a configuration to identify the atom. Atoms often will shift an electron from the predicted filling arrangement to create full or half-full d and f sublevels, which confer added stability on the atom.

The Periodic Table: Organization and Chemical Characteristics

The modern version of the periodic table was developed in the 1860s and 1870s by Dmitri Mendeleev, who ordered the elements into groups based on atomic weight, as well as known chemical and physical properties. Later, Henry Moseley refined this organization and based it on atomic number rather than atomic mass. Each region of the periodic table has a specific name. The rows on the table are also known as **periods**, and the columns as **groups** or **families**. The **representative (or main group) elements** are those elements whose configurations end with s or p electrons. The elements in the middle of the table are known as the **transition metals,** and they all have configurations that end with d electrons. The two rows at the bottom of the periodic table are known as **the rare earth elements** and comprise the top row, the Lanthanides, and the bottom row, the Actinides. These two periods are also known as inner transition metals, and they all have configurations that end with f sublevels.

The periodic table can also be represented in groups of "blocks" that describe the endings of the configurations, as in Figure 1.9.

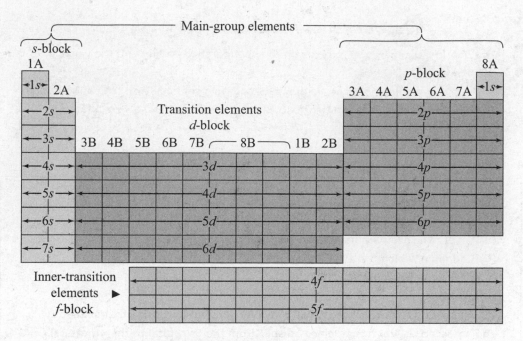

Figure 1.9. Blocks of the periodic table

This chart allows you to determine the ending of the configuration for an atom by its location on the periodic table. Chlorine is in the third period of the table in the fifth column of the p block, and its configuration ends in $3p^5$. Some other elements and their configuration endings are shown in Table 1.6.

Table 1.6 Sample Elements and Configuration Endings

Element	Ending
Sr	$5s^2$
Fe	$3d^6$
Sb	$5p^3$
Cs	$6s^1$

METALS, NONMETALS, AND METALLOIDS

The periodic table can be divided into elements based on their properties as metals or nonmetals as shown in Figure 1.10. Note the diagonal "staircase" consisting of B, Si, Ge, As, Sb, Te, and Po. These elements are known as **metalloids**, and they have properties intermediate to those of metals and nonmetals. There are many more metals than nonmetals or metalloids on the periodic table.

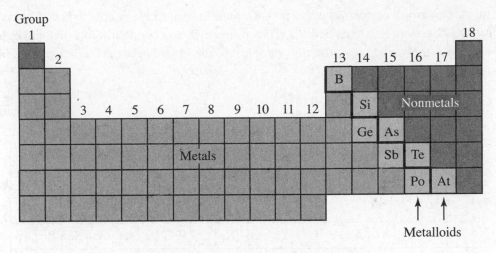

Figure 1.10. Metals, nonmetals, and metalloids

Metals tend to be lustrous, malleable (can be hammered into thin sheets), ductile (can be pulled into thin wires), and good conductors of heat and electricity. They are generally in a solid state at room temperature (except for mercury, Hg).

Nonmetals are often gases at room conditions. Solid nonmetals are often brittle and poor conductors.

Metalloids have physical properties that fall in between those of metals and nonmetals, while their chemical properties often depend on whether they are interacting with metals or nonmetals.

Some of the chemical properties of metals and nonmetals will be discussed later.

GROUPS OF THE PERIODIC TABLE

Group IA (or group 1 in the more modern labeling system) is known as the **alkali metals**. These are elements whose configurations all end in s^1, and they have one valence electron. They tend to be soft, silvery metals that are very reactive. Hydrogen is a nonmetal and is not considered a member of this family, even though it does have one valence electron.

Group IIA or 2 are **alkaline earth metals** with configurations that end in s^2, and they have two valence electrons. They are reactive, but generally less so than the alkali metals.

The **halogens** are in group VIIA (17) of the table. They have configurations that end in p^5, and all have seven valence electrons. Halogens are among the most reactive nonmetals.

Noble gases are the elements in group VIIIA (18). They are the least reactive elements on the table. Their completely full energy levels make them particularly stable and inert. They all have eight valence electrons (except He with only two valence electrons, which is a full first energy level).

The **transition metals** (d block) are the most common metals in our daily lives. These are elements whose configurations all end with d sublevels, and they typically have two valence electrons. They often have the ability to combine with other elements in a wide variety of combinations, owing to their partially filled d sublevels. These partially filled d sublevels are responsible for the many colors that compounds of transition metals have.

The **inner transition metals** are the two rows at the bottom of the periodic table, whose configurations end with f electrons. These two rows (the Lanthanides and the Actinides) are sometimes known as the Rare Earth elements.

The **oxygen group** consists of important elements in biological systems, especially oxygen and sulfur. These are elements with six valence electrons and configurations that end in p^4.

Figure 1.11 shows the regions of the periodic table described in the preceding paragraphs.

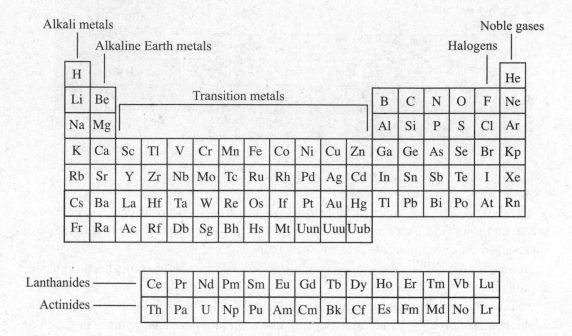

Figure 1.11. Named parts of the periodic table

Chemical Properties of the Elements: Periodic Properties

When the elements are arranged on the modern periodic table, many patterns and trends in their physical and chemical properties become apparent. Two principles predict and explain many of these properties.

1. The more protons there are in an atom's nucleus, the greater the attraction or "pull" on the electrons of the atom.
2. Electrons located farther away "feel" less pull from the nucleus and are held less tightly, making them easier to remove and thus more reactive.

CONFIGURATION ENDING AND VALENCE ELECTRONS

A quick look at an element's position in the periodic table allows you to determine the ending of its configuration and the number of valence electrons it has. This is important when looking at bonding, because atoms tend to gain or lose valence electrons so as to acquire a configuration that "matches" that of a noble gas.

For example, a bromine atom has a configuration that ends 4p^5 and has seven valence electrons. Bromine tends to gain one electron, which results in an extra electron (relative to the number of protons), thus forming a negative ion. A calcium atom with a configuration that ends 4s^2 and two valence electrons tends to lose two electrons, forming +2 ions with two fewer electrons than protons.

ATOMIC RADIUS

Atomic radius is defined as one-half the distance between nuclei of atoms just touching each other. It can also be thought of as the distance from the nucleus of the atom to the valence shell. As atoms go down a family, the atomic radius increases. This is because each successive row on the periodic table represents the use of an additional energy level, and thus the electrons will be located at a greater distance from the nucleus. The inner electrons will produce some shielding, reducing the pull on the electrons as well.

When atoms move across a period on the table, they get smaller. At first this may seem counterintuitive. Recall that positive protons attract negatively charged electrons. As you look across a period, the number of energy levels being used by the atoms remains constant. As the number of protons increases, there is a greater attractive pull on the electron cloud, resulting in a smaller atomic radius.

As a result, the largest atoms on the periodic table are found in the lower left section. This pattern for the representative elements is shown in Figure 1.12.

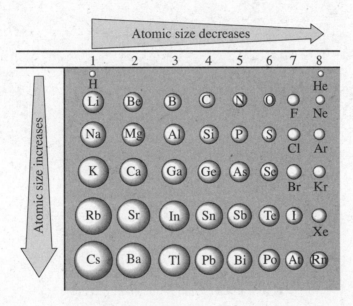

Figure 1.12. Trends in atomic radius

TIP

FRANCIUM AS A CONVENIENT REFERENCE POINT

Francium, the atom farthest down the table and farthest to the left, is the atom with the largest atomic radius.

FIRST IONIZATION ENERGY

First ionization energy, or ionization potential, is the amount of energy required to cause an atom to lose one valence electron when in the gaseous state. The more tightly held an electron is, the more energy will be required to remove it. First ionization energy decreases down a group because the atoms further down a group on the periodic table have valence electrons that are located a greater distance from the nucleus, and thus feel less pull from the nucleus. Across a row, first ionization energy increases because of an increased nuclear pull. The lowest values of first ionization energy are found in atoms on the lower left of the table (Cs, for example), and the highest belong to the noble gases and the halogens, with helium having the highest first ionization energy of all elements. Figure 1.13 shows this trend:

GROUP AND PERIOD TRENDS

Going down a group: an increasing distance from the nucleus, less nuclear pull, and more shielding

Going across a period: increased nuclear pull

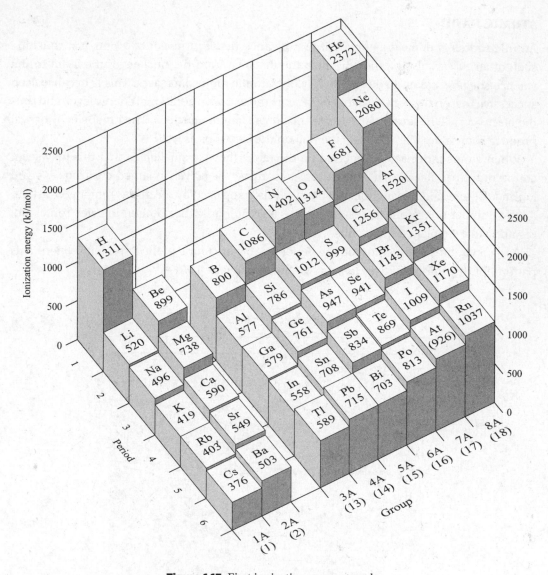

Figure 1.13. First ionization energy trends

Multiple Ionization Energies

It is also possible to cause an atom to lose more than one electron. We can measure the amount of energy needed for the removal of each successive electron. In general, it requires a greater amount of energy for the removal of each electron, because there will be a greater nuclear pull per electron. Also, once an atom has lost all of its valence electrons (and thus has a configuration that matches that of a noble gas), the amount of energy required increases dramatically. Based on these trends, one would expect the first two ionization energies of calcium or magnesium to be relatively low but the third one to be very high. For aluminum, the first three ionization energies would be relatively low (but increasing due to the proton/electron ratio) whereas the fourth one would be much higher.

METALS AND VALENCE ELECTRONS

Metals readily lose their valence electrons. Once those electrons have been lost, the metal is at a highly stable noble gas electron configuration.

ELECTRON AFFINITY

Electron affinity is the energy change associated with the gain of one electron by an atom in the gaseous state. The greater the nuclear pull, the greater the ability of an atom to gain an electron. The halogens have the highest electron affinity because when they gain an electron, an entire energy level is completed. The noble gases typically are not assigned values because their energy levels and sublevels are completely filled and they are already stable. The trend is shown by Figure 1.14.

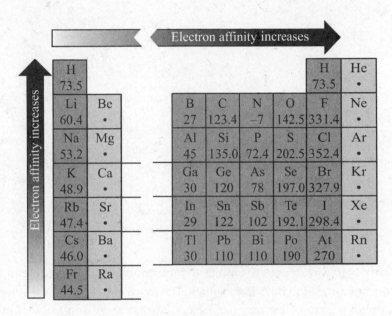

Figure 1.14. Electron affinity

The alkaline earth metals have very low electron affinities because they have configurations that end with s^2, and gaining an electron does not help them to complete a sublevel.

ELECTRONEGATIVITY

Electronegativity is a measure of the attraction an atom has for electrons in a bond. The greater the electronegativity, the greater the attraction or pull that atom exerts on bonded electrons. There are a number of electronegativity scales in use, the most common being the Pauling scale, which assigns the highest value to fluorine (see Figure 1.15). The lowest values are assigned to the alkali metals.

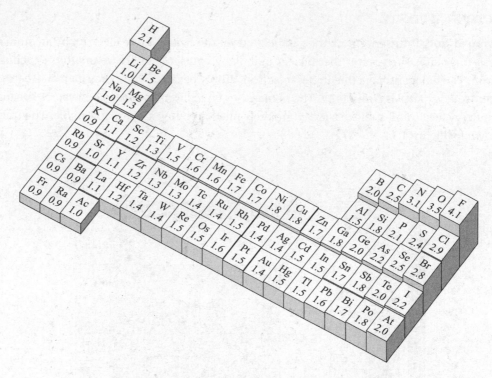

Figure 1.15. Electronegativity values. Note that fluorine, in the upper right corner, is assigned the highest value.

Electronegativity follows a pattern similar to ionization energy. Metals tend to have low values and nonmetals tend to have high values. The general trends are that electronegativity decreases down a group (electrons are located farther away and feel less pull from the nucleus) and increases across a period (greater nuclear pull). The noble gases are typically not assigned an electronegativity value because they are inert.

ELECTRONEGATIVITY

Electronegativity is very useful in predicting bonding patterns.

Metals: low electronegativity

Nonmetals: high electronegativity, with fluorine having the highest value

Noble gases: nonreactive with no electronegativity values

FRANCIUM AS A REFERENCE

Francium is a useful reference for these properties.

Atomic radius: largest

Electronegativity: lowest

METALLIC AND NONMETALLIC TRENDS

In general, the more active metals are found toward the left of the table. These are elements that tend to readily lose an electron, which means they have low ionization energies and electronegativities. The most active metal is cesium (there is not enough francium in the world to have actual data on it). Cesium most readily loses its one valence electron in reactions. Cesium will more easily lose a valence electron than rubidium or potassium because of its larger atomic radius, which locates the single valence electron at a greater distance, with less attraction, from the nucleus.

The most active nonmetals are the halogens (and fluorine in particular) because those are elements that are one electron away from a completely filled energy level. Nonmetals tend to readily gain valence electrons to complete their valence energy levels and to also hold onto the electrons they already have. This gives nonmetals properties such as high ionization energy and electronegativity.

TEST QUESTION

Moving across the periodic table from sodium to chlorine, which of the following periodic properties increases?

I. Atomic radius

II. Electronegativity

III. First ionization energy

(A) II only

(B) III only

(C) I and III only

(D) II and III only

(D) Going across any period on the table, the atomic radius decreases. This is primarily due to increased nuclear pull from the greater number of protons as the atomic number increases. Thus, choice I is incorrect, eliminating C. Both first ionization energy and electronegativity increase going across a period, making D the correct answer.

IONIC AND COVALENT BONDING

There are two general kinds of chemical bonds, ionic and covalent. In **ionic bonds**, electrons are transferred from one atom to another and fully charged ions are formed. In **covalent bonds**, electrons are shared between atoms. The sharing of electrons in covalent bonds may be even or uneven and will largely depend on the relative electronegativities of the two atoms involved in the bond. The **octet rule** is a general principle that states that atoms with 8 valence electrons (a configuration with a valence energy level that is ns^2np^6) are especially stable. This is the configuration of the noble gases (except He, which has a full first energy level, $1s^2$).

Ionic Bonds

Ionic bonds are formed by the interaction of electrically charged atoms or ions. They are also known as electrostatic bonds. The properties of ionic bonds can be explained by Coulomb's law. Many ionic compounds have similar general physical properties.

TIP

THE OCTET RULE

The octet rule is a very helpful guideline but many compounds violate it.

COULOMB'S LAW

Coulomb's law describes the force (attracting or repelling) between two charged objects. Coulomb's law is mathematically expressed by the equation

$$F = \frac{kQ_1Q_2}{d^2},$$

where k is a constant, Q_1 and Q_2 are the charges on the objects (in this case, ions), and d is the distance between them. This means that the larger the charges, the greater the force (an attractive force for objects with opposite charge and a repulsive force for objects with the same charge). The equation describes an inverse square law, which means as the distance increases, the force decreases, but by the distance squared.

INVERSE SQUARES

The equation for Coulomb's Law, above, is an example of an inverse square law. Force is inversely proportional to the square of the distance.

If the force at 2 mm is 18, what is the force at 6 mm?

The solution is below.

LATTICE ENERGY

Lattice energy is the change in energy that occurs when separated gaseous ions form an ionic solid. It can also be thought of as the energy released when a solid forms from its ions. In general, ions with greater charges have larger lattice energies and are harder to separate. Ions with larger radii have weaker lattice energies because they are separated by a larger distance, and the force of attraction is less.

FORMATION OF IONS

Ions are formed when atoms gain or lose electrons. Ionic bonds typically take place between atoms with large electronegativity differences, such as a metal and a nonmetal.

Metals tend to lose valence electrons. In doing so, they take on the configuration of (or become isoelectronic with) a noble gas. A calcium atom has the configuration $[Ar]4s^2$, and forms a positive ion or **cation**. Losing the two valence electrons gives calcium a charge of positive two (+2 or 2+) because the number of protons in the nucleus stays the same but there are now only 18, rather than 20, electrons. This imbalance between the number of protons and electrons leads to an ion, or charged particle, being formed. This positive ion is smaller than the atom because it uses only three energy levels, instead of the four used by the atom.

Negative ions, or **anions**, are formed when atoms gain enough electrons to complete their valence energy levels. An atom will gain as many electrons as needed to reach an octet, or eight valence electrons. For example, chlorine has the configuration $1s^22s^22p^63s^23p^5$. By gaining one electron, the configuration becomes $1s^22s^22p^63s^23p^6$,

INVERSE SQUARES SOLUTION

If the force at 2 mm is 18, what is the force at 6 mm?

When distance increases, force decreases by the square of the distance. The distance has increased by a factor of 3 (from 2 to 6). Force decreases by a factor of 3^2, or 9. A ninth of 18 is 2.

which is the same as argon's configuration. Thus, we say that the chlorine has become **iso-electronic** with argon. The number of protons has not changed, so the identity of the atom has not changed either. The additional electron now creates an imbalance between positive protons and negative electrons, resulting in a –1 charge. Extra electrons in the same energy level result in more repulsion in the valence shell, which tends to make anions larger than the atoms from which they form.

IONIC COMPOUNDS

Ionic compounds tend to be hard, brittle solids at room temperatures. They conduct electricity when dissolved or melted, but not when solid. They tend to form well-defined crystals.

Covalent Bonds

Covalent bonds join atoms with similar electronegativities. Covalent bonds can be nonmetal–nonmetal, metalloid–metalloid, or metalloid–nonmetal. In a covalent bond, each member of a pair of atoms exerts a pull on an electron pair located between the two atoms. This mutual attraction for the shared electrons constitutes the covalent bond. Covalent compounds typically have low melting points and they do not conduct electricity when dissolved or melted.

Covalent bonds are shared pairs of electrons. One pair of shared electrons produces a single bond, two pairs produce a double bond, and a triple bond consists of three pairs of electrons. The number of pairs of electrons being shared is called the bond order. Bonds with a higher order have a greater strength (bond energy) and are shorter in length. (See Table 1.7.)

Table 1.7 Bond Types, Lengths, and Strengths

Bond	Length (pm)	Energy (kJ/mole)
C – C	154	348
C = C	134	619
C ≡ C	120	849

Figure 1.16 shows the number of valence electrons (shown as dots) for atoms in the s and p blocks of the periodic table.

IA IIA IIIA IVA VA VIA VIIA VIIIA

H·   He:

Li·   Be: ·B·   ·C·   ·N·   ·O·   :F: :Ne:

Na·   Mg: ·Al·   ·Si·   ·P·   ·S·   :Cl: :Ar:

K·   Ca:

Figure 1.16. Dot formulas for representative elements

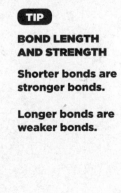

TIP

BOND LENGTH AND STRENGTH

Shorter bonds are stronger bonds.

Longer bonds are weaker bonds.

LEWIS DOT STRUCTURES

Dot formulas are used to show the number of valence electrons an atom has. In a valence electron dot formula, each valence electron of the atom is represented by a dot. Lithium with one valence electron would be the atomic symbol Li, with one dot to represent its one valence electron. Sulfur, with six valence electrons, is represented by the symbol S, with six dots.

The following steps can be used to write a Lewis dot structure for molecules.

1. Determine the total number of valence electrons in the molecule. For an ion, keep in mind that a positive ion has lost electrons (a +1 ion has lost one electron, a +2 ion has lost two electrons, and so on) and a negative ion has gained electrons.
2. Draw a skeleton in which you start with the assumption that each bond is a single bond. Less electronegative atoms tend to be central atoms. Hydrogen is never a central atom because it can only form one bond.
3. Calculate the number of electrons that remain.
4. Complete the octet (eight valence electrons) on all the outer atoms. Hydrogen has a full energy level with only two valence electrons.
5. Additional electrons go on the central atom. It is possible for the central atom to have an **expanded octet** or more than eight electrons.
6. If the central atom is "deficient" in electrons, use double or triple bonds to complete its octet.
7. Some atoms (especially Be and B) can be electron deficient.
8. Some atoms, such as those in the third period of the table, can have "expanded octets," with 10 or 12 electrons in the valence shell around the central atom.

Some examples of Lewis dot structures are shown in Figures 1.17 and 1.18. Water has the dot formula shown in Figure 1.17.

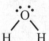

Figure 1.17. Lewis dot structure of water

The oxygen atom has two bonding pairs of electrons, each represented by a line. Recall that a bond is a pair of electrons and that the oxygen atom has two nonbonding pairs (sometimes called lone pairs).

Ammonia has the dot structure shown in Figure 1.18.

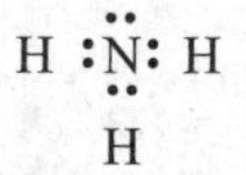

$$H \; :\!\overset{\cdot\cdot}{\underset{\cdot\cdot}{N}}\!: \; H$$
$$H$$

Figure 1.18. Lewis dot structure of ammonia

Some hydrocarbons with multiple bonds are shown in Figure 1.19. Note that hydrogen is never a central atom because it can only form one bond.

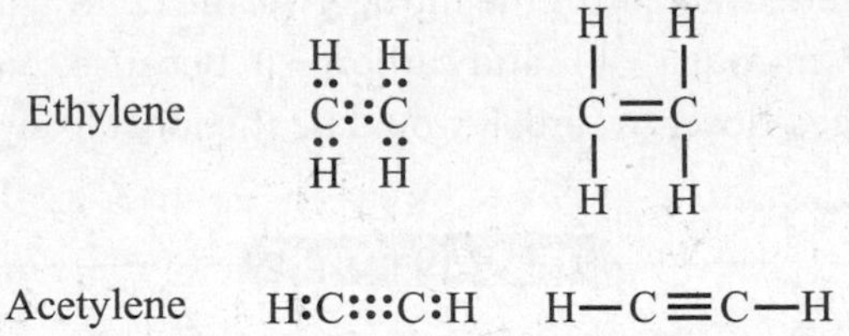

Ethylene

$$H:\overset{\overset{\displaystyle H}{|}}{\underset{\underset{\displaystyle H}{|}}{C}}::\overset{\overset{\displaystyle H}{|}}{\underset{\underset{\displaystyle H}{|}}{C} \qquad \overset{H \quad H}{\underset{H \quad H}{C=C}}$$

Acetylene $H:C:::C:H \qquad H—C\equiv C—H$

Figure 1.19. Dot structures of compounds with multiple bonds

Hydrogen cyanide, HCN, has the dot formula shown in Figure 1.20.

$$H—C\equiv N:$$

Figure 1.20. Lewis dot formula of hydrogen cyanide

Notice that the less electronegative carbon atom, and not the nitrogen atom, is in the center.

Figure 1.21 shows the dot formula for carbon dioxide. Again, note that the less electronegative atom is the central one.

$$:\ddot{O}=C=\ddot{O}:$$

Figure 1.21. Lewis dot structure of carbon dioxide

In carbon dioxide, each oxygen atom has a double bond to the carbon and two lone pairs (or nonbonding pairs).

Formal charge is a system for assigning a hypothetical charge to an atom in an ion or compound. In cases where it is possible to draw more than one Lewis dot structure, formal charge can help in determining the most likely (lowest energy) structure. In general, formal charges closer to zero are more likely to exist. Formal charge is calculated using the formula:

FC = # valence electrons – ½ (# bonding electrons) – # nonbonding electrons

The calculation is done for each atom in a compound. For example, in the molecule HCN, with a dot formula (Figure 1.22),

$$H—C\equiv N:$$

Figure 1.22. Hydrogen cyanide

the calculation would be as follows:

For the hydrogen atom: 1 valence electron – ½(2 bonding electrons) – 0 nonbonding electrons = 0

For the carbon atom: 4 valence electrons – ½(8 bonding electrons) – 0 nonbonding electrons = 0

For the nitrogen atom: 5 valence electrons – ½(6 bonding electrons) – 2 nonbonding electrons = 0

If the dot structure were drawn with the nitrogen as the central atom, the formal charges would be: hydrogen = 0, nitrogen = +1, and carbon = 0. Because the structure shown has all atoms with formal charges closer to zero, it would be the most likely structure.

TIP

FORMAL CHARGES

The closer the formal charges are to zero, the more likely that the structure exists.

TEST QUESTION

In a molecule of carbon monoxide, what are the formal charges on the two atoms?

(A) Carbon = 0, Oxygen = 0

(B) Carbon = +1, Oxygen = −1

(C) Carbon = −1, Oxygen = +1

(D) Carbon = 0, Oxygen = −1

(C) The sum of the formal charges of the two atoms must be zero, as carbon monoxide is a neutral compound. Carbon has four valence electrons, three bonds, and one lone pair (two nonbonding electrons), so the formal charge on the carbon atom is 4 − 3 − 2 = −1. Oxygen has 6 valence electrons, three bonds, and two nonbonding electrons (one lone pair). This makes the formal charge on the oxygen atom 6 − 3 − 2 = +1.

TIP

COMMON MOLECULAR GEOMETRIES TO KNOW

Know the geometries of carbon dioxide, water, and ammonia.

Valence Shell Electron Pair Repulsions (VSEPR) Theory is a model that uses Lewis dot structures to predict **molecular geometry**, that is, the three-dimensional shapes of simple molecules. The main concept is that electron pairs (bonding or nonbonding) have a negative charge and will arrange themselves in order to maximize the distance between them (like charges repel). To apply VSEPR, count the number of electron pairs around a central atom and then apply the information shown in Figure 1.23. In the case of molecules with lone pairs on the central atom, the shape describes only the atoms. You should memorize the shapes of certain simple, common molecules such as water, methane, ammonia, and carbon dioxide.

A summary of the geometries for two to six electron pairs around a central atom is shown in Figure 1.23.

In the case of molecules such as methane, water, and ammonia, there are four pairs of electrons around the central atom, but there are varying numbers of bonds and lone pairs. This gives rise to a tetrahedral geometry for the electron pairs but different geometries for the atoms.

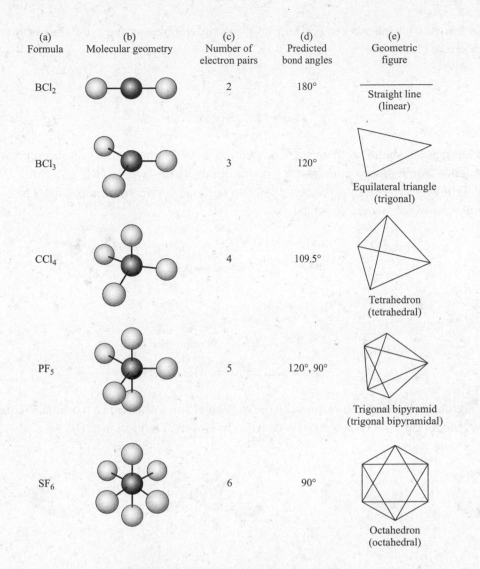

(a) Formula	(b) Molecular geometry	(c) Number of electron pairs	(d) Predicted bond angles	(e) Geometric figure
BCl_2		2	180°	Straight line (linear)
BCl_3		3	120°	Equilateral triangle (trigonal)
CCl_4		4	109.5°	Tetrahedron (tetrahedral)
PF_5		5	120°, 90°	Trigonal bipyramid (trigonal bipyramidal)
SF_6		6	90°	Octahedron (octahedral)

Figure 1.23. Common molecular geometries

TIP

CARBON AND BONDING

Carbon almost always forms four covalent bonds. The most common arrangement of bonds around a carbon atom is a tetrahedron.

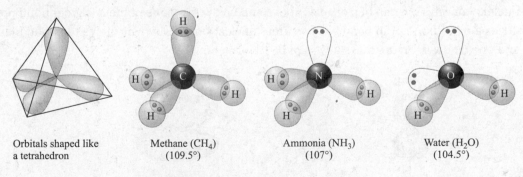

Orbitals shaped like a tetrahedron

Methane (CH_4) (109.5°)

Ammonia (NH_3) (107°)

Water (H_2O) (104.5°)

Figure 1.24. Tetrahedron-based molecules

TIP

LONE PAIRS

Lone pairs repel more than bonding pairs, causing shapes to be altered from the perfect tetrahedron and bond angles to be reduced.

In the case of methane, the molecule is tetrahedral in shape. Ammonia is trigonal pyramidal in shape, and water is bent or V-shaped.

Carbon dioxide has a central carbon atom and two double bonds around the carbon atom, as shown in Figure 1.25.

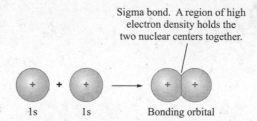

Figure 1.25. Carbon dioxide

It has a linear shape, as there are two "electron clouds" around the central carbon atom. **Valence bond theory** attempts to explain bonds as the overlapping of orbitals. In the model shown in Figure 1.26, the overlap of two s orbitals between the nuclei leads to a single orbital, known as a sigma (σ) orbital.

Sigma bond. A region of high
electron density holds the
two nuclear centers together.

1s   1s   Bonding orbital

Figure 1.26. Sigma bond formation

A **sigma bond** can also be formed by the overlap of an s orbital and a p orbital. Figure 1.27 shows the formation of a sigma bond between hydrogen and fluorine in HF.

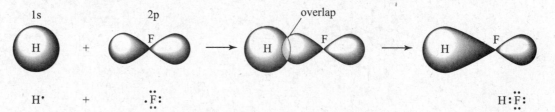

Figure 1.27. Sigma bond formation in HF

The overlap of two p orbitals can produce a sigma bond if the overlap is between the two nuclei. Sideways overlap of p orbitals above and below the plane of the σ (sigma) bond produces a π (pi) bond. A **pi bond** has two areas of electron density, one above the bond plane and one below it. Figure 1.28 shows a pi bond formation.

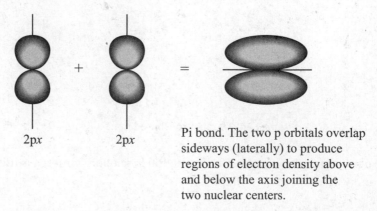

Pi bond. The two p orbitals overlap
sideways (laterally) to produce
regions of electron density above
and below the axis joining the
two nuclear centers.

Figure 1.28. Pi bond formation

A single bond is always a sigma bond. A double bond consists of a sigma bond and a pi bond. A triple bond consists of a sigma bond and two pi bonds.

As an example, the figure below shows a structural formula of 1-propene, which has 8 sigma bonds and 1 pi bond.

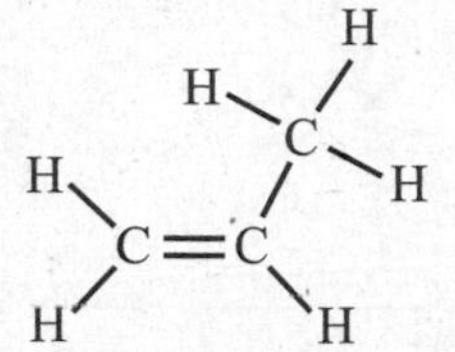

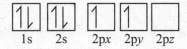

Figure 1.29. Sigma and pi bonds

Hybrid Orbitals

The sigma and pi bond description of molecules is very useful for the simplest of molecules. When molecules are more complex, the sigma and pi bond model becomes inadequate. Consider a molecule of methane being formed from one carbon atom and four hydrogen atoms. Each hydrogen atom has a configuration of $1s^1$, and one more electron would complete the first energy level. The carbon atom has a configuration of $1s^2 2s^2 2p^2$. The filling diagram for carbon is shown in Figure 1.30.

$$\boxed{1\downarrow}\ \boxed{1\downarrow}\ \boxed{1}\ \boxed{1}\ \boxed{}$$
1s 2s 2px 2py 2pz

Figure 1.30. Electron filling diagram for carbon

Experimental evidence shows that methane, CH_4, has four identical C–H bonds. A model of carbon with the ground state orbital diagram cannot explain this evidence. Instead, one can imagine the carbon atom simultaneously promoting one of the electrons from the 2s orbital to the 2p level, and then the 2s and 2p orbitals hybridizing to give four identical orbitals, each with one electron and the ability to form a bond.

Figure 1.31 shows the s orbital and the three p orbitals hybridizing to form four identical orbitals, labeled sp^3 for the orbitals from which they are formed, each with identical energy and a unique orientation.

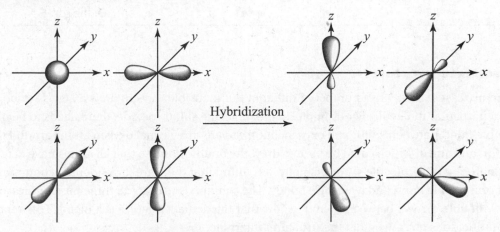

Figure 1.31. Orbital hybridization. One s orbital and three
p orbitals hybridize to form four identical sp^3 orbitals.

Any molecule with four electron clouds around the central atom, including water and ammonia, has this type of orbital hybridization. In a molecule such as formaldehyde, the central carbon atom has a double bond to the oxygen atom and single bonds to the hydrogen atoms. Figure 1.32 shows the sp^2 orbital hybridization thus formed.

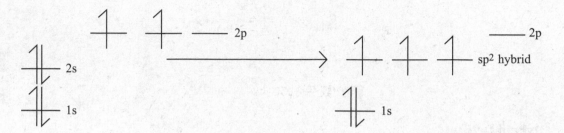

Figure 1.32. Formation of sp^2 hybrid orbitals

In general, a given number of electron pairs around a central atom has a specific orbital hybridization. In the case of the simplest molecules, this hybrid orbital model gives the same predictions as VSEPR theory (and is confirmed by experimental evidence). Such a model can also explain molecules in which the central atom either lacks an octet (electron-deficient molecules) or has an expanded octet. Table 1.8 summarizes this.

Table 1.8 Orbital Hybridization and Shape for Specific Numbers of Electron Pairs Around a Central Atom

Number of Electron Clouds Around a Central Atom (includes lone pairs and bonding pairs)	Orbital Hybridization	General Shape
2	sp	Linear
3	sp^2	Trigonal planar
4	sp^3	Tetrahedral
5	sp^3d	Trigonal bipyramidal
6	sp^3d^2	Octahedral

Resonance Structures

In many cases, there are a number of different but plausible ways to draw a Lewis structure for a particular molecule. For example, in the molecule sulfur trioxide, there needs to be one double bond between sulfur and oxygen, but there are three equal oxygen atoms around the sulfur, any one of which could be used to draw the double bond so that all atoms have octets. In analyzing the molecule experimentally, it is found that there are three identical bonds and not one double bond and two single bonds. The solution is to draw all three possibilities and draw double arrows between them to show that the actual structure is a blend. This representation does not mean that the structures alternate.

Figure 1.33. Resonance structures of sulfur trioxide. Lone pairs on O are not shown.

A better drawing, but one that does not fit as well with the Lewis dot structure model, is shown in Figure 1.34.

O
‖
S   143 pm
O 120° O

Figure 1.34. Sulfur trioxide

This drawing indicates that each bond is equivalent to $\frac{4}{3}$ of a bond. The experimentally measured bond length and bond energy of the S–O bonds in sulfur trioxide support this conclusion. In general, molecules that have multiple resonance structures (provided they follow the octet rule and have low formal charges) tend to be stable, because the charge around the atoms can be dispersed rather than concentrated. The three possible resonance structures for the nitrate ion (NO_3^{-1}) are shown in Figure 1.35.

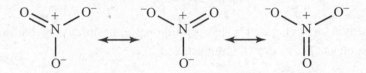

Figure 1.35. Nitrate ion resonance structures

A covalent bond in which both electrons in the bond originate in the same atom, rather than having each atom contribute one electron, is known as a **coordinate covalent bond**. Coordinate covalent bonds are typically found in the formation of a product of a Lewis acid–Lewis base reaction (which will be covered in more detail in the section on acids and bases). A **Lewis acid** is a substance that can accept a pair of electrons. Lewis acids are very often electron-deficient molecules such as BF_3 or $AlCl_3$. A **Lewis base** is a compound that can donate an electron pair. These compounds are very often molecules in which a central atom has a lone pair.

The reaction between BF_3 and NH_3 to form a single product is shown in Figure 1.36.

H   F   H F
| | | |
H — N: + B — F ⟶ H — N : B — F
| | | |
H   F   H F

Lewis Lewis
base   acid

Figure 1.36. A Lewis acid–base reaction

TIP

RESONANCE

A structure with several resonance forms allows charge to be spread over more atoms, increasing stability.

POLAR AND NONPOLAR BONDS (PARTIAL IONIC CHARACTER)

Polar bonds are bonds in which electrons are shared unevenly because one atom has a higher electronegativity and thus exerts a greater attractive force on the shared pair of electrons. In general, if a bond involves two atoms with electronegativity differences of less than 0.4, the pull each atom has on the shared electrons is close enough to equal that the bond is considered nonpolar (see below). Examples of **nonpolar** bonds include any bond between two identical atoms (such as H–H) and C–H bonds. If the electronegativity difference between the two atoms is greater than 1.8, the bond is more like an ionic bond in that one atom has a large enough pull for the electrons to be essentially transferred and not shared. Bonds with electronegativity differences between 0.4 and 1.8 are polar covalent.

In the case of a polar bond, the electrons in the bond are closer to the atom with a greater electronegativity and that atom has a partial negative charge, abbreviated δ^- (delta minus). The atom with the lower electronegativity has a slight "shortage" of electrons and is said to be δ^+ (delta plus). Another way to show this dipole is with an arrow, as in Figure 1.37. The greater the electronegativity difference between the two atoms, the greater the magnitude of the **dipole** or **dipole moment**.

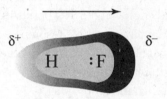

Figure 1.37. Dipole in HF

If identical atoms form a bond, it is always nonpolar (as in the case of diatomic oxygen, O_2, or a molecule such as Cl_2), as shown in Figure 1.38.

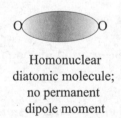

Homonuclear
diatomic molecule;
no permanent
dipole moment

Figure 1.38. Homonuclear diatomic molecule with no dipole

Another common example of nonpolar bonds is carbon–hydrogen bonding. These are extremely common in organic and biological molecules.

It is convenient to divide bonds into broad categories of ionic, polar covalent, and nonpolar covalent, as in Table 1.9.

Table 1.9 Electronegativity Difference and Bond Type

Electronegativity Difference	Bond Type
0.0–0.4	Nonpolar covalent
0.4–1.8	Polar covalent
>1.8	Ionic

Arrange these bonds from least to greatest ionic character.

I. carbon–hydrogen

II. oxygen–oxygen

III. sodium–oxygen

IV. oxygen–fluorine

(A) II, III, I, IV

(B) II, I, IV, III

(C) IV, II, I, III

(D) II, IV, I, III

(B) Glancing at the answer choices shows that three answers have III as the most ionic, so first check III. The bond between sodium and oxygen is an ionic bond and is the only ionic bond in the list, so it must be the most ionic in character of all the choices. This eliminates A as a possible answer. Any bond between a pair of identical atoms (such as oxygen–oxygen) has an electronegativity difference of zero and must be the least ionic. This narrows the possibilities to B and D. Carbon–hydrogen bonds are nonpolar and much lower in ionic character than oxygen–fluorine bonds.

In reality, it is more accurate to think of all bonds as having some ionic and some covalent character. As the electronegativity difference between the two atoms increases, the ionic character increases, and when a bond acts sufficiently ionic in terms of its properties, we find it convenient to label it ionic. A bond with 48% ionic character and a bond with 52% ionic character are very similar, even though one may be called polar covalent and the other ionic. A better way to think about bonds is as a continuum, as shown in Figure 1.39.

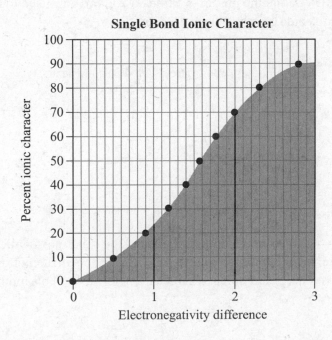

Figure 1.39. Electronegativity difference and percent ionic character of a bond

Two simple guidelines may help you predict the type of bond two atoms will make. First, a metal and a nonmetal will likely form an ionic bond. Second, the closer together on the periodic table two nonmetals or metalloids are, the less polar (more covalent) the bond will be. Thus, a bond between Na and F will be ionic, whereas a bond between F and P is likely to be polar covalent, and a bond between As and P is likely to be nonpolar covalent. More detailed calculations require a table of electronegativity values.

Just as an individual bond between a pair of atoms may have a charge imbalance and a dipole moment, so may a molecule. A **molecular dipole moment** depends on the geometry of the molecule and on the individual bonds in the molecule. For a diatomic molecule, the molecular polarity will equal the bond polarity. For a diatomic molecule such as HF (see Figure 1.37) the molecular dipole is the same as the bond dipole. In the case of carbon dioxide, there are two dipoles in the molecule, one for each C–O bond, but the two bond dipoles are equal in magnitude and yet opposite in direction, thus canceling each other out and producing a molecule with zero overall dipole moment.

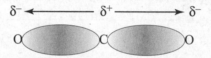

Figure 1.40. A symmetrical molecule where dipoles cancel

A water molecule has two polar bonds (O is much more electronegative than H), but they are not located in opposite directions (see Figure 1.41). In addition, one end of the water molecule has two lone pairs, which create still more charge imbalance. Dipoles are measured in units of Debye (D), but for the purposes of the MCAT, you only need to know how to tell whether or not a molecule is likely to have a dipole.

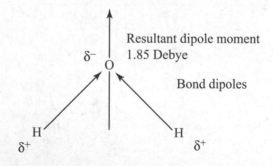

Figure 1.41. Molecular dipole in water

A molecule in which there are no lone pairs and all the bonds are identical almost always has no net dipole moment. A molecule with one or more lone pairs not oriented opposite each other (such as water or ammonia, see in Figure 1.42) has a dipole moment.

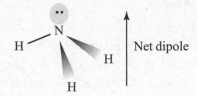

Figure 1.42. Molecular dipole in ammonia

The presence of a lone pair on the molecule does not automatically mean there is a molecular dipole. In the case of a square planar molecule such as XeF_4 (Figure 1.43), the two lone pairs are located opposite each other and will cancel each other.

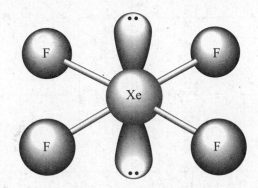

Figure 1.43. Lone pairs that are symmetrical will cancel

If a molecule contains a single lone pair, the molecule most likely has a dipole moment. Asymmetrical bonds around the central atom, as in the case of $CHCl_3$, also indicate the presence of a dipole moment.

STATES OF MATTER

The three states of matter one needs to understand for the MCAT are solids, liquids, and gases. Most gases have similar general properties that can be explained with the kinetic-molecular theory and the ideal gas concept. Solids and liquids, the condensed phases of matter, have properties that are largely determined by the intermolecular forces between their particles.

Gases

A gas is a state of matter with an indefinite shape and volume. Gases are compressible and are capable of flowing. Particles in a gas are relatively far away from each other and have fewer interactions, primarily as a result of fewer collisions. The behavior of gases can be described with the kinetic-molecular theory (KMT).

KINETIC-MOLECULAR THEORY

The **kinetic-molecular theory** describes the behavior of gases in terms of motion, collisions, and number of particles. From this theory, the basic laws that govern the properties of gases can be derived.

The Kelvin Temperature Scale

The temperature scale used in all calculations involving states of matter is the kelvin (or absolute) scale (Figure 1.44). A major advantage of the **kelvin scale** is that it shows a direct relationship between temperature and the average kinetic energy of molecules. At a temperature of 0 kelvin (absolute zero) there is no molecular motion at all. Absolute zero corresponds to –273°C. The relationship between kelvin and Celsius temperatures is:

$$K = °C + 273$$

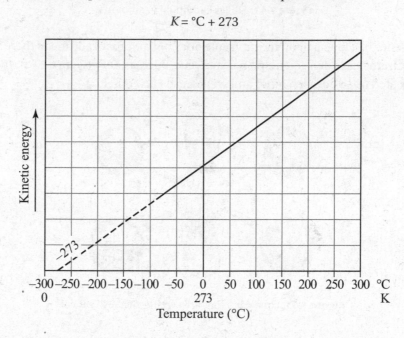

Figure 1.44. The kelvin scale

KELVIN TEMPERATURE

Every calculation involving gases requires the temperature to be in kelvin:

K = °C + 273

The main postulates of KMT are:

1. **GASES ARE COMPOSED OF PARTICLES WITH NEGLIGIBLE SIZE.** In a container of gas, almost all of the volume is empty space. Because the volume occupied by particles is so small, it can be ignored, which greatly simplifies calculations.

2. **PARTICLES MOVE RANDOMLY AT A WIDE VARIETY OF SPEEDS AND IN ALL DIRECTIONS.** The properties of a gas do not depend on direction.

3. **THERE ARE MINIMAL ATTRACTIVE OR REPULSIVE FORCES BETWEEN THE PARTICLES IN A GAS.** This means that particles move in straight lines until they collide with another particle, as shown in Figure 1.45.

4. **COLLISIONS BETWEEN PARTICLES ARE PERFECTLY ELASTIC.** This means that the total kinetic energy remains constant (or is conserved). A good example of an elastic collision is two steel spheres hitting each other. A piece of putty hitting a steel ball is an example of an inelastic collision, because some energy will go into changing the shape of the putty.

5. **AVERAGE KINETIC ENERGY ($KE = \frac{1}{2}mv^2$) OF A MOLECULE IS DIRECTLY PROPORTIONAL TO KELVIN (ABSOLUTE) TEMPERATURE.**

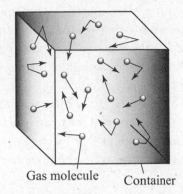

Gas molecule   Container

Figure 1.45. Particles of a gas move randomly in all directions

According to the KMT, pressure in a container is caused by collisions of particles with the walls of the container. A greater number of collisions or more energetic collisions lead to a greater pressure.

Gases that follow these postulates are said to behave ideally. Even though these postulates only approximate real-world conditions, they are very useful in almost every practical situation. Later in this chapter there will be a discussion of situations in which the ideal gas model is inaccurate enough to need modification. As the size of the container or the temperature of the particles vary, so will the number of collisions. This is a useful concept to remember.

Temperature is the average kinetic energy of a sample of gas particles. The molecules of these gas particles move with a wide range of speeds, described by the **Maxwell–Boltzmann distribution** of molecular speeds (Figure 1.46).

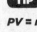

TIP

PV = nRT

The ideal gas assumptions almost always work on the MCAT. This equation is a REALLY important one for the MCAT!

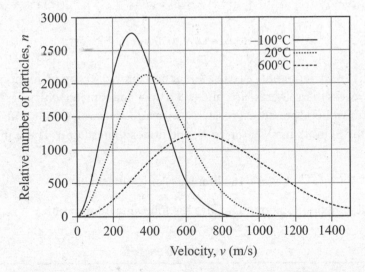

Figure 1.46. Maxwell–Boltzmann distribution of molecular speeds

The colder sample (–100°C) has some particles that move at very low speeds (far to the left) and some, with a greater kinetic energy, that move at high speeds (to the right). The average speed of the particles is toward the low end. At a higher temperature (600°C), molecules move with a wider range of speeds; however, the average particle moves with greater speed (and has greater kinetic energy) at 600°C than at 20°C. The pattern continues with the highest temperature on the graph. The average molecule moves faster and the range of speeds widens even more.

Gas **pressure** is measured with a **manometer**. A manometer works by comparing the pressure of a gas to a known pressure, using a column of mercury to indicate relative pressures. Closed manometers compare the pressure of a gas to that of a vacuum (zero particles = zero collisions = zero pressure). When the weight of the mercury column balances out the pressure from the gas, the two pressures are equal. The height of the mercury column can be measured and converted to other units. Other methods of measurement are used today, largely because of practical considerations and the toxicity of mercury.

There are different **types of manometers** (see Figure 1.47). In an open manometer, the pressure of the gas is compared to air pressure. The manometer indicates the pressure difference between the two sides.

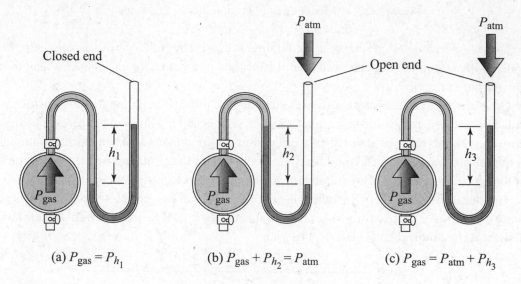

Figure 1.47. Manometers

In Figure 1.47, (a) represents a closed manometer, (b) an open manometer with gas sample pressure less than air pressure, and (c) an open manometer with gas sample pressure greater than atmospheric pressure. Pressure is measured in various units. The most common ones are kPa (the SI unit), mm Hg (or Torr), and atmospheres (atm). These units are related as follows:

$$1 \text{ atm} = 760 \text{ mm Hg (Torr)} = 101.3 \text{ kPa}$$

A typical manometer problem might give the following information.

Practice Question

A closed manometer connected to a sample of neon gas has a mercury height difference between the two arms of 575 mm Hg. What is the pressure of the gas in atm and kPa?

Solution: In a closed manometer the pressure of the gas is being compared to the closed end, which is a vacuum, and has a pressure of zero. This means that the height difference in mm Hg is one description of the pressure. To convert to the other units, the calculation would be:

$$P = 575 \text{ mm Hg} \times \frac{1 \text{ atm}}{760 \text{ mm Hg}} = 0.76 \text{ atm}$$

And $P = 575 \text{ mm Hg} \times \dfrac{101.3 \text{ kPa}}{760 \text{ mmHg}} = 77 \text{ kPa}$.

To solve for the pressure of a gas in an open manometer, you first have to decide if the gas pressure is greater or less than the atmospheric pressure. Then you should convert the height difference of the mercury to the appropriate unit to match the pressure unit for the atmospheric pressure, and add or subtract as needed.

Practice Question

In an open manometer, the mercury is higher by 180 mm on the side connected to a sample of helium gas. If the air pressure is 102 kPa, what is the pressure of the helium gas?

Solution: Because the mercury level is higher on the side connected to the helium, the pressure of the helium gas must be less than that of the atmosphere. First convert the pressure difference in mm Hg to kPa, which gives 24 kPa. Then subtract the 24 kPa from the 102 to give a helium gas pressure of 78 kPa.

A barometer is a manometer designed to measure the pressure of the atmosphere.

IDEAL GASES AND THE GAS LAWS

In working with problems involving gases, it is customary to compare the conditions of the gases to a specific reference, a set of conditions called **standard temperature and pressure** (**STP**). Standard pressure is 1 atm (or 760 mm Hg or 101.3 kPa) and standard temperature is 0°C or 273K.

The **empirical gas laws** allow us to relate factors such as temperature, volume, pressure, and number of moles to each other. By applying the concepts from KMT, these can be deduced logically, and all have been verified experimentally many times. These gas laws hold true for all gases under nearly all conditions.

According to **Boyle's law**, pressure and volume are inversely related (at constant temperature and number of moles). As more pressure is applied to a gas, the space between particles is compressed, as shown in Figure 1.48. The molecules themselves do not change size.

MANOMETERS

A manometer problem asks for a comparison of two sides, each with a push or pressure. The higher the pressure, the more the opposite side is pushed back.

PRESSURE UNITS

Be familiar with the common pressure units: atm, mm Hg, and kPa.

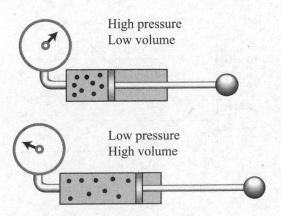

High pressure
Low volume

Low pressure
High volume

Figure 1.48. Pressure and volume

Boyle's law can be expressed as:

$$PV = \text{constant},$$

as shown in Figure 1.49, which shows the typical inverse relationship between pressure and volume.

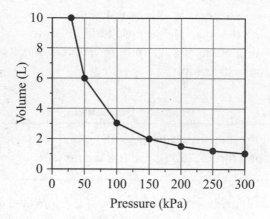

Figure 1.49. Boyle's law

Or, for situations where pressure and volume are changing:

$$P_1 V_1 = P_2 V_2$$

As the volume available to particles is decreased, collisions are more frequent, causing an increase in pressure.

Charles's law states that the volume of a gas is directly proportional to the absolute (kelvin) temperature, at constant pressure and number of moles. As a balloon is heated, the molecules gain kinetic energy and move faster. This leads to more collisions. To equalize the pressure, the balloon expands. If the container is inflexible, as would be true in a steel can, a different situation arises, represented by the following equation:

$$\frac{V_1}{T_1} = \frac{V_2}{T_2}$$

Figure 1.50 shows the situation graphically.

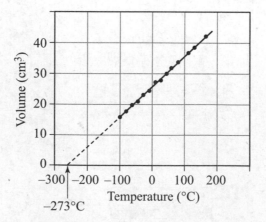

Figure 1.50. Volume and temperature

Theoretically, at 0 kelvin a gas would have zero volume. By extrapolating from measurements of gas volumes at different temperatures, the first determinations of absolute zero were made.

Gay-Lussac's law on pressure and temperature explains how, when a gas in a rigid container is heated, the particles move faster and collide more frequently, raising the number of collisions and the energy of the collisions, thus increasing the pressure (see Figure 1.51).

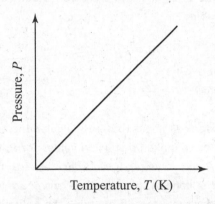

Figure 1.51. Pressure and temperature

> ## GAS LAW PATTERNS
>
> You don't need to know the gas laws by name.
>
> It is important to know that:
>
> P and V are inversely related
>
> P and T are directly related, as are V and T
>
> Each of these relationships can be derived from PV = nRT

The **combined gas law** allows us to determine what will happen when P, V, and T all change simultaneously. The combined gas law states:

$$\frac{P_1 V_1}{T_1} = \frac{P_2 V_2}{T_2}$$

It is common to convert a gas volume from one temperature and pressure combination to standard conditions (STP).

TIP

COMBINED GAS LAW

Know the combined gas law and the conditions that constitute STP.

Practice Question

A sample of Helium has a volume of 23.5L at 105kPa and 27°C. What volume would it have at STP?

$$\left(\frac{(105 \text{ kPa})(23.5\text{L})}{300\text{K}} \right) = \left(\frac{(101.3 \text{ kPa})(V_2)}{273\text{K}} \right)$$

Solution: Solving for V_2 gives $V_2 = 22.2$ L. The temperature must be in kelvin for all gas calculations.

GAS LAWS
AND KELVIN
TEMPERATURE

If a gas calculation
is not done in kelvin,
you'll end up trying
to divide by zero
for STP.

If P, V, or T is constant, then that factor cancels out and one of the named gas laws results. For example, if the temperature does not change, the equation reduces to $P_1 V_1 = P_2 V_2$, which is Boyle's law.

TEST QUESTION

What happens to the volume of a gas if the pressure is doubled and the absolute (kelvin) temperature is doubled?

(A) the volume is doubled

(B) the volume is halved

(C) the volume is unchanged

(D) the volume is quadrupled

(C) At first glance it might look as if this requires calculations, but no numbers are given. One solution would be to make up starting values for P, V, and T and then double the value of T and P and solve for V. Another way is to realize that doubling the pressure has the effect of halving the volume (P and V are inversely related) and doubling the temperature has the effect of doubling the volume (V and T are directly related). The net result of halving and doubling any number is no change.

The **ideal gas law** brings the concept of the number of moles of particles (symbolized as n) into the equation. As more gas molecules are added to a system, the number of collisions increases. P and n, then, are directly related. This equation can be written:

$$PV = nRT$$

R is the universal gas constant. It has the following values:

$R = 0.08206$ L atm/mole K
$R = 62.4$ L mm Hg/mole K
$R = 8.31$ L kPa/mole K

To use these values of R, volume must be in liters and temperature in kelvin.
You can use the ideal gas law in several ways.

Practice Question

Find the mass of oxygen gas (O_2) in a 32.8 L tank with a pressure of 45.0 atm and a temperature of 25°C.

Solution:

$$PV = nRT$$
$$(45.0 \text{ atm})(32.8 \text{ L}) = n(0.08206 \text{ L atm/mole K})(298 \text{ K})$$
$$= 60.4 \text{ moles} \times 32 \text{ g } O_2/1 \text{ mole } O_2 = 1930 \text{ g}$$

The ideal gas law can also be combined with the equation for density or molar mass to determine the molar mass of an unknown gas.

Practice Question

A sample of an unknown gas is vaporized in a 275 ml flask surrounded by 100.0°C water at standard pressure. The gas is cooled and condensed to a liquid and found to have a mass of 0.687 g. Determine the molar mass and the density of the gas.

Solution:

$$PV = nRT$$
$$(1 \text{ atm})(0.275 \text{ L}) = (n)(0.08206 \text{ L atm/mole k})(373 \text{ K})$$
$$n = 0.00898 \text{ moles}$$

$$\frac{0.687 \text{ g}}{0.00898 \text{ moles}} = 77 \text{ g/mole}$$

The density of the gas is 0.687 g/.275 L = 2.50 g/L.

You can use the ideal gas law to calculate the **molar volume of a gas and gas density**, that is, the volume that one mole of an ideal gas would have at standard temperature and pressure (STP). Solving for V gives 22.4 L, which is the molar volume of an ideal gas at STP.

Amadeo Avogadro determined that equal volumes of gases that are at the same temperature and pressure contain equal numbers of molecules. This is referred to as **Avogadro's hypothesis**. It means that the number of molecules (or moles) of a gas is directly proportional to the volume of the gas if the temperature and pressure are constant or that the number of molecules is directly proportional to the pressure if volume and temperature are constant (see Figure 1.52).

TIP

MOLAR VOLUME OF A GAS AT STP

Be able to recognize 22.4 L of a gas as 1 mole, 11.2 L as 0.5 mole, and 44.8 L as 2 moles, at STP.

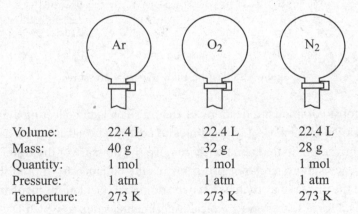

	Ar	O₂	N₂
Volume:	22.4 L	22.4 L	22.4 L
Mass:	40 g	32 g	28 g
Quantity:	1 mol	1 mol	1 mol
Pressure:	1 atm	1 atm	1 atm
Temperture:	273 K	273 K	273 K

Figure 1.52. Avogadro's hypothesis

TIP

AVOGADRO'S HYPOTHESIS

Equal volumes of gases (at the same T and P) have equal numbers of moles. Applications of Avogadro's hypothesis are common on MCAT questions.

> ## P, V, AND T PATTERNS
>
> P and V are inversely related.
>
> The following are directly related:
>
> P and T
>
> P and n
>
> V and T
>
> Many MCAT items test these patterns.

This means that in a chemical reaction, the mole ratio for chemicals (reactants or products) equals the volume ratio, as in the reaction below, showing the combustion of propane:

$$C_3H_{8(g)} + 5\,O_{2(g)} \rightarrow 4\,CO_{2(g)} + 5\,H_2O_{(g)}$$

If 10 L of propane react, 40 liters of carbon dioxide will be produced, along with 50 L of water vapor. This relationship applies only to gases. They need not be at standard conditions, but the comparison holds true only if they are at the same temperature and pressure.

In a mixture of gases, the pressure of each gas is independent of the others. This is known as **Dalton's law of partial pressures** (see Figure 1.53).

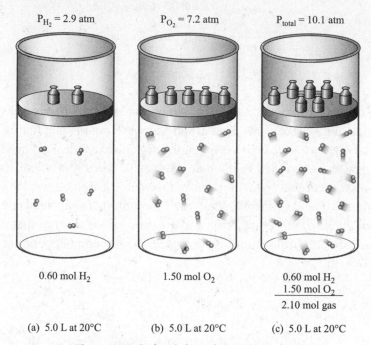

Figure 1.53. Dalton's law of partial pressures

One of the most common applications of Dalton's law is in collecting a gas over water, a common experimental method of generating and collecting a gas as a reaction product. It is usually more convenient to mathematically remove the pressure of the water vapor from the measured total by using water vapor pressures readily obtained from published data tables. The pressure of the dry gas may then be used in additional calculations involving gas pressures and/or volumes. Figure 1.54 shows a typical experimental setup in which Dalton's law would be applied.

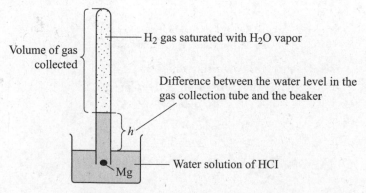

Figure 1.54. Collecting a gas over water

According to **Graham's law and gas diffusion and effusion–root mean square (RMS) speed of a gas,** the average speed of a molecule in a gas sample is given by the equation:

$$\mu_{rms} = \sqrt{\frac{3RT}{M}},$$

where R is the Universal Gas constant in SI units (8.31 J/mole K), T is the absolute (kelvin) temperature, and M the mass of a mole of gas in kilograms.

RMS SPEED OF A GAS MOLECULE

According to this equation:

The higher the temperature, the faster the molecules move.

The heavier the molecules, the slower they move on average.

The RMS speed of nitrogen gas at 25°C would be:

$$\mu_{rms} = \sqrt{3(8.31 \; \text{L} \cdot \text{kPa/mole} \cdot \text{K})(298 \; \text{K})/0.028 \; \text{kg/mole}} = 515 \; \text{m/s}$$

Looking at the equation, you should be able to determine that at higher temperatures, molecules have a great RMS speed (as predicted by the kinetic theory) and that heavier gases have a lower RMS speed at any given temperature. At the same temperature, molecules have the same average kinetic energy.

Diffusion in gases involves the random spreading out of gases, going from a higher concentration to a lower one (the same idea as diffusion of molecules in aqueous systems). **Effusion** is the passage of a gas through tiny orifices into an evacuated chamber. (See Figure 1.55.)

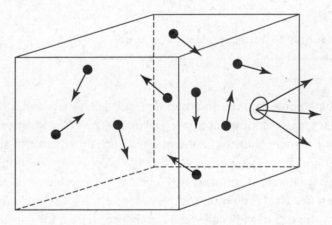

Figure 1.55. Effusion

In both cases, the rate is a function of the molar mass of the gas and the temperature. If two gases are compared at the same temperature, then **Graham's law** can be used to determine their relative rates of diffusion or effusion, which will depend only on their molar masses:

$$\frac{\text{rate of gas 1}}{\text{rate of gas 2}} = \frac{\sqrt{\text{molar mass of gas 2}}}{\sqrt{\text{molar mass of gas 1}}}$$

Practice Question

A gas effuses at a rate 6 times that of SF_6. What is the molar mass of the unknown gas?

$$\frac{\text{Rate of unknown gas effusion}}{\text{Rate of } SF_6 \text{ effusion}} = 6 = \frac{\sqrt{146.1}}{\sqrt{x}}$$

Solution: Solving for x gives 4.05, which suggests that the unknown gas is helium.

TIP

THE BOTTOM LINE ON RMS SPEED

At the same temperature, lighter gases move faster.

TIP

GRAHAM'S LAW

Graham's law does not calculate the actual speed of effusion or diffusion of a gas. It calculates relative rates only.

TEST QUESTION

Samples of neon gas and krypton gas are at the same temperature and pressure in a container with a small pore. In one hour, 20.0 ml of neon effuse through the pore. What volume of krypton will effuse during the same time?

(A) 5.0 ml

(B) 10.0 ml

(C) 40.0 ml

(D) 80.0 ml

(B) With any Graham's law calculation (effusion or diffusion), first decide which gas will effuse or diffuse faster. Because krypton has a molar mass of 84 g/mole and neon a molar mass of 20 g/mole, neon must effuse faster. This means that less krypton will effuse in the allotted time, making (A) and (B) the only plausible answers. Because Graham's law states that the relative rates depend on the square root of the molar mass ratio, krypton must effuse at about

$$\sqrt{\frac{20}{84}} \approx \sqrt{\frac{1}{4}} = \frac{1}{2}$$

This means that only 10 mL of krypton will effuse.

Real gases do have some volume, and their molecules do interact with each other. These facts make the ideal gas law slightly inaccurate. **Deviations from the ideal gas law** occur when (1) the molecules have more chances to interact with each other, which happens when they are closer together and are moving more slowly, and (2) the molecules are larger. Extremely high pressures (several hundred atm) and very low temperatures also make the ideal gas law inaccurate. The **van der Waals equation** compensates for this inaccuracy with one term that takes into account the size of molecules and another that takes into account the fact that attractions between molecules reduce the number of collisions and thus lower the pressure:

$$P = \frac{nRT}{V - nb} - \frac{n^2 a}{V^2}$$

correction for volume of molecules (decreases volume as a function of the number of molecules)

correction for molecular attraction (decreases pressure as volume decreases and the number of molecules increases)

In general, as molecules are closer together, collisions are more frequent and any intermolecular forces between molecules increase. At higher pressures (such as a few hundred atm) a gas will have a lower volume than would be predicted by the ideal gas law. At extremely high pressures the size of the particles is no longer negligible and the gas has a larger volume than would be predicted by the ideal gas law.

> **VAN DER WAALS EQUATION**
>
> If the *a* and *b* factors are both zero, which is what KMT suggests, this becomes the ideal gas law.

As the temperature of a gas decreases, the average molecular speed decreases and intermolecular forces become more significant, and the gas has a lower pressure than predicted by the ideal gas law.

In spite of its imperfections, the ideal gas law still serves a useful purpose, especially for quick estimates, and the elements of the kinetic molecular theory still hold true.

General Properties of Liquids and Solids

Liquids and solids are considered to be condensed phases of matter, as there is little space between particles. In a liquid, the molecules are able to move relatively freely (with some constraints due to intermolecular forces). Molecules in a liquid can evaporate from the surface. Bulk properties of liquids include having a definite volume but an indefinite shape, being able to flow, and being incompressible. Compare and contrast these with the bulk properties of a gas, which include having an indefinite shape and volume, being able to flow, and being compressible because of the large amount of available space between the particles.

INTERMOLECULAR ATTRACTIONS IN LIQUIDS

There are several attractive forces between molecules in liquids. Collectively, they are known as intermolecular forces. These forces tend to keep the molecules from separating from each other. As a result, intermolecular forces make it less likely that a molecule will evaporate. These forces are also responsible for determining whether molecules can interact (mix or dissolve) with each other.

Hydrogen bonding is a type of dipole–dipole interaction between a hydrogen atom bound to a highly electronegative atom with a lone pair of electrons (such as N, O, or F). Hydrogen bonding in water molecules is shown in Figure 1.56.

> **PROPERTIES OF LIQUIDS AND GASES**
>
> | Liquids | Gases |
> | --- | --- |
> | Definite volume | Indefinite volume |
> | Indefinite shape | Indefinite shape |
> | Able to flow | Able to flow |
> | Incompressible | Compressible |

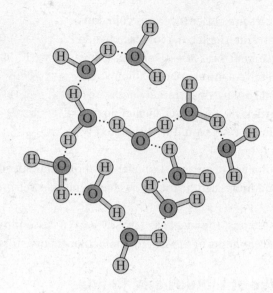

Figure 1.56. Hydrogen bonding in water

····· = hydrogen bond

TIP

HYDROGEN BONDS

Hydrogen bonding is of great importance in biological systems and is tested frequently on the MCAT.

Hydrogen bonding is responsible for many of the unique properties of water. These include a very high boiling point for such a low molar mass molecule, high specific heat capacity, low vapor pressure, high surface tension, and the fact that ice floats.

In molecules with dipole moments, oppositely charged ends of the molecules can exert attractive forces on each other. These **dipole interactions** are more effective when the molecules are compressed, as in solids and liquids, but much less so in gases, in which the molecules are farther apart. These attractive forces between polar molecules tend to result in higher boiling points and lower vapor pressures than nonpolar molecules of similar molar mass. An example of dipole–dipole interactions is shown in Figure 1.57.

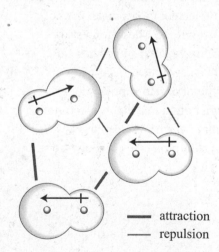

—— attraction
— repulsion

Figure 1.57. Dipole–dipole interactions

Although nonpolar molecules seem to have an even distribution of charges around the molecule, because of the random motion of electrons, at any given time the electrons may be unevenly distributed, leading to an "instantaneous dipole." This short-lived and weak dipole can allow molecules to attract each other. These attractive forces are collectively known as **London dispersion forces**. They are the forces that allow nonpolar molecules to exist as liquids. Without London dispersion forces, nonpolar liquids would have no interactions between their molecules and could not be liquefied. In general, London dispersion forces increase with molar mass and decrease with the compactness of the molecule. This means that for nonpolar molecules, such as hydrocarbons, the boiling point goes up with molar mass, and for isomers, a molecule with a longer chain has a higher boiling point. The instantaneous dipoles induce more dipoles in nearby atoms to create the attractive force. This is why larger molecules have stronger London forces, as they can be more easily induced into forming instantaneous dipoles.

Table 1.10 shows the formula, molar mass, and boiling point of several hydrocarbons.

Table 1.10 The Effect of Molar Mass on the Boiling Point of Hydrocarbons

Compound & Formula	Molar Mass (g/mole)	Boiling Point (°C)
Methane, CH_4	16	−164
Propane, C_3H_8	44	−42
Hexane, C_6H_{14}	84	69
Nonane, C_9H_{20}	128	151
Dodecane, $C_{12}H_{26}$	170	216

A molecule of pentane, $CH_3CH_2CH_2CH_2CH_3$ (molar mass = 72 g/mole) has a boiling point of 36°C whereas a molecule of 2,2-dimethylpropane (also molar mass 72 g/mole) has a boiling point of 9.5°C (see Figure 1.58).

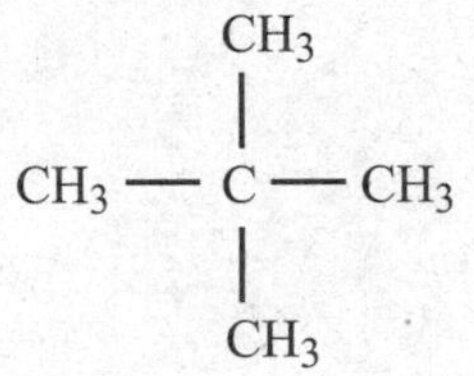

$$CH_3 - \overset{\displaystyle CH_3}{\underset{\displaystyle CH_3}{\overset{|}{\underset{|}{C}}}} - CH_3$$

Figure 1.58. A molecule of 2,2-dimethylpropane

The compact nature of this molecule lowers the magnitude of London dispersion forces, giving it a lower boiling point.

Which of following substances has the lowest boiling point?

(A) Calcium oxide, CaO

(B) Magnesium chloride, $MgCl_2$

(C) *n*-pentane, $CH_3(CH_2)_3CH_3$

(D) *n*-heptane, $CH_3(CH_2)_5CH_3$

(C) Choices A and B can be eliminated, as they are ionic compounds, which typically have very high melting and boiling points. The remaining choices are both hydrocarbons. In liquid hydrocarbons the main intermolecular forces between molecules are London dispersion forces, which are primarily dependent on molar mass. This means that *n*-heptane will have a higher boiling point, making choice C the correct answer.

Solids and Crystals

In a solid, the intermolecular forces are much stronger than in a gas or a liquid. This gives solids their rigid shapes and fixed or definite volumes. A solid may have a crystalline or an amorphous structure. In a crystalline solid, the atoms or ions are arranged in a repeated three-dimensional geometric array. The repeating unit is known as a **unit cell**. Common unit cells include cubic, face-centered cubic, and body-centered cubic (see Figure 1.59).

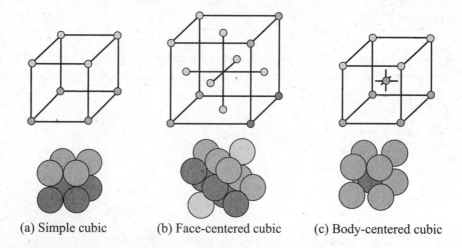

(a) Simple cubic   (b) Face-centered cubic   (c) Body-centered cubic

Figure 1.59. Common unit cells

Ionic solids have unit cells based on ions and the chemical formula of an ionic solid gives the ratio of ions in the compound. Metallic solids tend to be closely packed and have freely floating valence electrons (see Figure 1.60). These mobile valence electrons (sometimes called a "sea of electrons") allow metals to be malleable, ductile, and good conductors of heat and electricity.

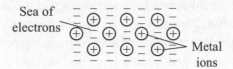

Figure 1.60. Electrons in metals

Amorphous solids have atoms rigidly held in place, but without a repeating unit of atoms. Glass is an example of an amorphous solid.

Phase Changes

Each state of matter can be converted into another via the absorption or release of heat energy as shown in Figure 1.61. The phase changes of melting, boiling, and sublimating are endothermic, whereas condensation, deposition, and freezing are exothermic changes.

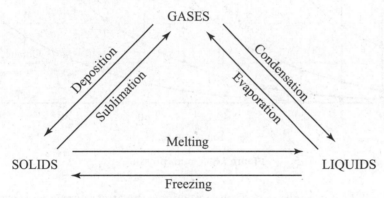

Figure 1.61. Phase changes

TIP

PHASE CHANGES

Know the names of each phase change, and also whether it is an endothermic or exothermic change.

VAPOR PRESSURE

In a closed container of a liquid, some surface molecules will have sufficient energy to overcome the intermolecular forces holding molecules together and will evaporate. Evaporated molecules form a vapor above the surface of the liquid. The measurement of the pressure they exert is called the vapor pressure. Eventually, enough molecules will enter the gas phase to cause condensation, and a balance or equilibrium will exist between the two processes. This **dynamic equilibrium** is shown below in Figure 1.62.

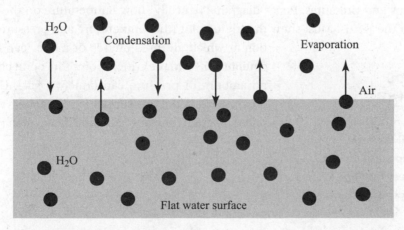

Figure 1.62. Dynamic equilibrium between evaporation and condensation

The vapor pressure of a liquid depends on the identity of the liquid and the temperature. For any liquid, a higher temperature results in greater average molecular motion and a higher vapor pressure, and stronger intermolecular forces result in lower vapor pressure. Figure 1.63 shows vapor pressure curves for four liquids. Note that at any temperature, the vapor pressure of pentane will be higher than that of the other liquids. This is because of the weaker intermolecular forces between pentane molecules.

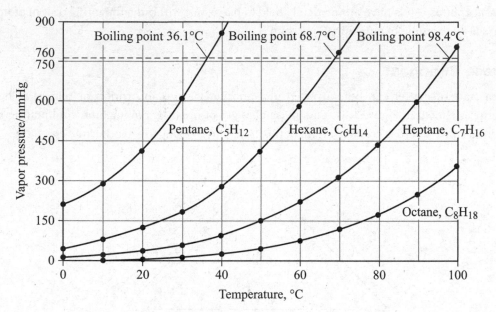

Figure 1.63. Vapor pressure

Any liquid will boil when its vapor pressure equals the atmospheric pressure above it. At standard pressure (1 atm, 101.3 kPa, or 760 mm Hg), the boiling temperature is known as the "normal" boiling point. At different atmospheric pressures, liquids will boil at different temperatures. In Figure 1.63, the normal boiling point of hexane is given as about 69°C. If the atmospheric pressure were lowered to 450 mm Hg, then the boiling point of hexane would be about 52°C. Liquids with strong intermolecular forces (such as water and alcohols with many hydrogen bonds) tend to have high boiling points and low vapor pressures.

PHASE DIAGRAMS

A phase diagram shows the state(s) of matter in which a substance will exist at specific temperatures and pressures. Phase diagrams typically show temperature on the x-axis and pressure on the y-axis. Most show the triple point (the temperature and pressure combination at which all three phases of matter can exist in an equilibrium) and the critical point (the point above which no amount of pressure can liquefy a gas). One atm of pressure (standard pressure) is usually shown as well. The phase diagram for carbon dioxide is shown in Figure 1.64.

> **HYDROGEN BONDS AND BOILING POINT**
>
> When comparing liquids, the one with the most hydrogen bonds will have the strongest intermolecular forces, the lowest vapor pressure, and the highest boiling points. Look for OH groups on carbons as "hydrogen bonding areas."

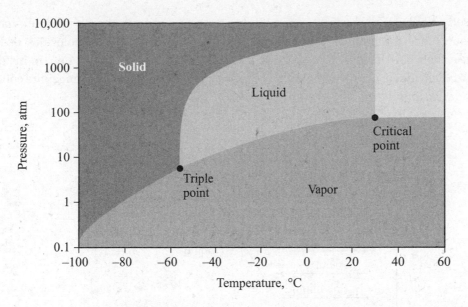

Figure 1.64. Phase diagram of carbon dioxide

In this phase diagram, the triple point of carbon dioxide is given as approximately −58°C and 5 atm and the critical temperature is 30°C. At one atmosphere of pressure, carbon dioxide cannot be a liquid. For any substance, no liquid can exist at a temperature below the triple point. The boundary lines between two phases show equilibria where melting, freezing, or boiling could be taking place. Note that the *x*- and *y*-axes may not be drawn to scale on a phase diagram.

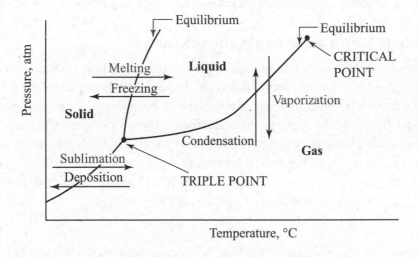

Figure 1.65. A phase diagram showing phase changes

TIP

PHASE DIAGRAMS

Be able to locate the triple point, critical point, and normal boiling and melting points on any phase diagram.

HEATING CURVES

A **heating curve** shows the phase of matter that a substance will have as it is warmed (as heat is added). The curve starts with the solid phase and then shows the result of increased temperature. Once sufficient energy has been added to overcome the intermolecular forces, the substance will melt, and while this phase change is taking place, the temperature remains constant. Once the substance has melted, the liquid molecules can absorb energy and move faster. Eventually, the molecules will change from a liquid to a gas throughout the liquid, as opposed to only on the surface. Again, during the phase change, the temperature remains constant. Once the liquid has boiled, the added energy goes to the molecules and they increase their kinetic energy. A typical heating curve is shown in Figure 1.66. If, instead of energy being added, energy is removed, a cooling curve results and the changes are condensing and freezing.

TIP

TEMPERATURE DURING A PHASE CHANGE

During a phase change the temperature remains constant.

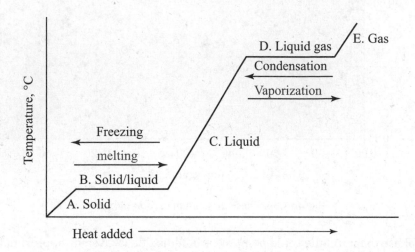

Figure 1.66. Heating curve

Colligative Properties

Colligative properties are properties of solutions that depend on the number of dissolved particles (ions or molecules) present, regardless of the type of particle.

LOWERING OF VAPOR PRESSURE (RAOULT'S LAW)

In a pure liquid, molecules can potentially evaporate from anywhere on the surface. When a solute is dissolved in a solvent, some fraction of the surface is taken up by the solute molecules, which causes the vapor pressure of the solvent to be lowered. The more moles of solute are dissolved, the more the vapor pressure decreases. If both substances in the mixture are volatile, then each will have a vapor pressure proportional to its mole fraction. A nonvolatile solute (such as salt or sugar) has no vapor pressure.

Raoult's law states that the vapor pressure of a solvent is equal to the mole fraction of the solvent ($X_{solvent}$) times the vapor pressure of the pure solvent ($P°$):

$$P_{vap} = (X_{solvent})(P°)$$

Raoult's law can also be used to calculate the amount that the vapor pressure is lowered by the addition of a solute:

$$\Delta P_{vap} = (X_{solute})(P°_{solvent})$$

The amount that the vapor pressure is lowered (ΔP_{vap}) is equal to the mole fraction of the solute times the vapor pressure of the pure solvent.

In a mixture of substances, each component has its own vapor pressure equal to the pure substance's vapor pressure times its mole fraction:

$$P_{total} = X_A P°_A + X_B P°_B$$

If either component is nonvolatile, then its contribution to the vapor pressure is zero, though it still reduces the vapor pressure of the other component.

BOILING POINT ELEVATION, FREEZING POINT DEPRESSION, AND APPLICATIONS

Adding a solute to a liquid will both raise the boiling point of the liquid and lower the freezing point. In each case, the change in the boiling or freezing point is proportional to the molality of the dissolved solute (times the van't Hoff factor, i, which represents the number of dissociated particles that come from each dissolved molecule). Each solvent has its own proportionality constant for this effect.

Molality is defined as moles of dissolved solute per kilogram of solvent. If one mole of sucrose is dissolved in one kilogram of water, a 1 m (1 molal) solution results.

The formula for the freezing point depression of a solution is:

$$\Delta T_f = iK_f m$$

For water, the value of K_f is 1.86°C/m. Constants such as this need not be memorized.

The formula for boiling point elevation is:

$$\Delta T_b = iK_b m$$

and for water the value of K_b is 0.512°C/m.

Practice Question

In 250 grams of water, 90 grams of glucose ($C_6H_{12}O_6$, molar mass = 180 g/mole) are dissolved. What are the freezing and boiling points of the solution?

Solution: 90 grams of glucose is 0.5 moles, so the molality of the solution is 0.5 moles/0.25 kg solvent = 2.0 m.

The boiling point elevation will be (0.512°C/m)(2 m) = 1.02°C. This means that the boiling point of the water will be raised from 100°C to 101.02°C.

The freezing point depression will be (1.86°C/m)(2 m) = 3.72°C so the solution will freeze at –3.72°C.

In the case of an ionic solute, an additional factor must be taken into account. Ionic substances separate into ions upon dissolving, so that the molality must be multiplied by the van't Hoff factor. For NaCl, $i = 2$, so the effect would be double that of glucose, a molecular substance. For $CaCl_2$, $i = 3$ and the effect is larger, which is why calcium and magnesium chloride are often used to prevent roads and driveways from freezing over in the winter. Each dissolved mole yields more particles in the solution, and these colligative properties depend only on the number of dissolved particles.

Which of the following aqueous solutions would have the highest boiling point?

(A) 0.20 m glucose

(B) 0.20 m NaCl

(C) 0.15 m CaCl$_2$

(D) 0.25 m sucrose

(C) The boiling point elevation in each case is described by the equation $\Delta T_b = iK_f m$. Because the solvent in each case is water, K_f is the same for each example. This means that the boiling point elevation is dependent only on i and the molality, m. Both glucose and sucrose are molecular substances and $i = 1$. NaCl is an ionic substance that dissolves in water to produce 2 ions and CaCl$_2$ produces 3 ions. It is the number of dissolved particles, whether they are ions or molecules, that is important. This makes C the correct answer. This is also the solution that would have the lowest freezing point.

ADDITION OF A SOLUTE TO A LIQUID

Adding a solute to a liquid widens the range between phases, making the boiling point higher and the freezing point lower. The antifreeze in a car is also "anti-boil."

OSMOTIC PRESSURE

If a semi-permeable membrane is placed between two solutions with different concentrations of solute, there will be a net movement of solvent molecules. The force that will oppose this motion is called the osmotic pressure, shown in Figure 1.67. The net flow of water is from the less concentrated solute or the pure solvent to the more concentrated side of the membrane. The weight of the extra liquid on one side (which is the volume of the liquid times its density), multiplied by the height difference represents the osmotic pressure of the solution.

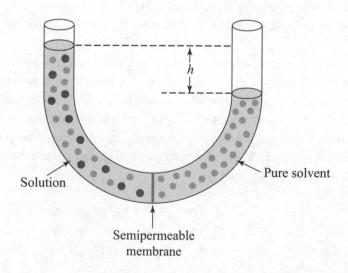

Figure 1.67. Osmotic pressure

The equation that describes the osmotic pressure is

$$\Pi = MRT,$$

where M is the molarity of the solution (measured in moles of solute per liter of solution), R is the gas constant (.0821 L · atm/mole K or 62.4 L · mm Hg/mole · K), and T is the absolute (kelvin) temperature.

The main use of osmotic pressure is in determining the molar mass of macromolecules, because their concentrations in solution would be too low to give a measurable change in freezing or boiling point.

Practice Question

A solution of a protein is made by dissolving 0.500 grams of protein in 100.0 ml of solution. The osmotic pressure is measured at 4.25 mm Hg at 25°C. Find the molar mass of the protein.

Solution:

$$4.25 \text{ mm Hg} = (M)(62.4 \text{ L} \cdot \text{mm Hg/mole} \cdot \text{K})(298 \text{ K})$$
$$M = 2.29 \times 10^{-4} \text{ M or } 2.29 \times 10^{-4} \text{ moles/L}$$
$$2.29 \times 10^{-4} M = \text{\# moles/0.100 L}$$
$$= 2.29 \times 10^{-5} \text{ moles}$$
$$0.500 \text{ g}/2.29 \times 10^{-5} \text{ moles} = 21{,}800 \text{ g/mole}$$

Colloids

A **colloid** is a dispersion of one substance in another. Fog is an example of a colloid, in which very small water droplets are the dispersed phase and air is the continuous phase. The particles in a colloid are larger than those in a true solution but are too small to be seen with a light microscope. The distinguishing feature of a colloid is that it exhibits the **Tyndall effect**, the scattering of light by the dispersed particles. An example of the Tyndall effect is when a beam from car headlights can be seen in a fog. The headlights do not create a visible beam in the air because molecules of nitrogen and oxygen are too small to scatter light, but the dispersed particles in a colloid are large enough to do so. An **emulsion** is a colloid in which one liquid is dispersed in another. Mayonnaise is an example of an emulsion.

STOICHIOMETRY

Stoichiometry is the branch of chemistry that deals with quantitative relationships in chemical reactions. Chemists apply stoichiometry to analyze unknown compounds and to predict the amounts of products that can be formed in chemical reactions.

Molecular Mass (Molecular Weight)

Just as an atom has a weight, so does a molecule. The weight of a molecule is simply the weight of the individual atoms that make up the molecule. For almost all calculations needed on the MCAT, you can safely round atomic weights to the nearest 0.1 amu, and in many cases, to the nearest whole number.

To find the molecular weight of NH_4Cl, the calculation would be:

$1 N = 1 \times 14.0 = 14.0$ amu
$4 H = 4 \times 1.0 = 4.0$ amu
$1 Cl = 1 \times 35.5 = 35.5$ amu
Molecular weight = 53.5 amu

When dealing with ionic compounds, it is more accurate to use the term "formula weight" because ionic compounds do not exist as discrete molecules but rather as large crystalline arrays of ions. The formula of an ionic compound represents the ratio of ions in a crystal of that compound but is not meant to suggest that there is an isolated unit of exactly that number of ions. NaCl does not contain a unit with one Na^+ ion and one Cl^- ion, but in any sample of NaCl, there will be a 1:1 ratio of sodium and chloride ions.

The Mole Concept

A **mole** is defined as the amount of a substance that has the same number of particles as exactly 12.0 grams of the isotope carbon-12. The number 6.02×10^{23} is known as Avogadro's number. One mole of a compound is defined as the molecular weight expressed in grams, rather than in amu. A single molecule of carbon dioxide has a mass of 44.0 amu, whereas a mole of carbon dioxide molecules has a mass of 44.0 grams. Carbon dioxide, then, has a **molar mass** of 44.0 grams. Once the molar mass of a substance is known, it is possible to convert between the number of grams and the number of moles.

> **AVOGADRO'S NUMBER**
>
> Be able to recognize Avogadro's number, 6.02×10^{23}, the number of particles in a mole of any substance. One-half mole is 3.01×10^{23}, and 2 moles is 1.204×10^{24}.

Practice Question

Find the mass of 3.2 moles of ammonia gas.

Solution: One mole of ammonia gas has a mass of 17.0 grams, so

$$(17.0 \text{ grams/mole}) \times 3.2 \text{ moles} = 54.4 \text{ grams}.$$

Practice Question

How many moles are in 22.2 grams of calcium chloride, $CaCl_2$?

Solution: $22.2 \text{ grams } CaCl_2 \times \dfrac{1 \text{ mole } CaCl_2}{111 \text{ g } CaCl_2} = 0.2 \text{ moles of } CaCl_2$

Percent Composition

The **mass percent** of a species is the mass of an element in one mole of the compound divided by the mass of one mole of the compound times 100. This can be determined either by using the chemical formula or experimental data.

Practice Question

What is the mass percent of silver in silver nitrate, $AgNO_3$?

Solution: Mass % Ag = $\dfrac{\text{mass of Ag}}{\text{mass of AgNO}_3} \times 100 = \dfrac{107.9\,\text{g}}{169.9\,\text{g}} \times 100 = 63.5\%$

Thus, in any sample of silver nitrate, 63.5% of the mass is due to silver atoms.

Practice Question

A sample of an iron and oxygen ore has a mass of 35.8 grams. The iron in the compound has a mass of 27.9 grams. What is the percent iron in the ore?

Solution: Mass Percent Iron = $\dfrac{\text{mass of Fe}}{\text{total mass}} \times 100 = \dfrac{27.9\,\text{g Fe}}{35.8\,\text{g total}} \times 100 = 78\%\ \text{Fe}$

Empirical and Molecular Formulas

The **empirical formula** is the simplest whole number ratio of atoms in a compound. The **molecular formula** is the actual whole number ratio of atoms in a molecule of a compound. Table 1.11 gives some examples.

Table 1.11 Molecular and Empirical Formulas

Molecular Formula	Empirical Formula
C_2H_6	CH_3
C_6H_6	CH
C_4H_{10}	C_2H_5
C_6H_{12}	CH_2

Some typical examples of problems involving empirical and molecular formulas are shown below.

Practice Question

A compound is analyzed and found to have a percent composition of 62.0% C, 10.3% H, and 27.6% O. What is the empirical formula of the compound?

Solution: Assume there are 100 grams of the compound so that the percent of each becomes grams. Then convert from grams to moles.

$$62.0\,\text{g C} \times \dfrac{1\,\text{mole C}}{12.0\,\text{g C}} \quad 10.3\,\text{g H} \times \dfrac{1\,\text{mole H}}{1.0\,\text{g H}} \quad 27.6\,\text{g O} \times \dfrac{1\,\text{mole O}}{16.0\,\text{g O}}$$

Moles C = 5.17 moles carbon

Moles H = 10.3 moles hydrogen

Moles O = 1.73 moles oxygen

TIP

NUMBERS INVOLVED IN EMPIRICAL FORMULAS

Look for small whole number ratios and be prepared to round. For example, 2.98 rounds to 3.

Divide each number of moles by the smallest number to give a ratio

$$\text{Carbon: } \frac{5.17}{1.73} = 3 \quad \text{Hydrogen: } \frac{10.3}{1.73} = 6 \quad \text{Oxygen: } \frac{1.73}{1.73} = 1$$

The empirical formula, then, is C_3H_6O. You can double check this by working the numbers in reverse.

Practice Question

A compound is determined to have an empirical formula of C_2H_6O and a molar mass of 138 g/mole. What is the molecular formula?

TIP

MOLECULAR AND EMPIRICAL FORMULA

The molecular formula may be the same as the empirical formula or it may be a whole number multiple of it.

Solution: Find the mass of one empirical formula unit. Because the molecular formula is a multiple of the empirical formula, divide the molar mass by the empirical formula unit mass. This ratio is multiplied by all the subscripts in the empirical formula to give the molecular formula.

One unit of C_2H_6O has a mass of 46 g/mole. $\frac{138}{46} = 3$, so the molecular formula is

$$3(C_2H_6O) = C_6H_{18}O_3.$$

The answer could be verified by confirming that this compound does have the proper empirical formula and molar mass.

TEST QUESTION

A substance is analyzed and found to have an empirical formula of CH_2 and a molar mass of 56g/mole. What is the molecular formula of the compound?

(A) C_2H_4

(B) C_3H_6

(C) C_4H_8

(D) C_5H_{10}

(C) All of the choices have an empirical formula of CH_2, so none can be eliminated by that criterion. Try each choice and see which comes out to a molar mass of 56 g/mole. A more efficient way is to use the fact that a unit of CH_2 has a mass of 14 g/unit so $\frac{56}{14} = 4$, which means that the empirical formula must be multiplied by 4 to give C_4H_8.

Density

The density of a substance is its mass per unit volume and is calculated by the formula

$$D = \frac{\text{mass}}{\text{volume}}$$

The most common units for mass are grams and kilograms. For volume, the units are milliliters (mL), centimeters cubed (cm^3), or liters (L). In any density problem, two of the terms must be supplied in order for the third term to be solvable. Remember that ml and cm^3 are equivalent.

For a solid or liquid, simply divide the mass by the volume to obtain the density. For a gas at STP the density is the mass of one mole of the gas (the molar mass) divided by the volume of one mole of the gas (22.4 L).

DENSITY OF GASES

At STP the density of argon gas is $\dfrac{39.9\,\text{g}}{22.4\,\text{L}}$ = 1.78 g/L. If the gas is at a different temperature and pressure, the volume can be determined by using the ideal gas law and then applying the density equation.

Practice Question

What is the density of argon gas at a temperature of 30°C and a pressure of 1.05 atm?

Solution: Solve for V: V = (1 mole)(0.0821 L · atm/mole · K)(303 K)/1.05 atm = 23.7 L

The density would be 39.9g/23.7 L = 1.68 g/L.

Chemical Equations

A chemical equation is a shorthand notation describing a reaction. In any chemical reaction, the starting materials are known as the reactants and the ending materials are the products. An arrow ($\rightarrow$) is used to show that a change or reaction has taken place. Chemists find it useful to categorize reactions into common types, even though the categories do not cover all of the nearly unlimited number of types of reactions that can occur.

PHYSICAL AND CHEMICAL CHANGES

A **physical change** does not result in the production of new substances. Examples include melting, freezing, and boiling.

A **chemical change or reaction** involves the conversion of the original chemicals into different products.

TIP

WORDS THAT INDICATE CHEMICAL REACTIONS

The words rusting, decomposing, oxidizing, forming, and burning are giveaway words that indicate chemical changes have taken place.

COMMONLY USED SYMBOLS

The table below shows some of the shorthand symbols used in writing chemical equations.

Table 1.12 Common Symbols Used in Chemical Equations

Symbol	Meaning
(s)	Solid
(l)	Liquid
(g)	Gas
(aq)	Aqueous or dissolved in water
$\rightarrow$	Yields, produces, or reacts to form
Δ	Heat

SUBSCRIPTS AND
COEFFICIENTS

Just as subscripts
are very often small
whole numbers, so
are coefficients.

BALANCING EQUATIONS

Chemical reactions are balanced using coefficients to adjust the numbers of reactants to products so that the law of conservation of matter is followed. Changing subscripts to balance an equation is not allowed as that would change the identity of a chemical, whereas changing a coefficient alters the amount of a substance but not its identity.

For example, in balancing the reaction $H_2O_{2(aq)} \rightarrow H_2O_{(l)} + O_{2(g)}$, the subscript on the H_2O cannot be changed to H_2O_2, as that would mean that the product would be hydrogen peroxide instead of water. Rather, a combination of coefficients such as the following could be used:

$$2H_2O_{2(aq)} \rightarrow 2H_2O_{(l)} + O_{2(g)}$$

This equation is balanced because each side has four hydrogen atoms and four oxygen atoms. Most inorganic reactions can be balanced by "inspection," with a quick look and some trial and error. The exception to this is oxidation–reduction (redox) reactions, which will be discussed later in this chapter.

TYPES OF CHEMICAL REACTIONS

For each of the main types of inorganic reactions, a short description and example are shown below.

SYNTHESIS

$A + B \rightarrow C$

In a **synthesis or combination reaction**, two or more reactants form a single product. The most common examples involve two elements combining to make one compound. A "generic" synthesis reaction would be: $A + B \rightarrow C$

$$2Na_{(s)} + Cl_{2(g)} \rightarrow 2NaCl_{(s)}$$

$$N_{2(g)} + O_{2(g)} \rightarrow 2NO_{(g)}$$

It is useful to keep in mind that some elements exist in nature in diatomic form (H_2, O_2, N_2, F_2, Cl_2, Br_2, and I_2). However, most of the other elements exist in monoatomic form in nature.

DIATOMIC ELEMENTS

Know the common diatomic elements.

H_2, O_2, N_2, Cl_2, Br_2, I_2, and F_2 exist in diatomic form when they are pure elements.

In a **decomposition reaction**, a single reactant breaks down into two or more products, very often elements. The most common ways to accomplish decompositions are with the addition of heat to a reactant or by passing an electric current through the liquid or aqueous form of the substance. A "generic" form of a decomposition reaction is: $A \rightarrow B + C$.

DECOMPOSITION

$C \rightarrow A + B$

$$2H_2O_{(l)} \rightarrow 2H_{2(g)} + O_{2(g)}$$

$$2Al_2O_{3(l)} \rightarrow 4Al_{(l)} + 3O_{2(g)}$$

> **SYNTHESIS AND DECOMPOSITION REACTIONS**
>
> Synthesis and decomposition reactions are opposites of each other.

In a **single displacement reaction (or replacement reaction)**, an element reacts with a compound to form a new ionic compound and a free element. The free element can either be a metal (in which case it will displace a metal) or a nonmetal (which displaces a nonmetal).

Most single displacement reactions are also oxidation–reduction reactions.

A generic single displacement reaction is A + BC → AC + B.

> **SINGLE DISPLACEMENT REACTION**
>
> A + BC → AC + B

$$Zn_{(s)} + CuSO_{4(aq)} \rightarrow ZnSO_{4(aq)} + Cu_{(s)}$$

$$2NaI_{(aq)} + F_{2(g)} \rightarrow 2NaF_{(aq)} + I_{2(s)}$$

Double displacement reactions involve "ion switching" between two different compounds. They are sometimes referred to as metathesis reactions. In many cases a solid product, known as a precipitate, is formed from two aqueous solutions. The generic double replacement reaction has the form AB + CD → AD + CB.

> **DOUBLE DISPLACEMENT**
>
> AB + CD → AD + CB

$$AgNO_{3(aq)} + KCl_{(aq)} \rightarrow KNO_{3(aq)} + AgCl_{(s)}$$

$$CaBr_{2(aq)} + Hg(NO_3)_{2(aq)} \rightarrow Ca(NO_3)_{2(aq)} + HgBr_{2(s)}$$

In a **combustion reaction**, a molecule reacts with oxygen gas to form carbon dioxide and water. To balance a combustion reaction, start by balancing the carbon atoms, followed by the hydrogen atoms, and finally, the oxygen atoms. If the oxygen coefficient comes out to a fraction, it is acceptable to either multiply all the coefficients by a factor that will yield whole numbers or to leave the oxygen as the fraction.

$$C_3H_{8(g)} + 5O_{2(g)} \rightarrow 3CO_{2(g)} + 4H_2O_{(g)}$$

$$C_6H_{14(l)} + 9.5O_{2(g)} \rightarrow 6CO_{2(g)} + 7H_2O_{(g)}$$

$$2C_6H_{14(l)} + 19O_{2(g)} \rightarrow 12CO_{2(g)} + 14H_2O_{(g)}$$

> **COMBUSTION REACTIONS**
>
> The products of a *complete combustion* are carbon dioxide and water. *Incomplete combustion* may produce CO instead of—or in addition to—CO_2.

Many displacement reactions involve aqueous solution of ions. Because ionic compounds in solution exist as aqueous ions, these reactions can also be written as **net ionic equations**, which show the ions that undergo changes in the reaction. Those ions that undergo no overall change are known as **spectator ions** and are left out of the final net ionic equation.

In the reaction between solutions of lead(II) nitrate and sodium chloride, the products are solid lead(II) chloride and aqueous sodium nitrate.

$$Pb(NO_3)_{2(aq)} + 2NaCl_{(aq)} \rightarrow PbCl_{2(s)} + 2\,NaNO_{3(aq)}$$

The equation can be written to show the chemical substances in their actual ionic form (called an overall ionic equation).

$$Pb^{+2}_{(aq)} + 2NO_3^{-1}_{(aq)} + 2Na^{+1}_{(aq)} + 2Cl^{-1}_{(aq)} \rightarrow PbCl_{2(s)} + 2Na^{+1}_{(aq)} + 2NO_3^{-1}_{(aq)}$$

Because the nitrate and sodium ions appear on both sides of the equation, they can be canceled out, and they are referred to as **spectator ions**.

The remaining substances are written in the net ionic equation:

$$Pb^{+2}_{(aq)} + 2Cl^{-1}_{(aq)} \rightarrow PbCl_{2(s)}$$

Reactions between acids and bases are usually double displacement reactions; however, because they are very common, they are also given the name **neutralization reactions**. In many neutralization reactions, an acid and base react to form an ionic salt and water:

$$acid + base \rightarrow salt + water$$

$$HCl_{(aq)} + KOH_{(aq)} \rightarrow KCl_{(aq)} + H_2O_{(l)}$$

$$H_2SO_{4(aq)} + 2\,LiOH_{(aq)} \rightarrow Li_2SO_{4(aq)} + 2\,H_2O_{(l)}$$

Balancing Redox Equations

One additional type of inorganic reaction involves oxidation and reduction, or the gaining and losing of electrons. When an atom undergoes a chemical process in which it gains electrons, the atom has been reduced. When an atom loses electrons, that atom has been oxidized. An easy way to remember this is to recall the phrase "Leo says Ger," which reminds you that "losing electrons is oxidation" (Leo) and "gaining electrons is reduction" (Ger). An oxidizing agent is a chemical species that accepts electrons (and is the species being reduced) whereas a reducing agent is an electron donor (and is the species being oxidized).

In order to understand and balance oxidation–reduction reactions (redox reactions), it is important to be able to recognize when an atom has been oxidized or reduced. This is done by assigning **oxidation numbers** to atoms in ions or molecules and noting when those oxidation numbers have been changed. Oxidation numbers are assigned based on the following rules (listed in order of priority):

1. The oxidation number of a free element is zero.
2. The oxidation number of a monoatomic ion is equal to the charge on the ion.
3. The oxidation number of an alkali metal (group 1 element) in a compound is +1.
4. The oxidation number of an alkaline earth metal (group 2 element) in a compound is +2.
5. The oxidation number of hydrogen in a compound or ion is +1. The only exception to this is in hydrides, where the hydrogen is combined with a group 1 or 2 element, in which case the oxidation number of the hydrogen is –1.

TIP

SPECTATOR IONS AND SOLUBILITY RULES

The spectator ions in reactions are often the ions whose compounds are soluble, such as nitrate, sodium, potassium, ammonium, and acetate.

TIP

LEO SAYS GER

Losing Electrons is Oxidation

Gaining Electrons is Reduction

6. The oxidation number of oxygen in an ion or compound is –2, except in peroxides, in which it is –1.
7. The oxidation number of a halide ion is –1 in a binary ionic compound.
8. The sum of all the oxidation numbers in a neutral compound is zero.
9. The sum of the oxidation numbers in an ion is equal to the charge of the ion.

Practice Question

Calculate the oxidation number of the S atom in the SO_3^{-2} ion.

Solution:
$$S + 3 (O) = -2$$
$$S - 6 = -2$$
$$S = +4$$

It is useful to include positive signs in oxidation numbers even though they are not needed.

Practice Question

Calculate the oxidation number of the Cr atom in $K_2Cr_2O_7$.

Solution:
$$2K + 2Cr + 7 (O) = 0$$
$$2(+1) + 2Cr = 7(-2) = 0$$
$$2Cr = 12$$
$$Cr = +6$$

TEST QUESTION

What is the oxidation number on the sulfur atom of the sulfite ion, SO_3^{2-}?
(A) +2
(B) +4
(C) +6
(D) +8

(C) The problem can be solved by recognizing that the sum of the oxidation numbers is equal to the charge on the polyatomic ion. This means that one sulfur atom plus four oxygen atoms add up to –2. Oxygen has an oxidation number of –2 in all cases except peroxides, where it is –1, and in O_2, where it is 0, like in all elements in their natural states.

$$S + 4(O) = -2$$
$$S + 4(-2) = -2$$
$$S - 8 = -2$$
$$S = +6$$

Failing to take into account the fact that the ion has a –2 charge would lead to the +8 answer.

To identify **oxidizing and reducing agents** in a chemical equation, it is necessary to determine which atoms have undergone oxidation and reduction. In the unbalanced example

$$Mn^{+2} + Br_2 \rightarrow MnO_4^{-1} + Br^{-1}$$

the oxidation numbers are as follows:

Mn on the reactants side = +2	Mn on the products side = +7
Br on the reactants side = 0	Br on the products side = –1

Mn was oxidized (from +2 to +7) and because the net increase was +5 (each Mn atom lost 5 electrons).

Br was reduced (from 0 to –1) and each Br atom gained 1 electron.

The oxidizing agent was Br_2 and the reducing agent was Mn^{+2}. Oxidizing and reducing agents are always reactants. A redox reaction does not need to be balanced to identify which atoms are oxidized and reduced and what the oxidizing and reducing agents are.

Once the atoms being oxidized and reduced have been identified, the redox reaction can be balanced. A systematic method such as the half-reaction method is used to balance a redox reaction. The example below shows how this method is applied.

$FeSO_4 + KMnO_4 + H_2SO_4 \rightarrow Fe_2(SO_4)_3 + MnSO_4 + H_2O + K_2SO_4$ (in acidic solution due to the sulfuric acid)

The net ionic equation is:

$$5Fe^{+2} + MnO_4^{-1} + 8H^{+1} \rightarrow 5Fe^{+3} + Mn^{+2} + 4H_2O$$

The oxidation number changes are:

$$\text{iron from +2 to +3 = oxidation}$$
$$\text{manganese from +7 to +2 = reduction}$$

All other ions (K^{+1} and SO_4^{-2}) are only spectators and are not needed to balance the equation. In balancing any redox reaction, both atoms and charge must balance.

$Fe^{2+} \rightarrow Fe^{3+}$ (iron is oxidized and each Fe atom loses 1 electron)

$MnO_4^{-1} \rightarrow Mn^{+2}$ (manganese is reduced and each Mn atom gains 5 electrons)

Separate the reaction into an oxidation half-reaction and a reduction half-reaction. Start balancing these half-reactions by identifying the number of electrons gained or lost. In the case of the iron oxidation half-reaction, the atoms are already balanced but the charge is not. To balance charge, add one electron on the right side:

$$Fe^{+2} \rightarrow Fe^{+3} + 1\ e^-$$

As there are no other atoms involved in this half-reaction, it is balanced.

Now balance the permanganate reduction half-reaction. Since Mn was reduced and each Mn atom gained 5 electrons, put $5e^-$ on the left side.

$$5e^- + MnO_4^{-1} \rightarrow Mn^{+2}$$

Then balance oxygen using water. Four water molecules are needed on the right.

$$5e^- + MnO_4^{-1} \rightarrow Mn^{+2} + 4H_2O$$

Then balance hydrogen by adding 8H+ to the left. You can do this because the reaction is taking place in acidic aqueous solution.

$$MnO_4^{-1} + 8H^{+1} + 5e^- \rightarrow Mn^{+2} + 4H_2O$$

Check to make sure that the half-reaction is balanced with respect to atoms and charge (1 Mn, 4 O, 8 H, and a +2 charge on each side).

Now there are two balanced half-reactions. The final step is to add these half-reactions, multiplying them by the appropriate coefficients so that the electrons cancel out. The easiest approach is to use the numbers of electrons in each half-reaction, which often results in finding the least common multiple of the number of electrons gained and lost so that the number of electrons gained equals the number of electrons lost. To have five electrons in both equations, multiply the first equation by 5:

$$5Fe^{+2} \rightarrow 5Fe^{+3} + 5e^-$$

and add both half-reactions to get

$$MnO_4^{-1} + 8H^{+1} + 5Fe^{+2} + 5e^- \rightarrow Mn^{+2} + 4H_2O + 5Fe^{+3} + 5e^-$$

Cancel out the electrons:

$$MnO_4^{-1} + 8H^{+1} + 5Fe^{+2} \rightarrow Mn^{+2} + 4H_2O + 5Fe^{+3}$$

The reaction is now balanced. Check to make sure that atoms and charges balance. In some cases, water and/or H+ ions may also cancel.

The following example shows how to balance an equation for a reaction in a basic solution.

$$Cr(OH)_3 + ClO_3^{-1} \rightarrow CrO_4^{-2} + Cl^{-1} \text{ (basic solution)}$$

First separate the reaction into two half-reactions and determine the number of electrons gained or lost for each atom that is oxidized or reduced. Cr goes from an oxidation number of +3 to +6, and each Cr atom is oxidized and loses 3 electrons, Cl goes from an oxidation number of +5 to –1, and each Cl atom is reduced and gains 6 electrons.

For the Cr half-reaction, first write the electrons included:

$$Cr(OH)_3 \rightarrow CrO_4^{-2} + 3e^-$$

Then add enough water to balance the oxygen atoms:

$$H_2O + Cr(OH)_3 \rightarrow CrO_4^{-2} + 3e^-$$

Then balance the hydrogen using H+. Even though the reaction takes place in a basic solution, start out as if it were acidic and make an adjustment later on.

$$H_2O + Cr(OH)_3 \rightarrow CrO_4^{-2} + 3e^- + 5H^{+1}$$

This half-reaction is now balanced in terms of both atoms and charge.
Use the same process for the Cl atom:

$$6e^- + 6H^+ + ClO_3^{-1} \rightarrow Cl^- + 3H_2O$$

Before combining the half-reaction, make sure that the electrons will cancel.

Double the first half-reaction and then combine the two:

$$6e^- + 6H^+ + ClO_3^{-1} + 2H_2O + 2Cr(OH)_3 \rightarrow 2CrO_4^{-2} + 6e^- + 10H^{+1} + Cl^- + 3H_2O$$

Cancel the 6 electrons from each side, 6 hydrogen ions from each side, and 2 water molecules on each side to give:

$$ClO_3^{-1} + 2Cr(OH)_3 \rightarrow 2CrO_4^{-2} + 4H^{+1} + Cl^- + H_2O$$

To make the solution basic, add as many OH^- ions as there are H^+ ions to each side, combine the H^+ and OH^- to make water, and then simplify for the water. In this case, add $4OH^-$ to each side:

$$\frac{ClO_3^{-1} + 2Cr(OH)_3 \rightarrow 2CrO_4^{-2} + 4H^{+1} + Cl^- + H_2O}{4OH^- + ClO_3^{-1} + 2Cr(OH)_3 \rightarrow 2CrO_4^{-2} + \underline{4H_2O} + Cl^- + \underline{H_2O}} \begin{matrix} + 4OH^- \quad\quad\quad\quad + 4OH^- \end{matrix}$$

To give the final answer of:

$$4OH^- + ClO_3^{-1} + 2Cr(OH)_3 \rightarrow 2CrO_4^{-2} + 5H_2O + Cl^-$$

There are other systems for balancing redox reactions, but the half-reaction method is reliable and consistent.

A **disproportionation reaction** is a special type of redox reaction in which the same element is both oxidized and reduced. In the reaction below, the chlorine atoms on the reactants side have an oxidation number of zero, whereas some on the products side have an oxidation number of –1 and others an oxidation number of +5. This means that some chlorine atoms have been oxidized and some reduced.

$$3Cl_2 + 6OH^{-1} \rightarrow 5Cl^{-1} + ClO_3^{-1} + 3H_2O$$
$$\uparrow \quad\quad\quad\quad \uparrow \quad\quad \uparrow$$
$$0 \quad\quad\quad\quad -1 \quad\quad +5$$

TIP

REDOX REACTIONS ON THE MCAT

MCAT questions are more likely to ask you to identify what is oxidized and reduced, and what the oxidizing and reducing agents are, rather than to ask you to balance a redox reaction.

Applications of Stoichiometry and Stoichiometric Calculations

After a reaction has been balanced properly, it is possible to use the ratios of the coefficients to make predictions about the amounts of chemicals that will be involved in a reaction. These amounts can be measured in terms of moles, molecules, grams, or liters. In any balanced equation, the ratio of the coefficients also gives the ratio of moles involved in the reaction.

MOLE–MOLE RATIOS

In the reaction below showing the oxidation of ammonia gas:

$$4NH_3 + 5O_2 \rightarrow 4NO + 6H_2O$$

TIP

CONVERT TO MOLES

When in doubt, convert to moles.

we can tell that for every 4 moles of ammonia, 5 moles of oxygen will react. There do not need to be exactly 4 moles of ammonia and 5 of oxygen, but they must be in that ratio. If 6 moles of ammonia react, then we could calculate the moles of oxygen as follows:

$$6 \text{ moles } NH_3 \times \frac{5 \text{ moles } O_2}{4 \text{ moles } NH_3} = 7.5 \text{ moles } O_2,$$

where the conversion factor $\frac{5}{4}$ comes from the coefficients of the balanced equation. In this example, 7.5 moles of oxygen would be reacted.

MASS–MASS PROBLEMS

Other useful applications of coefficient ratios (stoichiometric calculations) allow the mass (or volume) of product to be calculated based on a specific amount of reactant.

The equation below represents the combustion of butane gas.

$$2C_4H_{10} + 13O_2 \rightarrow 8CO_2 + 10H_2O$$

What mass of carbon dioxide can be formed from 100.0 grams of butane?

$$100.0 \text{ g C}_4H_{10} \times \frac{1 \text{ mole C}_4H_{10}}{58.0 \text{ g C}_4H_{10}} \times \frac{8 \text{ moles CO}_2}{2 \text{ moles C}_4H_{10}} \times \frac{44.0 \text{ g CO}_2}{1 \text{ mole CO}_2} = 303 \text{ g}$$

In a problem such as this, the units must cancel at each step, so that at the end of the problem, the unit matches the information you are asked to solve for. This is an example of using the factor label method, or dimensional analysis, to solve a problem.

A problem of this type can be solved for any substance, reactant, or product, provided the quantity of at least one chemical in the equation is known.

Practice Question

Given the equation

$$2NaClO_{3(s)} \rightarrow 2NaCl_{(s)} + 3O_{2(g)}$$

what mass of sodium chlorate is needed to produce 1.00L of oxygen gas at STP?

Solution: $1.00 \text{ L O}_2 \times \dfrac{1 \text{ mole O}_2}{22.4 \text{ L O}_2} \times \dfrac{2 \text{ moles NaClO}_3}{3 \text{ moles O}_2} \times \dfrac{106.5 \text{ g NaClO}_3}{1 \text{ mole NaClO}_3} = 3.17 \text{ g NaClO}_3$

TEST QUESTION

In the reaction of propane (molar mass = 44 g/mole) gas with oxygen to produce water vapor and carbon dioxide gas, what mass of water vapor can be produced from 22 grams of propane with excess oxygen?

$$C_3H_{8(g)} + 5O_{2(g)} \rightarrow 3CO_{2(g)} + 4H_2O_{(g)}$$

(A) 9 g

(B) 18 g

(C) 36 g

(D) 72 g

(C) A mass of 22 grams of propane is equivalent to 0.5 moles of propane. Note that the molar mass is provided and that the number of moles of propane is "convenient." Patterns such as this are common on the MCAT. Because there are 4 moles of water produced for every 1 mole of propane (from the coefficient ratio), there are 2 moles of water produced. The molar mass of water is 18 grams, making the correct answer 36 grams.

TITRATIONS

TIP

COMPLETION OF TITRATION

When the number of moles is the same for each reactant, the titration is complete.

A **titration** is a quantitative method of determining the concentration of an unknown solution by its reaction with a solution of known concentration. Two of the most common types of titrations are acid–base titrations (discussed later) and redox titrations. In most titrations, measured volumes of solutions are delivered into a reaction flask using a burette and the reaction proceeds until the specific indicator for the reaction undergoes a color change, which signals that the endpoint of the titration is reached. By knowing the volumes of solutions that reacted accurately, and by having one of the reactants in a solution of known concentration, it is possible to calculate the concentration of another reactant in that solution.

A typical example involves the reaction of purple permanganate ion solution with Fe^{+2} ions. When a stoichiometric ratio of permanganate ions has reacted, the solution goes from colorless to purple and endpoint has been reached. The balanced reaction is:

$$5Fe^{+2} + MnO_4^{-1} + 8H^{+1} \rightarrow Mn^{+2} + 5Fe^{+3} + 4H_2O$$

Practice Question

In an experiment, 38.65 ml of 0.265 M $KMnO_4$ solution reacted with 18.78 ml of Fe^{+2} solution. What was the molarity of the iron(II) ion in solution?

Solution: M = moles solute/L solution; therefore, the number of moles of MnO_4^{-1} that reacted are (0.265 moles/L)(0.03865 L) = 0.0102 moles MnO_4^{-1}.

The moles of Fe^{+2} can be found by using the stoichiometric ratio

$$0.0102 \text{ moles } MnO_4^{-1} \times \frac{5 \text{ moles } Fe^{+2}}{1 \text{ mole } MnO_4^-} = 0.0510 \text{ moles } Fe^{+2}$$

The concentration of Fe^{+2} is 0.0510 moles Fe^{+2}/0.01878 L = 2.72 M

You could also find the number of grams of iron in the sample as 0.0510 moles:

$$0.0510 \text{ moles } Fe^{+2} \times 55.8 \text{ g}/1 \text{ mole Fe} = 2.85 \text{ g } Fe^{+2}$$

LIMITING REAGENTS (OR LIMITING REACTANT)

TIP

RECOGNIZE A LIMITING REAGENT PROBLEM

Whenever the starting quantities of two reactants are given, that's a clue that the question will ask for the limiting reagent.

A balanced chemical equation shows the ratios in which substances react, but chemicals are not always present in those exact rations. This is analogous to making a simple sandwich, in which the "recipe" is two slices of bread for every slice of cheese. If the bread and cheese slices are in a ratio other than 2:1, then one starting material will run out first and it will not be possible to continue making sandwiches. Whichever starting material runs out in a chemical reaction is said to be the **limiting reagent**. Those chemicals that remain after the limiting reagent has been used up are said to be excess.

Practice Question

The synthesis of ammonia uses the Haber Process:

$$3H_2 + N_2 \rightarrow 2NH_3$$

If 20 grams of hydrogen react with 56 grams of nitrogen, what is the limiting reagent and how many grams of ammonia can be produced?

Solution: First convert grams of each reactant to moles:

$$56 \text{ grams of } N_2 = 2 \text{ moles of } N_2$$
$$20 \text{ grams of } H_2 = 10 \text{ moles of } H_2$$

Because hydrogen reacts with nitrogen in a 3:1 mole ratio, there have to be at least 3 times as many moles of hydrogen as nitrogen. In this case, there are 5 times as many moles of hydrogen. This makes nitrogen the limiting reagent. The 2 moles of nitrogen will react with 6 moles of hydrogen so that 4 moles of unreacted (excess) hydrogen will remain.

Two moles of nitrogen will produce 4 moles of ammonia, which is equivalent to 68 grams. The limiting reagent always determines the amount of product formed.

PERCENT YIELD

When calculating the amounts of substances in a chemical reaction, the yield is assumed to be 100%. This is, theoretically, the maximum amount of product that could be made from the reactant amounts given. In reality, less than the theoretical amount is formed and this amount is known as the actual yield. The ratio of the actual yield compared to the theoretical yield is called the percent yield, as is calculated by the formula:

$$\frac{\text{actual yield}}{\text{theoretical yield}} \times 100 = \% \text{ yield}$$

COEFFICIENTS AND RATIOS

Chemical reactions are always about mole ratios. If given grams, convert to moles. If asked for grams or liters, get moles first.

Practice Question

In the reaction $2NaClO_3 \rightarrow 2NaCl + 3O_2$, 50.0 grams of sodium chlorate react and 10.0 grams of oxygen gas are produced. What is the percent yield of the reaction?

Solution: First calculate the amount of oxygen gas expected from the reaction of 50.0 grams of $NaClO_3$.

$$50.0 \text{ g NaClO}_3 \times \frac{1 \text{ mole NaClO}_3}{106.5 \text{ g NaClO}_3} \times \frac{3 \text{ moles O}_2}{2 \text{ moles NaClO}_3} \times \frac{32.0 \text{ g O}_2}{1 \text{ mole O}_2} = 22.54 \text{ g O}_2$$

The percent yield is $\dfrac{10.0 \text{ g}}{22.54 \text{ g}} = 0.4436 \times 100 = 44.4\%$

If you know the percent yield with which a reaction takes place, you can use that to calculate the actual yield you will obtain from a given amount of reactants.

THERMOCHEMISTRY AND THERMODYNAMICS

Almost every chemical or physical process involves energy. The different forms of energy (heat, mechanical, chemical, potential, and kinetic) are interconvertible, and our ability to measure these forms of energy allows us to systematically study energy-related processes. Changes in energy can be used to predict which processes will happen naturally and how easily they can be made to take place.

HEAT AND TEMPERATURE

Temperature: average kinetic energy of a set of molecules

Heat: total thermal energy

Heat transfer is due to temperature differences.

Thermochemistry: Energy Changes in Chemical Reactions

Thermochemistry is the study of the heat changes involved in chemical reactions. Heat is a form of energy that can be transferred from one chemical system to another. This transfer occurs without the input of work, when heat spontaneously moves from a higher-temperature system to a lower-temperature system.

THERMODYNAMIC SYSTEMS AND STATE FUNCTIONS

A **system** is the particular part of the universe under study. Everything outside of the system is considered the **surroundings.** A system may be as small as a beaker with a chemical reaction taking place in it, or as large as a solar system.

When discussing heat and a system, if heat is absorbed (gained) by the system, then the heat change for the system is considered to be positive and the process is described as **endothermic**. The release of heat from a system is an **exothermic** process. This is demonstrated in Figure 1.68.

In an exothermic reaction, heat flows from the system to the surroundings.

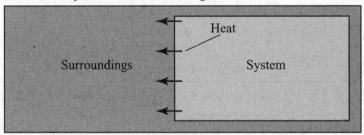

In an endothermic reaction, heat flows from the surroundings to the system.

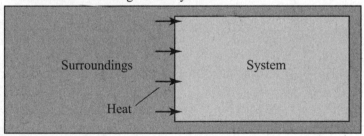

Figure 1.68. System and surroundings

A system may be isolated, in which case it undergoes no transfer of heat with its surroundings. This would be the case in a "perfect" thermos that keeps the temperature constant. A closed system can exchange heat with the surroundings but cannot exchange matter. An open system can exchange both heat and matter with the surroundings. Isothermal processes happen at a constant temperature and isobaric processes take place at a constant pressure.

A **state function** depends only on the current conditions of a system and not on how those conditions were reached (or the path used). State functions have the advantage of being easy to measure. Because very often we are interested in the changes a state function undergoes, we need to know only the initial and final states. It is not necessary to know anything about the conditions that may occur between the initial and final states.

CONSERVATION OF ENERGY AND UNITS OF ENERGY

The **law of conservation of energy** states that energy is neither created nor destroyed, but that it can be converted from one form to another. Scientists have developed many tools for measuring heat energy. In many thermochemical studies in which the energy of the system is converted into heat, energy changes are easily measured. The SI unit of energy is the joule (J), which is equal to $1 \ kg \cdot m^2/s^2$ or $1 \ N \cdot m$. This is also the unit of work (a force times a distance). All forms of energy (kinetic, potential, and electrical) have the same units. The unit calorie is also commonly used in heat measurements and calculations. One calorie is equal to 4.18 joules. The units kcal and kJ are often used as well.

ENDOTHERMIC AND EXOTHERMIC REACTIONS

An endothermic process is one in which heat is gained or absorbed by an object, whereas an exothermic process is one in which a system or object releases heat. An endothermic change is defined as having a positive change in heat energy, whereas an exothermic change is defined as a negative one. If you hold an ice cube in your hand, heat flows from your hand to the ice cube. The ice cube will absorb heat (endothermic for the ice cube) and your hand will lose or release heat (exothermic for your hand). Because energy is not created or destroyed, every time one part of the universe gains energy, some other part of the universe must have lost or released energy.

ENTHALPY

The most useful state function in the study of thermochemistry is **enthalpy**, which is the heat content of a system at a constant pressure. Enthalpy is symbolized as H and the change in the enthalpy of a system at constant pressure (such as in most aqueous processes) is symbolized by ΔH. Because enthalpy is a state function, in order to determine ΔH_{rxn} (the enthalpy change for a reaction), it is only necessary to know the initial and final states of the system. It is not necessary to know the path taken.

$$\Delta H_{rxn} = \Sigma \Delta H_{products} - \Sigma \Delta H_{reactants}$$

A positive value of ΔH indicates an endothermic process, whereas a negative value of ΔH indicates an exothermic process.

Standard Heats of Formation

One way to determine ΔH of a reaction is to use data tables that provide values of the standard enthalpies of formation of chemical compounds. These data tables have been constructed based on experimental data and allow ΔH calculations for processes that may be impractical to perform in lab settings because of cost or safety. This standard enthalpy of formation is abbreviated $\Delta H°_f$. The value of $\Delta H°_f$ for any pure element in its natural state is zero. An abbreviated table of $\Delta H°_f$ values is shown below, along with a sample calculation for $\Delta H°_{rxn}$.

TIP

THE $\Delta H°_F$ OF AN ELEMENT

The standard heat of formation of any element in its natural state is 0.

HEAT OF REACTION

For the combustion of propane, C_3H_8, the balanced chemical equation is

$$C_3H_{8(g)} + 5O_{2(g)} \rightarrow 3CO_{2(g)} + 4H_2O_{(g)}$$

The data for $\Delta H°_f$ for the compounds involved in the reaction are shown in Table 1.13. They would typically be provided in a larger data table with other thermodynamic properties.

Table 1.13 Heats of Formation of Some Substances

Substance	$\Delta H°_f$ (kJ/mole)
$C_3H_{8(g)}$	−101
$O_{2(g)}$	0
$CO_{2(g)}$	−393.5
$H_2O_{(g)}$	−242

Enthalpy is a state function; thus, one need only know the enthalpy of the products and the enthalpy of the reactants. The change or difference will be $\Delta H°_{rxn}$.

The total enthalpy of the products is

$$(3 \text{ moles})(-393.5 \text{ kJ/mole}) + (4 \text{ moles})(-242 \text{ kJ/mole}) = -2148 \text{ kJ}$$

The total enthalpy of the reactants is

$$(1 \text{ mole})(-101 \text{ kJ/mole}) + (5 \text{ moles})(0 \text{ kJ/mole}) = -101 \text{ kJ}$$

$\Delta H°_{rxn} = \Sigma \Delta H_{products} - \Sigma \Delta H_{reactants} = -2148 \text{ kJ} - (-101 \text{ kJ}) = -2047 \text{ kJ}$ per mole of propane combusted.

Use the following data table to calculate $\Delta H°_f$ for the reaction:

$$2\ C_4H_{10(g)} + 13\ O_{2(g)} \rightarrow 8\ CO_{2(g)} + 10\ H_2O_{(g)}$$

Substance	$\Delta H°_f$ (kJ/mole)
C_4H_{10}	–126
O_2	0
CO_2	–393.5
H_2O	–242

(A) +5316 kJ

(B) –5316 kJ

(C) +509.5 kJ

(D) –509.5 kJ

(B) Use the formula: $\Delta H_{rxn} = \Sigma\ \Delta H°_{products} - \Sigma\ \Delta H°_{reactants}$

8 moles [(–393.5 kJ/mole) + 10 moles (–242 kJ/mole)] – [2 moles (–126 kJ/mole) + 0)]
$$= –5316\ kJ$$

Choice A is the answer one would obtain if instead of doing the calculation as $\Delta H_{rxn} = \Sigma\ \Delta H°_{products} - \Sigma\ \Delta H°_{reactants}$ it had been done in reverse. Choices C and D are the answers one might obtain by not taking the coefficients into account.

A thermochemical equation is really a balanced chemical equation with an additional term that shows the change in heat. Just as there are ratios between moles of chemicals in a reaction, there are also ratios between the amount of heat absorbed or released by a reaction and the amounts of chemicals.

The formation of ammonia from hydrogen and nitrogen is an exothermic process that releases 92 kJ of heat energy. This can be written in two ways:

$$3H_2 + N_2 \rightarrow 2NH_3 + 92\ kJ$$
$$\text{or}$$
$$3H_2 + N_2 \rightarrow 2NH_3\ \Delta H = –92\ kJ$$

Each of these thermochemical equations tells us that for the formation of two moles of ammonia, there will be 92 kJ of heat energy released. The equations show that if 4 moles of ammonia were formed, 184 kJ of energy would be released, and if 20 moles of ammonia were formed, 920 kJ of energy would be released.

This information can be applied in concert with stoichiometric ratios as shown in the following example:

$$2NH_3 \rightarrow 3H_2 + N_2$$
$$\Delta H = +92\ kJ$$

The equation is said to have reversed, or "flipped," meaning it was multiplied by –1.

TIP

INTERPRETING HEAT IN A REACTION

These two equations are saying the same thing in slightly different ways. One is saying that 92 kJ of heat are released and the other that 92 kJ are produced.

A further extension of this would let us calculate the enthalpy change for the reaction

$$6NH_3 \rightarrow 9H_2 + 3N_2$$

as +276 kJ, which is the original reaction reversed and multiplied by 3.

HESS'S LAW OF HEAT SUMMATION

Hess's law states that the enthalpies of chemical reactions can be added to give enthalpies for new reactions. This is true because enthalpy is a state function. The most common application of Hess's law is the calculation of one reaction's enthalpy change based on the enthalpy changes of the other reactions that are given.

Practice Question

The enthalpy change for the reaction W(s) + C(s, graphite) → WC(s) is difficult to measure in a lab setting. Use the data below to determine the heat of reaction for the formation of tungsten carbide.

1. $2W_{(s)} + 3O_{2(g)} \rightarrow 2WO_{3(s)}$ $\Delta H = -1680$ kJ

2. $C_{(graphite)} + O_{2(g)} \rightarrow CO_{2(g)}$ $\Delta H = -394$ kJ

3. $2WC_{(s)} + 5O_{2(g)} \rightarrow 2WO_{3(s)} + 2CO_{2(g)}$ $\Delta H = -2392$ kJ

Solution: We multiply equation 1 by ½ to get:

$$W_{(s)} + \frac{3}{2} O_{2(g)} \rightarrow WO_{3(s)} \quad \Delta H = -840 \text{ kJ}$$

We leave equation 2 as is:

$$C_{(graphite)} + O_{2(g)} \rightarrow CO_{2(g)} \quad \Delta H = -394 \text{ kJ}$$

Reverse and halve equation 3:

$$WO_{3(s)} + CO_{2(g)} \rightarrow WC_{(s)} + \frac{5}{2} O_{2(g)} \quad \Delta H = +1196 \text{ kJ}$$

Adding them all gives:

$$W_{(s)} + C_{(graphite)} \rightarrow WC_{(s)} \quad \Delta H = -38 \text{ kJ}$$

BOND ENERGY AND CHEMICAL REACTIONS

Another way to determine the energy change involved in a chemical reaction is to use data tables of bond energies. **Bond energy** is the average amount of energy required to break one mole of a specific bond type in the gas phase. Energy is required (an endothermic process for the chemical bond) to break a bond. This means that bond energies are positive. Many types of bond energies have been measured and they are readily available in data tables. Bond energies can be used to estimate the energy changes in chemical reactions. For any chemical reaction:

$$\Delta H_{rxn} = \text{Total } \Delta H \text{ of bonds broken} - \text{Total } \Delta H \text{ of bonds formed}$$

Consider the balanced equation below:

$$H_{2(g)} + Cl_{2(g)} \rightarrow 2HCl_{(g)}$$

Figure 1.69 shows that the H–H bond and the Cl–Cl bond are being broken and that two H–Cl bonds are then formed.

$$H_{2(g)} + Cl_{2(g)} \rightarrow 2HCl_{(g)}$$

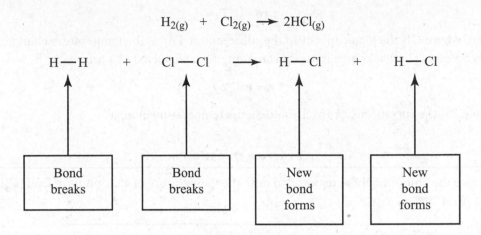

Figure 1.69. Breaking and forming bonds in a chemical reaction

The energies of these bonds are shown in Table 1.14.

Table 1.14 Sample Bond Energies

Bond	Energy (kJ/mole)
H–H	432
Cl–Cl	240
H–Cl	428

Calculate the energy change based on bond energies as follows:

(energy required to break an H–H bond + energy required to break a Cl–Cl bond)
– 2(energy required to form 2 H–Cl bonds) = (432 + 240) – (2 × 428) = –184 kJ

The reaction is exothermic.

Bond energies are based on average values and may vary slightly in specific molecules, but the calculation gives results that are in agreement with data from experiments involving heat changes in reactions.

CALORIMETRY AND MEASUREMENT OF HEAT CHANGES IN REACTIONS

A **calorimeter** is a device used to measure temperature changes in the surroundings during a chemical reaction. A simple calorimeter can be made out of nested Styrofoam coffee cups, because, for a short time period, they minimize the amount of heat exchanged between the reaction system and the surroundings. A calorimeter is treated as a thermally isolated system. For a reaction taking place in a calorimeter, one can say that the heat change for the chemicals involved, plus the calorimeter itself, plus any heat changes in the water if the reaction is aqueous, all add up to zero (that is, the system is thermally isolated). The symbol q is used for heat.

The heat capacity of a substance is the amount of heat required to raise the temperature of that substance by 1°C. The specific heat capacity is the amount of heat required to raise the temperature of 1 gram of a substance by 1°C.

When dealing with an object with a known heat capacity but an unknown mass, the equation

$$q = C\Delta T$$

is used, where C is the heat capacity of the substance and ΔT is the temperature change.

For an object with a known mass, the amount of heat involved in a process is

$$q = mC_p\Delta T$$

where C_p is the specific heat capacity and ΔT the temperature change.

Practice Question

Calculate the amount of heat required to raise the temperature of 45.6 grams of lead (C_p 0.14 J/g°C) from 20°C to 95°C.

Solution: $q = mC_p\Delta T$, so that $q = (45.6 \text{ g})(.14 \text{ J/g°C})(75°C) = 479$ J

Practice Question

When 12.1 grams of NaOH are dissolved in 50.0 grams of water in a calorimeter, the temperature of the water rises by 17°C. The specific heat capacity of water is 4.18 J/g°C and the heat capacity of the calorimeter is 145 J/°C. Find the heat of solution of NaOH per gram and per mole.

Solution: Treat the calorimeter and the water and the NaOH as an isolated system so that

$$q_{cal} + q_{H_2O} + q_{NaOH} = 0$$
$$(145 \text{ J/°C})(17°C) + (50.0 \text{ g})(4.18 \text{ J/g°C})(17°C) + q_{NaOH} = 0$$

Notice that the energy changes for the calorimeter and the water are both positive (endothermic) so that the energy change for the NaOH is exothermic.

$$q_{NaOH} = -6018 \text{ J}$$

so

$$\Delta H = -6018 \text{ J}/12.1 \text{ g}$$
$$= -497 \text{ J/g or } -497 \text{ J/g} \times 40 \text{ g/mole}$$
$$= -20 \text{ kJ}$$

Both the water and the calorimeter rose by 17°C.

A **bomb calorimeter** is a device used to measure the **heat of combustion** of a compound, typically a fuel. A typical bomb calorimeter is shown in Figure 1.70.

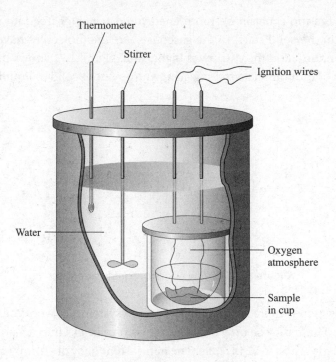

Figure 1.70. A bomb calorimeter

Practice Question

35.0 grams of benzene, C_6H_6 (molar mass = 78 g/mole), are ignited in a bomb calorimeter. The temperature of the calorimeter and its contents rises from 23.00°C to 30.17°C. The calorimeter has a heat capacity of 11.9 kJ/°C. Find the molar heat of combustion of benzene.

Solution:

$$q_{cal} + q_{benzene} = 0$$

$$(11.9 \text{ kJ/°C})(13.17°C) + q_{benzene} = 0, \text{ where } q_{benzene} = -157 \text{ kJ}$$

To get the molar heat of combustion: $\dfrac{-157 \text{ kJ}}{35.0 \text{ g}} \times \dfrac{78.0 \text{ g}}{1 \text{ mole}} = -350 \text{ kJ/mole}$

ENTROPY

Another feature of energy changes in chemical processes is entropy. **Entropy** is a measure of the disorder of a system. Another way to think of entropy is as the tendency of nature to disperse energy. The natural tendency of the universe is for entropy to increase, going from more organized to less organized. Entropy is a state function, so to calculate changes in entropy, only the final and initial states are needed.

$$\Delta S = S_{products} - S_{reactants}$$

At any given temperature, the entropy of a solid substance will be less than the entropy of the same substance as a liquid, which in turn will be less than the entropy of the substance in the gas state. In a solid, the particles are highly organized, as in a crystalline array. As more energy is added, the molecules have more energy and a greater freedom of motion in the liquid state than in the solid state. In the gaseous state, the molecules have almost no constraints on their motion and the entropy is higher still. Figure 1.71 shows how the organization and freedom of motion relate to increasing entropy from solid to liquid to gas.

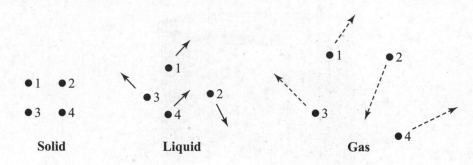

Figure 1.71. Entropy of solids, liquids, and gases

A disordered system is more likely than an ordered system, so over time, the entropy of a system increases. There may be only one way to organize bricks into a stable wall, but there are multiple ways for bricks to be in a pile. The natural tendency of entropy to increase can be overcome by the application of work to a system. A chemical system will be at its maximum entropy when it has reached equilibrium, its state of minimum energy.

The concept of entropy explains why, when two objects of different temperatures are placed in contact with each other, heat always goes from the hotter one to the colder one. This is nature's way of dispersing energy, rather than concentrating it.

Within the same state of matter, it is true that (1) larger molecules have greater entropy than smaller molecules, (2) larger collections of molecules have greater entropy than smaller collections of molecules, and (3) hotter molecules have greater entropy than cooler molecules. In a chemical reaction, clear signs that the entropy has increased include one or more of the following: (1) an increase in the number of moles of gas, (2) reactions in which decomposition has taken place, or (3) solids dissolving. For example, the reaction

$$NH_{3(g)} + HCl_{(g)} \rightarrow NH_4Cl_{(s)}$$

is a reaction with a negative change in entropy because gases are turning into a solid and solids have lower entropies than gases.

TIP

ENTROPY AND ARRANGEMENTS

The more ways that atoms or molecules can be arranged, the greater the entropy of the system.

TIP

INCREASING AND DECREASING ENTROPY

Entropy *increases* when the number of moles of gas increases.

Entropy *decreases* when the number of moles of gas decreases and when precipitates form.

This is a very important MCAT concept!

TEST QUESTION

Which of the following changes would involve an increase in entropy?

(A) $CO_{2(g)} \rightarrow CO_{2(l)}$

(B) $NH_{3(g)} + HCl_{(g)} \rightarrow NH_4Cl_{(s)}$

(C) $Pb^{+2}_{(aq)} + 2I^-_{(aq)} \rightarrow PbI_{2(s)}$

(D) $H_2O_{(l)} \rightarrow H_2O_{(g)}$

(D) Gases have much higher molar entropies than liquids or solids, so any process in which the number of moles of gas increases will exhibit an increase in entropy. Choices A and B show the opposite occurring. Choice C has ions combining to form a precipitate, also a decrease in entropy.

GIBBS FREE ENERGY

There are two main trends in chemical processes:

1. The tendency for energy to be minimized. The vast majority of chemical reactions are exothermic.

2. The tendency for entropy to be maximized.

Gibbs free energy (also known as Gibbs energy), G, is a state function that combines these two factors into a single function of great utility in thermodynamics.

$$\Delta G = \Delta H - T\Delta S$$

A small correction needs to be made to the equation if the temperature or the pressure is not constant but as a general guideline, the equation is always useful on the MCAT. Gibbs free energy represents the maximum amount of work that a system can do. The word *free* means available and does not refer to cost.

The most useful application of the Gibbs free energy equation is to predict the spontaneity of a chemical reaction. In thermodynamics, **spontaneous reactions** refer to processes that will take place without the addition of energy to the system. The phrase does not describe the rate or speed of the process. Examples of spontaneous processes include a ball rolling down a hill, food coloring mixing in water, and a hot object cooling when placed in a cold environment. The reverse of all of these processes can happen but requires the input of energy (pushing a ball up a hill, for example).

It is only the function ΔG that determines if a reaction is spontaneous. When information is available only about the value (or the sign) of ΔH or ΔS, the terms *favorable* and *unfavorable* are used. Negative values for ΔH are favorable, whereas positive values for ΔS are favorable.

Table 1.15 shows the possible signs of ΔH and ΔS and how they combine to give possible signs of ΔG, and thus indicate a reaction's spontaneity. Because the equation uses absolute (kelvin) temperature, T must be positive, so the $T\Delta S$ term has the same sign as ΔS.

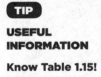

FAVORABLE VS. SPONTANEOUS

Negative energy changes and positive entropy changes are favorable, but it is the sign of ΔG that determines if a reaction is spontaneous.

Table 1.15 ΔG, ΔS, ΔH, and Spontaneity

	ΔG	ΔH	ΔS
Case 1	Always – and spontaneous	– (favorable)	+ (favorable)
Case 2	Depends on T	– (favorable)	– (unfavorable)
Case 3	Depends on T	+ (unfavorable)	+ (favorable)
Case 4	Always + and nonspontaneous	+ (unfavorable)	– (unfavorable)

USEFUL INFORMATION

Know Table 1.15!

Notice that when both the ΔH and ΔS terms are favorable, the reaction is spontaneous no matter what the temperature.

In the case of the two combinations in Table 1.15 for which one term is favorable and the other is not, the temperature determines which term matters more. The **effect of temperature on spontaneity** is such that the higher the temperature, the more the ΔS term matters because the ΔS term is multiplied by a larger number. Likewise, the lower the temperature, the greater the importance of the ΔH term, as the entropy term is multiplied by a smaller number. This means that in Case 2 in Table 1.15, at higher temperatures the unfavorable entropy terms become more important and the reaction becomes less spontaneous. In Case 3, at higher temperatures the favorable entropy terms become more significant and the reaction becomes more spontaneous.

Thermodynamics

Thermodynamics is the study of the motion of heat through the universe. Even though much of chemistry describes both microscopic and macroscopic properties of matter and energy, the science of thermodynamics is a macroscopic way of describing properties of systems and their surroundings. The laws of thermodynamics are based on mathematical descriptions of observations made over many decades.

ZEROTH LAW OF THERMODYNAMICS AND TEMPERATURE

The Zeroth law of thermodynamics is so called because it is considered fundamental to the study of heat, yet it was not established as a formal law until after the other laws of thermodynamics were discovered and explained. The Zeroth law states that two objects in thermal equilibrium (at the same temperature) must share a common state function, which is what we call temperature (see Figure 1.72).

> ### SPONTANEOUS PROCESSES
>
> The word *spontaneous* in a thermodynamic sense has nothing to do with speed. The speed of a reaction is the realm of kinetics, not thermodynamics. Iron rusting is a slow process but it is spontaneous. Thermodynamics tells what processes can happen, not how fast they can happen.

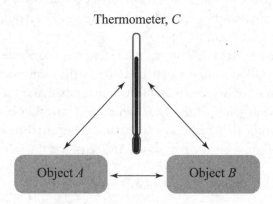

Figure 1.72. The Zeroth law of thermodynamics

Temperature is defined as the average kinetic energy of a group of molecules and is governed by the following equation,

$$KE_{avg} = \frac{3}{2}\, kT$$

where T is the absolute (kelvin) temperature and k is a constant. You can think of temperature as the average thermal energy of molecules, whereas heat is the total thermal energy of molecules. The minimum average kinetic energy of a group of molecules would be zero (in which case every molecule would have exactly the same motion). This is the basis of the kelvin, or absolute, temperature scale.

FIRST LAW OF THERMODYNAMICS

The first law of thermodynamics states that the total energy of the universe is constant. Any change in the energy of a system must be accompanied by a change elsewhere in the universe.

Interconversion of Energy Forms

Although the total energy of the universe must be conserved, the first law does not imply that energy must stay in the same form. One form of energy may be converted into another form, as long as the total energy remains the same. For example, energy stored in chemical bonds in gasoline may be released during a combustion reaction to create heat, which may be used to move a piston, which in turn may make a car move (kinetic energy). This process is demonstrated in Figure 1.73. The electromagnetic energy (light) from the sun may be stored as food energy, which we eat; it is this energy that allows us to do work. In thermodynamics, work and energy are interconvertible. If an object does work, it has less energy and if work is done on an object, the object has a greater energy. Because of this, the first law is often written as:

$$\Delta E = q + W \text{ (for work done on a system) and } \Delta E = q - W \text{ (for work done by a system)}$$

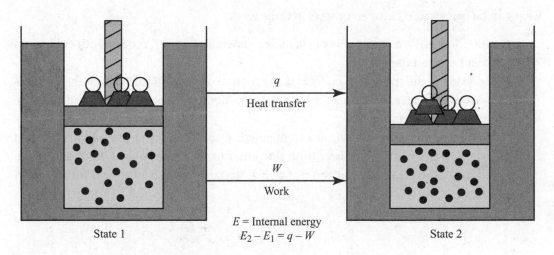

State 1

q
Heat transfer

W
Work

E = Internal energy
$E_2 - E_1 = q - W$

State 2

Figure 1.73. Heat and work

SECOND LAW OF THERMODYNAMICS

The second law of thermodynamics can be stated many ways. The most common statement of the second law is that the entropy of the universe must always increase. In a perfectly reversible process, the entropy of the universe can remain constant, but in the real world all processes lead to an increase in entropy of the universe. Another statement of the second law is that heat will spontaneously flow from a hotter object to a colder one, as shown in Figure 1.74.

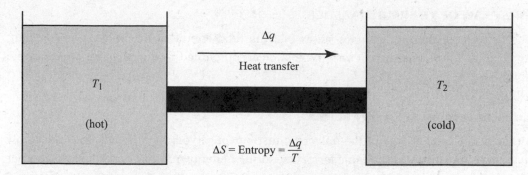

$$\Delta S = \text{Entropy} = \frac{\Delta q}{T}$$

Figure 1.74. The second law of thermodynamics

THIRD LAW OF THERMODYNAMICS

The third law of thermodynamics states that the entropy of a perfect crystal at 0 K would be 0. Absolute zero is not attainable. At absolute zero, the exact location and motion of every particle would be known because there would be no molecular motion of any kind (including vibrations of atoms).

HEAT TRANSFER

Heat can be transferred between objects in three ways:

TIP

HEAT TRANSFER

All heat transfer involves energy going from a hotter to a colder object.

1. **Conduction** is the transfer of heat via molecular collisions, and requires direct physical contact between the objects.
2. **Convection** is the transfer of energy via the motion of fluids (liquids or gases). Convection occurs because of differences in pressure or density. Ocean currents and wind are examples of convection.
3. **Radiation** is energy transfer via electromagnetic waves. Radiation, like all forms of heat transfer, always involves transfer from the hotter to the colder object. Radiation is the only type of heat transfer that can occur in a vacuum, and it is how heat from the sun reaches Earth.

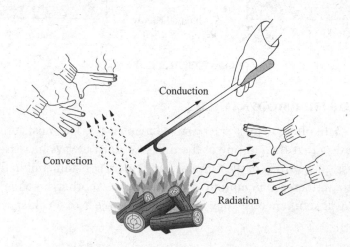

Figure 1.75. Modes of heat transfer

HEAT OF FUSION AND HEAT OF VAPORIZATION

Heat of fusion is the energy change associated with the melting or freezing of a substance. **Heat of vaporization** is the energy change associated with the boiling of a liquid. Heat of fusion and heat of vaporization can be described as energy change per gram or per mole.

Practice Question

30 grams of ice at 0°C was placed in 100 grams of water at 50°C in a calorimeter. Find the final temperature.

Solution: The following processes would take place. For simplicity, ignore any heat absorbed by the calorimeter in this example.

The heat of fusion of ice is 334 J/g. The specific heat capacity of liquid water is 4.18 J/g°C.

1. The ice would melt and the energy involved would be

$$q = (\Delta H_{fus})(m) = (334 \text{ J/g})(30.0 \text{ g}) = +10,020 \text{ J}$$

   (This has a positive value because the ice is absorbing energy from the warmer water.)

2. The ice that melted would warm up from 0°C to the final temperature

$$q = mC_p\Delta T = (30.0 \text{ g})(4.18 \text{ J/g°C})(T - 0°C)$$

   (This is also a positive number because the zero degree melted ice will also absorb water from the warmer water.)

3. The warm water will cool down to the same final temperature that the melted ice warmed up to.

$$q = mC_p\Delta T = (100.0 \text{ g})(4.18 \text{ J/g°C})(T - 50)$$

   (This is an exothermic process because the warm water is cooling down.)

The sum of the processes is zero:

$$q_{melt} \text{ ice} + q_{warm up melted ice} + q_{cool warm water} = 0$$

$$10,020 \text{ J} + (125.4 \text{ J/°C})(T) + (418 \text{ J/°C})(T - 50) = 0$$

A bit of algebra gives the answer as 20°C.

PV DIAGRAMS AND THE CARNOT CYCLE

Thermodynamics deals with work and heat. Work can be defined as a transfer of a form of energy other than heat. In physics, work is typically thought of as moving an object over a distance. The most common kind of work that a chemical system would do is *PV* work, or the expansion of a gas.

In 1824, Sadi Carnot proposed a heat engine that transferred heat from hotter to colder regions and used the energy transfer to do *PV* or expansion work. This was theoretically the most efficient engine possible. A **Carnot cycle** consists of four stages, shown in Figure 1.76.

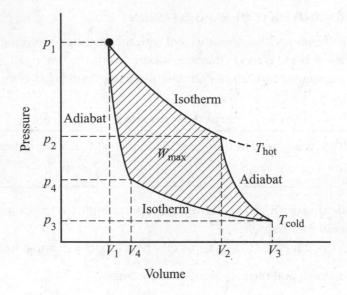

Figure 1.76. Carnot cycle

STEP 1 An isothermal (constant temperature) expansion of the gas at the hotter temperature

STEP 2 An adiabatic (no exchange of heat takes place) cooling as the gas expands and does work

STEP 3 An isothermal compression at the colder temperature

STEP 4 An adiabatic compression back to the original temperature

The total amount of work done is represented by the area bounded by the four curves. Carnot determined that the efficiency of a heat engine depends only on the temperatures of the two heat reservoirs and that the efficiency is

$$\varepsilon = 1 - T_c/T_h$$

This means that the greater the difference between the hot and cold temperatures, the more efficient the heat engine. If the cold reservoir could be made to reach absolute zero, the engine would have perfect (100%) efficiency.

In reality, no such perfectly efficient engine can be made, which is another way of stating the second law of thermodynamics. The heat engine is the basis of a refrigerator, although a refrigerator requires inputting energy to create temperature differences, rather than using temperature differences to perform work. Of course, Carnot's engine ignored friction, which always reduces efficiency.

KINETICS AND EQUILIBRIUM

Chemical **kinetics** is the study of the rates of reactions and the factors that affect these rates. Kinetics also deals with reaction mechanisms, the specific steps that lead to an overall reaction. Kinetics can use complex math, but the MCAT deals with kinetics in a more descriptive way.

Equilibrium is the state in which a reversible chemical reaction shows no net change in the concentration of any chemical species. This is the result of the forward and reverse reaction rates being equal to each other. Because the forward and reverse reactions are both occurring, this is an example of a dynamic process. The study of chemical equilibria helps determine ways in which to maximize the amounts of desired products in a reaction. Chemical equilibria are governed by the laws of thermodynamics.

Kinetics

Kinetics is the study of the rates of chemical reactions, the factors that determine reaction rates, and the mechanisms by which reactions occur.

REACTION RATES AND FACTORS AFFECTING REACTION RATES: COLLISION THEORY

Chemical reactions are the direct result of collisions of molecules. A useful way to think about how different factors affect the rates of reactions is by applying collision theory. **Collision theory** states that in order for a chemical reaction to occur between two (or more) molecules, several things must be true:

1. The molecules must collide with each other.
2. The molecules must collide with the proper orientation to allow a reaction to take place (see Figure 1.77).

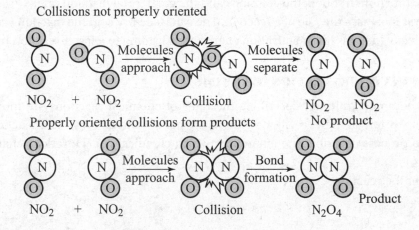

Figure 1.77. Orientation and collisions

3. The molecules must have sufficient energy to begin to break the bonds of the reactants. (See the section on activation energy below.)

Most collisions between molecules do not lead to formation of new substances. A collision that meets all three criteria above is called an **effective collision**.

The reaction rate of molecules is determined by the **effect of temperature**. At higher temperatures, molecules move more rapidly, leading to more collisions. A greater number of collisions leads to a faster reaction rate. Higher temperatures increase reaction rates and lower temperatures decrease rates. At a higher temperature, more molecules have sufficient energy to lead to an effective collision (see Figure 1.78).

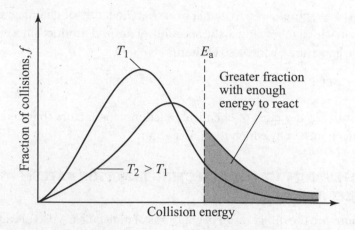

Figure 1.78. Temperature and reaction rates

The reaction rate of molecules is also determined by the **effect of pressure (for gaseous systems)**. At higher pressures, there are a greater number of molecules in a specific volume. More molecules means more collisions, which means that greater pressures increase reaction rates.

The **concentration** of reactants also affects the reaction rate. The greater the number of molecules, the more frequent the collisions and the greater the reaction rate.

A **catalyst** increases the rate of a reaction. The catalyst carries on the reaction via an alternative pathway that has lower activation energy, thus leading to a faster reaction rate.

CHANGES IN CONCENTRATION OVER TIME

The most common units for describing the rates of chemical reactions are moles/L/sec, sometimes written as moles $\cdot$ L^{-1} $\cdot$ s^{-1} (molarity per second or M/s). The reaction rate of a chemical process describes the amount by which chemical concentrations change every second.

Consider the reaction

$$a\text{A} + b\text{B} \rightarrow c\text{C} + d\text{D}$$

It is possible to describe the rate of the reaction in terms of any of the chemicals involved. Typically, the rate of the reaction will be described based on whichever chemical is easiest to measure. For the reaction above, the rate of the reaction can be described as:

$$\text{Reaction rate} = \frac{-1\Delta[\text{A}]}{a\Delta t} = \frac{-1\Delta[\text{B}]}{b\Delta t} = \frac{1\Delta[\text{C}]}{c\Delta t} = \frac{1\Delta[\text{D}]}{d\Delta t}$$

TIP

THE SYMBOL [X]

[X] means molar concentration of X.

where [X] means the molar concentration of chemical X. As the concentrations of reactants decrease over time, there is a negative sign in front of the change in the concentration of each reactant.

In the reaction

$$2\text{C}_4\text{H}_{10} + 13\text{O}_2 \rightarrow 8\text{CO}_2 + 10\text{H}_2\text{O},$$

if the rate of change of the concentration of carbon dioxide were 4.0 M/s, then the rate of change of water production would be 5.0 M/s and the rate of change of butane, C_4H_{10} would be -1.0M/s, with the negative sign indicating that its concentration was decreasing. Figure

1.79 shows how the concentrations of hydrogen (H), iodine (I), and HI would change for the reaction $H_2 + I_2 \rightarrow 2HI$.

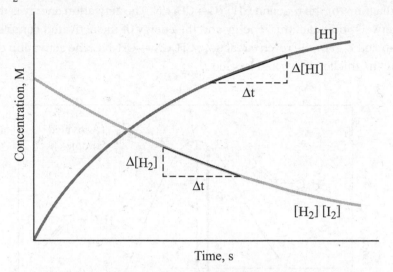

Figure 1.79. Concentrations of chemical species over time

Notice how the concentrations of the reactants, H_2 and I_2, decrease over time and at the same rate (they have the same coefficient) but the concentration of [HI] changes at a rate double that of the reactants.

TIP

CONCENTRATION CHANGES OVER TIME

For a reaction that starts with only reactants, the concentrations of reactants decrease over time and the concentrations of products increase.

TEST QUESTION

Consider the reaction:

$$3H_2 + N_2 \rightarrow 2NH_3$$

At a certain temperature and pressure, the change in the concentration of hydrogen gas is –0.60 M/s. What is the rate of increase in the concentration of ammonia, in M/s, under those same conditions?

(A) –0.40

(B) +0.40

(C) –0.30

(D) +1.20

(B) As the concentration of hydrogen gas is decreasing over time, and because ammonia is a product, it must be increasing in concentration. There are 2 moles of ammonia formed for every 3 moles of hydrogen reacted, so the ammonia is formed at a rate equal to $-\frac{2}{3}$ the rate at which hydrogen is reacted.

In 1889, Svante Arrhenius developed an equation that described the relationship between the rate of a chemical reaction and the temperature. This equation described the **activation energy**, the minimum energy of collision required for bonds to be broken and new substances to be formed. This energy is often thought of as a barrier between the initial energy of the reactants and the energy of an intermediate chemical formed during a reaction, called the **activated complex** or the **transition state**. This energy barrier is typically shown by means of an energy diagram, which shows the changes in the energy of a chemical system as a reaction proceeds from reactants, through the activated complex, to the products. Figure 1.80 shows the energy diagram for the reaction $CH_3NC \rightarrow CH_3CN$. The activation energy is the difference in energy between the reactants' energy and the energy of the activated complex, shown by the arrow labeled E_a. For the reverse reaction, $CH_3CN \rightarrow CH_3NC$, the activation energy would be shown by the thicker arrow and labeled $E_{a,rev}$.

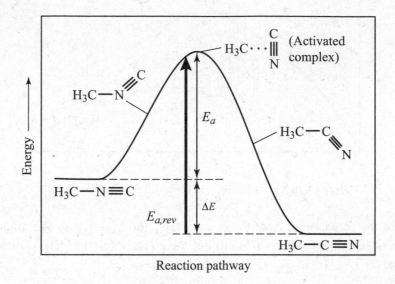

Figure 1.80. Activation energy

Activation energy is always a positive number because it is energy that must be put into a system (often by heating or adding energy in another form). The activation energy can be used to describe an energy barrier for a reaction in either the forward or the reverse direction.

The Arrhenius equation describes how the rate of a chemical reaction is affected by temperature. As the temperature rises, the number of molecules with enough energy to overcome the energy barrier (activation energy) increases, leading to a greater number of collisions and a greater number of effective collisions.

RATE LAWS: CONCENTRATION OF REACTANTS AND RATE LAW DETERMINATIONS BY EXPERIMENT

A **rate law** is a mathematical expression that shows how the rate of a chemical reaction depends on the concentrations of the reactants. A rate law can only be determined by experiment and not by looking at coefficient ratios. For the reaction:

$$A + B + C \rightarrow D$$

The generic rate law will have the form:

$$\text{rate} = k[A]^m[B]^n[C]^p$$

where $[A]$, $[B]$, and $[C]$ represent the concentrations of reactants A, B, and C, and m, n, and p are exponents (or orders) that are to be determined based on experimental data. The rate constant, k, is also determined based on experimental data. In the rate law for any reaction, every reactant must be included. The exponents m, n, and p are called the order of the reaction with respect to each reactant, and the sum of the exponents in the rate law is the overall order of the reaction. Rate law exponents are not the same as reaction coefficients. Rate law exponents are very often 0, 1, or 2, but may be negative or fractional. A sample rate law problem is shown below:

TIP

RATE LAW DETERMINATION

Rate laws can be determined only by experiment. The coefficients have no relationship to the order.

Determining the Rate Law from Experimental Data

In an experimental study of the reaction of acidified hydrogen peroxide and iodide ion to form triiodide ion and water, the following reaction takes place.

$$H_2O_2 + 3I^- + 2\,H^+ \rightarrow I_3^- + 2H_2O$$

A series of kinetic experiments provide the results shown in Table 1.16.

Table 1.16 Typical Data for a Rate Law Problem

Trial #	$[H_2O_2]$ (M)	$[I^-]$ (M)	$[H^+]$ (M)	Rate (M/s)
1	0.05	0.10	0.5	1.1×10^{-2}
2	0.10	0.10	0.5	4.4×10^{-2}
3	0.05	0.20	0.5	2.2×10^{-2}
4	0.05	0.10	1.0	1.1×10^{-2}

The initial rate law can be written as: rate = $k[H_2O_2]^m[I^-]^n[H^+]^p$

To solve for m, n, and p, find a pair of trials in which only one of the concentrations changes, with the others remaining constant. This allows the effect of the concentration of only that particular chemical on the reaction rate to be isolated. For example, in comparing trials 1 and 2, the concentration of hydrogen peroxide doubles, whereas the concentrations of iodide ion and hydrogen ion remain constant. Thus, any change in the reaction rate must be the result of changes in the concentration of hydrogen peroxide. Focusing only on factors that change gives the equation, rate = $[H_2O_2]^m$. Because the rate quadruples and the concentration of hydrogen peroxide doubles, the equation can be rewritten as $4 = 2^m$.

The terms for the other reactants and k do not change from trial 1 to trial 2, so they can be discounted in this calculation. Solving gives $m = 2$, so the order for hydrogen peroxide is 2 (or the reaction is second order with respect to hydrogen peroxide).

To solve for the order of I^-, compare trials 1 and 3 because only the rate and the $[I^-]$ change. Because the rate doubles and the concentration doubles (and k and other concentrations stay constant) $2 = [2]^n$ and $n = 1$, so the reaction's order is 1 for iodide ion. To solve for hydrogen ion, compare trials 1 and 4, where the hydrogen ion concentration doubles and the rate stays constant. This gives $1 = [2]^p$ and $p = 0$. The order of the reaction with respect to hydrogen ion is 0. The overall order of the reaction is 3(2 + 1 + 0). The overall rate law is:

TIP

EXPONENT REVIEW

Remember that $x^0 = 1$

$$\text{rate} = k[H_2O_2]^2[I^-]$$

To **solve for k, the rate constant**, select any trial, substitute in the values for the concentration and the rate, and solve for k.

Use trial 1:

$$1.1 \times 10^{-2} \text{ M/s} = k(0.05 \text{ M})^2(0.1 \text{ M})$$

$$k = \frac{1.1 \times 10^{-2} \text{ M/s}}{(0.05 \text{ M})^2(0.1 \text{ M})} \text{ or } \frac{1.1 \times 10^{-2} \text{ moles L}^{-1}\text{s}^{-1}}{(0.05 \text{ moles L}^{-1})^2(0.1 \text{ moles L}^{-1})}$$

Solving for k gives $k = 44 \text{ M}^{-2}/\text{s}$ or $44 \text{ M}^{-2}\text{s}^{-1}$ or $44 \text{ L}^2\text{moles}^{-2}\text{s}^{-1}$

> ### RATE LAW PROBLEM HINTS
>
> Rate law calculation problems are MCAT classics.
>
> Look for concentrations or rates to double, triple, and quadruple. Be able to predict the effect a change in the concentration of a reactant will have on the reaction rate.

If a reaction has the rate law, rate = $k[\text{H}_2]^2[\text{O}_2]$, then doubling the concentration of hydrogen will quadruple the reaction rate, whereas doubling the concentration of oxygen will double the rate of the reaction.

The value of k, the rate constant, is directly related to the reaction rate in the Arrhenius equation.

Each of the most common types of reaction orders (0, 1, and 2) gives a characteristic graph. For a zero-order reaction, a graph of [reactant] versus time gives a straight line with a slope equal to $[-k]$ (see Figure 1.81).

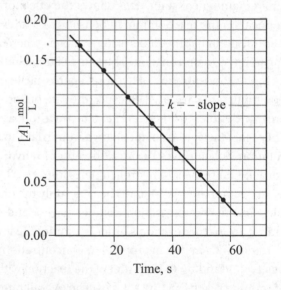

Figure 1.81. A zero-order reaction

For a first-order reaction, a graph of ln [reactant] versus time gives a linear plot with a slope equal to $-k$ (see Figure 1.82).

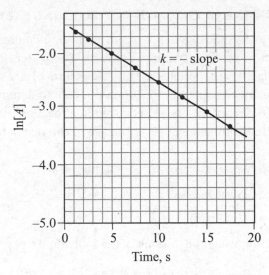

Figure 1.82. A first-order reaction

TIP

FIRST-ORDER REACTIONS

Be especially familiar with first-order reactions. They are important in many processes, such as radioactive decay and growth of bacteria.

For a second-order reaction, a graph of 1/[reactant] versus time gives a linear plot with a slope equal to k (see Figure 1.83).

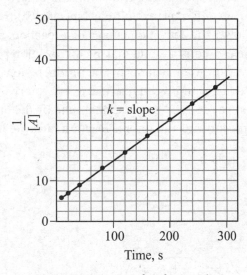

Figure 1.83. A second-order reaction

HALF-LIFE OF A FIRST-ORDER REACTION

For a first-order reaction, it is possible to quickly calculate the concentration of the reactant using the equation:

$$[A]_t = [A]_0 e^{-kt}$$

where $[A]_t$ is the concentration of A at any specific time and $[A]_0$ is the initial concentration of A. The rate constant, k, is the same one that would be calculated from the experimental data, and t is the time. The units of time in k and t must agree with each other. Solving this equation for an amount of A equal to half the original amount gives the relationship between the half-life of a first-order reaction and the rate constant of:

$$t_{1/2} = 0.693/k \text{ or } k = 0.693/t_{1/2}$$

REACTION MECHANISMS AND THE RATE-DETERMINING STEP

A **reaction mechanism** shows the detailed series of steps (or elementary reactions) through which reactants interact to produce the final products. These steps may produce reaction intermediates, chemicals that are produced and then consumed, and which therefore do not appear in the overall balanced equation. It is often possible to determine the relative rates of the individual steps in a reaction. The slowest step in a reaction mechanism is called the **rate-determining** or **rate-limiting** step. It is this stage in the reaction process that dictates the overall reaction rate.

For example, if the two elementary reactions of a process were:

1. $NO_2 + NO_2 \rightarrow NO + NO_3$ (slow step)
2. $NO_3 + CO \rightarrow NO_2 + CO_2$ (fast step)

Then the overall reaction would be the sum of the individual steps:

$$NO_2 + CO \rightarrow NO + CO_2$$

The reaction intermediate would be NO_3 because NO_3 is formed and then used up in the next step. The rate-limiting step would be the first one. The slowest elementary step determines the rate of the reaction.

A **catalyst** is a substance that speeds up a reaction without itself being used up. Catalysts alter the reaction mechanism and often exhibit high specificity for only a small number of reactants. Most catalysts lower the activation energy of a reaction, as shown in Figure 1.84, increasing the value of the rate constant and making the reaction proceed faster. A catalyst does not change the identity of the reactants or the products, nor the relative amounts of products and reactants at equilibrium. A catalyst (that is, enzyme) can be chemically changed during a reaction but must be returned to its original state by the end of the reaction. For a reversible reaction, both the forward and reverse reaction rates are increased.

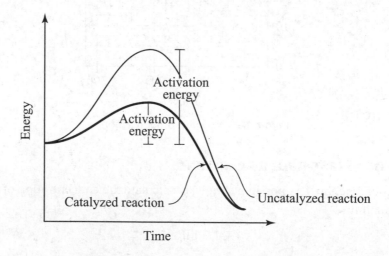

Figure 1.84. Catalytic effect on rate of reaction

A homogeneous catalyst exists in the same phase as the reactants, such as an aqueous acid solution catalyzing the reaction of two or more reactants dissolved in water.

A heterogeneous catalyst exists in a different phase than the reactants. The solid catalytic converter in an automobile exhaust system catalyzes the breakdown of gaseous nitrogen oxides from the engine.

Enzymes are protein catalysts that exhibit high specificity for only a small number of reactants. Most enzymes are proteins and many have the ability to increase the rate of a reaction by a factor of ten thousand to several million. The reactant for which an enzyme has high specificity is known as the substrate. Most enzymes are able to catalyze the reaction of only a single substrate or those with very similar structures. Enzymes act by making molecules adopt the most efficient orientation for reactions.

> **CATALYSTS**
>
> Catalysts don't change the products or the reactants, nor do they change the value of ΔH_{rxn} or ΔG_{rxn}. Catalysts are not consumed in the reactions that they catalyze.

TEST QUESTION

The chemical system below is known to follow second-order kinetics:

$$2 \, NO_2 \rightarrow O_3 + NO \text{ (slow)}$$
$$NO_3 + C \rightarrow NO_2 + CO \text{ (fast)}$$

What is the rate law for the overall reaction?

(A) rate = $k[NO_3][C]$

(B) rate = $k[NO_3]$

(C) rate = $k[NO_2]^2[NO_3]$

(D) rate = $k[NO_2]^2$

(D) The rate-limiting step is the slowest step in a reaction mechanism. It is this step that determines the rate law. The rate law must be based on the first step of the process, giving D as the correct answer. Choice C is a third-order mechanism and is not possible given the information in the problem.

Chemical Equilibrium

In most chemical reactions, we tend to think of starting with reactants and having all of the reactants converted into products. In many chemical systems, once sufficient quantities of products have been formed, it is possible for the reverse reaction to take place. A reaction in which the reactants are not completely converted into products is called a reversible reaction and is an example of an equilibrium system.

CRITERIA FOR EQUILIBRIUM

When a chemical system has reached equilibrium, certain conditions hold true:

1. The rates of the forward and reverse reactions are equal, as shown in Figure 1.85.

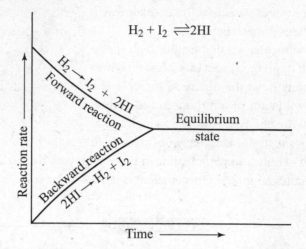

Figure 1.85. Forward and reverse reactions

2. The concentrations of all chemicals become constant, as seen in Figure 1.86. This does not mean, however, that the amounts of the chemicals are equal to each other.

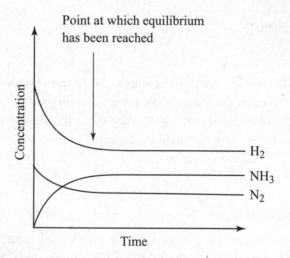

Figure 1.86. Concentrations of chemical species at equilibrium

3. Even though the amounts of all chemicals do not change, both the forward and reverse reactions continue to take place. Because the directions are opposite and the rates are equal, this is an example of a dynamic equilibrium.

DYNAMIC EQUILIBRIUM

A dynamic equilibrium also exists in a covered container of liquid in which the rates of evaporation and condensation are equal. Both processes are still going on, but at equal rates, so the liquid level stays constant.

THE LAW OF MASS ACTION AND EQUILIBRIUM CONSTANTS

For a reversible chemical equilibrium, the system will always reach a state in which the forward and reverse reaction rates are equal. Because the forward reaction rate depends only on the concentrations of the reactants and the reverse reaction rate on the concentrations of the product, it is possible to write a ratio of the two rates ($k_{forward}/k_{reverse}$). As both of these rates are constants, one can create a new constant that is the ratio of the two. This gives a ratio of the concentration of the products over that of the reactants. This is sometimes called the law of mass action.

For a reaction

$$a\text{A} + b\text{B} \leftrightarrow c\text{C} + d\text{D},$$

the law of mass action says that the **equilibrium constant** (K_{eq} or K_c) can be written as

$$K_{eq} = \frac{[C]^c [D]^d}{[A]^a [B]^b} \ .$$

Unlike with reaction rate calculations, the coefficients in this case are used as exponents. The symbol K_{eq} refers to the equilibrium concentrations of the chemicals in the reaction. In some cases the symbol K_c is used to refer to an equilibrium constant based on molar concentrations. An equilibrium constant can also be written in terms of the partial pressures of gaseous reactants or products, in which case the symbol K_p is used. In all cases, the numerical value of the equilibrium constant depends on temperature.

Two points should be kept in mind when working with equilibrium constants:

1. The ratio is always the concentration of each product raised to the power of its coefficient, divided by each reactant's concentration raised to the power of its coefficient.

2. Solids and liquids are not included in equilibrium constant expressions. The concentrations of liquids and solids (pure substances) are constant, so they are incorporated into the equilibrium constant. For the reaction:

$$\text{CaCO}_{3(s)} \leftrightarrow \text{CaO}_{(s)} + \text{CO}_{2(g)}$$

the equilibrium constant expression is $K_{eq} = [\text{CO}_2]$, with the solids being left out.

The **magnitude of K_{eq}** is significant in all equilibrium calculations. Because the ratio is given as products over reactants, a large value for an equilibrium constant ($K_{eq} > 1$) indicates that the equilibrium concentrations of products are greater than those of the reactants.

A small value of K_{eq} ($K_{eq} < 1$) indicates that at equilibrium the reactants predominate. An equilibrium constant value close to 1 indicates that there are roughly equal amounts of products and reactants at equilibrium.

The synthesis of ammonia is carried out via the following reaction:

$$3\text{H}_{2(g)} + \text{N}_{2(g)} \leftrightarrow 2\text{NH}_{3(g)}$$

The equilibrium constant $K_{eq} = \dfrac{[\text{NH}_3]^2}{[\text{H}_2]^3 [\text{N}_2]}$. If the equilibrium concentrations are [H$_2$] = 2.0M, [N$_2$] = 1.0 M, and [NH$_3$] = 6.0 M, then the value of the equilibrium constant would be $[6]^2/[2]^3[1] = 4.5$.

If the value of the equilibrium constant is given, along with some of the concentrations, then it is also possible to solve for the equilibrium concentration of a chemical.

TIP

MAGNITUDE OF THE EQUILIBRIUM CONSTANT

Know how to interpret the magnitude of K_{eq}. The larger the value, the greater the relative amount of products at equilibrium.

Q vs. K_{eq}

A variation of the equilibrium constant is the reaction quotient, Q, which measures the same concentrations but at any point in the reaction, not necessarily at equilibrium. For any reaction system, if $Q = K_{eq}$, then the system is at equilibrium and no further changes in concentrations of reactants or products will take place.

If Q is greater than K_{eq}, then the system has an excess of products relative to the equilibrium amounts, so the reverse reaction will increase in rate, using up products, forming reactants, and bringing the ratio closer to K_{eq}. If Q is less than K_{eq}, then the system has an excess of reactants (or a shortage of products), relative to the equilibrium rations and the forward reaction will take place, using up reactants and forming products. In any equilibrium calculation, all numbers must be positive because there can be no negative concentrations.

LE CHÂTELIER'S PRINCIPLE

TIP

LE CHÂTELIER'S PRINCIPLE

Le Châtelier's principle is applicable in many biological situations and is tested frequently on the MCAT.

A chemical system will reach equilibrium. Once at equilibrium, the concentrations of all chemicals remain constant. **Le Châtelier's principle** describes the changes a system will undergo if some change (referred to as a stress) is made to the equilibrium conditions (such as an increase or decrease in temperature, pressure, or the amount of a chemical). Le Châtelier's principle states that a system at equilibrium, when "stressed," will respond so as to regain equilibrium. Le Châtelier's principle does not work perfectly (there are a few exceptions), but it is a very useful and reliable guideline.

Effects of Changing Concentration

1. If a reactant is added to a system at equilibrium, then there will be an excess of reactants (in a Q vs. K_{eq} example, Q would be too small) so the system will respond with an increase in the forward reaction rate, forming more products and reestablishing the equilibrium ratio. Because the forward reaction is taking place, the response is sometimes referred to as a shift right. If a product is added, the reverse reaction will increase in rate, forming more reactants, or shifting left.

2. If a reactant is removed, the system will need to replace the reactant to reestablish equilibrium, so the reverse reaction will increase in rate (shift left). If a product is removed, the system will form more products by increasing the forward reaction rate (shift right).

TIP

If $Q < K$, the reaction shifts to the right.

If $Q = K$, the reaction is at equilibrium.

If $Q > K$, the reaction shifts to the left.

"SHIFTING" IN LE CHÂTELIER'S PRINCIPLE

Shift left means that the reverse reaction happens at a greater rate, forming more reactants and using up products.

Shift right means that the forward reaction takes place at a greater rate, using up reactants and forming products.

Pressure Changes

An increase in pressure will cause a shift to whichever side of the equilibrium has fewer moles of gas. In the ammonia synthesis reaction:

$$3\,H_{2(g)} + N_{2(g)} \leftrightarrow 2\,NH_{3(g)}$$

an increase in the pressure (often accomplished by decreasing the volume, an application of Boyle's law) will cause a shift to the right, because the product's side has two moles of gas and the reactant's side has four moles of gas. Note that this only applies to moles of gas. Adding an inert gas such as helium has no effect as it does not change the partial pressure of any gas. A decrease in the pressure will cause a shift toward the side with more moles of gas.

Temperature Effects

In applying Le Châtelier's principle, heat is treated as if it were a chemical substance. For example, consider the reaction:

$$2H_2 + O_2 \leftrightarrow H_2O + \text{heat}$$

Raising the temperature causes the system to shift to the left, which means that the reverse reaction increases in rate. Cooling the system would cause the forward reaction to increase in rate.

Le Châtelier's principle predicts the changes in the system when the equilibrium has been disturbed. The response continues only until equilibrium is reestablished.

Catalysts

A catalyst has no effect on the equilibrium of a system. Once a chemical system is at equilibrium, a catalyst has no effect. If a system is not at equilibrium, then because the catalyst lowers the activation energy in both the forward and reverse directions, equilibrium will be established faster.

The following example shows how Le Châtelier's principle might be applied:

$$N_2O_{4(g)} \leftrightarrow 2NO_{2(g)} + \text{heat}$$

Table 1.17 Examples of Le Châtelier's Principle

Stress to System	Response According to Le Châtelier's Principle
Add NO_2	Shift left
Add N_2O_4	Shift right
Remove NO_2	Shift right
Remove N_2O_4	Shift left
Raise temperature	Shift left
Lower temperature	Shift right
Increase pressure (or decrease volume)	Shift left
Decrease pressure (or increase volume)	Shift right
Add helium (or any inert gas)	No effect
Add a catalyst	No effect

Consider the equilibrium system:

$$2NOCl_{(g)} \rightarrow 2NO_{(g)} + Cl_{2(g)} \quad \Delta H = +500 \text{ kJ}$$

Which of the following would increase the equilibrium concentration of NOCl?

  I. raising the temperature

  II. raising the pressure

  III. increasing the concentration of NO

  IV. decreasing the concentration of Cl_2

  (A) I, II, and III only

  (B) II, III, and IV only

  (C) II and III only

  (D) II and IV only

(C) I is incorrect. For an endothermic reaction, raising the temperature increases the forward reaction rate, producing more products. II is correct, as a higher pressure favors the side of the reaction with fewer moles of gas, in this case the reactants. III is correct, as adding NO will shift the equilibrium to the left. The only answer that includes both II and III is C. Note that IV is also incorrect, as removing chlorine will shift the equilibrium to the right, forming more products.

THE EQUILIBRIUM CONSTANT, FREE ENERGY, AND SPONTANEITY

Just as the value of ΔG of a reaction can be used to predict whether a reaction is spontaneous or not, so can the value of the equilibrium constant. K_{eq} and ΔG are related by the following equation:

$$\Delta G = -RT \ln K \quad \text{or} \quad K = e^{-\Delta G/RT}$$

For the MCAT, it is important to know that a negative value of ΔG indicates a value of K_{eq} that is greater than 1 and means that the reaction is spontaneous. This can be summarized as shown in Table 1.18. These relationships are true for standard states (room temperature, 1 atm of pressure, and 1.0 M solutions).

TIP

K_{eq}, **SPONTANEITY, AND** ΔG

Understand the concepts in Table 1.18.

The MCAT will emphasize the concepts rather than actual calculations involving K_{eq} **and** ΔG**.**

Table 1.18 K_{eq}, ΔG, and Spontaneity

K	ΔG	Spontaneous?
< 1	>0	Nonspontaneous
>1	<0	Spontaneous
= 1	= 0	Does not apply

KINETIC AND THERMODYNAMIC CONTROL OF REACTIONS

Kinetics gives the rate of reactions and thermodynamics gives the equilibrium conditions. A reaction whose product formation is governed by the relative energies of the products and reactants is under thermodynamic control. A reaction whose product formation is governed by the activation energies of the possible reactions is under kinetic control. The issue of kinetic versus thermodynamic control arises when there is more than one possible pathway by which reactants can interact. If one possible pathway is significantly faster (because of having a lower activation energy) then that pathway or mechanism will be the one that takes place, even if there is a different mechanism that may be more energetically favorable.

SOLUTION CHEMISTRY

Most chemical reactions in cells take place among dissolved substances. Much of the chemistry of living things is based on ions and molecules whose concentrations are essential to proper cell function.

Solution Terminology

When referring to chemical solutions, it is important to always specify whether you are referring to the entire solution or to one specific component.

SOLUTION, SOLUTE, AND SOLVENT

A **solution** is a homogeneous mixture with a **solute** dissolved in a **solvent**. The most common and biologically important solutions are water-based, or **aqueous**. It is possible for a solution to have any number of solutes dissolved in the solvent. On the MCAT, solution examples consist of a single solute and a single solvent in almost all cases.

Solubility Curves

A solubility curve is a graph that shows the effects of temperature on the solubility of a substance. The graph typically shows the limits of solubility of the solute in 100 grams of solvent (usually water). The graphed line shows the amount of dissolved solute that will produce a saturated solution, one in which no more of that solute can be dissolved. If amount of solute dissolved is below this line,

> **HOMOGENEOUS AND HETEROGENEOUS**
>
> **Homogeneous:** uniform in composition throughout
> **Heterogeneous:** not uniform throughout

the solution would be unsaturated and would be capable of dissolving more of that solute. If the amount of solute dissolved is above the line, the solution would be supersaturated. This happens with only a few substances, typically hydrates, compounds that have water in their crystalline structures.

Figure 1.87 shows solubility curves for sodium chloride, $NaCl$, potassium iodide, KI, and potassium nitrate, KNO_3. A saturated solution of KI would have 180 grams of KI dissolved per 100 grams of water at 30°C. A solution with 120 grams of KI dissolved would be unsaturated and would be capable of dissolving an additional 60 grams of KI.

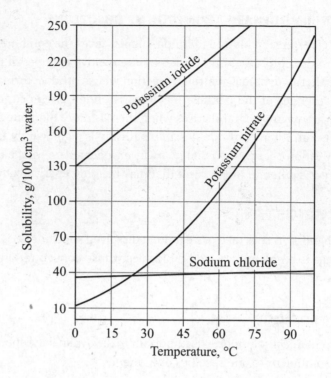

Figure 1.87. Solubility curves of ionic substances

Ions and Solubility Rules

An ion is an atom or a group of atoms with a charge. Cations are positively charged and anions are negatively charged. Ions of a single atom are known as monoatomic ions whereas those of more than one atom are polyatomic ions.

MONOATOMIC IONS

Monoatomic cations are named for the atom they are formed from. Some examples are listed in Table 1.19

Table 1.19 Common Monoatomic Cations

Sodium ion	Na^{+1}
Calcium ion	Ca^{+2}
Magnesium ion	Mg^{+2}
Aluminum ion	Al^{+3}
Potassium ion	K^{+1}

For elements with the capability of forming more than one ion (multivalent elements), a Roman numeral is used to indicate the charge of the ion. For the MCAT, these will include the common transition elements, tin, and lead.

When iron forms a +2 ion, it is called iron(II), and iron(III) is Fe^{+3}.

Monoatomic anions are named with the stem of the element and the ending "ide." Common examples are listed in Table 1.20.

Table 1.20 Common Monoatomic Anions

Chloride	Cl^{-1}
Bromide	Br^{-1}
Oxide	O^{-2}
Sulfide	S^{-2}
Hydride	H^{-1}

Some of the more common monoatomic ions and their relationships to the periodic table are shown in Figure 1.88.

TIP

MONOATOMIC IONS

Know the common monoatomic ions. Most charges can be deduced from the atom's location on the periodic table and the octet rule.

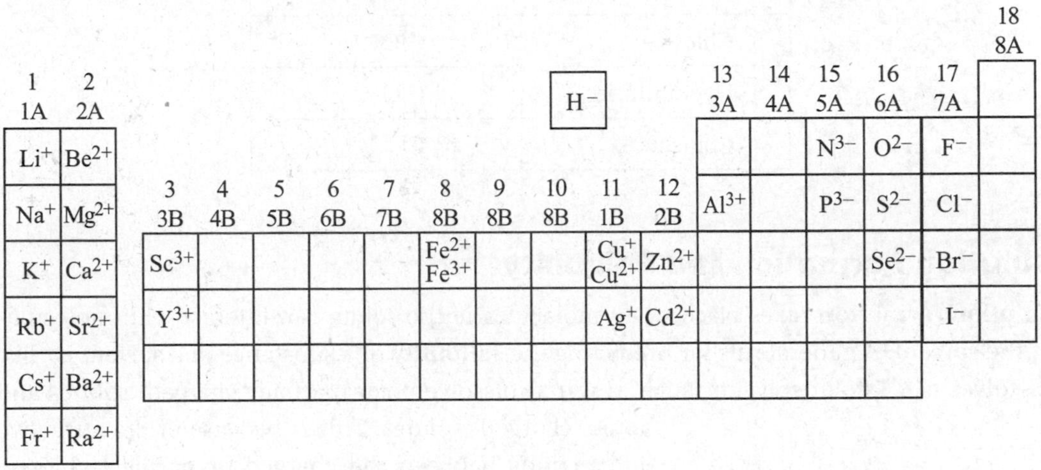

1 1A	2 2A	3 3B	4 4B	5 5B	6 6B	7 7B	8 8B	9 8B	10 8B	11 1B	12 2B	13 3A	14 4A	15 5A	16 6A	17 7A	18 8A
																H^-	
Li^+	Be^{2+}													N^{3-}	O^{2-}	F^-	
Na^+	Mg^{2+}											Al^{3+}		P^{3-}	S^{2-}	Cl^-	
K^+	Ca^{2+}	Sc^{3+}					Fe^{2+} Fe^{3+}			Cu^+ Cu^{2+}	Zn^{2+}				Se^{2-}	Br^-	
Rb^+	Sr^{2+}	Y^{3+}								Ag^+	Cd^{2+}					I^-	
Cs^+	Ba^{2+}																
Fr^+	Ra^{2+}																

Figure 1.88. Common monoatomic ions and their charges

POLYATOMIC IONS

Polyatomic ions are covalently bonded groups of atoms that have a charge on the entire unit. The most common polyatomic ions are listed in Table 1.21.

Table 1.21 Common Polyatomic Ions

Nitrate	NO_3^{-1}
Sulfate	SO_4^{-2}
Carbonate	CO_3^{-2}
Hydroxide	OH^{-1}
Phosphate	PO_4^{-3}
Acetate	$C_2H_3O_2^{-1}$ or CH_3COO^{-1}
Bicarbonate or hydrogen carbonate	HCO_3^{-1}
Chlorate	ClO_3^{-1}
Ammonium	NH_4^{+1}

Many other common ions are related to those listed in Table 1.21. For example, the nitrite ion is NO_2^{-1} and for many ions ending in *-ate*, there is a corresponding ion, with one less oxygen atom (but the same charge), ending in *-ite*.

There is another pattern of ions that is primarily found in the polyatomic ions of the halogen family. The ion with one more oxygen than chlorate is called perchlorate (*per-* is short for *hyper-*) and the ion with one less oxygen atom than chlorite is the hypochlorite ion (*hypo-* means below). Notice that the monoatomic ion ends with *-ide*.

Table 1.22 Ions Containing Chlorine

Perchlorate	ClO_4^{-1}
Chlorate	ClO_3^{-1}
Chlorite	ClO_2^{-1}
Hypochlorite	ClO^{-1}
Chloride	Cl^{-1}

Solution Formation and Solubility

Solution formation takes place when molecules of the solute can interact with molecules of the solvent. A general rule for predicting the **solubility** of a substance in a solvent is "like dissolves like." Polar solvents (such as water) dissolve polar (partially charged) solutes and ionic (charged) solutes. This is because of the attractive interactions between the charged or partially charged portions of the molecules or ions.

LIKE DISSOLVES LIKE

You can count on this rule of thumb.
Water is polar, salt is ionic (very polar), and hydrocarbons are nonpolar.

SOLVATION AND HYDRATION

For an ionic compound dissolving in water, each ion is surrounded (or **solvated**) by water molecules. A positive ion is surrounded by the partially negatively charged end of the water molecule (the oxygen atom) closest to the ion. A negative ion is situated so that the oppositely charged end of the water molecule (the partially positively charged hydrogens) is closest to the ion, as shown in Figure 1.89.

In water, the process of solvation is known as **hydration**, and the surrounding group of water molecules around the dissolved ion or molecule is known as a **hydration shell**. The number of water molecules surrounding a dissolved ion is called the **hydration number**.

Nonpolar solutes dissolve in nonpolar solvents via London dispersion forces, interactions between molecules formed by temporary dipoles caused by random fluctuations of electrons.

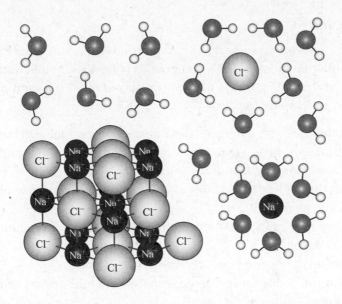

Figure 1.89. Solvation of sodium and chloride ions by water molecules

ELECTROLYTES

A compound that dissolves in water to form ions is called an **electrolyte**. Strong electrolytes produce large numbers of dissolved ions and include strong acids and bases, such as hydrochloric acid or sodium hydroxide, and soluble ionic compounds, such as sodium chloride. Weak electrolytes produce few ions when dissolved in water. Weak electrolytes are usually weak acids or bases, such as acetic acid or ammonia. A substance that produces no ions when dissolved is a nonelectrolyte and is typically a molecular substance or an insoluble ionic compound.

TIP

ELECTROLYTE STRENGTH

Whether a substance is a strong electrolyte, a weak electrolyte, or a nonelectrolyte depends on the number of ions produced when it dissolves, not the identity of the ions.

TEST QUESTION

Which of the following correctly pairs a substance with the type of electrolyte it is?

I. sodium acetate, strong electrolyte

II. acetic acid, weak electrolyte

III. sucrose, nonelectrolyte

(A) I only

(B) II only

(C) I and III only

(D) I, II, and III

(D) Sucrose is a nonelectrolyte. It is soluble in water because it is a polar compound but no ions form when it dissolves. Acetic acid is a weak acid and weak acids and bases tend to be weak electrolytes. Soluble ionic substances, such as sodium salts, are usually strong electrolytes.

Solubility Rules

The solubility of ionic compounds can be summarized by a small number of consistently reliable rules. These rules apply to ionic compounds being dissolved in water. The rules are applied in order so that rule 1 always has priority over another rule, and rule 2 always has priority over every other rule except rule 1.

1. All ionic compounds with a group 1 (alkali metal) ion are soluble in water.
2. All ionic compounds with ammonium ions as the positive ion are soluble in water.
3. All nitrate containing compounds are soluble.
4. All chlorides, bromides, and iodides are soluble, except for those of silver, lead(II), mercury(I), and mercury(II).
5. Sulfate compounds are soluble except those of calcium, strontium, barium, silver, mercury(I), and lead(II).
6. All oxides are insoluble, except as specified in rules 1 and 2.
7. Hydroxides are insoluble, except for those specified in rules 1 and 2 and calcium, strontium, and barium hydroxides.
8. Compounds of the ions carbonate, phosphate, and sulfide are insoluble, except as specified in rules 1 and 2.

TIP

THE MOST IMPORTANT SOLUBILITY RULES

The most important solubility rules are at the top of the list. Rules 1–4 are the most important.

Practice Question

Predict the solubility of potassium phosphide in water.

Solution: It will be soluble because of the potassium ion. If one of the ions in a compound is soluble, the other ion is not relevant in determining solubility.

THE HYDRONIUM ION

A hydrogen ion (H^+) rarely exists by itself in solution due to the high density of charge it would possess. Instead, the hydrogen ion will attach to a water molecule to form a hydronium (H_3O^+) ion, which spreads the positive charge over a greater number of atoms (Figure 1.90).

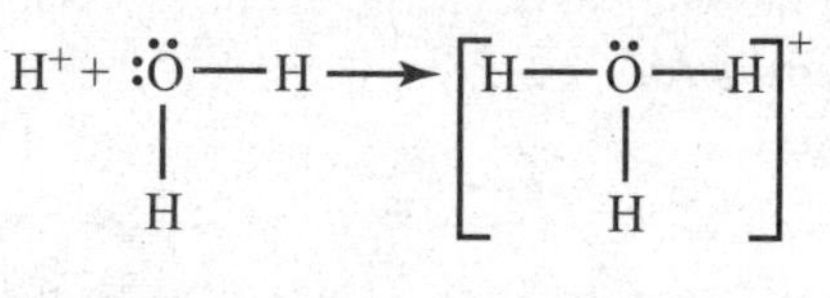

Figure 1.90. Hydronium ion formation

Factors Affecting the Solubility of Solids and Gases

The solubility of solids in water is generally affected only by the temperature of the water and the ionic substance being dissolved. The solubility of gasses is also affected by pressure.

SOLIDS

In general, the solubility of an ionic substance in water increases with increasing solvent temperature. The solubility of solids is unaffected by pressure.

GASES

Gases are generally more soluble at lower temperatures and are always more soluble at higher pressures. This relationship between gas solubility and pressure is known as Henry's law, which states that the solubility of a gas is directly proportional to the pressure applied. These solubility patterns for gases hold true regardless of the polarity of the solute.

Miscibility: The Mixing of Liquids

When discussing the mixing of two liquids, the terms **miscible** and **immiscible** are often used, rather than soluble and insoluble. Oil and water are immiscible in each other, whereas vinegar (acetic acid) and water are miscible in each other. The miscibility of liquids in each other follows the "like dissolves like" rule, just as it does for solids.

> **DISSOLVING SOLIDS AND GASES**
>
> Solids dissolve better at higher temperatures and gases dissolve better at lower temperatures and higher pressures. Soda has more dissolved carbon dioxide (it stays fizzy) when it is kept in the refrigerator (lower temperature) with the top on (higher pressure).

RELATIONSHIPS BETWEEN MOLECULAR STRUCTURE AND SOLUBILITY

For solubility in a polar solvent, such as water, the greater the ability of the solute to interact with water molecules, via hydrogen bonding, the greater the solubility. The solubility of some simple carboxylic acids is shown in Table 1.23.

Table 1.23 Solubility of Organic Acids in Water

Acid	Structure	Solubility in Water
Formic Acid	$HCOOH$	Completely miscible
Acetic Acid	CH_3COOH	Completely miscible
Hexanoic Acid	$CH_3(CH_2)_4COOH$	1.1 g/100 ml Water
Decanoic Acid	$CH_3(CH_2)_8COOH$	Insoluble

The COOH, or carboxylic acid, end of these molecules is polar and has the ability to form hydrogen bonds with water, allowing solubility. The hydrocarbon portion of these molecules is nonpolar and tends to make the molecule less soluble in water. The greater the portion of the molecule taken up by nonpolar hydrocarbon, the less soluble the molecule is in water. Similar patterns are found for the solubility of alcohols and other organic compounds.

These solubility patterns are reversed for a nonpolar solvent dissolving in water. Decanoic acid is the most soluble in hexane (C_6H_{14}). Formic acid is the least soluble.

Solution Concentration Units

Solution concentration can be described in several ways, each of which has uses in specific situations. The units needed for the MCAT are molarity (M), molality (m), mole fraction (χ), and mass percent.

MOLARITY

Molarity (M) is the number of moles of dissolved solute per liter of solution or

$$M = \frac{\text{moles solute}}{\text{L solution}}$$

If a solution is made by dissolving 5.80 grams of NaCl (molar mass = 58 g/mole) in a total volume of 0.25 L, then the molarity is

$$M = \frac{0.10 \text{ moles NaCl}}{0.250 \text{ L}} = 0.40 \text{ M}$$

> **MCAT MATH HINT**
>
> Notice how the 5.8 grams of solute conveniently become 0.1 moles when divided by the molar mass of NaCl. This is typical of the level of calculation needed on the MCAT.

Keep in mind that a final solution volume of 250 ml (or 0.25 L) is not the same as adding the salt to 250 ml of water.

MOLALITY

Molality (m) is the number of moles of solute per kilogram of solvent or

$$m = \frac{\text{moles solute}}{\text{kg solvent}}$$

The main advantage of using molality is that it does not vary with temperature, as molarity does (volumes change when substances are heated but mass does not). A solution made by dissolving 9.0 g glucose (molar mass = 180 g/mole) in 100 grams of water would be

$$m = \frac{0.050 \text{ moles glucose}}{0.1 \text{ kg water}} = 0.5 \ m$$

MOLE FRACTION

Mole fraction (χ) is equal to the number of moles of a substance divided by the total number of moles in the solution or

$$\chi = \frac{\text{moles component}}{\text{total moles in the solution}}$$

A solution made by mixing 0.6 moles of benzene and 0.9 moles of toluene would have a mole fraction of benzene of

$$\chi_{benzene} = \frac{0.6 \text{ moles benzene}}{1.5 \text{ moles total}} = 0.4\chi$$

and a mole fraction of toluene of 0.6. In any solution, the sum of the mole fractions of the components equals 1.0.

MASS PERCENT

The mass percent of a solution is the percentage of a solution's mass due to a specific component.

$$\text{Mass \%} = \frac{\text{mass of component}}{\text{total solution mass}} \times 100$$

A 3% sodium iodide solution would have 3 grams of NaI per 100 grams of solution. This means that 500 grams of the solution would consist of 15 grams NaI and 485 grams of water.

DILUTIONS

Very often one solution will be made by diluting a more concentrated (stock) solution. The equation that describes this is

$$M_1 V_1 = M_2 V_2$$

where M_1 is the stock solution molarity, V_1 the volume of stock solution used, M_2 the final solution molarity, and V_2 the final solution volume.

Practice Question

A chemist needs 600 ml of 1.5 M HCl. What volume of 9.0 M HCl is needed to make this solution?

Solution: $(9.0 \text{ M})(V) = (1.5 \text{ M})(600 \text{ ml})$ and $V = 100$ ml, so 100 ml of the concentrated HCl would be dissolved in enough water to form 600 ml total.

Solubility Product Constant

The solubility rules listed above are very good guidelines but they ignore the fact that even so-called insoluble ionic compounds are actually very slightly soluble. For an insoluble ionic compound such as silver chloride, there is an equilibrium between the solid and the dissolved ions:

SOLIDS AND EQUILIBRIUM CONSTANTS
Keep in mind that solids are not included when writing equilibrium constant expressions.

$$AgCl_{(s)} \leftrightarrow Ag^{+1}_{(aq)} + Cl^{-1}_{(aq)}$$

An equilibrium expression for this process can be written following the rules for writing equilibrium constants, namely that solids are not included in equilibrium expressions. This type of equilibrium constant, for a slightly soluble ionic compound, is known as a solubility product constant, or K_{sp}.

$$K_{sp} = [Ag^{+1}][Cl^{-1}]$$

SOLUBILITY PRODUCT CONSTANT CALCULATIONS

Tables containing the values of K_{sp} for many substances are available. For AgCl, the value of K_{sp} is 1.8×10^{-10}. This can be used to find the solubility of silver chloride in water on a molar basis and on a gram per liter basis. For AgCl,

$$1.8 \times 10^{-10} = [Ag^{+1}][Cl^{-1}]$$

but because the dissociation equation shows that the moles of silver and chloride ions are equal (but unknown), the expression becomes

$$1.8 \times 10^{-10} = x^2 \quad \text{and} \quad x = 1.34 \times 10^{-5} \text{ M}$$

TIP

K_{sp}

K_{sp} is a special case of an equilibrium constant. It never has a denominator.

> **MCAT MATH HINT**
>
> Quick estimate: $\sqrt{a \times 10^b} = \sqrt{a} \times 10^{b/2}$

Thus, the solubility of silver chloride in water is 1.34×10^{-5} moles/L, which equals 1.92×10^{-3} g/L.

If the solubility in moles per liter is known, the solubility product constant can be solved as shown below:

The solubility of lead(II) iodide in water at 25°C is 1.4×10^{-4} M. The value of K_{sp} can be calculated by writing a dissociation equation and a K_{sp} expression.

$$PbI_{2(s)} \leftrightarrow Pb^{+2}_{(aq)} + 2\,I^{-1}_{(aq)}$$

$$K_{sp} = [Pb^{+2}][I^{-1}]^2$$

TIP

MAGNITUDE OF K_{sp}

The smaller the value of K_{sp}, the less soluble the substance.

From the ion formation equation, the concentration of iodide ion is double that of the lead ion. If the molar solubility is 1.4×10^{-4} M, then the solubility of the iodide ion is 2.8×10^{-4} M (since there are two iodide ions for every one lead(II) ion) and

$$K_{sp} = (1.4 \times 10^{-4})(2.8 \times 10^{-4})^2 = 1.1 \times 10^{-11}$$

THE COMMON ION EFFECT AND SOLUBILITY

Thus far, we have discussed the solubility of an ionic compound in pure water. What happens if, instead of dissolving a substance such as lead(II) iodide in water, it is dissolved in a solution of sodium iodide, so that one of the ions of the salt is already present? Because the solution and the salt have an ion in common, the **common ion effect** will apply. This is really a special example of Le Châtelier's principle. The addition of an ion that is part of the equilibrium will tend to shift the equilibrium away from that ion.

In the lead(II) iodide example above, what would happen if there were already 0.1 M NaI in the solution? The sodium ions are not part of the overall equilibrium and they act as spectator ions. The ionization and equilibrium expressions are:

$$PbI_{2(s)} \leftrightarrow Pb^{+2}_{(aq)} + 2\,I^{-1}_{(aq)}$$
$$K_{sp} = [Pb^{+2}][I^{-1}]^2$$

Because the lead(II) ion concentration is not changed, its concentration is still represented by x, but the iodide ion concentration is $2x$ plus the 0.1 M from the addition of the sodium iodide.

$$K_{sp} = 1.1 \times 10^{-11} = (x)(0.1 + 2x)^2$$

If x is small (which is true for a slightly soluble compound), then $0.1 + 2x \approx 0.1$, and solving for x gives

$$\mathbf{1.1 \times 10^{-11} = (x)(0.1)^2}$$

where x is the solubility of lead(II) iodide, and in this situation $x = 1.1 \times 10^{-9}$ M. This is a quantitative way of saying that the equilibrium was shifted to the left, so the compound is less soluble, as Le Châtelier's principle would predict.

TIP

COMMON ION EFFECT

Knowing how the common ion effect works is more important on the MCAT than being able to do all of the calculations.

TEST QUESTION

The solubility product constant of silver bromide at 25°C is 9×10^{-13}. What is the molar solubility of silver bromide in a solution of 0.1 M sodium bromide?

(A) 3×10^{-12}
(B) 9×10^{-12}
(C) 3×10^{-7}
(D) 9×10^{-7}

(B) First write an equation describing the dissolving of AgBr:

$$AgBr_{(s)} \rightarrow Ag^{+1}_{(aq)} + Br^{-1}_{(aq)}$$

Then write a K_{sp} expression:

$$K_{sp} = 9 \times 10^{-13} = [Ag^{+1}][Br^{-1}]$$

The dissolving of silver bromide produces equal number of moles of silver ions and bromide ions and the concentration of bromide ions is already 0.1 M so this gives:

$$9 \times 10^{-13} = [x][0.1 + x]$$

As silver bromide is a sparingly soluble salt, $0.1 + x \approx 0.1$, giving:

$$9 \times 10^{-13} = (x)(0.1)$$

And x = solubility of silver bromide in moles/L = 9×10^{-12} M

TIP

Q vs. K_{eq}

This is an example of a Q versus K_{eq} problem. When the ion concentration product exceeds K_{sp}, the ions will precipitate out, shifting the equilibrium to the left.

MCAT MATH HINT

For ionic compounds of the form AB, the K_{sp} expression is $K_{sp} = [x]^2$; the molar concentrations of the positive ion (A) and the negative ion (B) are equal. For compounds of the form AB_2 or A_2B, the pattern gives

$$K_{sp} = 4x^3$$

Complex Ions: Formation and Solubility

A **complex ion** is an ion that contains a metal cation bonded to one or more small molecules or ions (such as NH_3, CN^-, H_2O, or OH^-). The ions or molecules surrounding the metal cation are known as **ligands**. The formation of a complex ion is a stepwise process, and each step has its own characteristic equilibrium constant. Complex ions are soluble in aqueous solutions because they are charged.

The attractive forces between the complex ions and water molecules occur because of ion–dipole intermolecular forces. The number of ligands that can surround the central metal ion is hard to predict, but a good guideline is that it is double the typical charge of the cation. Silver has a charge of +1. The most common number of ligands surrounding a silver ion in a complex ion is 2. Complex ion formation is indicated when the addition of a ligand causes an insoluble compound of a metal to redissolve. Complex ions of transition metals are very often colored.

Colloids and Suspensions

Colloids and suspensions are two additional types of mixtures. A solution is a homogeneous mixture with particles that stay mixed and cannot be separated by filtration methods. This is largely due to the small size of the dissolved ions or molecules in a true solution. A suspension is a heterogeneous mixture with particles large enough to separate based on gravity. The particles of a suspension can be separated by filtration.

A **colloid** is a homogeneous mixture in which the particles are larger than those of a solution, but small enough to be unaffected by gravity. Examples include aerosols (such as fog), foams (such as whipped cream), and emulsions (such as mayonnaise). The particles in a colloid are large enough to scatter light, a phenomenon known as the Tyndall effect. Seeing a beam from headlights in fog is an example of the Tyndall effect. The particles in a colloid can be attracted or repelled by the molecules in the medium in which they are dispersed. This attraction or repulsion can be based on charges or polarities of the colloidal particles and the dispersing medium. Even though colloidal particles are too small to separate by filtration, they can be made to coagulate by the addition of specific ions. A summary of the main features of solutions, suspensions, and colloids is shown in Table 1.24.

Table 1.24 Mixture Types

System	Solution	Colloid	Suspension
Particle size	$1 - 10^2$ pm	$10^2 - 10^5$ pm	Larger than 10^5 pm
Separate by filtration?	No	No	Yes
Shows Tyndall effect?	No	Yes	Yes
Homogeneous or heterogeneous?	Homogeneous	Homogeneous	Heterogeneous
Separates via gravity?	No	No	Yes
Example	Salt water	Fog	Muddy water

ACID–BASE CHEMISTRY

There are many important reactions in living systems that involve acid–base chemistry. Acids are chemicals that generally have sour tastes (although tasting is never an appropriate way to gain information about a chemical). Acids lower the pH of solutions and turn indicators into specific colors (litmus turns pink or red in the presence of an acid). They often react with carbonates or bicarbonates to produce carbon dioxide gas. Many metals react with acids to form hydrogen gas. Bases tend to raise the pH of solutions, taste bitter, turn litmus blue, and their solutions often have a slippery feel. All living organisms maintain a steady body pH via a series of chemical processes.

Arrhenius Theory

The oldest and simplest theory of acids and bases is the Arrhenius theory, which states that an acid is a chemical that dissolves in water and dissociates to produce hydrogen ions. An Arrhenius base is a substance that dissociates in water to produce hydroxide ions. However, the theory fails to explain acid–base chemistry in other solvents. It neither explains how a substance such as ammonia can be a base, nor the ability of a chemical to sometimes act as an acid and at other times, as a base.

Brønsted–Lowry Acids and Bases

The most widely used definition of acids and bases is the Brønsted–Lowry theory. In the Brønsted–Lowry theory of acids and bases, an acid is a substance that donates a hydrogen ion (or proton), and a base is a chemical species that accepts a hydrogen ion. An amphoteric substance is a chemical species that is capable of accepting a proton and acting as a base, or donating a proton and acting as an acid.

CONJUGATE ACID–BASE PAIRS

In the Brønsted–Lowry theory, acids and bases always appear in pairs, known as **conjugate acid–base pairs**. These acid–base pairs are related by the donation or acceptance of a proton, or hydrogen ion. The Brønsted–Lowry theory can explain acids and bases that do not have an H^+ or OH^- ion in their formulas, and it can describe acid–base chemistry in a variety of solvents. The examples below show conjugate acid–base pairs:

$$HCl + H_2O \leftrightarrow H_3O^+ + Cl^-$$

Acid Base Conjugate Acid Conjugate Base

HCl is an acid because it donates a hydrogen ion to the water. By accepting the proton, the water is acting as a base. The H_3O^+ (hydronium) ion is the conjugate acid because it is the original base with an extra proton. The chloride ion is now the conjugate base because it has the ability to accept a proton.

Water can act as an acid as in the following example:

$$NH_3 + H_2O \leftrightarrow NH_4^+ + OH^-$$

Base Acid Conjugate Acid Conjugate Base

TIP

CONJUGATE ACID-BASE PAIRS

Conjugate acid-base pairs differ by one hydrogen. The acidic form always has one more hydrogen and one more positive unit of charge.

In this case, the water donates a proton to the ammonia, making the water an acid and the ammonia a base. In the reverse direction, the ammonium ion donates a proton to the hydroxide ion.

It is common to define Brønsted–Lowry acid–base pairs so that the acid and base are always reactants and the conjugates always the products. A substance that has the ability to act as either a Brønsted–Lowry acid or base is said to be amphoteric. Water is an example of an amphoteric species, as are the bicarbonate (HCO_3^{-1}) and bisulfate (HSO_4^{-1}) ions.

Strong acids and bases have weak conjugates and weak acids and bases have strong conjugates.

Lewis Acid-Base Theory

The Lewis theory of acids and bases describes all acid–base reactions in terms of the donating and accepting of electron pairs. A Lewis acid is an electron pair acceptor and a Lewis base is an electron pair donor. Lewis acids are often electron-deficient molecules such as BF_3 or $AlCl_3$, and Lewis bases often are molecules with a lone pair of electrons on an atom, such as NH_3 or OH^-.

Self-Ionization of Water and K_w

Even though pure water is considered a nonelectrolyte, a small amount of water ionizes. This can be written as:

$$H_2O_{(l)} + H_2O_{(l)} \leftrightarrow H_3O^+_{(aq)} + OH^-_{(aq)}$$

The equilibrium constant expression is (recall that liquids are not included in equilibrium expressions):

$$K_w = [\mathbf{H_3O^+}] [\mathbf{OH^-}]$$

where the abbreviation K_w is simply the equilibrium constant for water. At room temperature this equilibrium constant has a value of 1×10^{-14} at 25°C, which means that in pure water at room temperature, the concentrations of hydronium and hydroxide ions are equal to each other, with a value of 1×10^{-7} M for each. In any aqueous solution at room temperature:

$$K_w = 1 \times 10^{-14} = [\mathbf{H_3O^+}] [\mathbf{OH^-}]$$

K_w is a constant at a given temperature, so an increase in hydronium ion concentration must be accompanied by a decrease in hydroxide concentration.

The pH Scale and the Relationships Between pH, pOH, [H_3O^+], and [OH^-]

Because the concentrations of hydronium and hydroxide ions vary greatly in solutions, a logarithmic scale is useful for describing the acidity or alkalinity of solutions. The definition of pH is:

$$\mathbf{pH = -log\ [H_3O^+]}$$

and the definition of pOH is

$$\mathbf{pOH = -log\ [OH^-]}$$

Figure 1.91 shows some common substances and their pH values.

TIP

MCAT MATH HINT: LOGARITHMS

Recall the basics of logs such as: log x^n = n log x and log 10^x = x.

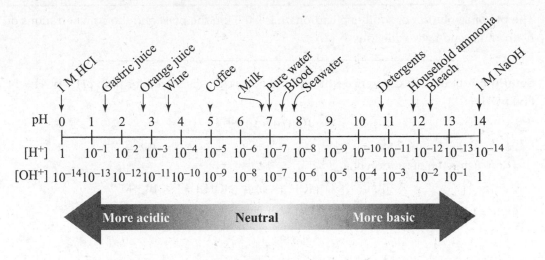

Figure 1.91. The pH scale

The pH scale generally is described as ranging from 0 to 14, but negative pH values as well as values greater than 14 are possible. At 25°C (room temperature) the pH of pure water is 7.0:

$$-\log(1 \times 10^{-7}) = 7.0$$

This gives some useful relationships:

$$1 \times 10^{-14} = [H_3O^+] [OH^-]$$
$$pH = -\log [H_3O^+]$$
$$pOH = -\log [OH^-]$$
$$pH + pOH = 14$$

Two other useful equations are:

$$[H_3O^+] = 10^{-pH} \quad \text{and} \quad [OH^-] = 10^{-pOH}$$

This means that for any solution, given either the pH, pOH, $[H_3O^+]$, or $[OH^-]$, it is possible to determine the other values.

Before showing how these calculations are done, it is useful to do a quick review on exponents.

For any number 10^x, $\log(10^x) = x$. This means that if $[H_3O^+]$ is 1×10^{-8} M, the pH is $-\log(1 \times 10^{-8}) = 8$.

If the concentration of the hydronium (or hydroxide) ion is of the form 1×10^{-x} M, then the pH (or pOH) will be x because the log of 1 is zero. If the value is not of this form, then a little estimating may be necessary.

For example, if the $[H_3O^+] = 3 \times 10^{-7}$ M, then the pH must be between 6 and 7 because 3×10^{-7} is between 1×10^{-6} and 1×10^{-7}. For almost all MCAT problems, this level of estimation will suffice.

The pH of a solution of sodium bicarbonate is 9.0. Find the pOH and the concentrations of hydronium and hydroxide ions.

Solution: It makes no difference which of the other terms is solved for first: pH + pOH = 14 and pOH = 5

$$[H_3O^+] = 10^{-pH}$$

So, $[H_3O^+] = 1 \times 10^{-9}$ M

Then, using the definition of K_w:

$$1 \times 10^{-14} = [H_3O^+][OH^-] \quad \text{and} \quad [OH^-] = 1 \times 10^{-5} \text{ M}$$

Figure 1.92 shows the relationships between each of these variables.

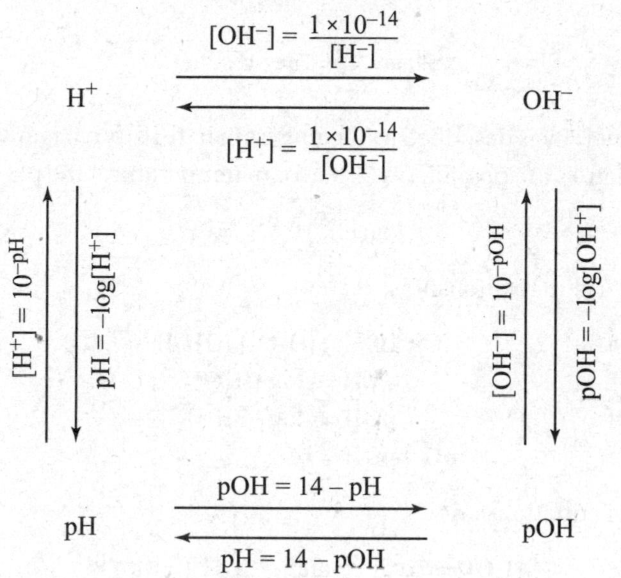

Figure 1.92. Mathematical relationships between pH, pOH, $[H_3O^+]$, and $[OH^-]$

Table 1.25 shows some selected values for these factors. Most general chemistry texts have a complete table for all pH values from 0 to 14.

Table 1.25 Relationships between pH, pOH, $[H_3O^+]$, and $[OH^-]$

pH	pOH	$[H_3O^+]$ (M)	$[OH^-]$ (M)
2	12	1×10^{-2}	1×10^{-12}
5	9	1×10^{-5}	1×10^{-9}
8	6	1×10^{-8}	1×10^{-6}
11	3	1×10^{-11}	1×10^{-3}
14	0	1×10^{-14}	$1 \times 10^0 = 1$

Notice that the pH and pOH columns add to 14 and the $[H_3O^+]$ and $[OH^-]$ columns multiply to 1×10^{-14}.

Strong Acids and Bases

A strong acid is defined as an acid that dissociates 100% in water. This means that the concentration of hydronium ion for a strong acid is equal to the original molar concentration of the acid. The common strong acids are listed in Table 1.26. For less common acids, any acid for which the number of oxygen atoms exceeds that number of hydrogen atoms by two or more is a strong acid, and can be considered to dissociate 100%. Thus, chloric acid, $HClO_3$, is a strong acid, but chlorous acid, $HClO_2$, is not. All strong acids are strong electrolytes.

Table 1.26 Common Strong Acids

HI	Hydroiodic acid
HCl	Hydrochloric acid
HBr	Hydrobromic acid
H_2SO_4	Sulfuric acid
HNO_3	Nitric acid
$HClO_4$	Perchloric acid

Practice Question

Find the pH of a 0.001 M solution of nitric acid.

Solution: Nitric acid is a strong acid. It is 100% ionized,

$$HNO_3 + H_2O \rightarrow H_3O^+ + NO_3^{-1} \qquad \text{or} \qquad HNO_3 \rightarrow H^+ + NO_3^-$$

Brønsted–Lowry Approach   Arrhenius Approach

so the concentration of H_3O^+ is 0.001 M or 1×10^{-3} M and the pH is 3.

TEST QUESTION

What is the approximate pH of a .0003 M solution of nitric acid?

(A) 3.0

(B) 3.7

(C) 4.0

(D) 9.0

(B) Nitric acid, HNO_3, is a strong acid, so it is 100% ionized in water. The concentration of hydronium ion will be 0.0003 M or 3×10^{-4} M. The pH will be $-\log(3 \times 10^{-4})$, which is equal to $4 - \log 3$. This makes the pH a bit less than 4. It is not necessary to know the value of the log of 3 to solve this. Choice D is a basic pH and is not possible as an answer.

A strong base is also a strong electrolyte, and it dissociates or ionizes 100%. If 0.1 mole of potassium hydroxide, a strong base, is added to water, to give a solution volume equal to 1.0 L, the molar concentration of KOH (and thus OH^-) is 0.1 M.

$$KOH \rightarrow K^+ + OH^-$$

Because $[OH^-] = 0.1$ M, the pOH is 1 and the pH is 13.

The strong bases are hydroxides of groups 1 and 2 on the periodic table. The most common strong bases are listed in the table below:

Table 1.27 Common Strong Bases

LiOH	Lithium hydroxide
NaOH	Sodium hydroxide
KOH	Potassium hydroxide
$Sr(OH)_2$	Strontium hydroxide
$Ca(OH)_2$	Calcium hydroxide
$Ba(OH)_2$	Barium hydroxide

STRENGTH VS. CONCENTRATION

For an acid, do not confuse concentration with strength. A solution of acetic acid, that is 1.0 M, has a pH of about 2.6. A solution of 0.001 M HCl has a pH of about 3.0. The strength of an acid refers to the fraction of acid ionized, whereas its concentration refers to the number of moles dissolved per liter.

Polyprotic Acids

Acids with more than one ionizable hydrogen atom are known as **polyprotic acids**. The most common polyprotic acids are sulfuric acid, H_2SO_4, a diprotic acid, and phosphoric acid, H_3PO_4, a triprotic acid. On the MCAT, the second and third hydrogens of polyprotic acids are weak enough to be ignored in calculations.

NORMALITY AND EQUIVALENT WEIGHT

An acid or base's **normality** (N) is its molarity multiplied by the number of hydrogen or hydroxide ions it can contribute to a reaction.

A 0.5 M solution of H_2SO_4 is 1.0 N
A 1.5 M solution of $Ca(OH)_2$ is 3.0 N
A 2.0 M solution of H_3PO_4 is 6.0 N

Equivalent weights and normality are independent of the strength of the acid or base. The **equivalent weight** is the mass of an acid or base that contributes 1 mole of either hydrogen or hydroxide ions.

The molar mass of sulfuric acid, H_2SO_4, is 98 g/mole. Because each molecule of sulfuric acid has two protons (it is a diprotic acid), the equivalent weight is $\frac{98}{2} = 49$ grams.

Weak Acids and Bases

Weak acids and bases are weak electrolytes and dissociate only slightly in aqueous solutions. The dissociation of a strong acid or base is considered to be 100% and can be represented by a nonequilibrium equation. Weak acids and bases result in equilibrium systems. The list of weak acids and bases is long and it is much easier to learn the rules for strong acids and bases (see above) and assume that an acid or base that is not strong must be weak. The most common weak base is ammonia, NH_3, and the common weak acids include hydrofluoric acid, HF, acetic acid, CH_3COOH, and any other organic acid.

For the weak acid HF, the ionization equation is:

$$HF + H_2O \leftrightarrow H_3O^+ + F^-$$

And the equilibrium expression, labeled K_a for an acid is:

$$K_a = \frac{[H_3O^+][F^-]}{[HF]}$$

The value of K_a (from tables) is 6.7×10^{-4}, so for a 1 M solution of HF, the equilibrium concentration of H_3O^+ and F^- are equal (call them "x") and the equilibrium concentration of HF is $1.0 - x$ M. For a weak acid, the amount of dissociation is small (recall the definition of a weak acid so that $1 - x \approx 1$. If the ratio $[HA]/K_a > 500$, then this approximation is valid. This gives:

$$6.7 \times 10^{-4} = \frac{(x)(x)}{1}$$

Solving for x gives: $x = \sqrt{6.7 \times 10^{-4}}$

A useful shortcut in this case is to estimate the square root of 6.7 and halve the exponent to give an answer of about 2.5×10^{-2} M for $[H_3O^+]$, leading to a pH of between 1 and 2, which is reasonable for an acid.

If the exponent is odd, for example 2.5×10^{-7}, then rewrite the expression as 25×10^{-8}. Take the square root of 25 and halve the exponent to get 5×10^{-4}.

On the MCAT, estimations and approximations such as this will work consistently.

For a weak base, a similar approach is used, but instead of solving for the hydronium ion concentration, solve for the hydroxide ion concentration, meaning that the K_w equation is needed as a last step.

> ### STRONG VS. WEAK ACIDS
>
> All weak acids and bases exist in an equilibrium between the ionized and the non-ionized forms. Strong acids and bases are essentially 100% ionized and are not in an equilibrium situation.

TIP

ORGANIC ACIDS

All carboxylic (organic) acids are weak acids and thus weak electrolytes. All organic bases are weak bases.

Practice Question

Find the pH of a 0.5 M solution of ammonia, with a $K_b = 1.7 \times 10^{-5}$.

Solution: First, write an ionization equation and a K_b (equilibrium expression for a base).

$$NH_3 + H_2O \leftrightarrow NH_4^+ + OH^-$$

$$K_b = \frac{[NH_4^+][OH^-]}{[NH_3]}$$

The concentrations of ammonium and hydroxide ions are equal (call them "x"), so:

$$1.7 \times 10^{-5} = \frac{[NH_4^+][OH^-]}{[NH_3]}$$

$$1.7 \times 10^{-5} = \frac{x^2}{0.5 - x}$$

Ammonia is a weak base, and only slightly ionized, so the equilibrium concentration of NH_3 $(0.5 - x)$ is ≈ 0.5, giving

$$1.7 \times 10^{-5} = \frac{x^2}{0.5}$$

Solving gives $x^2 = 8.5 \times 10^{-6}$ and x can be approximated as $\sqrt{8.5} \times 10^{-6/2}$ or 3×10^{-3} M. It is not possible to simply take the negative log of this number to get the pH because in this case $x = [OH^-]$. This means that $[H_3O^+]$ is expressed as:

$$[H_3O^+] = \frac{1 \times 10^{-14}}{3 \times 10^{-3}}$$

and the hydronium ion concentration is approximately 3.3×10^{-12} M and the pH a bit under 12, which is reasonable for a base.

MOLECULAR STRUCTURE AND ACID STRENGTH

The relative strengths of acids can be explained by referring to certain features of molecular structure.

1. The stronger the bond holding the hydrogen ion to the molecule, the less likely the hydrogen will be able to ionize (or the weaker the acid).
2. The more polar the bond, the more easily the hydrogen will be released (or the stronger the acid).
3. The more atoms over which the charge on the conjugate base can be spread, the more stable the anion formed (the stronger the acid).
4. For binary (non-oxygen containing) acids, the larger the anion, the less polar the bond; and the stronger the bond, the weaker the acid; the more stable the conjugate anion, the stronger the acid.

In terms of acid strength:

$$HF < HCl < HBr < HI$$
$$\text{and}$$
$$H_2O < H_2S < H_2Se < H_2Te$$

Even though all strong acids are considered to be 100% ionized, in reality a slightly higher percentage of HI molecules ionize than HCl molecules. The amount is not enough to matter when doing calculations. HF, however, is a weak acid because it has a stronger H–F bond as a result of the increased electronegativity of F.

For oxoacids, the pattern is different. Oxygen is a highly electronegative element, so electrons are drawn to the oxygen atoms, allowing the charge to be spread over more atoms. This means that the greater the number of oxygen atoms, the stronger the acid (or the more stable the conjugate anion). In terms of acid strength:

$$HClO < HClO_2 < HClO_3 < HClO_4$$

RECOGNIZING STRONGER OXOACIDS

More oxygen atoms = a stronger acid.

Salts and Hydrolysis

A **salt** is an ionic compound formed from the reaction of an acid and a base (see neutralization reactions below). Each salt consists of a positive ion and a negative ion. No matter how the salt was actually formed or obtained, it can always be thought of as having an acid ion and a base ion. The positive ion always comes from the base and the negative ion from the acid. The reaction of a salt with water to form acids or bases is called **hydrolysis**.

ACIDIC, BASIC, AND NEUTRAL SALTS

In working with salts, first determine whether it is a neutral, acidic, or basic salt. This is done by deciding of which acid and base the salt's ions are the conjugates.

Conjugates of acids have one less hydrogen atom and one less unit of charge, and conjugates of bases have one more hydrogen atom and one more unit of charge. The stronger the acid, the weaker the conjugate base and the stronger the base, the weaker the conjugate acid. Examples of salts and their acidic or basic nature are shown in Table 1.28.

Table 1.28 Common Salts and Their Acid–Base Properties

Compound	Formula	Positive Ion is the Conjugate of . . .	Negative Ion is the Conjugate of . . .	Acid/Base/ Neutral?
Sodium bromide	NaBr	NaOH (strong base)	HBr (strong acid)	Neutral
Ammonium nitrate	NH_4NO_3	NH_3 (weak base)	HNO_3 (strong acid)	Acidic
Sodium acetate	$NaC_2H_3O_2$	NaOH (strong base)	$HC_2H_3O_2$ (weak acid)	Basic
Lithium sulfate	Li_2SO_4	LiOH (strong base)	H_2SO_4 (strong acid)	Neutral
Ammonium fluoride	NH_4F	NH_3 (weak base)	HF (weak acid)	Need more info

To determine the acid–base nature of the ammonium fluoride, it is necessary to know the relative strengths of the acid and base of which the ions are conjugates. If both ions are conjugates of a strong acid or base, the salt is neutral because strong acids and bases are each completely ionized. If one ion is the conjugate of a strong acid or base and the other of a weak acid or base, the property of the salt is dictated by whichever is stronger, because a strong acid or base is always much more ionized than a weak one.

If each ion is the conjugate of a weak acid or base, it is necessary to know the exact K_a and K_b values. Whichever is greater will produce more ions. On the MCAT it is important to know the properties of salts shown in the first four examples of Table 1.28.

TEST QUESTION

Which of the following are acidic salts?

  I. NaCl

  II. NH_4NO_3

  III. $KC_2H_3O_2$

  (A) I only

  (B) II only

  (C) II and III only

  (D) I, II, and III

(B) Sodium chloride is the salt of a strong acid and a strong base, so it is a neutral salt. Answers A and D are out. Ammonium nitrate is the salt of a weak base (ammonia) and a strong acid (nitric acid), making it an acidic salt. Potassium acetate is the salt of a strong base (potassium hydroxide) and a weak acid (acetic acid), making it a basic salt. Only II is an acidic salt.

HYDROLYSIS CALCULATIONS

It is possible to calculate the pH of a salt solution by using the K_a or K_b value of the acids of which the salts ions are conjugates. Obviously, if the salt is neutral, the pH must be 7.

When a salt is dissolved in water, it dissociates into ions. The ions of a strong acid or base remain as spectator ions. Ions of weak acids or bases react with water in a process known as hydrolysis.

For example, if a solution of 0.1 M ammonium chloride (NH_4Cl) is dissolved in water, the salt will dissolve and the ion of the weak base (ammonia) will react with water. K_b for ammonia = 1.8×10^{-5}.

$$NH_4Cl \rightarrow NH_4^+ + Cl^-$$
$$NH_4^+ + H_2O \leftrightarrow NH_3 + H_3O^+$$

> **QUICK CHECK BEFORE DOING A pH CALCULATION**
>
> When you calculate the pH of a substance, decide first if it should be acidic, basic, or neutral. This will help catch common calculation errors and can also help eliminate choices from the questions.

Notice how the conjugate of the weak base reacts with water to produce a base.

The K_b for the second equation is:

$$K_b = \frac{[NH_3][H_3O^+]}{[NH_4^+]}$$

Multiplying both the top and bottom of the fraction and taking advantage of the fact that $[H_3O^+][OH^-] = K_w$ gives

$$K_b = \frac{K_w}{K_a}$$

For an acidic salt such as ammonium chloride, K_a for the acid, NH_4^+ is equal to:

$$K_a = \frac{K_w}{K_b}$$

which in this case is

$$K_a = \frac{1 \times 10^{-14}}{1.8 \times 10^{-5}}$$

which is 5.5×10^{-10}. This is sometimes called K_h, the hydrolysis constant.

$$5.5 \times 10^{-10} = \frac{[NH_3][H_3O^+]}{[NH_4^+]}$$

ESTIMATE!

Estimations and approximations such as this will work reliably on the MCAT.

The ammonium ion concentration is essentially 0.1 M, and the ammonia and hydronium ion concentrations are unknown but equal to each other. This gives

$$5.5 \times 10^{-10} = \frac{x^2}{0.1}$$

cross-multiplying and solving gives $x = [H_3O^+] \approx 7.5 \times 10^{-6}$ M and pH = $-\log (7.5 \times 10^{-6}) = 5.1$, a reasonable pH for an acidic salt.

Buffers

A **buffer** is a combination of a weak acid and a salt of that weak acid or a weak base and a salt of that weak base that resists a change in pH. This means that there must be an ion in common between the acid and the salt or the base and the salt. Examples of buffer solutions include sodium acetate in acetic acid and ammonium bromide in ammonia.

A solution made from sodium chloride and hydrochloric acid would not be a buffer solution. Although there is a common ion (Cl^-) the acid is strong, not weak.

A solution of ammonium chloride and acetic acid would not be a buffer solution because there is no common ion.

Consider a buffer system with hydrofluoric acid and sodium fluoride. The sodium ions will be spectator ions and can be ignored.

$$HF + H_2O \leftrightarrow F^- + H_3O^+$$

When a small amount of a base is added to the buffer, it can react with the H^+ ions forming water. This shifts the equilibrium to the right, forming more H^+ ions to replace those used up by reaction with the hydroxide ions from the NaOH. This restores the H^+ ion concentration, maintaining the original pH. When a small amount of HCl is added, the equilibrium shifts to the left, forming more of the HF, which is a weak acid. This maintains the original pH.

BUFFER CALCULATIONS AND THE HENDERSON–HASSELBALCH EQUATION

One of the most common calculations involving a buffered solution is to estimate the pH. Alternatively, the **Henderson–Hasselbalch equation** can be used to determine a "buffer recipe" to create a solution with a desired pH. The equation has one notation in it that needs explaining, and that is the term pK_a. Just as:

$$pH = -\log[H^+] \quad \text{and} \quad pOH = -\log[OH^-]$$

so,

$$pK_a = -\log K_a$$

There are several forms of this equation, some based on pK_a and some on pK_b, but the form below is consistently valid.

$$pH = pK_a + \log \frac{[\text{base}]}{[\text{acid}]}$$

In the case of a buffer made of a weak acid and its salt (which is a basic salt because it is formed from a weak acid and a strong base), the salt is the base. In the case of a buffer made from a weak base and an acidic salt, the more basic component is treated as the base. The point of maximum buffering will occur when the pH of a solution is approximately equal to the pK_a.

Because the pH depends on the log of the ratio of the base to the acid, adding water to a buffer has no effect on its pH. If a solution's volume were to double by the addition of pure water, the concentrations of the base and the acid would both be half, but the ratio of the two would be unchanged.

Practice Question

Determine the pH of a solution made from 0.2 M HF and 0.02 M NaF.

$$K_a \text{ for HF} = 6.7 \times 10^{-4}, \text{ and } pK_a = 3.17$$

Solution: First, it can be clearly seen that this is a buffer solution because it contains a weak acid and a salt of that weak acid.

$$pH = pK_a + \log \frac{[\text{NaF}]}{[\text{HF}]}$$

$$pH = 3.17 + \log \frac{[0.02]}{[0.2]}$$

$$pH = 3.17 - 1.0 = 2.17$$

Because the difference from the pK_a depends on the log of the ratio of the two components, it takes a very large amount of either acid or base to change the pH dramatically. The Henderson–Hasselbalch equation is most accurate when the amounts of acids, bases, salts, or water added to a buffer are relatively small. On MCAT buffer problems you can assume that the amounts are small.

NEUTRALIZATION REACTIONS

Neutralization reactions are reactions between acids and bases that produce salts and water. Examples of neutralization reactions are shown below:

Strong acid plus strong base $HCl + NaOH \rightarrow NaCl + H_2O$
Strong acid plus weak base $3H_2SO_4 + 2Al(OH)_3 \rightarrow Al_2(SO_4)_3 + 6H_2O$
Weak acid plus strong base $HF + LiOH \rightarrow LiF + H_2O$
Weak acid plus weak base $3HClO_2 + Al(OH)_3 \leftrightarrow Al(ClO_2)_3 + 3H_2O$

NEUTRALIZATIONS

Acid + Base → Salt + Water

In the case of ammonia, NH_3, a single product, an ammonium salt will be formed. Some books use NH_4OH, ammonium hydroxide, as the formula for ammonia dissolved in water, in which case the ammonium salt and water are formed.

$$NH_3 + HCl \rightarrow NH_4Cl \text{ or } NH_4OH + HCl \rightarrow NH_4Cl + H_2O$$

Titrations

A **titration** is a quantitative method of analyzing the concentration of an unknown solution by reaction with a solution of known concentration, called a standard. The most common type of titration is an acid–base titration. The titration example in Figure 1.93 shows the addition of a strong base to a strong acid. Because the base is being added to the acid, the pH starts out low and increases as more base is added. A graph showing the pH change as more base is added is called a titration curve.

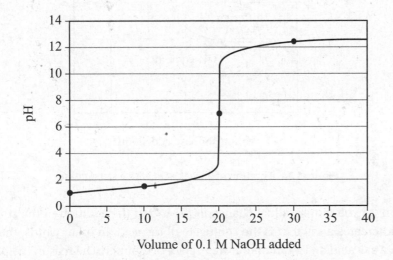

Figure 1.93. Titration of a strong acid with a strong base

The graph, or titration curve, in Figure 1.93 shows the change in pH as 0.1 M NaOH is added to 20.0 ml of 0.1 M HCl. Notice that at the midpoint, the graph is almost vertical, and that a very small volume of base causes a large change in the pH. The midpoint of this nearly vertical area is called the **equivalence point**. In this case, it occurs at a pH of 7.0, after 20.0 ml of base have been added. At this point, the moles of acid exactly equal the moles of base and because the reaction involves a strong acid and a strong base, the pH at the equivalence point is 7.0, or neutral. A titration involving the addition of a strong base to a strong acid starts at a low pH and increases. The equivalence point would also be at a pH of 7.0.

> ### EQUIVALENCE POINT
>
> At the equivalence point of a titration, the moles of acid equal the moles of base. The pH does not have to be 7.0, depending on the relative strengths of the acid and base.

TITRATION OF A WEAK ACID WITH A STRONG BASE

In this case, a strong base such as NaOH is added to a weak acid such as acetic acid. The titration curve is shown in Figure 1.94. Notice that there is a more gradual increase in the pH as the base is added and that the pH at the equivalence point is greater than 7.0.

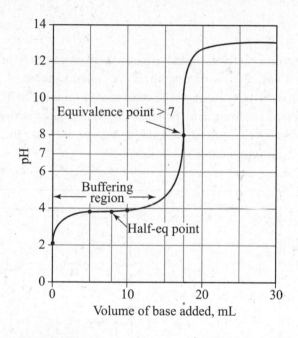

Figure 1.94. Titration of a weak acid with a strong base

The reason for the more gradual change in pH is that the addition of the strong base to the weak acid creates a salt that is the conjugate of the acid. In other words, there will be a solution of a weak acid and a salt of that weak acid, or a buffer. The reason the pH is greater than 7.0 at the equivalence point is that the salt formed when equal numbers of moles of acid and base have reacted is a basic salt. The pH range of the equivalence points of titrations involving strong and weak acids and bases is shown in Table 1.29. At the half-equivalence point, the pH = pK_a and the solution has its maximum buffering ability. This means that the concentration of the acid and its salt are equal.

Table 1.29 Equivalence Points of Titrations

Acid	Base	Equivalence Point
Strong	Strong	Neutral (7.0)
Strong	Weak	Acidic (<7.0)
Weak	Strong	Basic (>7.0)
Weak	Weak	Depends on relative strengths of acid and base

TITRATION OF A WEAK BASE WITH A STRONG ACID

In this situation, an acidic salt will be formed and the pH at the equivalence point will be less than 7.0 (the exact value will depend on the salt and its concentration). The point of maximum buffering (and minimum pH change) will occur when exactly half of the base has been neutralized by the acid.

TITRATION CALCULATIONS

Most titration calculations involve solving for the concentration of an unknown acid or base. The endpoint of a titration will be when the number of moles of acid and base are equal, which does not mean that the pH is neutral. The equation:

$$V_a N_a = V_b N_b$$

can be used to solve for the concentration of the unknown. V_a and V_b represent the volumes of acid and base (usually in ml), and N_a and N_b represent the normalities of the acid and base.

Practice Question

45.9 ml of 0.15 M H_2SO_4 are neutralized by 27.6 ml of sodium hydroxide, NaOH. What is the molarity of the base?

Solution:

$$V_a N_a = V_b N_b$$
$$(45.9 \text{ ml})(.30 \text{ N}) = (27.6 \text{ ml})(N_b)$$
$$N_b = .50 \text{ N}$$

Because each mole of NaOH has one mole of OH^- ions, the molarity is equal to 0.5M. The normality of .15 M sulfuric acid is 0.30 N, since each mole of sulfuric acid has two protons.

An unknown solution of a weak monoprotic acid is made by dissolving 1.0 g of the acid in 30.00 ml of water. The acid solution is titrated with 15.00 ml of 0.30 M calcium hydroxide. What is the molar mass of the acid?

(A) 55 g/mole

(B) 110 g/mole

(C) 220 g/mole

(D) 1100 g/mole

(B) At the endpoint of a titration (in this case the endpoint would occur at a basic pH), the moles of acid equal the moles of base. The number of moles of base used equals the volume of base multiplied by the normality (to account for the fact that each mole of $Ca(OH)_2$ has 2 moles of hydroxide ions). This means that there were (0.0150 L) × (0.30 moles/L) × (2 OH^-/mole) = 0.009 moles of OH^- reacted. The acid is monoprotic, so there must be 0.009 moles of acid in the 1.00 grams. Thus, one can say, 1.00 g/0.009 moles = 111 g/mole. Notice how the answers of 55 g/mole and 220 g/mole could easily result from not applying the fact that each mole of calcium hydroxide has two moles of hydroxide ions.

TIP

EQUIVALENCE POINT AND pH

The equivalence point does not always have a neutral pH. The pH depends on the type of salt formed.

INDICATORS AND pH DETERMINATION

The most common method for determining the pH of a solution is to use a pH meter. A pH meter works by using a selectively permeable electrode to create an ion concentration gradient and then converting this voltage to a pH. In some cases, a visual method is used, typically an acid–base indicator. **Acid–base indicators** are commonly used during titrations (see below). A well-known indicator is litmus, which is red in an acidic solution and blue in a basic solution. Other common indicators include phenolphthalein and bromothymol blue. The MCAT will not require you to know specific indicators, their colors, or the pH at which they undergo a color change. An indicator is usually a weak acid whose conjugate base is a different color.

TIP

INDICATORS

You don't need to memorize indicators, their colors, and pH transition points. Just understand what an indicator does and how it is used.

For example, if HIn is the formula for the indicator, then In^- is the formula for the conjugate base. If the indicator had a blue color and the conjugate had a yellow color, then whichever predominated in a solution would be the color seen. Typically when one form is present in a tenfold excess over the other, that color will be seen clearly.

Indicators are an application of Le Châtelier's principle. In the case of litmus:

$$HLit \quad \leftrightarrow \quad H^+ \quad + \quad Lit^-$$
$$\text{Red} \qquad\qquad \text{Colorless} \qquad \text{Blue}$$

When an acid is added to a solution of litmus, the equilibrium is shifted to the left and the red color is seen. When a base is added, this raises the pH, the concentration of hydroxide ion increases, and the concentration of hydrogen (hydronium) ions decreases, shifting the equilibrium to the right, forming the blue product.

The best indicator for an acid–base titration is one that undergoes a color change at the equivalence point. For example, in titrating ammonium hydroxide with hydrochloric acid, an acidic salt (ammonium chloride) is produced. An indicator such as bromcresol green, which changes color at a pH of about 4.8, would be appropriate. Because a small volume of titrant causes a large pH change near the equivalence point, the exact pH at the transition point of the indicator is not critical.

POLYPROTIC ACID AND BASE TITRATIONS

A polyprotic acid has more than one hydrogen atom available to react with the base. Each hydrogen atom has its own equivalence point. The graph in Figure 1.95 shows a titration curve for the titration of phosphoric acid, H_3PO_4, with sodium hydroxide. Notice that there are three equivalence points, one for each hydrogen.

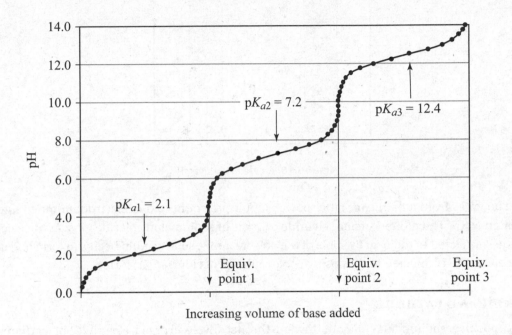

Figure 1.95. Polyprotic acid titration

REDOX TITRATION

A redox titration involves an oxidation–reduction reaction rather than an acid–base neutralization. It is possible to calculate the concentration of an unknown by comparing it with a known solution. The concentration of either the oxidizing or reducing agent must be known. In an acid–base titration, the reaction is monitored with either a pH meter or an acid–base indicator, whereas in a redox titration, either a potentiometer or a redox indicator is used.

ELECTROCHEMISTRY

Batteries have been used as a means of storing potential energy for over two hundred years. Electrochemical potentials exist across cell membranes and are heavily involved in cellular communication, nerve and muscle signaling, and many other biological processes. An **electrochemical cell** is a system in which electrodes are submerged in electrolytes, and in which a chemical reaction either results in or is a result of an electric current. Electrochemical cells that generate current are called voltaic or **galvanic cells**, whereas those that use electric current are called **electrolytic cells**.

Electrolytic Cells

An **electrolytic cell** is an electrochemical cell in which the reaction is driven by the application of electrical current. Electrolytic cells are widely used in the production of pure metals. A simple electrolytic cell is shown in Figure 1.96.

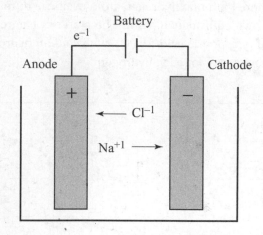

Figure 1.96. An electrolytic cell

TIP

For an electrolytic cell, just remember an ox and a red cat!

<u>ox</u>idation takes place at the <u>an</u>ode

reduction takes place at the <u>c</u>athode

The wires from a battery or other power supply are connected to electrodes dipped into molten NaCl. The molten sodium chloride consists of sodium and chloride ions. At the electrode connected to the negative pole of the power supply, solid sodium begins to form and at the electrode connected to the positive pole, bubbles of chlorine gas form.

ANODE AND CATHODE

The positive sodium ions migrate toward the negatively charged electrode, or **cathode**. Because the sodium ions are gaining electrons, they are being reduced. The process taking place at the negative electrode is

$$2Na^{+1} + 2e^- \rightarrow 2Na$$

The process taking place at the positive electrode, or **anode**, is

$$Cl^{-1} \rightarrow Cl_{2(g)} + 2e^-$$

The negative chloride ions migrate toward the positive electrode or anode. The chloride ions are losing electrons, so they are being oxidized.

TIP

OPPOSITE CHARGES ATTRACT

Plus moves toward minus.

Minus moves toward plus.

OXIDATION AND REDUCTION AND THE FLOW OF ELECTRONS

In all electrochemical cells, **oxidation** occurs at the anode and **reduction** takes place at the cathode. Electroplating of metals onto other surfaces is a common application of electrolysis, as is obtaining purified elements. Galvanizing is the process by which a metal such as zinc is plated onto or used to coat a more reactive metal.

In aqueous solutions of electrolytes, the reactions are not limited to the formation of pure elements. The products of electrolysis also include hydrogen or hydroxide ions, hydrogen or oxygen gas, or water.

TIP

LEO SAYS GER

Remember that LEO says GER; losing electrons is oxidation and gaining electrons is reduction.

Stoichiometry of Electrolysis and Faraday's Law

In the electrolysis of sodium chloride, when one mole of electrons reacts with one mole of sodium ions, one mole of elemental sodium is formed. Quantities of electrons cannot be weighed like quantities of compounds. Instead the amount of electrical current is measured. The charge on one mole of electrons is known as one Faraday. One Faraday is 96,500 coulombs of charge.

For any circuit with a flowing of electric current:

Electric charge = electric current × time current flows

Coulombs   =   Amperes   ×   seconds

When a solution of copper(II) sulfate is electrolyzed, copper metal is deposited at the cathode:

$$Cu^{+2}_{(aq)} + 2\,e^- \rightarrow Cu_{(s)}$$

Practice Question

If a current of 0.060 amperes is used for 5 hours, what mass of copper metal will be deposited?

Solution: The amount of charge was 0.060 amperes × 18,000 seconds = 1080 Coulombs. This gives $1080 \text{ Coulombs} \times \dfrac{1\text{ Faraday}}{96{,}500\text{ Coulombs}} = 0.0112$ Faradays (or 0.0112 moles of electrons).

$$0.0112 \text{ moles electrons} \times \frac{1\text{ mole Cu}}{2\text{ moles electrons}} = 0.00556 \text{ moles Cu}$$

$$0.00556 \text{ moles Cu} \times \frac{63.6\text{ g Cu}}{1\text{ mole Cu}} = 0.353 \text{ g Cu}$$

Galvanic (Voltaic) Cells

A **voltaic** or **galvanic** cell consists of two **half-cells** electrically connected to each other. Each half-cell is an oxidation or reduction reaction. A half-cell can be made by placing a strip of metal (an electrode) in an aqueous solution of its metal ion, such as a zinc strip in a zinc nitrate solution. In a galvanic cell, the two half-cells are connected through a **salt bridge** to allow an electric current to flow between the two electrodes. A salt bridge consists of a gel with an ionic compound dissolved in it. This allows for electron flow to complete a circuit but prevents the solutions from mixing. One metal will have a greater tendency to lose electrons than the other and a flow of electrons, or current, will result.

In any galvanic cell the electrode at which oxidation takes place is called the anode, and the electrode at which reduction takes place is the cathode. The definitions of anode and cathode are based on the gaining and losing of electrons, not whether the electrodes are positive or negative.

An example of two half-cells connected via a salt bridge is shown in Figure 1.97.

TIP

ELECTROLYTIC CELLS

Electrolytic cells convert electrical energy into chemical energy.

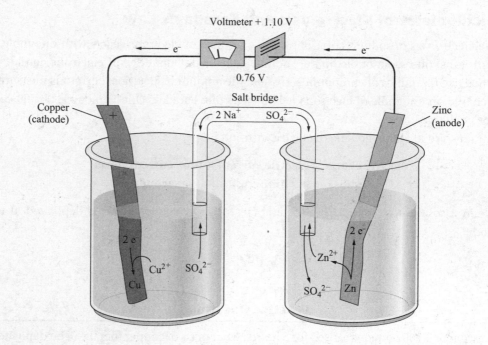

Figure 1.97. Galvanic cell

In this galvanic cell, electrons are flowing from the zinc anode (remember that electrons are lost at the anode) to the copper cathode. The voltmeter is not a necessary part of the cell, although a complete circuit is. Copper ions combine with electrons at the copper electrode, depositing copper metal and zinc metal to form zinc ions. The mass of the zinc electrode would decrease and the mass of the copper electrode would increase.

CELL NOTATION AND SHORTHAND

The following shorthand is used to describe the cell above.

$$Zn_{(s)} \mid Zn^{+2}_{(aq)} \parallel Cu^{+2}_{(aq)} \mid Cu_{(s)}$$

In this notation, the anode (oxidation half cell) is always written on the left and the cathode (reduction half cell) is always written on the right. The salt bridge is indicated by the symbol ‖.

The shorthand notation

$$Tl_{(s)} \mid Tl^{+1}_{(aq)} \parallel Sn^{+2}_{(aq)} \mid Sn_{(s)}$$

indicates a cell with a thallium anode and a tin cathode. The oxidation reaction at the anode is

$$Tl_{(s)} \rightarrow Tl^{+1}_{(aq)} + e^-$$

and the reduction at the cathode is

$$Sn^{+2}_{(aq)} + 2e^- \rightarrow Sn_{(s)}$$

By balancing the electrons (in this case doubling the thallium half-reaction) the overall reaction can be determined. A more detailed summary of a cell also specifies the concentrations of the aqueous species and the pressure of any gases that are involved.

REDUCTION POTENTIALS

Moving electrons through a wire requires the expenditure of energy or the performance of work. In moving water through pipes, the spontaneous process is for water to flow from a higher to a lower gravitational potential (downhill). For electrons, the comparable process is for electrons to move spontaneously from a higher **electrical potential** to a lower one. The potential difference is the difference in electric potential (electrical pressure) between two points. This potential difference is measured in **volts**. This means that

$$\text{electrical work} = \text{charge} \times \text{potential difference}$$

or

$$\text{joules} = \text{coulombs} \times \text{volts}$$

The maximum work that an electrical cell can do is given by the equation

$$W = -nFE_{cell}$$

where n is the number of moles of electrons in the balanced half-reactions, F is the Faraday constant, and E is the cell potential or voltage.

A cell has a voltage of 0.082 V and the balanced ionic equation is

$$Hg_2^{+2}{}_{(aq)} + 2H_{2(g)} \leftrightarrow 2\,Hg_{(l)} + 2\,H^+{}_{(aq)}$$

The two half-reactions are

$$Hg_2^{+2}{}_{(aq)} + 2e^- \rightarrow 2\,Hg_{(l)}$$

$$H_{2(g)} \rightarrow 2H^+{}_{(aq)} + 2\,e^-$$

Because each half-reaction involves the transfer of two electrons, $n = 2$.

The maximum work is 2 moles $e^- \times$ 96,500 C/mole $e^- \times$ 0.082 V = 1.6×10^4 J per mole of hydrogen gas.

Cell emf and Standard Electrode (emf) Potentials

An **electromotive force (emf)** is a measure of the chemical force of an electrochemical cell's reaction. The reaction actually takes place as two half-reactions; an oxidation and a reduction. The general forms of these are:

Reduced substance $\rightarrow$ Oxidized substance + ne^- (oxidation at the anode)

Oxidized substance + $ne^- \rightarrow$ Reduced substance (reduction at the cathode)

Each half-reaction contributes to the driving force of the reaction. These forces are called **potentials**, and the cell's emf is the sum of the two half-reactions' forces.

A **reduction potential** measures the tendency of an oxidized species to gain electrons and become reduced. The opposite process of a reduction half-reaction is an oxidation half-reaction. By convention, half-reactions are listed in tables according to their reduction potentials. The oxidation potential of a half-reaction is the opposite of the reduction potential.

TIP

OXIDATION AND REDUCTION

Every oxidation must be accompanied by a reduction.

**OXIDIZING AND
REDUCING AGENTS**

Substances that
are reduced act as
oxidizing agents.
Substances that
are oxidized act as
reducing agents.

In the galvanic cell shown in Figure 1.98, the two half-cells involve zinc and silver. The zinc is being oxidized and the silver is being reduced. The half-reactions for the cell are:

$$Zn_{(s)} \mid Zn^{+2}_{(aq)} \parallel Ag^{+1}_{(aq)} \mid Ag_{(s)}$$

$$Zn_{(s)} \rightarrow Zn^{+2}_{(aq)} + 2e^-$$

and

$$Ag^{+1}_{(aq)} + e^- \rightarrow Ag_{(s)}$$

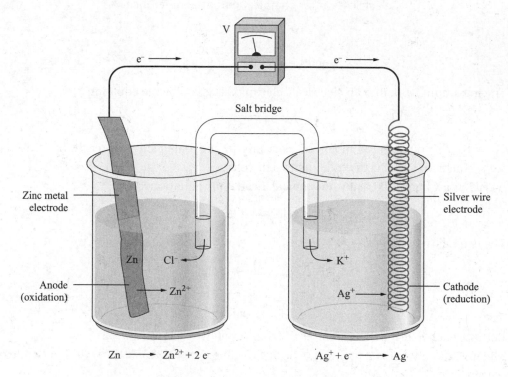

Figure 1.98. Zinc-silver galvanic cell

Because each reduction must be paired with an oxidation, two oxidations, as written above, cannot take place in the same cell. To get the cell potential (emf or voltage) the oxidation reaction must be reversed to give a reduction reaction. The cell voltage or emf will then be:

$$E_{cell} = E_{cathode} - E_{anode}$$

To get the numerical values of cell voltages, a table of standard reduction potentials is used. The table is written as reduction reactions. To get an oxidation reaction, the reaction must be reversed, which means the sign on the emf is reversed as well. For the reaction above, the emf values for the reduction reactions are:

$$Zn^{+2}_{(aq)} + 2e^- \rightarrow Zn_{(s)} \quad E = -0.76 \text{ V}$$

$$Ag^{+1}_{(aq)} + e^- \rightarrow Ag_{(s)} \quad E = +0.80 \text{ V}$$

To turn the Zn reaction into an oxidation (because zinc is the anode), reverse the reaction and the sign to get:

$$Zn_{(s)} \rightarrow Zn^{+2}_{(aq)} + 2e^- \quad E = +0.76 \text{ V}$$

The two half-reactions can then be combined to give 1.56 V. The silver reaction must be doubled to give two electrons. This does not affect the cell voltage.

The standard electrode potential is the electrical potential of a half-cell at 1 atm of pressure, 25°C and in 1.0 M solutions. Table 1.30 is an abridged version of the table of standard reduction potentials.

Table 1.30 Standard Reduction Potentials

Reduction Half-Reaction	Emf (V)
$Mg^{+2}_{(aq)} + 2e^- \rightarrow Mg_{(s)}$	−2.38
$Sn^{+2}_{(aq)} + 2e^- \rightarrow Sn_{(s)}$	−0.14
$Fe^{+3}_{(aq)} + 3e^- \rightarrow Fe_{(s)}$	−0.04
$2H^+_{(aq)} + 2e^- \rightarrow H_{2(g)}$	0.00
$Ag^{+1}_{(aq)} + e^- \rightarrow Ag_{(s)}$	+0.80
$Hg^{+2}_{(aq)} + 2e^- \rightarrow Hg_{(l)}$	+0.85
$F_{2(g)} + 2e^- \rightarrow 2F^-_{(aq)}$	+2.87

In all tables, cell emf's are compared to the hydrogen reduction potential, which is defined as 0.00 V at standard conditions.

Calculating a Cell Voltage

For an electrochemical cell involving tin and silver, the half-reaction with the more negative reduction potential (in this case the Sn) is reversed and the two half-reactions added. This is the same thing as

$$E_{cell} = E_{cathode} - E_{anode}$$

and in this case would give $E_{cell} = 0.80 \text{ V} - (-0.14 \text{ V}) = +0.94 \text{ V}$.

TEST QUESTION

Consider an electrochemical cell that uses lithium and iron:

$Li^+ + e^- \rightarrow Li$	$E° = -3.05 \text{ V}$
$Fe^{+2} + 2e^- \rightarrow Fe$	$E° = -0.44V$

What is the standard voltage for this cell?

(A) 2.61 V

(B) 3.49 V

(C) 5.61 V

(D) 6.54V

(A) Both half-reactions are given as reductions, so one of them (the more negative value) must be "flipped" to give an oxidation half-reaction. The fact that the lithium half-reaction must be doubled to make the electrons balance is not relevant to the voltage calculation.

Interpreting emf Values (Relating to K_{eq}, ΔG, and Spontaneity)

A cell voltage that is positive indicates a spontaneous reaction, as the cell is written. This means that a positive value is associated with a galvanic cell. A negative cell voltage indicates a nonspontaneous process, or an electrolytic cell, which requires the input of energy to make the reaction occur.

> **CELL VOLTAGE AND SPONTANEITY**
>
> Positive voltage = spontaneous (galvanic)
>
> Negative voltage = nonspontaneous (electrolytic)

TIP

APPLYING $\Delta G = -nFE$

Memorizing this equation is less important than understanding the significance of the positive and negative signs on the two terms.

A negative ΔG indicates that a reaction is spontaneous and a positive emf indicates that an electrochemical reaction is spontaneous. The equation that relates the two is:

$$\Delta G = -nFE$$

This means that both the free energy and the emf of a cell represent the maximum amount of work that can be done by the reaction at standard conditions.

Because a positive cell voltage indicates a spontaneous reaction, the following relationships exist:

If $K_{eq} = 1$, $\Delta G = 0$, $E^\circ = 0$, system is at equilibrium

If $K_{eq} < 1$, $\Delta G > 0$, $E^\circ < 0$, reaction is nonspontaneous

If $K_{eq} > 1$, $\Delta G < 0$, $E^\circ > 0$, reaction is spontaneous

Practice Question

Is the reaction $Al_{(s)} + Mg^{+2}_{(aq)} \rightarrow Mg_{(s)} + Al^{+3}_{(aq)}$ spontaneous at standard conditions?

$$Al^{+3}_{(aq)} + 3e^- \rightarrow Al_{(s)} \quad E^\circ = -1.66 \text{ V}$$

$$Mg^{+2}_{(aq)} + 2e^- \rightarrow Mg_{(s)} \quad E^\circ = -2.37 \text{ V}$$

Solution: To solve this problem, you must obtain the emf for each half-reaction, as written in the balanced equation. In the reaction, aluminum is oxidized, so the equation and the voltage must be reversed. This gives the following half-reactions:

$$Al_{(s)} \rightarrow Al^{+3}_{(aq)} + 3e^- \quad E^\circ = +1.66 \text{ V}$$

$$Mg^{+2}_{(aq)} + 2e^- \rightarrow Mg_{(s)} \quad E^\circ = -2.37 \text{ V}$$

TIP

GALVANIC VS. ELECTROLYTIC CELLS

Galvanic cells are spontaneous as written.

Electrolytic cells are nonspontaneous as written.

Adding the two half-reactions gives the overall reaction and a cell voltage of -0.71 V. As written, the reaction is not spontaneous, K_{eq} is less than one, and ΔG_{rxn} is positive. The reaction could happen as an electrolytic cell, with the input of energy. Note that because emf is an intensive property, it is not necessary to balance the overall equation in order to determine spontaneity.

EFFECT OF CONCENTRATION ON EMF VALUES

Up to now, all the calculations have been done assuming solution concentrations are at 1.0 M (one of the elements of standard conditions). In many situations, that is not the case. The Nernst Equation allows the cell emf to be calculated when concentrations are not standard.

Recall that the reaction quotient is an expression analogous to the equilibrium constant but is not necessarily at equilibrium. For a reaction

$$a\text{A} + b\text{B} \rightarrow c\text{C} + d\text{D}$$

$$Q = \frac{[\text{D}]^d [\text{C}]^c}{[\text{A}]^a [\text{B}]^b}$$

The Nernst equation is:

$$E_{\text{cell}} = E° - \frac{RT}{nF} \ln Q$$

TIP

THE SUPERSCRIPT SYMBOL °

The superscript ° indicates standard states.

SUMMARY

The general chemistry questions on the MCAT stress an understanding of the main concepts studied in a first-year inorganic chemistry course, and emphasize thinking and problem-solving. Many of the calculations on the MCAT can be worked out with estimations rather than attempting an exact answer. For example, in stoichiometric calculations, look for whole-number ratios. Therefore, if a substance such as sulfuric acid, H_2SO_4, has a molar mass of 98 g/mole, you can estimate 3 moles as 300 grams.

Be familiar with Avogadro's number and some common multiples of it (¼, ½, and 2 moles, for example) and the same for the molar volume of a gas at STP (22.4 L/mole). Look for inverse relationships, such as when pressure doubles, the volume is halved. It may not be necessary to know the names of the gas laws, but you should know what the laws state. For example, you should know Boyle's law, but it is not critical to remember that it is called Boyle's law.

By reviewing all the concepts in this chapter, paying attention to the test hints and tips, and working through the sample problems, you will be prepared for the general chemistry questions on the MCAT. All of the chemistry topics you will see on the MCAT have been covered and appear in sample questions.

> **DIRECTIONS:** This Chemistry test contains three passages. Each passage is followed by a series of questions. Read the passage, and then choose the one answer that is best. Some questions are not based on a passage or each other. If you are not sure of an answer, eliminate the answer choices that you think are wrong and choose one of the remaining answers. You can refer to the periodic table on page 36 at any time.

PASSAGE I

Extremophiles are bacterial species that live under conditions that would be fatal to most other organisms. Sulfur-metabolizing bacteria can use sulfur as an electron acceptor in the process of generating ATP. Among the chemicals that many extremophiles can live with and even depend on are those shown in Table 1.

Table 1 Chemicals that Extremophiles Can Tolerate

Name	Formula
Sulfur dioxide	SO_2
Methane	CH_4
Methanol	CH_3OH
Hydrochloric acid	HCl
Ammonia	NH_3
Iron(III) hydroxide	$Fe(OH)_3$
Carbon monoxide	CO

Some of these extremophiles can survive in pH ranges of greater than 10 and less than 3, conditions that would be lethal to the majority of cells. Some halophilic species can grow in salt concentrations of 0.3 M. Most analyses of the metabolic processes used by extremophiles come from carbon-14 and sulfur-33, isotopes used as tracers to follow metabolites from these bacteria.

1. Dissolving which of the chemicals from Table 1 in water would produce an alkaline (basic) environment?
   (A) $FeCl_3$
   (B) NH_3
   (C) CH_3OH
   (D) SO_2

2. Hydrogen bonding can allow which of the compounds from Table 1 to dissolve in water?

    I. CH_4

    II. CH_3OH

    III. NH_3

    (A) I only

    (B) II only

    (C) I and III

    (D) II and III

3. How does an atom of sulfur-33 differ from an atom of sulfur-32?

    (A) The sulfur-33 atom has one more neutron and has different chemical properties.

    (B) The sulfur-33 atom has one more electron and has different chemical properties.

    (C) The sulfur-33 atom has one more neutron and has the same chemical properties.

    (D) The sulfur-33 atom has one less neutron and has the same chemical properties.

4. A species of bacteria found in a 10 L solution that has 0.01 moles of HCl would be in an environment with what pH?

    (A) 0.001

    (B) 3.0

    (C) 10.0

    (D) 11.0

5. Which of the following has the same geometry as a carbon tetrachloride, CCl_4, molecule?

    (A) Silicon tetrafluoride

    (B) Xenon tetrafluoride

    (C) Sulfur tetrafluoride

    (D) Dinitrogen tetroxide

6. What would be the expected pH of the products of the reaction of equal volumes of 0.1 M solutions of hydrochloric acid and iron(III) hydroxide?

    (A) 1

    (B) 4

    (C) 8

    (D) 11

PASSAGE II

Scenario 1

In 1911, Ernest Rutherford performed a series of classic experiments in which he directed positively charged alpha particles (composed of two protons and two neutrons) at a thin sheet of gold foil. In his experiments, Rutherford observed that most of the alpha particles traveled through the gold foil unaffected but that a small portion of them deflected away at large angles. Rutherford used this experimental evidence to develop a new model of the atom, one in which a small positive nucleus occupied the center of the atom.

Scenario 2

The foil Rutherford originally used was gold, although he was able to replicate his results with other metal foils. The piece of gold Rutherford used had dimensions of about 5 cm $\times$ 4 cm and a mass of roughly 0.040 g. Gold has a density of 19.3 g/cm^3. By calculating the area of the foil and using the mass and density to determine the volume of the foil, it is possible to divide the volume in cm^3 by the area in cm^2 to get the thickness of the foil.

7. What results would Rutherford have obtained regarding the deflection of particles if he had directed neutrons toward the gold foil instead of alpha particles?
   (A) About the same fraction of neutrons would have been deflected because the size of the nucleus would not have changed.
   (B) A greater fraction of neutrons would have been deflected because neutrons have no charge and are unaffected by the neutral atoms of gold.
   (C) A smaller fraction of neutrons would have been deflected because neutrons are unaffected by the positive nuclei.
   (D) Most neutrons would have been able to enter the nucleus, forming different isotopes of gold.

8. Which of the following would not have been able to be substituted for gold in the Rutherford experiment?
   (A) Silicon
   (B) Platinum
   (C) Copper
   (D) Silver

9. What is the approximate thickness of the gold foil used by Rutherford?
   (A) 1×10^4 cm
   (B) 1×10^{-4} cm
   (C) 1×10^{-2} cm
   (D) 1×10^{-6} cm

10. A student determines the thickness of a foil of aluminum as 1×10^{-3} cm. Aluminum atoms have an atomic radius of about 100 pm (1×10^{-10} m). Approximately how many atoms thick is the foil?

(A) 2×10^5

(B) 1×10^5

(C) 5×10^4

(D) 2×10^3

11. The nucleus of the atom is best described as:

(A) small (compared to the total volume of the atom) and positive.

(B) small (compared to the total volume of the atom) and negative.

(C) large (compared to the total volume of the atom) and positive.

(D) large (compared to the total volume of the atom) and negative.

PASSAGE III

Many artificial flavorings are made by esterification. These reactions are widely used in the food and cosmetics industries.

Experiment 1

In a trial, a food chemist combined 0.500 grams of ethyl alcohol (molar mass = 46 g/mole) with 0.750 grams of butyric acid (molar mass = 88 g/mole) in a 100.0 ml volume in the presence of a sulfuric acid catalyst to produce ethyl butyrate (molar mass = 116 g/mole), which gives the flavor and aroma of pineapples.

The reaction is as follows:

$$CH_3CH_2OH_{(aq)} + CH_3CH_2CH_2COOH_{(aq)} \xrightarrow{H^+} CH_3CH_2CH_2COOCH_2CH_{3(aq)} + H_2O_{(l)}$$

Experiment 2

In this experiment, the chemist varied the concentrations of starting materials and found the relative amounts of products and reactants formed in order to determine the equilibrium constant.

12. What is the molarity of the butyric acid in the solution at the start of the experiment?

(A) 0.0085 M

(B) 0.066 M

(C) 0.085 M

(D) 0.66 M

13. Which of the following is the expression for the equilibrium constant (K_{eq}) for the reaction shown above?

(A) $$\frac{[CH_3CH_2CH_2COOCH_2CH_3][H_2O]}{[CH_3CH_2OH][CH_3CH_2CH_2COOH]}$$

(B) $$\frac{[CH_3CH_2CH_2COOCH_2CH_3]}{[CH_3CH_2OH][CH_3CH_2CH_2COOH]}$$

(C) $$\frac{[CH_3CH_2OH][CH_3CH_2CH_2COOH]}{[CH_3CH_2CH_2COOCH_2CH_3][H_2O]}$$

(D) $$\frac{[CH_3CH_2CH_2COOCH_2CH_3]}{[CH_3CH_2OH]+[CH_3CH_2CH_2COOH]}$$

14. Increasing which of the following would result in the formation of the greatest amount of ethyl butyrate?
(A) Water, H_2O
(B) Ethyl butyrate, $CH_3CH_2CH_2COOCH_2CH_3$
(C) Sulfuric acid, H_2SO_4
(D) Butyric acid, $CH_3CH_2CH_2COOH$

15. In analyzing the reaction, it is found that the reaction is first order with respect to each reactant. The rate constant, k, would have what units?
(A) $M \, sec^{-1}$
(B) sec^{-1}
(C) $M^{-1}sec^{-1}$
(D) $M^{-2} \, sec^{-1}$

16. What mass of ethyl butyrate will be formed in the reaction?
(A) 0.986 g
(B) 1.26 g
(C) 1.76 g
(D) 2.25 g

The following questions do not refer to a descriptive passage and are not related to each other.

17. Given the following data:

$Zn^{+2} + 2e^- \rightarrow Zn_{(s)}$ $E° = +.76V$
$Au^{+3} + 3e^- \rightarrow Au_{(s)}$ $E° = +1.50 \text{ V}$

What is the cell electrode potential for the reaction below?

$2Au^{+3} + 3Zn_{(s)} \rightarrow 2Au_{(s)} + 3Zn^{+2}$

(A) −0.74 V
(B) +0.74 V
(C) + 2.26 V
(D) + 5.28 V

18. If the volume of a gas at 3.0 atm and 27°C is 450 ml, what volume will the gas occupy at 6.0 atm and 327°C?
(A) 225 ml
(B) 450 ml
(C) 900 ml
(D) 2700 ml

19. Some characteristics of the hydrogen halides are summarized in the table below.

Compound	Boiling Point (°C)	State of Matter at Room Temperature and Pressure
HF	+20	liquid
HCl	−85	gas
HBr	−67	gas
HI	−35	gas

Which of the following best explains the differences in states of matter and boiling point between hydrogen fluoride and the other substances?
(A) Fluorine is the smallest halogen, so the hydrogen and fluorine atoms are closer together.
(B) Fluorine is the most electronegative atom, so the HF bond is stronger.
(C) HF can undergo hydrogen bonding.
(D) Fluorine atoms use only s and p orbitals to form bonds, whereas the other halogens can use available d orbitals.

20. Which of the following is the most electronegative?
    (A) Hydrogen
    (B) Oxygen
    (C) Carbon
    (D) Bromine

21. When an electron in a hydrogen atom emits a photon and moves from the fourth energy level to the second energy level, a photon of blue-green (486 nm) light is emitted. Which of the following electron transitions would result in the emission of a photon of red light?
    (A) 3 to 2
    (B) 5 to 2
    (C) 5 to 1
    (D) 6 to 1

22. Which of the following pairs of chemicals would produce a buffer?
    (A) HCl and NaCl
    (B) HCl and HF
    (C) HF and NaF
    (D) NaF and NaOH

ANSWER KEY

1. B		**6.** B		**11.** A		**16.** A		**21.** A	
2. D		**7.** C		**12.** C		**17.** B		**22.** C	
3. C		**8.** A		**13.** B		**18.** B			
4. B		**9.** B		**14.** D		**19.** C			
5. A		**10.** C		**15.** C		**20.** B			

ANSWERS EXPLAINED

1. **(B)** Ammonia is a weak base. Sulfur trioxide is an acidic anhydride, which means that when it reacts with water, it forms an acid. Methanol has an OH group, but on an organic molecule this makes it an alcohol and not a base. $FeCl_3$ is an acidic salt.

2. **(D)** Alcohols, such as CH_3OH, can interact with water via hydrogen bonds. Ammonia, NH_3, a polar molecule, can interact with water through hydrogen bonds. Methane, CH_4, a nonpolar molecule, cannot interact with water. The presence of a hydrogen atom by itself does not mean that a compound can form hydrogen bonds.

3. **(C)** The number after the name of the isotope is the mass number. Because isotopes differ in number of neutrons, a sulfur-33 atom has a mass number one greater than sulfur-32 because it has one more neutron. Isotopes of an atom have the same chemical properties.

4. **(B)** The molarity of the solution is 0.01 moles divided by 10 L, or 0.001 M. Hydrochloric acid is a strong acid and is 100% dissociated in water. This makes the hydronium ion concentration 1×10^{-3} M and the pH equal to $-\log(1 \times 10^{-3}) = 3.0$.

5. **(A)** The geometry of a molecule depends on the number of bonds and lone pairs around the central atom. Both silicon tetrafluoride (SiF_4) and methane have 4 bonds and no lone pairs. The other compounds may have 4 bonds, but the presence of lone pairs gives them a different geometry.

6. **(B)** The reaction of HCl and $Fe(OH)_3$ will produce water and $FeCl_3$, iron(III) chloride, an acidic salt. The pH of this salt will be above that of the pure acid but well below the neutral pH of 7.0.

7. **(C)** Because neutrons have no charge, they would not be repelled as they came very close to the nucleus. Only those neutrons that actually hit the nucleus would be deflected. Because the nucleus is very small, the odds of this event taking place are very small.

8. **(A)** A malleable metal that can be made into very thin foils is needed for this experiment.

9. **(B)** Estimating the density of gold as 20 g/cm^3, the volume of the gold foil is equal to the mass of the foil (0.04 g) divided by the density (20 g/cm^3). This gives a volume of 0.002 cm^3. Because volume is equal to length times width times height, and the area of the foil is given (20 cm^2), the height (or thickness) is 0.002 cm^3/20 $cm^2 = 0.0001$ cm or 1×10^{-4} cm.

10. **(C)** The number of atoms is equal to the total thickness divided by the diameter (not radius) of a single atom, which equals 1×10^{-3} cm or $(1 \times 10^{-5}$ m)/$(2 \times 10^{-10}$ m), yielding 5×10^4 atoms.

11. **(A)** The passage states that the nucleus of the atom is positively charged and takes up a very small portion of the total size of the atom.

12. **(C)** The molarity of the solution is the number of moles of butyric acid per liter. The number of moles of butyric acid is

$$0.75 \text{ g} \times \frac{1.0 \text{ mole}}{88 \text{ g}} = 0.0085 \text{ moles}/0.1 \text{ L} = 0.085 \text{ moles/L or } 0.085 \text{ M}$$

13. **(B)** The equilibrium constant for a system is the concentration of each product raised to the power of its coefficient over the concentration of each reactant raised to the power of its coefficient. Liquids and solids are not included in equilibrium constant expressions.

14. **(D)** This is an application of Le Châtelier's principle. Increasing the concentration of one of the reactants will shift the equilibrium to the right, producing more ethyl butyrate.

15. **(C)** The reaction is first order with respect to both butyric acid and ethyl alcohol, making it second order overall. The units for a second order reaction's rate constant are $M^{-1}\text{sec}^{-1}$.

16. **(A)** Because the mass of each reactant is given, this is a limiting reagent problem. Butyric acid is the limiting reagent because there are fewer moles of this reactant and the two reactants are in a one-to-one ratio.

$$0.75 \text{ g butyric acid} \times \frac{1 \text{ mole butyric acid}}{88 \text{ g}} \times \frac{1 \text{ mole ethyl butyrate}}{1 \text{ mole butyric acid}} \times \frac{116 \text{ g ethyl butyrate}}{1 \text{ mole ethyl butyrate}}$$

$$= 0.98 \text{ g ethyl butyrate}$$

17. **(B)** The less positive reaction must be "flipped around" and the sign of its voltage reversed before adding the two equations.

18. **(B)** The doubling of the pressure would halve the volume, whereas the doubling of the kelvin temperature (from 300 K to 600 K) would double the volume, resulting in no net change.

19. **(C)** Hydrogen bonding increases the attractive forces between molecules, making them less likely to evaporate or boil. The other statements are factually correct (F is the most electronegative element and the smallest halogen) but they do not explain the high boiling point, which depends on intermolecular forces.

20. **(B)** The most electronegative atoms tend to be in the upper right of the table (excluding the noble gases), with F having the highest value.

21. **(A)** Red light has a lower energy than blue-green light, so the electron transition must involve less energy than from $n = 4$ to $n = 2$. Transitions to energy level 1 are part of the Lyman series and tend to emit UV light, which is more energetic.

22. **(C)** A buffer is produced from a mixture of a weak acid or base and a salt of that weak acid or base, so that there is a common ion.

For online practice, go to
http://barronsbooks.com/tp/mcat

Physics 2

- → MATH AND UNITS OF MEASUREMENT
- → MOTION, FALLING BODIES, AND PROJECTILES
- → FORCES (INCLUDING FRICTION)
- → MASS AND WEIGHT
- → WORK, ENERGY, AND POWER
- → TORQUE AND EQUILIBRIUM
- → FLUIDS
- → MECHANICAL WAVES AND SOUND
- → SIMPLE HARMONIC MOTION
- → ELECTROSTATICS
- → DC CIRCUITS
- → CAPACITANCE
- → ELECTROMAGNETISM
- → REFLECTION, REFRACTION, POLARIZATION, AND DIFFRACTION
- → MIRRORS AND LENSES
- → ATOMS AND NUCLEI

Achieving success on MCAT Physics questions requires a good grasp of concepts and the ability to do any required mathematics rapidly and accurately. Physics is more mathematics-oriented than chemistry or biology. Therefore, the chapter begins with a math review.

MATH AND UNITS OF MEASUREMENT
Math Strategies

You cannot use a calculator on the MCAT. However, most calculations on the test are simple enough that they do not require a calculator. If you find yourself trying to do involved calculations, look for another approach. Strategies such as estimation and simplification can lead you to the correct answer. Many powerful math strategies are covered in the introduction to this book.

> **3-4-5 RIGHT TRIANGLE**
>
> Remember the 3-4-5 right triangle, with the side of length 5 as the hypotenuse:
>
> $$3^2 + 4^2 = 5^2$$
>
>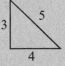

Standard Deviation

Without a calculator it is very difficult to calculate the classic standard deviation. However, an approximate standard deviation can be found rather quickly. Take the following data points: 2.97, 2.99, 3.01, and 3.03. Adding them and then dividing the total by the number of data points (4) gives an average of 3.00. Adding up the deviations between the average and each point—0.03, 0.01, 0.01 and 0.03—and dividing by the number of data points produces a "standard deviation" of 0.02. This is not the classic standard deviation calculation but it is a good approximation and probably all you would need for any exam question. The answer written in standard deviation format is 3.00 ± 0.02. The percentage error is just 2 parts in 300, or 0.7% error.

A good round number to remember is that for a normal distribution of data, 68% of the data lie within one standard deviation of the mean. Also, 95% of the data lie within two standard deviations and 99.7% lie within three standard deviations.

Significant Figures

In doing calculations, keep to the appropriate number of significant figures. Simply put, if data you are given is reported to three significant figures, use three or possibly four significant figures to do calculations. When the calculations are complete, present the answer to three significant figures. In the problem above on standard deviation, the answer is expressed correctly because it reflects significance in the original data to the second decimal place.

Working with Units

CANCELING UNITS

If you multiply $\frac{2}{3} \times \frac{3}{5}$, the 3's canceled because there is 3 on top and 3 on the bottom. In the same way, units can cancel. $\frac{60 \text{ miles}}{\text{hour}} \times \frac{24 \text{ hours}}{\text{day}}$ yields units of miles per day. The units *hours* have canceled out. Consider the following:

$$\frac{550 \text{ miles}}{\text{hour}} \frac{5280 \text{ feet}}{\text{mile}} \frac{1 \text{ meter}}{3.28 \text{ feet}} \frac{1 \text{ hour}}{60 \text{ min}} \frac{1 \text{ min}}{60 \text{ sec}} = 246 \text{ meters/sec}$$

By carefully identifying and factoring out units, you can avoid many errors. Double check what units your answer should be in. If, for example, you are trying to calculate velocity, the answer must be in units of distance over units of time, such as kilometers over hours.

TEST QUESTION

A mass of 20,000 g has an acceleration of 400 cm/s². The net external force is:

(A) 0 N

(B) 50 N

(C) 80 N

(D) 8 million N

(C) You should switch to units that will produce an answer in newtons. Rewrite 20,000 g as 20 kg and 400 cm/s² as 4 m/s². Notice that the multiplication (*ma*) is much easier, giving 80 kg · m/s², which is 80 N. The answer is C.

COMMON UNITS

Units are usually written in SI (the International System of Units, the modern standardization of the metric system), also called the m-kg-s system, and have the basic units of meter, kilogram, and second. Occasionally quantities are written in the c-g-s system: centimeter, gram, and second. Table 2.1 defines the basic units and some derived units. Velocity is an example of a derived unit, meters/second, or m/s.

Table 2.1 SI Units

Unit	Name and Symbol	Equivalent
Length	meter (m)	
Mass	kilogram (kg)	
Time	second (s)	
Force	newton (N)	$kg \cdot m/s^2$
Energy	joule (J)	$N \cdot m$
Momentum		$kg \cdot m/s$
Power	watt (W)	J/s
Charge	coulomb (C)	
Potential	volt (V)	J/C
Current	ampere (A)	C/s
Resistance	ohm (Ω)	V/A
Capacitance	farad (F)	C/V
Magnetic field	tesla (T)	$N/A \cdot m$

Table 2.2 lists common metric prefixes that should be committed to memory:

Table 2.2 Common Metric Prefixes

Prefixes	Value	Standard Form	Symbol
Tera	1,000,000,000,000	10^{12}	T
Giga	1,000,000,000	10^9	G
Mega	1,000,000	10^6	M
Kilo	1000	10^3	k
deci	0.1	10^{-1}	d
centi	0.01	10^{-2}	c
milli	0.001	10^{-3}	m
micro	0.000001	10^{-6}	μ
nano	0.000000001	10^{-9}	n
pico	0.000000000001	10^{-12}	p

Graphing

CARTESIAN COORDINATE SYSTEM

You should be able to recognize the shapes of the graphs of certain common equations on a Cartesian coordinate system. Table 2.3 shows various algebraic functions, the general shapes of their graphs, and hints for rapidly graphing or visualizing the function. Figure 2.1 illustrates some of these shapes.

Table 2.3 Equations and Their Graphs

$y = mx + b$	**Straight line:** Slope m, y-intercept b.
$y = ax^2 + bx + c$	**Parabola:** The basic parabola $y = x^2$ opens upward, is symmetric about the *y-axis* and has minimum at $(0, 0)$. The a changes the shape (sharper or flatter), the c moves the curve up or down, and the b moves the curve left or right.
$y = x^3$	**Cubic curve:** The y increases rapidly with increasing x, and decreases rapidly with decreasing x.
$y = x^{\text{higher power}}$	**Higher power curves:** Even power curves look like parabolas. Odd power curves look like cubic curves.
$(x - a)^2 + (y - b)^2 = r^2$	**Circle:** The basic circle; $x^2 + y^2 = r^2$ is centered about the origin and has radius r. The form shown is for a circle centered at (a, b).
$\dfrac{x^2}{a^2} + \dfrac{y^2}{b^2} = 1$	**Ellipse:** This is a circle stretched in the x or y direction depending on the constants. The x's and y's may be written in the $(x - a)$ or $(y - b)$ form.
$\pm ax^2 \mp by^2 = c$	**Hyperbola:** Note the different signs for the terms. Hyperbolas consist of two parts that open either up and down or right and left.

Relationships involving logarithms or exponents can often be graphed using a system other than the Cartesian coordinate system.

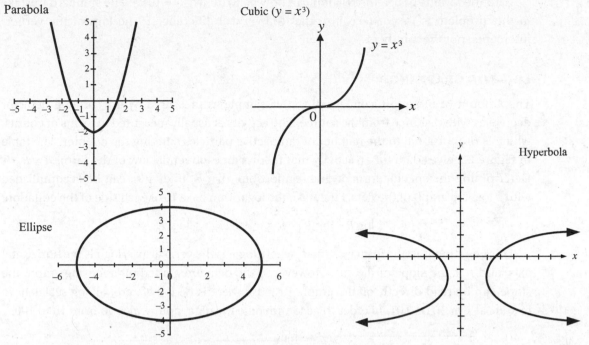

Figure 2.1. Illustrations of four graphs

LOG–LINEAR GRAPHING

For a mathematical relation of the form $y = 10^{\lambda t}$, graphing on what is known as log–linear paper has certain advantages. The 10^{λ} can be written as 2^{α} or e^{β} or any number raised to a power. Using 10 is convenient for the next step of taking the logarithm to the base 10 of both sides.

$$\log_{10} y = \lambda t \log_{10} 10 \quad (\log_{10} 10 = 1) \quad \log_{10} y = \lambda t$$

Graphing log y versus t produces a line of slope λ. When the four data points in the table are graphed on log-linear graph paper, that is, y versus t, the resulting line will have slope λ (see Figure 2.2).

TIP

NATURAL LOGS

Log base e is the natural log, symbol ln.

The value of e is close to 2.7.

t	y
0.5	1.6
1.0	2.5
1.5	4.0
2.0	6.3

$$\text{slope} = \frac{\log 8 - \log 2}{1.5}$$

$$\text{slope} = \frac{0.6}{1.5} = 0.4$$

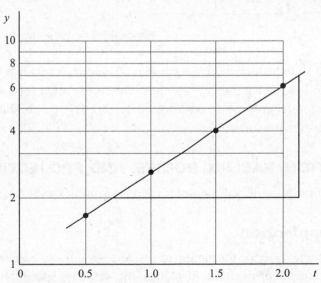

Figure 2.2. Log–linear graph

With the λ value of 0.4, the relation can now be written as $y = 10^{0.4t}$. The standard mistake in this problem is to not recognize that the vertical difference is the logs of the vertical intercepts, not the numbers.

LOG–LOG GRAPHING

The amount of radiation from a radioactive sample as measured by a fixed-area detector decreases with distance from the source. The activity is usually measured in terms of counts, which is proportional to the number of radioactive particles entering the counter. The table in Figure 2.2 gives data for an activity that follows an exponential law of the form, $R = R_0 r^n$. Determining the specific form of this relationship, that is, finding n, can be accomplished with a log–log graph of the data. First, take the logarithm base 10 of each side of the equation.

$$\log R = \log R_0 + \log r^n = n \log r + \log R_0$$

This equation is in the form $y = mx + b$, where $\log R$ is the vertical axis, $\log r$ is the horizontal axis, and n is the slope of the line. However, if the data are plotted on a log–log graph, the slope can be read directly off the graph. Because there is no log of zero, all log scales have to start at 1 or 10 or 0.01. In order to accommodate the data, both scales go from 10 to 100.

Counts	Distance
100	10 cm
25	20 cm
11	30 cm

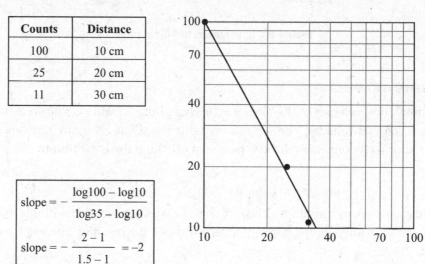

$$\text{slope} = -\frac{\log 100 - \log 10}{\log 35 - \log 10}$$

$$\text{slope} = -\frac{2 - 1}{1.5 - 1} = -2$$

Figure 2.3. Log–log graph

The slope as shown on the graph is –2, and the specific relationship is $R = R_0 r^{-2}$, making this an inverse square law, which is what is expected for a spherically symmetric radiator being intercepted by a fixed-area detector. The graph shows that a distance of 15 cm produces a little over 50 counts.

MOTION, FALLING BODIES, AND PROJECTILES

This topic requires the most math of all the physics sections.

Linear Motion

In order to describe the motion of a particle (whether a baseball, a golf ball, or gas molecules) the concepts of **position**, **displacement**, **velocity**, **speed**, and **acceleration** are important. The change in position is called **displacement**.

DISPLACEMENT

Displacement is the shortest distance between the starting point and the ending point of a particle or body. Displacement is different from distance traveled. If a person travels 3 miles north and then 4 miles east, the total distance traveled is 7 miles, but the displacement, or distance from initial position to final position, is 5 miles. Displacement is a vector.

VELOCITY AND SPEED

Velocity is defined as the displacement between two points divided by the time taken to travel between the points. Velocity is a vector quantity, meaning it has both magnitude and direction. Speed is a scalar, meaning it has magnitude only.

Vectors are quantities that have both magnitude and direction. For example, a velocity would be specified as 300 km/hr north or 300 km/hr at an angle of 30 degrees north of east. **Scalars** are quantities that include only magnitude. Speed would be simply 300 km/hr. For an object traveling in a circle (for example, the moon orbiting Earth), the speed may be constant but the velocity is changing because the direction of motion is changing.

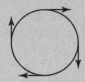

CHANGING MOTION

Changing motion has changing velocity.

An object in circular motion can have a constant speed, but it has changing velocity because velocity is a vector. When adding vectors, the vector sum is not the simple addition of the magnitudes of the vectors.

TEST QUESTION

A force of 3 N acts north on an object and a force of 4 N acts east. What is the magnitude of the resultant force?

(A) 7N

(B) 5N

(C) 1N

(D) –1N

(B) In this case, you would use the Pythagorean theorem to find the hypotenuse of the triangle. The resultant force is 5 N. The answer is B.

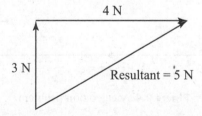

VECTORS AND SCALARS

Vectors: velocity, acceleration, displacement

Scalars: speed, distance, mass, time

ACCELERATION

Acceleration is defined as the difference in velocity divided by time. On the MCAT, problems involving acceleration will deal only with constant acceleration. You will not see problems in which acceleration is not constant. There are four equations governing constant acceleration (**kinematic** equations) and they should be memorized.

1. $v = v_0 + at$

2. $x - x_0 = \dfrac{v_0 + v}{2} t$

3. $x - x_0 = v_0 t + (1/2)at^2$

4. $v^2 = v_0^2 + 2a(x - x_0)$

In these equations, v represents velocity, a is acceleration, t is time, and x is position. The first three equations involve time, and the fourth one is a combination of the others with time eliminated. A subscript 0 (zero) indicates an initial velocity or initial position of zero. A v or x without a subscript 0 is the final velocity or position.

Acceleration Equations Using Time. The following are some problems that use the three equations involving time.

Practice Question

Consider a car that accelerates from rest to 60 m/s in 7.5 s. Find the assumed constant acceleration and the distance traveled.

Solution: First diagram the situation. Diagrams are very helpful. They need not be elaborate. They need to contain just the information that helps in solving the problem. Figure 2.4 is an example.

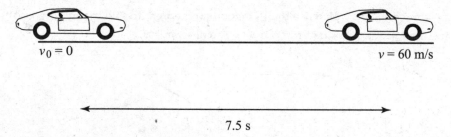

$v_0 = 0$ $v = 60$ m/s

7.5 s

Figure 2.4. Acceleration problem

To find the acceleration: We know the initial and final velocities (v_0 and v) and the time, t. We need to find a. The first equation contains all of these variables.

$$v = v_0 + at$$

$$60 \text{ m/s} = v_0 + a(7.5 \text{ s})$$

$$a = \frac{60 \text{ m/s}}{7.5 \text{ s}} = 8.0 \text{ m/s}^2$$

TIP

FROM REST

The phrase *from rest* means that the initial velocity is zero in the kinematic equations.

The distance can be calculated from:

$$x = x_0 + v_0 t + \frac{1}{2}at^2$$

$$x = 0 + 0 + \frac{1}{2}(8.0 \text{ m/s}^2)(7.5 \text{ s})^2$$

$$x = 225 \text{ m}$$

Alternatively use:

$$v^2 = v_0^2 + 2a(x - x_0)$$

$$\frac{(60 \text{ m/s})^2}{2(8.0 \text{ m/s}^2)} = (x - x_0)$$

$$x - x_0 = 225 \text{ m}$$

Here is another problem that requires calculating the stopping distances for a car.

Practice Question

A vehicle traveling at 10 m/s stops over a distance of 25 m when the brakes are applied. Assuming the deceleration is a constant value, find the magnitude of deceleration.

Solution:

$$v^2 = v_0^2 + 2a(x - x_0)$$
$$0 = 100 + 2a(25)$$
$$a = -2 \text{ m/s}^2$$

The negative sign in the equation indicates deceleration.

Practice Question

A greyhound is one of the fastest land animals. Suppose a greyhound is racing in a 620-meter race. It starts from rest in the starting box and reaches a speed of 20 m/s over a time of 2 seconds. The greyhound then maintains this speed for the rest of the race. The heart rate of a racing greyhound can reach 300 beats per minute.

1. Find the distance traveled by the greyhound in the first 1.5 seconds.
2. How many heartbeats does the greyhound have during the time it is running at top speed?

Solution:

1. To find the distance traveled, use the formula

$$x - x_0 = \frac{v_0 + v}{2} t$$

$$x - 0 = \left(\frac{0 + 20}{2}\right) 2$$

$$x = 20 \text{ m}$$

The greyhound traveled 20 m in the first 1.5 seconds.

2. Since the greyhound traveled 20 meters in the first 2 seconds and the total distance is 620 meters, we know that it needs to travel another 600 meters. The question states that the greyhound maintains a speed of 20 m/s for the rest of the race, which is a constant speed. To find the time, we just use

$$\text{speed} = \frac{\text{distance}}{\text{time}}$$

$$20 \text{ m/s} = \frac{600 \text{ m}}{t}$$

$$t = \frac{600 \text{ m}}{20 \text{ m/s}}$$

$$t = 30 \text{ s}$$

Since the heart rate is 300 beats per minute for half a minute, the answer is 150 heartbeats.

Acceleration Equations without Time. All the examples so far have involved time. However, sometimes the only way to get started on a problem is to use the one **equation of motion that does not contain time** as a parameter.

Practice Question

A dog jumps straight up to a height of 0.8 m. What is the initial velocity of the dog and how long is it in the air?

Solution: Diagram the situation similarly to Figure 2.5.

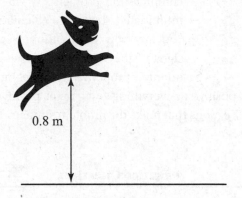

0.8 m

Figure 2.5. Initial velocity

Be careful of the signs! If the dog jumps up with a positive velocity, it reaches maximum height while under a negative (down) acceleration. Keeping the signs correct in motion problems is most important. Small sign mistakes can make your results very wrong. To get started on the problem, realize that the dog leaves the ground with a certain velocity (up), and at the top of the jump it has zero velocity. This zero velocity comes about because of the downward acceleration. Write:

$$v^2 = v_0^2 + 2a\,(x - x_0)$$

$$0^2 = v_0^2 + 2\,(-10\text{ m/s}^2)(0.8\text{ m})$$

$$v_0 = 4.0\text{ m/s}$$

To find the time the dog takes to get to the top of his jump (0 final velocity) use

$$v = v_0 + at$$

$$0 = 4.0\text{ m/s} - 10\text{ m/s}^2 t$$

$$t = 0.4\text{ s}$$

The dog leaves the ground with velocity 4.0 m/s and is in the air 0.8 s (up and down).

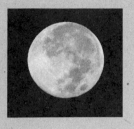
Falling Bodies

Falling body problems are one category of constant acceleration problems. Because they are easy to visualize, falling body problems offer the best opportunity for mastering constant acceleration. For MCAT purposes, consider the acceleration of gravity to be 10 m/s².

In falling body problems, and in constant acceleration problems in general, there are two things to keep in mind that will make the problems easier. First, some problems are worded in such a way that it is difficult to see how to complete the problem. When this happens, do not be intimidated. Try some calculations and see if they give you any new information. Second, keep the algebraic signs of the velocities, acceleration, and displacements oriented properly. This does not mean to always orient everything to the right as positive or everything going up as positive. It means looking at the problem and setting up directions that make the problem simpler. This skill is especially useful in projectile problems.

Practice Question

A ball is falling from the top of a 34-meter tall building. How long does it take the ball to reach the ground? What is the velocity of the ball when it reaches the ground?

Solution: Diagram the situation as in Figure 2.6 and associate the appropriate equations on the diagram.

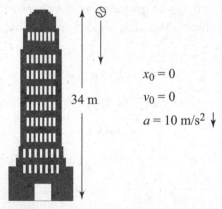

34 m

$x_0 = 0$
$v_0 = 0$
$a = 10$ m/s² ↓

Figure 2.6. Acceleration due to gravity

In this problem it is important to orient the coordinate system so that the origin is at the top of the building. This orientation makes displacement, velocity, and acceleration all positive in the down direction. If you were to place the origin of the coordinate system on the ground and make the displacement positive in the upward direction, the ball would start at +34 m and move in the negative direction. The velocity and acceleration would also be negative. This would make the problem harder.

Use a kinematic equation to find the time to reach the ground,

$$x = x_0 + v_0 t + (1/2)at^2$$

$$34 \text{ m} = 0 + 0t + (1/2)(10 \text{ m/s}^2)t^2$$

$$t = 2.6 \text{ s}$$

and similarly the velocity when it reaches the ground.

$$v = v_0 + at$$

$$v = 0 + (10 \text{ m/s}^2)(2.6 \text{ s}) = 26 \text{ m/s}$$

A safer calculation of velocity is from the equation relating velocity, acceleration, and displacement.

$$v^2 = v_0^2 + 2a(x - x_0)$$

$$v^2 = 0 + 2(10 \text{ m/s}^2)(34 \text{ m})$$

$$v = 26 \text{ m/s}$$

This is a safer calculation because it uses original information. If you made a mistake in calculating t and used the incorrect number in the next equation, then that calculation of the velocity would be incorrect. Using an equation that requires original information is the safer way to proceed.

Adding an initial velocity to the ball falling from the top of a building adds an interesting complication to the problem.

Practice Question

A ball is thrown up from the top of a 40-meter tall building with an initial velocity of 10 m/s.

1. How long does it take for the ball to rise to its maximum height and return to the roof level (on the way down)?
2. What is the maximum height above the building?

Solution: The origin for the coordinate system is best placed at the top of the building (Figure 2.7). The final displacement is down, the velocity when the ball hits the ground is down, and the acceleration is down. For this reason, the most convenient positive direction is down.

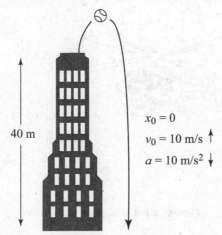

40 m

$x_0 = 0$
$v_0 = 10 \text{ m/s} \uparrow$
$a = 10 \text{ m/s}^2 \downarrow$

Figure 2.7. Acceleration due to gravity, with a variation

The question about the time for the ball to rise to maximum height and return to the roof (level) is best done in two parts. The ball starts up at 10 m/s and goes to 0 m/s at maximum height. Use a simple velocity relation to find this time.

$$v = v_0 + at$$

$$0 = -10 \text{ m/s} + (10 \text{ m/s}^2)t$$

$$t = \frac{10 \text{ m/s}}{10 \text{ m/s}^2} = 1.0 \text{ s}$$

The flight must be symmetric. The acceleration is the same, and the fourth equation works on the way up and on the way down to the roof level. The time to go to maximum height is 1 second and the time to return to the roof level is 1 second. The velocity on the way down is numerically equal to the initial upward velocity. The maximum height is derived from the velocity equation without the time.

$$v^2 = v_0^2 + 2a(x - x_0)$$

$$0^2 = (-10 \text{ m/s})^2 + 2(10 \text{ m/s})(x - x_0)$$

$$x - x_0 = -\frac{100 \text{ m/s}^2}{20 \text{ m/s}^2} = -5.0 \text{ m}$$

It makes sense for x to be negative because we defined the downward direction as positive and x is an upward height.

Another popular falling body problem is one in which something is being dropped from a rising or falling platform, such as a camera or bottle of champagne from a balloon or helicopter.

Practice Question

You are in a helicopter rising at a constant velocity of 8 m/s. At a height of 40 meters, you drop your camera. If it takes 3.7 seconds for the camera to hit the ground, what is the height of the helicopter when the camera hits the ground?

Solution: Diagram the problem, as in Figure 2.8, taking the origin of the coordinate system at the point at which the camera leaves the helicopter and the positive direction down, and label the initial conditions.

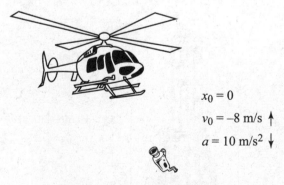

$x_0 = 0$

$v_0 = -8 \text{ m/s} \uparrow$

$a = 10 \text{ m/s}^2 \downarrow$

Figure. 2.8. Falling body problem

It takes 3.7 seconds for the camera to reach the ground. In this 3.7 seconds, the helicopter moves up (8 m/s)(3.7 s) = 30 m. The helicopter is 40 + 30 = 70 m above the ground when the camera hits the ground.

Projectile Motion

In projectile problems the motion is analyzed in two perpendicular directions, one oriented in the direction of the acceleration and the other perpendicular to the first. Projectile motion (trajectory) is parabolic. Understanding the symmetry property of parabolas is essential to understanding projectile motion.

The equations needed for projectile problems are the kinematic equations of motion used in the above sections. The coordinate systems must be arranged so the acceleration is a constant nonzero value in one direction and zero in the other direction.

Practice Question

A soccer ball is kicked at 30° with respect to the horizontal at an initial velocity of 12 m/s. Find the range, maximum height, and time of flight.

Solution: Diagram the problem as in Figure 2.9 and take the origin of the x-y coordinate system at the point where the ball is kicked. This is a good place to set $t = 0$.

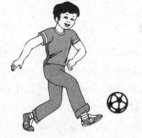
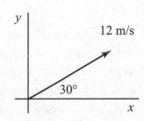
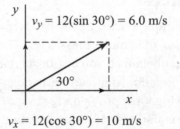

Figure 2.9. Projectile motion

The acceleration due to gravity is in the (negative) y-direction and there is no acceleration in the x-direction. The velocity components are as calculated in Figure 2.10. Now write the equations for acceleration, velocity, and position in the two directions.

$$a_x = 0 \qquad\qquad a_y = -10 \text{ m/s}^2$$

$$v_x = 10 \text{ m/s} \qquad\qquad v_y = 6.0 \text{ m/s} - \frac{1}{2}(10 \text{ m/s}^2)t$$

$$x = (10 \text{ m/s})t \qquad\qquad y = (6.0 \text{ m/s})t - (5.0 \text{ m/s}^2)t^2$$

As with most kinematics problems, calculate the time of flight first. The time of flight comes out of the equation for y, and is obtained by setting y equal to zero, corresponding to the ball on the ground, and solving for t.

$$0 = 6t - 5.0t^2 = t(6 - 5.0t)$$

The time is 0 as the ball is just leaving the ground, and at 6/5.0 = 1.2, the ball is back on the ground. The time of flight then is 1.2 seconds.

TIP

PERPENDICULAR COMPONENTS

The x- and y-components of velocity are independent of one another. A change to one component cannot affect a perpendicular component.

The range, the distance the ball travels in the x-direction is equal to the value of x at 1.2 s or

$$x\big|_{1.2} = (10 \text{ m/s})(1.2 \text{ s}) = 12 \text{ m}$$

The maximum height occurs when v_y is zero.

$$0 = 6 - 10t$$

$$t = \frac{6}{10} = 0.60$$

This produces a value for t of just one-half of the time of flight. This is one of the symmetry properties of parabolas. The time for maximum height is one-half the time of flight for any parabolic motion. The height at this point is from the $y = \ldots$

$$y\big|_{t=0.6s} = (6.0 \text{ m/s})(0.6 \text{ s}) - (5.0 \text{ m/s}^2)(0.6 \text{ s})^2 = 1.8 \text{ m}$$

Review the steps through the problem and note how the coordinate system is set up and then how the six equations of motion are written.

Review all the problems, paying particular attention to the procedure. Projectile problems are not difficult if the coordinate system is made for convenience in doing the problem and the acceleration, velocity, and position statements are written for each direction.

FORCES (INCLUDING FRICTION)

In the previous section we reviewed the relationships between position, velocity, and constant acceleration. Now we will consider the forces that produce constant acceleration.

Forces

In simple terms, forces cause masses to accelerate. To be more precise, it is unbalanced forces that make masses accelerate. The basic law is $F = ma$, where F is understood as an unbalanced force. Constant forces produce constant accelerations, the only kind of acceleration that can be handled with the equations of motion. The general strategy for solving force problems is to relate a force to an acceleration through $F = ma$ and then apply the equations of motion to determine velocities and positions.

ATWOOD'S MACHINE

A simple force problem involving masses and a pulley system is known as an Atwood's machine. This simple two-mass, one-pulley system is a good problem for reviewing forces.

Practice Question

For the system shown below, find the acceleration and the tension (force) in the cord.

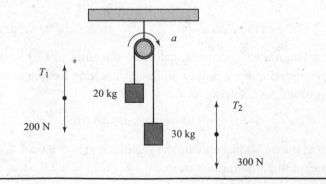

Solution: Looking at the figure and ignoring the force vectors, estimate that the system moves clockwise (because the mass on the right is larger). As systems become more complicated, estimation is less likely to be correct. In forces without friction—as long as you are consistent in writing the $F = ma$ equations—an incorrect estimate of the direction of motion will simply result in a negative acceleration, which tells you that the motion was in the other direction.

Now construct the force vectors. The force of gravity acts down on each of the masses so add the vectors

$$(10 \text{ m/s}^2)(20 \text{ kg}) = 200 \text{ N}$$

$$(10 \text{ m/s}^2)(30 \text{ kg}) = 300 \text{ N}$$

There is tension in the cord that is constant throughout the cord and acts in an upward direction on both masses. A tension is a force and if a force meter were inserted anywhere in the cord, it would read the same in both directions. Add these (force) tension vectors to the diagram and label them T_1 and T_2. In this problem it is not necessary to label the tensions with two distinct labels, but it helps in keeping track of the equations and is a good habit to develop for more complicated problems. Add an arrow indicating your best guess as to the direction of the acceleration.

If the acceleration is clockwise, then the 20 kg mass goes up and the 30 kg mass goes down. For this assumption, write the unbalanced force equations for the two masses.

$$T_1 - 200 \text{ N} = (20 \text{ kg})a$$

$$300 \text{ N} - T_2 = (30 \text{ kg})a$$

Study these equations of motion and follow the logic of how they are written, especially the algebraic signs. A mistake here is probably your only source of error in the problem.

Now, $T_1 = T_2$, so add the equations to obtain

$$100 \text{ N} = (50 \text{ kg})a$$

$$a = 2.0 \text{ m/s}^2$$

The tension in the string is from either equation. Use

$$T = 200 \text{ N} + (20 \text{ kg})(2.0 \text{ m/s}^2) = 240 \text{ N}$$

INCLINED PLANES

Many force problems involve inclined planes.

Single inclined planes. The problem below involves a single inclined plane.

Practice Question

Find the acceleration and the tension in the cord for a simple 30° inclined plane with 30 kg and 50 kg masses connected over a pulley as shown in the figure below.

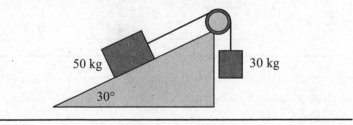

Solution: Guessing at the direction of the acceleration is not as simple in this problem. A wrong guess will be revealed by a negative result, so simply make a best guess for now. Choose counterclockwise as the direction of acceleration and proceed with the force vectors. The 30 kg mass presents no problem. For the 50 kg mass we need the component of the gravitational force down the plane. This is something unique to inclined plane problems. The force vectors are as shown in the **free body** diagram in Figure 2.10. The term *free body diagram* is used to describe a diagram in which (1) simple shapes or dots are used to represent an object and (2) all the forces acting on the object are drawn as vectors.

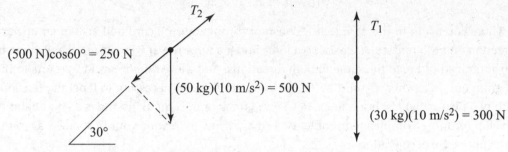

Figure 2.10. A free body diagram

Start construction of this diagram with the 500 N gravitational force. The component of the 500 N down the plane is 250 N. Assuming the counterclockwise rotation, write:

$$250 \text{ N} - T_2 = (50 \text{ kg})a$$

$$T_1 - 300 \text{ N} = (30 \text{ kg})a$$

Again, $T_1 = T_2$, so add the two equations.

$$-50 \text{ N} = (80 \text{ kg})a$$

$$a = -0.62 \text{ m/s}^2$$

The negative sign means the acceleration is clockwise. Now find the tension in the cord.

$$T = 300 \text{ N} + (30 \text{ kg})(-0.62 \text{ m/s}^2) = 281 \text{ N}$$

Double inclined planes. Now consider double inclined planes.

Practice Question

A double inclined plane with 30° and 45° angles and 20 kg and 35 kg masses is arranged as in the figure below. What is the acceleration of the system and what is the tension in the cord?

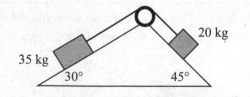

Solution: Take the rotation direction to the left and write the force vector diagrams. Place the force vectors due to gravity (the 200 N and 350 N forces) first, then calculate the components down the incline (Figure 2.11).

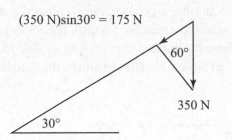

(350 N)sin30° = 175 N

60°

350 N

30°

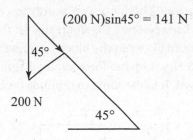

(200 N)sin45° = 141 N

45°

200 N

45°

Figure 2.11. Force vector diagram 1

Now add the tension in the cord and draw another force vector diagram (Figure 2.12).

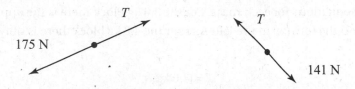

T

175 N

T

141 N

Figure 2.12. Force vector diagram 2

Remember that the rotation is assumed to the left, and write the unbalanced force causing the acceleration of each of the masses. Add the two equations to eliminate the tension, and calculate the acceleration.

$$175 \text{ N} - T = (35 \text{ kg})a$$

$$T - 141 \text{ N} = (20 \text{ kg})a$$

$$34 \text{ N} = (55 \text{ kg})a$$

$$a = 0.62 \text{ m/s}^2$$

The tension in the cord is

$$T = 141 \text{ N} + (20 \text{ kg})(0.62 \text{ m/s}^2) = 153 \text{ N}$$

BLOCK PROBLEMS

Block and cord problems. Two blocks connected by a cord with one block pulled by an accelerating force present an interesting variation on force problems.

Practice Question

Two masses with a cord between them are pulled by a force F of 25 N as shown in the following figure. What is the acceleration of the system and what is the tension in the cord between the blocks?

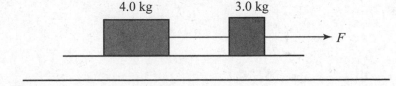

4.0 kg   3.0 kg

F

TIP

ANGLE OF INCLINE

If the angle of incline is specified with respect to the horizontal, the component of weight acting parallel to the surface of the plane is *mg sinθ.*

Solution: There are two points to consider before starting any calculations. First, the two blocks accelerate together; that is, they have the same acceleration. Second, the tension in the cord between the blocks is probably different from the applied force. For an applied force of 25 N, set up the force vector diagram as shown in Figure 2.13. The tension in the cord is as shown. It is the same magnitude on both blocks.

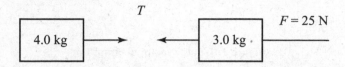

Figure 2.13. Force vector diagram

Write $F = ma$ equations for each mass. For the 3.0 kg block there is the applied force of 25 N to the right and the tension to the left. And for the 4.0 kg block there is only the tension to the right.

$$T = (4.0 \text{ kg})a$$

$$25 \text{ N} - T = (3.0 \text{ kg})a$$

Adding the two equations produces the statement that the applied force of 25 N acts to accelerate both masses. This statement allows calculation of the acceleration and then, using the first equation, the tension in the cord.

$$25 \text{ N} = (7.0 \text{ kg})a$$

$$a = \frac{25 \text{ N}}{7.0 \text{ kg}} = (3.6 \text{ m/s}^2)$$

$$T = (4.0 \text{ kg})(3.6 \text{ m/s}^2) = 14 \text{ N}$$

Multiple-block problems. Variations of this type of problem involve three or more blocks, multiple blocks on a double inclined plane, and multiple blocks with the accelerating force supplied by a mass that is hanging and is acted on by gravity. The key concepts for these problems are that (1) the accelerating force, whatever it may be, pulls all the masses together and (2) the tensions between the various blocks are different. Knowing this, set up force vector diagrams for each block, using all the tensions, and solve the equations.

Only one block pushed. In another type of force problem, only one block is pushed by an applied force. An example is shown in Figure 2.14.

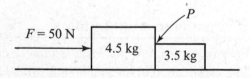

Figure 2.14. One block pushed by an applied force

Practice Question

TIP

$F = ma$

It takes more force to accelerate 8 kg than it does to provide the same acceleration to 3.5 kg.

One block of 4.5 kg mass is in contact with another block of 3.5 kg mass, with the two being pushed in the direction of larger block to smaller block with a force of 50 N on the larger block. What is the acceleration of the system and the force between the blocks?

Solution: In this situation, both blocks accelerate together, so the $F = ma$ statement for the system is straightforward. However, the force P between the blocks is not the same as the applied force. If it were, the smaller mass block would accelerate away from the larger mass ($F = ma$), a situation that clearly does not happen. The applied force accelerates both blocks, so write:

$$50 \text{ N} = (8.0 \text{ kg})a$$

$$a = 6.2 \text{ m/s}^2$$

The force, P, between the blocks is the force to make the 3.5 kg block accelerate at this rate.

$$P = (3.5 \text{ kg})(6.2 \text{ m/s}^2) = 22 \text{ N}$$

The analysis for this type of problem is much like that for blocks pulled by cords between them. First, find the acceleration of the system, and then work on the tensions in the cords or force between the blocks.

Frictional Forces

Adding frictional forces to force problems makes them more complicated. The following two points will help.

1. Frictional forces are less than or equal to μN, the coefficient of friction times the normal force (the force perpendicular to the surface).
2. Frictional forces always oppose the motion.

Friction is encountered in many problems. The discussion here serves to illustrate some of the techniques and some of the pitfalls typically encountered in working problems involving frictional forces.

The simplest illustration of frictional force is pulling a box along a floor.

Practice Question

Place a 4.0 kg or 40 N block on a floor where the coefficient of friction between block and floor is 0.6, and apply a 180 N force to push the block as shown in the figure below. Calculate the acceleration of the box. In working friction problems, be careful not to mix newtons and kilograms.

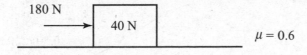

180 N

40 N

$\mu = 0.6$

Solution: The force to the right is 180 N and the frictional force to the left has a maximum value of 24 N (0.6 times 40 N). The applied force is greater than the frictional retarding force. Therefore, the unbalanced force to the right is 156 N. The block accelerates to the right at 156 N over 4.0 kg, or 39 m/s^2.

A single inclined plane with friction involves most of the features found in friction problems.

Practice Question

A single 30° inclined plane with coefficient of friction 0.50 has a 30 kg mass on the incline and a 60 kg hanging mass, as shown in the following figure. What is the acceleration of the system?

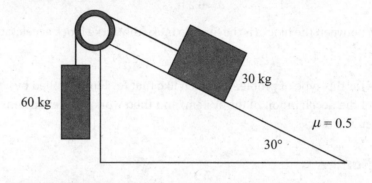

Solution: First resolve the force components for the 30 kg mass into forces down the plane and normal to the plane (Figure 2.15).

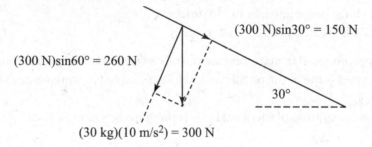

Figure 2.15. Force components

Draw the force vector diagram for the 60 kg mass attached to the cord. Assume counterclockwise rotation and draw the vector diagram for the 30 kg mass. If the system is moving counterclockwise, the frictional force must be down the incline (Figure 2.16).

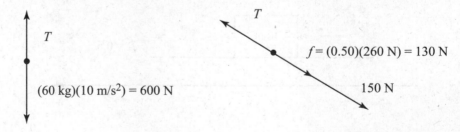

Figure 2.16. Force vector diagram

Now write the equations.

$$600 \text{ N} - T = (60 \text{ kg})a$$

$$T - 130 \text{ N} - 150 \text{ N} = (30 \text{ kg})a$$

$$320 \text{ N} = (90 \text{ kg})a$$

$$a = 3.6 \text{ m/s}^2$$

A positive acceleration shows that this is the correct solution. If the acceleration had been chosen as clockwise, then the vector diagram would have been as in Figure 2.17.

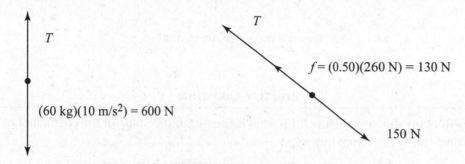

Figure 2.17. Vector diagram

And the equations would have been

$$T - 600 \text{ N} = (60 \text{ kg})a$$

$$150 \text{ N} - 130 \text{ N} - T = (30 \text{ kg})a$$

$$-580 \text{ N} = (90 \text{ kg})a$$

$$a = -6.4 \text{ m/s}^2$$

A negative result for acceleration means that the acceleration direction was chosen incorrectly. Be careful with this in friction problems. You cannot just say the system acceleration is in the other direction because if it does accelerate in the other direction, the frictional force has to be reversed and the acceleration recalculated. For example, with a negative result, such as –6.4 in this case, the correct answer is not necessarily 6.4 in the other direction. Furthermore, in certain cases, such as when the forces involved are not enough to overcome the friction, the coefficient of friction is greater or the angle of the forces different, the system will not move. If the acceleration comes out negative for both directions, this is an indication that the system will not move.

Some friction problems will ask not for the acceleration or tension in the cord but for the minimum coefficient of friction to prevent the system from moving. A typical problem of this type involves a block on a friction surface, with a cord to a wall and with an additional weight on the cord, as shown in Figure 2.18.

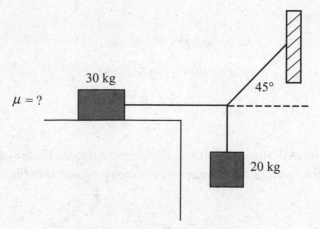

Figure 2.18. Friction block problem

Practice Question

For the situation shown in Figure 2.16, what is the minimum value of the coefficient of friction to keep the system from moving?

Solution: In this situation there are two tensions, T_2 in the horizontal cord and T_1 in the cord going from the junction of the cords up to the wall. The force vectors shown in Figure 2.19 are for a static situation but they are determined in much the same way as for earlier examples.

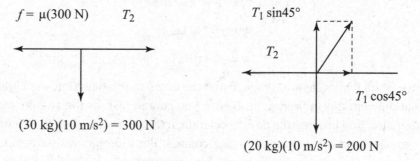

Figure 2.19. Force vectors

Using these diagrams, write the equations.

$$T_1\sin45° = 200 \text{ N}$$

$$T_1 = \frac{200 \text{ N}}{\sin45°} = 283 \text{ N}$$

At this point, it should be easy to see that $T_1\sin45° = T_1\cos45° = 200 \text{ N} = T_2$. So the calculation of the friction coefficient is

$$\mu(300 \text{ N}) = 200 \text{ N}$$

$$\mu = 0.67$$

The minimum coefficient of friction to prevent the system from moving is 0.67.

Gravitation

The basic law of gravity prescribes the force one mass exerts on another. For two masses the attraction between them is given by

$$F = G\frac{m_1 m_2}{r^2}$$

where G is a universal constant, m_1 and m_2 are the masses, and r is the separation of their centers. In SI units, the gravitational constant $G = 6.7 \times 10^{-11}$ N·m²/kg. The gravitational force is an action-reaction force acting along the line connecting the centers of the two masses.

The force of attraction for a relatively small mass on Earth is

$$F = G\frac{m_{earth}}{r_{earth}^2}m = (10 \text{ m/s}^2)m \text{ or } mg$$

The term **weight** refers to this gravitational force at the surface of Earth. A 90 kg person exerts a 900 N force on Earth's surface.

Practice Question

What is the gravitational force between two 6.0 kg balls of 0.20 m diameter when they are touching?

Solution:

$$F = G\frac{m_1 m_2}{r^2} = 6.7 \times 10^{-11} \text{ N} \bullet \text{m}^2/\text{kg}^2 \frac{(6.0 \text{ kg})^2}{(0.20 \text{ m})^2} = 6.0 \times 10^{-8} \text{ N}$$

When working force problems, follow the general procedure used in the examples above.

1. Draw a rough diagram of the situation.
2. Make a separate drawing of the force vectors as they are given or as they are calculated in the course of working the problem.
3. If friction is involved, the calculation is almost always for maximum frictional force. Do not forget that in some problems the direction of the frictional force might have to be reversed, and sometimes friction prevents a system from moving.

MASS AND WEIGHT
Definitions

Mass and **weight** are not the same thing. Consider the definitions below.

The **mass** of an object is loosely defined as the quantity of matter in the object. Operationally, mass is the property that determines the acceleration in the equation $F = ma$. The units of mass are the kilogram (most popular) or the slug. Slug is the mass unit in the British system and is encountered only rarely.

Weight is a force. Consider the example of the weight of a mass on Earth's surface. A mass of 1 kg has a weight of 10 N or 2.2 lb on the surface of Earth. The relationship of mass to weight on Earth's surface follows from the equation $W = mg$, where g is the acceleration due to gravity.

To add to the confusion of weight and mass, if you ask people from Europe or Asia their weight, they will give you an answer in kilograms. If you ask the same question of people from North America or the United Kingdom, they will give you an answer in pounds. One has given the answer in mass units and the other in weight or force units. For even more confusion, in the United States, gold is bought by the gram and rabbit food by the pound!

The easiest example for understanding mass and weight is with the weight of a person standing on Earth.

Practice Question

In the figure below, what is the weight (force) that this 80 kg person exerts on the surface of Earth?

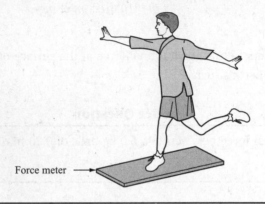

Force meter ⟶

Solution: The weight of the person is the force between the person and Earth or

$$W = mg = (80 \text{ kg})(10 \text{ m/s}^2) = 800 \text{ N}$$

Perhaps this illustrates why people might prefer to say that they weigh 80 kg, instead of 800 N!

Apparent Weight

The best example of apparent weight is what you feel in an accelerating elevator. Accelerating up in an elevator, you feel an additional force between your feet and the floor of the elevator. With a little experimenting you can say that you feel lighter when accelerating downward, heavier when accelerating upward, and normal when the elevator is moving at constant velocity. This acceleration affects the force you exert on the floor of the elevator and leads to what is called *apparent weight*.

Consider the 80 kg person from the above example in an upward accelerating elevator as shown in the figure below. What is the apparent weight of this person?

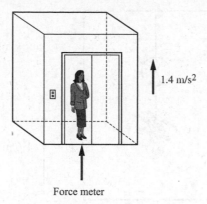

1.4 m/s²

Force meter

(A) 688 N

(B) 800 N

(C) 912 N

(D) 1030 N

(C) The apparent weight of this person is 800 N, already calculated for standing on the surface of Earth, plus the additional weight due to the elevator accelerating up. The apparent weight of this person then—that is, the number that would be read by the force meter—is:

$$W = (80 \text{ kg})(10 \text{ m/s}^2) + (80 \text{ kg})(1.4 \text{ m/s}^2) = 800 \text{ N} + 112 \text{ N} = 912 \text{ N}$$

If the elevator is accelerating downward, you feel lighter. Do this apparent weight calculation a little differently. Simply subtract the downward acceleration from the acceleration due to gravity.

$$W = m \, (g - a) \, (80 \text{ kg})(10 - 1.4) \text{ m/s}^2 = 688 \text{ N}$$

In apparent weight problems the main source of error is in getting the signs wrong. To keep this straight, remember the elevator: accelerating upward, you feel heavier (the force meter reads higher) and accelerating downward, you feel lighter (it reads lower).

The correct answer is C.

Practice Question

A 12 kg plant is hanging in an elevator that is accelerating up at 1.6 m/s^2 on the surface of Mars, where the acceleration due to gravity is 3.7 m/s^2. What is the tension in the cord?

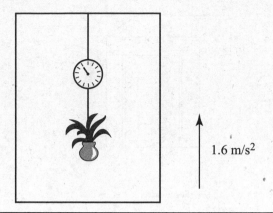

1.6 m/s^2

Solution: In this problem, the tension in the cord is due to the gravity on Mars and the acceleration. Again, think about what happens to the tension when the elevator accelerates up. The tension increases, so

$$W = (12 \text{ kg}) (3.7 + 1.6) \text{m/s}^2 = 63.6 \text{ N}$$

There is another category of apparent weight problem that has to do with sliding down poles or climbing up ropes.

Practice Question

A 70 kg firefighter slides down a pole at an acceleration of 3.0 m/s^2. What is the additional force he exerts on the pole in the downward direction? Take the weight of the pole as 500 N. What is the total force exerted by the pole and firefighter on the ground?

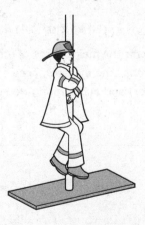

TIP

FREE FALL

In free fall, where the acceleration of the firefighter would be 10 m/s^2, there would be no increased force at the bottom of the pole.

Solution: The acceleration is less than that due to gravity and the firefighter is holding on to the pole or, in other terms, is exerting a force through the pole onto the floor. Remember the way elevators work and follow the logic of the problem. The pole by itself exerts a force between pole and floor of 500 N. If the 70 kg firefighter just held on to the pole, the increase in force at the bottom of the pole would be 700 N, for a total of 1200 N. But the firefighter is not holding on to the pole but accelerating down it.

The additional force then must be somewhere between zero and 700 N. A very small acceleration compared to gravity would mean a small decrease in this additional force whereas a large acceleration would mean a large decrease in the 700 N force. The decrease from 700 N has to be the mass of the firefighter times the acceleration or $(70 \text{ kg})(3.0 \text{ m/s}^2) = 210 \text{ N}$ so the increased force due to the firefighter sliding down the pole with 3.0 m/s^2 acceleration is 700 N – 210 N = 490 N. The total force between pole and floor is then 990 N.

In apparent weight problems, considering extreme situations can keep you from making mistakes. If the firefighter is in free fall and accelerating at 10 m/s^2, there is no compression in the pole. If the firefighter is holding tight to the pole, the firefighter's entire weight adds to the force at the bottom of the pole. A modest acceleration means nearly all the weight of the firefighter is transferred to the force between pole and floor.

The analysis just described can be used in what are known as rope climbing problems. In designing a habitat for an orangutan, suppose the designer specifies a climbing rope that has a breaking strength of 500 N. The designer reasons that since the orangutan is 35 kg, or 350 N, the rope is more than sufficient for the orangutan to climb. The situation is shown in Figure 2.20.

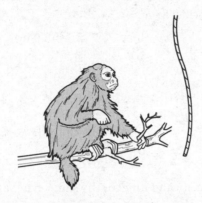

Figure 2.20. A rope climbing problem

However, considering that an orangutan can accelerate up a rope as fast as 6.0 m/s^2, this rope may not be sufficient. As the orangutan accelerates up the rope, there is an additional tension in the rope beyond the 350 N weight of the animal. The calculation of the additional weight due to acceleration up the rope indicates that the total tension could be as high as

$$W = (10 + 6.0)\text{m/s}^2 \ (35 \text{ kg}) = 560 \text{ N}$$

This is beyond the design strength for the rope and clearly will not support the orangutan when it accelerates up the rope.

Practice Question

Consider a 55 kg person in an elevator moving down at a constant velocity of 12 m/s. The elevator is brought to rest with uniform acceleration over 20 m. What is the force between the person and the elevator during the deceleration?

Solution: The 55 kg person moving down in the elevator at a constant velocity experiences normal weight. A force meter between the person and the floor of the elevator would read

$$mg = (55 \text{ kg})(10 \text{ m/s}^2) = 550 \text{ N}$$

When the elevator is brought to rest under the constant acceleration, the force meter will read more than 550 N and by an amount equal to 55 kg times the acceleration. Find the acceleration from the motion equation $v^2 = v_0^2 + 2a(x)$.

$$0^2 = (12 \text{ m/s})^2 + 2a(20 \text{ m})$$

$$a = -\frac{144 \text{ m}^2/\text{s}^2}{40 \text{ m}} = -3.6 \text{ m/s}^2$$

We now have to add 3.6 m/s^2 to the acceleration of gravity, 10 m/s^2, to get the total acceleration for the force on the floor of 13.6 m/s^2. With this acceleration the force exerted on the floor is

$$W = (55 \text{ kg})(13.6 \text{ m/s}^2) = 748 \text{ N}$$

Here is one final insight for problem-solving. On the moon or Mars, where the acceleration due to the local gravity is much less than on Earth, events seem to move slower. The value of g for Mars is 3.7 m/s^2. If an astronaut working on a Martian residence drops a 2.0 kg tool 8.0 m to the Martian surface, the velocity with which the tool hits the surface is, according to the equations of motion, specifically $v^2 = v_0^2 + 2a(x)$.

$$v^2 = 0^2 + 2(3.7 \text{ m/s}^2)(8.0 \text{ m})$$

$$7.7 \text{ m/s}$$

And the time is from

$$v = v_o + at$$

$$7.7 \text{ m/s} = (3.7 \text{ m/s}^2)t$$

$$t = 2.1 \text{ s}$$

Contrast this with the velocity and time for the same event on Earth.

$$v^2 = 0^2 + 2(10 \text{ m/s}^2)(8.0 \text{ m})$$

$$v = 12.6 \text{ m/s}$$

$$v = v_0 + at$$

$$12.6 \text{ m/s} = (10 \text{ m/s}^2)t$$

$$t = 1.3 \text{ s}$$

WORK, ENERGY, AND POWER

You have now reviewed kinematics—the relationship between position, velocity, and acceleration for a mass point—and force, specifically that unbalanced forces make masses accelerate. The next concept for review, **work**, is needed in order to solve problems involving nonconstant forces, forces over a distance, or forces that are time-dependent.

Work

Work is defined simply as force times displacement. More specifically, mechanical work is the component of an applied force in the direction of the displacement times the displacement. The force in a direction parallel to the movement is the only component of the force that contributes to work. Keep in mind that a force such as friction can oppose motion and that you need to calculate the amount of work needed to overcome friction. And also remember that if you push on a large stone and do not move it, then no work is done.

Work can be expressed as the product of the vector *F* times the displacement vector *s* times the cosine of the angle between the force and the displacement.

$$W = F(s \cos \theta)$$

The units of work and energy are N-m (newton-meters), which is equivalent to a joule (J). A joule is the amount of work performed in exerting a force of 1 newton over a distance of 1 meter. Stored energy is also expressed in joules.

A good basic work problem involves moving a box a certain distance along a surface, as shown in the following problem.

Practice Question

If a 70 N force is applied horizontally to a 20 kg mass, moving it (horizontally) 30 m, what is the work performed?

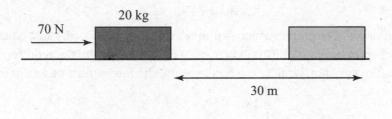

Solution: The work performed by this horizontal force is

$$W = F \cdot s = (70 \text{ N})(30 \text{ m}) = 2100 \text{ N} \cdot \text{m} = 2100 \text{ J}$$

Now try this more complex work problem.

Practice Question

A 30 N force is applied to a 30 kg mass at an angle of 20° to the horizontal with the mass moving horizontally 8.0 m. What is the work done?

Solution: Diagram the problem as in Figure 2.21, with particular attention to the component of the force in the direction of the motion.

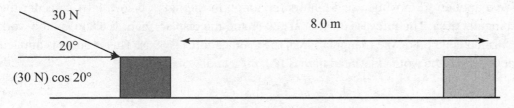

Figure 2.21. A work problem

Work is the force in the **direction of the displacement** times

$$W = (30 \text{ N})(\cos 20°)(8.0 \text{ m}) = 226 \text{ N} \cdot \text{m} = 226 \text{ J}$$

The following problem adds friction.

Practice Question

Find the force applied at 26° above the horizontal necessary to pull a 200 kg crate at constant speed along a surface with coefficient of friction 0.5. Then find the work performed for a 30 m displacement.

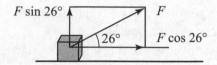

Solution: The constant speed requirement is the key to this problem. For constant speed, the applied force in the direction of the displacement must equal the frictional retarding force. So first find the normal force, which is the weight of the block minus the up component of the applied force.

$$N = mg - F\sin 26°$$

The frictional retarding force, which is μ times this (normal) force, must equal $F\cos 26°$, the horizontal component of the applied force. This is dictated by the requirement of constant velocity. For constant velocity (no acceleration) the forces must be balanced.

$$\mu(mg - F\sin 26°) = F\cos 26°$$

$$\mu mg = F(\cos 26° + \mu \sin 26°)$$

$$0.5(200 \text{ kg})(10 \text{ m/s}^2) = F(0.90 + 0.22) = 1.12F$$

$$F = 893 \text{ N}$$

The horizontal component of this 893 N force applied over the 30 m displacement of the block is the work performed.

$$W = Fx \cdot s = (893 \text{ N})\cos(26°)(30 \text{ m}) = 26{,}800 \text{ J}$$

It could also be said that this is the work performed by the frictional force.

The definition of work as the product of force in the direction of displacement times that displacement can be represented graphically.

Practice Question

A force applied to moving a sled follows the graph in the figure below. First consider the rectangular area. The force is constant at 120 N and the displacement is 0.8 m, so the work performed is 96 J. For the triangular area, the average force is 60 N. This average is applied over 0.2 m. So the work associated here is 12 J, for a total work of 108 J.

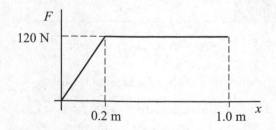

Another way of looking at the above problem is to say that the work is equal to the area under the line of the graph. In this case, the area consists of a rectangle and a triangle, the areas of which can be calculated by length times width (0.8×120) and by one-half base times height ($\frac{1}{2} \times 0.2 \times 120$), respectively. However, if the graph were a curve or an irregular area, it would not be possible to measure it directly. Instead, the area could be approximated by breaking it up into many small rectangles.

In summary, if a force can be graphed as force versus distance (displacement), then the work done is the area under the curve.

The following problem involves the work done by the gravitational force.

Practice Question

A 4.0 kg mass slides down an inclined plane a vertical distance 2.0 m as shown in the figure below. What is the work done?

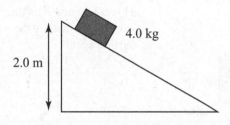

Solution: The definition of work is the force in the direction of the displacement. In this problem the force is acting down, so the displacement in the down direction is the one that is significant in calculating the work. The work performed on the mass by the gravitational force is

$$W = (4.0 \text{ kg})(10 \text{ m/s}^2)(2.0 \text{ m}) = 80 \text{ J}$$

Notice that we do not have to calculate the component of gravity acting along the incline plane. For the work done by gravity, the amount of work is independent of the path taken.

Energy

For problems involving mechanical systems, it is helpful to consider both potential and kinetic energy. There are other forms of energy—for example, electrical energy, which is stored in an electric or magnetic field—and these are encountered in the study of electricity and magnetism.

For the MCAT, it is important to be able to distinguish potential and kinetic energy. As an illustration, consider a mass on the surface of Earth. To raise the mass to a height, h, under the effect of gravity, the work performed is mg times the height, h. At this height, the mass is said to have potential energy equal to mgh. If the mass is dropped, the gravitational force acts to give it a velocity and the mass takes on kinetic energy equal to $(\frac{1}{2})mv^2$. Energy is **potential** by virtue of position and **kinetic** by virtue of velocity. If a mass is not moving, it does not have translational kinetic energy.

POTENTIAL ENERGY

Potential energy can also be thought of as the potential to do work.

The term *conservative force* is used to describe a force where the work done by the force is independent of the path taken. For a "nonconservative force," the amount of work done does depend on the path taken. Gravity is an example of a conservative force, whereas friction is a nonconservative force.

Calculate the potential energy associated with a 20 kg mass 6.0 m above the surface of Earth.

Solution: The energy is clearly potential and equal to the work performed to raise the 20 kg the 6.0 m. Near the surface of Earth the gravitational force of *mg* is constant, so the work is this force times the vertical distance. In this case, work is done on the mass by an outside agent raising it in the gravitational field as shown in Figure 2.22.

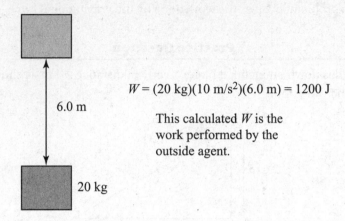

$$W = (20 \text{ kg})(10 \text{ m/s}^2)(6.0 \text{ m}) = 1200 \text{ J}$$

This calculated *W* is the work performed by the outside agent.

Figure 2.22. Potential energy of a raised 20 kg mass

This work performed is equal to the potential energy, which would be written as

$$PE = mgh = (20 \text{ kg})(10 \text{ m/s}^2)(6.0 \text{ m}) = 1200 \text{ J}$$

Now calculate the kinetic energy associated with this 20 kg mass moving with a velocity of 36 m/s.

$$KE = \frac{1}{2}mv^2 = \frac{1}{2}(20 \text{ kg})(36 \text{ m/s})^2 = 12960 \text{ J}$$

Work–Energy

The concept of work being translated into energy or energy being manifest as work is a very important problem-solving tool. Problems using work–energy analysis can be viewed as *goes into* problems. The phrase *goes into* simply and accurately describes the process of work going into or becoming energy and vice versa.

If a 20 kg box is pushed 30 m by a 70 N force, the work performed is 2100 J. Using work–energy, this work must be manifest as velocity:

$$2100 \text{ J} = \frac{mv^2}{2}$$

$$v^2 = \frac{4200 \text{ J}}{20 \text{ kg}}$$

$$v = 14.5 \text{ m/s}$$

The velocity could have been calculated with the equations of motion using the acceleration produced by the force acting over the distance involved.

Practice Question

Determine the force used and the work performed for a 1.5 g bullet traveling at 400 m/s that strikes and penetrates a block of wood 0.12 m before coming to rest.

Solution: The work performed in stopping the bullet is the average retarding force of the wood times the distance over which the average retarding force acted. The amount of work must equal the kinetic energy of the bullet just before it struck the block. This initial kinetic energy *goes into* the average retarding force applied over the stopping distance.

$$\frac{mv^2}{2} = F_{avg}\,x$$

$$F_{avg} = \frac{mv^2}{2x} = \frac{(1.5 \times 10^{-3}\ \text{kg})(400\ \text{m/s})^2}{2(0.12\ \text{m})} = 1000\ \text{N}$$

The work performed in stopping the bullet is (1000 N)(0.12 m) = 120 J, which is also the total kinetic energy of the bullet.

Now consider the work performed by a force proportional to displacement, such as the force encountered in elongating or compressing a spring. Calculate the work performed by the nonconstant $F = (3.0\ \text{N/m})x$ force applied over a distance (displacement) from 0 to 1.2 m. Graph the force versus distance relationship in Figure 2.23.

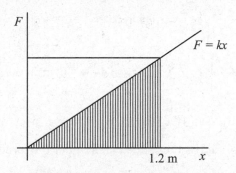

Figure 2.23. Force versus distance

Since the force is linear, the average force over any displacement, x, is $kx/2$.

The work performed, the product of average force times displacement, is $kx^2/2$.

This is also the area under the $F = kx$ curve between 0 and x. This is the area of a right triangle with base 1.2 m and height $F = (3.0\ \text{N/m})(1.2\ \text{m}) = 3.6\ \text{N}$.

The work is

$$W = \frac{kx^2}{2} = (3.0\ \text{N/m})\frac{(1.2\ \text{m})^2}{2} = 2.2\ \text{J}$$

Understanding that the work is represented by the area under the curve is very helpful in doing this problem. It is important, in general, in understanding work calculations.

Practice Question

Consider a race car making a left turn. The 180 lb/in right front spring compresses from 3 inches of compression to 8 inches of compression. Find the amount of work performed on this spring during this left turn.

Solution: This unit of force per length is standard for describing car springs. The force law is $F = kx$, the law typical of springs. This law is known as **Hooke's law**. The work is $W = kx^2/2$, taking into consideration the initial compression of 3 inches. The work performed is the area under the curve from 3 inches to 8 inches, as shown in Figure 2.24.

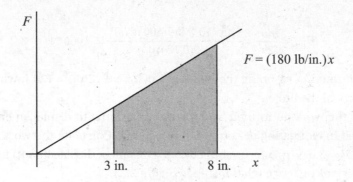

Figure 2.24.

$$W = \frac{kx^2}{2}\bigg|_{x=8} - \frac{kx^2}{2}\bigg|_{x=3} = \frac{(180\ \text{lb/in})}{2}[(8\ \text{in})^2 - (3\ \text{in})^2]$$

$$W = 4950\ \text{lb-in} = 412\ \text{lb-ft}$$

Picturing the work performed as the shaded area under the force versus distance curve is a helpful visual aid.

Practice Question

Stretching a Hooke's law spring 6.0 cm requires 15 J of work. What is the spring constant and the work required to compress the spring 8.0 cm?

Solution: First, whether stretching or compressing a Hooke's law spring, the constant is the same. So find the constant using

$$W = \frac{kx^2}{2}$$

$$15\ \text{J} = \frac{k(0.06\ \text{m})^2}{2}$$

$$k = \frac{30\ \text{J}}{0.0036\ \text{m}^2} = 8300\ \frac{\text{N}}{\text{m}}$$

Now, find the work to compress the spring 8.0 cm.

$$W = \frac{kx^2}{2} = \frac{8300}{2\,m}(0.080\,m)^2$$
$$W = 27\,J$$

Often it is easier to analyze friction problems with a work–energy approach than to use an approach that looks at forces and accelerations leading to equations of motion.

Practice Question

A 20 kg block slides 14 meters (slant distance) down a frictionless 30° inclined plane and then encounters a friction surface with friction coefficient 0.60 as diagrammed below. Analyze the problem using work-energy, and determine where the block comes to rest.

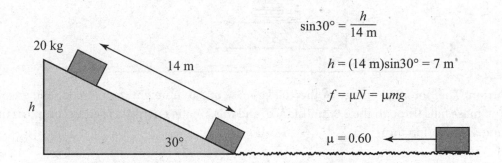

$$\sin 30° = \frac{h}{14\,m}$$

$$h = (14\,m)\sin 30° = 7\,m$$

$$f = \mu N = \mu mg$$

$$\mu = 0.60$$

Solution: The simple work–energy type statement of this problem is the following. The potential energy of the block at the top of the plane *goes into* kinetic energy at the bottom of the plane and this kinetic energy *goes into* doing work against friction. The work due to friction is the constant force μmg over a distance L. In equation form

$$mgh\Big|_{\text{top of the plane}} = \frac{mv^2}{2}\Big|_{\text{bottom of the plane}} = \mu mgL\Big|_{\text{after coming to a stop}}$$

and solving for L

$$L = \frac{v^2}{2\mu g} \text{ or } L = \frac{h}{\mu}$$

Using the second equation for L is the best choice. It is simpler and it relies on less calculated information. This is a good example of how the *goes into* approach simplifies the problem. Rather than calculating the initial potential energy and then perhaps the kinetic energy at the bottom of the plane, a work–energy approach allows the answer to be calculated directly.

$$L = \frac{h}{\mu} = \frac{7.0\,m}{0.60} = 12\,m$$

Another classic work–energy problem involves a **mass** dropping onto a spring. The question concerns the compression of the spring and the final resting place of the **mass**.

Practice Question

A 100 kg mass is dropped a distance of 2.0 meters onto a Hooke's law spring ($F = -kx$) with spring constant 2000 N/m, as in the figure below. Given that the energy stored in a spring is $kx^2/2$, find how much the spring is compressed.

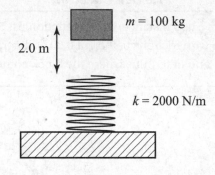

Solution: The potential energy of the 100 kg mass at 2.0 m height *goes into* kinetic energy as the mass falls through the 2.0 m distance, and this kinetic energy is used to compress the spring. In equation form

$$mgh = \frac{1}{2}mv^2 = \frac{kx^2}{2}$$

$$x = \sqrt{\frac{2mgh}{k}} = \sqrt{\frac{2(100 \text{ kg})(10 \text{ m/s}^2)(2 \text{ m})}{2000 \text{ N/m}}} = \sqrt{2} \text{ m} = 1.4 \text{ m}$$

If the mass were gently placed on the spring, the compression could be calculated as the solution of the force of the mass acting down and the force of the spring acting up. In equation form this would be a force balance statement.

$$mg = kx \quad \text{or} \quad x = \frac{mg}{k}$$

$$x = \frac{(100 \text{ kg})(10 \text{ m/s}^2)}{2000 \text{ N/m}} = 0.50 \text{ m}$$

Practice Question

A glider pilot attempting to do a loop dives to attain sufficient speed to prevent falling out of the loop. The proposed flight path is shown in the figure below. At what height, h, must the glider start in order to not fall out of the loop? Express your answer in terms of R, the radius of the circle.

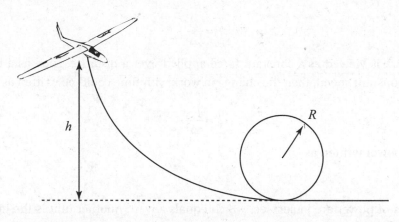

Solution: The problem is solved with energy analysis. At the bottom of the loop, the glider must have sufficient energy to climb the diameter of the loop and provide the mv^2/r force to keep the glider moving in a circle. This mv^2/r force must equal or exceed mg. Write a statement relating this velocity to mg.

$$\frac{mv_{top}^2}{R} = mg$$

$$\text{so} \quad v_{top} = \sqrt{Rg}$$

Taking the zero of mechanical energy at the bottom of the loop, the energy statement for not falling out of the loop is: The kinetic energy at entry (the bottom of the loop) has to equal the potential energy to rise $2R$ plus the energy to keep the glider moving in the circle.

$$E_{bottom} = \frac{mv_{top}^2}{2} + 2mgR = \frac{mgR}{2} + 2mgR = \frac{5}{2}mgR$$

This energy at the bottom comes from the glider diving through a distance h, and, therefore, the glider has to have mgh of potential energy. Set this mgh equal to the required minimum energy and solve for h.

$$mgh = \frac{5}{2}mgR$$

$$\text{so } h = 2.5R$$

The total potential energy at the start of the dive is converted to mechanical energy at the bottom. This mechanical energy is used by the glider to climb the $2R$ and also provides the glider with sufficient velocity to provide the mv^2/r force.

TIP

CONSISTENT UNITS

An equation cannot mix units by adding forces (units of newtons) and energy (units of joules).

Power

Power is the rate of doing work or the rate of energy transfer. In other words, power is the amount of work done in a given amount of time. Power can be calculated as the work performed, measured in joules, divided by the time to perform that work. In equation form this is

$$P = \frac{\Delta W}{\Delta t}$$

If the work is viewed as a constant force applied over a distance, such as a boat or car moving at constant speed, then the change in work with time could be written as

$$P = \frac{F \Delta x}{\Delta t}$$

and the power written as

$$P = F \cdot v$$

The units of power are joules/sec, which equals a watt. Another unit is the horsepower, defined as 746 W or 550 ft-lb/sec.

Practice Question

A 60 kg person walks up a 10 meter tall hill in 3 minutes. What is the average power output?

Solution: The average power output of this person is the work performed over the time. In equation form, the average power is

$$P = \frac{\Delta W}{\Delta t}$$

The work performed is the same as the change in energy. There is no need to calculate forces acting over a distance. Use the potential energy equivalent for the work performed. Work performed equals change in potential energy. Substitute mgh for ΔW.

$$P = \frac{mgh}{\Delta t} = \frac{(60 \text{ kg})(10 \text{ m/s}^2)(10 \text{ m})}{180 \text{ s}} = 33 \text{ W}$$

Sometimes a problem requires knowing **peak** or **instantaneous power** along with average power.

Practice Question

A pile driver exerts a constant force of 2000 N over a distance of 15 cm for 0.12 s, with this force exerted once per second. Find the instantaneous power and average power exerted by the pile driver.

Solution: The work performed while the force is being exerted is

$$W = F \cdot s = (2000 \text{ N})(0.15 \text{ m}) = 300 \text{ J}$$

The instantaneous power is the power delivered while the pile driver is exerting this large force on the pile.

$$P = \frac{W}{t} = \frac{300 \text{ J}}{0.12 \text{ s}} = 2500 \text{ W}$$

The instantaneous power is different from the power required to run the pile driver. In a pile driver a motor winds up a cable, lifting the large mass that is allowed to drop on the pile. The motor supplies the 300 J of work necessary to raise the mass every second; that is, the motor supplies a small amount of power over a relatively long time to give the mass potential energy. When the mass is dropped, the stored potential energy is delivered to the pile in a very short (instantaneous) time. The electric motor that winds up the cable and lifts the heavy mass needs only to supply 300 J per second, but it may do so for thousands of seconds.

$$P_{\text{avg}} = \frac{300 \text{ J}}{1 \text{ s}} = 300 \text{ W}$$

Practice Question

A motorboat towing a water skier exerts a constant 2000 N while traveling at a constant speed of 15 m/s. Find the average power exerted by the motorboat.

Solution: The general formula for power is

$$P = \frac{\Delta W}{\Delta t} = \frac{F \cdot \Delta s}{\Delta t} = Fv$$

In this situation, power is force times velocity, so

$$P = (2000 \text{ N})(15 \text{ m/s}) = 30,000 \text{ W}$$

TORQUE AND EQUILIBRIUM

Simply stated, the momentum associated with a moving mass is the product of mass times velocity. In general, the momentum of a mass is an indication of the amount of force, applied over space or time, it would take to stop that mass.

Force can be written as a change in momentum divided by a change in time. Momentum is a vector. As with velocity, it has a direction as well as a magnitude. Calculations based on momentum can provide an easy approach to problems that involve interactions of multiple forces, problems in which a force varies, or problems in which the individual forces are unknown. MCAT momentum questions will ask about both the momentum of a mass moving in a straight line (**linear momentum**) and momentum of a mass moving in a circle around a central point, such as with a wrench turning a nut (**angular momentum**).

CENTER OF MASS

Consider a dumbbell with equally sized weights on either end of a rod. The center of mass is exactly halfway between the two ends—the midpoint of the rod. If the weight on the left of the dumbbell is replaced by a heavier one, the center of mass would now be closer to the left end.

What if the rod had various sized weights placed along it? How would the center of mass be determined?

Solution: First, create a coordinate line that runs through all of the masses and establish an origin (zero point). For each mass, multiply the mass times the distance from the zero point. Then add together all of these products (mx, where x is the distance from zero). Finally, divide the result by the sum of all of the masses. The formula is

$$x_{cm} = \frac{\sum\limits_i m_i x_i}{\sum\limits_i m_i}$$

The summation in the numerator is the sum of the product of each mass times its position in x, and the denominator is simply the sum of all the masses.

For a three-dimensional situation, this summation has to be done in three directions. Fortunately, most center-of-mass problems are in one dimension, or at the most two and many have symmetry properties that can be used to advantage. Center of mass problems can be solved more accurately if the coordinates are chosen carefully.

Practice Question

Two masses, each 20 kg, are separated by 4 m. Where is the center of mass?

Solution: Place one mass at unit 1 and the other at unit 5 as shown in Figure 2.25.

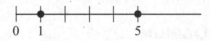

Figure 2.25.

The formal definition of the center of mass is

$$x_{cm} = \frac{(20 \text{ kg})(1) + (20 \text{ kg})(5)}{(20 \text{ kg}) + (20 \text{ kg})} = \frac{120}{40} = 3$$

The center of mass is at 3 units, halfway between the masses.
Redo the problem with a 40 kg mass at unit 5.

$$x_{cm} = \frac{(20 \text{ kg})(1) + (40 \text{ kg})(5)}{(20 \text{ kg}) + (40 \text{ kg})} = \frac{220}{60} = 3.7$$

Now the center of mass is closer to the 40 kg mass, as it should be.

Angular Systems

Angular, or rotational, systems are systems in which there is a rigid lever (for example, a wrench) that is fixed at one end (such as around a nut to be tightened) and to which a force is applied at the other end (a hand pushing the wrench in order to tighten the nut).

BASIC CONCEPTS

Lever arm. In this example, the length of the wrench is an important variable. A certain force applied to a short wrench will have a much different effect than the same force applied to a very long wrench. The length of the wrench is referred to as the **lever arm**. Even though the term *lever arm* may sound like it refers to the wrench itself, it actually refers to the length of the wrench. In general terms, lever arm is the distance from the fixed center of rotation to the point at which the force is applied. If you were to push the wrench from its midpoint instead of from its end, the lever arm would be the distance from the nut to the point at which you are pushing. It would not be the length of the entire wrench.

Distance in radians. If you were to put a pencil at the endpoint of a wrench and push the wrench one full revolution, the pencil would draw a circle. In general, a rigid lever pushed around a fixed center point moves in a circle. Because of this, the distance that the endpoint of the lever travels is usually measured in radians, instead of in linear units (cm or m). This means that the velocity of the endpoint of the wrench must be expressed in radians per second, rather than in meters per second. If the wrench is pushed with an accelerating force, acceleration has to be measured in radians per second squared.

Special terms for angular systems. Angular systems use different terminology than do linear systems for concepts such as mass, force, momentum, kinetic energy, velocity, and acceleration. Most of the corresponding terms have different units. (See Table 2.4.) You can refer to these corresponding terms throughout this section.

Table 2.4 Linear and Angular Terminology

Term in Linear Systems	Corresponding Term in Angular (Rotational) Systems
Mass (kg)	Moment of Inertia ($kg \cdot m^2$)
Force $\left[\dfrac{kg \cdot m}{s^2}\right] = N$	Torque ($N \cdot m$. This is *not* joules.)
Linear Momentum $\dfrac{kg \cdot m}{s}$	Angular Momentum $\dfrac{kg \cdot m^2}{s}$
Kinetic Energy (J)	Kinetic Energy of Rotation (Rotational Energy) (J)
Velocity $\left[\dfrac{m}{s}\right]$	Angular Velocity $\left[\dfrac{radian}{s}\right]$
Acceleration $\left[\dfrac{m}{s^2}\right]$	Angular Acceleration $\left[\dfrac{radian}{s^2}\right]$

Torque

In angular (rotational) systems, the concept of torque is parallel to the concept of force in linear systems. How hard one pushes on the wrench (force) affects how strongly the nut is turned (torque). However, the force is not the only factor that affects how strongly the nut is turned. The length of the wrench is also important. A newton (N) of force applied at the end of a long wrench will produce more turning (torque) than that same newton of force applied to a short wrench.

The exact relationship is that torque is force times lever arm. This means that the units will be newtons times meters (N·m). In a linear system, N · m is the same as joules. However, in a rotational system, torque must be labeled as N · m, not as joules.

Another definition of torque is the product of the force perpendicular to a line drawn from the center of rotation to the point at which the force is applied times this lever arm. The situation is shown in Figure 2.26. Because displacements and forces are described by vectors, the formal definition of torque involves vectors. However, for MCAT purposes, the appropriate force can be considered the one perpendicular to the wrench (or other rigid body) at its end (or other point at which the force is applied).

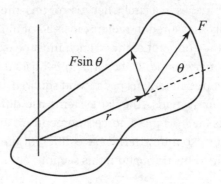

Figure 2.26. Torque

If you push a wrench in a direction that is exactly perpendicular to the wrench, then all of the force that you applied, for example 240 N, is applied to the torque (240 times the lever arm.) However, if the force that is applied to the end of the wrench is not at right angles to the wrench, then only the component of that force that is perpendicular to the lever arm contributes to the torque.

In Figure 2.26, the lever is represented by the arrow labeled r, with the fixed center at the origin of the axes. The lever arm, then, is the distance, r. A force, F, is being applied at the end of the lever but at an angle, θ. The portion of F that acts in the perpendicular direction is $F \sin \theta$.

WHY $F \sin \theta$?

In the example in Figure 2.26, break the vector that represents F (the one at θ degrees) into horizontal and vertical components. The horizontal component is represented by the dotted line. The vertical component is represented by the solid line perpendicular to r, which is the component we want to determine. This is $F \sin \theta$.

The torque, T, is the portion of the force in the perpendicular direction ($F \sin \theta$) times the lever arm, r:

$$T = rF \sin \theta$$

For an applied force at 240 N and 0.70 m and an angle of 30°, the torque is

$$T = (240\ \text{N})(0.70\ \text{m})\sin 30° = 84\ \text{N} \cdot \text{m}$$

Torque is a vector. Although it is calculated by multiplying the force times the lever arm, the direction of the torque vector is perpendicular to the plane in which the force and lever arm lie. In Figure 2.26, the force and lever arm are in the plane of the page. The torque vector comes perpendicularly out of the page; it follows the right-hand rule. With your fingers extended in the direction of r, naturally rotate your fingers in the direction of F. Your extended thumb then points in the direction of the torque.

Practice Question

After a sports injury, a patent's leg is placed in traction, as shown in the figure below. The physician has requested that a 142 N force be applied horizontally to the leg.

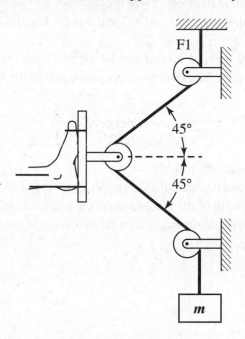

1. What mass, m, must be used for the object hanging from the massless cable?
2. What is the force, $F1$, exerted by the cable on the ceiling?
3. What is the force of friction between the patient and the bed?

Solution:

1. The force diagram for this situation is shown below.

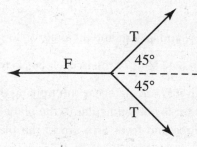

$$F = 2T\cos 45°$$
$$\cos 45° = 0.71$$
$$142\ N = 2T(0.71)$$
$$142\ N = T(1.42)$$
$$T = 100\ N = mg = m(10\ m/s^2)$$
$$m = 10\ kg$$

Note that the tension in the lower cable is equal to the tension in the upper cable. You should also remember that both sin 45° and cos 45° equal 0.71. The required mass is 10 kg.

2. Remember that the upward force must be equal to the downward force since the system is in equilibrium. The downward force is equal to the weight of the mass:

$$w = mg$$
$$w = (10\ kg)(10\ m/s^2)$$
$$w = 100\ N$$

So the upward force equals 100 N.

3. Since there is a horizontal force of 142 N pulling on the patient's foot, there must be an equal and opposite force of friction acting on the patient from the bed. The result is no net force in the horizontal direction. The force of friction between the patient and the bed equals 142 N.

Practice Question

A man is holding a ball with his forearm horizontal as shown in the diagram below. The lifting force F_B is provided by the biceps muscle and acts upward at a distance of 5 cm from the elbow joint pivot point, labeled P. The center of mass of the man's forearm is 20 cm from the pivot P. The center of mass of the ball is 40 cm from P. The downward force on the elbow is labeled F_E.

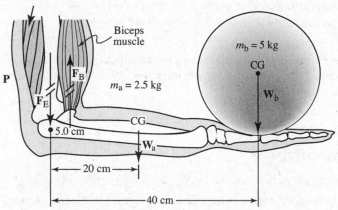

1. What is the force F_B applied by the biceps muscle?
2. What is the downward force on the elbow, F_E?

Solution:

1. Use the principle of moments. The clockwise moment caused by the weight of the patient's arm plus the weight of the ball must be equal to the counterclockwise moment provided by the force in the biceps muscle. This is equivalent to saying that the net torque is zero. Use $F = mg$, where $g = 10$ m/s^2, to approximate the force.

$$\tau = Fd$$
$$F_B(5 \text{ cm}) = (25 \text{ N})(20 \text{ cm}) + (50 \text{ N})(40 \text{ cm})$$
$$F_B(5 \text{ cm}) = 500 \text{ N} \cdot \text{cm} + 2000 \text{ N} \cdot \text{cm} = 2500 \text{ N} \cdot \text{cm}$$
$$F_B = 500 \text{ N}$$

The force F_B applied by the biceps muscle is 500 N.

2. To find F_E, use the equilibrium condition that the sum of all the forces acting upward must equal the sum of all the forces acting downward.

$$\text{Forces acting upward} = \text{Forces acting downward}$$
$$25 \text{ N} + 50 \text{ N} + F_E = 500 \text{ N}$$
$$F_E = 425 \text{ N}$$

The downward force on the elbow, F_E, is 425 N.

Joint deterioration and damage to the tendons in the elbow, such as tennis elbow, can result from repetitive motion while holding a tennis racket. The physical cause of this may be best described as:

(A) due to the pressure caused by holding the racket on the elbow joint.
(B) due to the large lever arm of the weight of the racket from the elbow joint.
(C) due to the large force of the weight of the racket.
(D) due to the velocity with which the racket is moved.

(B) Pressure, force, and velocity are not really important factors. A very large torque is the problem. That very large torque is caused by the racket's center of mass being far from the elbow joint.

ANGULAR MOMENTUM

Angular momentum is defined as the linear momentum of a mass point (mv) times the lever arm (r). As with torque, angular momentum is a vector, but in most problems the angle between r and mv is a right angle, so vectors and angles between r and mv are not a problem.

Angular momentum, L, can be expressed as follows.

$$L = r(mv)$$

TIP

RADIAN

The radian is a unitless quantity.

Consider the units. Linear momentum, mv, is expressed as kg $\cdot$ m/sec. When this is multiplied times the lever arm (in meters), the result is kg $\cdot$ m^2/sec. Linear momentum and angular momentum, then, have different units.

The angular momentum of a 20 kg mass rotating at a radius of 0.50 m with angular velocity of 12 rad/s has an angular momentum of ($v = r\omega$)

$$L = (20 \text{ kg})(0.50\text{m})^2(12 \text{ rad/s}) = 60 \text{ kg} \cdot \text{m}^2/\text{s}$$

ANGULAR VELOCITY AND ANGULAR ACCELERATION

Angular velocity and angular acceleration are the rotational counterparts of linear velocity and linear acceleration. They are calculated in much the same way as their linear counterparts (distance over time and distance over time squared, respectively) except that the distance is not measured in meters but rather in radians.

Consider a point traveling along the circumference of a circle with a radius of 5 m. If the distance that the point travels in 1 second is known in meters, for example 15 m, then the velocity in linear terms would be 15 m/sec. To express this as an angular velocity, the distance in meters must be converted into radians. One radian is by definition the length of the radius. In this case, it takes 5 meters to make 1 radian. Dividing the number of meters by the number of meters per radian gives radians.

$$15 \text{ m/sec} \times 1 \text{ rad}/5 \text{ m} = 3 \text{ rad/sec}$$

The formula for angular velocity, then, is $v/r = \omega$, where ω is angular velocity. This formula allows you to calculate the angular velocity if you know the linear velocity. If you know the angular velocity, it can be converted to the linear velocity by $v = r\omega$. In other words, if the velocity is 3 radians per second and a radian (the length of the radius, r) is 5 meters long, then the velocity is 15 meters per second.

Similarly, for angular acceleration, the acceleration expressed in meters per second squared can be multiplied by radians per meter (which is the same as 1/radius) to give radians per second squared.

$$a/r = \alpha,$$

where α is the angular acceleration. This can also be written as $a = r\alpha$.

MOMENTS OF INERTIA

Force and momentum are related via mass and acceleration. In a similar manner, torque and angular momentum are related by inertia and angular acceleration. Recall that in the study of motion, the movement of a mass point around a circle at radius r is $s = r\theta$, with s the arc length and θ the angle turned through. This leads to the relationship, $v = r\omega$, with ω the angular velocity, and to $a = r\alpha$, with α the angular acceleration.

If in Figure 2.26, the force is applied to a mass point, then the torque is r times the mass of the point and its linear acceleration.

$$T = rF = rma = rm(r\alpha) = (mr^2)\alpha$$

The quantity mr^2 is called the moment of inertia. For a mass point, the moment of inertia is simply the mass times r^2. For a hoop of mass, m, rotated about its center, the moment of inertia is also mr^2. For several mass points, it is just the sum of mr^2 for all the mass points. The values for the moment of inertia for more complicated shapes have been worked out and tabulated. In any test, any moment of inertia other than for a mass point would be given in the problem. The relationship between torque, moment of inertia (I), and angular acceleration then is

$$T = I\alpha$$

and in words: Torques make (masses with) moments of inertia angularly accelerate.

Looking at Figure 2.26 again, write the angular momentum as

$$L = r(mv) = r(mr\omega) = (mr^2)\omega = I\omega$$

The angular momentum of a rotating body or collection of mass points is the total moment of inertia times the angular velocity. Angular momentum, like linear momentum, is conserved, and this provides a powerful law for analyzing problems.

BOWLING

A good bowler gets a lot of rotation on the ball. This angular momentum is then transferred to the pins, creating a very violent pin action capable of clearing all the pins in one shot!

Practice Question

Two 6.0 kg mass points are separated by a 1.2 m rod. The mass of the rod is negligible. If the axis of rotation is moved from the middle to a point 0.20 m from one of the masses, by what percentage does the moment of inertia change?

Solution: Start by finding the moment of inertia of the system about an axis perpendicular to their line of centers and at the midpoint, as in Figure 2.27.

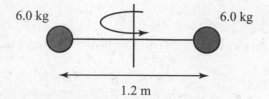

Figure 2.27. Moment of inertia

$$I = 2mr^2 = 2[(6.0 \text{ kg})(0.60 \text{ m})^2] = 4.3 \text{ kg} \cdot \text{m}^2$$

Now calculate the inertia about an axis perpendicular to their line of centers and 0.20 m from one mass as shown in Figure 2.28.

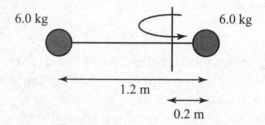

Figure 2.28. Inertia about an axis

$$I = (6.0 \text{ kg})(0.20 \text{ m})^2 + (6.0 \text{ kg})(1.0 \text{ m})^2 = 0.24 \text{ kg} \cdot \text{m}^2 + 6.0 \text{ kg} \cdot \text{m}^2 = 6.24 \text{ kg} \cdot \text{m}^2$$

Moving the axis of rotation closer to one mass increases the moment of inertia by roughly 50%.

In Figure 2.27, a 600 N · m torque is applied by means of a force of 100 N tangent to the circle of rotation of the masses. This is a torque of 600 kg · m²/s². This torque makes the masses with moment of inertia 4.3 kg · m² accelerate according to

$$T = I\alpha \quad \text{or} \quad \alpha = \frac{T}{I} = \frac{600 \text{ kg} \cdot \text{m}^2/\text{s}^2}{4.3 \text{ kg} \cdot \text{m}^2} = 140 \text{ 1/s}^2$$

Practice Question

A cylinder of mass 300 kg and radius 0.15 m revolves around a horizontal axis through the center of the cylinder. A cord wrapped around the cylinder is pulled with a constant force of 60 N. For a cylinder rotated about its central axis, the moment of inertia is $I_{\text{cylinder}} = (\frac{1}{2})MR^2$. The situation is shown in the figure below.

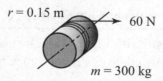

Find the angular acceleration of the cylinder.

Solution: First, calculate I for the cylinder.

$$I = \frac{1}{2}(300 \text{ kg})(0.15 \text{ m})^2 = 3.4 \text{ kg} \cdot \text{m}^2$$

The force applied at right angles to the radius supplies a torque to produce rotation.

$$T = (60 \text{ N})(0.15 \text{ m}) = 9.0 \text{ kg} \cdot \text{m}^2/\text{s}^2$$

The angular acceleration is

$$\alpha = \frac{T}{I} = \frac{9.0 \text{ kg} \cdot \text{m}^2/\text{s}^2}{3.4 \text{ kg} \cdot \text{m}^2} = 2.6 \text{ 1/s}^2$$

KINETIC ENERGY OF ROTATION

The general expression for the kinetic energy of a moving mass point is $mv^2/2$. If $v = r\omega$, then the kinetic energy associated with it is

$$KE = \frac{mv^2}{2} = \frac{mr^2\omega^2}{2} = \frac{I\omega^2}{2}$$

This gives a **kinetic energy of rotation**, expressed in terms of angular velocity or moment of inertia. Kinetic energy of rotation is also called **rotational energy**.

Looking at the figure in the previous problem, calculate the kinetic energy of the rotating cylinder if the angular rotation is 50 1/s².

$$KE = \frac{3.4 \text{ kg} \cdot \text{m}^2}{2}(50 \text{ 1/s})^2 = 4250 \text{ J}$$

To generate this much energy with linear motion, the 300 kg cylinder would need to be moving at 5.3 m/s.

> ### SLIDING VERSUS ROLLING
>
> A ball sliding down an inclined plane (without rolling) reaches the bottom faster than if it were rolling. In the case of sliding, the gravitational potential energy goes *into* only one form—the translational kinetic energy. In the case of rolling, the gravitational potential energy must go into two forms—the translational kinetic energy and the rolling. The addition of the rolling energy means the translational kinetic energy is less.

SUMMARY OF ANGULAR SYSTEMS

In angular (rotational) motion problems, the key is to think in terms of moment of inertia, angular velocity, and angular acceleration. It is important to be clear on the difference between these concepts and their linear counterparts. Memorize the definition of the radian, which is $\theta = s/r$, arc length (s) over radius (r). This statement can be rewritten as $s = r\theta$, which means that multiplying the number of radians times the radius gives the arc length.

FLUIDS

To master MCAT problems that involve fluids, review these important fluid concepts:

- Density, Specific Gravity, and Buoyancy
- Pressure
- Gauge Pressure versus Absolute Pressure
- Hydraulics
- Manometers
- Fluid Dynamics
- Viscosity and Flow
- Bernoulli Equation

Density, Specific Gravity, and Buoyancy

Density is the measure of how much mass is packed into a given volume. An object that has 10 grams of mass in a cubic centimeter is denser than an object that has 6 grams in a cubic centimeter. Density is calculated as mass per unit volume, or $\rho = \frac{m}{v}$. Many MCAT problems refer to the density of water, which is 1 g/cm^3 or 1000 kg/m^3.

It is sometimes easier to describe the density of an object by comparing it with something familiar, such as water. **Specific gravity** is, by definition, the ratio of the density of a substance to the density of water. Silver has a specific gravity of 10.5, which means that for equal volumes, silver has 10.5 times the mass of water. In other words, silver is 10.5 times denser than water.

Buoyancy is the property of a liquid that causes it to buoy up, or reduce the weight of, an object immersed in it. It is easier to carry a rock when it is in a swimming pool, compared to when the rock is on dry land, because the water is buoyant. It partially supports the weight of the rock, making it seem to weigh less. Buoyancy is the measure of how much of the rock's weight is supported.

Imagine that a swimming pool is completely full and that you then slowly lower a rock into it. A certain amount of water will overflow to accommodate the volume of the rock. This is called the displaced water. The amount of space that the displaced water occupies (its volume) is the same as the space that the rock occupies (its volume). Note, though, that they have different masses.

Buoyancy can be thought of as the upward force that the water exerts on the rock. A force is defined as a mass times an acceleration. The mass in this case is the mass of the displaced water (not the mass of the rock). In effect, buoyancy measures the amount of force that the displaced water is exerting on the rock. The acceleration in this situation would be gravity. The buoyant force is expressed by **Archimedes's principle: A body partially or completely immersed in a liquid is buoyed up by a force equal to the weight of the liquid displaced.** In other words, the force is the mass of the displaced liquid times the acceleration of gravity.

Suppose that the mass of the displaced liquid is not known but the volume of it and the density of it are known. If there were 3 cubic centimeters of water and given that water has

VOLUMES OF IRREGULAR OBJECTS

A rock usually has an irregular shape. How could its volume be calculated? In the example of the rock and the swimming pool, if you collect the water that was displaced and put it into a beaker, you can directly measure its volume. Because the amount of space that the rock takes up is the same as the amount of space that the displaced water took up, the volume of the displaced water is also the volume of the rock.

a density of 1 gram for every cubic centimeter, you can calculate that there are 3 grams of water. In other words, the density (g/cm^3) times the volume (cm^3) yields the mass (grams).

Buoyant force, then, can be expressed either as the mass of displaced liquid times gravity ($F = ma$) or as density times volume (which gives mass) times gravity.

$$BF = \rho g V$$

where ρ is the density of the liquid displaced, g is the gravitational constant, and V is the volume of liquid displaced. Note that the buoyant force has the unit of newtons, which is the same as mg.

In many instances, the buoyant force is measured as a mass loss, which can be expressed as

$$\Delta m_B = \rho V$$

Consider a cube of aluminum with a volume of 10 cm³ and a density of 2.7 g/cm³. In air, the aluminum "weighs" (2.7 g/cm³) × (10 cm³) = 27 g. The buoyant force experiment is shown in Figure 2.29.

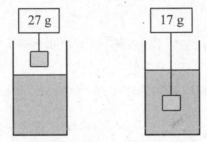

Figure. 2.29. Buoyant force

When the block is submerged, 10 cm³ of water will be displaced. The displaced water has a mass of (1 g/cm³) × (10 cm³) = 10 g. Thus the apparent "weight," or mass, of the aluminum in water is reduced by 10 g (27 g – 10 g) to an apparent 17 g.

A classic, and rather difficult, problem involving buoyancy and Archimedes's principle is determining the metal content of a supposedly gold statue (Figure 2.30).

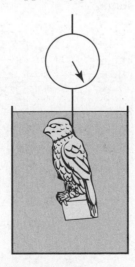

Figure 2.30. A classic buoyancy problem

The statue is attached to a spring scale and lowered into a cylinder of water. The statue is observed to weigh 42 N out of the water and 30 N when submerged in the water. Is the statue gold? The density of gold is 19,000 kg/m³. The buoyant force is the difference between the 42 and 30 N forces. This 12 N buoyant force equals

$$12 \text{ N} = \rho_{water} \cdot g \cdot V_{statue}$$

Remember that the volume of the statue is the same as the volume of the displaced water. Either one can be used in the above equation. The density of an object (kg/m³) times the volume of the object (m³) gives the mass (kg) $\rho V = m$.

So, solving for volume, the volume of the statue is related to the density of the statue:

$$V_{statue} = \frac{m_{statue}}{\rho_{statue}} = \frac{42 \text{ N}/10 \text{ m/s}^2}{\rho_{statue}}$$

Note that the actual weight of the statue, 42 N, is used, not the apparent weight. Now substituting in the previous equation:

$$12 \text{ N} = \rho_{water} \cdot g \frac{42 \text{ N}/10 \text{ m/s}^2}{\rho_{statue}} = \rho_{water} \frac{42 \text{ N}}{\rho_{statue}}$$

and solving for the density of the statue:

$$\rho_{statue} = \rho_{water} \frac{42}{12} = (1.0 \times 10^3 \text{ kg/m}^3)(3.5) = 3.5 \times 10^3 \text{ kg/m}^3$$

Since the density of gold is 19×10^3 kg/m³, the statue is not gold. It is either hollow or is a layer of gold over a lighter metal.

Pressure

Pressure in a fluid is defined as the amount of force (N) exerted on a unit area (m²). The unit of pressure is the pascal (1 pascal = 1 N/m²). Atmospheric pressure is 1.01×10^5 Pa.

The pressure at a depth, h, in an open container of fluid is the pressure at the top of the liquid plus the weight (force) of the column of fluid, as depicted in Figure 2.31. The weight of the column of fluid is calculated by multiplying the density of the fluid times the acceleration of gravity times the height of the column.

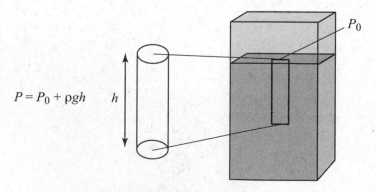

$$P = P_0 + \rho g h$$

Figure 2.31. Pressure in a fluid

Find the pressure in the deep end of a pool where the depth is 7.0 m.

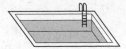

Solution: The pressure at the bottom of the pool is the pressure at the top of the pool (atmospheric) plus the ρgh for the water. Atmospheric pressure (top of the pool) is 1.01×10^5 Pa. At the bottom of the pool the pressure is

$$P = P_0 + \rho gh$$

$$P = 1.01 \times 10^5 \text{ Pa} + (1000 \text{ kg/m}^3)(10 \text{m/s}^2)(7.0 \text{ m})$$

$$P = 1.01 \times 10^5 \text{ Pa} + 7.0 \times 10^4 \text{ Pa} = 1.70 \times 10^5 \text{ Pa}$$

$$P = 1.70 \times 10^5 \text{ Pa} \frac{1 \text{ atm}}{1.05 \times 10^5 \text{ Pa}} = 1.68 \text{ atm}$$

In pressure problems, sometimes information is given in terms of Pascals (Pa) and sometimes in terms of atmospheric pressure (atm), 1 atm being 1.01×10^5 Pa. Sometimes it is written as 101 kPa.

Gauge Pressure versus Absolute Pressure

The pressure in an automobile tire is typically measured with a pressure gauge. When the tire is flat, the gauge reads zero. However, the air that is inside the tire is actually at atmospheric pressure, not at zero pressure. The pressure gauge is, in fact, reading the difference between the inside and outside pressures. This is called **gauge pressure**.

Pressure is an absolute number, and gauge pressure is a difference in pressure. In the previous problem, the gauge pressure at the bottom of the pool, with respect to the top of the pool, is 0.68 atm, whereas the absolute pressure is 1.68 atm.

Hydraulics

Hydraulics is based on **Pascal's principle: An increase in pressure applied to a closed liquid container is transmitted throughout the liquid**. The most popular use of this principle is in a two-piston hydraulic system in which the force to move one piston is multiplied by the area ratio of the two pistons. Figure 2.32 shows an application of Pascal's principle:

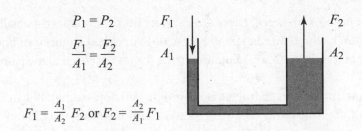

$$P_1 = P_2$$

$$\frac{F_1}{A_1} = \frac{F_2}{A_2}$$

$$F_1 = \frac{A_1}{A_2} F_2 \text{ or } F_2 = \frac{A_2}{A_1} F_1$$

Figure 2.32. Pascal's principle

In the system in Figure 2.32, a force, F_1, is applied to the left column, which has a relatively small area. This creates a pressure throughout the whole system that is equal to the force over the area, F_1/A_1. If F_1 is 200 N and A_1 is 5 m², then the pressure would be 40 Pa.

Because this is the pressure throughout the system, the pressure at the right-hand surface is also 40 Pa. If the area, A_2, is 10 m² (twice that of A_1), what force would be exerted at that surface?

$$P = F_2/A_2$$

$$40 \text{ Pa} = F_2/10 \text{ m}^2 \text{ or } F_2 = 10 \text{ m}^2 \times 40 \text{ Pa or } F_2 = 400 \text{ N}$$

Thus, a force of 200 N applied to the small surface area results in a force of 400 N on the larger surface area. A doubled surface area results in a doubled force.

Practice Question

The small piston of a hydraulic jack has a radius of 1.0 cm. The large piston has a radius of 2.5 cm. What force must be applied to the small piston to produce a force of 1500 N, the force necessary to lift the front or side of a car?

Solution: The pressure is constant everywhere, so

$$\frac{F_1}{A_1} = \frac{F_2}{A_2}$$

$$F_1 = \frac{A_1}{A_2} F_2 = \frac{\pi(1.0 \text{ cm})^2}{\pi(2.5 \text{ cm})^2}(1500 \text{ N}) = 240 \text{ N}$$

where F_1 is the force of the small piston, F_2 is the force of the large piston, and A_1 and A_2 are the areas of the small and large pistons. Notice that the problem gives radii, not the areas, for the circular regions. An MCAT question may try to trap you into thinking that a doubled radius would give a doubled force. However, the radius must be squared to calculate the area (πr^2), so a doubled radius will result in a quadrupled force. Multiplying the radius by 3 results in a force that is 9 times greater.

Manometers

A **manometer** measures pressure. There are a variety of manometers especially constructed for various purposes, and they all depend on gas pressures and columns of liquid. The most popular manometer is the mercury manometer, the device first used to measure atmospheric pressure.

A mercury manometer is constructed by first filling an approximately 1 m long (closed at one end, open at the other end) tube with mercury and inverting the tube in a container of mercury as shown in Figure 2.33. Note that the column of mercury is being maintained by the external pressure of the air. As the outside atmospheric pressure changes, the height of the column will change. The pressure at point A is the same as at point B because they are at the same level.

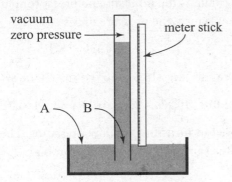

Figure 2.33. A mercury manometer

This pressure is the atmospheric pressure of 1.01×10^5 Pa. There is no air in the top of the tube and hence no pressure. If the atmospheric pressure increases, the height of the column (measured by the meter stick) will increase. This pressure is counterbalanced by the weight of the column of mercury. The pressure in a column of liquid is ρgh with ρ the density of mercury, g the gravitational constant, and h the height of the column. This allows calculation of the height of the mercury column. In this calculation, we use more accurate values of atmospheric pressure, mercury density, and "g" value.

$$p = \rho gh \quad or \quad h = \frac{p}{\rho g} = \frac{1.01 \times 10^5 \text{ N/m}^2}{(13.6 \times 10^3 \text{ kg/m}^3)(9.8 \text{ m/s}^2)} = 760 \text{ mm}$$

This is the measured value of the mercury column on a good day. Atmospheric pressures are usually given in terms of millimeters of mercury and written as 760 mmHg. Note the following equivalencies in pressure units:

$$1.01 \times 10^5 \text{ Pa} = 760 \text{ mmHg} = 760 \text{ Torr}$$

Mercury, and the unit mmHg, is used for pressure measurements like this because it is a liquid and has a high density. Torr is also sometimes used in place of mmHg. The typical blood pressure cuff gives pressure in mmHg. Note that a water manometer, in which the liquid has a much lower density of 1000 kg/m^3, would be nearly 14 meters tall!

Practice Question

Using a U-tube manometer (see the figure below), determine the gas pressure that produces a 0.20 m height difference in the U-tube.

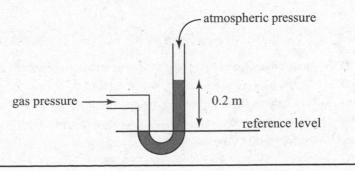

Solution: The pressure of the gas pushes the mercury up the right side of the manometer tube. The pressure at the reference level is the applied gas pressure and must be equal to the pressure at the top of the column (the atmospheric pressure) plus the pressure due to the column of mercury. In formula form the pressure of the gas is

$$p_g = p_0 + \rho g h$$

$$p_g = 1.01 \times 10^5 \text{ Pa} + (13.6 \times 10^3 \text{ kg/m}^3)(10 \text{ m/s}^2)(0.2 \text{ m})$$

$$p_g = 1.01 \times 10^5 \text{ Pa} + 2.7 \times 10^4 \text{ Pa} = 1.28 \times 10^5 \text{ Pa}$$

Manometers are also used to measure very low pressures. The analysis of low pressure manometers is very much the same as in the previous problem.

Fluid Dynamics

A fluid flowing through a pipe of variable cross section flows faster in the smaller cross section area than in the larger cross section area (Figure 2.34). With fluid dynamics, in a system with continuous flow, the product of the cross-sectional area times the velocity must be the same at all points.

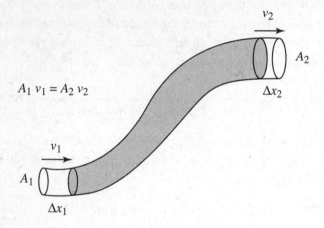

Figure 2.34. Fluid flowing through a pipe

The mass flow equation is:

$$A_1 v_1 = A_2 v_2$$

One result of this equation is that if a cross-sectional area is doubled, the velocity must be halved to maintain the same product. If, at one point, Av is 40 m² × 60 m/sec, then at a point with an 80 m² area, Av would be 80 m² × 30 m/sec.

CONTINUITY

This mass flow equation is also called the continuity equation. Another example of continuity is in electrical circuits, for which all the current going into a junction must equal all the current exiting the junction. In the case of both water and electricity, if continuity did not hold, water or charge would build up in a certain spot. This does not happen in a system with continuous flow.

The units for Av, as in 80 m² × 30 m/sec, are m³/sec. Cubic meters per second is a measure of the rate of flow, or **volume flow rate**, the volume of liquid that flows per a given time period. Av, then, is volume flow rate, which is constant for a continuous flow system.

The volume flow statement can be written as shown below, with the left side representing the rate of flow and the right side showing that it is the product of area and velocity.

$$\frac{\Delta V}{\Delta t} = Av$$

Practice Question

A simple syringe is an excellent example of a fluid flow problem. Consider a syringe with a body radius of 0.20 cm and a needle radius of 0.050 cm. If the plunger in the syringe is moved at the rate of 1.0 m/s, what is the speed of the fluid in the needle?

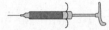

Solution: This is a flow problem, for which

$$A_1 v_1 = A_2 v_2$$

Be sure to notice that you have been given radii, not areas! Plug in the numbers that will calculate the areas, and plug in the known velocity, v_1.

$$\pi(0.20 \text{ cm})^2(1.0 \text{ m/s}) = \pi(0.050 \text{ cm})^2 v_2$$

$$v_2 = \left(\frac{0.20}{0.05}\right)^2 (1.0 \text{ m/s}) = 16 \text{ m/s} = 1600 \text{ cm/s}$$

According to this model, the flow rate, $\Delta V/\Delta t$, is the cross-sectional area of the needle times the velocity.

$$\frac{\Delta V}{\Delta t} = A_{\text{needle}} \; v_2 = \pi(0.050 \text{ cm})^2(1600 \text{ cm/s}) = 12.6 \text{ cm}^3/\text{s}$$

The problem above is an idealized situation. In reality, the viscosity of a liquid affects the flow rate so that for small radius pipes (including the hypodermic needle), the mass flow equation is not accurate.

Viscosity and Flow

Viscosity is a measure of the internal friction in a fluid. The internal frictional forces that result from viscosity oppose the relative motion of one part of the fluid with respect to other parts. When a fluid flows over a surface, the fluid right next to the surface moves very slowly, and the fluid farther away from the surface moves more quickly. The viscosity of a fluid is defined as the stress to strain ratio. The units of viscosity are N·s/m², which can be thought of as force times time, then divided by area.

The viscosity unit, called the poise, is defined as 10^{-1} N·s/m². Low viscosity fluids flow easily, whereas high viscosity fluids do not. Lubricants are high viscosity fluids that move slowly and readily stick to surfaces. The flow rate for a viscous liquid through a pipe is given by **Poiseuille's law**

$$\frac{\Delta V}{\Delta t} = \frac{\pi}{8}\left(\frac{R^4}{\eta}\right)\left(\frac{p_1 - p_2}{L}\right)$$

where η is the viscosity, R the radius of the pipe, p_1 and p_2 the pressure difference, and L the length of the pipe. For small diameter pipes, if all other factors are equal, the flow is limited by the diameter of the pipe. Going back to the syringe problem, consider a needle with length 4.0 cm, radius 0.050 cm, and the viscosity as the viscosity of water, 1.8×10^{-3} N · s/m². In order to solve the problem, we must know the pressure applied by the syringe, and that requires knowing the force and the area over which the force is applied. Take the force as 5.0 N. For a 0.20 cm radius barrel, the pressure is

$$p = \frac{F}{A} = \frac{5.0 \text{ N}}{\pi(0.20)^2} = 40 \text{ N/cm}^2 = 4 \times 10^5 \text{ N/m}^2$$

Since the atmospheric pressure is 1×10^5 N/m², the pressure difference is 3×10^5 N/m².

$$\frac{\Delta V}{\Delta t} = \frac{\pi}{8}\left[\frac{(5 \times 10^{-4} \text{ m})^4}{1.8 \times 10^{-3} \text{ N} \cdot \text{s/m}^2}\right]\left[\frac{3 \times 10^5 \text{ N/m}^2}{4 \times 10^{-2} \text{ m}}\right] = 1.0 \times 10^{-4} \frac{\text{m}^3}{\text{s}}$$

TEST QUESTIONS

Arteries have elastic, muscular walls to withstand high pressures. Pressure in the arteries is relatively constant throughout their length. The pressure in arteries is greater than that in arterioles. As blood flows through an arteriole, the pressure drops as a function of distance traveled. An individual capillary has a very small cross section compared to an arteriole, yet the pressure in the capillary is lower than that in an arteriole.

1. The pressure does not drop as blood flows through the arteries because:
   (A) the flow rate is constant throughout the artery.
   (B) the velocity of the blood is high.
   (C) the oxygen content of the blood is high.
   (D) the lumen of arteries is so large that blood does not encounter resistance.

2. The pressure drops as blood passes through arterioles because:
   (A) arterioles are farther from the heart than arteries.
   (B) the pressure drop for a viscous fluid is greater for a smaller cross-sectional area.
   (C) a drop in pressure is needed to satisfy Bernoulli's equation.
   (D) the flow rate increases.

3. The pressure is lower in capillaries as compared to arterioles because:
   (A) the diameter of capillaries is less.
   (B) capillaries are farther from the heart.
   (C) the total cross-sectional area of all the capillaries is greater than that of arterioles.
   (D) the pressure must be lower at the entrance to a capillary compared to the end of the capillary to satisfy Poiseuille's law.

1. **(D)** Constant flow rate, high velocity, and oxygen content are not related to a pressure drop. Pressure drop occurs because of resistance with the walls, which depends on the radius. We are essentially looking at Poiseuille's law and saying that smaller radius leads to more resistance. This is similar to electricity, where wires with smaller cross-sectional areas have higher resistance.

2. **(B)** This is the same concept as stated in the answer to question 1. Blood is a viscous fluid. The drop in pressure is due to resistance as the fluid interacts with the walls of the arterioles. Bernoulli's equation deals with the relationship between pressure and velocity. However, it does not consider the viscosity of a fluid producing an energy loss because of this resistance.

3. **(C)** Although an individual capillary has a smaller cross section than an individual arteriole, if you add up the cross sections of ALL the capillaries, it is far greater than the total cross section of all the arterioles leading into capillaries. Choice D is not correct because the pressure is lower at the end of a capillary, not at the entrance. The term $P_1 - P_2$ in Poiseuille's law shows that pressure is lost by a viscous fluid as the fluid encounters friction while flowing.

LAMINAR FLOW

Laminar flow is the condition in which the fluid next to a surface is at nearly zero velocity, with the velocity increasing smoothly as it moves away from the surface. There is a flow speed, however, at which the flow becomes chaotic. The transition from laminar, in which the flow velocity is nearly zero at the surface, to turbulent flow is very sharp. Paddle a canoe through water slowly and the flow is laminar. Increasing the speed of the canoe leads to downstream turbulence. The flow is going from laminar to turbulent.

SURFACE TENSION

Another phenomenon associated with forces and liquids is **surface tension**. Dip a loop of wire into a soapy water solution and a film of liquid forms in the loop. This can also be done with a U-shaped piece with a slider on the arms of the loop. If the slider is moved, the force on the slider divided by the length of the slider is used as a measure of the surface tension. Interestingly, the molecules on the surface are not actually being stretched farther apart. Rather, the molecules are migrating from the interior of the film to the surface, thus making the surface larger (Figure 2.35).

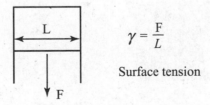

$$\gamma = \frac{F}{L}$$

Surface tension

Figure 2.35. Surface tension

Bernoulli Equation

To better understand the concept of mass flow, consider the effect of differences in pressure and differences in elevation, the details of which are shown in Figure 2.36. Applying work and energy to the flow leads to the **Bernoulli equation**.

$$p_1 + \rho g y_1 + (1/2)\rho v_1^2 = p_2 + \rho g y_2 + (1/2)\rho v_2^2$$

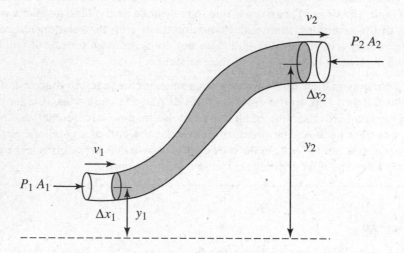

Figure 2.36. Bernoulli equation

Practice Question

Apply the Bernoulli equation to water leaking from a tank (shown in the figure below) of 2.0 m radius and water height of 3.0 m. The leak is from a hole of 1.5 cm radius and is located 2.6 m down from the level of the water. What is the speed of the water leaving the tank and what is the volume flow rate of the leak?

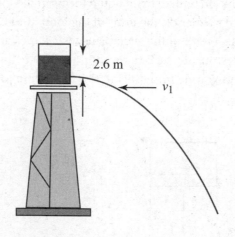

Solution: This problem involves using the flow equation and the Bernoulli equation. Apply the flow equation first. A_2 and v_2 are the cross section and velocity of the top surface of the water.

$$A_1 v_1 = A_2 v_2$$

$$\pi (1.5 \times 10^{-2} \text{ m})^2 v_1 = \pi (2.0 \text{ m})^2 v_2$$

$$v_1 = \left(\frac{2}{1.5 \times 10^{-2}} \right)^2 v_2 = 1.8 \times 10^4 v_2$$

Although the flow equation does not provide a specific answer, it does provide important information. The velocity of the top surface is insignificant compared to the velocity of the water leaking out of the tank, allowing us to set $v_2 = 0$ in the Bernoulli equation. This information applied to the Bernoulli equation is a big help in solving this problem.

$$p_1 + \rho g y_1 + (1/2)\rho v_1^2 = p_2 + \rho g y_2 + (1/2)\rho v_2^2$$

Subscript 2 refers to the top of the water. The flow calculation has shown that the velocity at the top surface is insignificant compared to the velocity of the leaking stream, so this term can be neglected.

Further, the pressure at the top and bottom is essentially the same. The 2.6 m column of water is insignificant compared with the atmospheric pressure. Therefore, the pressure terms can be neglected. These approximations are most important in being able to do this problem. With $v_2 = 0$ and $p_1 = p_2$, the Bernoulli equation reduces to

$$\rho g y_1 + (1/2)\rho v_1^2 = \rho g y^2$$

$$v_1^2 = 2g(y_2 - y_1)$$

$$v_1 = \sqrt{2(9.8 \text{ m/s}^2)(2.6 \text{ m})} = 7.1 \text{ m/s}$$

And the flow from the leak is

$$\frac{\Delta V}{\Delta t} = A_1 v_1 = \pi (1.5 \times 10^{-2} \text{ m})^2 (7.1 \text{ m/s}) = 5.0 \times 10^{-3} \text{ m}^3/\text{s}$$

MECHANICAL WAVES AND SOUND

Mechanical waves travel in a medium. The properties of the wave, such as wavelength and speed, are determined by the medium and the excitation method. There are two types of mechanical waves: **transverse** and **longitudinal**.

Transverse waves are waves for which the motion producing the wave is perpendicular to the direction of the wave. If you start a wave on a stretched rope by shaking it up and down, the pieces of the rope move up and down as the wave moves along the rope.

In **longitudinal** waves, the individual pieces of the object move in the same direction as the wave. If a spring is compressed, for example, the compression wave and the parts of spring travel in the same direction.

Transverse Waves on Ropes

Transverse waves are the waves you will encounter most on the MCAT, and they are the easiest to visualize. A simple transverse wave on a rope is shown in Figure 2.37. The image on the left is a snapshot of the rope and the image on the right depicts the wave with the parameters used to describe the motion.

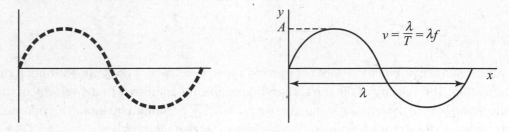

Figure 2.37. A transverse wave on a rope

The peaks and valleys on the wave are called **crests** and **troughs**. Any two points along a wave that have the same height, speed, and direction are said to be **in phase**.

- The **wavelength**, λ, is the length of one wave.
- The **amplitude**, A, of the wave is its maximum height measured from a center line.
- The **period**, T, of the wave is the time for one oscillation, or the time for one wavelength to pass a specific point
- The **frequency**, f, is the inverse of the period. It is given as the number of cycles (wavelengths) per second. This unit is Hz.

In the transverse wave it is easy to see that the period is the time for one complete wavelength to pass a certain point. It is also the time for any piece of the string to make a full round trip starting from the center line and going up and down and back to the center line.

The wave travels at a velocity of one wavelength for each T (period) seconds. The period also defines the frequency as in $T = 1/f$ or $f = 1/T$. Because the velocity of the wave is wavelength over the period, it is also wavelength times frequency.

$$v = \frac{\lambda}{T} = \lambda f$$

Frequency has the units of one over seconds, but rather than writing $1/s$, it is more common to use the units hertz, abbreviated **Hz**.

> **PHASE**
>
> The concept of phase can also refer to two or more different waves. Two waves are in phase if their crests line up. Such a condition would cause constructive interference. If the waves were 180 degrees out of phase this would cause destructive interference (a crest lining up with a trough).

Figure 2.38 is a snapshot of a wave traveling to the right on a rope. Looking at the figure, the amplitude is 0.2 m and the wavelength is 0.6 m. If it takes 0.4 s for the entire wave to pass a point, then the period is the 0.4 s. The frequency, which is the reciprocal of the period, is 2.5 Hz.

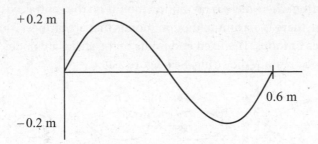

Figure 2.38. Measuring a wave

The velocity of the wave, or perhaps more correctly the velocity of a point on the wave traveling to the right, is the wavelength divided by the period or the wavelength times the frequency.

$$v = \frac{\lambda}{T} = \frac{0.6 \text{ m}}{0.4 \text{ s}} = 1.5 \text{ m/s} \quad \text{or} \quad v = \lambda f = (0.6 \text{ m})(2.5 \text{ Hz}) = 1.5 \text{ m/s}$$

In the next example, illustrated in Figure 2.39, consider a wave traveling to the right and also how the specific points P and Q behave as the wave moves in time.

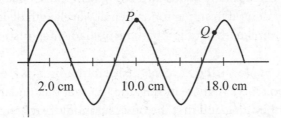

Figure 2.39. A wave moving in time

Based on the graphic, the wavelength is 8 cm. Given a velocity of 2.0 m/s, use the basic $v = \lambda f$ relationship to find the frequency. (Remember to convert 8.0 cm to 0.08 m.):

$$v = \lambda f \quad \text{or} \quad f = \frac{v}{\lambda} = \frac{2.0 \text{ m/s}}{0.08 \text{ m}} = 25 \text{ Hz}$$

The wave is moving to the right, so the crest at P is moving to the right and the piece of the wave depicted by P will move toward the center line of the wave. The same is true for point Q.

Standing Waves on Strings

If a string is fixed at both ends, then plucking the string will produce a sinusoidal wave. When the wave reaches a fixed point, it will reflect back in the other direction. The waves moving to the right will be canceled out by the waves reflecting back to the left. The result is a wave that stays in a constant position. Such a wave is called a **standing**, or **stationary**, **wave**. Both transverse and longitudinal waves can occur as standing waves.

To create a standing wave, the wave moving in the first direction and the wave moving in the opposite direction must match in amplitude and wavelength/frequency. If two people hold either end of a jump rope and move the ends up and down, there is usually an irregular pattern of interference. However, if they move the ends at exactly the same frequency and amplitude, a standing wave will be created and the rope will appear to be stationary.

Positions on a string where there is no motion (points on the central axis) are called **nodes**, and positions where there is maximum motion (points that are farthest from the central axis) are called **antinodes** or **loops**. The fixed endpoints of the string are nodes. It is also possible for other nodes to occur along the string. See Figure 2.40.

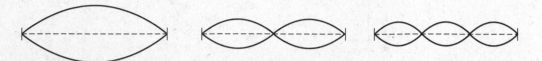

Figure 2.40. Nodes along a string

Consider a string that is 1 meter long and fixed at both ends. If the ends are the only nodes, then a wave is produced that has the maximum length for this length of string, such as in the leftmost example in Figure 2.40. The wavelength for this wave is twice the length of the string, in this case 2 meters. This wave is called the **fundamental harmonic**. If there is a node in the center of the string, at the 0.5 meter point, the length of each wave will be exactly one-half of the fundamental, as in the center example. This is called the second harmonic. The rightmost example shows waves with exactly one-third the wavelength of the fundamental. This is the third harmonic. There can be many nodes on a string with shorter and shorter wavelengths, but all wavelengths are derived from the fundamental wavelength divided by an integer. In a vibrating string, the amplitudes of other than the fundamental (first) vibrating mode drop off dramatically.

The frequencies (as opposed to the wavelengths) of the harmonics are all integral multiples of the fundamental frequency. Mathematically, the fact that the fundamental wavelength is twice the length, L, of the string and that the other harmonic wavelengths are integral fractions of the fundamental can be expressed by $\lambda = 2L, L, 2L/2, 2L/3 \ldots$ or

$$\lambda_n = \frac{2L}{n} \ (n = 1, 2, 3, \ldots)$$

Likewise for a specific velocity, the allowed frequencies are

$$f_n = \frac{v}{\lambda_n} = n\frac{v}{2L} \ (n = 1, 2, 3, \ldots)$$

Operationally, the speed of the wave is the wavelength divided by the period. However, the speed is controlled by the thickness of the string and tension on it. Common experience dictates that waves move faster as the tension in the string is increased and that the speed on a lighter string is faster than on a heavier string under the same tension.

For a string with mass per unit length μ and under tension (force) F, the wave speed can be determined solely from these two factors by

$$v = \sqrt{\frac{F}{\mu}}$$

Note that force divided by (mass per length) gives the following units:

$$\frac{\dfrac{kg \times m}{sec^2}}{\dfrac{kg}{m}} = \frac{kg \times m}{sec^2} \times \frac{m}{kg} = \frac{kg \times m \times m}{kg \times sec \times sec} = \frac{m^2}{sec^2}$$

Taking the square root will give m/s, which is speed. Note that increasing the force increases the speed, whereas increasing the mass per unit length decreases the speed. These concepts make the formula easier to remember.

The wave speed for a 2.0 m string with mass 0.050 kg under tension of 200 N is

$$v = \sqrt{\frac{F}{\mu}} = \sqrt{\frac{200 \ kg \cdot m/s^2}{(0.050 \ kg)/(2.0 \ m)}} = 89 \ m/s$$

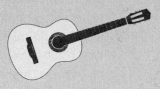

GUITAR STRINGS

On an acoustic guitar there are usually 6 strings that vary in thickness. The lower pitch notes come from the thicker strings and the higher pitch (frequency) notes come from the thin strings. The guitar is tuned by adjusting the tension in each string. Tightening a string increases the frequency of the sound.

Practice Question

The string of a cello is tightened so as to produce the concert pitch of A (440 Hz) when it is bowed, that is, set in sinusoidal motion. The length of the string is 0.60 m and the mass is 2.0 g. How much must the cello player shorten the string to play a 660 Hz note?

Solution: The tension in the string is adjusted so as to produce the 440 Hz frequency. The fundamental frequency is produced with the string length equal to a half wavelength (the fundamental wavelength is twice the length of the string), so the velocity on the string is

$$v = \lambda f = (1.2 \ m)(440 \ Hz) = 528 \ m/s$$

The tension remains the same, as does the mass per unit length, so the $v = \lambda f$ relationship holds. Simply insert the new frequency and find the appropriate wavelength.

$$528 \ m/s = \lambda \ (660 \ Hz) \quad or \quad \lambda = 0.80 \ m$$

The length of string to produce this fundamental frequency is 0.40 m, so the cellist has to shorten the string by 0.20 m.

Longitudinal Waves in Springs

Longitudinal waves are found in springs, and in air and solids. A snapshot view of a wave traveling along a spring is shown in Figure 2.41.

Figure 2.41. A wave traveling along a spring

For longitudinal waves there is no up and down motion leading to crests and troughs. Rather, the motion is back and forth in the direction of the wave, so the corresponding terms are **compressions** and **rarefactions**. The amplitude, wavelength, period, frequency, and velocity relationships are much the same as those in the transverse wave.

If a longitudinal wave is propagated down an air-filled tube or pipe, the wave will be reflected in much the same manner as waves on a stretched string are reflected, thus setting up standing waves in the pipe. Many musical instruments rely on vibrating columns of air to produce musical sounds. Organ pipes are a simple example. You can see this easily by blowing across the top of a bottle and noting the different frequency of sound excited as you change the level of liquid. This is a "closed at one end–open at the other end" pipe set into resonance. Organ pipes are set into resonance in much the same way. The possible resonant wavelengths (and frequencies) correspond to maximum **displacement** (motion in the direction of the wave) of the air at the open end of the pipe and no displacement at the closed end of the pipe. Depending on whether the pipes are "open one end–closed at the other" or "open both ends," the various allowed wavelengths can be determined as shown in the following depictions.

First consider a "closed at one end–open at the other end" pipe. The first wavelength that can be supported in this pipe is one for which there is no displacement at the closed end and there is displacement at the open end. This situation is depicted in Figure 2.42. In this situation, the closed end of the pipe is a node and the open end of the pipe is an antinode. This means that the air is free to vibrate at the open end of the tube while it does not vibrate at the closed end of the tube. The pipe length corresponds to a quarter of the wavelength and the pipe resonates at this wavelength (four times its length).

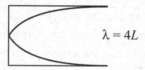

$$\lambda = 4L$$

Figure 2.42. First wavelength from a "closed at one end–open at the other end" pipe

The next possible wave is depicted in Figure 2.43. In this case, there is one node occurring in the pipe, along with the node at the closed end. The additional node makes this a second harmonic. The length of the pipe corresponds to three-quarters of a wavelength for the second harmonic.

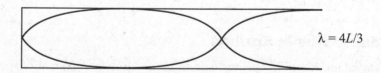

$$\lambda = 4L/3$$

Figure 2.43. A second harmonic

This process can be carried on producing the fundamental, the second harmonic, the third harmonic, and so on.

Now consider an "open at both ends" pipe. In this situation, there is displacement of the air at both ends of the pipe. This situation is depicted in Figure 2.44. The pipe length for this fundamental resonance corresponds to a half wavelength. Note that because neither end is a node, there is only one node here and it is in the interior of the pipe.

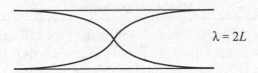

$\lambda = 2L$

Figure 2.44. Wavelength from an "open at both ends" pipe

The next possible wave is depicted in Figure 2.45. With two interior nodes, this is the second harmonic. In this case, the length of the pipe corresponds to a full wavelength (the wavelength of the fundamental, divided by 2).

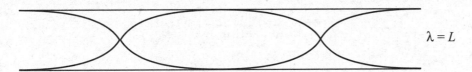

$\lambda = L$

Figure 2.45. The second harmonic

Again, the fundamental wave for the open at both ends pipe is followed by the second harmonic, third harmonic, and so on.

TEST QUESTION

What is the first (fundamental) resonant frequency of an 85 cm long pipe open at one end and closed at the other end? Take the speed of sound as 340 m/s.

(A) 100 Hz

(B) 200 Hz

(C) 300 Hz

(D) 400 Hz

(A) The view of the wave is shown in the figure below. The open end is depicted as having maximum displacement and the closed end as having zero displacement. The speed of sound is given as 340 m/s.

$\lambda = 4L$

Drawing sketches like this is the best way to keep from getting confused in resonant pipe problems. If you sketch the situation, the wavelength for resonance is clearer. The length of the pipe corresponds to one-fourth of a wavelength, so the resonant wavelength for the pipe is 4(0.85 m) = 3.4 m, and the resonant frequency is from

$$v = \lambda f \quad \text{or} \quad f = \frac{v}{\lambda} = \frac{340 \text{ m/s}}{3.4 \text{ m}} = 100 \text{ Hz}$$

The correct answer is A. The wrong answers are the higher harmonics.

Find the resonant frequency of an "open at both ends" pipe of length 0.90 m. Both ends of this pipe have maximum displacement. The displacement situation is as shown in the figure below. It is essential that you draw diagrams like this for resonating pipe problems.

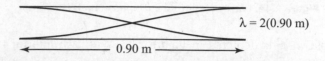

$$\lambda = 2(0.90 \text{ m})$$

0.90 m

Solution: Note that 0.90 m corresponds to half a wavelength. So the fundamental resonance has wavelength 1.8 m.

$$f = \frac{v}{\lambda} = \frac{340 \text{ m/s}}{1.8 \text{ m}} = 189 \text{ Hz}$$

An "open at both ends" pipe has two successive resonances at 567 Hz and 850 Hz. Refer to the graphics above for the possible displacement situations.

Solution: The possible resonant wavelengths for an "open at both ends" pipe is

$$\lambda_n = \frac{2L}{n} \ (n=1,2,3,\ldots).$$

Check the wavelength versus length relationship for the pipes shown in the figures above. To find out whether the frequencies are first and second harmonics, second and third harmonics, or higher, take the first wavelength as n and the next as $n + 1$, producing two equations in one unknown. Velocity is given as 340 m/s, the speed of sound in air.

$$340 \text{ m/s} = \frac{2L}{n}(567 \text{ Hz}) \quad \text{and} \quad 340 \text{ m/s} = \frac{2L}{n+1}(850 \text{ Hz})$$

Setting the velocities equal,

$$\frac{567}{n} = \frac{850}{n+1} \quad \text{or} \quad 567n + 567 = 850n \quad \text{or} \quad n = 2$$

So these frequencies correspond to the second and third harmonics. The second harmonic corresponds to a pipe length equal to one wavelength, so find the wavelength.

$$\lambda = \frac{v}{f} = \frac{340 \text{ m/s}}{567 \text{ Hz}} = 0.60 \text{ m}$$

Therefore, the pipe is 0.60 m long.

Beat Frequencies

A **beat** is an interference between two sounds of slightly different frequencies. The **beat frequency** is the difference between the two frequencies. The frequencies must be close, within about 20 Hz, in order for this effect to be easily perceivable. For example, if a piano player in a band plays the note of A at 440 Hz and a guitarist plays a note at 442 Hz, they would hear the waves become constructive and destructive twice per second as the two tones came in and out of phase. Thus, they would hear a beat frequency of 2 Hz.

HUMAN HEARING

The range of human hearing is 20 Hz to 20,000 Hz. As people get older, or if hearing is damaged, the high frequency end of hearing tends to diminish.

Sound Transmission

Sound is a longitudinal wave. In air, the sound wave is produced by the back and forth motion of individual air molecules moving in the direction of the wave. A good visual image of sound waves is to picture how the sound of a drum gets to your ears. When the drum head is struck, it vibrates and sets the air next to the drumhead in motion. View air as thin slices of collections of molecules that vibrate about an equilibrium position. This back and forth motion of the drumhead is transmitted from one slice of molecules to the next slice of molecules through the air, and in this way the wave travels out from the drumhead. Vibrating air molecules cause adjacent air molecules to also vibrate at the same frequency. Your ear intercepts only a very small portion of the moving air but it is enough to set your eardrum in motion. The vibrations in the air actually move out in spheres but you are only interested in the small column of air between you and the drumhead.

The compression and rarefaction of the air is depicted in Figure 2.46. A longitudinal wave on a spring (slinky) is shown for comparison. The compressions and elongations of the spring as the wave travels along it are comparable to the compressions and rarefactions of the air in the tube. The wave for pressure is shown as the sinusoidal wave superimposed on the depiction of the density of molecules.

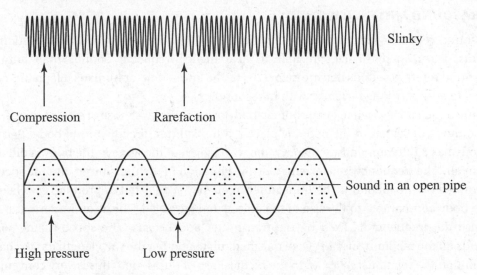

Figure 2.46. Longitudinal wave in spring and air column

For a transverse wave on a rope, the individual pieces of the rope move up and down as the wave moves along the rope. For a longitudinal wave in air, the individual air molecules move back and forth about an equilibrium position as the sound wave passes by. Because of this transmission mechanism, sound requires a medium such as air. Sound cannot be transmitted in vacuum or space because there are no particles to displace. Sound, however, can be transmitted in solids and liquids, and because the molecules are closer together than in air, the speed of sound in liquids is higher than in air and even higher in metallic solids. In air the speed of sound is affected by temperature, the temperature being a measure of how close the air molecules are (at higher temperature, molecules move faster, which results in higher sound speed). In air the speed of sound is around 340 m/s. In water the speed is around 1500 m/s and in steel around 5000 m/s.

The production of sound by a vibrating drumhead was described earlier. The compressions and rarefactions produced are depicted in Figure 2.46, with a sine wave superimposed.

For a single frequency vibration, as envisioned with the vibrating drumhead, the compressions and rarefactions take on this sinusoidal appearance as shown. Even a source as simple as a drumhead, however, has more than one vibration. Instruments such as a violin, with an unusually shaped sound box, produce many different frequencies. So when a violinist bows the string, the string is set into a vibration that has many different frequency waves moving up and down the string, producing sound waves at different frequencies and different amplitudes. These different frequency waves are suppressed or enhanced by the shape of the sound box of the violin. This unique mix of frequencies is what makes one instrument sound different from another. In a symphony orchestra when the conductor calls for tuning, the concertmaster plays concert A on the violin, and as the other instruments play the same note (frequency) it is obvious that each instrument, although playing concert A, sounds different. This difference is due to the mix of frequencies other than the fundamental ones, which are the result of the unique shapes of the other instruments.

A pure frequency can be obtained by using a tuning fork, a U-shaped device that, when struck, vibrates with a specified frequency. Piano tuners use these tuning forks to tune the strings of a piano. Physics students use them to produce pure frequencies for studying resonance in pipes.

ULTRASOUND AND INFRASOUND

Ultrasound refers to sounds that are beyond 20,000 Hz, the upper limit of detection for humans. Dogs, in particular, are able to hear higher frequency sounds than humans. Infrasound refers to sounds that are below 20 Hz, the lower limit for humans. Elephants communicate over very long distances with infrasound.

Ultrasound can be used to image human body parts, especially those of a developing fetus. The sound is delivered to the body by placing a transmitter directly on the body. Because the body has a different density than air, the wavelength of the wave in the body is different than in air. The frequency is determined by the vibration of the transmitter and the speed is determined by the medium. The transmitter frequency is adjusted to produce wavelengths in the body comparable to the size of the objects to be imaged. This is an important point. Because the frequency is fixed by the transmitter and because the speed of the sound depends on the medium, in going from one medium to another the wavelength has to change to maintain the relationship $v = \lambda f$. In the medical use of ultrasound, this is very convenient. Ultrasound imaging has a very low probability of causing damage, which makes it preferable to X-rays for studying internal body parts.

TIP

RESOLUTION OF ULTRASOUND

The resolution of ultrasound depends on the wavelength. Smaller wavelengths are able to get a good image of smaller features.

Suppose in an ultrasound apparatus, high-frequency sound is used to image objects in body tissue. The source of sound is a 4.5 MHz transmitter placed on the body tissue. The physical properties of the tissue, basically density and elasticity, produce a wave speed of 1600 m/s. The choice of frequency for the source produces a wavelength for the sound in the body.

The wavelength follows from the basic relationship, $v = \lambda f$ or $\lambda = v/f$.

$$\lambda_{tissue} = \frac{1600 \text{ m/s}}{4.5 \times 10^6 \text{ Hz}} = 0.00036 \text{ m}$$

The wavelength is a fraction of a centimeter, making it ideal to image objects of roughly this size. The comparable wavelength for this source in air shows a much smaller wavelength.

$$\lambda_{air} = \frac{340 \text{ m/s}}{4.5 \times 10^6 \text{ Hz}} = 0.000076 \text{ m}$$

Intensity and Inverse Square Law

Sound waves transport energy. Most sound sources radiate in a spherically symmetric pattern whereas most detectors are small-area, flat devices. Thus, in sound there are two measures of power: (1) the total power of a source and (2) the **intensity**, the power per unit area at a certain distance from the source. The intensity can be calculated if the total power and the distance from the source are known. It helps to imagine that the sound produced at the source radiates out in three dimensions on the surface of a sphere and that the total power of the sound is distributed evenly around that spherical surface area. Consider that you are standing r meters from a sound source. The intensity at the point you are standing is the total power divided by the surface area of a sphere with radius r. This can also be stated by saying that the intensity times the surface area of a sphere of radius equal to the distance from the source is the total power.

$$P_{total} = I(4\pi r^2)$$

Calculate the intensity at 8.0 m for a spherically symmetric source with a total power output of 10 W. The intensity at 8.0 m is

$$I = \frac{10 \text{ W}}{4\pi(8.0 \text{ m})^2} = 0.012 \text{ W/m}^2$$

The human ear is responsive to sound intensities over a dynamic range of roughly 10^{10}. Also, the human perception of loudness is such that increasing the intensity by a factor of 10 effectively doubles the loudness. This property of the human ear suggests that intensity should be measured on a logarithmic scale. The logarithmic scale is called the decibel scale. It is defined with a base intensity roughly equivalent to a sound level that is just audible to the human ear, $I_0 = 1.0 \times 10^{-12}$ W/m^2 as

$$\beta = (10 \text{ dB})\log\frac{I}{I_0}$$

Sound levels described as so many dB are a measure of the log of the relative intensity of that sound compared to I_0. Sometimes dB is a relative term. Increasing the sound level by a factor of 10 increases the perception of loudness by a factor of 2.

TIP

AMPLITUDE VERSUS INTENSITY

The amplitude of a wave and its intensity are not the same thing. Intensity is proportional to amplitude squared.

The Doppler Effect

The apparent increase or decrease in frequency of a sound when the source or observer are moving toward or away from one another is known as the Doppler effect. If the source and observer are moving toward one another (either because the source is moving, the observer is moving, or both), then the apparent frequency is increased compared to when both are stationary. If the source and observer are moving away from one another, then the frequency is decreased. The general formula covering all cases of source or observer or both moving is

$$f' = f\frac{v \pm v_0}{v \mp v_s}$$

In this formula, f represents the source frequency and f' the frequency heard by the observer. In the fraction, v_o represents the velocity of the observer, meaning the person hearing the sound. The term v_s represents the velocity of the source, or whatever is emitting the sound. In the numerator, the $\pm$ indicates the movement of the observer. The top or *positive* sign should be used for an observer moving *toward* the source. The bottom or *negative* sign should be used for an observer moving *away* from the source. In the denominator, the top and bottom signs are reversed. The *top* sign (in this case negative) should be used for the source moving *toward* the observer. And the *bottom* sign (in this case positive) should be used for the source moving *away* from the observer. Notice that if either the source or the observer moves toward the other, a greater frequency results. If either the source or the observer moves away from the other, a lower frequency results.

Practice Question

A train sounding a whistle at a frequency of 400 Hz is moving toward a stationary observer at a speed of 100 m/s, as depicted in the diagram below. Assume the velocity of sound in air to be 300 m/s. Find the frequency that is heard by the observer.

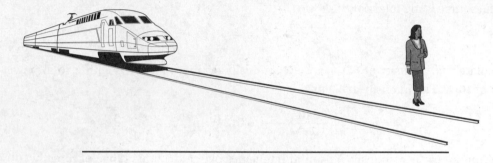

Solution: The apparent frequency heard by the stationary observer is

$$f' = (400 \text{ Hz})\frac{300 \text{ m/s} + 0}{300 \text{ m/s} - 100 \text{ m/s}} = (400 \text{ Hz})\frac{3}{2} = 600 \text{ Hz}$$

The numerator shows the term 300 m/s + 0 because the velocity of the observer is zero. The velocity of the source is subtracted in the denominator because the source is moving toward the observer.

TEST QUESTIONS

An echocardiogram uses ultrasound to determine the speed and direction of blood flow in an artery. A transducer both emits and receives ultrasonic waves. It is placed at an angle of 60° with respect to the blood flow direction as shown below.

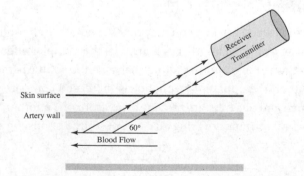

The transducer transmits a frequency, f_t, and receives back a Doppler-shifted frequency, f_r. The difference in these frequencies is used to determine the speed of the blood inside the artery. The speed of sound in air is 330 m/s, the speed of sound in blood is 1500 m/s, and the velocity of the blood is v.

1. What is the correct formula for the Doppler-shifted frequency?

   (A) $fr = ft\left(\dfrac{1500}{1500 + v\cos 60}\right)$

   (B) $fr = ft\left(\dfrac{1500}{1500 + v\sin 60}\right)$

   (C) $fr = ft\left(\dfrac{1500}{1500 - v\cos 60}\right)$

   (D) $fr = ft\left(\dfrac{1500}{1500 - v\sin 60}\right)$

2. The figure above shows a straight path for the ultrasound when traveling through air, skin, and blood. In reality, the direction of the ultrasound changes as it enters the blood because:
   (A) the frequency changes when the medium of propagation changes.
   (B) the speed changes when the medium of propagation changes.
   (C) there is absorption of ultrasound in the blood but not in the air.
   (D) there is interference from other sound waves created by the blood flow.

3. As the transducer is moved along the artery, the velocity of the blood is found to be less. Possible reasons for this are:

   I. the artery is larger in the new region.
   II. there is hemorrhaging of the artery in the new region.
   III. the pressure gradient in the new region is lower.

   (A) I only
   (B) I and II only
   (C) II and III only
   (D) I, II, and III

1. **(A)** The Doppler-shifted frequency is less than the transmitted frequency since the blood is moving away from the detector. So we are looking for a denominator that is greater than the numerator (choice A or B). The component of the blood velocity parallel to the direction of the waves changes the frequency. This is the cosine component.

2. **(B)** When a wave goes from one medium to another, the frequency remains constant. However, the speed changes, which causes a refraction or bending of the light when going from one medium to the other.

3. **(D)** Based on the Bernoulli equation, a larger cross-sectional area in the artery and lower pressure gradient reduce blood velocity. Hemorrhaging causes blood loss, which also reduces the pressure gradient.

SIMPLE HARMONIC MOTION

Simple harmonic motion is motion with a regular (periodic) cycle, such as the oscillation of a mass on a spring, the rotation of a point moving at constant angular speed, or small amplitude pendulum motion. The parameters characterizing the motion are the period (the time for one complete cycle), the frequency (the reciprocal of the period, namely the number of cycles per unit of time), and the amplitude (the maximum excursion from the equilibrium point). Period is measured in seconds and frequency is measured in reciprocal seconds, or Hertz (Hz).

Mass–Spring System

The mass–spring system consists of a mass, m, and a spring with spring constant k that oscillates at a certain amplitude and frequency. The spring is assumed to be a Hooke's law spring. A Hooke's law spring is a spring for which the restoring force (the force that returns the spring to its original position) is proportional to the displacement (the amount that the spring is stretched). If the spring is stretched a certain distance, the restoring force will be a particular value. If the distance stretched is doubled, the restoring force doubles. The statement governing the force is $F = -kx$. The k has the units of N/m or kg/s^2 and the minus sign indicates that the force is always opposite the displacement. The x represents the displacement (how far the spring was stretched from equilibrium. If the spring constant is 3 N/m, for example, then a stretch of 1 m will result in a force of 3 N that is pulling the spring back in the opposite direction (toward the original equilibrium point.)

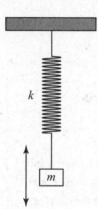

The up and down motion is described by a sinusoidal function of the form

$$x = A \sin \frac{2\pi t}{T} = A \sin 2\pi ft = A \sin \omega t$$

The functional relationship is sinusoidal using the sine function with A, the amplitude of the motion. In the equation, x represents the distance from equilibrium at time, t, during one cycle. Because it takes T seconds to make a cycle, the fraction t/T represents the fraction of the cycle that has passed. Therefore, t ranges from 0 to T. At the same time, the angle for which the sine is being taken ranges from 0 to 2π radians (0 to 360 degrees.) Thus the expression $2\pi t/T$ tells what fraction of 2π (a full circle) has taken place.

In the equation above, $A \sin 2\pi ft$, is derived from the fact the $1/T$ is equal to frequency. The expression $2\pi f$ that results represents a measure called **angular frequency**, represented by the variable ω. The formula indicates that angular frequency can be thought of as frequency times 2π, the number of radians in a circle. Angular frequency can also be derived directly from the mass and the spring constant, $\omega = \sqrt{k/m}$.

The position of an oscillating mass is given by $x = (0.020 \text{ m})\sin(4.2 \text{ rad/s } t)$. Looking at the general expression for a mass in simple harmonic motion, the amplitude of the oscillation is 0.020 m. The angular frequency ω is 4.2 1/s so the frequency and period can be calculated.

$$\omega = 4.2 \text{ 1/s} \quad \text{so} \quad f = \frac{4.2}{2\pi \text{ s}} = 0.67 \text{ 1/s} \quad \text{and} \quad T = 1.5 \text{ s}$$

A mass–spring system consisting of a 2.5 kg mass and a spring of constant 5.5 N/m as shown in Figure 2.47 is set into oscillation. The mass and the spring constant provide the angular frequency, and then the frequency and the period.

$$\omega = \sqrt{\frac{k}{m}} = \sqrt{\frac{5.5 \text{ N/m}}{2.5 \text{ kg}}} = 1.5 \text{ Hz} \quad f = \frac{1}{2\pi}\sqrt{\frac{k}{m}} = 0.24 \text{ Hz} \quad T = 4.2 \text{ s}$$

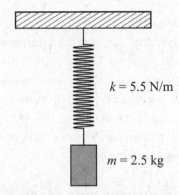

$k = 5.5$ N/m

$m = 2.5$ kg

Figure 2.47. A mass–spring system

Position, Velocity, and Acceleration

Graphs of position, velocity, and acceleration can be drawn for anything in simple harmonic motion. The three graphs in Figure 2.48 show position, velocity, and acceleration as functions of time. Two simple observations help to understand these curves. The velocity of the motion is zero at the extremes. The acceleration is at maximum at the extremes in displacement. The equation $F = -kx$ dictates that the force and hence the acceleration of the mass be greatest when x is maximum.

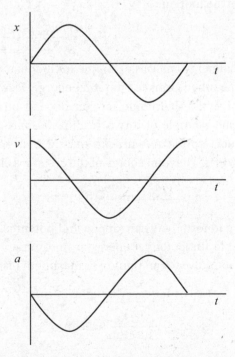

Figure 2.48. Position, velocity, and acceleration as functions of time

The top curve is the displacement. It is a sine wave and shows that the mass moves from equilibrium to maximum positive displacement and continues through one cycle of the sine curve. The middle curve is the velocity. The velocity is maximum in the up direction at the start. The velocity slows until maximum displacement, where it is zero, and then starts negative and continues on as the cosine curve. The bottom curve is for acceleration, which shows zero for zero displacement and then goes negative as the spring is compressed on the upward displacement, going back to zero again as the mass passes through equilibrium. The acceleration curve follows this negative sine curve.

Energy Analysis of Simple Harmonic Motion

In simple harmonic motion, it is obvious that when the spring is fully compressed or elongated, the velocity is zero, indicating zero kinetic energy. However, in these extreme situations, all the energy associated with the motion is stored as potential energy in the spring. In simple harmonic motion, energy is passed back and forth between kinetic energy, which is maximum at equilibrium when the velocity is a maximum, and potential energy, which is maximum when the spring is fully compressed or elongated. Because the kinetic energy is $mv^2/2$, the total energy of the system can be written in terms of maximum velocity. Also since the potential energy is $kx^2/2$, the total energy of the system can be written in terms of the amplitude of the motion.

$$E_{\text{total}} = \frac{mv_{\text{max}}^2}{2} = \frac{kA^2}{2}$$

Energy analysis of simple harmonic motion is based on one or the other forms for the total energy. Examples of energy analysis of simple harmonic motion depend on the initial information. One example of this is to find the maximum displacement of a mass–spring system with mass 2.2 kg, spring constant 1.0 N/m, and maximum velocity 0.20 m/s. The total energy of the system is either

$$\frac{kx_{\text{max}}^2}{2} \text{ or } \frac{mv_{\text{max}}^2}{2}$$

The energy passes back and forth between kinetic and potential, with the kinetic energy at maximum velocity equal to the potential energy at maximum displacement. Using this energy equivalence statement, solve for amplitude or maximum displacement.

$$(1.0 \text{ N/m})x_{\text{max}}^2 = (2.2 \text{ kg})(0.20 \text{ m/s})^2$$

$$x_{\text{max}}^2 = \frac{2.2 \text{ kg}}{1.0 \text{ N/m}}(0.20 \text{ m/s})^2$$

$$x_{\text{max}} = 0.30 \text{ m}$$

Consider the example of a mass–spring system with mass 0.50 kg, period 0.10 s and amplitude 0.020 m. The energy of the system is either

$$\frac{kx^2_{max}}{2} \quad \text{or} \quad \frac{mv^2_{max}}{2}$$

In this problem, mass, amplitude, and period are given, so it will take some creativity to find the energy. Note that $\omega = \sqrt{k/m}$, so $m\omega^2 = k$. Now the total energy can be written as

$$E = \frac{m\omega^2 A^2}{2} \quad \text{with} \quad \omega = \frac{2\pi}{T} = \frac{2\pi}{0.10 \text{ s}} = 20\pi \text{ Hz}$$

so

$$E = \frac{(0.50 \text{ kg})(20\pi/\text{s})^2(0.020 \text{ m})^2}{2} = 0.39 \text{ J}$$

Simple harmonic motion problems also can be encountered in more conventional energy analysis problems.

Practice Question

A 0.20 kg pellet traveling at 20 m/s is fired into a mass (spring system) at rest, as shown in the figure below. The pellet sticks to the 2.0 kg mass, which is attached to a horizontal spring of force constant 100 N/m. The system then oscillates without friction. What is the amplitude of the oscillation?

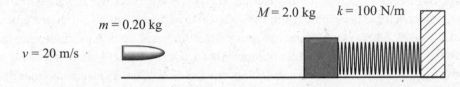

$M = 2.0$ kg $k = 100$ N/m

$m = 0.20$ kg

$v = 20$ m/s

Solution: The problem looks to be appropriate for energy analysis. However, a conservation of momentum approach is needed for the part of the problem in which the pellet goes into the block.

Momentum is conserved in the collision between the pellet and the large mass so write:

$$mv = (m + M)V,$$

where V is the velocity of the pellet and mass. Calculate V.

$$V = \frac{m}{m+M}v = \frac{0.20 \text{ kg}}{2.20 \text{ kg}}(20 \text{ m/s}) = 1.8 \text{ m/s}$$

The pellet comes to rest in the large mass before the two masses together can move any significant distance, so the total energy of the system is

$$E_t = \frac{1}{2}(m+M)V^2 = \frac{1}{2}(2.20 \text{ kg})(1.8 \text{ m/s})^2 = 3.6 \text{ J}$$

Using the displacement form of the total energy,

$$E_t = \frac{kx_{max}^2}{2}$$

$$3.6\ \text{J} = \frac{(100\ \text{N/m})x_{max}^2}{2}$$

$$x_{max} = 0.27\ \text{m}$$

ELECTROSTATICS

Electrostatics is the study of electrical charges that are either stationary or are moving very slowly. **Static electricity** is the buildup of charges on the surface of objects. This buildup can either leak away slowly or discharge quickly.

Charge Transfer

Charge transfer, the transfer of electrical charges from one object to another, is the phenomenon that is readily observed when a balloon is rubbed on hair. The rubbing action causes negative charges to accumulate on the balloon and positive charges to accumulate in the hair. Removing the balloon from the hair isolates these charges. When the balloon is brought back close to the hair, the hair will be attracted to the balloon. Technically, the balloon is equally attracted to the hair, but because hair moves easily, its movement toward the balloon is obvious. If the hair and the balloon are left in contact, the charges will equalize.

In static electricity experiments, rubbing a glass rod with a silk cloth produces a positive charge on the rod, whereas an ebony rod and animal fur combination produces a negative charge on the rod. Atoms in the rod are composed of a positively charged nucleus with orbiting electrons. In the glass and silk combination, the rubbing transfers electrons from the rod to the cloth, leaving the rod with a net positive charge. Atoms that have gained or lost an electron in this process become **ions** and are either positively or negatively charged.

With these charged rods it is easy to do some simple static electricity experiments. If a glass rod is rubbed with silk, the rod becomes positively charged. With the charged rod, charge can be transferred to bits of paper arranged on an insulating surface. The bits of paper will repel one another, indicating that the similarly charged bits of paper repel one another or, simply, like charges repel. A more convincing experiment can be done with lightweight spheres that conduct electricity. The spheres are hung close to one another as illustrated in Figure 2.49.

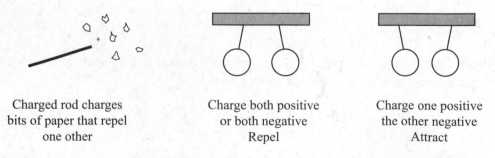

Charged rod charges
bits of paper that repel
one other

Charge both positive
or both negative
Repel

Charge one positive
the other negative
Attract

Figure 2.49. A static electricity experiment

In the image in the center, both spheres have been given the same charge (either positive–positive or negative–negative.) They repel each other. In the image on the right one sphere has been given a negative charge and the other a positive charge. They attract each other.

Induction

Charged bodies can be used to charge other bodies, not necessarily by touching and transferring some charge but by induction, that is, causing charges to move about on the other body. This is best understood by using a charged rod and an initially neutral uncharged metallic rod. Place the metallic rod on an insulating stand. Then bring a charged rod toward one end of this metallic rod. This causes a rearrangement of the charge with the originally uncharged metallic piece becoming oppositely charged in the vicinity of the charging rod.

This inducing of a charge by one object on another object, without touching, is called **induction**. Consider the sequence depicted in Figure 2.50.

If a positively charged rod is brought near one end of an initially uncharged metallic rod that is resting on an insulated stand, the electrons at that end of the uncharged rod will move toward the charged rod, leaving that end negatively charged and leaving the far end positively charged. Touching or grounding the opposite end of the metallic rod results in positive charge being drained off and, with the removal of the positively charged rod, a net negative charge on the metallic rod. This process using a charging rod and metallic rod is shown in Figure 2.50.

> ### ATTRACTION BY INDUCTION
>
> A positively charged rod can attract a neutral metal sphere that is not grounded. Why? Electrostatic induction will cause negative charges to move to the side of the sphere closest to the rod, producing an attraction.

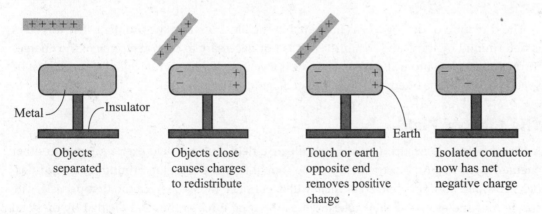

Figure 2.50. Induction

Coulomb's Law

Coulomb's law describes the interactions between static electrical charges on objects. It is the basic force law for charges. The force acts along the line connecting the two charges and is repulsive for like charges and attractive for opposite charges.

$$F = \frac{1}{4\pi\varepsilon_0} \frac{q_1 q_2}{r^2}$$

In the formula above, r is the straight line distance between the two charges, q_1 and q_2. The quantity $\frac{1}{4\pi\varepsilon_0}$ is a constant (the **Coulomb constant** or **Coulomb force constant, k_e**) and has value $\frac{1}{4\pi\varepsilon_0} = 9.0 \times 10^9$ N $\cdot$ m^2/C^2, with $\varepsilon_0 = 8.9 \times 10^{-12}$ C^2/N $\cdot$ m^2. The force is proportional to the product of the charges divided by the square of the distance between them with this constant. This law defines the coulomb (C) of charge. With each charge, one coulomb and a separation of one meter, the constant makes the force come out equal to one newton. One coulomb is equivalent to the charge on 6.25×10^{18} electrons. Two charges in line provide an excellent example of the application of Coulomb's law.

Practice Question

Find the force on $q_1 = 3.0 \times 10^{-6}$ C placed 0.20 m from $q_2 = -2.5 \times 10^{-6}$ C, as shown in the figure below.

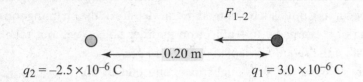

$$q_2 = -2.5 \times 10^{-6} \text{ C} \qquad\qquad\qquad\qquad q_1 = 3.0 \times 10^{-6} \text{ C}$$

Solution: The force is attractive or toward q_2 and has magnitude

$$F_{1-2} = \frac{1}{4\pi\varepsilon_0}\frac{q_1 q_2}{r^2} = 9.0 \times 10^9 \, \frac{\text{N}\cdot\text{m}^2}{\text{C}^2} \frac{(-2.5 \times 10^{-6} \text{ C})(3.0 \times 10^{-6} \text{ C})}{(0.20 \text{ m})^2} = -1.7 \text{ N}$$

The quantity $\dfrac{1}{4\pi\varepsilon_0}$ is a single constant, sometimes written as k.

The direction of the force is as indicated in the illustration in the problem. The direction is determined by the + and – charges so it is not necessary to carry the signs of the charges through the calculations. Because the force is a vector, the magnitude and direction must be specified, but this is often best done with a diagram or words.

The Electric Field

A charged particle is surrounded by an **electric field** and this field exerts a force on other charged particles. An electric field can be thought of as the region around a charged particle in which another charged particle will experience the force from the first particle. The strength of the electric field is measured as the total force of the field divided by the total charge. A force of 6000 N and a charge of 2 C would yield an electric field with a strength of 3000 N/C. The strength of an electric field, then, is the amount of force per unit of charge.

$$E = F/q$$

The electric field is a vector in the direction a positive charge would move in the field. Electric field vectors must be added as vectors. The unit of electric field is the N/C or Volt/meter. Written in analog with Coulomb's law

$$E = \frac{1}{4\pi\varepsilon_0}\frac{q}{r^2}$$

This force between charges makes them move. Isolated charges experience this force from other charges. The direction of the force is radially outward from a positive charge and radially inward to a negative charge. The term *radially* refers to radiating out in all directions from the central point of a sphere. The electric field is depicted by lines with arrows showing the direction of the field, defined as the direction a positive charge would move in that field. Schematically, the strength of the field is represented by the density of these lines of force. For isolated positive and negative charges, the electric field lines go from the positive charge to the negative charge.

A simple example of an electric field problem is two charges on a line, as illustrated in the following problem.

Practice Question

Find the electric field to the right and left (but not between) two charges and along the line joining them, for two charges of $+q$ and $+2q$, separated by a distance, d. Neglecting the field between them simplifies the problem and allows you to see all the features of electric field calculation.

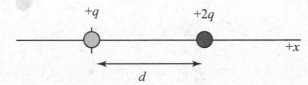

Solution: Place the origin at the $+q$ charge. First consider the field to the right of the $+2q$ charge. The field due to the $+q$ and the $+2q$ is to the right. This is the direction a positive charge would move.

$$E_q = \frac{1}{4\pi\varepsilon_0}\frac{q}{x^2} \qquad E_{2q} = \frac{1}{4\pi\varepsilon_0}\frac{2q}{(x-d)^2}$$

So, the total field to the right of the $+2q$ charge is

$$E = \frac{q}{4\pi\varepsilon_0}\left[\frac{1}{x^2} + \frac{2}{(x-d)^2}\right] \quad x > d$$

Now consider the field to the left of the $+q$ charge. The field is to the left in this region.

$$E_q = \frac{1}{4\pi\varepsilon_0}\frac{q}{x^2} \qquad E_{2q} = \frac{1}{4\pi\varepsilon_0}\frac{2q}{(-x+d)^2} = \frac{1}{4\pi\varepsilon_0}\frac{2q}{(|x|+d)^2}$$

Note that the squared term for $+2q$ uses the absolute value for x. At any distance $-x$ to the left of $+q$ the distance from the $+2q$ is the absolute value of x plus d. So the total field to the left of the $+q$ charge is

$$E = \frac{q}{4\pi\varepsilon_0}\left[\frac{1}{x^2} + \frac{2}{(|x|+d)^2}\right] \quad x < 0$$

Electric fields are often set up between plates or between plates and small spheres. The following problem illustrates what goes on in such an electric field.

TIP

PARALLEL PLATES

The electric field between parallel plates is uniform.

An electric field of 1.0×10^4 V/m = 1.0×10^4 J/C·m is established between plates separated by 10 cm. An electron is released from the negative plate and moves to the positive plate. What is the acceleration of the electron, the velocity at the opposite plate, the kinetic energy at the opposite plate, and the time for the electron to move from one plate to the other?

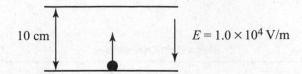

Solution: The force on the electron is eE, and this force makes the mass (the electron) accelerate.

$$a = \frac{eE}{m} = \frac{(1.6 \times 10^{-19} \text{ C})(1.0 \times 10^4 \text{ J/C·m})}{9.1 \times 10^{-31} \text{ kg}} = 1.8 \times 10^{15} \text{ m/s}^2$$

The electron starts from zero velocity at the positive plate, so v is from the basic kinematic equation

$$v^2 = v_0^2 + 2a(x - x_0)$$
$$v^2 = 0^2 + 2(1.8 \times 10^{15} \text{ m/s}^2)(1.0 \times 10^{-1} \text{ m})$$
$$v = 1.9 \times 10^7 \text{ m/s}$$

The total energy is kinetic.

$$\frac{1}{2}mv^2 = \frac{1}{2}(9.1 \times 10^{-31} \text{ kg})(3.6 \times 10^{14} \text{ m}^2/\text{s}^2) = 1.6 \times 10^{-16} \text{ J}$$

The time for the trip is from another basic kinematic equation

$$x = v_0 t + \frac{1}{2}at^2$$

$$t = \sqrt{\frac{2x}{a}} = \sqrt{\frac{2(1.0 \times 10^{-1} \text{ m})}{(1.8 \times 10^{15} \text{ m/s}^2)}} = 1.0 \times 10^{-8} \text{ s}$$

Alternatively, the energy can be obtained in eV. The electron falls through a voltage of 1.0×10^3 V, so it has an energy of 1.0×10^3 eV. Remember that 1 eV is equivalent to 1.6×10^{-19} joule.

$$10 \times 10^3 \text{ eV} \cdot 1.6 \times 10^{-19} \text{ J/eV} = 1.6 \times 10^{-16} \text{ J}$$

Gauss's Law

Gauss's law is a very calculus concept-oriented law, but Gauss's law problems can be understood without resorting to involved calculus-type mathematical operations.

Gauss's law starts with the concept of flux. Flux is a property of vector fields. The field lines are a construct to aid in understanding electric fields, and are envisioned as lines indicating the direction a positive charge would move in the field. The strength (intensity) of the field is measured by the density, or number per area, of field lines.

Consider a problem in which an *E* field of 1.0×10^3 N/C is normal to a flat surface with area 12 cm² as shown in Figure 2.51.

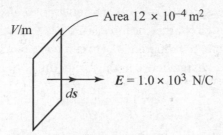

V/m — Area 12×10^{-4} m²

ds

$E = 1.0 \times 10^3$ N/C

Figure 2.51. Flux

The vector, *E*, and a surface element, *ds*, have zero angle between them, so the flux is simply

$$\phi_E = (1.0 \times 10^3 \text{ N/C})(12 \times 10^{-4} \text{ m}^2) = 1.2 \text{ N} \cdot \text{m}^2/\text{C}$$

This flux number represents the density of flux lines normal to the surface. Although this is a calculus definition, the representation of the flux in terms of field strength and area is quite simple.

The specific Gauss's law relates the flux out of a closed surface to the charge contained. The equation for charge enclosed by a sphere is

$$q = \varepsilon_0 E(4\pi r^2)$$

Practice Question

Determine the electric field on a sphere of radius 0.10 m containing a charge of 1.0×10^{-6} C placed at its center.

Solution: Note that the symmetry in the problem makes *E* a constant over the sphere. Applying Gauss's law:

$$q = \varepsilon_0 E(4\pi r^2)$$

$$E = \frac{q}{4\pi\varepsilon_0} \frac{1}{r^2} = (9.0 \times 10^9 \text{ N} \cdot \text{m}^2/\text{C}^2) \frac{1.0 \times 10^{-6} \text{ C}}{(0.10 \text{ m})^2} = 9.0 \times 10^5 \text{ N/C}$$

Thus, electric fields at any distance from charges can be calculated with this formula and they are radially out from the charge. For multiple charges these fields add as vectors.

Electric Potential

In mechanics, force analysis of problems works well when the force is a constant. When the force is not a constant, the concepts of work and energy are used. In an electric field, for example the field surrounding a charge, the force is not a constant and the concept of **electric potential** is needed. The potential difference between two points A and B is defined as the work to move a unit positive charge between the two points.

$$V_B - V_A = \frac{W_{AB}}{q_0}$$

Electric potential is a scalar. For convenience in calculating a specific electric potential, one point is taken at infinity and is assigned the arbitrary potential of zero. The unit of electric potential is the **volt** (V), equal to a joule per coulomb or work per charge. The electric potential near a positive charge is positive. It takes positive work to move a unit positive charge from infinity (zero potential) into the vicinity of a positive charge. In the vicinity of a charge the electric potential is given by

$$V = \frac{q}{4\pi\varepsilon_0}\frac{1}{r}$$

For a large number of charges the voltages add as scalars, which make for an easier calculation compared with working with electric field vectors. For a collection of charges the potential at any point is the scalar sum of the contribution of each charge.

$$V = \sum_n V_n = \frac{1}{4\pi\varepsilon_0}\sum_n \frac{q_n}{r_n}$$

Electric field and electric potential are related by

$$E = -\frac{\Delta V}{\Delta s}$$

Another important concept is that of the **electron-volt** (eV). One eV is equivalent to 1.6×10^{-19} joule. An electron that has fallen through one volt of electric potential is said to have 1 eV of energy.

Consider the potential 0.25 m away from a single charge of -5.0×10^{-6} C, as illustrated in Figure 2.52.

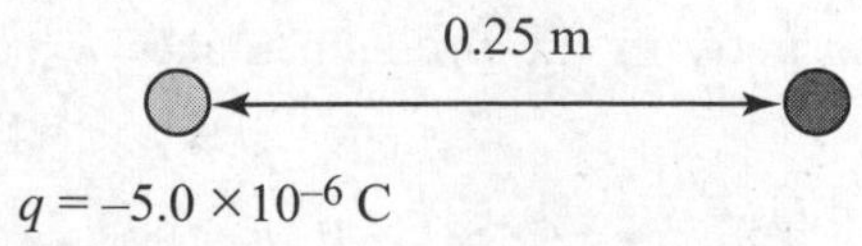

$$q = -5.0 \times 10^{-6} \text{ C}$$

Figure 2.52. Electrical potential

$$V = \frac{1}{4\pi\varepsilon_0}\frac{q}{r} = -(9.0\times10^9 \text{ N}\cdot\text{m}^2/\text{C}^2)\frac{5.0\times10^{-6} \text{ C}}{0.25 \text{ m}} = -180\times10^3 \text{ J/C} = -1.80\times10^5 \text{ V}$$

The potential is negative because negative work has to be done to move a unit positive charge from infinity to 0.25 m away from a negative charge.

Practice Question

For the situation shown in the figure below, find the electric potential 1.0 cm perpendicular (and opposite the negative charge) from the line joining two charges, $q_1 = -5.0 \times 10^{-9}$ C and $q_2 = 2.0 \times 10^{-9}$ C, separated by 3.0 cm.

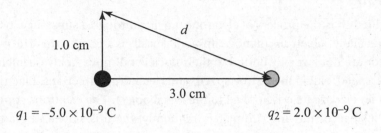

$q_1 = -5.0 \times 10^{-9}$ C $q_2 = 2.0 \times 10^{-9}$ C

Solution: First find the distance from q_2 to the point in question.

$$d^2 = 1^2 + 3^2 = 10 \text{ cm}^2 \qquad d = \sqrt{10} \text{ cm}$$

The most difficult part of this problem is keeping the signs correct. The potential due to q_1 is negative.

$$V_1 = \frac{1}{4\pi\varepsilon_0}\frac{q_1}{r} = -(9.0 \times 10^9 \text{ N·m}^2/\text{C}^2)\frac{5.0 \times 10^{-9} \text{ C}}{1.0 \times 10^{-2} \text{ m}} = -4.5 \times 10^3 \text{ V}$$

The potential due to q_2 is positive.

$$V_2 = (9.0 \times 10^9 \text{ N·m}^2/\text{C}^2)\frac{2.0 \times 10^{-9} \text{ C}}{\sqrt{10} \times 10^{-2} \text{ m}} = 570 \text{ V}$$

The total potential is

$$V = V_1 + V_2 = -3930 \text{ V}$$

Practice Question

Consider a spherical drop of water of radius 0.20 mm carrying a charge of 4.0×10^{-12} C. What is the potential at the surface of this drop of water?

Solution:

$$V = \frac{1}{4\pi\varepsilon_0}\frac{q}{r} = (9.0 \times 10^9 \text{ N·m}^2/\text{C}^2)\frac{4.0 \times 10^{-12} \text{ C}}{2.0 \times 10^{-4} \text{ m}} = 180 \text{ V}$$

DC CIRCUITS

The study of DC circuits starts with an understanding of electric conduction, current, batteries, and resistance.

Conduction

Electric **conduction** is the process of electrons moving through a substance, usually a metal. A material that allows electrons to move through it easily is a **conductor**. The outer electrons in a conductor are not strongly bound to their nuclei and move freely through the material at a very high speed, called **mean free speed**, and in random directions. Electric conduction occurs when an electric field is applied to the metal object. The electrons continue to move rapidly, but instead of moving completely randomly, there is slow and gradual **drift** in a particular direction (the direction opposite of the applied field). This **drift velocity** is small compared to the mean free speed.

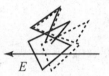

Drift Velocity

The motion of each electron in a current is influenced by the drift velocity, the mean free speed, the mean free path length (the length between collisions with the massive ion cores in the metal), and the relaxation time (the time between collisions). The drift velocity is determined by the applied field. The other parameters are determined by the material and physical conditions such as temperature and pressure.

Current

Current is the flow of charge. The charges can be positive (ions) or negative (electrons). In metallic circuits it is the electrons that move. In electric theory the convention is that current is in the direction of flow of positive charge. Thus, electron flow is in the opposite direction to conventional current flow. In a wire, the electric current is the amount of charge passing a cross section of a wire each second. The mathematical relationship is written in terms of charge and time, Q and t or Δq and Δt, where Q is charge and I is current.

$$I = \frac{Q}{t} \text{ or } i = \frac{\Delta q}{\Delta t}$$

The unit of current is the ampere, defined as a coulomb per second passing a cross section of the conductor (A = C/s).

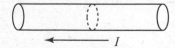

Current can be measured in terms of total charge or in terms of actual numbers of electrons passing a cross section of a conductor as depicted in Figure 2.53. An electron current of 1.0×10^{15} electrons passing a cross section of wire every second produces a certain current.

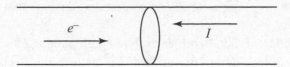

Figure 2.53. Electrons passing a cross section of a conductor

The charge per electron is 1.6×10^{-19} C/electron, so the current in the wire is

$$I = \frac{1.0 \times 10^{15} e}{s} \times \frac{1.6 \times 10^{-19} \text{ C}}{e} = 1.6 \times 10^{-4} \text{ C/s} = 1.6 \times 10^{-4} \text{ A}$$

Remember that the current direction is opposite to the electron flow, as illustrated in Figure 2.53.

The **current density** is defined as the current per cross-sectional area. For a current of 50 A in a wire of 0.50 cm diameter, the current density is

$$j = \frac{i}{A} = \frac{50 \text{ A}}{\pi (0.25 \times 10^{-2} \text{ m})^2} = 2.5 \times 10^6 \text{ A/m}^2$$

The amount of charge in a length of wire is the product of the number density of charge carriers (electrons) times the charge per carrier times the volume, where the volume can be written as the cross-sectional area times a length, or $q = nAle$. In the presence of an electric field, the time for this charge to move the length, l, is this length divided by the drift velocity, $t = l/v_d$. The current, $\Delta q/\Delta t$, is written in as

$$i = \frac{\Delta q}{\Delta t} = \frac{nAle}{l/v_d} = nAev_d$$

For a typical metallic wire conductor, the density of electron charge carriers is 8.0×10^{25}/m^3. If the wire has cross-sectional area of 1.0×10^{-4} m^2 and a current of 5.0×10^{-2} A, the drift velocity is given by

$$v_d = \frac{i}{nAe} = \frac{5.0 \times 10^{-2} \text{ A}}{(8.0 \times 10^{25} \text{ } e/\text{m}^3)(1.0 \times 10^{-4} \text{ m}^2)(1.6 \times 10^{-19} \text{ C}/e)} = 3.9 \times 10^{-5} \text{ m/s}$$

This drift velocity is a very slow velocity.

Batteries

Batteries are composed of two distinct materials that differ in their affinity for attracting electrons. Because of this difference, electrons move between the two poles of the battery. The affinity of a material for attracting electrons is called **electronegativity**.

Two probes of different metals—for example, copper and zinc—placed in a fruit such as an orange, form a battery. The liquid in the orange provides a medium through which charges can move from one metal probe to the other. The difference in electronegativity causes electrons to move from one probe to the other. In this way, the battery can be viewed as a device that "pumps" charges.

The typical dry cell battery has a zinc cylindrical electrode and a pressed carbon rod center electrode. Their 1.5 V electronegativity difference is the dry cell voltage. The medium between the carbon rod and zinc cylinder in a dry cell is a paste rather than a liquid. This paste is an **electrolyte**, meaning a substance containing free ions that make the substance electrically conductive.

There are many different metal and electrolyte combinations for making a battery. An automotive battery is quite different from a flashlight battery, but the principle is the same. A schematic of a typical dry cell battery is shown in Figure 2.54.

TIP

BATTERIES

Batteries placed in a series produce the sum of the two voltages, whereas batteries set in parallel give the same voltage.

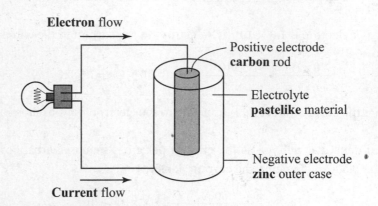

Figure 2.54. A typical dry-cell battery

Resistance and Resistivity

RESISTANCE

Resistance is a measure of the degree to which the movement of electrons is inhibited. The relationship between resistance, voltage, and current is given as $V = IR$ or $R = V/I$. If a fixed voltage is applied to a resistor, then a higher resistance results in a lower current and vice versa. The unit of resistance is the **ohm**, which is a volt per ampere ($\Omega = V/A$). In Figure 2.55, consider the battery voltage to be 1.5 V and the current to be 0.6 A. The resistance of the lightbulb is

$$R = \frac{V}{I} = \frac{1.5\,\text{V}}{0.6\,\text{A}} = 2.5\,\Omega$$

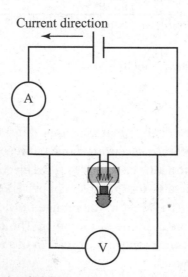

Figure 2.55. Resistance in a lightbulb. Note that the direction of conventional current flow is shown by the arrow. In this diagram, the 1.5 V battery supplies current to the lightbulb. The current is measured with the ammeter, and the voltage "across" the lightbulb is measured with the voltmeter. The ratio of V to I is the resistance of the lightbulb.

Lightbulb filaments increase in resistance with increasing temperature, which is typical of metals. When the light is first switched on, the filament is cold, has low resistance, and draws a large current. The large current heats the filament, which increases in resistance and reduces current. As the current goes down, the heating effect lessens until an equilibrium is reached.

Resistors are very common circuit elements. The simplest resistor is a coil of wire, usually wound on a ceramic or carbon rod. Depending on what it is mixed with and how hard it is, compressed carbon resistors can be made over a very wide range of values.

RESISTIVITY

When an electron leaves the battery and enters the conductor, that electron does not flow through the wire and come out the other end. Rather, in moving just slightly in one direction, it causes the nearest electrons to also move slightly in that direction. Electrons move relatively slowly through a conductor, effectively drifting at slow speeds. The relatively free electrons experience an electric field that accelerates them in a direction opposite the field. They accelerate until they crash into an ion core, at which point they momentarily stop and begin the acceleration again. This stopping can be thought of as the conductor's **resistivity** to the movement of electrons.

The more frequently an electron collides with an ion core, the more resistivity it will experience. The number of collisions per second is determined by the mean free speed (how fast the random motion of the electron is). The mean free speed is determined primarily by properties of the material (what it is made of, temperature, pressure). A given material at a given temperature and pressure will have a specific resistivity.

Resistance and resistivity are not exactly the same thing. Consider two pieces of copper wire. The first is 1 m long and has a cross-sectional area (thickness of the end of the wire) of 4π mm^2. The second is 3 m long and has a cross-sectional area of 9π mm^2. Both have the same resistivity because they are made of the same material and are at the same temperature and pressure. The total resistance for each wire, however, will be different because of the different lengths and cross-sectional areas.

Resistance, R, and resistivity, ρ, are related by the equation $R = \rho\,(l/A)$, where l is length and A is cross-sectional area. Resistance increases with the length and decreases with cross-sectional area. This means that a longer piece of wire has more resistance. However, it also means that a thicker wire has less resistance, which may seem counterintuitive. You can think of a thicker wire as offering the electrons multiple paths of equal resistance, which leads to less overall resistance. The units of resistivity are ohm-meter ($\Omega \cdot$ m).

The resistivity of nichrome, a nickel-chrome combination that is very stable at high temperatures in air, is $100 \times 10^{-8}\ \Omega \cdot$ m. This material is the preferred wire for electric toasters and heaters of all sorts.

METER RESISTANCES

A voltmeter has high resistance so as not to divert current away from what is being measured, because it is placed in parallel in a circuit. An ammeter has very low resistance. It is placed in series in a circuit, and a large resistance would cause a voltage drop across the meter.

A nichrome heater is constructed of 12 m of nichrome wire with cross section 2.0×10^{-7} m². Determine the resistance of the wire and the current in the heater when it is connected to a 120 V source.

Solution: First calculate the resistance of the 12 m length of wire. Use the resistivity value given above.

$$R = \rho\frac{l}{A} = (100 \times 10^{-8}\,\Omega\cdot\text{m})\,\frac{12\,\text{m}}{2.0 \times 10^{-7}\,\text{m}^2} = 60\,\Omega$$

Now the current is

$$I = \frac{120\,\text{V}}{60\,\Omega} = 2.0\,\text{A}$$

Batteries, Work, and *emf*

In a battery, work is performed on a charge as it moves through the battery, thus raising the potential energy of the charge. When connected to an external circuit, this potential energy is expended as the charge travels out of the battery, through the circuit, and back to the battery (see Figures 2.54 and 2.55). The ability of the battery to do work on the charge passing through it is called the **electromotive force (*emf*)**. This electromotive force is measured in volts. A 12-volt battery can perform 12 joules of work on each coulomb of charges passing through it. The battery is said to have an *emf* of 12 volts.

A battery connected to a load with resistance R, causes a current to flow that follows the $V = IR$ relation. For the current through the load, the drop in potential across the load is the same as the gain in potential for the charge moving through the battery. This is a conservation of energy statement. The gain in energy within the battery is equal to the energy dissipated outside the battery.

Real batteries have internal resistance associated with the charge moving through the battery. The voltage at the terminals of a battery with no load is the *emf* of the battery. When the battery is connected to a load, current flows and because of the internal resistance of the battery, the voltage at the terminals drops. In circuits, batteries are usually depicted as a voltage source in series with an internal resistance. For a battery with an *emf* (the rated or no load voltage) of 12 V and internal resistance of 0.40 Ω connected to a 20 Ω resistor, the terminal voltage and voltage across the load can be calculated. Figure 2.56 shows how a real battery is portrayed in a circuit. The dashed line encloses the battery.

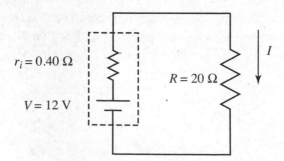

$r_i = 0.40\,\Omega$

$R = 20\,\Omega$

$V = 12\,\text{V}$

I

Figure 2.56. A battery in a circuit

The current is

$$I = \frac{12 \text{ V}}{20.4 \text{ }\Omega} = 0.59 \text{ A}$$

And the voltage across the load is

$$V_R = IR = (0.59 \text{ A})(20 \text{ }\Omega) = 11.8 \text{ V}$$

The terminal voltage is the *emf* minus the voltage drop for the internal resistance.

$$\text{Terminal voltage} = (12 \text{ V}) - (0.59 \text{ A})(0.40 \text{ }\Omega) = 11.8 \text{ V}$$

Power

The voltage across any load is a measure of the work that can be performed on the charges passing through the load, volt = joule/coulomb. The current through the load is the amount of charge per time, A = coulomb/sec. The product of the voltage and the current has the units of joule/sec, which is the definition of power measured in **watts**. Because of the Ohm's law relationship, the power can be written in terms of any two of the three parameters—voltage, current, and resistance.

$$P = VI = \frac{V^2}{R} = I^2 R$$

The easiest form to use is usually *VI*. The expression $I^2 R$ is called the joule heating form. In many instances, this power calculation gives the power dissipated in a resistor. In the nichrome wire calculation, the power dissipated by the nichrome wire as heat is

$$P = I^2 R = (2.0 \text{ A})^2 (60 \text{ }\Omega) = 240 \text{ W}$$

Resistors

RESISTORS IN SERIES

As circuit elements, resistors in series add linearly as illustrated in Figure 2.57. In a series arrangement, the current through each resistor is the same.

$$R = R_1 + R_2$$

Figure 2.57. Resistors in series

TIP

POWER TRANSMISSION

In order to get the least amount of loss from heating of the wires, it is best to transmit electrical power at high voltage and low current so that the I^2R power loss is minimized.

Two resistors, 30 Ω and 40 Ω, are placed in series with a 10 V source as shown in the following illustration.

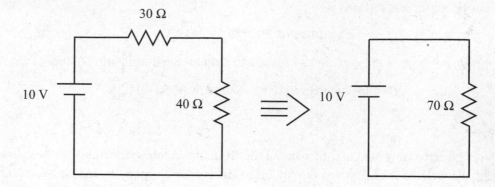

What is the equivalent resistance (and circuit), the total current from the source, and the current and voltage drop for each resistor?

Solution:

$$R = R_1 + R_2 \qquad R = 40\ \Omega + 30\ \Omega = 70\ \Omega$$

The total current is

$$I = \frac{V}{R} = \frac{10\ \text{V}}{70\ \Omega} = 0.14\ \text{A}$$

Because the resistors are in series, the current is the same in both. The voltage on each is

$$V = IR \qquad V_{30} = (0.14\ \text{A})(30\ \Omega) = 4.3\ \text{V} \qquad V_{40} = (0.14\ \text{A})(40\ \Omega) = 5.7\ \text{V}$$

The voltage across the two resistors adds up to the source voltage, as it should.

RESISTORS IN PARALLEL

If three resistors are placed in parallel, as shown in Figure 2.58, and a voltage is applied to this combination, the voltage across each resistor is equal to the applied voltage with the current in each resistor determined by $V = IR$ for that resistor. In a parallel arrangement, the voltage on each resistor is the same. The resistors add in a reciprocal manner:

$$\frac{1}{R_{eq}} = \frac{1}{R_1} + \frac{1}{R_2} + \frac{1}{R_3} + \ldots$$

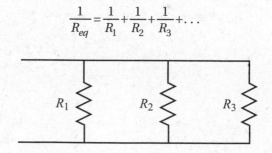

Figure 2.58. Resistors in parallel

Find the current in each resistor, the equivalent resistance, and equivalent circuit for the combination of 3.0 Ω, 3.5 Ω, and 4.0 Ω resistors placed in parallel with 10 V applied, as shown in the following diagram.

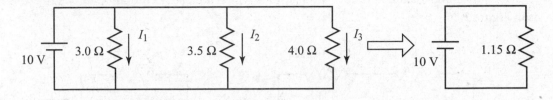

Solution: The current in each resistor is

$$I_1 = \frac{10\text{ V}}{3.0\text{ }\Omega} = 3.3\text{ A}\quad I_2 = \frac{10\text{ V}}{3.5\text{ }\Omega} = 3.0\text{ A}\quad I_3 = \frac{10\text{ V}}{4.0\text{ }\Omega} = 2.5\text{ A}$$

so the total current is 8.8 A.

The equivalent resistance is

$$\frac{1}{R_{eq}} = \frac{1}{3.0\text{ }\Omega} + \frac{1}{3.5\text{ }\Omega} + \frac{1}{4.0\text{ }\Omega} = \frac{14}{42\text{ }\Omega} + \frac{12}{42\text{ }\Omega} + \frac{10.5}{42\text{ }\Omega} = \frac{36.5}{42\text{ }\Omega}\quad R_{eq} = \frac{42}{36.5}\text{ }\Omega = 1.15\text{ }\Omega$$

The equivalent resistance calculated using this fraction approach is fast and convenient if the resistance numbers are small, as they will be on the MCAT. The current calculated from the equivalent circuit is the same as before (with slight rounding error from our fraction addition).

$$I = \frac{10\text{ V}}{1.15\text{ }\Omega} = 8.7\text{ A}$$

SERIES-PARALLEL COMBINATION RESISTORS

Series-parallel resistor combinations are best learned by example. The first step is to find the equivalent resistance for the parallel combination. Combining this with the other series resistor is fairly easy. Consider the series-parallel resistor combination connected to 50 volt source as shown in Figure 2.59.

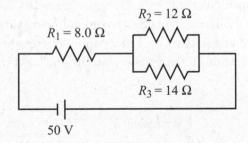

Figure 2.59. A series-parallel resistor combination

The first step in analyzing this circuit is to find the equivalent resistance, R_4, of the parallel combination.

$$\frac{1}{R_4} = \frac{1}{R_2} + \frac{1}{R_3} = \frac{1}{12\,\Omega} + \frac{1}{14\,\Omega} = \frac{26}{14 \cdot 12\,\Omega} \quad \text{or} \quad R_4 = \frac{168\,\Omega}{26} = 6.5\,\Omega$$

The equivalent resistance is now two resistors, which are easily combined to one resistor as in Figure 2.60.

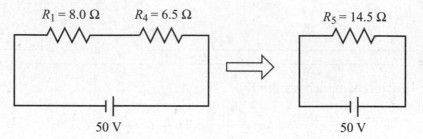

Figure 2.60. Two resistors combine into one

Now it is necessary to work backward to find the voltage and current in all the resistors. The 50 V across the 14.5 Ω produces a total current of (50/14.5) A = 3.4 A. This 3.4 A flows through the 8.0 Ω resistor, producing a voltage drop across this resistor of (3.4 A)(8.0 Ω) = 27.2 V. This means that there are (50 – 27.2) V = 22.8 V across the parallel combination. The 22.8 V across the 12 Ω resistor produce an I_2 of (22.8/12) A = 1.9 A.

Similarly for the 14 Ω resistor, the current I_3 is (22.8/14) A = 1.6 A. The currents in the two parallel resistors add up, within round-off error, to the total current in the circuit. This working backward and keeping everything labeled in the process is important in getting the correct answer to a perhaps obscure question, such as "What is the power dissipated in the 12 Ω resistor?" With the information available, the power is most easily calculated from the $P = VI$ form, so $P_{12} = (22.8\ \text{V})(1.9\ \text{A}) = 43\ \text{W}$.

CAPACITANCE

Capacitance is a measure of the ability to store charge. This is done through a **capacitor**, an arrangement of conducting surfaces on which charge can be stored. The capacitance of the arrangement is the amount of charge that can be stored per volt of potential difference between the surfaces. In mathematical terms the capacitance is $C = Q/V$, where Q is charge. The unit of capacitance is the **farad**, defined as a coulomb/volt. Although capacitors can be concentric cylinders, concentric spheres, or even separate spheres, the most convenient shape to use in understanding capacitors is the parallel plate arrangement shown in Figure 2.61.

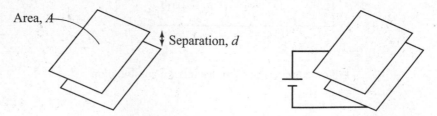

Figure 2.61. Parallel plate arrangement

The capacity of this parallel plate arrangement is measured by the amount of charge that can be stored on the plates. A battery connected to these plates can be viewed as a charge pump that pumps positive charge on one plate and negative charge on the other plate. In Figure 2.61 the graphic on the right shows the plates connected to a battery. As the battery pumps charge on the plates, the first bit of charge goes on with little effort, but as the amount of charge on the plate increases, the mutual repulsion of like charges makes it more and more difficult to add charge. At a certain point no more charge can be added. The capacitor has reached its capacity for that voltage.

If the plate area is increased, the capacitance is increased. If the plates are moved closer together, the mutual attraction between the opposite charges allows for more charge to be stored. The capacity of a parallel plate arrangement is proportional to the area of the plates (more area means more charge) and inversely proportional to the separation (more separation means less charge). With the appropriate constant,

$$C = \frac{k\varepsilon_0 A}{d}$$

where ε_0 is the permittivity of free space and has the value 8.9×10^{-12} F/m and k is the dielectric constant, which is 1 for air or a vaccum.

Capacitors are made by rolling a sandwich consisting of thin metallic sheets and a "dielectric" material that maintains a small but constant separation and has an effective permittivity greater than free space, making for a higher capacitance. This increased permittivity is given in terms of a multiplier called the dielectric constant. For polystyrene, a very popular insulating material for rolled capacitors, the dielectric constant is 2.6. A rolled capacitor might have a spacing of 1.0×10^{-4} m, a width of 2.0 cm, and a length of 50 m. Using polystyrene for the dielectric the calculation of the capacitance gives

$$C = \frac{2.6(8.9 \times 10^{-12} \text{ F/m})(2.0 \times 10^{-2} \text{ m})(50 \text{ m})}{1.0 \times 10^{-4} \text{ m}} = 2.3 \times 10^{-7} \text{ F} = 0.23 \text{ µF}$$

Because of their ability to store charge, capacitors play an important role as circuit elements.

CAPACITORS IN PARALLEL

Capacitors placed in parallel add in a linear manner. In the parallel plate capacitor, the capacitance is proportional to the surface area. Placing capacitors in parallel is equivalent to increasing the total surface area.

Practice Question

Find the equivalent capacitance, equivalent circuit, and charge situation for a 12 µF capacitor placed in parallel with an 8 µF capacitor and an applied voltage of 100 V as shown in the diagram below.

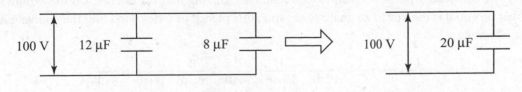

Solution: The capacitors in parallel add linearly so the equivalent circuit is as shown. The applied voltage is 100 V, so the charge can be determined from the capacitance.

$$q_{12} = C_{12}V = (12\,\mu F)(100\,V) = 12 \times 10^{-4}\,C$$

$$q_8 = (8\,\mu F)(100\,V) = 8 \times 10^{-4}\,C$$

$$q_{20} = (20\,\mu F)(100\,V) = 20 \times 10^{-4}\,C$$

The total charge on the two parallel capacitors equals the charge on their equivalent.

CAPACITORS IN SERIES

Capacitors placed in series add in the reciprocal manner. This is the opposite of what is true for resistors.

Arrangement	Capacitor	Resistor
Series	Add reciprocally	Add linearly
Parallel	Add linearly	Add reciprocally

Practice Question

Find the equivalent capacitance, equivalent circuit, and charge situation for a 10 μF capacitor placed in series with a 15 μF capacitor, and 100 V applied as shown in the diagram below.

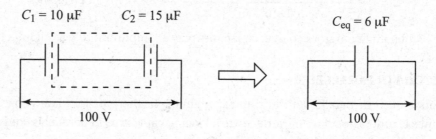

Solution: The capacitors in series add in the reciprocal manner. The equivalent circuit is as shown. The voltage on the two capacitors is not the same, but the charge on them is the same.

Look at the capacitor plates enclosed in the dashed line. There is no connection to the battery, so the total charge in this enclosed area must add to zero. Simply put, for a negative charge on the one plate of C_1, there must be a numerically equal positive charge on the directly connected plate of C_2 and vice versa. Recognizing that the charges on these plates must be equal is the key to an analysis of capacitors placed in series. First find the equivalent capacitance.

$$\frac{1}{C_{eq}} = \frac{1}{C_1} + \frac{1}{C_2} = \frac{1}{10\,\mu F} + \frac{1}{15\,\mu F} = \frac{3}{30\,\mu F} + \frac{2}{30\,\mu F} = \frac{5}{30\,\mu F} = \frac{1}{6\,\mu F}$$

This equivalent capacitor is shown in the diagram. The charge can now be calculated from $q = CV$.

$$q = (6\ \mu F)(100\ V) = 6 \times 10^{-4}\ C$$

The charges are the same, allowing calculation of the voltage on each capacitor. That the voltages add up to the 100 V applied is evidence that the charges on the equivalent and each single capacitor are the same.

$$V_1 = \frac{6 \times 10^{-4}\ C}{10\ \mu F} = 60\ V \quad V_2 = \frac{6 \times 10^{-4}\ C}{15\ \mu F} = 40\ V$$

ELECTROMAGNETISM

Electromagnetism is one of the fundamental forces of nature and governs the interactions of charged particles both in ordinary matter and on a subatomic level. The MCAT will test concepts of magnetism and electromagnetic fields.

Magnetism

Magnetic material called magnetite or lodestone occurs in nature. Pieces of magnetite that are free to rotate align themselves with the large magnetic field of Earth. A study of this orientation phenomena and the attraction/repulsion of individual magnets lead to the idea of magnetic poles. Earth itself is a giant magnet with north (N) and south (S) poles. Magnets can induce magnetism in certain other materials such as soft iron when they are placed close together. This is what causes attraction between magnets and initially unmagnetized iron pieces. Any magnet that is free to move, such as a compass needle, orients with one pole pointing to what we refer to as the N pole of Earth.

> **CUTTING A MAGNET**
>
> If you cut a permanent magnet in half, in the middle between the south and north poles, you do not get isolated poles. The original poles stay the same, and the end that you cut becomes the opposite pole.

The magnetic unit is the **tesla** (T) which is a N/A·m. The tesla is related to the smaller magnetic unit, the **gauss** (1 tesla = 10^4 gauss). The intensity (flux) of the magnetic field is the **weber** (1 Wb = 1 T · m²).

Moving Charges in a Magnetic Field

A magnetic field, whether naturally occurring or produced electrically, exerts a force on a *moving* charge. This force is a vector force $F = qv \times B$, where B is the strength of the magnetic (B) field. If a particle with negative charge, mass, and velocity is injected into a B field, with orientation as shown in Figure 2.62, the force is at right angles to the velocity and the particle moves in a circle. A positively charged particle would move in a counterclockwise circle. The force is *always* at right angles to the velocity and for right angles has magnitude qvB. This force provides the (centripetal) mechanical force required to move a mass in a circle, that is, the mv^2/r force.

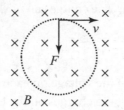

The crosses are the tails of arrows representing the B field.

Figure 2.62. A magnetic (B) field

An electron would move in a circle, indicated by the dashed line in the figure, and with a radius calculated by equating the force on the moving charge (due to the magnetic field) to the mechanical force required to make a mass move in a circle

MAGNETIC FORCE

The magnetic force only occurs if the charge is moving, with a component of the velocity perpendicular to the field. If a charge is stationary, there is no magnetic force. Also, if the charge is moving in the direction of the magnetic field, there is no force.

$$qvB = \frac{mv^2}{r} \quad \text{with} \quad r = \frac{mv}{qB}$$

Taking the electron velocity as 4.0×10^7 m/s, the charge and mass of the electron, and a field of 0.50 T, the radius is

$$r = \frac{9.1 \times 10^{-31} \text{ kg} \cdot 4.0 \times 10^7 \text{ m/s}}{1.6 \times 10^{-19} \text{ C} \cdot 0.50 \text{ T}} = 4.6 \times 10^{-4} \text{ m}$$

The Mass Spectrometer

A **mass spectrometer** measures the ratio of mass to charge for a charged particle. The results of mass spectrometry can be used to find the mass of particles, to evaluate what elements are present in a compound, or to determine the structure of complex molecules. The essential components of the mass spectrometer are shown in Figure 2.63.

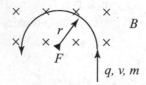

Figure 2.63. A mass spectrometer

The mass spectrometer identifies ions, which are positively charged. With the injection velocity as shown, the ions circle to the left. The detecting scheme is typically an array of sensors that display the relative intensity of each ion as it strikes the individual detectors. The ions are accelerated by a voltage, V, and acquire energy, qV, before entering the magnetic field. This energy must be equal to their kinetic energy, $mv^2/2$. Combining this with the equation relating the magnetic force to the centripetal force, the mass of the ion is

$$m = \frac{qB^2r^2}{2V}$$

For a singly charged ion accelerated through 4120 V that travels in a circle of radius 3.5×10^{-2} m in a 1.0 T field, the mass is

$$m = \frac{(1.6 \times 10^{-19}\ \text{C})(1.0\ \text{T})^2 (3.5 \times 10^{-2}\ \text{m})^2}{2(4120\ \text{V})} = 2.4 \times 10^{-26}\ \text{kg} \approx 14\ \text{amu}$$

This is the mass of carbon-14.

The *B* Field Around a Wire

A magnetic (*B*) field surrounds a current-carrying wire and this magnetic field is tangent to circles concentric about the wire. The orientation of the field, *B*, and the current, *I*, is shown in Figure 2.64. The direction of the field is determined by a right-hand rule. Place your hand with thumb in the direction of the current and your fingers naturally indicate the direction of the field.

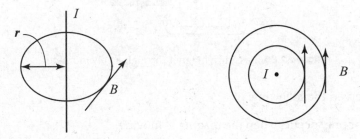

Figure 2.64. The *B* field around a wire

The strength of the *B* field is given by

$$B = \frac{\mu_0 I}{2\pi r}$$

For a wire carrying 100 A, the field tangent to a circle about the wire at 1.0 cm radius is

$$B = \frac{(4\pi \times 10^{-7}\ \text{Wb/A} \cdot \text{m})(100\ \text{A})}{2\pi (1.0 \times 10^{-2}\ \text{m})} = 2.0 \times 10^{-3}\ \text{T}$$

The Solenoid

When a loop of a current-carrying wire is wrapped into a circle, the field inside the loop is concentrated. As more loops are added, the field inside the loop becomes stronger. Wrapping the wire as shown in Figure 2.65 produces a solenoid, a device with a highly concentrated magnetic field along the axis of the winding. The dots at the top of the solenoid indicate the current coming out of the page and the crosses indicate the current going into the page. The strength of the magnetic field inside the solenoid depends on the current and the number of turns per unit length *N*.

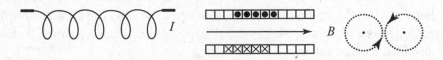

Figure 2.65. A solenoid

Solenoids are very useful and are used in door bells, door latches, circuit breakers, and many other devices. When activated, the solenoid becomes a magnet and can open or close a metal latch, among other things.

Faraday's Laws

There are two Faraday laws that you should know for the MCAT.

FIRST FARADAY LAW

The first law is derived from an experiment in which a magnet is passed through a loop of wire and a current is observed in the loop with a galvanometer. The arrangement is shown in Figure 2.66. A galvanometer is used because it reads current in either direction.

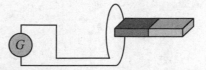

Figure 2.66. Passing a magnet through a galvanometer

Faraday observed the following:

1. The current only occurs when the magnet is moving.
2. The current is proportional to the strength of the magnet and the speed.
3. The direction of the current (in the galvanometer) depends on the N-S orientation of the magnet.

SECOND FARADAY LAW

Faraday's second law is much like the first. However, rather than passing a magnet through a coil, a second coil attached to a battery generates a field normal (perpendicular) to the plane of both coils in much the same manner as the field generated in a solenoid. This changing magnetic field in the generating coil has the same effect as physical motion of a magnet. The arrangement is shown in Figure 2.67.

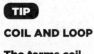

COIL AND LOOP

The terms coil and loop are interchangeable. You may see either one.

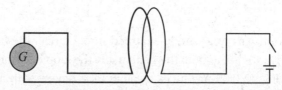

Figure 2.67. Faraday's second law

The right-hand part of the setup shows a battery, switch, and coil. The left-hand part shows the galvanometer (round element on the left) and the sensing loop. When the switch is closed, current flows and the sensing loop will register a current. As the current continues to flow in the right-hand circuit, the sensing loop stops showing a current. The current only flows in the sensing loop as the current in the right-hand loop *changes*. When the switch is closed, the sensing loop will once again show a current.

The following are Faraday's observations:

1. Current in the sensing coil is observed during the time when the switch is opening or closing.

2. No current is observed in the galvanometer when the switch is left open (no current) or closed (steady current).

3. The induced current is proportional to the number of turns in either coil and the rate of change of current in the driving coil.

When the switch in the inducing circuit is closed, a magnetic field is created by the change in current and that field can be viewed as magnetic lines more or less perpendicular to the coil and passing through the detecting coil. This changing field induces a current in the detecting coil. The coupling of the coils can be enhanced by adding a soft iron core.

Lenz's Law

Faraday's observations involved using one magnetic field (either a magnet or a coil with current) to induce a magnetic field in another circuit. What is a little harder to understand is the direction of the induced current. This direction is explained by **Lenz's law: A changing magnetic field in a coil induces a current in the coil in a direction such that the magnetic field produced by this current *opposes* the change in the field that created it.** In other words, when magnetic field 1 induces magnetic field 2 in a coil, the two fields are in opposite directions (opposing each other.)

The moving magnet and the inducing coil both act to create a magnetic field in the induced coil. If the magnetic field is increasing in the induced coil, the coil produces a current in a direction so that the magnetic field produced by the induced current opposes the magnetic field that created it.

LENZ'S LAW

Make sure you understand this concept clearly. It is a popular MCAT topic.

REFLECTION, REFRACTION, POLARIZATION, AND DIFFRACTION

Light is understood today to be electromagnetic in nature. In the study of light, it is sometimes helpful to characterize light by its electromagnetic properties and sometimes by other properties, such as properties of waves. For example, diffraction is best understood by looking at light as waves. Polarization is best understood through electromagnetic properties. In early studies, light was thought to behave as rays. A "ray" model is helpful for understanding reflection and refraction. It is important, though, to understand that light rays are only a conceptual construct.

Reflection and Refraction

In the study of reflection and refraction, light is viewed as traveling in rays, with the ray representing a thin beam of light. This view is also convenient for mirrors and lenses. Reflection and refraction of rays are shown in Figure 2.68.

When light encounters an interface between different media—for example, air and water—part of the incident light is reflected and part is refracted. Note that the angles are always measured from the normal, the perpendicular to the interface between the two media, shown by the dotted line.

Reflection follows this rule: The angle of incidence is equal to the angle of reflection as measured from the normal, or $\theta_i = \theta_i'$.

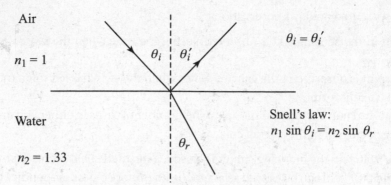

Figure 2.68. Reflection and refraction

The refracted ray, the transmitted portion of the incident ray, is at an angle dictated by Snell's law, as written in Figure 2.68. The subscripted n_1 and n_2 are the indices of refraction for air and water. There are indices of refraction for all materials. Air has an index of 1 and all other indices are greater than 1. The indices of refraction determine the angle for the refracted wave (the one that enters the new medium) and also are a measure of the speed of light in the medium. The index, n, for any material is the ratio of the speed of light in air c to the speed of light in the indexed material, $n = c/v$. Refraction follows Snell's law relating the incident and refracted angles: $n_1 \sin \theta_i = n_2 \sin \theta_r$.

Practice Question

Find the angles of reflection and refraction for a beam of light from air incident on the surface of ethyl alcohol ($n = 1.36$) at an angle of 55° as shown in the figure below. Also determine the speed of the light in ethyl alcohol.

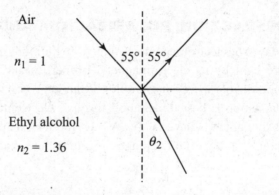

Solution: The angle of reflection, measured from the normal, is equal to the angle of incidence, or 55°. The angle of refraction is from Snell's law: $n_1 \sin \theta_1 = n_2 \sin \theta_2$.

$$(1) \sin 55° = (1.36) \sin \theta_2$$

$$\sin \theta_2 = \frac{\sin 55°}{1.36} \quad \theta_2 = 37°$$

The speed of light in ethyl alcohol is the speed of light in air divided by the refraction index for ethyl alcohol: $v = c/n = 3.0 \times 10^8 \text{ m/s} / 1.36 = 2.2 \times 10^8 \text{ m/s}$.

Total Internal Reflection

If conditions are right, a light ray hitting an interface between one medium and another may be bent at such a sharp angle that it goes back into the first medium, at a new angle. This is called **total internal reflection**. Among other applications of this principle, total internal reflection makes fiber optics possible. A light beam carrying coded information injected nearly parallel to the fiber axis will be internally reflected down the fiber and can be detected at the other end. Any bends in fiber optic cable must be gentle so as not to have the light contact the fiber–air interface at less than the critical angle.

Consider the factors that determine the angle at which light will be bent. When a light ray goes from a low index material to a higher index material, the ray is bent *toward* the normal. When a light ray goes from a higher index material to a lower index material, the ray is bent *away* from the normal. The left side of Figure 2.69 shows the general bending of light when the ray goes from the higher index medium (for example, water) to the lower index medium (for example, air).

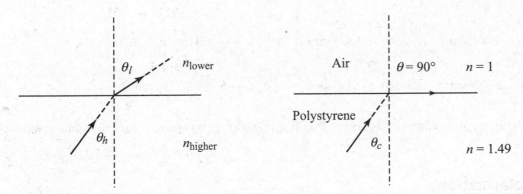

Figure 2.69. Total internal reflection

In some cases (depending on the index difference and original angle), the refracted wave can be bent to 90° (shown on the right in Figure 2.69). It is even possible for the ray to be reflected back into the original (higher index) medium. Setting $\theta_l = 90°$ produces what is known as the **critical angle**, the angle beyond which the light ray is reflected back into the higher index material. The right side of the figure shows the critical angle for light going from polystyrene ($n = 1.49$) to air. The refraction follows Snell's law $n_{higher} \sin \theta_h = n_{lower} \sin \theta_l$, which, for this case, is

$$(1.49) \sin \theta_c = (1) \sin 90° \qquad \sin \theta_c = \frac{1}{1.49} \qquad \theta_c = 42°$$

In a fiber optic cable, the index is higher than for air, so light injected reasonably close to parallel to the axis of the fiber will be internally reflected as it travels down the fiber.

Dispersion

The term **dispersion** refers to the prism effect, the separation of various wavelengths of light passing through a prism. The separation results because the index of refraction for a medium varies with wavelength. If light that includes multiple wavelengths enters a medium such as a prism, the different wavelengths will be refracted at different angles. For example, the index of refraction for fused quartz is 1.470 for 400 nm wavelength light and 1.455 for 800 nm light.

TIP

TOTAL INTERNAL REFLECTION

Total internal reflection only occurs if light is going from a high index to a low index material, never the other way around.

The difference in refraction angle between 400 nm (blue) light and 800 nm (red) light for an incident angle of 40° is shown in Figure 2.70.

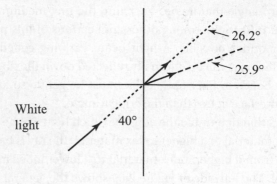

Figure 2.70. Dispersion

Using Snell's law,

For 400 nm $(1)\sin 40° = (1.470)\sin\theta_b$ $\sin\theta_b = \dfrac{1}{1.470}\sin 40°$ $\theta_b = 25.9°$

For 800 nm $(1)\sin 40° = (1.455)\sin\theta_b$ $\sin\theta_b = \dfrac{1}{1.455}\sin 40°$ $\theta_r = 26.2°$

The angular difference is only 0.3°, but it is sufficient to create a very dramatic rainbow effect.

Polarization

Light waves are composed of sinusoidally oscillating electric and magnetic fields at right angles to one another, and each oscillating field is perpendicular to the direction of the wave. The direction of the wave is along the x-axis. The plane of the electric field is along the y-axis, and the plane of the magnetic field is along the z-axis. This orientation is shown in Figure 2.71.

For most common light sources (for example, the sun and lightbulbs), the electric vectors are randomly oriented in space. Polarization is described in terms of electric vectors. Polarized light means light with all the electric vectors aligned in the same direction. Certain materials, called **Polaroids**, can filter light so that only electric vectors in one direction pass through. Polaroid sun glasses are made of a Polaroid with the molecules all aligned in a certain direction providing the appropriate filtering.

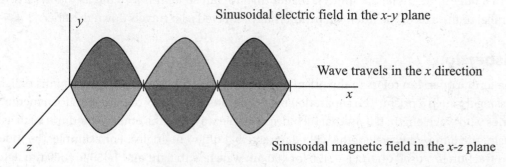

Figure 2.71. Polarization: Traveling electromagnetic wave

Light reflected at the air–water (or any other) interface is more or less polarized depending on the angle of incidence and the indices of refraction of the two media. When randomly polarized light is incident from air onto water, the reflected beam is of lower intensity and at least partially polarized, with the electric field direction parallel to the reflecting surface. The transmitted (refracted) beam has a diminished intensity and is partially polarized by the reduction of the electric field parallel to the reflecting surface.

The angle of incidence for complete polarization of the reflected beam occurs when the angle between reflected and refracted beams is 90°. The reflected beam is polarized with the electric vector parallel to the surface of the water. Figure 2.72 illustrates this situation for a beam that is traveling from air into water. The solid dots indicate an electric vector into and out of the page. The double-ended arrows indicate an electric vector in the plane of the page.

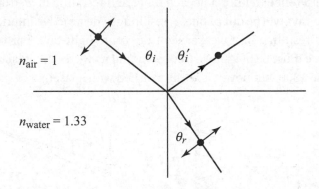

Figure 2.72. Complete polarization of a beam traveling from air into water

Brewster's law states that for complete polarization, the refracted ray and the reflected ray must form a right angle. Based on the diagram, this means $\theta_r + \theta'_i = 90°$ ($\theta_i = \theta'_i$).

Snell's law requires that

$$n_{air} \sin\theta_i = n_{water} \sin\theta_r \text{ but } \theta_r = 90° - \theta_i \text{ and } \sin\theta_r = \sin(90° - \theta_i) = \cos\theta_i, \text{ so}$$

$$n_{air} \sin\theta_i = n_{water} \cos\theta_i \text{ and } \tan\theta_i = \frac{n_{water}}{n_{air}}$$

The critical step is a trigonometric identity. In equation form, Brewster's law, when light passing through air is reflected and refracted from water, is

$$\tan\theta_i = \frac{n_{water}}{n_{air}} = \frac{1.33}{1} \quad \theta_i = 53°$$

The angle of incidence (angle of polarization), θ_i, is known as **Brewster's angle**.

People looking out over a body of water can notice that there is a glare at about 53° from the normal. The electric vector of the light wave is polarized horizontally. Polaroid sunglasses, for which the Polaroid is oriented to remove the horizontal electric field component, greatly reduce the glare. Many automobile windows contain a Polaroid coating to reduce glare. If you wear sunglasses inside the automobile and turn your head sideways so that the direction of the Polaroids in the sunglasses and the automobile window are crossed, you will notice that your view darkens, as less light is allowed through. Do not try this while driving.

Diffraction

Diffraction refers to what happens to light when it hits an obstacle. Diffraction is best understood by viewing light as waves. The following experiments, Young's double slit experiment (circa 1800) followed by a single slit diffraction experiment, illustrate what you need to know about diffraction for the MCAT.

DOUBLE-SLIT INTERFERENCE

Coherent monochromatic (single color) light, usually from a laser, is directed onto a double slit (two slits separated by a distance, d) with the intensity pattern displayed on a screen, as illustrated in Figure 2.73. Because the light is coming through two different openings, there will be two rays of light. At some points the rays will be in phase with each other, resulting in constructive interference (reinforcing each other and resulting in a stronger light ray). At other points the two rays will be out of phase, resulting in destructive interference (canceling each other out and resulting in a weaker light ray or no light ray). For the experiment to work, the light source must be of a single frequency and its waves must be in phase. This was difficult for Young in 1800, but now it is easily satisfied with a laser.

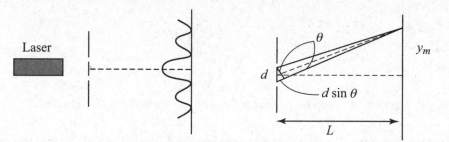

Figure 2.73. Double-slit interference

Directly opposite the center of the slits, the light from the two slits travels the same distance, L, so a bright spot (fringe) appears there. Now consider a point away from the center of the screen. Notice that the light from the upper slit does not have to travel as far as the light from the lower slit. The two beams travel different distances along their path to a given point. The difference between the lengths of the two paths, the **path difference**, determines how the two beams interact.

When the path difference is one-half of a wavelength, there is **destructive interference** (the two waves cancel each other out), and a dark area appears on the screen. This same situation occurs for path differences of $\frac{1}{2}, \frac{3}{2}, \frac{5}{2}$, and so on, of a wavelength. When the path difference is an integral number of wavelengths, there is **constructive interference** (the two waves amplify each other) and bright regions appear on the screen. Referring to Figure 2.73, the criteria for bright fringes is

$$d \sin \theta = m\lambda \quad \text{for} \quad m = 0, 1, 2 \ldots$$

The distance to the mth fringe, y_m on the graphic, divided by the slits-to-screen distance is equal to $\tan \theta$. And for a small θ, $\tan \theta = \sin \theta = \theta$. From the figure, $\tan \theta = \dfrac{y_m}{L}$, and adding the bright fringe criteria, $\sin \theta = \dfrac{m\lambda}{d}$, the formula relating wavelength, slit width, separation on the screen, and fringe number, called order, is

$$\frac{y_m}{L} = \frac{m\lambda}{d}$$

Practice Question

In a Young's experiment with slits separated by 10 μm and illuminated by coherent 550 nm light, what is the angle in radians and degrees for the first bright fringe?

Solution: Refer to Figure 2.73 and note that for the first bright fringe, the path length difference is one wavelength. This means,

$$d\sin\theta = \lambda \text{ so } \sin\theta = \frac{\lambda}{d} = \frac{550 \times 10^{-9} \text{ m}}{10 \times 10^{-6} \text{ m}} = 55 \times 10^{-3} = 0.055$$

$$\theta = \sin^{-1} 0.055 \text{ and } \theta = 3.1°$$

For such a small angle, $\sin\theta = \theta$, so the angle in radians is 0.055.

SINGLE-SLIT DIFFRACTION

A similar phenomenon occurs when there is a single slit. Coherent monochromatic light incident on a single slit of width a, which is 100 to 1000 wavelengths wide, produces a diffraction pattern on a screen. The symbols are changed to help avoid confusion with the double-slit diffraction analysis. The experiment is shown in Figure 2.74.

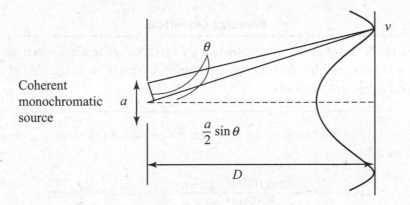

Figure 2.74. Single-slit diffraction

For analysis, the slit is viewed as divided in half. Light from near the top of the upper half and light from near the top of the lower half when out of phase by a half wavelength produce a dark fringe. The dark fringe criterion is used in single slit diffraction analysis. The criteria for the dark fringe is

$$\frac{a}{2}\sin\theta = \frac{\lambda}{2} \text{ or } \sin\theta = \frac{\lambda}{a}$$

The general formula for the dark fringes is

$$\sin\theta = \frac{m\lambda}{a} \text{ for } m = \pm1, \pm2, \ldots$$

Note on the diagram that the point on the central axis (dotted line) has maximum brightness. Going up or down from that point, the light fades in brightness until a dark fringe is reached. Above the upper dark fringe and below the lower dark fringe, the light intensity increases again. This area between the first bottom dark fringe and first upper dark fringe (between the line D and point v in the diagram) is called the **central maximum**.

Referring to Figure 2.74 and using the same approximation as before (that $\sin\theta = \tan\theta = \theta$ for small angles), gives the equation:

$$\frac{v_m}{D} = \frac{m\lambda}{a}$$

USE DIAGRAMS

In diffraction problems, it is very easy to get confused and use the wrong formula. Making a diagram helps a lot!

Do not attempt to memorize formulas for bright and dark fringes for single- and double-slit situations. MCAT questions on this topic will usually include the formula, if needed. Understand the concepts and how to apply the formulas.

Practice Question

Light from a He-Ne laser of 633 nm is incident on a 0.02 cm wide slit. Determine the width of the central maximum (the distance between the dark fringes on either side of the central maximum) on a screen 3.0 m away.

Solution: First find the distance to the first dark fringe with a rearranged general formula. Refer to Figure 2.73.

$$v_1 = \frac{1\lambda D}{a} = \frac{1(633 \times 10^{-9} \text{ m})(3.0 \text{ m})}{2.0 \times 10^{-4} \text{ m}} = 9.5 \times 10^{-3} \text{ m} = 0.95 \text{ cm}$$

The width of the central maximum (first dark fringe up to first dark fringe down) is twice this value, or 1.90.

MIRRORS AND LENSES

To master mirrors and lenses it is important to learn (1) definitions of real and virtual images, (2) rules for determining magnification, and (3) rules for determining whether objects, images, and focal points are positive or negative. Doing problems is not difficult if you have the rules written out in front of you. On a test, however, it is easy to scramble the rules, so the best way to approach test questions about mirrors and lenses is to amass experience in doing the problems. With enough experience, you can at least get started correctly and then remember your way through the problem. Because of this approach, there is more than the usual number of illustrative examples in this section. The best way to learn, however, is to keep redoing these and similar problems until the procedures are clear in your mind.

Mirrors

If you face a plane mirror holding a book in front of you with the word PHYSICS on the cover, you will see the words written backwards in the mirror. This property of mirrors is called **lateral inversion,** which means turned from side to side. The word AMBULANCE is often written backwards (laterally inverted) on the front of an ambulance so that drivers in front of the ambulance can read the word in their rear view mirrors.

If you comb your hair to the right while standing in front of a mirror, the person in the mirror (your image) is upright and appears to be combing his or her hair to the left (**right to left inversion**). If you point at the mirror, the image points back at you. This is called **front to back inversion**.

In studying mirrors, it is common to use the concept of rays, or pencil-like beams of light. These rays are not really beams of light. They are geometric constructs to help in understanding mirrors.

Figure 2.75 depicts what you see if you look at an object in a mirror. As you look in the mirror, the image you see is a **virtual image**. In a virtual image, the light does not physically come from the image itself. In other words, the light is not coming from where the image appears to be (for example, three feet behind the mirror) but from the surface of the mirror. A **real image** is one for which the light comes from or passes through the image. The virtual image appears as far in back of the mirror as the real image is in front of the mirror.

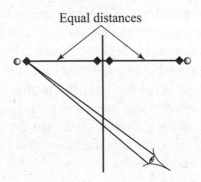

Equal distances

Figure 2.75. Looking at an object in a mirror

A light source (the ball in Figure 2.75) is 5.0 cm in front of a plane mirror. Determine where the observer sees the image and whether it is real or virtual.

Solution: Referring to Figure 2.75, the image appears 5.0 cm behind the mirror. It is a virtual image because the light showing the image does not come from the image. It comes from the object.

To summarize, plane mirrors (1) reverse images right to left, (2) display front to back inversion, (3) present images upright, and (4) can be used to show virtual images.

CONCAVE (CONVERGING) SPHERICAL MIRROR

In analyzing curved mirrors, there are four parameters to consider: (1) the object distance, o, (2) the image distance, i, (3) the radius of curvature, R, and (4) the focus, f. The focus is the point on the center line of the mirror at which all parallel rays incident on the mirror will be focused. The sign convention for all mirrors is given below.

SIGN CONVENTION FOR MIRRORS

o is positive if object is in front of the mirror

o is negative if object is in back of the mirror

i is positive if the image is in front of the mirror

i is negative if the image is in back of the mirror

f is positive if the center of curvature is in front of the mirror

f is negative if the center of curvature is in back of the mirror

---

The relationship between the parameters for the mirror is given by what is called the **lens maker's formula**.

$$\frac{1}{o} + \frac{1}{i} = \frac{1}{f}$$

When trying to solve a problem, the relationships between the object distance, image distance, and focus for the spherical mirror are most easily seen by drawing rays. Consider a concave spherical mirror having a 20 cm radius of curvature with an object placed 30 cm along the center line mirror, as shown in Figures 2.76 and 2.77. First draw the rays to locate the image. In Figure 2.76, the center of curvature, the radius, is marked C. The focus is one-half the radius ($f = R/2$). All incident parallel rays go through the focus.

Draw a ray across the top of the object, parallel to the center line of the mirror. This ray is reflected through the focus and is illustrated on the left of Figure 2.76. Draw another ray across the top of the object passing through the focus. This ray is reflected parallel to the center line and is on the right of the diagram.

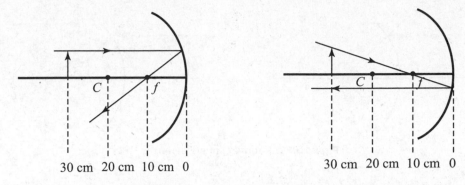

Figure 2.76. A concave spherical mirror (1)

The intersection of these two rays, as shown in the left of Figure 2.77, is the top of the image. The image is drawn on the right.

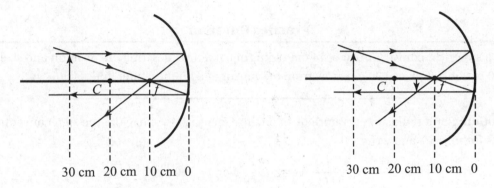

Figure 2.77. A concave spherical mirror (2)

Using the lens maker's formula the image distance can be calculated.

$$\frac{1}{o}+\frac{1}{i}=\frac{1}{f} \Rightarrow \frac{1}{30}+\frac{1}{i}=\frac{1}{10} \Rightarrow \frac{1}{i}=\frac{1}{10}-\frac{1}{30}=\frac{3}{30}-\frac{1}{30}=\frac{2}{30}=\frac{1}{15}$$

The image distance is 15 cm, which seems to match the scale in the drawing. As a visual check, note from the drawing that o, i, and f are all on the same side of the mirror and must have the same algebraic sign. This sign-checking scheme is very helpful in mirror and lens problems. The triangle whose base is the line from the top of the object to the mirror is similar to the triangle whose base is the line from the top of the image to the mirror. Thus, their heights are in proportion to their bases, so the magnification $M = h'/h$ (object over image) equals $-(i/o)$. The magnification of this image is $M = -(15/30) = -(1/2)$. The minus sign indicates that the image is inverted.

CONVEX (DIVERGING) SPHERICAL MIRROR

The calculating rules for image height and magnification are the same for convex mirrors as for concave ones. The rules for drawing the rays and finding the image are, however, slightly different. The ray drawing procedure is illustrated in Figure 2.78.

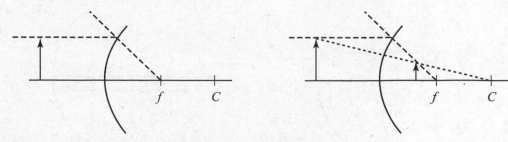

Figure 2.78. A convex spherical mirror

In the left-hand drawing in Figure 2.78, draw a ray across the top of the object parallel to the center line of the mirror. This ray is reflected from the convex surface as if it came from the focus.

In the right-hand drawing above, draw a ray between the center of curvature and the top of the object. The intersection of these rays locates the top of the image as shown.

Practice Question

For a spherical convex mirror of 14 cm radius of curvature, describe the position and size of a 4.0 cm object placed 30 cm away from the mirror and on the center line.

RADIUS OF CURVATURE

For a spherical mirror, the radius of curvature has a magnitude that is twice the focal length.

Solution: For a radius of curvature of 14 cm, the focus is at 7 cm. Note the sign convention rules for mirrors and write

$$\frac{1}{30 \text{ cm}} + \frac{1}{i} = -\frac{1}{7 \text{ cm}} \text{ or } i = -10 \text{ cm}$$

Again, as a visual check, note that the object distance and focus must have opposite algebraic signs, as they do in the calculation. The magnification is

$$M = -\frac{i}{o} = -\frac{(-10)}{(40)} = 0.25$$

The image is 0.25 × 4.0 cm = 1.0 cm high. It is erect, virtual, and appears to come from a point 10 cm from the lens and on the same side as the object.

Lenses

Lenses are either converging or diverging. In **converging** lenses, rays from infinity are refracted on entrance and exit from the lens in such a way that they are focused at one spot, the focus of the lens. The rays converge. Converging lenses act like two prisms placed base-to-base. In diverging lenses, rays from infinity are refracted on entrance and exit from the lens so they appear as if they came from a focus. **Diverging** lenses act like two prisms placed point-to-point. Converging and diverging lenses are shown in Figure 2.79. For lenses, real images are the ones formed on the side opposite the object and virtual images are ones formed on the same side as the object.

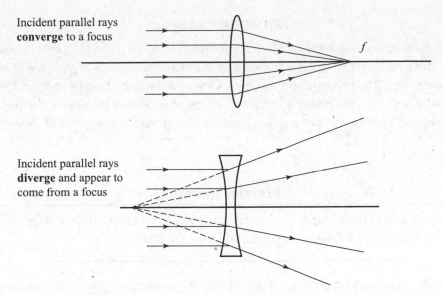

Incident parallel rays **converge** to a focus

Incident parallel rays **diverge** and appear to come from a focus

Figure 2.79. Converging and diverging lenses

SIGN CONVENTION FOR LENSES

o is positive if object is in front of the lens

o is negative if object is in back of the lens

i is positive if the image is on the opposite side of the
   lens from the object

i is negative if the image is on the same side of the lens
   from the object

f is positive for a converging lens

f is negative for a diverging lens

The same formula relating object and image distances and focus for mirrors is also valid for lenses. The ray drawing rules for locating images is different for lenses than for mirrors. They are simpler and most people find them easier to apply.

RULES FOR LOCATING LENS IMAGES BY DRAWING RAYS

1. A ray parallel on one side passes through the focus on the other side.

2. A ray through the focus will emerge parallel on the other side.

3. A ray through the center is not diverted.

Two rays are sufficient to locate the image, and rules 1 and 3 are generally the easiest to apply.

Practice Question

A converging lens of focal length 12 cm forms an image of an object placed 20 cm on one side of the lens. Draw the rays using the rules and locate the image.

Solution: In Figure 2.80 the top ray is drawn parallel to the center line and is focused by the lens to pass through *f*. The bottom ray goes through the focus on the same side as the object and is made parallel to the center line by the lens. The third ray, the one with no arrows, passes through the center of the lens without diversion. All three rays intersect to fix the top of the image.

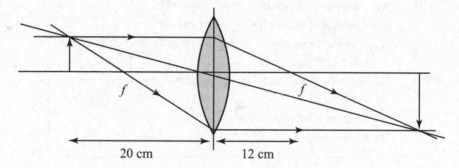

Figure 2.80. A converging lens

Use the lens maker's formula, remembering that, for a converging lens, *f* is positive. Also note that the object is in front of the lens and the image is in back of the lens, so

$$\frac{1}{o} + \frac{1}{i} = \frac{1}{f} \;\Rightarrow\; \frac{1}{20} + \frac{1}{i} = \frac{1}{12} \;\Rightarrow\; \frac{1}{i} = \frac{1}{12} - \frac{1}{20} = \frac{5}{60} - \frac{3}{60} = \frac{2}{60} = \frac{1}{30}$$

The image distance is 30 cm.

Practice Question

A diverging lens has a focal length of 14 cm. Characterize the image of a 4.0 cm object placed 40 cm from the lens.

Solution: The situation and rays are shown in Figure 2.81.

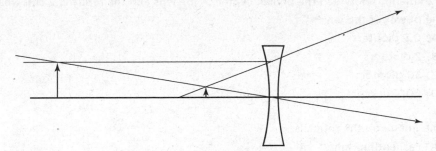

Figure 2.81. A diverging lens

Draw the first ray across the top of the object and parallel to the center line and refract it in the diverging lens, extending the line through the focus. The focus is the point from which the ray appears to come. Next, draw a ray from the top of the image through the center of the lens. The intersection of these rays locates the top of the image.

Now apply the lens maker's formula to find the image distance.

$$\frac{1}{o}+\frac{1}{i}=\frac{1}{f} \implies \frac{1}{40}+\frac{1}{i}=-\frac{1}{14} \implies i=-13$$

The focal length is negative because this is a diverging lens. The image distance is negative because it is on the same side of the lens as the object. The magnification is $M = -i/o = -(-13/40) = 0.325$.

The image is 0.325×4.0 cm $= 1.3$ cm high erect, virtual, and appears to come from a point 13 cm from the lens and on the same side as the object.

TEST QUESTIONS

The diagram shows light entering the eye from a distant object and being focused by the lens onto the retina.

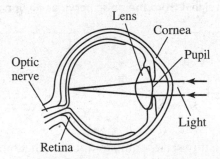

The power of a converging lens is sometimes described in the unit of diopters and uses the equation $P = \frac{1}{f}$, where P is the power in diopters and f is the focal length in meters.

1. What feature of the diagram indicates that the eye is looking at a distant object?

   (A) The light rays converge on the retina.

   (B) The light rays entering the eye are parallel.

   (C) The light rays are centered vertically on the retina.

   (D) The light rays inside the eye form an isosceles triangle.

2. If the length between the optical center of the lens and the retina is 2 cm, what is the power of the lens?
   (A) 0.5 diopters
   (B) 2 diopters
   (C) 50 diopters
   (D) 500 diopters

3. The image on the retina is:
   (A) real and upright.
   (B) virtual and inverted.
   (C) diminished and virtual.
   (D) real and inverted.

1. **(B)** If an object was close to the eye, the rays would be diverging as they enter the eye. Parallel rays of light coming from an object are an indication that the object is far away. Light rays converge on the retina as long as the eye is able to focus on the object.

2. **(C)** Use the formula for the diopter. Remember to convert 2 cm to 0.02 m.

$$P = \frac{1}{f}$$

$$P = \frac{1}{0.02 \text{ m}}$$

$$P = 50 \text{ diopters}$$

The focal length of the lens is defined as the point where rays converge on one side if the light rays are parallel on the opposite side.

3. **(D)** An image is real if it can be focused on a screen, which in this case is the retina. In addition, a converging lens creates and inverted image. The brain is able to reinterpret the electrical signal from the optic nerve as an upright image.

ATOMS AND NUCLEI

Scale

Atoms and nuclei exist on a tiny scale, compared to the phenomena of our daily lives. The size of an atomic nucleus is on the order of 10^{-14} m. Atoms, including the orbit radius for the electrons, are in the range of 10^{-10} m. The interatomic spacing in solids is double the atomic radius.

Hydrogen Atom

This section will deal with a stable (Bohr) model for the simplest atom, hydrogen. A basic property of the hydrogen atom is the atomic spectra, which are a collection of specific wavelength lines in the visible region that have a unique orderly relationship to one other. These spectral lines are produced when the hydrogen gas is subjected to electric fields sufficient to tear electrons out of their normal orbits. The presence of these lines and their specific wavelengths is explained by the Bohr model for hydrogen.

The orbiting electrons require a center-directed force to make them move in a circle. This force is the coulomb force between the negatively charged electrons and the positive charge in the nucleus. If the line spectra are based on discrete energy differences, then the energy associated with these orbits has to be discrete. In other words, the orbits cannot be continuous. They must be at specific radii. This requirement is handled by assigning angular momenta to the electrons having specific integer values of the Planck constant, $n(h/2\pi)$.

The allowed radii for hydrogen are given by

$$r_n = \frac{h^2 \varepsilon_0}{\pi m e^2} n^2 \quad \text{or} \quad r = a_0 n^2 \quad \text{with} \quad a_0 = 0.05 \text{ nm}$$

where $n = 1$ corresponds to the first allowed electron orbit radius, $n = 2$ corresponds to the second allowed electron orbit radius, and so on. The first electron orbit radius is 0.05 nm, with succeeding radii written as indicated above.

The mechanics of the motion dictate that the energy associated with these allowed orbits be written as

$$E_n = -\frac{13.6 \text{ eV}}{n^2}$$

The energy differences that lead to the emission spectral lines agree with this formula, and the arrangement of the lines fits with this 1 over n^2 sequence. The negative sign fits with the way electric potential is defined. For a positive and negative charge, the closer the charges are to one another, the greater the energy required to remove the electron to infinity. Think of it as the electrons falling into a potential well. For higher n's the energy is less negative. This makes it easier to understand the light spectra of the atom. If an electron is knocked out of orbit and it falls back into either the $n = 1$ or $n = 2$, or any other state, then the energy difference appears as radiation with this energy being some fraction of the 13.6 eV.

Further, transitions between the various allowed energy levels produce spectral lines that are unique to the hydrogen atom. Identifying the difference in energy with hf, an expression for the frequencies of allowed spectra, can be written in terms of the energy differences as

GAS SPECTRA

Each gas has specific spectral lines corresponding to the electronic transitions. Certain transitions have a higher probability of occurring when an electric field is applied to "excite" the gas. Neon has strong transitions in the red, whereas argon has strong green transitions.

$$f = \frac{E_i - E_f}{h} = \frac{13.6 \text{ eV}}{h} \left[\frac{1}{n_f^2} - \frac{1}{n_i^2} \right]$$

These frequencies are experimentally verified, and observation of these lines is part of many undergraduate laboratory experiments. The wavelengths are given by adding $c = \lambda f$ to the formula

$$\frac{1}{\lambda} = \frac{13.6 \text{ eV}}{hc} \left[\frac{1}{n_f^2} - \frac{1}{n_i^2} \right]$$

The Quantum Numbers

The hydrogen atom theory works well for hydrogen and other single electron orbiting atoms, providing a model for the spectral lines and a wavelength relationship for the lines that agrees with observation of the spectra. The n's that came about because of the quantization of the angular momentum of the orbiting electrons became known as the principal quantum numbers.

As an example of how to make these calculations, find the first three orbit radii for the hydrogen atom. The orbits follow from

$$r_n = (0.05 \text{ nm}) n^2 \quad n = 1, r_1 = 0.05 \text{ nm} \quad n = 2, r_2 = 0.20 \text{ nm} \quad n = 3, r_3 = 0.45 \text{ nm}$$

The formula for the first three allowed energies of the orbiting electrons in hydrogen yields energies of

$$E_n = -\frac{13.6 \text{ eV}}{n^2}$$

$$E_1 = -\frac{13.6 \text{ eV}}{1^2} = -13.6 \text{ eV} \quad E_2 = -\frac{13.6 \text{ eV}}{2^2} = -3.4 \text{ eV} \quad E_3 = -\frac{13.6 \text{ eV}}{3^2} = -1.51 \text{ eV}$$

Notice that as n increases, the energies get closer and closer together and approach zero. Because the energies get closer together, the observed spectral lines also get closer together, forming what is called the head of the spectral series. In the spectral observation, a reasonably low pressure of hydrogen gas is subjected to an electric voltage sufficiently high to cause the electrons to be torn from the atoms. The electrons falling back into orbits and rearranging between orbits produces the spectral lines. There are a series of lines associated with the $n = 1$ state and another for the $n = 2$ state, and so on. The lines associated with the higher n value series are hard to see because at the low energy differences involved, it is hard to visually separate out the individual lines.

The spectral lines are caused by transitions between energy levels, and the wavelengths of these transitions are according to the formula for $1/\lambda$. The sample calculation of a wavelength is for the $n = 1$ and $n = 3$ transition. This choice gives a visible wavelength.

$$\frac{1}{\lambda} = \frac{13.6 \text{ eV}}{hc} \left[\frac{1}{n_f^2} - \frac{1}{n_i^2} \right] \quad \text{and for } n = 1 \text{ and } 3$$

$$\frac{1}{\lambda} = \frac{13.6 \text{ eV}}{(9.14 \times 10^{-15} \text{ eV} \cdot \text{s})(3.0 \times 10^8 \text{ m/s})} \left[\frac{1}{1^2} - \frac{1}{3^2} \right] \Rightarrow \lambda = 227 \text{ nm}$$

TIP

ISOTOPES

Common MCAT problems involving isotopes include carbon dating, uranium in nuclear fission, hydrogen in nuclear fusion, and radon for problems involving radioactive gas.

Nuclei

Nuclei are conveniently viewed as a collection of neutrons and protons. A proton has a positive charge equal in magnitude to the charge on the electron. The number of protons in the nucleus (the **atomic number**) defines the properties of the atom. In other words, it determines which element the atom is. Neutrons have no charge. The number of protons, Z, plus the number of neutrons, N, gives the mass number, $A = Z + N$.

The mass number and atomic number can be shown along with the letter symbol for the element, such as $^{14}_{6}C$, where 6 is the atomic number (number of protons) and 14 is the mass number. For the carbon nucleus just described, there are more neutrons than protons. The element, carbon in this case, is defined by the number of protons (charge carriers). In writing the symbol for an element, the atomic number is often left off because the element defines the number of protons. Both $^{14}_{6}C$ and $^{12}_{6}C$ represent carbon. The difference is that the first has two extra neutrons, making it heavier. The form with 6 protons and 6 neutrons is the most common form. The form with 6 protons and 8 neutrons is called an isotope of carbon. Isotopes have the same number of protons as the most common form of the element, but they have a larger number of neutrons.

The masses of neutrons and protons are given in terms of atomic mass units (amu or u). 1 amu is equal to 1.66×10^{-27} kg. This unit is based on the mole. A mole of carbon-12 (^{12}C) is 12 g and contains Avogadro's number (6.02×10^{23}) of molecules. Putting the number of grams (12) over Avogadro's number yields grams per molecule, namely the weight of each atom, as in this case the molecule is the atom.

The Binding Energy

It would seem that the mass of the nucleus should be the sum of the masses of the protons and neutrons. However, this is not the case. The mass of a nucleus is, in fact, less than the sum of the masses that make up that nucleus. This mass difference is manifest as energy. Using the famous $E = mc^2$ formula, the missing mass (m) times c^2 equals the energy equivalent of the missing mass and is called the **binding energy** of the nucleus. The binding energy represents the amount of energy necessary to take apart a nucleus. Atom smashing machines routinely use particles with MeV of energy, 100 thousand times the energy to remove an electron from its orbit.

Fission and Fusion

The $^{235}_{92}U$ atom spontaneously decays into two smaller nuclei. The total binding energies of these resulting nuclei is smaller than the binding energy of the original atom. This type of decay process is known as a **fission reaction**, fission referring to a splitting. The difference in energy (the amount of binding energy lost in the process) appears as heat. Nuclear power plants use this heat energy. In the power plant, neutrons released by the decay of U_{235} atoms bombard other U_{235} atoms and accelerate the decay process beyond what would otherwise be the spontaneous decay rate. The amount of heat released is controlled by reducing the number of neutrons in the pile of uranium. The neutrons are absorbed, usually with carbon rods, thus regulating the number of decays and amount of heat produced. If the nuclei are packed close together, then the neutrons released in the spontaneous decay induce further decays and a large amount of energy is released in a short period of time (an explosion.)

If two nuclei are brought together, a **fusion reaction** is possible. With the correct selection of nuclei, the binding energy of the fused product can be lower than the binding energy of the original components. In this case, energy is released.

Nuclear Forces

The periodic table shows that as the number of particles in the nucleus increases, the ratio of neutrons to protons increases. The protons have the same charge and repel one another. The larger number of neutrons serves to separate them and act as a "nuclear glue." The nuclear residents (protons and neutrons) are packed closely together in seeming defiance of the coulomb repulsion. This indicates that the forces holding the nucleus together must be very

TRANSURANIC ELEMENTS

Elements with atomic numbers greater than that of uranium (92) are usually not stable. The most noteworthy of these is probably plutonium, used in nuclear reactions. Plutonium was first manufactured by bombarding uranium with deuterons (a hydrogen nucleus that has both a neutron and a proton in the nucleus).

strong and of very short range. In fact, the nuclear particles are packed so close together that the density of nuclei is 10^{13} times the density of gold!

The periodic chart does not go to infinity. At a certain size, large elements tend to be unstable and decay. Their decay is usually in the form of stable particles, such as helium nuclei, being emitted, accompanied by stray particles or electromagnetic radiation. There are three kinds of nuclear decay products: α particles (2 neutrons and 2 protons, which are basically a helium nucleus), β particles (either electrons or positrons, which are positively charged electrons), and γ particles (electromagnetic radiation, typically high-energy X-rays). Very large nuclei often decay through a chain of different nuclei, with the decay stopping at lead. Some of the decay times are short and some of them are long.

Radioactive Decay

Nuclear decay is measured by the number of decay products per second. The historically first unit of activity was the Curie (Ci), which is equivalent to 3.7×10^{10} decays per second. This is the activity of 1 g of a radioactive radon isotope. The smaller and more popular activity unit is the Becquerel (Bq), which is equivalent to 1 decay per second.

Although it is not possible to predict when a particular nucleus will decay, it is possible to predict the decay rate of a large collection of nuclei. The decay rate is the number of decays per unit of time. This rate is proportional to the number of nuclei in a sample or simply the amount of material that is decaying. Simply put, the more material, the more decays. In equation form, the activity or decay rate is written as

$$R \text{ or } A = \frac{\Delta N}{\Delta t} = \lambda N$$

The proportionality constant λ is positive for growth and negative for decay. In a nuclear decay situation, the decaying material and the decay product are known as the parent-daughter materials, and the process is known as parent-daughter decay. While the amount of parent material is declining, the amount of daughter material is growing. The solution to this equation is

$$N = N_0 e^{\lambda t}$$

One popular measure of decay is by specification of the half-life of the material, that is, the time for half the original material to decay. In mathematical terms, this means reworking the equation with $N = N_0/2$ and specifying t at $T_{1/2}$. This produces the equation

$$\frac{N_0}{2} = N_0 e^{\lambda T_{1/2}} \quad \text{or} \quad \frac{1}{2} = e^{\lambda T_{1/2}}$$

This equation is solved by taking natural logarithms of both sides. The logarithm of $\frac{1}{2}$ is $-\ln 2$ and the natural logarithm of the exponential function is $T_{1/2}$ and, with a little rearranging, the expression for the half-life is

$$\ln \frac{1}{2} = \lambda T_{1/2} \quad \text{and} \quad T_{1/2} = \frac{-\ln 2}{\lambda}$$

Strontium-90, or ^{90}Sr, is a product of nuclear fission. It appears in nuclear fuel waste and in fallout from nuclear testing or explosions of nuclear reactors. The decay constant is 0.024 1/yr and the decay product is yttrium, which decays in a few hours. The decay of strontium to yttrium is accompanied by a high energy electron and the yttrium decay is also accompanied by a high energy electron. The half-life of ^{90}Sr can be calculated from the formula given above. The constant λ is inherently negative.

$$T_{1/2} = \frac{-\ln 2}{-0.024 \; 1/\text{yr}} = 28.8 \text{ yr}$$

^{90}Sr is a radioactive material that is routinely monitored in the environment, appearing most readily in milk. The half-life of 28.8 years means that anyone who ingests this material and retains it will receive all the radioactive decay products during their lifetime. Radioactive materials that decay rapidly may cause damage to the body that cannot be repaired, and radioactive materials with very long half-lives will produce little radiation over a lifetime and cause little damage. ^{90}Sr is dangerous because it is radioactive over an extended period and yet decays quickly enough to expose people to significant radiation.

If the amount of decaying material decreases according to an exponential law, then the amount of radiation per second should follow the same law. The number of counts per minute then follows

$$R = R_0 r^n$$

The number of counts of radiation of a sample is measured by an ionization tube. The ionization tube contains a gas and electrodes at a low potential. When a radiation particle enters the tube, it knocks an electron off a gas atom, creating a current in the tube. Thus, the number of counts is proportional to the number of nuclear particles entering the ionization tube.

In a typical laboratory experiment, the detector tube is moved away from the source and the number of counts recorded. The decrease in counts with distance is given in the table in Figure 2.82. The counts drop off according to a law of the form shown.

$$R = R_0 r^n$$

Counts	Distance
100	10 cm
25	20 cm
11	30 cm

Figure 2.82.

The number of counts decreases with distance, r, so n will be negative. The problem is to first find n and then determine the number of counts at 5 cm. A graphing approach is usually used to solve the problem. Take the base 10 logarithm of both sides of the equation.

$$\log R = \log R_0 + \log r^n = n \log r + \log R_0$$

This equation is in the form $y = mx + b$, where $\log R$ is the vertical axis, $\log r$ is the horizontal axis, n is the slope of the line, and $\log R_0$ is the intercept on the vertical axis. Now set up a table for calculating the points on a linear graph (Figure 2.83).

log R	log r
$\log 100 = 2$	$\log 10 = 1$
$\log 25 = 1.4$	$\log 20 = 1.3$
$\log 11 = 1.04$	$\log 30 = 1.48$

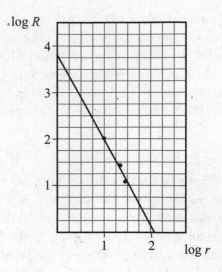

Figure 2.83. Calculating points on a linear graph

The slope of this graph is approximately 2, so take the exponent $n = 2$. The intercept is around 3.8, which makes R_0 roughly 6000. To find the activity at 5 cm, find $\log 5 = 0.70$ on the graph, giving $\log R = 2.5$ and $R = 350$. Before hand calculators, this was the way such problems were solved.

SUMMARY

For the MCAT, you need to be familiar with basic physics concepts. This chapter reviewed the major topics and concepts needed for the MCAT. You should be familiar with basic math strategies for physics questions, including the elements of standard deviation, significant figures, working with units, and graphing. Review linear motion, projectile motion, motion of falling bodies, and time delay.

Be sure you are confident with the concept of forces, in general, and with frictional forces and gravitation. Review mass and weight, focusing on definitions and apparent weight. Also carefully review work, energy, power, and work–energy.

Many aspects of fluids will be tested on the MCAT. Thoroughly review density, specifc gravity, and bouyancy. Make sure you understand pressure (guage and absolute), hydraulics, manometers, fluid dynamics, viscosity and flow, and the Bernoulli equation. Equally important is the area of mechanical waves and sound. Be sure you understand transverse waves on ropes, standing waves on strings, longitudinal waves in springs, beat frequencies, sound transmission, intensity and the inverse square law, and the Doppler effect. Be familiar with the fundamental concepts of simple harmonic motion, which include mass–spring systems, position, velocity and acceleration, and the energy analysis of simple harmonic motion.

Carefully review electrostatics. Be confident with the concepts of charge transfer, induction, Coulomb's law, the electric field, electric potential, and Gauss's law. Likewise, be sure to review DC circuits, including conduction, current, batteries, resistance and resistivity, work and emf, power, and resistors. Review the following subtopics within electromagnetism: magnetism, moving charges in a magnetic field, the mass spectrometer, the B-field around a wire, the solenoid, Faraday's laws, and Lenz's law.

The physics of light is an important MCAT topic. Be sure you are confident with reflection, refraction, polarization, and diffraction, as well as the concepts of total internal reflection. Review the concepts of concave and convex spherical mirrors, lenses, and the sign conventions for mirrors and lenses.

Finally, there are some important concepts related to atoms and nuclei that you should master. Review the chapter sections on scale, the hydrogen atom, quantum numbers, nuclei, binding energy, fission and fusion, nuclear forces, and radioactive decay.

To get the most out of the physics chapter, go through it at least three times completely. In addition, whenever you have trouble with a physics question on a practice MCAT, come back to the part of the chapter that reviews the concept that you missed. By using both of these methods, you will build up your physics knowledge and at the same time master the concepts that are not clear to you now.

> **DIRECTIONS:** This Physics test contains four passages. Each passage is followed by a series of questions. Read the passage, and then choose the one answer that is best. Some questions are not based on a passage or each other. If you are not sure of an answer, eliminate the answer choices that you think are wrong and choose one of the remaining answers. You can refer to the periodic table on page 36 at any time.

PASSAGE I

The electric current in a metal is the result of the motion of electrons. In the metal, electrons that are not tightly bound to an atom have a random motion with a mean free speed on the order of 10^6 m/s. In the presence of an electric field, this motion is altered slightly so as to produce a net motion opposite the direction of the field. This motion is called the drift velocity and is on the order of 10^{-4} m/s. The random motion is determined by the temperature of the metal. The electrons move in a straight line until they encounter an ion core, where they are stopped, and then continue in a different direction. It is during the motion between these collisions that the electron "drift" leads to the current. Each material has an inherent resistivity, which is a material property. This resistivity for metals is on the order of 10^{-8} ohm-meters.

The ohm is the unit derived from the operational relationship between voltage and current in a resistor, $V = IR$. The ohm is equivalent to volt/ampere. The resistance of a particular piece of wire is calculated as the resistivity times the length of the wire divided by the cross-sectional area of the wire. Resistors are widely used in electronic circuitry, and whereas their resistance depends on basic material properties, their behavior as circuit elements depends on how they are used. A single resistor placed in series with a battery follows the $V = IR$ rule. Two resistors placed in series with a battery divide the battery voltage but have the same current through them. Series resistance is added in a linear fashion. Two resistors placed in parallel have the same voltage across them but divide the current. Parallel resistors add in a reciprocal manner, where one over the equivalent resistance is equal to one over one resistance plus one over the other resistance. The $V = IR$ relations are used to determine the voltage and currents in each situation.

1. An electron enters one end of a 10-meter metallic current-carrying conductor. How long does it take for this electron to reach the other end of the wire?
   (A) It is instantaneous.
   (B) 1 sec
   (C) hours
   (D) 3.0×10^{-7} s

2. What is the resistance of a 4-meter long wire with a resistivity of 2×10^{-8} $\Omega \cdot$ m and a cross section of 8×10^{-7} m^2?
   (A) 8×10^{-7} Ω
   (B) 1×10^{-8} Ω
   (C) 0.1 Ω
   (D) 100 Ω

3. Two 17.3 Ω resistors are placed in series with a 20 V battery. What is the voltage across each resistor?
   (A) 10 V
   (B) 40 V
   (C) 17.3 V
   (D) 20 V

4. Two resistors of different values are connected in parallel to a battery. Which of the following statements is correct?
   (A) The current is greater in the larger resistor.
   (B) The voltage is greater across the larger resistor.
   (C) The current is greater in the smaller resistor.
   (D) The voltage is greater across the smaller resistor.

5. What unit is given to the product of voltage and current?
   (A) Joule
   (B) Watt
   (C) Ohm
   (D) Newton

6. For pieces with the same dimensions, a piece of metal A has a higher resistance than a piece of metal B. Which statement is NOT true?
   (A) Metal A has a higher resistivity.
   (B) For a given voltage, metal A has a lower current.
   (C) A wire made of metal A can be made to match the resistivity of a wire made of metal B by increasing its cross sectional area.
   (D) Metal A consumes less power.

The following questions do not refer to a descriptive passage and are not related to each other.

7. An object of mass 2 kg is thrown straight upward with a velocity of 10 m/s. Neglecting air resistance and taking the acceleration of gravity to be 10 m/s^2, how high does the object go?
   (A) 5 m
   (B) 10 m
   (C) 100 m
   (D) 200 m

8. Which of the following statements about sound and light waves is/are true?

   I. They are both transverse waves.
   II. They both require a medium to travel.
   III. They both slow down when going from air to water.

   (A) I only
   (B) I and II
   (C) III only
   (D) None are true.

PASSAGE II

A man has suffered a cardiac arrest. A defibrillator is used to deliver an electrical shock in order to restore the normal rhythm of the heart. The purpose of the electricity is so that the rhythm of the heart can be reestablished by the body's natural pacemaker in the sinoatrial node of the heart. The placement of the paddles on the man's body is shown below.

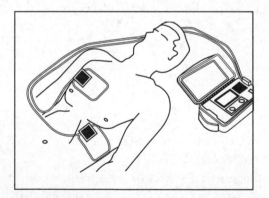

A medical emergency response team arrives on the scene. An electrocardiogram reader is first used to diagnose the cardiac condition. A paramedic uses a manual external defibrillator on the man. The paddles must make good electrical contact with the skin. So the paramedic first applies a liquid conducting gel to the patient's chest so that the total resistance through the body is about 20 ohms. The paramedic determines that 200 joules of electrical energy must be used and sets the voltage to 600 volts. A circuit diagram for the defibrillator is shown below.

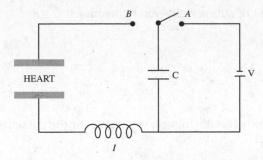

First the switch is moved to position *A*, which charges capacitor *C* by connecting it to voltage source *V*. Once the capacitor is fully charged, the switch is moved to position *B* and the capacitor discharges the electrical energy to the heart through inductor *I*.

9. When designing the capacitor of the defibrillator, the engineers wanted to increase the amount of charge that could be stored by increasing the capacitance. Which modification would provide an increase of capacitance?
    (A) Increasing the spacing between the plates of the capacitor
    (B) Decreasing the area of the capacitor plates
    (C) Increasing the dielectric constant between the capacitor plates
    (D) None of the above

10. The discharging curve for the capacitor is shown below.

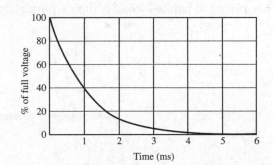

Time (ms)

(A)

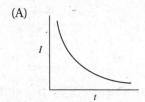

(C)

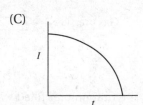

(B)

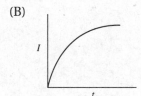

(D)

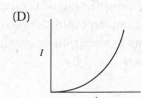

11. What is the amount of charge delivered to the man?
    (A) 0.33 coulombs
    (B) 3 coulombs
    (C) 6 coulombs
    (D) 10 coulombs

12. What part of the body has the highest resistance for the current?
    (A) Muscle tissue
    (B) Skin
    (C) The heart itself
    (D) Connective tissue

13. The 200 joules of energy are delivered to the patient with a discharge time of 5 ms. How much power is delivered to the patient over the first 2 ms of this time?
    (A) 40 W
    (B) 100 W
    (C) 40,000 W
    (D) 200,000 W

The following questions do not refer to a descriptive passage and are not related to each other.

14. Two 2 Ω resistors are placed in parallel. What is their equivalent resistance?
    (A) 1 Ω
    (B) 2 Ω
    (C) 4 Ω
    (D) 1/2 Ω

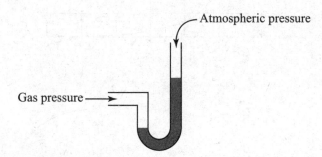

15. For the U-tube manometer filled with mercury in the figure above, the gas pressure is:
    (A) lower than atmospheric pressure.
    (B) higher than atmospheric pressure.
    (C) the same as atmospheric pressure.
    (D) unknown.

PASSAGE III

Rollerblading is a popular sport in which skaters test their skills in specially designed arenas. The challenge involves traveling down steep inclines and skating up walls on the opposite side. Figure 1 shows an arena with three sections. A 65 kg skater starts at point A, at height R, and travels down to the ground level along a frictionless semicircular path with radius R. The skater then travels a distance $2R$ along a flat, rough surface between points B and C, where the coefficient of friction, representing the ratio of the frictional force to his weight, is 0.20. There is a lot of sound generated from the friction with the rough surface. After passing point C, the skater again encounters a frictionless semicircular wall of radius R and rises to a height represented by point D. During the trip from A to D, the skater simply coasts with the supply of gravitational potential energy he started with at point A.

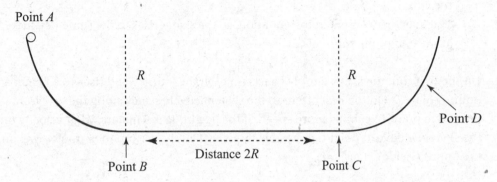

Figure 1. A rollerblading arena

16. The amount of gravitational potential energy that the skater has at point D is:
    (A) $mgR - mgR/2$
    (B) $mgR - 0.2mgR$
    (C) $mgR - 0.2mg2R$
    (D) $2mgR - 0.2mgR$

17. Point D is lower than Point A because:
    (A) the skater lost energy to sound and heat from point B to point C, and lost energy due to gravity from point A to point B, and lost energy due to gravity from point C to point D.
    (B) the skater lost energy to sound and heat from point B to point C and lost energy due to gravity from point C to point D.
    (C) the skater lost energy to sound and heat from point B to point C.
    (D) The skater lost energy to gravity from point C to point D.

18. Sound travels at 340 m/s. There is a wall at a distance $4R$ away from point B. How long after reaching point B does the skater begin to hear the echo from this wall?
    (A) $8R/340$ m/s
    (B) $8R(340$ m/s$)$
    (C) $4R/340$ m/s
    (D) $4R(340$ m/s$)$

19. If the distance, R, is 5 meters, then the amount of kinetic energy the skater has at point C is
    (A) 1300 joules
    (B) 1950 joules
    (C) 2600 joules
    (D) 3250 joules

20. On the next attempt, the skater puts on a backpack that has a mass of 10 kg. Which of the following will be true?
    (A) The skater will have a greater velocity at point B.
    (B) There will be a greater coefficient of friction between point B and point C.
    (C) Because of the extra mass, the skater will rise to a greater height at the end of the run.
    (D) The mass cancels out in the equation, so the skater rises to the same height at the end of the run.

21. On the first run, the skater simply coasts through the journey and rises to a height at point D of $0.6R$. On the next attempt, the skater actively skates along the way from point B to point C, gaining more speed. If the height, R, is 5 meters, what velocity must the skater achieve at point C to be able to make it all the way up the 5-meter wall on the opposite side?
    (A) 4 m/s
    (B) 6 m/s
    (C) 8 m/s
    (D) 10 m/s

PASSAGE IV

The heart of a radio transmitter or receiver is the oscillator. In mechanics, a mass hanging from a spring is set in oscillation by a small displacement, with the mass moving up and down at a frequency determined by the mass, m, and the stiffness of the spring, k. In electricity, the current in an inductor–capacitor circuit oscillates at a frequency determined by the values of inductance, L, and capacitance, C, according to $f = 1/2\pi\sqrt{LC}$. The analogous systems are shown in Figure 1.

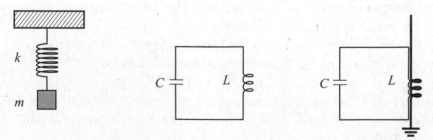

Figure 1. A mass–spring system and an inductor–capacitor circuit

In the oscillator, the voltage and current oscillate sinusoidally in much the same manner as the mass–spring system. The oscillating current in the inductor induces a current in the concentrically wound coil that is connected to an antenna. This induced current causes electrons to oscillate up and down in the antenna. This current produces a magnetic (B) field that is tangent to circles concentric around the antenna. And this oscillating B field, along with the oscillating E field in the up and down direction, produces an electromagnetic wave moving out from the antenna. This is a basic radio signal.

This signal is detected by another antenna and, as the wave passes the receiving antenna, the E and B fields lead to current in that antenna and in another oscillator tuned to oscillate at the same frequency. It is through the E and B field wave that the oscillations of the transmitter are transmitted through the air to the receiver. The speed of the wave is $c = 3.0 \times 10^8$ m/s, which is the speed of all electromagnetic waves and is the ratio of E/B.

The simplest way to communicate with this radio is to turn it on and off. A series of long and short (dots and dashes) signals coded for letters of the alphabet (Morse code) allows the transmitter to communicate with a receiver tuned to the appropriate frequency. No one can hear the electromagnetic wave, so this wave is modulated by an audio signal that is detected at the receiver. Time varying modulation of the amplitude of the oscillating wave by a voice allows broadcast and detection of the spoken word at the receiver. Tuning of the receivers is accomplished by changing the L or C of the receiver to match the transmitter.

22. The speed of radio waves is determined by:
    (A) the density and resilience of the air.
    (B) the ratio of L/C.
    (C) the ratio of E/B.
    (D) multiplying the speed of sound by 100.

23. Why are radio receiving antennas oriented to detecting the E part of the wave rather than the B part of the wave?
    (A) The E field is much larger than the B field.
    (B) There is no B component in the wave.
    (C) The E field is in the direction of the wave and is easily detected.
    (D) The B field always points toward the ground.

24. A transmitter in the radio band broadcasts at 60,000 kHz. What is the appropriate length of the associated wave?
    (A) 60,000 m
    (B) 5 m
    (C) 0.1 m
    (D) 300 m

25. In most situations involving transmitters and receivers, the transmitter is at a fixed frequency and the receiver is tunable within a range to best match the transmitter frequency. How can a receiver be tuned?
    (A) Vary the inductance.
    (B) Vary either the inductance or capacitance.
    (C) Vary the length of the antenna.
    (D) Vary the capacitance.

26. If an oscillator circuit is made with an inductor of 2×10^{-3} H and a capacitor of 8×10^{-5} F, approximately what is the oscillating frequency?
   (A) 1600 Hz
   (B) 60,000,000 Hz
   (C) 400 Hz
   (D) 8 Hz

27. For a radio wave moving through the air, which of the following best describes the orientation of the E and B fields and the direction of the wave for a radio wave moving through the air?
   (A) E and B are at right angles and in a plane normal to the direction of the wave.
   (B) E and B are in the direction of the wave.
   (C) E is at a right angle to the direction of the wave.
   (D) B is at a right angle to the direction of the wave.

The following questions do not refer to a descriptive passage and are not related to each other.

28. A block 5 cm by 10 cm by 16 cm is made of material with density 5 g/cm^3. What is the minimum pressure that the block can exert if it is placed flat on a table?
   (A) 2500 N/m^2
   (B) 5000 N/m^2
   (C) 8000 N/m^2
   (D) 11,000 N/m^2

29. The index of refraction of water is 1.3. If a ray of light comes from air and enters water at a 0-degree angle of incidence (perpendicular to the surface of the water), then:
   (A) the light is both refracted and slows down.
   (B) the light is only refracted.
   (C) the light only slows down.
   (D) the light is neither refracted nor does it slow down.

ANSWER KEY

1. C	**6.** C	**11.** A	**16.** C	**21.** D	**26.** C
2. C	**7.** A	**12.** B	**17.** C	**22.** C	**27.** A
3. A	**8.** D	**13.** D	**18.** A	**23.** A	**28.** A
4. C	**9.** C	**14.** A	**19.** B	**24.** B	**29.** C
5. B	**10.** A	**15.** B	**20.** D	**25.** B	

ANSWERS EXPLAINED

1. **(C)** At a drift speed of 10^{-4} m/s it would take hours to move a meter, assuming that the same electron could be followed through metal.

2. **(C)** The resistance is the resistivity times the length divided by the cross section. The calculation comes out 0.1 Ω.

3. **(A)** Because the resistors are equal, the voltage is divided equally.

4. **(C)** The smaller resistor has the greater current, $V = IR$.

5. **(B)** The unit resulting from the product of joule/coulomb times coulomb/sec is joule/sec, which is a power unit (work per time) and is the definition of the watt.

6. **(C)** Resistivity is an inherent property and cannot change because of the dimensions of the wire. Only resistance changes with the dimensions.

7. **(A)** The object has 100 J of kinetic energy ($0.5 \, mv^2$), which translates to gravitational potential energy, $mgh = 20$ N (h) = 100 J.

8. **(D)** Sound is a longitudinal wave. Light does not need a medium to travel. Sound speeds up when it goes from air to water.

9. **(C)** Capacitance is given by the equation $C = \dfrac{k\varepsilon_0 A}{d}$. Increasing the capacitance is accomplished by increasing the dielectric constant k, not by increasing the spacing d or decreasing the area A.

10. **(A)** Use the equation $V = IR$. The body has some resistance. However, the equation shows that the higher the voltage, the higher the current. So the current curve has the same shape as the voltage curve.

11. **(A)** Voltage is equal to joules/coulomb. The voltage given in the passage is 600 volts, and the energy is 200 joules.

$$600 \text{ V} = \frac{200 \text{ J}}{\text{charge}}$$
$$\text{charge} = 0.33 \text{ coulombs}$$

12. **(B)** Dry skin typically has a resistance above 10,000 ohms. The conducting gel is absorbed into the skin and provides a low-resistance path inside the body. Tissues, muscles, and the heart have relatively low resistance due to their high water content.

13. **(D)** Power = $\dfrac{\text{energy}}{\text{time}}$ where time is in seconds. Dividing the total energy by 5 ms results in 40,000 W. However, the shape of the discharge curve given in question 10 shows that much higher voltage and higher current exist in the first 2 ms compared to the last 3 ms. Therefore, we look for a value much higher than 40,000 W.

14. **(A)** Resistors add as $1/R$ when in parallel.

15. **(B)** It must be higher than atmospheric pressure in order to push up the column of mercury on the other side.

16. **(C)** $mgR - 0.2mg2R$. The skater starts at point A with gravitational potential energy mgR. None is lost on the way down or up the frictionless semicircle. Work done vs. friction along the flat distance $2R$ is the force of friction times the distance $2R$. The force of friction is the coefficient of friction (0.2) times the weight (mg). This quantity of energy is lost.

17. **(C)** The only place where energy is lost is along the path from B to C. The other paths are frictionless. There is no energy lost to gravity, only to the sound and heat due to friction.

18. **(A)** The sound must travel a distance $4R$ to the wall and then $4R$ back to the skater for a total distance of $8R$. Speed = distance/time. Time = distance/speed. So the time is $8R/340$ m/s.

19. **(B)** The skater starts with energy, $mgR = 65$ kg(10 m/s^2)(5 m) = 3250 J. Along the path from point B to point C, the skater loses an amount of energy equal to 0.2(65 kg)(10 m/s^2)(10 m) = 1300 J. This leaves 3250 – 1300 = 1950 J.

20. **(D)** For choice A the kinetic energy is greater, but only because of the mass. The velocity will be the same because masses cancel in the conservation of energy statement ($mgh = \frac{1}{2}mv^2$). Choice B is not correct since the force of friction may change, but the coefficient of friction does not depend on weight. It is a constant. Answer D is true since mass appears at every stage of the conservation of energy statement for the trip ($mgh = mgR - 0.2(mg2R)$), where h is the height on the opposite side.

21. **(D)** The skater's kinetic energy at point C must be equal to his gravitational potential energy at the top of the climb. So $\frac{1}{2}mv^2 = mgh$, and $v = 10$ m/s

22. **(C)** The speed of the waves is E/B.

23. **(A)** The E field is equal to the speed of the waves times the B field. $E/B = c$.

24. **(B)** Use $c = \lambda f$ 3.0×10^8 m/s = $\lambda(6.0 \times 10^7$ Hz) $\lambda = 5$ m

25. **(B)** The frequency of an oscillator depends on inductance and capacitance only. Varying either one changes the frequency.

26. **(C)** The calculation can be done approximately, using $f = 1/2\pi\sqrt{LC}$. The product $(2 \times 10^{-3})(8 \times 10^{-5}) = 16 \times 10^{-8}$ has square root 4×10^{-4}. Add 2π, and the frequency is approximately 10,000 over 25 or 400 Hz.

27. **(A)** In a broadcast antenna, the electric field is vertical, and the magnetic field is horizontal, and the wave moves away from the antenna in a direction perpendicular to the plane formed by these fields.

28. **(A)** The mass of the block found from density = M/V is 4 kg. This is 40 N. Use the largest possible area to get minimum pressure, or 16 cm $\times$ 10 cm.

29. **(C)** Since the light is perpendicular to the surface, there is no angle of refraction, but the speed is still lower.

For online practice, go to
http://barronsbooks.com/tp/mcat

Biology

3

→ CELL BIOLOGY

→ CELL METABOLISM AND ENZYMES

→ MICROBIOLOGY

→ DNA AND PROTEIN SYNTHESIS

→ EUKARYOTIC CELL REPLICATION: THE CELL CYCLE, MITOSIS,
   AND CYTOKINESIS

→ MEIOSIS AND GENETIC VARIABILITY

→ GENETICS

→ POPULATION GENETICS AND HARDY-WEINBERG EQUILIBRIUM

→ EVOLUTION

→ HUMAN ANATOMY

→ DEVELOPMENTAL BIOLOGY

Biology is the foundation of medicine and is heavily tested on the MCAT. For the most part, the MCAT tests your understanding of concepts and relationships in biology. However, test takers are expected to know a certain amount of detail as well. Carefully review both the concepts and details in this chapter.

CELL BIOLOGY

Cells were first observed by Anton van Leeuwenhoek and Robert Hooke in the seventeenth century shortly after the invention of the microscope. During the next century, other observers noted the ubiquity of cells in plants and animals, leading to the development of the **cell theory**. The cell theory holds that:

1. All living things are made of cells.
2. Cells are the fundamental unit of life.
3. All cells come from other living cells.

The third tenet of the cell theory was the most difficult to establish because it rejected the widely held concept of **spontaneous generation**, the idea that life can emerge from nonlife. The cell theory also clearly established a method for determining living from nonliving things. Cells are the fundamental unit of life. Thus, a single cell has all the necessary components of a living thing. For example, cells are the smallest entity capable of independent reproduction, of metabolism, and of maintaining a stable internal environment (**homeostasis**) in the midst of a variable external environment. Individual cells respond to their environments. Populations of cellular organisms adapt and evolve.

Cells may exist as single-celled (**unicellular**) organisms, such as bacteria and many protists. Individual cells may congregate in colonies, or they may specialize at the cellular level into an assemblage of distinct cell types, as in sponges. Alternatively, they may form the highly specialized tissues of a complex **multicellular** organism.

Cell size is measured in micrometers (μm). Most cells are too small to be viewed without a light microscope. Bacterial cells measure a few micrometers in diameter, with the smallest being less than 1 μm. Most plant and animal cells are between 10–100 μm in diameter. The largest cells are visible with the naked eye. They include the eggs of vertebrates, which can be up to 12 cm in diameter, and elongated nerve and muscle cells, which in large animals may reach several meters in length.

Cell Structure

All cells have the same basic structure, consisting of an exterior **plasma membrane**, an interior **cytosol**, **ribosomes**, and **genetic material**. The plasma membrane (or cell membrane) regulates the passage of materials into and out of the cell. The cytosol is a watery medium in which dissolved solutes undergo essential reactions of metabolism. Ribosomes are large molecules involved in the synthesis of proteins. The genetic material is **deoxyribonucleic acid**, or **DNA**. The DNA is responsible for transmitting hereditary material and for controlling cellular activities via protein synthesis. Based on their structure, cells are classified as either **prokaryotic** or **eukaryotic**.

Prokaryotic Cells

Prokaryotic cells are the smallest cells, found only in bacteria and the evolutionarily distinct single-celled Archaea. They have ribosomes and DNA but lack nuclei and other membrane-bound organelles. Instead, all metabolic processes occur in the cytoplasm. Their DNA is a single circular molecule attached to the plasma membrane. Prokaryotic cell replication occurs by binary fission.

Generalized Eukaryotic Cells

Eukaryotic cells are larger and more complex than prokaryotic cells. They are found in a wide diversity of organisms, ranging from single-celled, aquatic protists to plants, fungi, and animals, including humans. Eukaryotes have membrane-bound intracellular organelles and multiple linear DNA molecules enclosed in a membrane-bound nucleus. Eukaryotic cells replicate by the processes of mitosis and cytokinesis. Figures 3.1 and 3.2 show typical eukaryotic animal and plant cells.

CYTOSOL

The **cytosol**, or intracellular fluid, is a complex mixture of water, small molecules such as oxygen, dissolved ions, and macromolecules. The cytosol occupies a region of the cell called the **cytoplasm**, which consists of cytosol and suspended substances such as cytoskeletal elements and organelles. Water makes up roughly 70% of the cytosol, acting as the solvent of the cell. Proteins make up an additional 20% or more of the volume, giving the cytosol a consistency that ranges from a low-viscosity liquid to gel. In both prokaryotes and eukaryotes, the cytosol is a medium for the chemical reactions of metabolism.

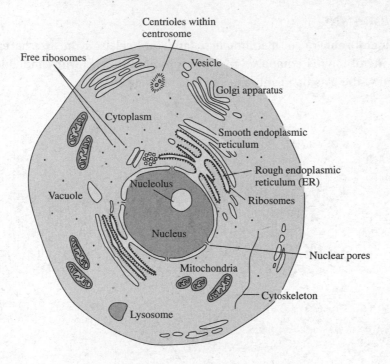

Figure 3.1. Typical eukaryotic animal cell

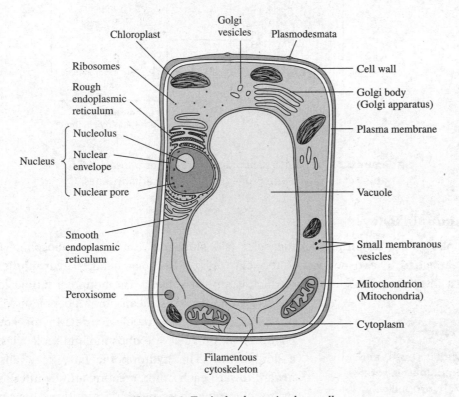

Figure 3.2. Typical eukaryotic plant cell

PLASMA MEMBRANE

The **plasma membrane** (or cell membrane) separates the cell from the external environment. The plasma membrane is composed of a **phospholipid bilayer** with embedded proteins. Figure 3.3 shows the plasma membrane and its components.

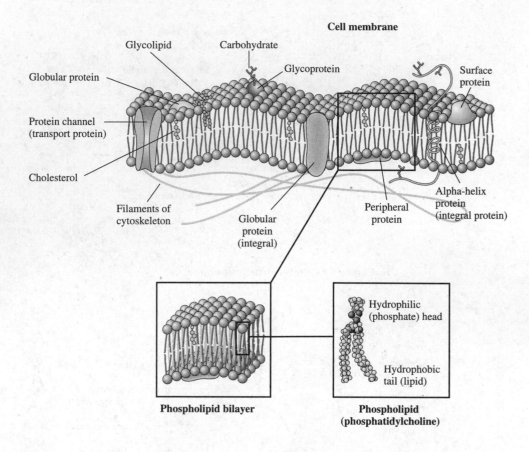

Figure 3.3. The plasma membrane, showing the phospholipid bilayer and associated proteins, lipids, and carbohydrates

Phospholipid Bylayer

Phospholipids are **amphipathic** molecules (see sidebar) with a polar phosphate group "head" attached to two nonpolar fatty acid "tails." The polar head is **hydrophilic**. This means it dissolves readily in water, which is a polar solvent. The nonpolar fatty acid tails are **hydrophobic**. This means they do not dissolve in water and, in fact, are repelled by it. In the aqueous environment of a cell, the phospholipid molecules form a double row. The hydrophobic fatty acid tails face inward toward each other, creating an oily interior. The hydrophilic phosphate heads face outward toward the extracellular and the intracellular solutions. In addition to phospholipids, other amphipathic molecules in the membrane include **glycolipids** (lipids bonded to carbohydrates) and **sterols** such as cholesterol (animals) or ergosterol (fungi and protists).

AMPHIPATHIC

From the Greek words *amphis* (both) and *pathia* (love), the word amphipathic refers to a molecule that is both hydrophilic (water loving) and hydrophobic (water fearing.) In phospholipid molecules, one end is hydrophilic and the other hydrophobic.

Membrane Proteins

Membrane proteins are proteins attached to the cell membrane. Amphipathic proteins are embedded in the lipid layer as either transmembrane proteins or peripheral proteins. **Transmembrane proteins** are a type of **integral membrane protein** that extend completely across and remain permanently embedded in the membrane. In contrast, **peripheral proteins** may project from either side of the membrane. They are weakly bound to phospholipids or to integral proteins by noncovalent attractions.

These proteins may act as **transport proteins**, allowing water, ions, and other dissolved solutes to cross the membrane. They may also act as membrane receptors. **Membrane receptors** are proteins that carry branching oligosaccharide chains on the outside (**exoplasmic**) surface of the cell. These side chains act as binding sites for signal molecules.

The carbohydrate side chains attached to membrane proteins (**glycoproteins**) and glycolipids of the phospholipid bilayer form an outer halo of carbohydrate called a **glycocalyx** that surrounds the cell. The side chains within the glycocalyx are unique to every individual. These side chains serve as binding or recognition sites for signaling molecules important in cell adhesion, cell–cell recognition, and cell signaling. (See Cell–Cell Communication on page 328.)

Fluid Mosaic Model

According to the **fluid mosaic model** of membrane structure, a cell membrane is a mosaic of proteins and phospholipids, with protein molecules floating like icebergs in a lipid sea. Phospholipids and proteins slide easily past each other in constant lateral movement within the membrane depending on the degree of fluidity. Membrane fluidity depends on temperature, on the degree of saturation of the fatty acids chains, and on the amount of embedded cholesterol. Membranes with phospholipids composed of unsaturated fatty acids are more fluid than those with saturated fatty acids because the double bonds between the carbons in unsaturated fatty acids cause the carbon chains to kink. This kinking keeps the fatty acids from packing together tightly, increasing fluidity. Large amounts of the steroid cholesterol reduce membrane fluidity because cholesterol molecules interfere with phospholipid movement. However, cholesterol can also help keep membranes from solidifying at low temperatures. Cholesterol can make up 50 percent of the volume of some cell membranes.

Membrane Permeability

Because the area surrounding cells consists mostly of water, the lipid layer of the cell membrane forms a water-repellent boundary that limits the entry and exit of water-soluble molecules. The embedded membrane proteins can act as gates for the transport of polar molecules and can restrict or allow passage of materials. The cell membrane is considered to be **selectively permeable**, or **semipermeable**. The cell membrane regulates and restricts which molecules dissolved in water (**solutes**) enter and leave the cell.

Factors that determine the permeability of the membrane include the size, charge, and polarity of solute molecules. Small, uncharged particles and nonpolar, hydrophobic molecules have no difficulty crossing the lipid layer. Charged particles such as ions and large, polar molecules such as proteins and polysaccharides cannot cross except through regulated protein channels. The movement of materials across the membrane occurs through both **passive transport** and **active transport**.

IMPORTANT TERMS FOR SOLUTIONS

Solution: A **solute** (substance dissolved) plus a solvent (dissolving agent). In living things, water is the universal solvent.

Tonicity: A term for the relative solute concentration of a solution.

Isotonic solutions: Relative term for two solutions that have the same dissolved solute concentration. The net movement of water will be equal in both directions between isotonic solutions.

Hypotonic solution: Relative term for a solution that has less dissolved solute than another solution. The net movement of water by osmosis will be out of a hypotonic solution.

Hypertonic solution: Relative term for a solution that has more dissolved solute than another solution. The net movement of water by osmosis will be into a hypertonic solution.

Passive Transport

Passive transport of materials across a membrane does not require any energy expenditure by the cell. The kinetic energy of the molecules themselves drives the movement of materials. Passive transport can occur by simple diffusion, osmosis, or facilitated transport.

Simple diffusion of particles occurs when the random kinetic energy causes particles to bounce randomly off one another in all directions. Because more frequent collisions occur in areas of higher concentration, the net movement of particles is from high concentration to low concentration, down a concentration gradient. This results in particles becoming equally distributed, reaching equilibrium. In living cells, substances that are small or nonpolar can readily cross the phospholipid bilayer and enter or leave the cell by simple diffusion. The passage of oxygen into the cell and carbon dioxide out of the cell occurs by simple diffusion.

Osmosis is a special case of simple diffusion. In biological systems, osmosis specifically refers to the movement of water across a semipermeable membrane. Water moves by diffusion down a concentration gradient from a region of high concentration to a region of low concentration. Water is at its greatest concentration as pure water, with no dissolved solutes. The addition of solutes decreases the effective concentration of water. When a semipermeable membrane separates two regions with differing concentrations of solute, the net movement of water will be down its own concentration gradient, from high concentration of water to low. Consequently, water will flow by osmosis from a low concentration of solute (**hypotonic**) toward a high concentration of solute (**hypertonic**).

Osmotic pressure is the pressure generated by the presence of solutes (water-soluble molecules) dissolved in water. A solution with a higher concentration of solutes has a higher osmotic pressure. Water flows from regions of low osmotic pressure (low solute, high water concentration) toward regions of high osmotic pressure (high solute, low water concentration). Osmotic pressure can therefore be thought of as a negative or pulling pressure. A solution with high osmotic pressure pulls water from more dilute solutions.

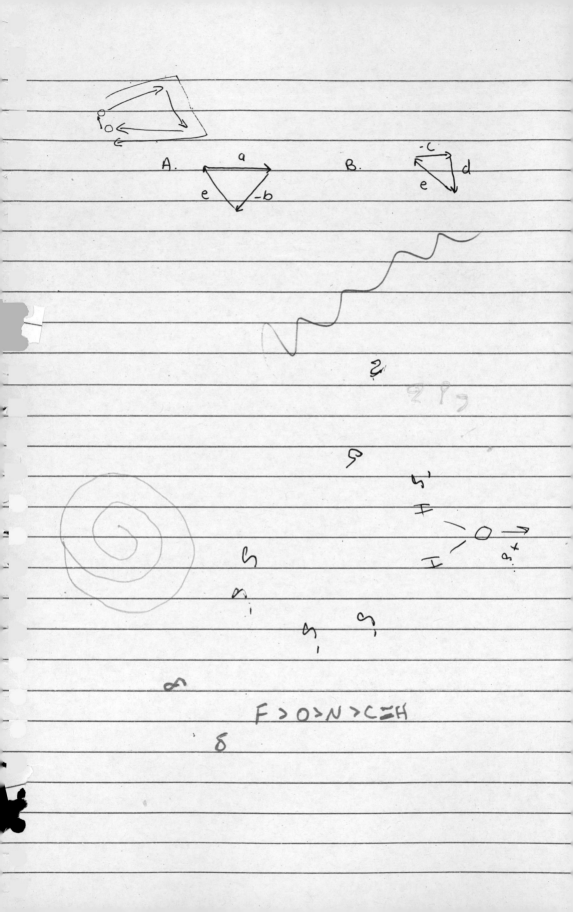

A.

a

e   -b

B.   -c

e   d

F > O > N > C≡H

A membrane that lets water through but does not let dissolved solutes through can result in dramatic changes in water volume on either side of the membrane. If the concentration of solutes (osmotic pressure) is higher on one side of the membrane, the net flow of water will continue toward the more concentrated solution until the hydrostatic pressure of water building up on that side counterbalances the osmotic pressure or until the membrane ruptures. This is shown in Figure 3.4.

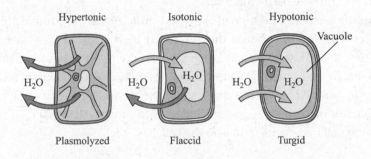

Figure 3.4. Net movement of water by osmosis in a plant cell placed in hypertonic, isotonic, and hypotonic environments

Placing plant or animal cells into distilled water results in a dramatic example of osmosis. Water moves by osmosis from the distilled water into the hypertonic (higher concentration of solutes) cytosol. In plants with a rigid cell wall, the cell does not burst. Instead, the plant cell experiences an increase in **turgor pressure** as it swells. A red blood cell placed into distilled water, in contrast, will rupture (**hemolyze**) because the cell membrane cannot withstand the pressure of the influx of water. Placing the same cells into a hypertonic (higher concentration) salt solution will have the opposite effect. Both cells will lose water. The cytoplasm of the plant cell will shrivel and shrink away from the cell wall (**plasmolyze**). The red blood cell will shrivel (**crenate**).

In **facilitated diffusion**, the third type of passive transport, solute molecules cross the lipid bilayer through transport proteins, which act as gates or carriers. As with all passive transport, facilitated diffusion is a spontaneous process in which no energy is expended by the cell. The two types of transport proteins used in facilitated diffusion are channel proteins and carrier proteins.

Channel proteins are amphipathic transmembrane molecules with a region of hydrophilic (water-loving) amino acids on the interior. This region provides a passageway for water and small ions. Although water molecules are small enough to cross the lipid bilayer by simple diffusion, their polarity inhibits this transport. The ability of water to cross cell membranes is greatly enhanced by the presence of **aquaporins**, which are integral membrane proteins found in animals, plants, and bacteria. Aquaporins have a central pore just large enough for water molecules to pass through in single file. Water and other small hydrophilic molecules can move into and out of the cell, but charged molecules cannot enter.

Channel proteins called **ion channels** allow the passage of charged ions across a membrane. Ion channels are composed of either one or a group of several integral membrane proteins surrounding a water-filled pore. The charge of the ion or the width of the channel at its narrowest point determines which type of ions can pass. In many ion channels, an outside stimulus is needed to open the channel. Such channels are referred to as **gated**. Ion channels may be **voltage gated**, which means they require an electrical stimulus or a change in electric potential in order to open. Ion channels may also be **chemically gated**, also called **ligand gated**. These ion channels require the binding of another molecule to open or close.

Examples of gated ion channels include sodium, potassium, and calcium channels important in nervous and muscle tissue function.

Carrier proteins are a second type of transport protein. Carrier proteins bind to solutes and undergo a conformational change that physically carries the solute molecule across the membrane. When the solute molecule is released on the other side of the membrane, the carrier protein returns to its original shape. Examples include the carrier proteins involved in the facilitated diffusion of glucose across the cell membrane. These glucose transporter proteins bind to glucose molecules, triggering a change in protein shape that "flips" the bound glucose across the cell membrane and into the cell.

DRINKING SEAWATER?

Why should you not drink seawater?

Is it possible to drink too much fresh water?

What would be the consequence?

TIP

LIGAND

The term *ligand* refers to a substance that binds to a biological molecule, usually to trigger a signal.

Active Transport

Active transport is the movement of substances across a membrane in a way that requires the expenditure of cellular energy. Typically this involves movement of substances against their concentration gradients. This process requires the investment of cellular energy in the form of adenosine triphosphate (ATP), the energy molecule of the cell. Like facilitated diffusion, active transport relies on carrier proteins to move substances across the membrane. An example is the sodium-potassium pump, which moves sodium and potassium ions against their concentration gradients across the plasma membrane.

The **sodium-potassium pump** consists of a carrier protein, the enzyme Na^+-K^+-ATPase, which transports sodium (Na^+) and potassium (K^+) ions in opposite directions across the plasma membrane. Sodium binds to the ATPase on the cytoplasmic side of the membrane. This triggers the protein to hydrolyze the terminal phosphate group of an ATP molecule, converting ATP to ADP. The phosphorylation of the protein provides the energy for a conformational (shape) change in the protein. The change in shape results in pumping the sodium out of the cell, where it is released. In its current conformation, the carrier protein now has a higher affinity for extracellular K^+, which binds to the carrier protein and triggers the release of the phosphate group. The protein reverts to its original conformation, releasing the potassium into the cell and once again regaining a high affinity for Na^+ (see Figure 3.5).

The sodium-potassium pump transports 3 sodium ions out of the cell for every 2 potassium ions pumped into the cell. Consequently, potassium concentrations are high within the cell whereas sodium concentrations are high in the extracellular space.

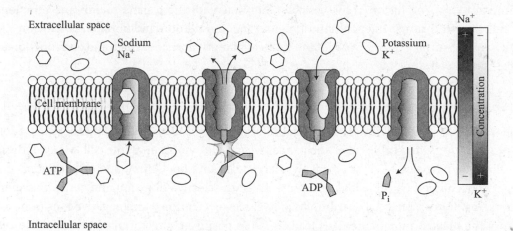

Figure 3.5. Sodium-potassium pump

Active transport is also required to transport large, polar molecules and large particles which cannot cross the plasma membrane by means of diffusion or carrier proteins. These substances must cross the membrane by the mechanism of **bulk transport**, either endocytosis or exocytosis.

Endocytosis is the process by which large substances are brought into the cell. **Exocytosis** is the process by which large substances are released from the cell. Both processes involve the use of **transport vesicles**, which are membrane-bound sacs that surround the substance to be exported or imported.

Endocytosis occurs in 3 ways: phagocytosis (cell eating), pinocytosis (cell drinking), and receptor-mediated endocytosis. In **phagocytosis**, the plasma membrane forms extensions called pseudopodia (false feet) to surround a particle that is outside of the cell. The pseudopodia engulf the particle in a pocket of membrane that pinches off as it is pulled into the cell. This pinched-off pocket of membrane becomes a large transport vesicle called a vacuole. Once inside the cell, other vesicles called **lysosomes**, carrying digestive enzymes, fuse with the membrane of the vacuole. The particle is then digested.

In **pinocytosis** (cell drinking), the cell membrane folds inward (**invaginates**) to suck extracellular fluid and its solute contents into a pouch. This pouch then breaks off in the cell as a vesicle. The cell uses pinocytosis to sample the contents of extracellular fluid.

Receptor-mediated endocytosis allows the cell to take in particular substances regardless of their concentration outside of the cell. Receptor proteins are located in depressions in the plasma membrane. These proteins have binding sites to which only specific substances can bind. Once a substance binds to the site, the membrane pockets inward, carrying the membrane receptors and their bound molecule or ion (**ligand**) into the cell inside a transport vesicle. The receptor proteins are then released from the bound ligands, and the proteins return to the plasma membrane.

ACTIVE TRANSPORT SUMMARY

I. Sodium-potassium pump

II. Bulk transport

    A. Endocytosis

    B. Exocytosis

Exocytosis is essentially the reverse process of endocytosis. Substances manufactured within the cell are packaged into a membrane-bound transport vesicle. The vesicle then fuses with the plasma membrane and expels its contents. Exocytosis is used by cells in the digestive, endocrine, and nervous systems to secrete digestive enzymes, hormones, and neurotransmitters. The fusion of the vesicle membrane with the plasma membrane functions in cell growth through the addition of membrane. In addition, membrane proteins on the inner vesicle surface become part of the extracellular membrane surface and can function as receptors in cell signaling.

Membrane Potential

The semipermeability of the plasma membrane allows cells to maintain a high concentration of proteins, ions, and other polar substances within the cytoplasm of the cell. Many of these are charged particles, such as positively charged sodium, potassium, and calcium ions and negatively charged chloride ions and proteins. Both selective diffusion and active transport of ions result in an unequal distribution of positive ions (**cations**) and negative ions (**anions**) across the plasma membrane. This leads to a net positive charge on the outside of the cell membrane and a net negative charge on the inside, a separation of charge that results in a voltage gradient called the **membrane potential**. This charge difference applies only at the membrane. Overall, the cell and the extracellular fluid are electrically neutral.

The difference in charge between the interior of the membrane and the exterior results in a **resting membrane potential** that ranges from –50 to –100 millivolts (mV). The negative sign of the resting potential indicates that the inside of the cell is negatively charged compared with the outside. In addition, the large differences in concentration of the ions create a chemical gradient. Together, the membrane potential and the chemical gradient combine to form an **electrochemical gradient** across the membrane.

Electrochemical gradients store chemical and electrical energy as potential energy that is available to do work. Consequently, the membrane potential reflects the ability of the cell to do work across the membrane. Membrane potential is important in the functioning of the muscular and nervous systems and in cellular processes such as the cotransport of metabolic substances across membranes.

Cell–Cell Communication

Cells can communicate with each other by direct contact or through either local- or long-distance signaling molecules. The plasma membrane contributes to cell–cell communication through the binding of molecules to receptors on the outer surface of the membrane, initiating a cellular response or signal. These receptors include glycolipids and glycoproteins in the glycocalyx, both of which have carbohydrate side chains projecting into the extracellular medium. The side chains act as receptors (binding sites) for signal molecules. When a signaling molecule binds to a specific membrane receptor, it triggers a conformational (shape) change in the receptor molecule, leading to a cellular response. This response may be direct, such as the opening of an ion channel within a membrane protein. This response may also be indirect, such as the activation of an enzyme through a series of intermediaries.

> Signaling molecules include the sphingolipids, a group of glycolipids associated with cell membranes. Defects in sphingolipid metabolism can result in genetic disorders such as Tay-Sachs disease, a progressive deterioration of brain function caused by a harmful buildup of membrane-derived sphingolipids in brain neurons.

Autocrine signaling occurs when a signal molecule produced by a cell binds to receptors on the plasma membrane of the same cell. Cells that employ autocrine signaling are found in the immune system.

Juxtacrine signaling occurs between cells that are in direct physical contact with each other, such as across cell junctions. Juxtacrine signaling is important in cell differentiation during development and in the transmission of electrical signals in cardiac cells.

Paracrine signaling involves chemical messengers that send signals over short distances between nearby cells. Examples include neurotransmitters that transmit electrochemical signals between neurons and target cells, cytokines that function in the immune system, and growth factors that trigger cell division and cellular differentiation during development.

Endocrine signaling involves hormones (chemical messengers) that function in long-distance communication by traveling through the bloodstream to target cells. Hormones may bind to membrane receptors or may cross the plasma membrane to bind with receptors within the target cell.

The process by which the binding of an extracellular signal molecule is converted to an intracellular response is termed **signal transduction**. Signal transduction frequently involves a sequence of metabolic steps (comprising a **pathway**), with each step triggering the next in the sequence. Such an indirect metabolic pathway is referred to as a **signal transduction cascade** or **metabolic cascade**. The presence of multiple intermediaries in a transduction cascade allows for amplification and feedback loops as well as for propagation of the signal.

One major type of signal transduction pathway is the **phosphorylation** of a chain of protein intermediates by **protein kinase** enzymes. This pathway uses energy from the hydrolysis of ATP to fuel multiple conformational changes among proteins in the transduction sequence, ultimately transferring a phosphate group to activate an enzyme and trigger the cellular response.

Another important type of signal transduction pathway is mediated by **G-protein coupled membrane receptors**. Both protein kinase enzymes and G-protein coupled membrane receptors may act through **second messengers**, which carry out the intracellular response. In a signal transduction cascade, the extracellular signal molecule is a first messenger. The binding of the first messenger initiates a conformational change in the membrane receptor. This conformational change activates intracellular second messengers such as calcium ions or the nucleoside monophosphate cyclic AMP to activate a target protein and trigger a **cellular response** (see Figure 3.6). The cellular response to a second messenger is frequently the activation of an enzyme, the opening of an ion channel, or the transcription of a gene.

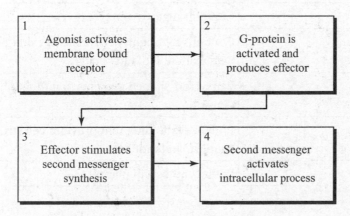

Figure 3.6. The second messenger mechanism

RIBOSOMES

Ribosomes are molecules of protein and ribonucleic acid (ribosomal RNA) that are responsible for protein synthesis in the cell. Ribosomes are found in all cells, including prokaryotic cells. They may occur as free ribosomes in the cytoplasm or they may bind to membranes of intracellular organelles, such as the endoplasmic reticulum and nucleus. Ribosomes are composed of two subunits, one large and one small. Prokaryotic ribosomes are typically 70S, or svedberg units, a characterization based on the rate of sedimentation in a centrifuge. The two subunits are 30S and 50S. (Note that these do not add up to 70.) The larger ribosomes of eukaryotes are 80S, with 40S and 60S subunits. Each subunit is composed of both ribosomal RNA (rRNA) and protein, with RNA providing the basic structure of the subunit. When the ribosome is not synthesizing protein, the two subunits separate. It has recently been shown that the RNA component of a ribosome functions as a **ribozyme**, or RNA enzyme, during protein synthesis.

CYTOPLASMIC ORGANELLES

In addition to the plasma membrane and free ribosomes shared with prokaryotes, eukaryotic cells contain membrane-bound organelles, specialized structures that perform a specific function within the cell. Most eukaryotic organelles are membrane-bound, which means they are surrounded by a membrane of similar composition to the plasma membrane. Table 3.1 shows some major eukaryotic organelles and their functions.

Table 3.1 Major Eukaryotic Organelles and Their Functions

Organelle	Function
Nucleus	Control center of cell; location of DNA
Nucleolus	Location of RNA and ribosome assembly within the nucleus
Mitochondria	Cellular respiration; ATP production
Rough endoplasmic reticulum	Protein synthesis; ribosome attachment
Smooth endoplasmic reticulum	Lipid synthesis; detoxification of drugs and toxins
Golgi apparatus	Packaging and transport of proteins and lipids
Vacuole	Storage of water, food, and wastes
Lysosome	Contains digestive enzymes
Peroxisome	Contains hydrogen peroxide and oxidative enzymes; beta oxidation of fatty acids
Centrioles	Pair of rod-shaped proteins that function in cell division
Cytoskeleton	Protein scaffolding that provides cell structure, support, and motility
Chloroplast	Photosynthesis in plants

The function of the **nucleus** is to house the DNA and to act as the command center of the cell, controlling cell replication and protein synthesis. The nucleus consists of a **nuclear membrane** and an interior region of **nucleoplasm**, which contains the DNA, as well as a circular region called the **nucleolus**. The DNA in eukaryotic cells is organized into linear **chromosomes**. The nucleoplasm of the nucleus contains a cytoskeletal support network called the **nuclear lamina**.

The **nuclear membrane** (nuclear envelope) is a double membrane composed of two phospholipid bilayers that separate the interior of the nucleus (nucleoplasm) from the cytoplasm of the cell. These two membrane layers are separated by a narrow space except at certain points where they are fused to form nuclear pores. These pores are protein-gated channels that regulate the passage of materials into and out of the nucleus. Messenger and ribosomal RNA (ribonucleic acid) pass through the nuclear pores, carrying information from the DNA to the cytoplasm. Proteins synthesized in the cytoplasm enter the nucleus through the pores. The outer layer of the nuclear membrane, which may be embedded with ribosomes, is continuous with other membrane-bound organelles in the cytoplasm, such as the endoplasmic reticulum.

The **nucleolus** is the site of rRNA synthesis and ribosome assembly. It is visible with a light microscope as a darkly staining body inside the nucleus. A nucleus may contain more than one nucleolus, depending on the type of cell.

Eukaryotic chromosomes consist of **chromatin**, a complex of DNA and protein (see Figure 3.7). Eight different proteins can combine with DNA to form chromatin. These proteins are **histones**, positively charged proteins that bind to the negatively charged phosphate backbone of DNA. The linear DNA wraps around a histone protein, much like thread on a spool. This process forms **nucleosomes**, DNA wrapped around 8 histone proteins to form the basic structural unit of chromatin. Nucleosomes, in turn, are further wrapped, and the DNA is looped and twisted to form **DNA supercoils**. This packaging allows the DNA, which may be over a meter long, to fit inside the nucleus. Ultimately, highly coiled (condensed) DNA takes the form of linear chromosomes, compact molecules of DNA that are visible on stained slides of dividing cells.

Chromatin may be in the form of **euchromatin** or **heterochromatin**. Euchromatin, found in both prokaryotes and eukaryotes, is loosely coiled DNA that is actively involved in gene expression. Heterochromatin, in contrast, is an inactive form of DNA. It is tightly coiled and is found only in eukaryotes. The dense coiling converts the DNA to one of two inactive forms—**constitutive** (permanently inactive) or **facultative** (temporarily inactive). Conversion of heterochromatin is an important mechanism for regulation of gene expression in eukaryotes.

Chromosome means "colored body." This term was originally applied to the dark structures visible in stained slides of dividing eukaryotic cells. These structures are highly condensed DNA molecules that have replicated before cell division, resulting in two identical **sister chromatids** joined at a constricted region called a **centromere**. As a result, such duplicated chromosomes appear X-shaped. When eukaryotic cells are not undergoing cell division, the DNA is unduplicated and is loosely coiled as chromatin, not condensed into chromosomes. Prokaryotic cells lack chromatin and instead have a circular DNA molecule called a **genophore**. However, the term chromosome is widely used to refer to the DNA molecules of both eukaryotic and prokaryotic cells during all stages of the cell cycle.

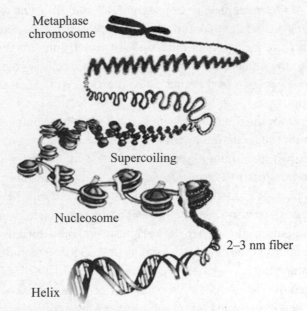

Metaphase
chromosome

Supercoiling

Nucleosome

2–3 nm fiber

Helix

Figure 3.7. Chromatin structure

Mitochondria (singular: **mitochondrion**) are cylindrical organelles that produce energy for the cell by the process of aerobic cellular respiration. Like the nucleus, mitochondria are surrounded by a double membrane. Most eukaryotic cells, including plant cells, possess mitochondria. These organelles convert the chemical energy obtained through photosynthesis and glycolysis into usable energy in the form of ATP.

MITOCHONDRIA

The mitochondria are the location of **aerobic respiration** within the cell. The citric acid cycle occurs within the matrix. The proteins of the electron transport chain and ATP synthesis are embedded in the inner mitochondrial membrane.

The double membrane of each mitochondrion consists of an outer membrane, an intermembrane space, and an inner membrane that encloses a viscous interior **matrix**. The outer mitochondrial membrane has numerous protein channels called **porins** that make the membrane permeable to small molecules. However, larger proteins must cross by active transport. The inner membrane, in contrast, is highly impermeable. The inner membrane folds inward through the matrix to form **cristae** (singular: **crista**). These are compartments that greatly increase the surface area of the inner membrane, where aerobic respiration and ATP synthesis takes place. The large surface area of the cristae serves to enhance energy production, as shown in Figure 3.8.

Mitochondria, along with chloroplasts essential for photosynthesis in plant cells, contain a small amount of DNA in individual, circular chromosomes like the chromosomes of prokaryotes. Mitochondria also have their own ribosomes, which resemble those of prokaryotes. This evidence, along with the presence of a double membrane, has led to the **endosymbiotic hypothesis**. This hypothesis states that mitochondria originated as prokaryotes that were engulfed and incorporated (by endocytosis) into an ancestral eukaryotic cell. Most proteins in the mitochondria originate from the cell nucleus and are imported from the cytoplasm.

However, some mitochondrial proteins are coded for by mitochondrial DNA and are translated by way of mitochondrial ribosomes and enzymes within the mitochondrial matrix.

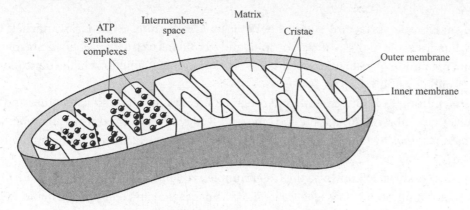

Figure 3.8. Mitochondrion

Unlike nuclear DNA, mitochondrial DNA is transmitted solely by the mother through the egg, or ovum. Sperm cells contain relatively small numbers of mitochondria compared with egg cells, and the egg typically destroys the mitochondria in sperm during fertilization. So no paternal mitochondria are transmitted to the embryo, though extremely rare exceptions have been reported. The transmission of mitochondrial DNA from mother to child is a form of **cytoplasmic** (**extranuclear**) **inheritance** because mitochondrial genes occur outside the nucleus and replicate independently of nuclear DNA.

The **endoplasmic reticulum (ER)** is a network of membranes and flattened, fluid-filled sacs called **cisternae** that weaves throughout the cytoplasm, connecting the outer nuclear membrane to the plasma membrane. The endoplasmic reticulum plays a role in protein and lipid synthesis as well as in intracellular transport. Endoplasmic reticulum may be either rough or smooth.

The membrane surface of **rough endoplasmic reticulum (RER)** is dotted with ribosomes, giving it a rough appearance. The RER is the major site of protein synthesis in eukaryotic cells. Protein synthesis is initiated by free ribosomes in the cytosol. During protein synthesis, proteins are tagged with a short sequence of amino acids called a **signal sequence** or **targeting peptide,** which determines the protein's ultimate destination in the cell.

Depending on the signal sequence, protein synthesis may be completed in the cytoplasm or the ribosome-protein complex may be **cotranslationally translocated** to the RER membrane. From there, the newly synthesized protein may pass into the **lumen** (cisternal space) of the endoplasmic reticulum or remain embedded in the membrane. Proteins that pass into the lumen are folded into the correct three-dimensional conformation with the assistance of **chaperone** proteins. They may also be modified into glycoproteins through the addition of carbohydrate side chains. Then they are wrapped in membranous transitional vesicles for transport to the **Golgi body**, an organelle that will further process or export the protein.

Proteins that remain embedded in the RER membrane may be used in **membrane biosynthesis**. In this case, the rough endoplasmic reticulum not only synthesizes membrane

> The mutation rate of mitochondrial DNA (mtDNA) is rapid compared to nuclear DNA, and the accumulation of neutral mutations is assumed to be fairly constant over time. Consequently, mitochondrial DNA has been used as a **molecular clock** to determine the time of divergence between different species and populations. Mitochondrial DNA is also useful in forensics and in determining ancestry through the female line.

proteins but also the phospholipids necessary to generate new membrane. New membrane is transferred throughout the cell as transport vesicles bud off the ER and fuse with other cellular membranes.

The membrane surface of **smooth endoplasmic reticulum (SER)** lacks attached ribosomes. It plays a role in the synthesis of lipids and steroids as well as in carbohydrate metabolism and regulation of calcium concentration. In the liver, SER functions in the detoxification of drugs and alcohol.

The membranes of both smooth and rough ER are continuous with each other and with the nuclear membrane. Rough ER and smooth ER may be converted from one type to the other as ribosomes become bound to or released from the surface, depending on the needs of the cell.

The **Golgi body**, also known as the Golgi complex or Golgi apparatus, is a network of flattened, membrane-bound sacs (cisternae). It is the packaging and shipping center of the cell, taking proteins or lipids synthesized in the endoplasmic reticulum and further modifying them before they are sent to their final destinations. Proteins and lipids coming from the endoplasmic reticulum pass into the Golgi body by means of transport vesicles. In the Golgi body, proteins and lipids may be further modified by **glycosylation** (addition of sugars), **phosphorylation** (addition of phosphate groups), or other forms of **posttranslational modification** that may help direct a protein to its final destination. Once processing is completed, products are incorporated into membrane-bound, secretory vesicles. These vesicles pinch off and travel through the cytoplasm to fuse with the plasma membrane, releasing their contents outside the cell. Golgi bodies are particularly abundant in the cells of the digestive and respiratory tracts and in other tissues that involve secretion.

Lysosomes break down the cell's waste products. They are membrane-bound vesicles filled with **hydrolytic** digestive enzymes in a highly acidic (pH 5) medium. Lysosomes contain proteins synthesized by the rough ER and packaged by the Golgi body. These proteins are capable of breaking down other proteins, polysaccharides, and nucleic acids. Instead of exporting their contents from the cell like secretory vesicles, lysosomes remain in the cytoplasm in order to fuse with transport vesicles obtained by phagocytosis to digest or destroy the contents. Lysosomes are also known as suicide sacs for their role in programmed cell death (**apoptosis**). When a cell dies, the membranes of the lysosomes disintegrate and release digestive enzymes that rapidly break down cell components. Apoptosis is important during development when tissues must be broken down and in programmed cell death of aged or defective cells. (See also Apoptosis, page 402.)

Vacuoles are large, fluid-filled, membrane-bound vesicles with a variety of functions. In plant and fungal cells and in some protists, vacuoles are important in maintaining osmotic balance. Vacuoles are also used by cells to store food and waste. They also function in both endocytosis and exocytosis.

Peroxisomes are spherical vesicles containing enzymes for oxidative metabolic processes such as the beta oxidation of fatty acids. A by-product of these reactions is hydrogen peroxide, a strong oxidant that is toxic to the cell. Peroxisomes contain the enzyme catalase to break down hydrogen peroxide into oxygen and water. The hydrogen peroxide can also be used by the peroxisome in the breakdown and detoxification of other substances. Peroxisomes are not associated with other membranous vesicles within the cell and are capable of self-replicating by absorbing materials from the cytoplasm.

CYTOSKELETON

Eukaryotic cells are given shape, support, and structure by an internal **cytoskeleton** (cell skeleton) of protein fibers. The cytoskeleton also plays a critical role in intracellular transport of materials, cell adhesion, and cell movement. The components of the cytoskeleton include microfilaments, intermediate filaments, and microtubules.

Microfilaments are also known as **actin filaments**. They are composed of two thin threads of the protein **actin** that twist around each other to form linear cables or networks. The actin filaments have pulling (tensile) strength and, along with thick filaments of myosin protein, form the contractile machinery of muscle cells. Microfilaments help maintain the shape of the cell by forming a mesh support system on the inside of the cell membrane. Microfilaments participate in cell division through the formation of the **cleavage furrow** in animal cells. Microfilaments are involved in cell-cell interactions, in the formation of pseudopodia and microvilli, and in **cytoplasmic streaming**, the movement of materials and organelles within the cytoplasm of the cell.

Intermediate filaments are intermediate in size between microfilaments and microtubules. They are composed of a diverse group of proteins, which gives them considerable variation in form. Intermediate filaments work with microtubules and microfilaments to provide a structural matrix in the cytoplasm. They include the structural protein keratin, the principal protein making up hair, nails, and skin. Intermediate filaments are also involved in intracellular transport and cell-cell junctions. Intermediate filaments are one of the main components of the **nuclear lamina**, the cytoskeletal matrix inside the nucleus.

Microtubules, the largest cytoskeletal elements, are hollow tubes composed of the protein **tubulin**. Microtubules function in the intracellular transport of organelles and materials. Two subunits (alpha and beta) of the tubulin polypeptide form a basic dimer from which the microtubule polymer is assembled. Tubulin dimers wrap around each other in a helix to form the hollow tube. Dimers can be added or removed in order to lengthen or shorten the microtubule. Because of their ability to lengthen and contract, microtubules can generate force to push or pull materials apart. Microtubules provide a structural support system in the cytoplasm. They can also work with motor proteins to function in intracellular transport, cell division, and cell locomotion.

Cilia and **flagella** are specialized structures composed of differing arrangements of microtubules that propel substances across cell surfaces or contribute to cell motility (movement). Flagella are long, whiplike bundles of microtubules that project from the cell membrane to propel spermatozoa or single-celled protists through a liquid medium. Cilia are much shorter clusters of microtubules that typically occur in groups on the external surface of a membrane. Their rapid beating can propel mucus across the membrane, as in respiratory epithelia, or can allow the cell to move. Cilia also participate in cell signaling and signal transduction.

The functional unit of motile cilia and flagella consists of a central core or skeleton (**axoneme**) and a **basal body**. The axoneme is composed of a ring of 9 pairs of microtubules arranged lengthwise around 2 central microtubules in what is referred to as a **9 + 2 arrangement** (see Figure 3.9). Microtubule pairs are joined by cross-linking **dynein** proteins, which act as molecular motors. The axoneme is firmly attached to the cell by the basal body of 9 clusters of 3 microtubules. When the dynein proteins of a microtubule pair form cross-linkages in an ATP-powered reaction, the axoneme

POLYMERS

Polymers are complex molecules built out of repeating subunits (building blocks). Polymers have the advantage of being able to store additional subunits or to donate subunits.

microtubules pull on each other and bend. The result is a wavelike motion of the flagellum that can propel the cell.

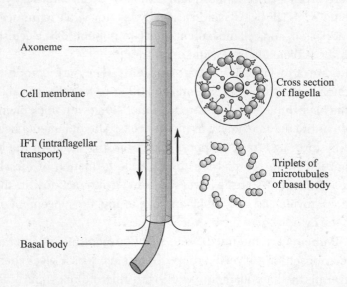

Figure 3.9. Flagellum

Centrioles resemble the basal bodies of cilia and flagella in the triplet arrangement of 9 sets of microtubules. Centrioles are short, paired structures found in the **centrosome** of animal cells. The centrosomes function as **microtubule organizing centers (MTO)** of the mitotic spindle during cell division.

EXTRACELLULAR COMPONENTS AND INTERCELLULAR JUNCTIONS

Cells secrete a variety of substances outside the cell membrane to aid in support, cell signaling, cell-cell recognition, and intercellular adhesion.

Plants, fungi, prokaryotes, and some protists produce a **cell wall** that is outside of the cell membrane. The cell wall supports and protects the cell. In plants, this cell wall is composed primarily of fibers of **cellulose**, a polysaccharide carbohydrate. The cell walls of prokaryotes and fungi are structurally different and will be discussed in later sections.

The **extracellular matrix (ECM)** is the network of materials outside of the cells that provides a supportive framework for the cells and tissues. It is also a key element in connective tissues such as blood, cartilage, and bone. The ECM occupies the **interstitial matrix** between cells and forms the **basement membrane**, which anchors and underlies epithelial tissues.

The ECM contains a complex variety of proteins that contribute to cell interactions and tissue formation. One of these proteins is **collagen**, the protein that forms connective tissue and the most abundant protein in the human body. Other ECM proteins include glycoproteins such as **proteoglycans**, which are heavily glycosylated proteins attached to **glycosaminoglycans** (mucopolysaccharides). Proteoglycans are associated with collagen in the matrix of connective tissue. Another ECM protein is **fibronectin**, which binds the ECM to **integrin** proteins in the plasma membrane. Fibronectin provides a communication pathway between the internal environment of the cell and the extracellular matrix.

Cells that adhere to one another to form tissues in multicellular organisms rely on a variety of **intercellular junctions**. In animal cells, the primary intercellular junctions are gap junctions, tight junctions, and desmosomes.

Gap Junctions

Gap junctions connect the cytoplasm of adjacent cells across a gap of interstitial space by means of integral membrane protein channels (see Figure 3.10). The proteins act as hollow conduits, maintaining continuity between the cytoplasm of adjacent cells. Gap junctions allow chemical and electrical signals to be transmitted quickly because they provide a direct passageway for ions and small molecules. For example, the electrical signal passing between cardiac cells in the heart travels through gap junctions to allow all cardiac cells to contract simultaneously.

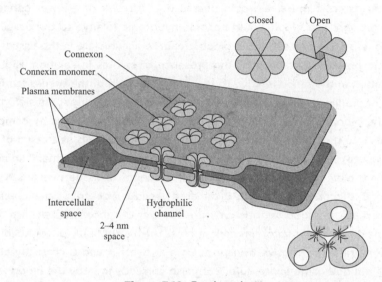

Figure 3.10. Gap junction

Tight Junctions

In tight junctions, the adjacent plasma membranes of two cells are fused together, with no space in between, by a network of membrane proteins that anchor on microfilaments in the cytoskeleton. Tight junctions form a waterproof seal to prevent the transport of extracellular fluids and solutes across a tissue layer. For example, cells lining the blood vessels that supply the brain are joined by tight junctions to prevent harmful substances in the blood from crossing into cerebrospinal fluid, contributing to the **blood-brain barrier**.

Desmosomes

Desmosomes are dense cellular adhesions that act as protein anchors or spot welds to hold cells together in tissues. Transmembrane proteins anchored to intermediate filaments of keratin in the cytoplasm bind together with proteins of other cells, spanning a wide intercellular gap. Desmosomes hold cells together in tissues, including muscle cells in cardiac and skeletal muscle and the epithelial cells bound in sheets to form the epidermis.

The protein albumin is produced by the liver. Albumin constitutes 50% of the protein content of the blood and contributes significantly to plasma colloid osmotic pressure. A low serum albumin level due to chronic liver failure will result in:

(A) a decrease in the osmotic pressure of the blood, resulting in an accumulation of fluid in the hypotonic blood plasma.

(B) an increase in the osmotic pressure of the blood, resulting in an accumulation of fluid in the hypertonic blood plasma.

(C) a decrease in the osmotic pressure of the blood, resulting in an accumulation of fluid in hypertonic interstitial fluid.

(D) diffusion of cytoplasmic anionic proteins into the bloodstream.

(C) Plasma osmotic pressure would decrease as a result of a lower concentration of blood protein. The blood would become hypotonic relative to the tissues. Water would move by osmosis out of the bloodstream to accumulate in the tissues.

Osmotic pressure is caused by the presence of solutes in solution. High protein concentration in the blood relative to the interstitial fluid of the tissues leads to high osmotic, or "pulling," pressure in the bloodstream. Under normal physiological conditions, the blood is hypertonic to the tissue fluid and water flows by osmosis from the tissues into the blood. If osmotic pressure in the blood falls as a result of lowered protein (solute) levels, the blood becomes hypotonic to the interstitial fluid and water flows from the blood back into tissues, causing edema, or tissue swelling.

Answer B is incorrect and can be eliminated because it describes an increase, rather than a decrease, in blood osmotic pressure. Answer D is incorrect because polar and charged particles such as proteins cannot cross the hydrophobic phospholipid bilayer of cell membranes by passive transport. Both answers A and C correctly describe a decrease in blood osmotic pressure. Both also correctly identify the blood plasma or interstitial fluid as hypotonic and hypertonic, respectively. However, answer A can be eliminated because fluid moves by osmosis from hypotonic solutions to hypertonic solutions and therefore would not accumulate in the hypotonic blood plasma.

CELL METABOLISM AND ENZYMES

The chemical reactions of metabolism are an essential characteristic of life.

Types of Metabolic Reactions

Every cell needs to generate usable cellular energy via the breakdown of complex macromolecules (**catabolic reactions**) and to drive the synthesis of new biomolecules (**anabolic reactions**). Catabolic and anabolic pathways are linked, one set powering the other. The energy required by the cell is ultimately provided by the energy stored in chemical bonds by photosynthesis or chemosynthesis. The breakdown of these bonds releases **Gibbs free energy** (ΔG), which is the energy available to do work within the cell. In living systems, this energy is captured by the molecule **adenosine triphosphate**, or **ATP**. Catabolic reactions are **exergonic** processes that produce ATP, resulting in a negative change in free energy (ΔG) because products are at a lower energy state than reactants. Anabolic reactions are

endergonic, requiring ATP. Anabolic reactions result in a positive ΔG because products have a higher energy level than reactants.

Exergonic reactions that release free energy are **spontaneous reactions**. However, most of these reactions would take years to occur at the temperatures and pressures found within living cells. In order for any chemical reaction to take place, bonds must be broken before new ones can be formed. This creates an energy barrier, or **activation energy (E_a)**, that must be overcome before a reaction can continue spontaneously. For example, logs in a fireplace can burn spontaneously but only if friction is applied to light the match and provide the initial E_a. At high enough temperatures and pressures, collisions between molecules occur forcefully enough to exceed the activation energy barrier and to allow the substrate to pass through the higher-energy transition state to form products. However, living things cannot withstand high temperatures due to the effect of temperature on the hydrogen bonding of proteins and nucleic acids.

In living organisms, activation energy can be overcome chemically through catalysts. The primary catalysts available for metabolism are enzymes.

Enzymes as Catalysts

Enzymes are proteins that act as biological catalysts to lower activation energy, as shown in Figure 3.11. Enzymes allow exergonic reactions (catabolism) to proceed spontaneously at lower temperatures. They also catalyze endergonic anabolic reactions that use ATP. Enzymes participate in chemical reactions but are not chemically altered or consumed during the reactions.

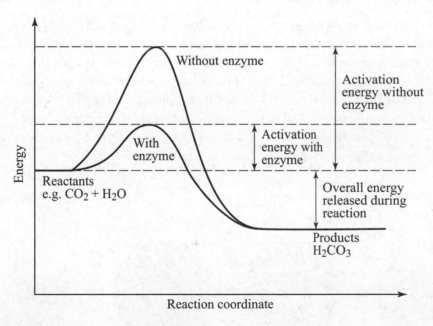

Figure 3.11. Enzymes as catalysts

ENZYME STRUCTURE AND FUNCTION

Enzymes are complex, three-dimensional polypeptides twisted into a highly specific tertiary conformation by interactions between amino acid R-group side chains. Enzymes catalyze reactions by binding with a reactant, or **substrate**. The binding of the substrate to the enzyme usually occurs through weak molecular interactions, such as ionic and hydrogen bonding, resulting in an **enzyme-substrate complex**. The binding of the enzyme causes a change in the substrate to allow breakage or formation of bonds. After products are formed, the enzyme detaches and becomes available to catalyze another reaction.

MECHANISMS OF CATALYSTS

The enzyme-substrate complex lowers the activation energy to favor the breakage of existing bonds in the substrate and the formation of new bonds. This can happen in various ways.

1. The binding of the enzyme puts strain on bonds within the substrate molecule, allowing them to break more readily.
2. The enzyme places two or more substrates into the correct physical orientation to initiate a reaction.
3. The enzyme creates a more favorable microenvironment for the required reaction. For instance, the enzyme may modify the pH in the active site by incorporating acidic amino acid side chains.
4. The enzyme participates directly in the reaction by forming temporary bonds that aid in the conversion of substrate to product.

When the reaction is complete, the enzyme separates from the products and the active site returns to its original conformation. Enzymes are not consumed during catalysis. A single enzyme can catalyze multiple reactions each second.

ACTIVE SITE VS. INDUCED FIT

One model proposed for enzyme function, the **active site** (or **lock and key**) hypothesis, compared the fit of the enzyme and the substrate with a lock and key mechanism. This model assumed a static enzyme structure (lock) that was exactly fit to the particular conformation of a specific substrate (key). More recent evidence suggests that enzymes change shape on binding the substrate, leading to the **induced fit** hypothesis. According to this model, the enzyme changes shape on binding to better fit the substrate into the active site. Induced fit gives enzymes the flexibility to bind to substrates with some degree of variation in size and shape. The induced fit process is illustrated in Figure 3.12.

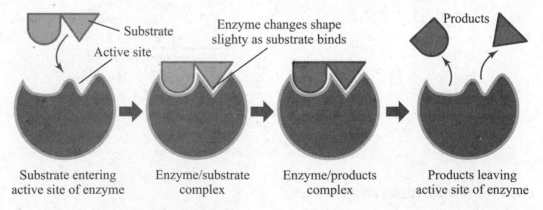

Figure 3.12. Induced fit (Adapted from a work by Tim Vickers.)

ENZYME SPECIFICITY

Because of the shape and molecular structure of the active site, enzymes are specific to a particular type of substrate. Many enzymes are highly specific, binding only with a single substrate. Other enzymes are less specific and can bind to a range of substrates with similar functional groups, side chains, or types of chemical bonds. Cells require thousands of different enzymes to accommodate the diversity of substrates involved in cellular metabolism.

COFACTORS AND COENZYMES

In some cases, enzymes need to be activated by nonprotein **cofactors**. Cofactors can include metal ions (such as iron, zinc, or magnesium) or organic molecules. An enzyme bound with a required cofactor is called a **holoenzyme**. An enzyme without the cofactor it requires is a nonfunctional **apoenzyme**. The term *holoenzyme* can also refer to an enzyme consisting of several independent enzyme subunits that have come together as a functional unit, as in the holoenzyme complex DNA polymerase.

Cofactor molecules can be either permanently or reversibly bound. Permanently bound molecules typically have covalent bonding. These cofactors are called **prosthetic groups**. Reversibly bound cofactors are called **coenzymes**.

Coenzymes, such as ATP, NAD, and coenzyme A, transfer organic subunits to enable catalysis. These subunits include phosphate groups and hydrogen ions. Coenzymes also include **water-soluble vitamins** such as the B-complex vitamins thiamine and niacin. For this reason, vitamin deficiency can have a drastic effect on cellular metabolism. Unlike enzymes, coenzymes are physically altered during the course of the reaction. Because of this, they can also be called **second substrates**. Coenzymes are not as specific as enzymes and can assist a wide variety of different enzymes. They are continually regenerated for reuse by the cell.

ENZYME KINETICS

The general reaction of an enzyme is

$$E + S \leftrightarrow ES \leftrightarrow E + P,$$

where E = enzyme, S = substrate, ES = enzyme–substrate complex, and P = product.

The rate at which an enzyme converts substrate to product, or **enzyme activity**, is determined by **saturation kinetics**. Enzyme activity increases linearly as the amount of substrate (S) increases until the number of available active sites starts to become limiting. At this point, the reaction rate continues to increase slightly but at a much slower rate. When every enzyme is binding and releasing substrate molecules at its maximum rate (V_{max}), the enzyme is saturated with substrate and the reaction curve levels out. Any further increase in substrate concentration will have no effect on the reaction rate.

The reaction rate, V_1, is given by the Michaelis–Menten equation:

$$V_1 = \frac{V_{max}[S]}{\{K_m + [S]\}}$$

The **Michaelis–Menten constant**, K_m, is another measure of an enzyme's activity (see Figure 3.13). K_m is defined as the substrate concentration that generates a reaction rate that is 1/2 of the maximum reaction velocity (V_{max}) for a particular enzyme. The higher the value of K_m, the more substrate that is required for an enzyme to achieve a given reaction rate. Because each enzyme has a specific K_m for a given substrate, K_m can be used to compare the binding affinity of different enzymes for the same substrate. An enzyme with a higher K_m than another requires more substrate to achieve the same reaction rate and therefore has less ability to bind the substrate. Lower K_m values mean higher binding affinity and, consequently, a higher reaction rate.

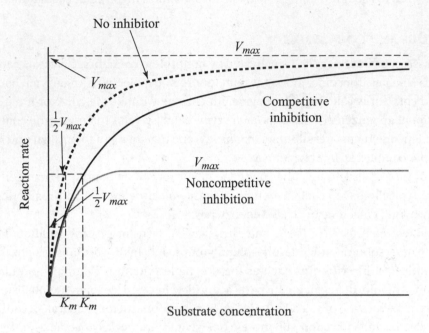

Figure 3.13. The Michaelis–Menten curve of an enzyme reaction

EFFECT OF TEMPERATURE AND pH ON ENZYME ACTIVITY

An enzyme's activity is affected by environmental conditions. Changes in temperature or pH can break hydrogen bonds between side chains and alter the shape of the enzyme, affecting the ability of the active site to bind to a specific substrate. The optimal range of environmental conditions for each enzyme is determined by the location and function of the enzyme within an organism. An enzyme subjected to temperature or pH outside its optimal range will exhibit a lower activity due to disruption of its three-dimensional structure and ultimately may be **denatured** and cease to function.

CONTROL OF ENZYME ACTIVITY

Enzymes can be either inhibited or activated by nonenzyme substances called **enzyme regulators**. These regulators typically act by changing an enzyme's shape or by blocking the active site. Enzyme regulators that increase the action of an enzyme (**enzyme activators**) are less common than inhibitors. **Enzyme inhibitors** can be either **reversible** or **irreversible**. Many metabolic poisons, such as nerve gas, are irreversible enzyme inhibitors. Most biological enzyme inhibitors are reversible. Types of enzyme inhibitors include competitive, uncompetitive, noncompetitive, and mixed.

Enzyme Inhibition

Competitive inhibitors are substances that are structurally similar enough to a substrate to compete with the substrate for the active site. When these inhibitors bind to an enzyme, they prevent the substrate from binding. The degree of inhibition depends on the relative concentrations of inhibitor and substrate. A higher concentration of the competitive inhibitor results in greater inhibition of the enzyme. Competitive inhibition also depends on the relative affinity of the enzyme for each substrate (K_m). Substrates with a lower Michaelis constant, K_m, and a higher binding affinity will outcompete other substrates for binding sites. Competitive inhibitors do not alter V_{max}. Because competitive inhibition creates a situation in which inhibitors either compete with the substrate for the active site or prevent the substrate from binding, competitive inhibition can be overcome by increasing the concentration of substrate. (See Figure 3.13.)

Competitive inhibition occurs when two similar substrates are present, but only one at a time can bind to the enzyme. Other types of inhibition include uncompetitive inhibition, noncompetitive inhibition, and mixed inhibition. These inhibitors typically bind to an **allosteric** site on the enzyme, a site outside or near the active site. Allosteric binding either blocks the substrate from binding or alters the conformation of the enzyme–substrate complex to impair the conversion of substrate to product.

Uncompetitive inhibition occurs only in the presence of substrate because these inhibitors bind to the enzyme–substrate complex. Since uncompetitive inhibitors bind allosterically when the substrate is already bound, they do not compete with the substrate for the active site and do not need to resemble the substrate. Uncompetitive inhibition slows the conversion of substrate to product, lowering V_{max}. Because the enzyme remains attached to the substrate but does not form product, uncompetitive inhibition lowers K_m and raises the apparent binding affinity of the enzyme. Uncompetitive inhibition occurs more readily at high substrate concentrations.

> Ethylene glycol, a component of antifreeze and brake fluid, is sweet-tasting but highly toxic when ingested. It acts as a competitive inhibitor of ethanol. If ethylene glycol poisoning is suspected, ethanol can be administered as an antidote. Increasing the concentration of the substrate ethanol will reduce competitive inhibition by ethylene glycol.

Noncompetitive inhibition occurs when an inhibitor can bind to an enzyme regardless of whether substrate is present. Noncompetitive inhibitors bind to an allosteric site on an enzyme whether or not substrate is already in the active site. Neither interferes with the binding of the other. Noncompetitive inhibition prevents the enzyme from undergoing conformational change necessary for conversion of substrate to product. Substrate binds to the enzyme, but the binding of the inhibitor prevents catalysis. If the concentration of the inhibitor is raised to saturation levels, enzyme activity will cease. Noncompetitive inhibition occurs at both low- and high-substrate concentrations. (See Figure 3.13.)

Mixed inhibition is similar to noncompetitive inhibition; however, the binding of the inhibitor can affect the binding affinity of the substrate and vice versa, lowering binding affinity and raising K_m. Noncompetitive inhibition can be considered a form of mixed inhibition. Both mixed inhibition and noncompetitive inhibition lower V_{max}. In noncompetitive inhibition, K_m is unchanged, whereas in mixed inhibition, K_m is increased as a reflection of decreased binding affinity.

FEEDBACK REGULATION

As an enzyme catalyzes a reaction, one of the by-products of the reaction—either an immediate product or a downstream product—can act as a regulator of that enzyme. This creates a feedback mechanism. In **feedback inhibition**, a product of a reaction or chain of reactions inhibits an enzyme that catalyzes its production. As the concentration of product increases, the activity of the enzyme decreases. For example, ATP acts as a feedback inhibitor of several enzymes in the glycolytic reaction pathway that generates ATP.

ALLOSTERIC ACTIVATION AND COOPERATIVITY

In contrast with enzyme inhibitors, some enzyme regulators activate or enhance the function of enzymes. Enzyme activators commonly bind to an allosteric site and change the conformation of an enzyme such that it can more readily bind substrate. Another form of allosteric regulation is **cooperativity**. In this case, the substrate itself acts to regulate the binding of additional substrate. Substrate can bind to more than one binding site on an enzyme. When substrate is bound to one site, the shape of the enzyme alters to increase the likelihood that additional substrate will bind at its other sites. This phenomenon is called **positive cooperativity**. The binding of substrate can also make the conditions less favorable for binding at other sites. This is called **negative cooperativity**.

ALLOSTERIC ENZYMES

Allosteric enzymes are enzymes with multiple binding sites for substrate or other regulatory molecules that allow for allosteric regulation and cooperativity. Because they are regulated by multiple factors, allosteric enzymes do not follow Michaelis–Menten kinetics. Instead, the reaction curve for allosteric enzymes is sigmoidal, showing a transition between low-affinity and high-affinity binding states. Although not technically an enzyme, hemoglobin is a protein that behaves as an allosteric enzyme. It exhibits cooperativity in binding oxygen and a sigmoidal reaction curve.

COVALENT MODIFICATION

In addition to allosteric inhibition or activation, enzymes can also be regulated by **covalent modification**. Common forms of covalent modification include phosphorylation or dephosphorylation of R-group side chains on amino acids such as serine or tyrosine. For example, the enzymes actyltransferase and deacetylase, which regulate gene expression through histone acetylation, are themselves regulated by phosphorylation and dephosphorylation by protein kinase and phosphatase enzymes.

Enzymes can also be covalently modified by proteolytic cleavage, the breaking of peptide bonds to remove a peptide or amino acid. A newly synthesized enzyme can remain in an inactive precursor state called a **zymogen**. Digestive enzymes are generally produced as zymogens to prevent tissue damage. For example, the protease enzyme pepsin is produced as an inactive zymogen (pepsinogen) in the pancreas. Once pepsin is excreted into the intestine, it is converted to an active state through proteolytic cleavage by protease enzymes in the duodenum.

ENZYME CLASSIFICATION

Enzymes are classified and named by the types of reactions they catalyze. Traditionally, enzymes have been given common names with the suffix -*ase* added to the name of their particular substrate or to their mode of action. For example, the enzyme **amylase** acts on the substrate amylose. The enzyme **ATP synthase** catalyzes the synthesis of ATP. Exceptions to this rule include enzymes such as **pepsin** and **trypsin**, which break down protein in the digestive tract, and **renin**, which acts as a protease and hormonal regulator in the kidneys. Enzymes have also been put into groups by their actions. For example, **kinases** are a group of enzymes that transfer phosphate groups from high-energy donor molecules such as ATP to a substrate.

More recent formal classification attempts to standardize naming. This system gives an enzyme the designation EC and then assigns enzymes to one of six numbered categories based on the type of reaction. The category number is followed by numeric designations that provide additional information on the catalyzed bond. Table 3.2 describes the six EC categories of enzymes based on reaction type.

Table 3.2 Categories of Enzymes Based on Reaction Type

Group Number	Category Name	Type of Reaction Catalyzed	Examples by Common Name
EC 1	Oxidoreductases	Oxidation/reduction reactions; transfer electrons or H and O atoms	Oxidase, Dehydrogenase
EC 2	Transferases	Transfer of a functional group between substrates	Kinase, Polymerase, Phosphorylase
EC 3	Hydrolases	Cleavage of a substrate by hydrolysis, the addition of water	Nuclease, Protease, Lipase, Phosphatase
EC 4	Lyases	Non-hydrolytic bond formation or cleavage of functional groups, particularly of C–C, C–O, C–N, or C–S bonds	Decarboxylase, Synthase, Aldolase
EC 5	Isomerases	Rearrangement of a molecule from one isomer to another	Isomerase
EC 6	Ligases	ATP-fueled joining of substrates by formation of C–C, C–O, C–S, or C–N bonds	DNA Ligase, Synthetase

Basic Metabolism

The principal metabolic pathway for generating energy for the cell is **cellular respiration**. In the presence of oxygen, the overall reaction for cellular respiration is the breakdown of glucose to release carbon dioxide and water via **aerobic respiration**:

$$C_6H_{12}O_6 + 6O_2 + \rightarrow 6CO_2 + 6H_2O + \text{Chemical energy} + \text{Heat}$$

This reaction is essentially the reverse of photosynthesis, which uses light energy to convert carbon dioxide and water into glucose and oxygen. The oxidation of glucose is an exergonic combustion reaction that yields 686 kcal (kilocalories) of energy per mole of glucose. Some of this energy is lost as heat. However, some energy is trapped in the chemical bonds of a variety of transition molecules and, ultimately, in the molecule adenosine triphosphate (ATP). The breakdown of a single glucose molecule by aerobic cellular respiration yields a total of 38 ATP. ATP is the principal energy source for the cell, providing fuel for metabolic processes.

STRUCTURE OF ATP

Adenosine triphosphate is composed of the nitrogenous base adenine linked to a ribose sugar (an adenine nucleoside), with three phosphate groups attached. The phosphate groups are joined to the adenine nucleoside by **phosphorylation**, a condensation reaction carried out by **protein kinase** enzymes. Removal of a phosphate group, or **dephosphorylation**, is carried out by **phosphatase** enzymes. The three phosphate groups are connected by two very high energy bonds. When these bonds are cleaved, a large amount of energy is released.

In this reaction, ATP is hydrolyzed to **ADP** (**adenosine diphosphate**) plus an inorganic phosphate group (P_i).

$$ATP + H_2O \rightarrow ADP + P_i$$

ATP can also be hydrolyzed to **AMP** (**adenosine monophosphate**) plus a pyrophosphate group (PP_i).

$$ATP \rightarrow AMP + PP_i$$

ADP may also be hydrolyzed to AMP (adenosine monophosphate). Each phosphate group hydrolyzed from ATP under cellular conditions releases –13 kcal/mol. Figure 3.14 shows the structure of ATP, ADP, and AMP.

ADP and AMP can be converted back to ATP. The process of ATP being broken down to release energy and built back up to store energy is analogous to the functioning of a rechargeable battery. ATP is referred to as the energy currency of the cell because of its ability to couple exergonic with endergonic reactions. ATP serves as the link between catabolic and anabolic pathways, capturing the energy of cellular respiration to provide energetic "payment" for biosynthesis, membrane transport, and other energetically costly metabolic and cellular processes.

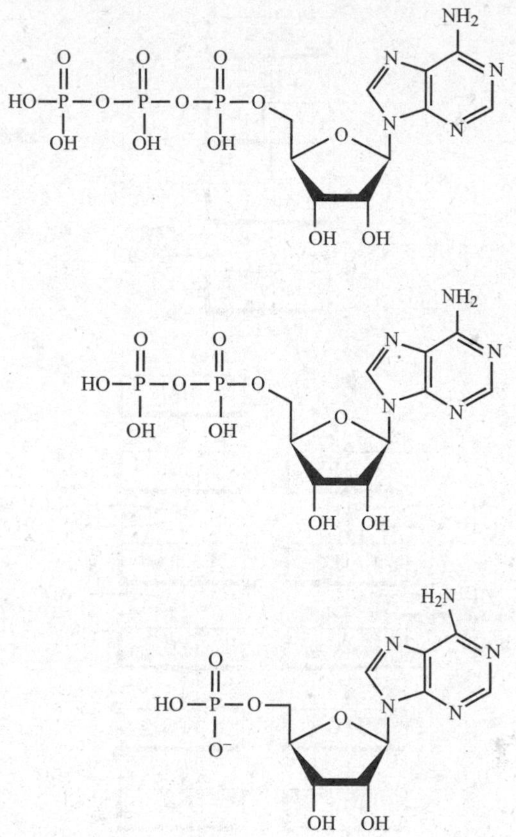

Figure 3.14. ATP molecule (top), ADP molecule (middle), and AMP molecule (bottom)

GENERATION OF CELLULAR ENERGY

The synthesis of ATP ultimately depends on the transfer of energy in the form of electrons from a molecule such as glucose to a more electronegative electron receptor such as oxygen in a series of oxidation reduction reactions. Electrons, accompanied by a proton, H^+, "fall" down an energy gradient as they are transferred from one intermediate to the next. In the process, the coenzymes NAD^+ (nicotinamine adenine dinucleotide) and $FADH^+$ (flavin adenine dinucleotide) act as electron carriers. In the presence of oxygen as a terminal electron receptor, the cell undergoes **aerobic cellular respiration**, which involves three metabolic processes: glycolysis, the citric acid cycle, and the electron transport chain.

Glycolysis

Glycolysis, or "sugar splitting," involves the conversion of 1 molecule of the 6-carbon sugar glucose into 2 molecules of 3-carbon pyruvate, yielding a net energy gain of 2 ATP (see Figure 3.15). In addition, 2 NAD^+ molecules are reduced to 2 NADH, picking up electrons that can be used in subsequent metabolic pathways for additional ATP synthesis. Glycolysis occurs in the cytoplasm of the cell. It is an anaerobic process that does not require oxygen. Glycolysis prepares the way for either aerobic or anaerobic respiration.

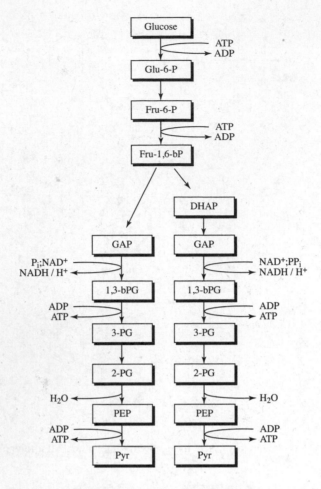

Figure 3.15. Overview of glycolysis

Step 1: Phosphorylation of glucose. As a glucose molecule is transported across the cell membrane, it is immediately phosphorylated by the enzyme **hexokinase**, which transfers a phosphate group from ATP to form **glucose-6-phosphate** (G-6-P). This step is shown in Figure 3.16. This requires an initial energy input of 1 ATP. The phosphorylation of glucose traps glucose within the cell, keeps the concentration of free glucose low, and activates glucose to enter glycolysis.

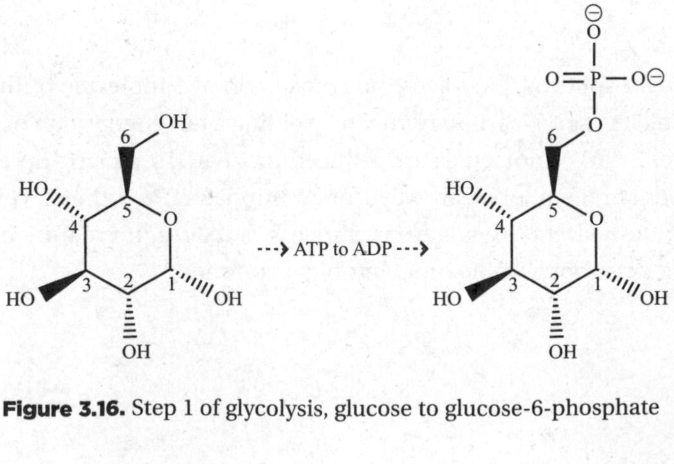

Figure 3.16. Step 1 of glycolysis, glucose to glucose-6-phosphate

Step 2: Glucose to fructose. Next, glucose-6-phosphate is converted to its isomer **fructose-6-phosphate** (F-6-P) by the enzyme **isomerase** (see Figure 3.17).

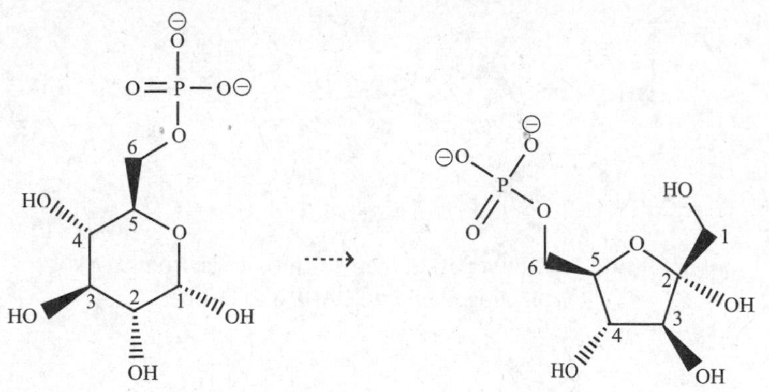

Figure 3.17. Step 2 of glycolysis, glucose-6-phosphate to fructose-6-phosphate

Step 3: Second phosphorylation. A second ATP is expended to phosphorylate fructose-6-phosphate, forming **fructose 1,6-bisphosphate**, a symmetrical molecule with phosphate groups on each end (see Figure 3.18). The enzyme in this reaction, **phosphofructokinase**, is subject to feedback inhibition by ATP and citrate. Phosphorylation of F-6-P commits the substrate to enter the glycolytic pathway. Therefore, feedback regulation of phosphofructokinase controls the rate of glycolysis.

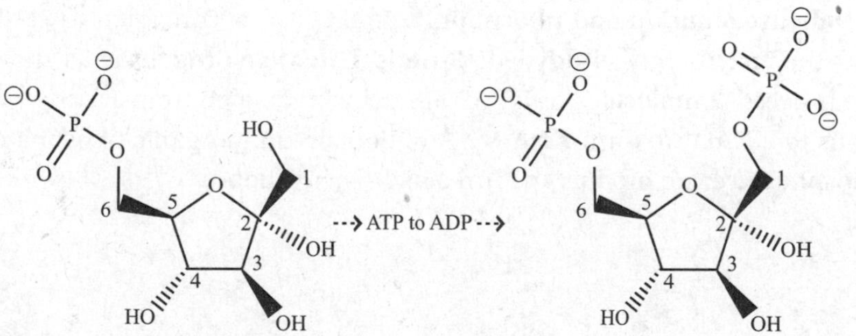

Figure 3.18. Step 3 of glycolysis, fructose-6-phosphate to fructose 1,6-bisphosphate

Step 4: Split into two sugars. The enzyme aldolase splits fructose 1,6-bisphosphate into two 3-carbon isomers, the triose phosphates **GADP** (gylceraldehyde 3-phosphate, or phosphoglyceraldehyde) and **DHAP** (dihydroxyacetone phosphate). DHAP is immediately converted by **triose isomerase** (**TPI**) into GADP. Two molecules of GADP now enter the next step of glycolysis for every 1 glucose molecule entering the pathway, resulting in a doubling of the products of each of the following steps. Step 4 marks the end of the energy-investment phase of glycolysis. The remaining half of the glycolytic pathway repays the 2 ATP invested and generates a net energy gain of 2 additional ATP. Figures 3.19 and 3.20 break down this step of glycolysis into two parts.

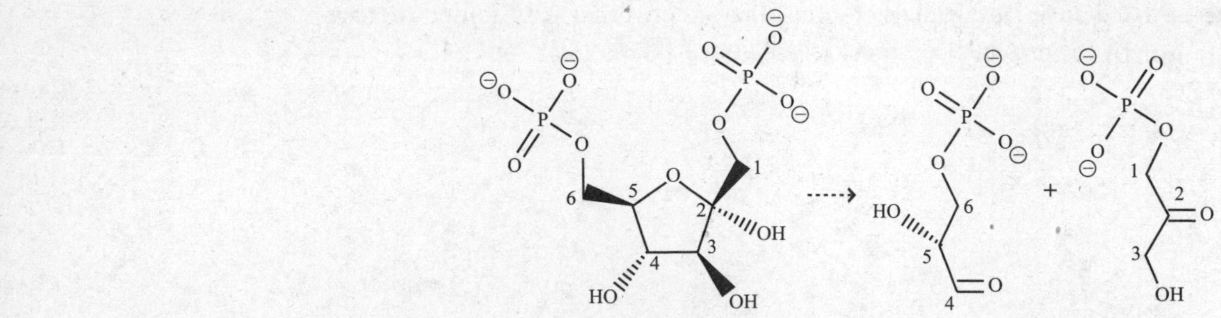

Figure 3.19. First part of Step 4 of glycolysis, fructose 1,6-bisphosphate into GADP and DHAP

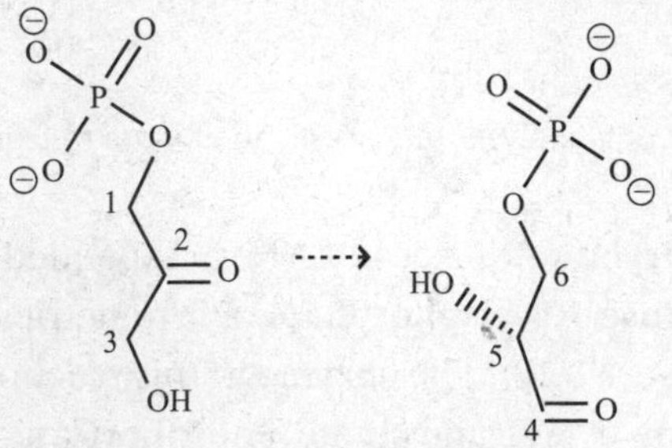

Figure 3.20. Second part of Step 4 of glycosis, DHAP is converted to GADP, resulting in 2 molecules of GADP

Step 5: Dehydrogenation and phosphorylation. GADP is converted to 1,3-bisphosphoglycerate by the enzyme **glyceraldydyde 3-phosphate dehydrogenase** as shown in Figure 3.21. In the process, 2 molecules of DHAP are dehydrogenated, transferring hydrogen ions and electrons to 2 NAD$^+$ to form 2 NADH. Additionally, an inorganic phosphate is added to each bisphosphoglycerate product to form a high-energy bond.

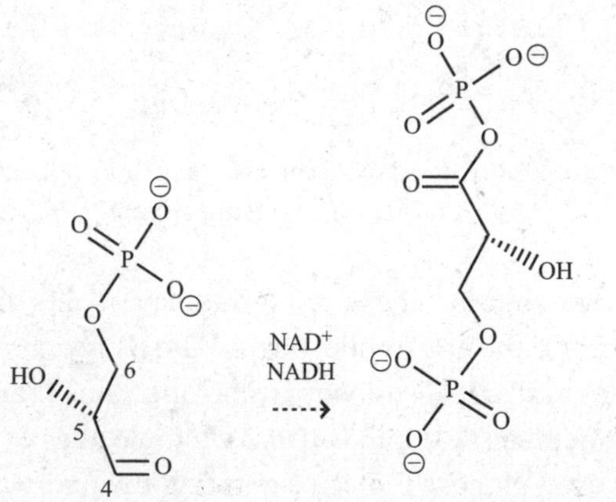

Figure 3.21. Step 5 of glycolysis, GADP to 1,3–bisphosphoglycerate

Step 6: Transfer of phosphate to create ATP. Two 1,3-bisphosphoglycerate molecules are converted to 3-phosphoglycerate. In the process, the high-energy phosphate of each substrate molecule is transferred to ADP, forming 2 ATP molecules (see Figure 3.22). The transfer of an inorganic phosphate group from an intermediate molecule to ADP to form ATP is called **substrate-level phosphorylation.** This is the first of two substrate-level phosphorylation steps that occur in glycolysis. Because this step depends on the availability of ADP, it is another rate-limiting step. When the ATP concentration is high and the ADP concentration is low, glycolysis does not proceed. As of this step, the 2 ATP molecules that were consumed in the preparatory phase have been paid back.

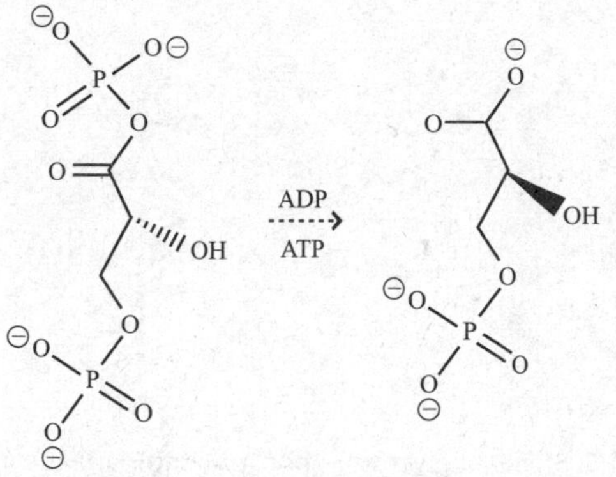

Figure 3.22. Step 6 of glycolysis, 1,3-bisphosphoglycerate to 3-phosphoglycerate

Step 7: Shift of phosphate group. The two 3-phosphoglycerate substrates are rearranged to 2-phosphoglycerate by a shift of the phosphate group as shown in Figure 3.23.

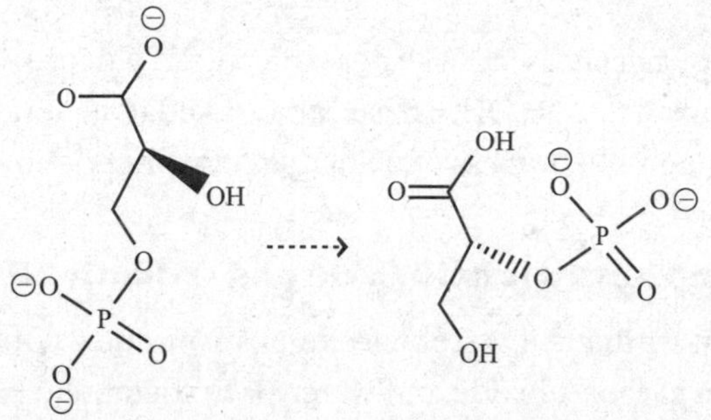

Figure 3.23. Step 7 of glycolysis, 3-phosphoglycerate to 2-phosphoglycerate

Step 8: Production of phosphoenolpyruvate. A molecule of water is removed from each 2-phosphoglycerate molecule to form two phosphoenolpyruvate (PEP) molecules (see Figure 3.24).

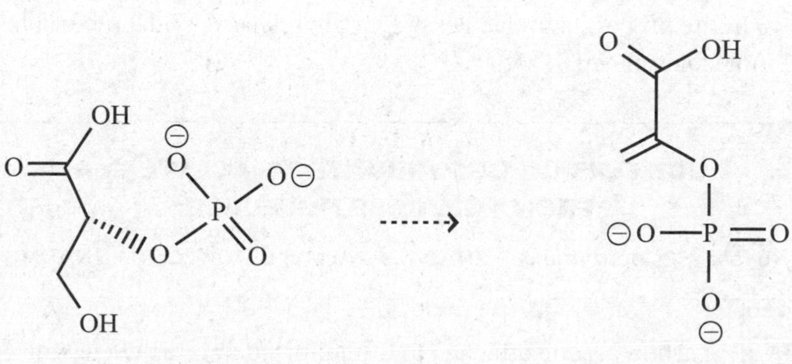

Figure 3.24. Step 8 of glycolysis, 2-phosphoglycerate to phosphoenolpyruvate

Step 9: ATP and pyruvate. The enzyme pyruvate kinase catalyzes the transfer of the phosphate group from each PEP molecule to ADP as shown in Figure 3.25. This process forms 2 pyruvate molecules and 2 ATP molecules in another substrate-level phosphorylation, which is regulated by the availability of ADP. The reaction has resulted in a net surplus of 2 ATP molecules.

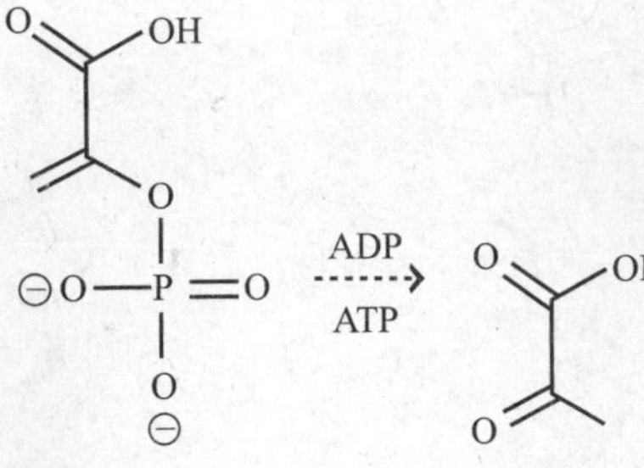

Figure 3.25. Step 9 of glycolysis, phosphoenolpyruvate to pyruvate

---

THE OVERALL REACTION FOR GLYCOLYSIS

Glucose + 2ADP + 2P$_i$ + 2NAD$^+$ → 2Pyruvate + 2ATP + 2NADH + 2H$^+$ + 2H$_2$O

The net energy yield of glycolysis is 2 ATP per molecule of glucose. In addition, 2 molecules of NAD$^+$ have been oxidized to 2 NADH. These can be used to generate additional ATP in the presence of oxygen through the process of oxidative phosphorylation.

Aerobic Respiration: The Citric Acid Cycle and Oxidative Phosphorylation

When oxygen is present in the cell, aerobic cellular respiration converts the pyruvate produced by glycolysis into carbon dioxide and water. Two metabolic pathways are involved in aerobic respiration: the citric acid cycle and oxidative phosphorylation. In prokaryotes, these pathways occur in the cytoplasm with glycolysis. In eukaryotes, aerobic respiration takes place within the mitochondria.

Pyruvate decarboxylation. In eukaryotes, the 2 pyruvate molecules produced by glycolysis are actively transported across both mitochondrial membranes to the inner matrix, where they are decarboxylated to acetyl coenzyme A (CoA) by a complex of pyruvate dehydrogenase enzymes. In the process, 2 molecules of CO$_2$ are released, and 2 molecules of NAD$^+$ are reduced to 2 molecules of NADH.

CONVERSION OF PYRUVATE TO ACETYL CoA
FROM 1 GLUCOSE MOLECULE

2Pyruvate + 2Coenzyme A + 2NAD$^+$ → 2Acetyl CoA + 2CO$_2$ + 2NADH + 2H$^+$

Acetyl CoA, a 2-carbon acetate attached to the sulfur-containing coenzyme A, then enters the citric acid cycle, also known as the **tricarboxylic acid cycle (TCA)** or the **Krebs cycle**.

Citric acid (Krebs) cycle. In this cycle, acetyl CoA is combined with the 4-carbon molecule oxaloacetate to form the 6-carbon molecule citrate. Citrate is then broken down in a series of steps, releasing 2 molecules of CO_2 and transferring electrons to the electron carriers NAD^+ and $FADH^+$ to form 3 NADH and 1 $FADH_2$ molecules per cycle. Water added in two different steps is split to provide hydrogen ions for the electron acceptors. In some animal cells, 1 molecule of guanosine diphosphate (GDP) is phosphorylated to guanosine triphosphate (GTP), which can be used to synthesize 1 ATP via substrate-level phosphorylation. Finally, oxaloacetate is regenerated by the cycle, combining with a new molecule of acetyl CoA to start the cycle again. Figure 3.26 shows the citric acid (Krebs) cycle in detail.

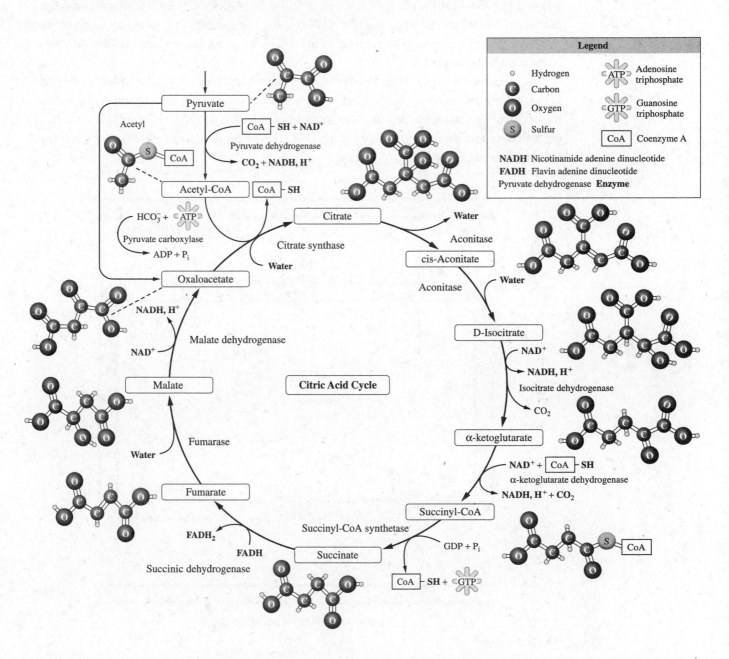

Figure 3.26. Citric acid (Krebs) cycle

REACTION EQUATION FOR TWO TURNS
OF THE CITRIC ACID CYCLE

$$2\text{Acetyl CoA} + 6\text{NAD}^+ + 2\text{FAD}^+ + 2\text{GDP} + 2\text{P}_i + 2\text{H}_2\text{O} \rightarrow$$
$$4\text{CO}_2 + 6\text{NADH} + 6\text{H}^+ + 2\text{FADH}_2 + 2\text{GTP} + 2\text{Coenzyme A}$$

Because a single molecule of glucose results in 2 molecules of acetyl CoA, two turns of the citric acid cycle are necessary to oxidize 1 molecule of glucose to carbon dioxide. Thus, the net energy yield of the citric acid cycle for 1 molecule of glucose is 2 GTP plus the electrons carried by NADH and $FADH_2$. The GTP molecules can be used for energy or can be converted to ATP. Most of the energy generated by aerobic respiration is produced by the next step, oxidative phosphorylation.

The electron transport chain and oxidative phosphorylation. The next series of reactions is carried out by enzymes embedded in the inner mitochondrial membrane. They involve the transfer of electrons from the electron carriers NADH and $FADH_2$ through a chain of oxidation-reduction reactions (see Figure 3.27). This series of reactions is called the **electron transport chain**.

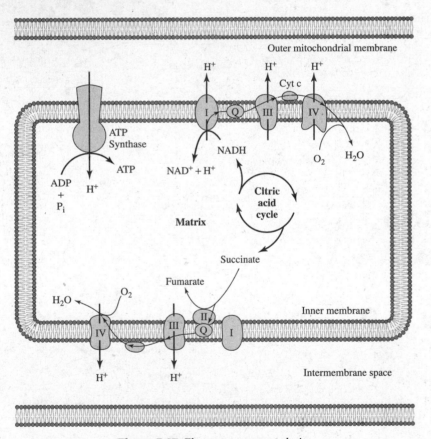

Figure 3.27. Electron transport chain

The electron receptors within the electron transport chain include **cytochrome** proteins. These proteins incorporate an iron-containing heme group as both a prosthetic group (tightly bound cofactor) and an electron acceptor. Each electron acceptor is alternately reduced and then oxidized as it accepts and then donates electrons. Electrons travel down a free-energy gradient, passing from a less electronegative receptor to a more electronegative receptor, until they are finally passed to the terminal electron receptor, oxygen, which combines with hydrogen ions to form water.

The change in free energy caused by the "fall" of electrons is coupled with the transport of H^+ ions, pumping H^+ ions across the inner mitochondrial membrane into the inner membrane space. Hydrogen ions cannot cross back over the membrane because of their charge and the selective permeability of the phospholipid bilayer. As a result, positive charge accumulates in the intermembrane space, creating a region of low pH. The electrochemical gradient formed across the membrane can now be coupled with ATP synthesis in a process called **chemiosmosis**.

In chemiosmosis, the high concentration of H^+ ions in the intermembrane space generates a **proton-motive force** to do molecular work in the cell. The return of H^+ ions down a concentration gradient through a transmembrane channel protein drives the phosphorylation of ADP to ATP. This channel protein is the enzyme **ATP synthase**, a multiunit enzyme composed of 4 subunits and that acts as a molecular rotor. As hydrogen ions bind to each subunit, the ions trigger rotational movement of the rotor mechanism, allowing H^+ to be pumped across the membrane. At the same time, the turning of the rotor activates catalytic regions in the matrix that convert ADP and inorganic phosphate to ATP. Because this phosphorylation of ADP takes place along with the redox reactions of the electron transport chain, this ATP synthesis is known as **oxidative phosphorylation**. In contrast, substrate-level phosphorylation of ATP occurs during glycolysis and the citric acid cycle.

Once ATP is synthesized within the matrix, it is exported to the cytoplasm across the inner and outer mitochondrial membranes by the enzyme **ATP-ADP translocase**. This enzyme couples the transport of ATP out of the cell with the transport of ADP into the cell. If ADP levels outside of the cell are low, then ADP will be slow to enter the mitochondrial matrix. As ATP cannot be synthesized in the absence of ADP, ATP production will slow or stop. Once ATP production stops, ADP levels outside the cell will increase, resulting in positive feedback to increase ATP production and transport.

The energy yield of oxidative phosphorylation is 2 to 3 ATP molecules for every $NADH + H^+$ entering the electron transport chain and 2 ATP molecules for each $FADH_2$. Therefore, oxidative phosphorylation produces a total of 32 to 34 ATP molecules. The total energy produced by aerobic respiration, including glycolysis, is therefore 36 to 38 ATP from each molecule of glucose.

Anaerobic Respiration

The electron transport chain requires a molecule at the end of the chain that can accept an electron. In most organisms, oxygen is the final electron acceptor. Some bacteria, however, have the ability to use electron acceptors other than oxygen, such as nitrate, sulfate, and elemental sulfur. The bacteria can generate ATP in an anaerobic environment. None of the alternate electron receptors, however, are as efficient as oxygen. Examples of bacteria that use anaerobic respiration include those that cause gas gangrene and those living in undersea volcanic vents.

NET MOLECULAR AND ENERGETIC RESULTS OF AEROBIC RESPIRATION

Process	ATP Produced Directly by Substrate-Level Phosphorylation	Reduced Coenzyme	ATP Produced by Oxidative Phosphorylation	Total
Glycolysis	Net 2 ATP	2 NADH	4 to 6 ATP	6–8
Oxidation of pyruvate	--------	2 NADH	6 ATP	6
Krebs cycle and electron transport chain	2 ATP	6 NADH + 2FADH$_2$	18 ATP 4 ATP	24
			Total	36–38

Fermentation

If oxygen is absent, cells can continue to generate ATP via glycolysis using the process of fermentation. Fermentation differs from anaerobic respiration in that fermentation does not use either the citric acid cycle or the electron transport chain. There are two main fermentation pathways: alcohol fermentation and lactic acid fermentation. Both pathways use a terminal electron receptor other than oxygen. The only ATP molecules generated are the two produced by substrate-level phosphorylation in glycolysis. Oxidative phosphorylation cannot occur in the absence of oxgyen.

Alcohol fermentation is carried out by species of bacteria and yeast that convert the pyruvate generated by glycolysis to ethanol and carbon dioxide. Pyruvate is converted to acetaldehyde by the removal of carbon dioxide. Acetaldehyde is then reduced to ethanol by NADH. In the anaerobic pathway of alcohol fermentation, acetaldehyde replaces oxygen as the terminal electron receptor. Alcohol fermentation is used to make alcoholic beverages, such as beer and wine, as well as bread and many other fermented food products. The CO_2 produced by alcohol fermentation provides the bubbles in beer and enables bread to rise.

Lactic acid fermentation is an alternate anaerobic pathway in which pyruvate itself acts as the terminal electron receptor. NADH reduces pyruvate directly to lactate (the ionized form of lactic acid). In the process, NADH is oxidized to NAD^+, which is needed for glycolysis. Lactic acid metabolism occurs in some bacteria and fungi. It also occurs in human muscle cells in high-performance situations, such as during sudden exertion or vigorous exercise when the supply of oxygen is insufficient to meet metabolic demand.

Alternate Energy Sources

Carbohydrates are the primary metabolic energy source. However, fats and proteins can also be metabolized and used for energy.

The primary carbohydrate energy source in humans is glucose, which makes up more than 90% of blood sugar. The glucose molecules that enter glycolysis can come directly from food. They can also be derived from the breakdown of complex carbohydrate storage molecules such as glycogen (animals) and starch (plants). Monosaccharides other than glucose can be converted either to glucose or to other substances that can be used in glycolysis. For example, when sucrose (table sugar) is hydrolyzed into the monomers glucose and fructose, fructose is phosphorylated to fructose 1-phosphate and then hydrolyzed to DHAP and glyceraldehyde 3-phosphate. In this way, it can enter step 5 of glycolysis.

Oxidation of fats. Fats are high-energy molecules that yield considerably more ATP per mole than glucose. Fat molecules are broken down into glycerol and fatty acid chains. Each of these components can be used as energy sources. For example, the 3-carbon **glycerol** is converted to glyceraldehyde 3-phosphate (GADP), which can enter glycolysis.

Fatty acids are transported to the mitochondrial matrix where they go through **beta oxidation**. Beta oxidation involves the oxidation of the carbon backbone of the fatty acid. This is followed by dehydrogenation and hydration reactions and, ultimately, the cleavage of 2-carbon acetyl CoA molecules from the end of each fatty acid chain. The acetyl CoA molecules then enter the citric acid cycle. For each acetyl CoA produced, the dehydrogenation reactions of beta oxidation also generate 1 NADH and 1 $FADH_2$ that can proceed directly to oxidative phosphorylation. Fatty acids are a major source of energy for skeletal muscle engaged in sustained aerobic activity.

Oxidation of amino acids. Dietary proteins are hydrolyzed by digestive enzymes that break the peptide bonds linking amino acids. Amino acids then undergo **deamination**. During this process, the amino group is removed and converted to urea, which is excreted by the urinary tract. The remaining carbon backbone is modified in various ways depending on the R-group side chain and is ultimately converted to an intermediate of the citric acid cycle.

In cases of severe malnutrition, the body can use structural proteins as an energy source, resulting in emaciation and wasting of muscle tissue.

ANABOLIC PATHWAYS

Anabolic pathways create more complex molecules from simpler ones. Anabolic pathways require the input of energy. If a glucose molecule is transported into a cell that has sufficient ATP, it may enter a pathway that is an alternative to glycolysis. The molecule may then be converted to an energy storage molecule such as glycogen or starch.

Intermediates in glycolysis can be used in anabolic biosynthesis. Half of the required amino acids can be made in the citric acid cycle. Pyruvate can be converted to glucose via **gluconeogenesis**, the reverse of glycolysis. Acetyl CoA can be converted to fatty acids for lipid synthesis.

The enzyme pyruvate dehydrogenase (PDH) is the first subunit of the pyruvate dehydrogenase complex (PDC), a multiunit enzyme that catalyzes the conversion of pyruvate to acetyl CoA during pyruvate decarboxylation. Pyruvate dehydrogenase binds the cofactors thiamine pyrophosphate (TPP) and Mg^{2+} and is allosterically inhibited by acetyl CoA, NADH, and ATP. Disruption of PDH activity as a result of thiamine deficiency or inherited metabolic disorders can lead to:

(A) increased production of lactic acid with no corresponding increase in ATP production.

(B) high levels of citrate exported to the cytoplasm, resulting in inhibition of glycolysis.

(C) a decrease in the beta oxidation of fatty acids.

(D) decreased ATP production as a result of a decrease in pyruvate synthesis.

(A) Lactic acid production would increase as glycolysis and lactic acid fermentation become the primary pathways of cellular respiration.

Failure of the PDC complex to convert pyruvate to acetyl CoA can shut down aerobic cellular respiration in the mitochondria since acetyl CoA is the entry molecule leading to the citric acid cycle and oxidative phosphorylation. Answer B can be eliminated because citrate is the product of the first step of the citric acid cycle, which would be inhibited by the decrease in acetyl CoA. Answer C can be eliminated because beta oxidation, or the breakdown of fatty acids to yield acetyl CoA, would increase as lipids replace carbohydrates as the fuel for the citric acid cycle. Answer D can be eliminated because although ATP production will decrease significantly, the reason for the decline is the disruption of aerobic respiration. Glycolysis will still occur, and pyruvate will continue to be produced in the cytoplasm. Instead of entering the citric acid cycle, pyruvate will be converted to lactic acid by the fermentation pathway necessary to regenerate the oxidized NAD^+ necessary for glycolysis. Because substrate-level phosphorylation does not occur during fermentation, the conversion of pyruvate to lactic acid will not provide additional ATP.

MICROBIOLOGY

The study of microbiology involves the study of prokaryotic cells, fungi, and viruses. Note that fungi are not currently covered on the MCAT outline.

Prokaryotic Cells

Prokaryotes include two highly divergent lineages of single-celled organisms: the domains Eubacteria and Archaea. The Eubacteria include familiar bacteria such as *Escherichia coli*, *Streptococcus*, *Staphylococcus*, and other medically important species. The Eubacteria also include the free-living, photosynthetic cyanobacteria such as blue-green algae. The Archaea have only recently been identified as entirely distinct from bacteria based on differences in DNA sequence, biomolecular structure, and enzyme pathways. Archaean prokaryotes have been found in extreme habitats such as deep-sea vents and hot springs. Methane-producing species are found in the digestive tract of humans and ruminants.

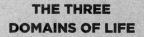

THE THREE DOMAINS OF LIFE

Archaea
Bacteria
Eukaryota

All prokaryotes are unicellular, occurring as single cells or in colonies. Prokaryotes exhibit a variety of shapes and are described as either **coccus** (spherical), **bacillus** (rod shaped), or **spirillus** (spiral). They may be further classified based on whether they occur singly, as pairs (*diplo-*), in straight chains (*strepto-*), or as branching clusters (*staphylo-*). Figure 3.28 shows the shapes of several types of prokaryotes.

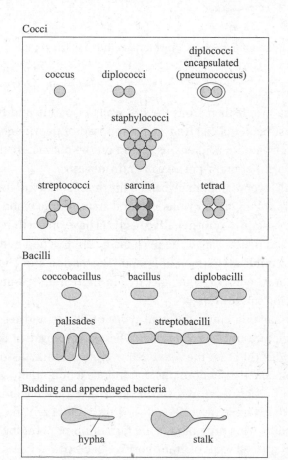

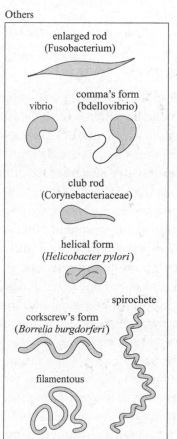

Figure 3.28. Shapes of bacteria

PROKARYOTIC CELL STRUCTURE

Prokaryotic cells consist of a cell wall, a plasma membrane, cytosol, a nucleoid region, ribosomes, and a cytoskeleton, as shown in Figure 3.29. Prokaryotic cells are much smaller than eukaryotic cells. All metabolism occurs in the cytosol. Because of their small size, prokaryotic cells can rely on diffusion and lack the complex membrane-bound organelles of eukaryotes.

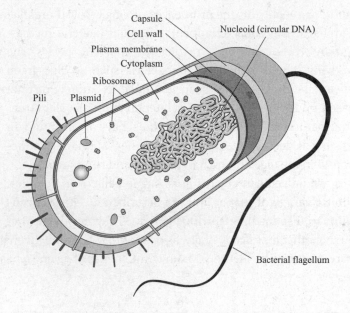

Figure 3.29. Prokaryotic cell (Adapted from a work by Mariana Ruiz Villarreal.)

Cell Wall

The cell walls of bacteria and archaea are distinct from the cell walls of plants and fungi, which contain cellulose or chitin. Most bacterial cell walls are composed of **peptidoglycan**, a polysaccharide cross-linked with short amino acid chains. Based on the characteristics of their cell wall, bacteria are classified as either gram-positive or gram-negative.

Gram-positive bacteria have a thick layer of peptidoglycan on the outer surface of the cell wall. This thick layer causes the cell to retain crystal violet dye and stain purple when subjected to a procedure known as a Gram's stain. **Gram-negative bacteria** have only a thin layer of peptidoglycan located in a fluid-filled region called the **periplasm**, sandwiched between the inner (plasma) membrane and an outer membrane of lipopolysaccharide and channel proteins. Gram-negative bacteria do not retain crystal violet dye from a Gram's stain and appear pink or red due to the underlying safranin stain.

Gram-positive and gram-negative bacteria cause different types of illness and respond differently to drugs based on the structure of their cell walls. When gram-negative bacteria infect a host, the lipopolysaccharides (LPS) on the outer cell wall membrane dissociate from the bacterial cell. These LPS molecules are **endotoxins** that induce a potentially severe inflammatory response that can lead to high fever and shock. Gram-negative bacteria are also resistant to certain antibiotics that target the cell wall. For example, gram-negative bacteria are less susceptible to penicillin. This drug targets the formation of peptidoglycan cross-linkages, which are abundant in the cell walls of gram-positive bacteria.

The cell walls of archaea differ from those of bacteria. In general, most archaea lack peptidoglycan in their cell walls and therefore stain as gram-negative.

Glycocalyx

Some prokaryotes produce a **glycocalyx** (sugar coat) of carbohydrate or protein on the outer surface of their cell walls. This glycocalyx can be a thick capsule that protects pathogenic species from the host's defenses as well as from some antibiotics. The glycocalyx can also form a **slime layer** that enables cells to adhere to a substrate or to one another during the formation of bacterial assemblages (**biofilms**).

Fimbriae, Pili, and Flagella

Fimbriae are thin protein filaments that extend from a prokaryotic cell to aid their attachment to other cells or to the substrate. Fimbriae are used by some species of pathogenic bacteria to attach themselves to their host. **Sex pili** are similar to fimbriae but are longer extensions used to attach two cells together for the process of conjugation. This process is described in "Genetic Variation in Prokaryotes."

Some types of prokaryotes have one or more **flagella** on their outer surface to allow movement. Prokaryotic flagella are smaller than eukaryotic flagella and differ in structure. A bacterial flagellum consists of a whiplike filament of the protein **flagellin** embedded in the cell wall and plasma membrane. The filament is attached to a basal apparatus, or ion-driven motor, by a hooklike swivel. This swivel rotates the flagellum in a corkscrew motion. The energy to move the flagellum is provided by a proton gradient, or **proton motive force**. This proton gradient is produced when hydrogen ions are actively transported across the flagellar membrane. The flow of ions back into the cell through ion channels provides the energy needed to rotate the flagella in either direction. The motion of the bacterium may be random, or it may be toward or away from a chemical signal (**positive chemotaxis** and **negative chemotaxis**, respectively).

Plasma Membrane and Cytoplasm

The plasma membrane of prokaryotes is composed of a semipermeable phospholipid bilayer with integral and peripheral proteins. Glycolipids and cholesterol are absent, although a diverse array of fatty acids allows for the regulation of membrane fluidity. Although true membrane-bound organelles are absent in prokaryotes, the plasma membrane may form intracellular extensions in some photosynthetic and nitrifying bacteria, allowing for additional surface area for membrane-associated enzymes.

Free ribosomes in the cytosol coordinate protein synthesis. The ribosomes of bacteria and Archaea differ from each other and from eukaryotic ribosomes in size and nucleotide sequence. Because of this, antibiotics such as tetracycline can specifically target bacterial RNA without affecting human host cells. Bacterial cells are now known to contain cytoskeletal elements homologous to the microfilaments, microtubules, and intermediate filaments of eukaryotic cells.

Nucleoid Region

Prokaryotes lack a membrane-bound nucleus. Instead, prokaryotic DNA is located in the **nucleoid region** of the cytoplasm and is attached to the plasma membrane. The DNA is a single, circular molecule in a complex with protein. The nucleosomes and histone proteins associated with eukaryotic chromosomes are absent. Prokaryotic DNA is also distinguished by the presence of smaller, extrachromosomal rings of DNA called **plasmids**, which replicate separately and can be transferred from cell to cell.

REPRODUCTION IN PROKARYOTES

Prokaryotes do not undergo mitosis and lack mitotic apparatus. Instead, they reproduce by **binary fission**. Once the circular DNA molecule is duplicated, the cell membrane elongates, causing the two attached DNA copies to pull apart. Then the cell wall and cell membrane pinch inward and divide the cell into two halves, each of which becomes a daughter cell. Binary fission is a form of asexual reproduction that results in daughter cells that, in the absence of mutation or the other processes described below, are copies of each other and of the parent cell.

Prokaryotic reproduction occurs extremely rapidly under optimal conditions. Some bacteria can divide by binary fission in under half an hour. This **exponential growth** occurs when resources are not limiting and can result in billions of offspring from a single cell within a 24-hour period.

GENETIC VARIATION IN PROKARYOTES

Although bacterial reproduction is asexual, genetic variability arises through mutation. Once a mutation appears, it can be passed among individuals of the same or of different species by **horizontal gene transfer**. Horizontal transfer can occur by **conjugation**. This process occurs when two bacteria of different mating strains exchange DNA via cellular extensions called sex pili. Bacteria may also take up DNA from fragments left by dead bacteria in the external environment, a process called **transformation**. Finally, bacterial viruses called bacteriophages (or phages) can transfer DNA as they infect new cells, a process called **transduction**. Because of the rapidity of bacterial reproduction, novel genetic traits, such as antibiotic resistance, can spread rapidly within and between species.

ANTIBIOTIC RESISTANCE

One of the most medically important mutations in bacteria is the development of antibiotic resistance. Genes that confer resistance to antibiotics are frequently **transposons**, mobile genetic elements that can move from place to place in the genome. Transposons in bacteria frequently jump between the bacterial chromosome and plasmid DNA. Plasmids, in turn, can be transferred between bacteria of the same or even different species, contributing to the spread of antibiotic resistance or other associated genes through horizontal gene transfer.

The spread of antibiotic resistance in bacteria is further promoted through natural selection. When an antibiotic is applied, most of the bacteria are destroyed. However, a few may carry genes that give them some degree of resistance to the antibiotic. Those few quickly multiply, particularly if the antibiotic is stopped prematurely, resulting in a new population against which the antibiotic is no longer effective. This process of natural selection can lead to widespread antibiotic resistance in environments in which antibiotics are in heavy or continuous use. In addition, horizontal gene transfer can cause resistance to spread even among unrelated species of bacteria.

ENDOSPORE FORMATION

In adverse environmental conditions, some prokaryotes can form a tough structure that can remain biologically inactive and nonreproductive for long periods. Such a structure is called an **endospore**. Endospores can withstand extreme temperature or environmental fluctuations and can remain dormant for centuries. Extremely high temperature and pressure, such as when autoclaving lab instruments, are needed to kill the endospores of bacteria. Bacteria that form endospores include *Bacillus* and *Clostridium* species that cause anthrax, tetanus, and botulism.

AEROBIC VERSUS ANAEROBIC METABOLISM

Prokaryotes generate cellular energy by metabolic pathways that occur within the cytoplasm. **Aerobes** are species that utilize oxygen as the terminal electron acceptor in aerobic cellular respiration (see "Generation of Cellular Energy").

Prokaryotes that are capable of surviving in the absence of oxygen are **anaerobes**. Prokaryotes that use aerobic cellular respiration pathways when oxygen is present but are capable of switching to fermentation or anaerobic respiration if oxygen becomes unavailable are **facultative anaerobes**. Anaerobic respiration involves the use of nitrate, sulfate, or inorganic sulfur as the ultimate electron acceptor in the place of oxygen. **Obligate anaerobes** rely exclusively on fermentation or anaerobic pathways. Obligate anaerobes can exist only in the absence of oxygen. To these species, oxygen is a metabolic poison. The bacterium that causes botulism, *Clostridium botulinum*, is an obligate anaerobe.

> ### FACULTATIVE VERSUS OBLIGATE
>
> *Facultative* means "I can."
> *Obligate* means "I must."

TIP

FACULTATIVE VERSUS OBLIGATE

Facultative anaerobic organisms can use oxygen when it is present. Obligate anaerobic organisms die in the presence of oxygen.

BACTERIAL SYMBIOSIS: PARASITIC OR COMMENSAL?

Only a small proportion of bacteria cause disease. Most bacteria are free-living. Bacteria that live on or in another organism are said to be **symbiotic** (*sym* means together; *bio* means life.) Bacteria that cause disease are **parasitic**, taking the energy and resources from another host organism and causing harm. Most symbiotic bacteria live on or in a host without causing harm (**commensal**). Sometimes they actually benefit the host (**mutualistic**.) There are more bacterial cells in and on a human body than there are human cells, and yet in a healthy person these bacteria do not cause disease. Instead, the normal commensal bacterial flora aid in digestion, are a source of B vitamins, and may discourage the growth of parasitic, pathogenic bacteria. When these commensal bacteria are destroyed during administration of antibiotics, harmful bacterial species can become established. Alternatively, some strains of commensal bacteria, such as the intestinal species *E. coli*, can become pathogenic under certain conditions.

Viruses

Viruses are complexes of nucleic acids and proteins that straddle the divide between living and nonliving things. Because viruses are not cells, they are not considered to be alive. They are incapable of independent metabolism or reproduction. Like living organisms, however, viruses can undergo evolution. By natural selection, they can adapt to a particular host environment, immune response, or drug regimen. All viruses are infectious agents. They are obligate parasites—parasites that cannot live independently of their host. Viruses are parasitic on the metabolic and reproductive machinery of other cells.

VIRUS STRUCTURE

A virus particle outside of a host cell is called a **virion**. Viruses are extremely small, approximately 20 to 200 nm in diameter. The largest viruses barely reach the size of the smallest of bacteria. Most viruses cannot be seen with a light microscope. Because they are not cells, viruses lack a cell membrane. They have no organelles or nucleus. However, viruses do contain a sequence of nucleic acid, either **DNA** or **RNA**, that encodes the viral genome. The nucleic acid is enclosed in a protein coat (**capsid**) composed of protein subunits (**capsomeres**). Capsomeres can be arranged into a variety of helical, icosahedral, or complex structures. Capsids, in turn, may have an outer **envelope** of protein and phospholipids. These are derived in part from the cell membrane of the host cell and in part from proteins and glycoproteins coded for by viral genes. The viral envelope aids in penetration of the host's immune system, which is made easier because the envelope materials are derived from the host. Viral envelopes are particularly common in animal viruses, such as herpes and influenza viruses.

Bacteriophages (viruses that infect bacteria) have a particularly complex structure that includes an icosahedral capsid with a protein tail sheath and tail fibers that function to inject the viral DNA directly into the host cell. Figure 3.30 shows 3 different types of viruses.

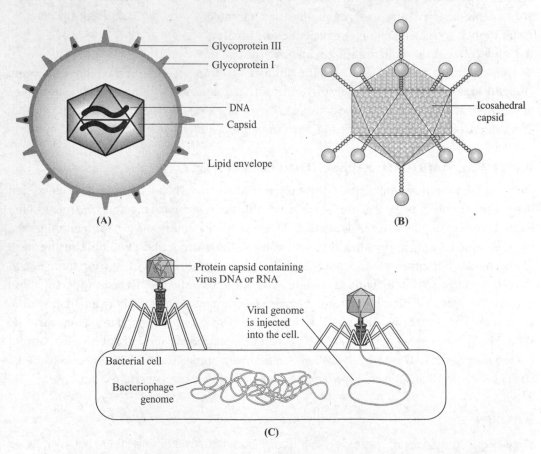

Figure 3.30. Examples of viruses. Herpesvirus (A), Adenovirus (B), Bacteriophage (C) (A, adapted from a work by Gérard Cohen; B, from a photo by Dr. Richard Feldmann, National Cancer Institute; and C, from a work by Graham Colm)

VIRAL HOST RANGE

Viruses infect every form of life, including bacteria, Archaea, animals, plants, protists, and fungi. Most viruses are highly host specific, meaning that they are capable of infecting only a limited range of host species. A few viruses, such as West Nile virus, have a broad host range. The potential of a virus to infect a cell is determined by interactions between proteins on the surface of the virus and receptors in the cell membrane of the host. Viruses can develop mutations that allow them to switch hosts. Avian flu and H1N1 influenza are examples of influenza viruses that typically infect wild birds and other animal species but that have developed mutant strains that can infect humans. The 1918 Spanish flu epidemic that killed more than 40 million people worldwide was an influenza strain that may have originated in birds or pigs. The HIV virus that causes AIDS originated in primates. Viruses may also be limited to a particular type of cell in multicellular organisms. For example, HIV specifically targets T lymphocytes of the immune system.

VIRAL GENOME

Viral nucleic acid in a virion can be in the form of double-stranded DNA (dsDNA), single-stranded DNA (ssDNA), double-stranded RNA (dsRNA), or single-stranded RNA (ssRNA). The DNA may be in the form of a single circular molecule, such as occurs in bacteria, or as one or more linear molecules.

If RNA is used to encode genes, it can act directly as an mRNA template, can be used to synthesize mRNA, or can be used as a template to synthesize a DNA molecule via reverse transcription. **Reverse transcription** is used by **retroviruses** such as HIV, the causative agent of AIDS (Acquired Immune Deficiency Syndrome). Retroviruses enclose the enzyme **reverse transcriptase** in the viral capsid to enable the synthesis of a DNA molecule from viral RNA once the retrovirus enters a host cell. In this transcription pathway, information flow is initially the reverse of the typical transfer from DNA to RNA.

VIRAL LIFE CYCLES

Viruses function by inserting their nucleic acid into a host cell and using the host cell to express viral genes. Host cell metabolic processes are co-opted to synthesize viral nucleic acids and proteins, assembling new viruses that are then released to infect other cells. This general process may follow several different pathways depending on the type of virus and the environmental conditions.

Bacteriophage Reproduction

Bacteriophage life cycles show alternation between an actively infectious lytic cycle and a dormant lysogenic cycle. In the **lytic cycle**, bacteriophages use their protein tails as injectors to insert their genes into a host bacterial cell. Tail fibers recognize specific receptors on the bacterial membrane and bind to the cell. The tail sheath contracts and injects viral DNA through the bacterial cell wall into the cytoplasm. Viral genes are then translated by the host cell. One of the gene products is an enzyme that degrades host cell DNA. Other viral genes code for the production of viral capsid and tail piece proteins using amino acids, ATP, and enzymes supplied by the host. The viral DNA is also replicated by the cell.

Once viral proteins and DNA self-assemble into new viruses, the host cell bursts (**lyses**), and newly synthesized bacteriophages are released to infect other cells. This life cycle pathway is called a lytic cycle because it results in the lysis, or bursting, of the host cell. Viruses that utilize the lytic cycle are **virulent** bacteriophages that cause the death of the host.

In the **lysogenic cycle**, bacteriophage genes remain dormant within the host genome. When a bacteriophage injects its genetic material into a bacterial cell, a piece of viral nucleic acid containing the viral genome is spliced into the host DNA. The virus suppresses expression of its own genes. However, the viral genome, or **prophage**, is replicated with each replication of the host bacterial cell. This cycle allows bacteriophage replication without destroying the host cell and allows the spread of prophage genomes within the bacterial population. In the presence of an appropriate environmental signal, viruses may convert from a lysogenic cycle to a lytic cycle—multiplying themselves and destroying the host cells. Bacteriophages that are capable of both cycles are called **temperate phages**. Figure 3.31 shows the lytic cycle, the lysogenic cycle, and the conversion from a lysogenic to a lytic cycle.

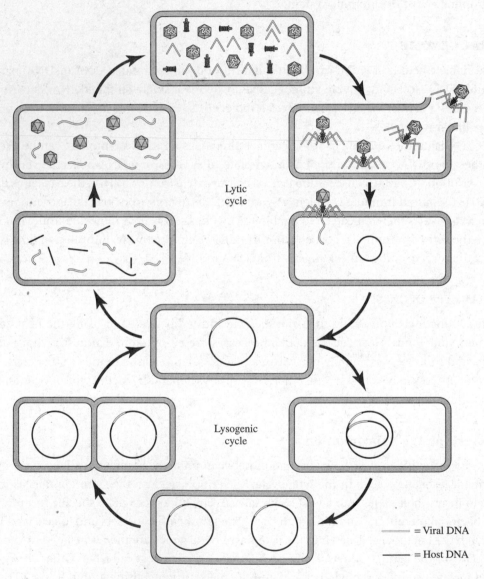

Figure 3.31. Relationship of the lytic and lysogenic cycles of viral reproduction in a plant cell

Some lysogenic viruses may alter the gene expression of their host. In a process called **lysogenic conversion**, prophage genes may result in the expression of a toxin in an otherwise nonvirulent bacterium. For example, lysogenic conversion is responsible for the transformation of a benign strain of *Escherichia coli*, a bacterium normally found in the human intestine, into a virulent strain responsible for outbreaks of food poisoning. Cholera and diphtheria are both bacterial diseases caused by prophage-induced toxins.

Bacteriophage Transduction/Horizontal Gene Transfer

DNA viruses are capable of transferring genes from one host to another host, a process called **transduction**. Transduction by bacteriophages can occur in the lytic cycle when a piece of degraded DNA from the host cell is accidentally incorporated with the DNA of the viral capsid during capsid assembly.

Alternately, a prophage in the lysogenic cycle may incorporate bacterial DNA that is then excised and carried with the virus when the lytic cycle is initiated. Transduction is a form of **horizontal** or **lateral gene transfer**, allowing the rapid spread of an advantageous mutation, such as antibiotic resistance, through a bacterial population.

Animal Virus Reproduction

Animal viruses are classified into six categories based on the form and function of their nucleic acid. RNA viruses in particular are very diverse in animals and plants. Many animal RNA viruses and some animal DNA viruses are encased in an envelope derived from components of host cell membrane. Viral glycoproteins on the outer surface of the envelope bind to receptors on the outer surface of the host cell. The capsid gains entry into the host by fusing the viral envelope with the host's plasma membrane or by endocytosis.

Once inside the host cell, the viral nucleic acid either is integrated into the host DNA or remains as RNA in the cytoplasm, where it codes for the production of new viral proteins. Capsid proteins are synthesized in the cytoplasm. Viral glycoproteins, which are synthesized in the endoplasmic reticulum and Golgi apparatus, are transported in vesicles to the plasma membrane. Viral capsids self-assemble around copies of viral nucleic acid and then bud off of the host cell, surrounded by envelopes derived from the host plasma membrane. This budding of enveloped viruses off of the cell membrane occurs without destroying the host cell. Examples of enveloped RNA viruses include influenza viruses, HIV, and the coronaviruses, which are a major cause of the common cold.

Prions and Viroids

Prions and viroids are subviral particles capable of causing infectious or genetic disease. Prions are proteins located in the brain and other tissues. Under normal circumstances, they may play a role in the development of long-term memory. The misfolding of these proteins from alpha helices to beta pleated sheets triggers conformational changes in other prions, resulting in the accumulation of abnormal protein and degeneration of neural tissue. For example, **bovine spongiform encephalopathy** (**BSE**, or **mad cow disease**) is a fatal, neurodegenerative disorder of cattle that can be transmitted to humans through the consumption of contaminated meat. In humans the disease is fatal. The symptoms are similar to **Creutzfeldt-Jakob disease** (**CJD**), a genetic disorder caused by a mutation in a prion coding gene.

Viroids are short sequences of circular, single-stranded RNA. They can cause infectious disease in plants. Viroids are noncoding RNA sequences that lack the protein coat typical of

RNA viruses. Like viruses, they take over the host cell's reproductive machinery and replicate autonomously. They act as catalytic ribozymes, which can regulate a host plant's gene expression. Viroids are spread between plants through mechanical contact or insect vectors.

TEST QUESTION

Escherichia coli is a rod-shaped, gram-negative bacterium found as a commensal and occasional pathogen in the digestive tract of humans, domestic animals, and wildlife. One pathogenic strain, *E. coli* O157:H7, causes severe hemorrhagic diarrhea and can lead to death from kidney failure and hemolytic anemia caused by the destruction of red blood cells. The toxicity of this strain is linked to lambda bacteriophage genes embedded within the bacterial genome. These genes code for an enterotoxin called Shiga-like toxin in the outer lipopolysaccharide coat of the bacterium. Shiga-like toxin triggers an inflammatory response and blocks protein synthesis in host cells, leading to cell death. The presence of genes for Shiga-like toxin within the genome of *E. coli* O157:H7 suggests that at some point in the past, the *E. coli* strain:

(A) was transformed by another bacterium during a lysogenic cycle.

(B) was transduced by another bacterial strain during conjugation.

(C) was transformed by a virus carrying bacterial genes.

(D) was transduced by a bacteriophage.

(D) The *E. coli* strain is carrying genes of a lambda phage, or bacteriophage, a virus that infects bacteria. The lambda phage has inserted bacteriophage genes into the bacterial genome, a process called *transduction*.

Answers A and C can be eliminated because neither uses the term *transduction*. Additionally, the term *transformation*, which refers to bacterial uptake of DNA directly from the environment, is used incorrectly. Answer A is also incorrect because only viruses undergo lysogenic life cycles, not bacteria. Of the two remaining answers, only answer D uses the term *transduction* correctly to refer to a process carried out by a virus.

DNA AND PROTEIN SYNTHESIS

Deoxyribonucleic acid (**DNA**) is the biological macromolecule that encodes genetic information. Each cell contains a complete set of DNA molecules that encode all information required by the organism. This information is passed from one cell to another during cell replication and is responsible for the transmission of hereditary traits between generations. DNA also controls cellular activities through its role in protein synthesis. DNA and its companion molecule, **RNA** (**ribonucleic acid**) belong to a class of biological macromolecules known as **nucleic acids**. Nucleic acids are polymers composed of repeated subunits called **nucleotides**.

Structure of Nucleotides

Nucleotides are building blocks, structurally independent units that can combine in different sequences to create nucleic acid polymers. Each nucleotide is composed of three subunits: a 5-carbon (**pentose**) **sugar**, a **phosphate group**, and a **nitrogenous base** (see Figure 3.32). The sugar and phosphate group of a nucleotide can form covalent bonds with adjacent nucleotides to form polynucleotides, which are nucleic acids.

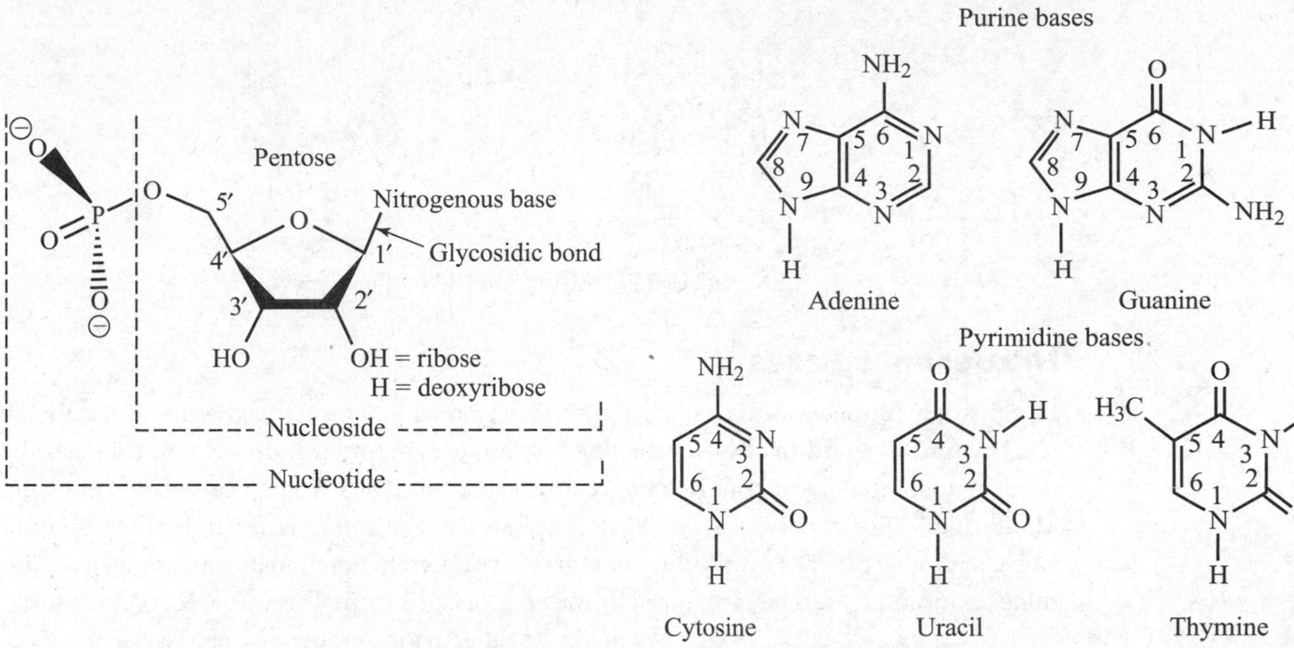

Figure 3.32. Nucleotide structure; a nucleotide is composed of a phosphate group, pentose sugar, and single- or double-ringed nitrogenous base

Nucleotides that incorporate the pentose sugar **ribose** are called **ribonucleotides**. Ribonucleotides make up RNA. They are found in molecules such as adenosine triphosphate (ATP) and cyclic adenosine monophosphate (**cyclic AMP**). Nucleotides that incorporate the pentose sugar **deoxyribose** are called **deoxyribonucleotides**. DNA is formed from chains of deoxyribonucleotides. Deoxyribose is formed when a hydroxyl group is removed from the $2'$ carbon of ribose.

> **BUILDING BLOCKS**
>
> Pentose sugar + Nitrogenous base = Nucleoside
>
> Phosphate group + Pentose sugar + Nitrogenous base = Nucleotide
>
> Nucleotide + Nucleotide + Nucleotide . . . = Nucleic acid

Positional Nomenclature

The 5-carbon pentose sugar of a nucleotide forms a pentagonal ring with an oxygen atom at the apex (see Figure 3.33). The carbon atoms are numbered by convention with carbon number one (referred to as $1'$ or "one prime") attached to the nitrogenous base and the remaining carbons numbered sequentially away from the oxygen atom. Note that the $5'$ carbon is not part of the ring but projects out of it, bonded to a terminal phosphate group. The $3'$ carbon carries a terminal hydroxyl (–OH) group, which becomes the attachment site for additional nucleotides during polynucleotide formation and strand elongation.

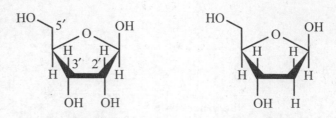

Figure 3.33. The pentose sugar molecules of the nucleic acids RNA and DNA, ribose (*left*) and deoxyribose (*right*)

Nitrogenous Bases

Five possible nitrogenous bases can occur in nucleotides: **adenine** (A), **guanine** (G), **cytosine** (C), **thymine** (T), and **uracil** (U). The first four are present in DNA. In RNA, uracil takes the place of thymine. Nitrogenous bases are composed of hexagonal rings of carbon and nitrogen. These rings differ in various ways. First, the rings differ in the number and arrangement of single or double bonds. Second, different rings have different functional groups attached. Thymine, for example, can be recognized by the presence of a methyl group ($-CH_3$).Third, nitrogenous bases differ in the number of rings. Two of the bases, adenine and guanine, are double-ringed molecules, known as **purines**. The other three bases are single-ringed **pyrimidines** (see Figure 3.32).

Structure of DNA

In 1953, James Watson and Francis Crick published a model describing the three-dimensional structure of DNA. According to the **Watson-Crick model**, DNA is formed of two strands of polynucleotides. The strands are joined by hydrogen bonds between the nitrogenous bases of each strand. The two strands spiral around the central axis, forming a **double helix**, as shown in Figure 3.34. On each strand, the 3′ carbon of a deoxyribose is joined to the phosphate group of the 5′ carbon of another nucleotide via dehydration synthesis. This forms a strong, covalent **phosphodiester bond**. The sequence of phosphodiester bonds forms a backbone of sugar-phophate-sugar-phosphate on each strand. The nitrogenous bases of each nucleotide strand extend outward from this sugar-phosphate backbone toward the bases of the opposite strand. The second strand, running in the opposite direction, is **antiparallel**. This means that the 3′ end of one strand is paired with the 5′ end of the opposite strand. The resulting molecule twists in on itself in a right-handed direction to form a helical double chain of nucleotides.

The structure of the DNA double helix can be compared with that of a spiral staircase. The railings of the staircase are two sugar-phosphate chains, facing opposite directions. Strong covalent bonds between each sugar and the phosphate group support the vertical railings. The horizontal steps of the staircase are the pairs of nitrogenous bases, one from each nucleotide, held together by weak hydrogen bonds.

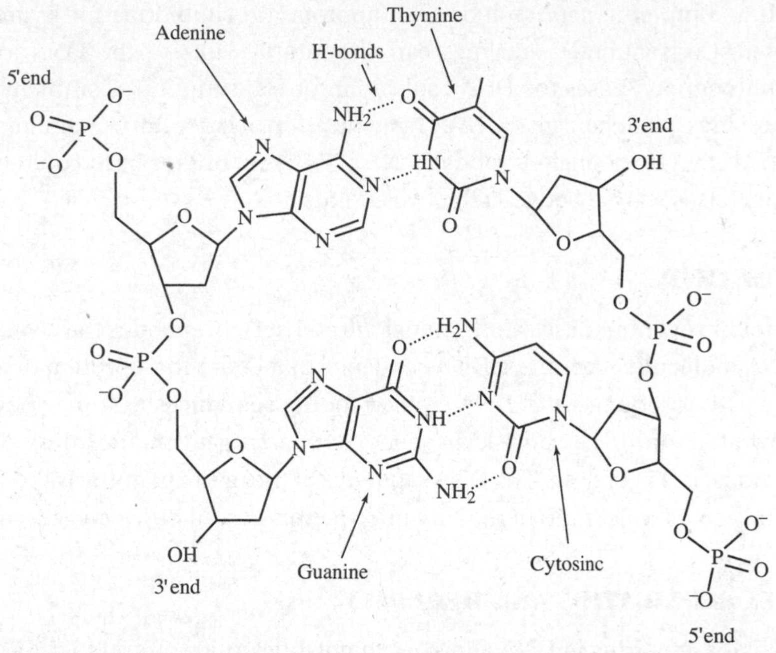

Figure 3.34. DNA double helix structure (Adapted from: Madeleine Price Ball)

The orientation of the antiparallel strands is indicated by the orientation of the sugar molecules. On one side, both the oxygen atom and the 5′ carbon face upward, with the 5′ carbon attached to a phosphate group at the top of the chain of nucleotides. At the bottom of this same chain, the 3′ carbon and its attached hydroxyl (–OH) group face downward, and the 3′ carbon is not attached to the phosphate group of another nucleotide. This is referred to as the **5′-3′ strand**. The opposite strand has its 3′ carbon atom and hydroxyl group on top, and the oxygen and 5′ carbon and terminal phosphate group face downward. This is referred to as the **3′-5′ s**trand.

Complementary Base Pairing

The two strands are joined by hydrogen bonds between their nitrogenous bases. However, each nitrogenous base can form bonds with only a specific complementary base. In this **complementary base-pairing** system, adenine bonds with thymine via two hydrogen bonds (**A=T**) and guanine bonds with cytosine by three hydrgon bonds (**G≡C**). In RNA, the base uracil replaces thymine as the complementary base to adenine (**A=U**). A double-ringed purine always pairs with a single-ringed pyrimidine. Therefore, the width of the DNA molecule remains constant. Because of complementary base pairing, the amount of adenine in a DNA molecule equals the amount of thymine and the amount of guanine equals the amount of cytosine. This relationship is known as one of **Chargaff's rules**. The ratio of G≡C to A=T complementary base pairs, however, varies among species. In addition, this **GC content**, or the proportion of the total number of G and C bases in the DNA, can vary between different regions of DNA within a single genome. DNA with higher GC content is more stable.

The hydrogen bonds that join complementary bases together are relatively weak. As a result, the DNA strands are easily separated, or **denatured**, into single-stranded DNA by enzymes or by changes in temperature or pH. These same hydrogen bonds can also spontaneously reform between complementary nucleotides, allowing single-stranded DNA to

reanneal with a complementary strand when appropriate conditions for hydrogen bonding are restored. Consequently, enzymes can temporarily "unzip" the DNA to reveal the sequence of nitrogenous bases for DNA replication or transcription. Complementary base pairing also provides a mechanism for **DNA hybridization**, a laboratory technique that forms double-stranded DNA from single-stranded DNA of different origins based on the number of complementary bases shared between the two strands.

Function of DNA

The sequence of nitrogenous bases along a single strand of DNA encodes the genetic information of the DNA molecule. A **gene** is a DNA sequence that codes for a protein or a regulatory RNA molecule. Other sequences of DNA are **noncoding sequences** that may have a regulatory or unknown function. The entire DNA sequence of an organism, including all genes and noncoding regions, is its **genome**. The DNA sequence of the entire genome is the "instruction manual" for the cell as well as the hereditary information passed between generations.

ROLE IN CELL REPLICATION AND HEREDITY

Complementary base pairing in DNA allows each polynucleotide strand to act as a template for the synthesis of a second, complementary strand and provides a mechanism for DNA replication. DNA replication occurs before a cell is duplicated so that each daughter cell will receive an identical set of genetic instructions. DNA must also be replicated in meiosis in order for parents to pass genetic information to their offspring.

ROLE IN PROTEIN SYNTHESIS

The active role of DNA in a cell is to direct protein synthesis, or **gene expression**. By controlling which proteins are expressed at which times, DNA exerts control over all aspects of cellular growth, development, and metabolism.

ORGANISMAL DIVERSITY

The variation in the order of nitrogenous bases of DNA sequences results in genetic differences among individuals, populations, and species. Ultimately, this variation accounts for the diversity of all living things.

DNA Replication

One of the valuable contributions of the Watson-Crick model was to provide an insight into how DNA is replicated. During replication, DNA uncoils and the strands of DNA are pulled apart. Each strand then serves as the template for the construction of a new, complementary strand. The two identical DNA molecules that result are composed of one original strand and one new strand. Hence, DNA replication is considered to be **semiconservative**. In other words, one strand of the new DNA molecule is new, and the other strand is conserved from the original molecule, as shown in Figure 3.35.

DNA REPLICATION IN PROKARYOTES

Much of the initial knowledge about the process of DNA replication was obtained from observations of DNA replication in prokaryotes. In most prokaryotic cells, such as the bacterium *E. coli*, DNA is a single, circular chromosome located in the nucleoid region of the cytoplasm. The circular chromosome is attached to the internal surface of the cell membrane. The cytoplasm of a bacterial cell often contains smaller circular DNA molecules called **plasmids**, which are capable of replicating independently of the bacterial chromosome. Prokaryotic DNA is **supercoiled** to fit into the nucleoid region by the **topoisomerase** enzyme **DNA gyrase**. This enzyme introduces counterclockwise twists or, **negative supercoils**, into the circular DNA molecule.

Replication of the DNA of the circular bacterial chromosome begins at one specific sequence of nucleotides called the **origin of replication**. First, the double helix is unwound by **DNA helicase** enzymes. Next, the hydrogen bonds holding complementary bases together are denatured, and the strands separate. The strands are held apart by single-stranded binding (**SSB**) proteins. Topoisomerase enzymes cut and rejoin the DNA to aid uncoiling. Two Y-shaped **replication forks** form at the origin of replication and proceed in opposite directions, unzipping the DNA molecule along a replication bubble. This is termed **bidirectional replication**.

As the DNA molecule unwinds, a short **RNA primer** is synthesized by **DNA primase** at the replication fork. This primer provides a starting sequence for DNA synthesis and will eventually be replaced with DNA. The enzyme **DNA polymerase III** then binds to the RNA primer and travels along the replication fork. DNA polymerase III synthesizes a new complementary strand of nucleotides along one of the original template strands.

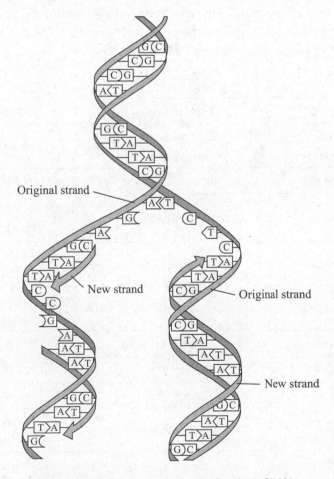

Figure 3.35. Semiconservative replication of DNA

DNA polymerase III adds nucleotides to the 3′ end of a complementary strand in the form of **deoxynucleoside triphosphates** (dNTPs). These dNTPs are dATP, dGTP, dCTP, and dTTP. Two of the phosphate groups on each dNTP are hydrolyzed via a dehydration synthesis reaction to provide the energy for the formation of a new phosphodiester bond. DNA polymerase III can only add nucleotides to the free hydroxyl group on the 3′ end of each previous nucleotide and therefore can synthesize a new strand in only the 5′–3′ direction.

This directionality of synthesis results in differences in the direction of DNA synthesis between the antiparallel DNA strands. On the 3′–5′ strand of the template DNA (the **leading strand**), replication proceeds continuously along the replication fork. DNA polymerase III creates a complementary strand in the 5′–3′ direction. On the **lagging strand** (the 5′–3′ strand), DNA replication is **discontinuous**. After binding to a RNA primer sequence on the lagging strand, DNA polymerase moves backward to synthesize a short strand of roughly 1000 nucleotides called **Okazaki fragments**. New RNA primers are added as the replication fork elongates. DNA polymerase continues to synthesize short Okazaki fragments from these multiple primers. Eventually, Okazaki fragments are joined together into a continuous complementary strand. DNA polymerase I removes the primer sequences and replaces them with DNA. The enzyme **DNA ligase** joins the fragments together. Because of the continuous replication on the leading strand and discontinuous replication on the lagging strand, DNA replication is said to be **semidiscontinuous**.

The rate of DNA replication in prokaryotes is approximately 100,000 nucleotides per minute, proceeding in both directions. To achieve this rate of replication, the DNA molecule must uncoil at a rate of approximately 10,000 revolutions per minute. In *E. coli*, the entire genome of over 4 million base pairs can be replicated in under an hour. Table 3.3 describes the various enzymes involved in DNA replication.

Table 3.3 Enzymes Involved in DNA Replication

Enzyme	Type of Cell	Function
DNA gyrase (topoisomerase)	Prokaryotes, some eukaryotes	DNA supercoiling
DNA helicase	Bacteria, eukaryotes	Unwinds DNA double helix
DNA primase	Bacteria, eukaryotes	Synthesis of RNA primer at replication fork
DNA Polymerase I	Bacteria	Excises and replaces RNA primer sequences with DNA
DNA Polymerase III	Bacteria	Synthesis of complementary DNA strand in 5′–3′ direction
Polymerase α	Eukaryotes	DNA replication
Polymerase ε	Eukaryotes	DNA replication
Polymerase δ	Eukaryotes	DNA replication
DNA ligase	Bacteria, eukaryotes	Joins Okazaki fragments of lagging strand

DNA REPLICATION IN EUKARYOTES

The linear chromosomes of eukaryotes contain vastly more DNA than the single prokaryotic chromosome. A diploid human cell has approximately 6 billion base pairs. This DNA is wound around histone proteins in nucleosomes into chromatin to fit the DNA of 46 linear chromosomes into the nucleus.

Prokaryotic and eukaryotic organisms have similar mechanisms for DNA replication. However, some differences occur between the replication of linear eukaryotic DNA and replication of the single circular chromosome of prokaryotes. (See Figure 3.36.)

Multiple Origins of Replication

Eukaryotic chromosomes have multiple origins of replication. Replication bubbles initiated at multiple origins proceed in both directions simultaneously and eventually fuse together, allowing the linear chromosomes to be replicated much more rapidly than if replication started at a single origin. Nevertheless, a eukaryotic cell copies fewer than 10,000 nucleotides per minute. This replication rate is 10 times slower than that of prokaryotes. Replication of the entire genome requires many hours.

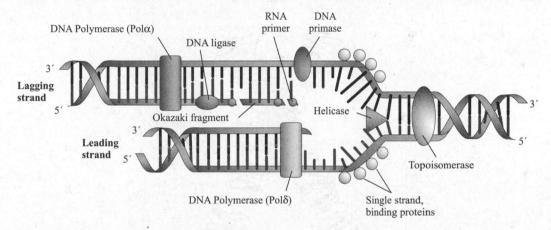

Figure 3.36. DNA replication in eukaryotes

Telomeres

In a linear eukaryotic chromosome, DNA polymerase proceeding in a 5′–3′ direction cannot replicate the last RNA primer sequence on the terminal end of the lagging strand. The 3′ strand of the newly synthesized DNA molecule has fewer nucleotides than the opposite 5′ strand once the terminal RNA primer is removed. Consequently, the 3′ end of a chromosome gets shorter with each replication. This has been termed the **end replication problem**.

To compensate, eukaryotic chromosomes have regions of short, repetitive sequences of nucleotides called **telomeres** at their tips. Telomeres serve only as space holders. At the end of each replication cycle, a telomere is lost rather than a critical piece of DNA. Some eukaryotic cells, such as germ cells, also have a special enzyme, **telomerase**, to add additional repetitive sequences of nucleotides to their 3′ ends after each replication. This prevents the loss of sequences and retains genetic information to be transmitted to subsequent generations.

Somatic cells lack telomerase. Once telomeres have been removed through repeated replication, chromosomes in somatic cells lose critical information with each additional replication. The length of the telomeres sets the limit on the number of times a cell can divide, and the loss of telomeres is associated with aging on a cellular level. Telomeres also act as a cap to prevent the ends of chromosomes from combining with other chromosomes, a process that can lead to cancer.

Centromeres

Centromeres are constricted regions of the eukaryotic chromosome containing noncoding, repetitive sequences of nucleotides, frequently called **satellite DNA**. When eukaryotic chromosomes replicate, the two new chromosomes synthesized from the original double-stranded DNA molecule remain attached at the centromere as sister chromatids until the copies can be separated during mitosis or meiosis, as shown in Figure 3.37. The repetitive sequences of DNA in both centromeres and telomeres are typically highly condensed as inactive **heterochromatin**.

Okazaki Fragments

In eukaryotes, discontinuous replication on the lagging strand results in much shorter Okazaki fragments. The Okazaki fragments of eukaryotes contain an average 100–200 nucleotides instead of 1000–2000 nucleotides in prokaryotes.

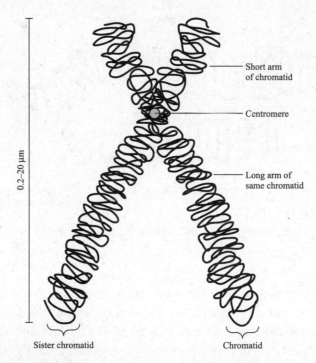

Figure 3.37. A duplicated chromosome consisting of two DNA copies (chromatids) joined at the centromere

DNA Polymerases

DNA polymerases are the enzymes that join nucleotides into a DNA strand. More than ten DNA polymerase enzymes have so far been identified in eukaryotes, in contrast to five identified for prokaryotes. The eukaryotic polymerases involved in DNA replication include polymerase α, polymerase ε, and polymerase δ.

REPAIR DURING REPLICATION

Because complementary base pairing strictly limits which nitrogenous bases can combine, DNA replication is highly accurate. However, errors occur in roughly 1 in 100,000 nucleotides. Various enzymes proofread and repair the DNA as it is being replicated. As a result, the final error rate is only 1 in 10 billion nucleotides.

The primary group of enzymes involved in proofreading and repair during DNA synthesis is the DNA polymerase complex. As each nucleotide is added to the growing strand, DNA polymerase checks it for mismatches against the original template, proofreading the DNA. An enzyme with this capability is called a **3′–5′ exonuclease**. If an error is detected, the enzyme excises the incorrect nucleotide and replaces it before allowing DNA synthesis to continue. A common error is the substitution of the base uracil, normally found in RNA, for thymine.

MUTATIONS

If an error that occurs during DNA replication is not corrected, it can result in a **mutation**, which is an alteration of the nucleotide sequence of DNA. Mutations are discussed on pages 408–411.

REPAIR OF MUTATIONS

Mutations can be repaired in several ways, including mismatch repair, base excision repair, and nucleotide excision repair. The method used depends on the type of mutation.

Mismatch Repair (MMR)

Bases that were incorrectly paired during DNA replication and escape correction by DNA polymerase can be repaired by the mismatch repair pathway. Single base mutations can also be repaired by mismatch repair. In this pathway, **MUT enzymes** (for mutation enzymes) compare the original DNA template with the newly synthesized strand. The original template is identified by the presence of **methylation**. When a mismatch is found, the enzymes nick the DNA strand by cleaving a phosphodiester bond. Once MUT enzymes nick the strand to be repaired, **helicase** enzymes unwind the DNA and an **exonuclease** removes the affected region. A correct replacement is synthesized by **DNA polymerase** and the strand is reannealed by **DNA ligase**.

Base Excision Repair (BER)

Like mismatch repair, the BER group of pathways can be used to excise and replace an incorrect base formed as a result of mutation. A variety of enzymes called **DNA glycosylases** are specialized to remove specific bases, such as a uracil incorrectly incorporated opposite adenine. This base excision creates an abasic site (**AP site** = apurinic/apyramidic site) at the nucleotide where the base was removed. An **AP endonuclease** enzyme nicks the sugar-phosphate backbone of the affected strand, exposing a 3′ end for the attachment of DNA polymerase. DNA polymerase and DNA ligase replace the defective AP site with one that matches the DNA template.

SINGLE NUCLEOTIDE POLYMORPHISMS (SNPs = "SNIPS")

Snips are random mutations in a single nucleotide that occur in 1% or more of the human genome in either coding or noncoding regions of the DNA. Snips may result from substitutions, insertions, or deletions. Variation in snip sequences reflects genetic differences among individuals. Snips are used as genomic markers and are currently under investigation for use in the development of personalized medicine.

Nucleotide Excision Repair (NER)

In a situation where damage to the nucleotide sequence is severe enough to distort the double helix, nucleotide excision repair provides a mechanism to cut and repair multiple nucleotides at a time. Nucleotide excision repair is a significant repair pathway for damage from ultraviolet radiation. This particular type of damage can trigger the formation of thymine dimers (covalent bonds joining two thymines) that disrupt the helical structure of DNA (see Figure 3.38). The enzymes UVrA, UVrB, and UVrC excise the affected nucleotide sequence. Then DNA polymerase and DNA ligase replace the damaged strand. Defects in the nucleotide excision repair pathway can result in the genetic disorder **xeroderma pigmentosum**, which causes skin to become hypersensitive to sunlight and highly susceptible to skin cancer.

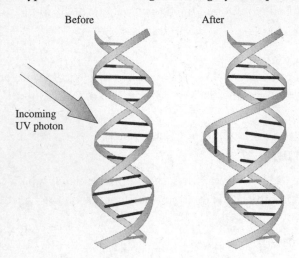

Figure 3.38. Formation of thymine dimers

Protein Synthesis

DNA is the ultimate source of information in a cell. The sequences of nitrogenous bases form a code for storing information. This code is expressed in the cell through the synthesis of protein.

CENTRAL DOGMA

The overall flow of information in the cell goes from DNA to RNA to protein. This information flow is termed the **central dogma** of biology.

CENTRAL DOGMA

DNA → RNA → protein

TRANSCRIPTION AND TRANSLATION

A DNA sequence that codes a protein or regulatory molecule is a **gene**, the basic unit of genetic information. The process of synthesizing a protein or regulatory molecule from information stored in DNA is **gene expression**. Gene expression leading to protein synthesis involves two processes, transcription and translation. In **transcription**, the DNA sequence of a gene is read by enzymes to make an RNA copy, or RNA transcript. In **translation**, the

RNA transcript serves as a template to guide the linkage of amino acids into a protein.

STRUCTURE OF RNA

Unlike the DNA double helix, RNA is a **single strand** of ribonucleotides. RNA contains the pentose sugar **ribose** instead of the deoxyribose sugar found in DNA. RNA also contains the nitrogenous base **uracil** instead of thymine. The single-stranded polynucleotide chain can fold upon itself to form hairpin loops and helical regions where areas of complementary AU and GC bases form cross-linkages.

A cell produces several different forms of RNA. Some forms of RNA are directly involved in protein synthesis. Other types of RNA act as regulatory molecules or enyzmes.

Messenger RNA (mRNA)

mRNA is the RNA that is synthesized directly from a DNA template in the nucleus of the cell. It is a single strand of nucleotides that is complementary to one strand of the DNA, the template strand. After transcription, mRNA leaves the nucleus to direct protein synthesis at the ribosomes, as shown in Figure 3.39.

Transcription, or rewriting, involves the conversion of genetic information from one type of nucleic acid to another. During transcription, the language of nucleic acids remains the same.

DNA → RNA

Translation is the conversion of information between two languages, from the language of nucleic acids to the language of proteins.

RNA → amino acid → protein

RETROVIRUSES

Retroviruses encode their information as RNA and are capable of reverse transcription. Their information transfer proceeds initially from RNA to DNA, which is an exception to the central dogma.

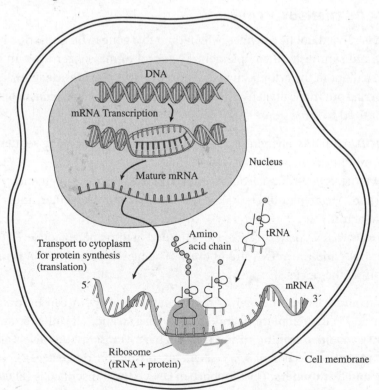

Figure 3.39. mRNA interaction

Ribosomal RNA (rRNA)

rRNA is one of the primary components of ribosomes, the complex two-subunit macromolecules that assemble amino acids into proteins. rRna is involved in the decoding of mRNA and interacts with transfer RNA.

Transfer RNA (tRNA)

Transfer RNA is a short sequence of RNA that transports amino acids to the ribosome and binds to a complementary sequence on the messenger RNA.

Noncoding RNA

Ribosomal RNA and transfer RNA are examples of **noncoding RNA**, or RNA that does not code for protein. Other types of noncoding RNA include **small nuclear RNAs** (**snRNAs**) in bacteria, **small interfering RNA** (**siRNA**), and **micoRNAs**. These and other noncoding RNAs play critical roles in posttranscriptional RNA splicing and as regulators of gene expression.

> **RIBOSOMES = RIBOZYMES**
>
> Recent evidence has shown that ribosomal RNA and other forms of noncoding RNA can act as enzymes to catalyze biological reactions. Such **catalytic RNAs** are also called **ribozymes**. A linear RNA molecule can form a three-dimensional tertiary structure through interactions between complementary bases. This tertiary structure is similar to the tertiary structure of protein enzymes.

MECHANISM OF TRANSCRIPTION

Transcription is carried out by enzymes, which bind to a gene to be transcribed, separate the DNA strands, and synthesize a complementary strand of messenger RNA. In bacteria, this process is carried out in the cytoplasm by the enzyme **RNA polymerase**. In eukaryotes, transcription is carried out in the nucleus by **RNA polymerase II**. The mechanism of transcription can be summarized in three steps.

1. **INITIATION.** An RNA polymerase binds to the beginning of a gene sequence, the DNA uncoils, and the strands separate.
2. **ELONGATION.** Free RNA nucleotides match up with their complementary bases on the DNA strand. Sugar-phosphate linkages join nucleotides together into an elongating molecule of mRNA.
3. **TERMINATION.** RNA polymerase reaches the end of the gene sequence. Hydrogen bonds between DNA and the mRNA strand break. The newly formed mRNA is processed and moves out of the nucleus.

Template strand. Genes on either of the two strands of DNA can be transcribed. The transcribed strand is the **template strand**, or **antisense strand**. The other strand is the **nontemplate**, **sense strand**, or **coding strand** (see sidebar). Transcription travels along the DNA template strand in the direction of 3'–5', called, by convention, **downstream**.

Promoters and terminators. The sequence of DNA to be transcribed is called a **transcription unit**. A transcription unit consists of a **promoter** sequence, which binds to RNA polymerase, the DNA sequence to be transcribed, and a **terminator** sequence, which signals the end of transcription. In eukaryotes, an adenine-rich DNA base sequence called a **polyadenylation signal** replaces the terminator region.

Step 1. Initiation. In prokaryotes, the RNA polymerase is an inactive **core enzyme** consisting of several subunits. In order to be activated as a functional holoenzyme to initiate transcription, RNA polymerase must bind to a protein **transcription initiation factor** called a **sigma factor.** A variety of sigma factors can bind to RNA polymerase to regulate the transcription of different genes in response to varying environmental conditions. The activated RNA polymerase then binds directly to the promoter sequence of the specific gene to be transcribed.

RNA POLYMERASE ACTIVATION AND TRANSCRIPTION INITIATION IN PROKARYOTES

RNA polymerase core enzyme + Sigma factor = RNA Polymerase holoenzyme (complete, or active, enzyme)

Activated RNA Polymerase → Binds to Promoter to Initiate Transcription

In eukaryotes, **transcription factors** must bind to the promoter site before RNA polymerase can bind. Transcriptions factors are proteins characterized by **DNA binding domains**, which allow them to bind to specific sequences of DNA within the promoter. In some genes, the promoter is a **TATA box,** a sequence of nucleotides usually starting with TATAAA on the template (non-coding) strand of DNA. In eukaryotes, the complex of RNA polymerase and transcription factors bound to a promoter is called a **transcription initiation complex**.

TRANSCRIPTION INITIATION IN EUKARYOTES

Transcription Factors + RNA Polymerase II → Bind to Promoter = Transcription Initiation Complex

RNA polymerase then uncoils the DNA molecule and denatures the hydrogen bonds holding the strands together, "unzipping" the DNA. In eukaryotes, this process involves the unwrapping of DNA from the histone protein complexes that make up nucleosomes.

Step 2. Elongation. RNA polymerase moves down the DNA template from **3′ to 5′**, synthesizing a single strand of complementary mRNA antiparallel to the DNA template. (See Figure 3.40.) The mRNA transcript elongates by the addition of ribonucleoside triphosphate molecules (rATP, rGTP, rCTP, rUTP) to the 3′ end, so that synthesis occurs in the 5′ to 3′ direction. Hydrolysis of two of the phosphate groups on these molecules to pyrophosphate (PP_i) provides energy for the formation of phosphodiester bonds of the sugar-phosphate backbone between nucleotides. The DNA double helix is continuously unwound and then rewound as RNA polymerase moves along the template strand. Multiple RNA polymerase enzymes can transcribe the same DNA template at a time, making multiple copies of mRNA.

Step 3. Termination. When RNA polymerase reaches the terminator sequence or the polyadenylation sequence, it is triggered to release the mRNA transcript and end transcription. Completed mRNA transcripts may be several hundred to several thousand nucleotides in length.

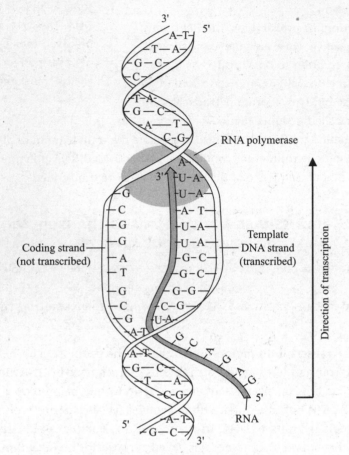

Figure 3.40. Transcription

Errors in transcription. RNA polymerase can proofread the mRNA and identify and correct errors in the growing mRNA transcript. However, RNA polymerase does not proofread as efficiently as does DNA polymerase. Defective copies of mRNA are degraded by **exonucleases**, enzymes that remove nucleotides from the end of a polynucleotide chain.

Posttranscriptional Modification in Eukaryotes

The most significant difference between prokaryotic and eukaryotic RNA synthesis is that in eukaryotes, the mRNA transcript must be modified before it can be translated into protein. This is called **posttranscriptional modification**. Two specific modifications are modifications to the ends of the molecule and RNA splicing.

Modification of 5′ and 3′ ends. Newly synthesized eukaryotic mRNA is called a **primary transcript** or **pre-mRNA**. A **5′ cap** and a **poly-A tail** are added to this primary transcript. The 5′ cap is a guanine nucleotide attached to the 5′ end of the primary transcript by means of a triphosphate linkage. The poly-A tail is a long sequence of up to several hundred adenine nucleotides. The tail is added to the 3′ end of the pre-mRNA after the 5′ untranslated region (5′ UTR).

Both the 5′ cap and the poly-A tail protect the pre-mRNA from breakdown by exonuclease enzymes before the pre-mRNA can exit the nucleus. The end caps also help transport the pre-mRNA out of the nucleus and help bind the mRNA to the ribosomes.

RNA splicing. Before the primary transcript of mRNA can exit the nucleus, it must undergo **RNA splicing** as shown in Figure 3.41. Large regions of eukaryotic pre-mRNA are noncoding **introns** that must be removed before translation. The remaining coding regions, the **exons**, are then spliced back together to form the **mature mRNA** transcript.

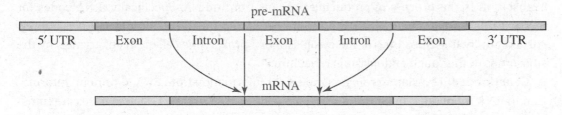

Figure 3.41. RNA splicing of pre-mRNA to generate mature mRNA transcript

The beginning of each intron is marked by a short nucleotide sequence that provides a binding site for **small nuclear ribonucleoproteins** (**snRNPs** = "snurps"), which are complexes of protein and catalytic RNA that aid in RNA splicing in the nucleus. The snRNPs bind with additional proteins to form a **spliceosome**, a large protein/RNA complex that forms a loop in the mRNA transcript, excises the intron, and joins the remaining exon ends together. In other words, snRNPs "snip" the introns. The intron sequences are degraded by exonucleases in the nucleus.

Alternative RNA splicing. In normal RNA splicing, the introns are removed and the exons are spliced together in their original order. In many cases, the exons may be spliced together in a new order. This is called **alternative RNA splicing** or **differential RNA splicing**. In this way, a single transcribed gene can code for more than one protein, depending on the order in which the exons are spliced together. In humans, fewer than 30,000 genes code for more than 2 million proteins. More than 75% of human genes are alternatively spliced.

Remember the difference between introns and exons: exons get to exit the nucleus.

Mature mRNA Transcript

The mature mRNA transcript, which now consists of only exons in the coding region, exits the nucleus through nuclear pores and proceeds to the ribosomes, where it undergoes translation into protein.

Functional and Evolutionary Importance of Introns

Fewer than 1.5% of the 3 billion base pairs of the haploid human genome end up in mature mRNA transcripts that are translated into protein. Introns and the other noncoding regions make up more than 98% of human DNA. Many introns contain sequences that code for regulatory or catalytic RNAs, which play a critical role in gene expression and regulation. However, most noncoding DNA is composed of mobile elements and repetitive DNA.

One significant mobile element is the **transposon** (jumping gene). Transposons are repetitive sequences of DNA that are capable of copying themselves and moving about in the genome. The number and position of transposons is highly variable among individuals and can be used for **DNA fingerprinting** in forensic and paternity analysis. Transposons also include **interspersed elements** such as the **Alu sequence** of 300 bases that is repeated over a million times in human DNA.

Repetitive DNA was initially considered to be junk DNA with no discernable function. However, noncoding repetitive sequences contribute to the genetic diversity of organisms and may play a role in evolution.

Translation

Translation is the process of producing proteins from mRNA. Specifically, RNA codes for amino acids, and amino acids are then combined into proteins by ribosomes. Translation is carried out by free ribosomes in the cytoplasm of a prokaryotic cell or, in eukaryotes, by the ribosomes of the rough endoplasmic reticulum.

Genetic code. Translation converts molecular information from RNA to protein. Information in RNA is encoded by the four nitrogenous bases A, U, C, and G. These bases are translated into 20 different amino acids by the **genetic code** (see Figure 3.42). The genetic code is composed of sequences of three RNA nucleotides, called **triplet codons**, that code for a particular amino acid. In addition, the codon AUG, which codes for the amino acid methionine, is an initiation, or **start codon**, in eukaryotes. The codons UAA, UAG, and UGA are termination, or **stop codons**. Start and stop codons signal the ribosome to begin or end translation. Because the four nucleotides in RNA can be combined in up to 64 triplet combinations, each amino acid, start codon, or stop codon can be coded for by more than one triplet.

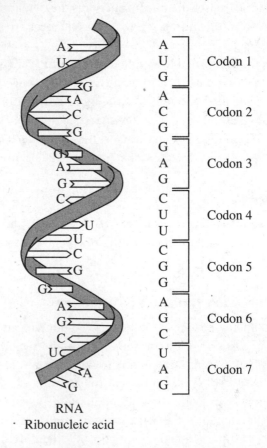

RNA
Ribonucleic acid

Figure 3.42. Triplet codons of nitrogenous bases in mRNA

Figure 3.43 shows the genetic code of RNA. The DNA-based genetic code would be identical with the exception that "T" would replace "U." Whereas the RNA-based genetic code corresponds to the 5'–3' sequence of bases in a molecule of mRNA, the DNA-based genetic code corresponds to the base sequence of the nontemplate, 5'–3' (**sense**) strand of DNA. The genetic code is virtually universal among living things. The same codons specify the same amino acids in organisms as diverse as bacteria, fungi, plants, and humans.

GENETIC ENGINEERING

Because the genetic code is universal, genes from one organism can be transferred to a very different organism through **genetic engineering** and still produce the same protein. For example, genetically modified corn has been created through the insertion of a bacterial gene coding for Bt toxin, a systemic insecticide produced by the bacterium *Bacillus thuringensis.* The Bt toxin incorporated into the corn genome is expressed as protein in all cells of the plant, providing pest resistance.

		2nd base						
		U		**C**		**A**		**G**
1st base	**U**	UUU	Phenylalanine	UCU	Serine	UAU	Tyrosine	UGU	Cysteine
		UUC	Phenylalanine	UCC	Serine	UAC	Tyrosine	UGC	Cysteine
		UUA	Leucine	UCA	Serine	UAA	*Stop*	UGA	*Stop*
		UUG	Leucine	UCG	Serine	UAG	*Stop*	UGG	Tryptophan
	C	CUU	Leucine	CCU	Proline	CAU	Histidine	CGU	Arginine
		CUC	Leucine	CCC	Proline	CAC	Histidine	CGC	Arginine
		CUA	Leucine	CCA	Proline	CAA	Glutamine	CGA	Arginine
		CUG	Leucine	CCG	Proline	CAG	Glutamine	CGG	Arginine
	A	AUU	Isoleucine	ACU	Threonine	AAU	Asparagine	AGU	Serine
		AUC	Isoleucine	ACC	Threonine	AAC	Asparagine	AGC	Serine
		AUA	Isoleucine	ACA	Threonine	AAA	Lysine	AGA	Arginine
		AUG	Methionine (*Start*)	ACG	Threonine	AAG	Lysine	AGG	Arginine
	G	GUU	Valine	GCU	Alanine	GAU	Aspartic acid	GGU	Glycine
		GUC	Valine	GCC	Alanine	GAC	Aspartic acid	GGC	Glycine
		GUA	Valine	GCA	Alanine	GAA	Glutamic acid	GGA	Glycine
		GUG	Valine	GCG	Alanine	GAG	Glutamic acid	GGG	Glycine

Figure 3.43. The RNA-based genetic code

Table 3.4 shows a sequence of DNA with six triplets of bases. The second row shows how these bases are coded for by mRNA. The third row shows the resulting amino acids and stop or start codes. For example, AGA codes for arginine. An MCAT question that tests codons will give you the information you need. You do not need to memorize the codons and amino acids.

Table 3.4 DNA Bases Converted to Codons and Then to Amino Acids

Phase	Codons 1 Through 6					
DNA template strand (3′–5′)	TAC	TCT	GAA	TTA	GAT	ATC
Transcription mRNA transcript (5′–3′)	AUG	AGA	CUU	AAU	CUA	UAG
Translation	Start	Arginine	Leucine	Asparagine	Leucine	Stop

Wobble Pairing. The genetic code allows different mRNA codons to specify a single amino acid through complementary binding to a tRNA molecule. In binding to tRNA, the nucleotide at the third (3′) base position in the mRNA codon can violate Watson–Crick base pairing rules without altering the specified amino acid. For example, an adenine in mRNA could bind to a guanine on the complementary tRNA. This is called **wobble pairing**. Because of wobble pairing and codon variation, the genetic code is considered to be a **degenerate code** in which the 20 amino acids can be specified by more than one codon.

Reading frame. The **reading frame** of the DNA and mRNA bases is critical to gene expression. Each base triplet or codon must be read in the appropriate order, from the 5′ start codon, to result in the correct sequence of amino acids. If the reading frame is shifted by even a single base, an entirely different polypeptide may result, or transcription may fail to initiate or to terminate appropriately. As an analogy, altering the reading frame of "the boy came home" might result in "theb oyca meh ome."

Such a **frameshift** can result from a point mutation in the DNA. For example, the insertion or deletion of a base changes the reading frame. This may create **missense codons**, which result in the substitution of one amino acid for another, altering the polypeptide chain. Alternatively, point mutations may result in a premature mRNA stop codon, or **nonsense codon**, resulting in an incomplete or nonfunctional protein. For example, deletion of the fourth nucleotide in the mRNA sequence AUG-CUA-GAU-UAG results in the frameshift AUG-UAG-AUU-AG, with a nonsense stop codon (UAG) replacing the second triplet. Nonsense codons also include those that do not code for an amino acid.

Structure of tRNA. Transfer RNA (tRNA) consists of a short sequence of approximately 80 nucleotides. Noncovalent attractions between regions of complementary bases form a two-dimensional structure of three hairpin loops in a cloverleaf arrangement. The three-dimensional structure is an "L" shape that allows the tRNA to bind with the ribosome. Figure 3.44 shows the structure of tRNA.

At the end of one of the loops is a sequence of three nucleotides called an **anticodon**. During translation, the anticodon binds with the corresponding codon of mRNA. At the opposite side of the tRNA molecule is the free 3′ end with an amino acid attachment sequence that binds a specific amino acid. Because it can bind both nucleotides and amino acids, tRNA acts as a translator for the conversion of nucleic acids to proteins.

Transfer RNA is transcribed in the nucleus and then travels through nuclear pores to the cytoplasm. To serve its function in protein synthesis, the tRNA molecule must bind to a matching amino acid at the 3′ attachment site. A tRNA molecule with its amino acid attached is called an **aminoacyl-tRNA** and is also referred to as **charged tRNA**. A group of enzymes called **aminoacyl-tRNA synthetases** are responsible for attaching the correct amino acid to a tRNA. There are 20 of these enzymes, corresponding to each of the 20 amino acids. Once a tRNA molecule has given up (**discharged**) its amino acid to a polypeptide, it can be recharged with another amino acid and continue to function.

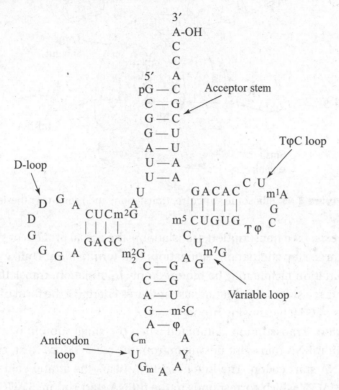

Figure 3.44. Transfer RNA (tRNA)

Structure of ribosomes. The translation of the genetic code into amino acids takes place in the ribosomes (see Figure 3.45). Ribosomes are composed of **two subunits**, one large and one small. Each subunit is composed of both rRNA and protein, with rRNA providing the basic structure of the subunit and acting as a ribozyme. Prokaryotic ribosomes are typically somewhat smaller than eukaryotic ribosomes. Ribosomal subunits are synthesized in the nucleus and exported through nuclear pores to the cytoplasm, endoplasmic reticulum, or nuclear membrane. When the ribosome is not synthesizing proteins, the two subunits are separate.

During translation, the small ribosomal subunit binds to an mRNA molecule. The large ribosomal subunit has three binding sites for tRNA. When the ribosomal subunits come together, they bring the mRNA and tRNA into close contact. An incoming charged tRNA molecule with an anticodon matching the codon of mRNA binds to the first binding site on the large ribosomal subunit, the **A site** (for aminoacyl-tRNA). From the A site, it is moved to the adjacent **P site**, where its corresponding amino acid is removed and is joined to amino acids deposited by the previous tRNAs, forming a growing polypeptide chain. Finally, the tRNA molecule freed of its amino acid leaves the ribosome from the **E site** through an exit tunnel in the large subunit. Once translation is completed, the assembled polypeptide also exits the ribosome through the exit tunnel.

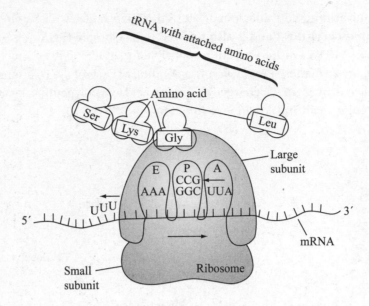

Figure 3.45. Ribosome structure, translation, and protein synthesis

Protein synthesis. Like transcription, translation—the actual process of synthesizing proteins—involves three steps: initiation, elongation, and termination. Unlike transcription, in which protein initiation factors may be required only in initiation, translation requires protein factors in all three stages. Translation also requires energy in the form of the high-energy phosphate bonds of GTP (guanosine triphosphate).

Step 1. Initiation. Transcription is initiated when the small subunit of a ribosome binds to the 5′ end of an mRNA transcript upstream from the start codon. Next, an **initiator tRNA** binds to the mRNA start codon. The initiatior tRNA bears the amino acid methionine and an anticodon 3′ UAC 5′ which corresponds to the mRNA start codon, 5′AUG 3′. The initiator tRNA locks into the starting position on the mRNA and provides a methionine as the first amino acid of the new polypeptide chain.

The large ribosomal subunit binds with the small subunit. This binding requires the assistance of protein **initiation factors** and the hydrolysis of GTP. The combination of both ribosomal subunits with mRNA, initiator tRNA, and protein initiation factors is called the **translation initiation complex**. At the start of translation, the initiator tRNA is bound to the mRNA start codon at the P site of the ribosome, and the A site is open to receive the aminoacyl tRNA (charged tRNA) that will match the next (downstream) codon of mRNA.

Step 2. Elongation. During the next step, elongation, the mRNA feeds through the ribosome in the 5′–3′ direction. New aminoacyl-tRNA molecules move through the ribosome one at a time. First, a charged tRNA binds to an mRNA codon at the A site. Then the aminoacyl-tRNA translocates to the P site, where the amino acid is removed and bound to the growing polypeptide. Finally, the molecule exits as tRNA from the E site. Each addition of amino acid and translocation of tRNA requires protein **elongation factors** as well as energy from the hydrolysis of GTP.

Step 3. Termination. The termination of translation is signaled when the mRNA stop codon enters the ribosome. Because there is no amino acid that corresponds to a stop codon, protein **release factors** bind to the stop codon and add a molecule of water instead of an amino acid to the C-terminus of the polypeptide at the P site. This process requires energy in the form of GTP. The addition of a water molecule triggers the release of the polypeptide from the ribosome. The translation complex then is disassembled and the ribosomal subunits separate.

Polyribosomes. In both prokaryotes and eukaryotes, more than one ribosome at a time may translate the same mRNA transcript to speed translation, forming strings of ribosomes called polyribosomes.

Coupling of transcription and translation. In prokaryotes, transcription and translation both occur in the cytoplasm and are coupled. RNA polymerase begins transcribing the circular molecule of DNA. As soon as the 5′ end of the mRNA transcript is free of the DNA template, ribosomes bind the mRNA and begin translation. As a result, proteins can be rapidly synthesized and distributed throughout the cell. In eukaryotes, transcription and translation are not coupled because mRNA must be posttranscriptionally modified to remove introns and must exit the nucleus before translation can begin.

Posttranslational modification of polypeptides. After the translation process is completed, the newly formed polypeptides may undergo further modification (posttranslational modification) before becoming functional. Posttranslational modification can include the removal of the initial methionine from the polypeptide chain or the cleavage of portions of the polypeptide chain to convert an inactive preprotein or zymogen to an active protein. For example, proinsulin is synthesized as a single polypeptide that must undergo cleavage and modification to form two subunits joined by a sulfide bridge, the active form of insulin. Other posttranslational modifications of proteins include glycosylation, methylation, and phosphorylation. In eukaryotes, posttranslational modification may occur in the cytoplasm or within the rough endoplasmic reticulum or Golgi body.

REGULATION OF GENE EXPRESSION

Transcription and translation are strictly regulated in biological systems so that genes are expressed only in the proper amounts and at the proper times. Multiple feedback pathways provide for **up-regulation** (**gene activation** or **induction**) and **down-regulation** (**gene repression**) of genes and gene products. For example, certain genes may be expressed at only certain times during development. Genes may also be activated or silenced to allow specific cell types to perform specific functions in a multicellular organism. Regulatory control mechanisms prevent unregulated metabolic processes that can disrupt homeostasis and lead to metabolic disorders and cancer.

Prokaryotic Gene Regulation

A common pathway for gene expression in prokaryotes is the **operon**. An operon consists of several structural genes in series, along with an upstream regulatory **promoter** and **operator**. When the operon is activated, it allows for simultaneous coordinated expression of all the structural genes on a single mRNA molecule. The concept of an operon was developed as the **Jacob–Monod model** of gene regulation, based on research on the **lac operon**, a set of genes in *E. coli* bacteria that code for enzymes necessary to digest lactose. These genes, *lacZ*, *lacY*, and *lacA*, code for β-galactosidase and β-galactoside enzymes, which catalyze the breakdown of lactose and the transport of lactose into the cell. Figure 3.46 shows the reaction pathway of lactose breakdown and the structure of the lac operon.

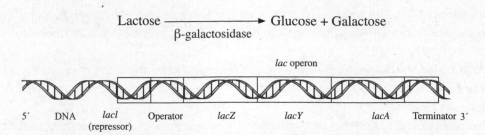

Figure 3.46. The lac operon transcription pathway in *E. coli*

The lac operon exhibits two forms of gene regulation, gene repression and positive control. These regulatory mechanisms prevent the bacterial cell from synthesizing enzymes when the substrate is absent or when a preferred energy source is available.

Gene repression. The lac operon genes are activated only when lactase is present and glucose levels are low. When lactose is absent, the lac operon is turned off through **gene repression** by a nearby repressor gene, *lacl. Lacl* codes for a protein that binds to the operator sequence of the lac operon and blocks transcription by RNA polymerase. When lactose is present and glucose is low, an isomer of lactose, allolactose, binds to the repressor protein and reduces its affinity for the operator. RNA polymerase can then bind to the promoter and proceed to transcribe the lac structural genes. The lac operon is an example of an **inducible operon** because transcription of the operon is normally repressed, a form of **negative control**. The substrate lactose acts as an effector protein to induce transcription.

Positive control. Even if lactose is present, the lac operon genes will not be transcribed if the preferred energy source, glucose, is available. This form of transcriptional regulation is called **positive control**. Positive control requires the presence of an activator molecule that binds to an inducer protein, which, in turn, binds to DNA to promote transcription. In the lac operon, **cyclic AMP** (**cAMP**) is an activator molecule. When cAMP is present, it binds to **catabolite activator protein** (**CAP**), a DNA binding protein, to form a **CAP–cAMP complex**. Binding of the CAP–cAMP complex to the lac operon promoter region in turn increases the affinity of RNA polymerase for a second binding site on the promoter. As a result, positive control by the CAP–cAMP complex enhances transcription of the lac operon. However, when glucose is present, cAMP levels are low. The reduction in the CAP–cAMP complex reduces the binding affinity of RNA polymerase and reduces lac operon transcription.

> **REGULATORY CONTROL OF LAC OPERON**
>
> **Glucose absent, lactose present:** high lactose levels, high cAMP, Lac operon transcribed
>
> **Glucose present, lactose present:** high lactose levels, low cAMP, Lac operon not transcribed

Eukaryotic Gene Regulation

In eukaryotes, genes are not organized into operons. Instead, gene regulation includes the removal of introns and alternative RNA splicing, which allows for a single region of DNA to code for multiple proteins (see page 383). In addition to RNA splicing, eukaryotic gene regulation includes the regulation of chromatin structure, transcriptional regulation, and post-transcriptional gene regulation by noncoding RNA.

Regulation of chromatin structure. In eukaryotes, the coiling of DNA is a mechanism for regulating gene expression because genes in more tightly coiled regions are less accessible for transcription.

DNA is wrapped around histones into nucleosomes, which form the basic building blocks of chromatin. Chromatin may in turn be further coiled or supercoiled to further condense the DNA. Genes that occur in tightly condensed regions of chromatin, such as heterochromatin, are inaccessible for transcription. For a gene to be expressed, the chromatin must be unwound to expose the DNA for transcription.

Chromatin can be either uncoiled or more tightly coiled by several processes. Chromatin can be uncoiled (exposing regions of DNA for transcription) by adding acetyl groups to the N-terminus of histone proteins in nucleosomes, a process called **histone acetylation**. Chromatin can be more tightly coiled by **deacetylation** and **methylation** of histones, effectively silencing the gene by preventing transcription. The conversion of chromatin to tightly wound heterochromatin results in the deactivation of any associated genes. This deactivation can be passed from cell to cell during cell division and from one generation to the next in a form of **epigenetic inheritance**, the inheritance of acquired traits that are not encoded by the sequence of bases in the DNA. Epigenetic inheritance caused by modifications to chromatin during development can contribute to phenotypic differences between genetically identical organisms such as identical twins. Epigenetic inheritance may also affect the risk of cancer and cardiovascular disease in offspring through several generations.

DNA methylation. Methylation of cytosine or adenine bases in DNA is another critically important means of gene regulation that acts by affecting chromatin structure. DNA methylation can act epigenetically to stabilize a particular pattern of gene expression through multiple mitotic divisions, providing a means of turning genes off and on as necessary during development and cell differentiation. Methylated bases interact with proteins to deacetylate histones, condense DNA, and silence gene expression. In adult mammalian cells, approximately 70% of cytosine bases are methylated. DNA methylation is also a defense against viral DNA and mobile genetic elements and is responsible for deactivating regions of repetitive DNA into heterochromatin (see Figure 3.47).

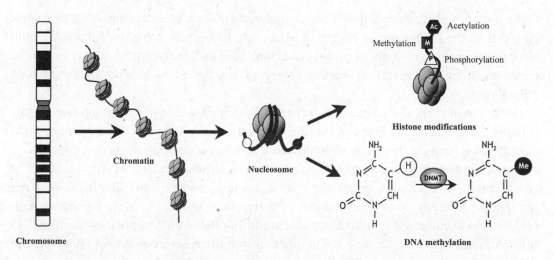

Figure 3.47. DNA regulation through DNA methylation and histone modification

Transcriptional regulation. In eukaryotic cells, a group of **DNA binding proteins** called **transcription factors** must bind to the promoter to start transcription (see Figure 3.48). In order for transcription factors to bind, the DNA must be arranged so that the promoter region is brought into proximity with separate regions of noncoding DNA called **control elements**. Control elements may be located near the promoter (proximal control elements) or at some distance away within an intron or on a different region of the chromosome (distal control elements). Approximately a dozen control element sequences may be arranged in different combinations for different genes. A group of distal control elements is called an **enhancer**. A group of genes on the same chromosome or different chromosomes may have copies of the same enhancer, allowing for **coordinate control of gene expression**.

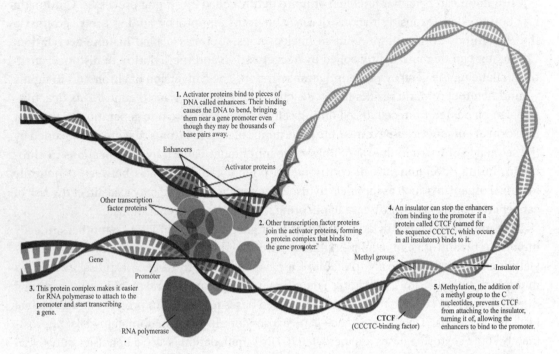

Figure 3.48. Transcription factors of eukaryotic cells. Note that this drawing provides a simplified perspective of DNA structure. Promoters, enhancers, and insulators can be hundreds of base pairs long.

To initiate transcription, specific transcription factors called **activators** bind to control elements in the enhancer and trigger DNA bending proteins to bring the enhancer region close to the promoter. **Mediator proteins** can then bind with transcription factors to link the enhancer and promoter regions together to form a transcription initiation complex with RNA polymerase.

Inhibition of transcription can also occur through **repressor proteins** that interact directly with the DNA. These repressor proteins can bind with control elements to inhibit transcription directly. These can also indirectly inhibit transcription by promoting histone deacetylation.

Gene regulation by noncoding RNA. The role of noncoding RNA in the regulation of gene expression is a rapidly expanding area of genetic research. Noncoding RNAs are short sequences of single- or double-stranded RNA that bind to mRNA. These regulatory molecules include **microRNA (miRNA)**, **small interfering RNA (siRNA)**, **piwi-interacting RNA (piRNA)**, and others. Noncoding RNAs function in posttranscriptional **RNA silencing** and **RNA interference** to prevent the translation of target mRNA. They bind to complementary sequences on mRNA and degrade or cleave the mRNA to prevent translation. Alternatively, they may block the binding of mRNA to the ribosome. Still other noncoding RNAs regulate gene expression through histone modification and other modification of chromatin structure. When noncoding RNAs block the translation of regulatory transcription factors they can act as downregulators of gene expression, affecting entire complexes of genes. Others act as upregulators and activators by binding to a promoter sequence to enhance transcription.

One of the primary functions of noncoding RNAs is to protect the cell from retroviruses and transposons. Some types of microRNAs are involved in regulation of the cell cycle, and malfunctioning miRNA may play a role in the development of cancer and heart disease.

Recombinant DNA and Biotechnology

Recombinant DNA (**rDNA**) has been altered through genetic engineering to combine two or more sources of DNA, creating a DNA sequence that does not occur in nature. Recombinant DNA technology has been used to produce synthetic insulin and growth hormone, to create transgenic crops designed to resist herbicides and crop pests, and to provide gene therapy for treating genetic disorders. Cells containing recombinant DNA are said to have been **genetically modified** through the process of **genetic engineering**. Organisms containing recombinant DNA are called **genetically modified organisms** (**GMOs**).

PRODUCING RECOMBINANT DNA

Creating recombinant DNA requires the use of restriction endonucleases, or **restriction enzymes**, which are derived from bacteria. Bacteria use restriction enzymes as a defense against viral infection, chopping up invading viral DNA into small pieces. These enzymes can be applied in biotechnology to cut a DNA molecule at a specific sequence of nucleotides. For example, the restriction enzyme *Eco*R1 will cut the DNA strand everywhere it encounters the following sequence:

$$5' \text{ G} \,|\, \text{A A T T C} \; 3'$$
$$3' \text{ C T T A A} \,|\, \text{G} \; 5'$$

Note that the vertical lines indicate where cuts would take place.

*Eco*R1 will cut both strands of the sequence shown in Figure 3.49 between the bases G and A, as shown by the marker lines. Because the strands are antiparallel, the ends of cut strands will be offset. The projecting bases on the 5′ ends are called **sticky ends**. The cut DNA strands can be mixed with other sources of DNA that have been cut by the same restriction enzyme, and all the sticky ends will be complementary to one another. In this way, two different sources of DNA can be recombined by the attraction between their sticky ends. The ends are then joined by DNA ligase (Figure 3.49).

GENETIC MODIFICATION

Recombinant DNA can be inserted into target cells by several means. **Transformation** involves the addition of foreign DNA into self-replicating bacterial plasmids, as shown in Figure 3.49. The plasmids are then reinserted into bacterial cells. As the bacteria replicate, they reproduce not only their own DNA but also the inserted sequence. Bacteria capable of taking up DNA from their environment, or **exogenous DNA**, are said to be **competent**. Typically, a marker, such as a gene for antibiotic resistance, is used to identify and isolate recombinant bacterial cultures. Bacteria may also take up exogenous DNA directly from the environment or through bacterial conjugation. **Transduction** is the insertion of exogenous DNA into bacteria by a bacteriophage virus.

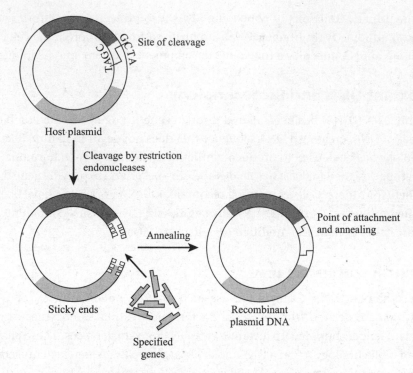

Figure 3.49. Producing recombinant plasmid DNA

Introduction of foreign DNA into a eukaryotic cell is termed **transfection**. Both transformation and transfection can be accomplished by mechanical or chemical means. These include the application of DNA in a calcium phosphate solution, the use of an external electric field to perforate the cell wall or membrane, the use of DNA-containing liposomes, or the use of a **gene gun** to shoot DNA directly into a target eukaryotic cell.

GENE CLONING

Gene cloning is the process of using recombinant DNA technology to make identical copies of a gene within living cells. In molecular cloning, the gene of interest is cut out of the source DNA by restriction enzymes and recombined with vector DNA. Vectors may be bacterial plasmids or bacteriophage DNA. The recombinant DNA is then inserted into bacterial cells. When the bacterial host cells replicate, they will replicate the gene insert. In this way, the inserted gene can be copied rapidly or amplified. Gene cloning is used to amplify a gene for study or to express and purify large quantities of protein coded for by the gene insert. Cloned genes are frequently maintained in gene or DNA libraries (see below.)

> ### CLONING OF HUMAN INSULIN
>
> Biosynthetic insulin for treatment of diabetes can be manufactured by recombinant DNA technology. The gene for insulin is cloned into *E. coli*. The bacteria then express the gene to produce human insulin, which is harvested for medical use.

DNA LIBRARIES

A **DNA library** consists of a set of fragments of DNA that are maintained in culture within the genome of a host organism, such as *E. coli*. The DNA to be maintained in a library is cut into various sized fragments by restriction enzymes. These fragments are cloned into a pool of genetically modified bacteria that replicate the inserted fragments along with their own DNA. The cultured bacteria collectively maintain the DNA library of the entire set of fragments.

DNA libraries can be composed of **genomic DNA** or **cDNA** (**complementary DNA**). A **genomic DNA library** consists of the entire genome of an organism that is maintained as a collection of spliced restriction fragments in a culture of host cells. Alternatively, a DNA library may contain only DNA sequences of the expressed genes from a given tissue. To obtain DNA only from genes that are actively expressed, an mRNA transcript is used to synthesize complementary DNA, or cDNA. In cDNA cloning, the retroviral enzyme **reverse transcriptase** synthesizes a single-stranded cDNA copy from the mRNA template. Then DNA polymerase converts the single-stranded cDNA into double-stranded cDNA. Because the mRNA transcript contains only exons, the cDNA copy contains only those DNA sequences that are being expressed by the cell. The complementary DNA is then spliced into bacterial plasmids using molecular cloning techniques as described above.

DNA libraries function as a repository and source of target DNA sequences. The library can be screened for clones containing desired sequences. For example, target DNA can be marked with a gene for antibiotic resistance, and the library can be screened by antibiotic selection. DNA libraries are used to study which genes are expressed in different tissues, to identify genes that produce particular proteins, and to analyze gene expression and gene function.

GEL ELECTROPHORESIS AND SOUTHERN BLOT

DNA sequences can be compared through the use of gel electrophoresis and Southern blot. In **gel electrophoresis**, restriction enzymes are used to cut the DNA at specific sequences of bases called restriction sites. DNA fragments are then transferred to an agarose or polyacrilymide gel and subjected to electric current, the process of gel electrophoresis (*electro* means charge; *phoresis* means carry). Negatively charged DNA fragments will migrate through the gel toward the positive pole with smaller fragments traveling faster and farther than larger fragments, causing segregation of DNA fragments by size. The DNA on the gel is visualized using stain or radioactive marker probe to reveal a pattern of bands of different densities and distances which correspond to the DNA fragments of different lengths. (See Figure 3.50.)

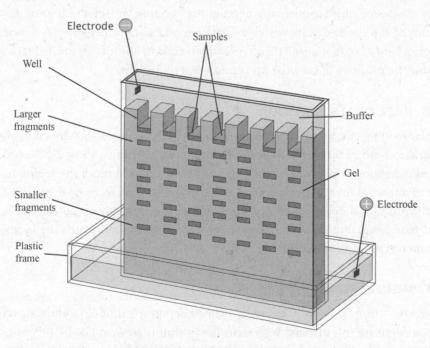

Figure 3.50. Gel electrophoresis

In a **Southern blot**, the DNA fragments are transferred from the electrophoresis gel to a membrane and then probed for a particular gene or target sequence. First, the DNA bands are treated to denature the DNA into single strands. Then the single-stranded DNA is hybridized with a labeled single-stranded DNA probe that will bind to complementary sequences on the membrane. The membrane is then treated to allow visualization of the hybridized bands, indicating the size and position of the target DNA sequences.

Electrophoresis and Southern blot can be used to screen for a particular gene or to determine the number of copies of a gene in a genome.

ANALYZING GENE EXPRESSION AND GENE FUNCTION

While the Southern blot uses electrophoresis to separate DNA, the **northern blot** is a similar technique used to separate fragments of mRNA. Northern Blot is used to analyze how much mRNA is being produced by different genes in different cells or tissues. Other techniques to analyze gene expression include **microarrays** and **serial analysis of gene expression** (SAGE), which allow for the screening of transcripts from thousands of genes expressed simultaneously in a particular tissue. These techniques are useful for comparing patterns of gene expression between tissues and during different times of development. Once active genes are identified in a tissue, their function can be analyzed through gene deletion or inhibition of gene expression. For example, "**knockout**" mice genetically engineered to lack a particular gene are studied to determine the effect of the missing gene on phenotype and behavior.

DNA SEQUENCING

DNA sequencing involves determining the sequence of nitrogenous bases of a single gene, a region of DNA, or an entire genome. DNA sequencing involves separating the strands of a region of DNA and synthesizing a new complementary strand using labeled nucleotides. The labeled strands of DNA are then separated and analyzed on an electrophoresis gel using X-ray film, fluorescent emissions, or other techniques. Automated high-throughput sequencing now allows for rapid sequencing of an entire genome within a matter of days or hours. The ability to rapidly and inexpensively sequence genes or entire genomes is essential to the developing field of personalized medicine, which aims to identify an individual's genetic risk factors for the purpose of targeted prevention and treatment.

POLYMERASE CHAIN REACTION

Molecular cloning can amplify DNA in cell culture. DNA can also be cloned in vitro through **polymerase chain reaction**, or **PCR**. PCR can rapidly amplify a short DNA sequence. DNA is heated to separate the strands, and primers are inserted to mark the region to be copied. The temperature is lowered, and a DNA polymerase enzyme from heat-resistant bacteria is used to synthesize a complementary strand. Once the strand is complete, the temperature is raised again, causing the new strand to separate from the template. The cycle is repeated many times to amplify the DNA.

DNA HYBRIDIZATION

DNA hybridization involves the use of heat to separate complementary strands of DNA, which can then be re-annealed with DNA from another source. As the mixture cools, DNA strands will bind together at regions of complementary bases. Hybrid DNA can be used as a **probe** for specific sequences of DNA within the genome. DNA hybridization has also been used to examine evolutionary relationships between organisms. When marked DNA of a known sequence is hybridized with unknown DNA, the annealed strands will reveal the location of specific DNA sequences, allowing rapid determination of the unknown sequence structure.

STEM CELLS

Stem cells are unspecialized cells that have the capacity to divide indefinitely and differentiate into a variety of cell and tissue types. Stem cells are found in embryos, in umbilical cord blood and amniotic fluid, and in some adult tissues. The stem cells of a blastula embryo inner cell mass are **totipotent**, having the ability to differentiate into all cell types, including into a complete organism. After four days of development, embryonic stem cells differentiate into **pluripotent** cells, capable of generating cells of all tissue types except for the extra-embryonic membranes. These pluripotent cells eventually differentiate further and become **multipotent** stem cells that can give rise only to cells within a single tissue type. Most adult stem cells are multipotent.

Research into the therapeutic use of stem cells has examined their use as a source of readily-dividing undifferentiated cells, which could be used to repair and replace damaged tissue. The harvest of embryonic stem cells for this purpose has raised ethical concerns. However, pleuripotency has been successfully induced in adult stem cells, resulting in **induced pleuripotent stem cells**, which have characteristics similar to embryonic stem cells. These induced stem cells, in turn, have been cultured and transplanted to regenerate cells such as neurons. Stem cell therapy is currently used as a treatment for leukemia and is a potential therapy for brain and spinal cord injury, Parkinson's disease, Alzheimer's disease, burn injuries, and other conditions that require cell regeneration and tissue replacement.

PRACTICAL APPLICATIONS OF DNA TECHNOLOGY

DNA technology is being developed for an ever-increasing number of applications in our society. Gel electrophoresis and DNA fingerprinting techniques are used to identify people for paternity analysis and forensics. Recombinant DNA and gene cloning are used in genetic engineering to produce transgenic crops (GMOs) that increase yields, resist herbicides and agricultural pests, or produce pharmaceutical drugs ("**pharming**"). Designer microbes can be engineered to break down environmental toxins or produce biofuels. Medical applications of DNA technology include gene therapy for treating genetic disorders, stem cell therapy to repair or replace damaged tissues and organs, the production of recombinant or synthetic insulin and growth hormone, and the development of personalized medicine, among a rapidly expanding list of other possibilities.

SAFETY AND ETHICS OF DNA TECHNOLOGY

The use of DNA technology is not without safety and ethical issues. Although genetically modified foods have been shown in many studies to be substantially equivalent to traditional crops, their safety continues to be questioned. A plan to produce a nutritionally enhanced soybean by incorporating genes from Brazil nuts was abandoned after the transgenic soy was found to be potentially allergenic. Other GMO crops have been modified to contain systemic pesticides, which may contribute to the decline of pollinators. Drug pharming poses the risk of drug-producing genes escaping into crops intended for food. Similarly, transgenic animals and plants may alter ecosystems if they escape into the wild.

Ethical issues raised by developing biotechnology have been raised about the feasibility and desirability of cloning humans or extinct animals, the use of fetal cells for research, and the use of patient DNA or cell cultures obtained without consent. Although genetic screening of embryos may be highly useful for identifying genetic disorders during pregnancy, genetic screening could also give parents the option of selecting embryos for particular traits such as sex or hair or eye color. Also, the availability of individual genetic profiles may aid in the development of personalized medicine, but the dissemination of such information to insurers or other agencies could raise privacy concerns.

TEST QUESTION

The genetic code refers to:

(A) the sequence of amino acids in a protein.

(B) the sequence of nucleotides in a DNA molecule.

(C) the relationship between mRNA triplet codons and amino acids.

(D) the sequence of nitrogenous bases in mRNA.

(C) The genetic code is the relationship between the codons, or triplet sequences of nitrogenous bases in mRNA, and the amino acids they code for in translation. The molecule tRNA acts as the translator of the code by bearing specific amino acids to bind to specific mRNA codons at the ribosome. The genetic code can be represented by a table showing the amino acid specified by each particular mRNA codons.

EUKARYOTIC CELL REPLICATION

Eukaryotic cells progress through a life cycle, or cell cycle, from one cycle of cell division to the next. Regulation of the cell cycle is critical to proper growth and development. In multicellular organisms, defects in the cell cycle and unregulated cell division lead to cancer.

The Cell Cycle

The **cell cycle consists** of several stages, including cell growth, DNA replication, and cell division. The cell cycle is typically represented as a circle. The time between cell divisions is called the **generation time** of a cell. Generation times vary greatly between different types of cells. Bacteria have extremely rapid generation times, doubling their numbers in less than half an hour. Eukaryotic cells may have generation times of many hours or days.

INTERPHASE (G_1, G_0, S, G_2)

A cell that is not currently dividing is said to be in **interphase**. During interphase, the cell grows, carries out normal activities of cellular metabolism, and replicates its DNA for future cell division. Cells spend most of their lives in interphase. Interphase can be broken into three subphases, called the **first gap** (**Gap 1** or G_1), **synthesis** (**S**), and the **second gap** (**Gap 2** or G_2). A newly created cell enters G_1, during which it grows and synthesizes RNA and proteins. At some point, the cell is triggered to begin synthesizing copies of its DNA. This stage is the S (synthesis) phase. After the S phase, the cell enters G_2, the second gap phase. During both G_1 and G_2, the cell grows, undergoes RNA and protein synthesis, and performs its normal functions. The amount of time a cell spends in each gap phase varies among different types of cells and different types of organisms.

During the two gap phases, the G_1 and G_2 **checkpoint** or **restriction point mechanisms** regulate cell division. Cell checkpoints prevent damaged cells from continuing on to cell division, and healthy cells from dividing inappropriately. Cells that pass all checkpoints continue through the cell cycle and, after G_2 of interphase, enter the first stage of mitosis.

Cells that do not pass the checkpoint (and, therefore, will not divide further) may go into **growth arrest**, entering a Gap 0 or G_0 phase. Certain types of cells remain in G_0 for extended periods. These include nerve, muscle, liver, and cardiac cells. Liver cells can exit G_0 and return to the cell cycle in the case of liver damage or injury. Damaged or mutated cells that are arrested from further cell division at regulatory checkpoints typically undergo apoptosis, or programmed cell death.

> ### DNA IN INTERPHASE
>
> Although interphase chromatin is not condensed into darkly staining chromosomes, the term chromosome may still be used by convention in reference to the number of DNA molecules in a cell, regardless of the stage in the cell cycle. True condensed chromosomes are visible only during the stages of mitosis and meiosis.

Interphase Chromatin

During interphase, chromosomes are not condensed as darkly staining bodies. Instead, DNA remains in the form of chromatin. Interphase chromatin can be loosely wrapped or tightly coiled. Loosely coiled DNA, or euchromatin, exposes regions of the DNA to allow for transcription and gene expression. Tightly coiled heterochromatin is not accessible for transcription. Under a light microscope, interphase chromatin appears as a granular material in the nucleus, with the darkly staining heterochromatin concentrated near the nuclear membrane.

When the DNA is replicated during the S phase, the DNA copies, or sister chromatids, join at the centromere of a duplicated chromosome. Each sister chromatid is attached to a cluster of proteins called a **kinetochore**, which is linked to the centromere. Kinetochores facing opposite directions bind the sister chromatids together and act as attachment points for microtubules during mitosis. Sister chromatids are also bound together by **cohesin** proteins that run the length of each chromatid.

By convention, DNA replication and the formation of duplicated chromosomes does not change chromosome number. A human cell in G_1 has 46 unduplicated chromosomes, which belong to 23 homologous pairs. In G_2, the same cell still has 46 chromosomes and 23 homologous pairs, although the chromosomes are now duplicated chromosomes, each consisting of two sister chromatids.

> ### CENTROMERE
>
> When a chromosome replicates before cell division, two identical copies called **sister chromatids** are temporarily joined together at the centromere into a single, X-shaped duplicated chromosome. The location of the centromere can vary along the length of the chromosome between different homologous pairs.

Mitotic Spindle

The **mitotic spindle** or **spindle apparatus** ultimately separates the chromosomes into the daughter cells during mitosis. The spindle is composed of microtubules, proteins, and centrosomes. During mitosis, centrosome pairs organize the mitotic spindle. During the S phase of interphase, centrosome replication occurs at the same time as DNA replication, paving the way for mitosis to occur after G_2.

SISTER CHROMATIDS VERSUS HOMOLOGOUS CHROMOSOMES

Sister chromatids and homologous chromosomes are not the same. Sister chromatids are identical copies of the same DNA molecule, joined at the centromere of a single duplicated chromosome. Homologous chromosomes, in contrast, are different molecules of DNA. In a pair of homologous chromosomes, one chromosome comes from the father and one from the mother. During cell division, a homologous pair is visible as two stained dyads of similar size and shape. Because of their different source, homologous chromosomes look similar but carry slightly different versions of the same genes.

MITOSIS AND CYTOKINESIS

The mitotic (M) phase of the cell cycle includes mitosis and cytokinesis. Mitosis is division of chromosomes. Cytokinesis is the division of cytoplasm. Mitosis has four stages: prophase, metaphase, anaphase, and telophase. Figure 3.51 summarizes the process of mitosis, and Figure 3.52 illustrates the process in more detail.

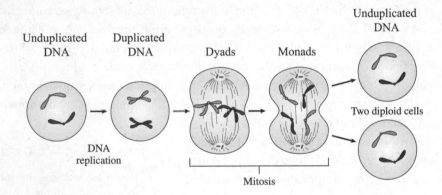

Figure 3.51. Summary of mitosis

Prophase

At the beginning of prophase, tightly coiled, duplicated chromosomes condense and become visible under a light microscope as **dyads**, condensed, darkly staining, X-shaped structures in the nucleus. The nuclear membrane and nucleolus disappear. The mitotic spindle begins to form as microtubules grow outward from each centriole pair, forming a star-shaped array called an **aster**. Centrosomes are pushed apart by the growing spindle apparatus.

Metaphase

By metaphase, the nucleus has disappeared. Dyad chromosomes are lined up along the metaphase plate (midline of the cell). The centrosomes have reached the opposite poles of the cell. Spindle microtubules extending from the asters are attached to the kinetochores of each sister chromatid. Other spindle fiber microtubules remain unattached, overlapping microtubules from the opposite side.

Anaphase

During anaphase, the sister chromatids of duplicated chromosomes are pulled apart to form separate, unduplicated chromosomes, or **monads**. Cohesin proteins joining sister chromatids are broken apart by enzymes. Motor proteins powered by ATP guide the chromatids along the spindle microtubules toward the centrosomes. The spindle fibers connected to each kinetochore shorten by depolymerization. At the same time, unattached microtubules lengthen and push against adjacent microtubules, extending the cell. Consequently, the newly formed monad chromosomes move toward opposite poles of the cell.

Telophase and Cytokinesis

In telophase, monad chromosomes reach opposite poles of the cell and decondense back into unduplicated chromatin. The nuclear membrane reforms around each new nucleus, and the cytoplasm divides by cytokinesis. In animal cells, cytokinesis occurs when the plasma membrane of the cell invaginates, forming a **cleavage furrow** that splits the cell in two. The cleavage furrow is formed by a band of actin microfilaments and myosin protein. This band constricts around the cell.

In plant cells, cytokinesis involves the formation of a **cell plate**. Transport vesicles from the Golgi body fuse together and deposit material for the formation of a new cell wall down the midline of the cell. When the cell plate fuses with the plasma membrane, the original cell is divided in two.

Mitosis results in two daughter cells that are identical to the parent cell and identical to each other. Daughter cells have the same number of chromosomes and the same number of homologous pairs as the parent cell. Mitotic cell division creates new cells for growth, repair, and the development of a fertilized egg into a multicellular adult. Some eukaryotes, such as protists and fungi, use forms of mitotic cell division for asexual reproduction.

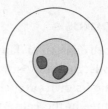

Interphase

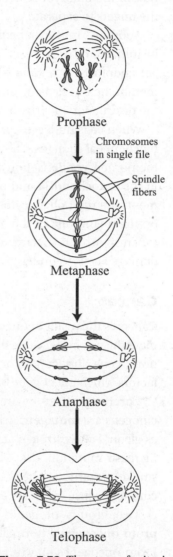

Prophase

Chromosomes in single file

Spindle fibers

Metaphase

Anaphase

Telophase

Figure 3.52. The steps of mitosis: (1) Prophase; (2) Metaphase; (3) Anaphase; (4) Telophase

---

BIOSIGNALING AND FEEDBACK IN MITOSIS

Mitosis must be tightly regulated to coordinate the timing of spindle assembly and disassembly, chromosome movement, sister chromatid separation, and cytokinesis. Critical enzymes involved in on/off feedback regulation and biosignaling during this process are **protein kinases** and **mitotic phosphatases**.

Apoptosis

The cell division of damaged cells is arrested by mitotic checkpoints. These cells are triggered to undergo apoptosis, or programmed cell death. A cell that is damaged or infected may initiate its own programmed cell death, or cell suicide, triggered by the release of caspase enzymes in the cell. Apoptosis may be initiated as a result of membrane or DNA damage from ionizing radiation, free radicals, viral infection, or other sources of stress. Apoptosis is a normal process during development and cell differentiation. For example, during the formation of the embryonic hand, cells between developing fingers undergo apoptosis, allowing the fingers to separate.

Apoptosis may also be triggered by extrinsic signals from other cells. For example, it can be initiated by the direct binding of immune system cells. Cytotoxic T lymphocytes may trigger apoptosis by a variety of mechanisms, including binding to "death receptors" in a cell membrane or releasing enzymes (granzymes) that activate intracellular caspases to initiate the destruction of virus-infected cells.

When cells undergo apoptosis, they follow a characteristic pattern of morphological and biochemical changes. These include shrinkage, development of buds or "blebs" on the outer membrane, condensation and rupture of the nucleus, and increased membrane permeability in the mitochondria and other organelles, terminating in the rupture of the cell. Cell fragments are then phagocytosed by other cells attracted to "death signal" molecules displayed on the membrane of the dying cell. Programmed cell death does not initiate an inflammatory response and occurs without causing damage to adjacent cells. The failure of genetically damaged cells to undergo apoptosis can lead to cancer.

Cancer

Cancer is the result of uncontrolled cell division due to the malfunctioning of genes that regulate the cell cycle. Gene malfunction can be caused by genetic factors, such as point mutations, gene duplication, or chromosomal translocation. It can also be caused by epigenetic factors which affect gene expression, such as alterations in DNA methylation.

Carcinogens are environmental factors that are capable of causing cancer. Many carcinogens are **mutagens**, which directly damage the DNA. However, other carcinogens, such as alcohol and estrogen, are nonmutagenic factors that overstimulate cell division and thus increase mutation risk. Carcinogens include ultraviolet and ionizing radiation, tobacco smoke, hazardous chemicals, and viruses. In humans, viral infection is the second-most common cause of cancer after tobacco.

Two groups of genes are generally involved in cancer development. One group, **proto-oncogenes**, normally codes for proteins involved in cell growth and cell division. Proto-oncogenes may be converted into cancer-causing **oncogenes**, which actively promote cell division by transcribing proteins such as growth factors. Oncogenes stimulate cells to divide excessively.

Another group of genes, called **tumor-suppressor genes**, normally act as checkpoints to prevent inappropriate cell division, even when oncogenes are present. Tumor-suppressor genes activate DNA repair processes in damaged cells and can arrest the cell cycle to allow for repair. If the DNA cannot be repaired, tumor-suppressor genes trigger programmed cell death, or apoptosis.

The development of cancer typically involves the accumulation of multiple mutations in both oncogenes and tumor-suppressor genes, leading to an increase in cancer risk with age.

Cancer cells can also result when the gene for the production of telomerase enzyme is activated. When this happens, the string of telomeres is not shortened after each cell division and the cells divide indefinitely. An interesting example of indefinite cell division caused by an active telomerase enzyme is seen in cells in the tissue culture line HeLa. HeLa cells were derived from a cancerous lesion taken from a patient in the 1950s and continue to be used as an immortal cell line for medical and genetic research.

TEST QUESTION

The tumor suppressor protein p53 is an important regulator of the cell cycle in multicellular organisms, acting to prevent uncontrolled cell division, tumor formation, and cancer. In humans, p53 is encoded by the *TP53* gene located on chromosome 17. The protein acts as a transcription factor that activates or represses genes in damaged cells to arrest the cell cycle, activate DNA repair proteins, and, in severely damaged cells, initiate apoptosis, or programmed cell death. In a healthy cell, p53 is continuously produced and broken down by binding to the protein Mdm2, which targets p53 for degradation. When a cell is subject to environmental stress such as UV radiation, a protein kinase–mediated signal cascade triggers the phosphorylation of the p53 N-terminus, preventing Mdm2 from binding and increasing p53 levels. Other protein coactivators acetylate the p53 C-terminus to expose the DNA binding region, enabling p53 to bind to target DNA.

A nonsense mutation in the DNA binding region of *TP53* would:

I. originate from an error in translation.
II. result in a functional mRNA transcript but a truncated protein.
III. lead to cancer in cells with one or more mutations in an oncogene.
IV. result in growth arrest and apoptosis.

(A) I and II only
(B) III only
(C) II and III only
(D) II and IV only

(C) Options II and III are both correct. A nonsense mutation in the TP53 gene would result from a base substitution during DNA replication that leads to a misplaced stop codon in the intact mRNA transcript. Option I can be eliminated because a mutation in the TP53 gene would occur during DNA replication, not during translation. Option II is correct because the nonsense mutation would not interfere with transcription. However, when the mRNA transcript is translated by the ribosome, the resulting protein would be truncated and nonfunctional. Option III is correct because cancer develops as a result of mutations in both proto-oncogenes and tumor-suppressor genes. A mutant oncogene stimulates inappropriate cell division. A mutant tumor-suppressor gene fails to repair the damaged oncogene and allows the cell cycle to proceed uncontrollably.

Option IV can be eliminated because a nonfunctional, mutant p53 protein would lose the ability to arrest the cell cycle and initiate programmed cell death in damaged cells.

MEIOSIS AND GENETIC VARIABILITY

To reproduce sexually, multicellular eukaryotes must produce specialized sex cells, or **gametes**, that transmit half of each parent's genetic information to the next generation. **Meiosis** is the process of gamete formation (see Figure 3.54).

Asexual versus Sexual Reproduction

Many multicellular organisms are capable of **asexual reproduction**. These organisms include protists, plants, and fungi, as well as animals such as sea anemones, hydra, and a few vertebrates. However, most multicellular eukaryotes undergo some form of **sexual reproduction**. Whereas asexual reproduction results in identical copies of the parent cell, sexual reproduction recombines the genetic material of two different parents to form offspring that differ from the parents and from each other. As a result, organisms that reproduce sexually have two copies of each chromosome, one copy from each parent. Sexual reproduction may offer offspring a better chance for survival in environments that are changing or unpredictable.

Meiosis and Ploidy

Sexual reproduction involves the combining of male and female gametes. **Meiosis** is the process of gamete formation, in which each parent's genome is reduced by half. Each gamete carries half the number of chromosomes and, consequently, half the number of genes of the parent cell. The parent cells, with two copies of each chromosome, are said to be **diploid (2n)**. Chromosomes occur in **homologous pairs**. Gametes are **haploid (n)**, carrying only one of each chromosome and lacking homologous pairs. Male gametes are **spermatozoa (sperm)**, and female gametes are **ova** (eggs). When an egg and sperm combine during fertilization, they form a single-celled, diploid **zygote**, or fertilized ovum, with homologous pairs of chromosomes. The zygote then divides by mitosis to form a multicellular embryo and, ultimately, an adult organism.

In animals, gametes are produced by **germ cells** located in the **gonads**, or sex organs. Germ cells are generalized cells that do not differentiate into specialized tissues during development. All other cells in the body except gametes are **diploid somatic cells**, a term that refers to any cell that is not a germ cell or gamete.

Human somatic cells are diploid, with 46 chromosomes, or 23 homologous pairs ($2n = 46$). Human haploid gametes have 23 chromosomes ($n = 23$). The homologous pairs in diploid cells include 22 pairs of **autosomes** and one pair of **sex chromosomes** (the X and Y **chromosomes**). The sex chromosomes in humans are the only pair of homologous chromosomes that are different in size and shape. The Y chromosome in males has significantly fewer genes than the larger X chromosome. Figure 3.53 shows a **karyotype**, or composite photograph of ordered homologous pairs of chromosomes, from a human somatic cell.

> ### DIFFERENT NUMBERS OF CHROMOSOMES
>
> Different species have different numbers of chromosomes. The fruit fly *Drosophila melanogaster* has a diploid number of 8 and a haploid number of 4 ($2n = 8$, $n = 4$). The adder's tongue fern has a diploid number of 1200 ($2n = 1200$, $n = 600$), the largest known number of chromosomes.

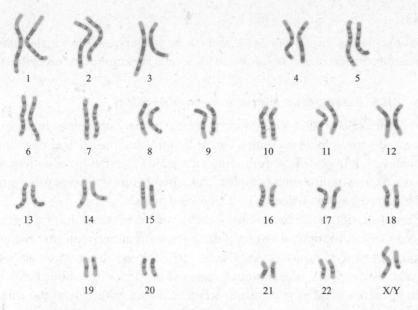

Figure 3.53. Karyotype of a human male showing 46 chromosomes in 23 homologous pairs

Meiosis

During meiosis, germ cells in the gonads produce gametes by undergoing a process of cell division similar to mitosis. Unlike mitosis, meiosis involves two rounds of cell division, **meiosis I** and **meiosis II**. (See Figure 3.54.)

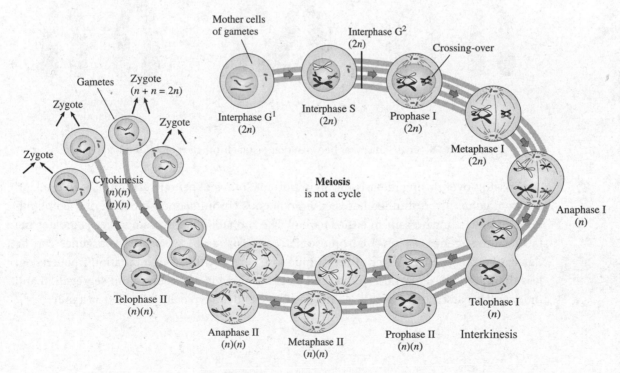

Figure 3.54. Steps of meiosis

MEIOSIS I

The phases of Meiosis I are prophase I, metaphase I, anaphase I, and telophase I. These phases are similar to the phases of mitosis, with several very important exceptions.

Synapsis and Crossing-Over: Genetic Recombination

Prophase I of meiosis I is similar to mitotic prophase in that duplicated chromosomes condense into dyads, the spindle apparatus begins to form, and the nuclear membrane disappears. In meiosis I, homologous chromosomes are joined together by a complex of proteins and RNA called the **synaptonemal complex**. This joining process, or **synapsis**, forms pairs of dyads called **tetrads**. Synapsis does not occur during mitosis.

During synapsis, nonsister chromatids of each dyad in the tetrad may undergo **crossing-over**, or **genetic recombination**, when pieces of maternal and paternal chromatids are exchanged between chromosomes (see Figure 3.55). Two nonsister chromatids cross over and form a **chiasma** (plural: **chiasmata**), a region of overlap. Chromatids break at the chiasma and are reannealed to the nonsister strand. Cohesion proteins at the chiasmata are important in holding dyads together in a tetrad.

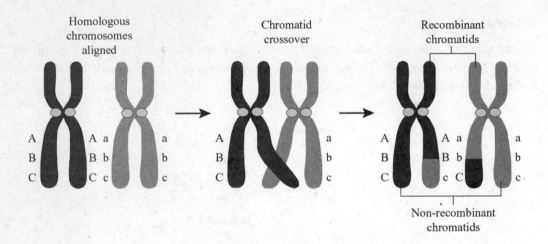

Figure 3.55. Single crossover between non-sister chromatids of a homologous pair

Crossing-over during meiosis I is an important source of genetic variation. Maternal and paternal genes are reshuffled between homologous chromosomes, creating new combinations of genes not present in either parent. The probability of crossing-over is greater the farther apart genes are on a chromosome. The distance between any two genes can be determined by the frequency of recombination. Genes with a recombination frequency of less than 50% are said to be **linked**. Linked genes provide an exception to segregation and independent assortment as they do not segregate and are typically inherited as a unit.

Reduction Division

At metaphase I, tetrads line up along the metaphase plate. During anaphase I, homologous chromosomes are separated. Meiosis I is also called the **reduction division** because it reduces the number of chromosomes by half. The two daughter cells produced by meiosis I are now haploid, containing either the maternal or paternal chromosome of each homologous pair. Upon completion of meiosis I, daughter cells enter **interkinesis**, a stage similar to interphase but without an S phase of DNA replication.

Segregation

The separation of homologous chromosomes during anaphase I results in the segregation of maternal and paternal alleles into different daughter cells. Each gamete produced by meiosis therefore contains either the maternal allele or the paternal allele of each gene but not both. The terms *maternal* and *paternal* refer to the source of the alleles in the parents of the organism undergoing meiosis. Both sperm and ova carry maternal and paternal alleles of different genes. In genetics, the **principle of segregation** (Mendel's first law) refers to the separation of maternal and paternal alleles during gamete formation.

Independent Assortment

During metaphase I, homologous pairs of chromosomes (tetrads) line up randomly. There is an equal probability that either a maternal homologue or a paternal homologue will line up on a given side of the metaphase plate. As a result, the probability that either the paternal or maternal allele of any given gene will be incorporated into any gamete is 50%. Also, the alignment of one chromosome pair is independent of the alignment of any other chromosome pair. Therefore, genes located on different chromosome pairs assort independently into gametes, and genes are inherited independently of one another. This is the basis for the **principle of independent assortment** (Mendel's second law). An exception to this rule occurs for linked genes, which occur on the same chromosome. In the absence of recombination, linked genes are inherited together.

MEIOSIS II

Meiosis II is similar to mitosis except with half the number of chromosomes. In prophase II, the nuclear membrane and the nucleoli disappear. During metaphase II, nonhomologous dyads line up single file along the metaphase plate. Sister chromatids are pulled apart by the spindle apparatus at anaphase II, separating dyads into monads. The nuclear membrane reforms during telophase II, and cytokinesis II generates four **haploid daughter cells**, or **gametes**. Gametes contain a varied combination of maternal and paternal alleles. They also differ from each other and from the parent cell.

Table 3.5 Differences Between Meiosis and Mitosis

	Mitosis	Meiosis
Number of divisions	1	2
Number of daughter cells	2 somatic cells	4 gametes
Ploidy of daughter cells	Diploid	Haploid
Prior DNA replication	Yes	Yes
Chromosomes line up at metaphase plate	Yes	Yes
Separating chromosomes	Dyads to monads	Tetrads to dyads to monads
Crossing over/recombination	No	Yes
Interkinesis	No	Yes
Parent cell type	Somatic cells	Germ line cells of gonads
Purpose	Replicate copies of diploid cells for growth, repair, development	Produce genetically distinct haploid gametes for sexual reproduction

Meiosis and Other Factors Affecting Genetic Variability

The recombination of genes from two different parents in sexual reproduction produces highly variable offspring. In addition, the genetic recombination between maternal and paternal alleles that occurs during meiosis I further increases the number of potential variations. Finally, mutations that occur during DNA replication and meiosis provides the ultimate source of new genetic variation in a population.

MUTATION

Mutations are changes to a DNA sequence that provide a source of novel genetic variation between individuals. Mutations can occur during DNA replication as mistakes in complementary base pairing. Mutations can also occur spontaneously by exposure to **mutagens** such as ultraviolet radiation, viruses, ionizing radiation such as X-rays, and certain chemicals, such as metabolic free radicals or environmental toxins. Mutations can also result from mobile sequences of DNA called **transposons** that can "jump" from one position in the genome to another. If the mutation is not corrected, it may result in the death or malfunction of the cell. Mutations can also result in unregulated cell division, leading to cancer.

Mutations that are not corrected can be passed on through mitotic cell division in somatic cells. Mutations that occur during meiosis can be passed to offspring. If a mutation belongs to a gene that codes for a protein, the protein may or may not be affected, depending on the type and location of the mutation. Most mutations are **silent**, meaning they have no effect. A small percentage of mutations are harmful, and an even smaller percentage may be beneficial.

Mutations can involve the alteration of a single base, of a gene sequence, or of an entire chromosome. A mutation involving a single nitrogenous base is called a point mutation. Point mutations may be substitutions, insertions, or deletions.

Substitution Mutations

A **substitution mutation** occurs when one base is substituted for another. When a purine is replaced by a purine or a pyrimidine replaced by a pyrimidine, the substitution is called a **transition**. When a purine replaces a pyrimidine or vice versa, the substitution is a **transversion**. A base substitution that does not result in a change in the amino acid sequence of a protein is called a **silent mutation**. However, a substitution in a coding region that replaces one amino acid for another results in a **missense mutation** that may result in a protein with an incorrect conformation and impaired function. If a substitution results in a premature **stop codon**, such as when the stop codon UAA replaces UAC in an RNA molecule, the resulting **nonsense mutation** produces a nonfunctional, truncated protein.

Insertion and Deletion Mutations

Substitution mutations involve replacing an existing base with a different base. **Insertion mutations** and **deletion mutations** involve adding or removing bases. A base that is inserted into or deleted from a nucleotide sequence results in a **frameshift mutation**. A frameshift alters the reading frame of the DNA and leads to the expression of a protein with a completely different amino acid sequence downstream from the insertion or deletion. Mobile genetic elements such as transposons are the primary cause of insertions. Point deletions result in **abasic sites**, which are locations on a DNA molecule where a nitrogenous base is missing. Point deletions may be either spontaneous or induced by environmental mutagens.

Types of Chromosomal Mutations

Mutations may also be caused by an alteration in the size or number of chromosomes as a result of errors during crossing-over or segregation. These types of mutations are called chromosomal mutations. Figure 3.56 shows some examples.

GENE DUPLICATION

Gene duplication results in more than one copy of a gene on a chromosome. This duplication can occur because of unequal crossing over, errors during DNA replication, viral transfer, or failure of chromosomes to separate competely during meiosis. Duplication of a coding gene results in an increase in the protein product and amplification of gene expression.

GENE DELETION

Large regions of a chromosome may be deleted, resulting in a loss of any associated coding genes.

CHROMOSOMAL INVERSION

A section of chromosome is inverted end to end, causing the same genes to be present in reverse order. Most human chromosomal inversions have few deleterious effects.

CHROMOSOMAL TRANSLOCATION

Genes may be exchanged between nonhomologous chromosomes. Translocations may result in significant alteration in gene expression due to changes in proximity between gene promoters and enhancer regions.

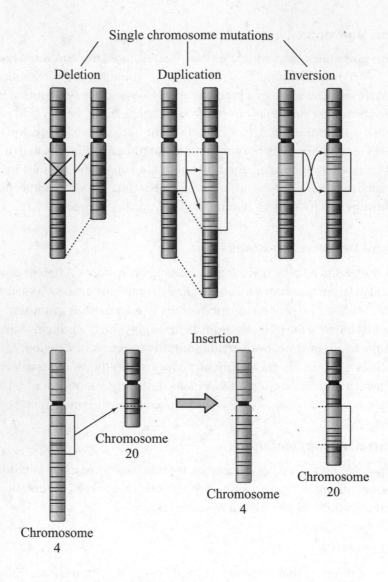

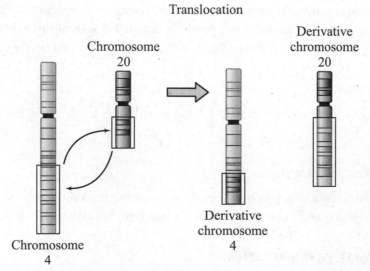

Figure 3.56. Types of single chromosome mutations

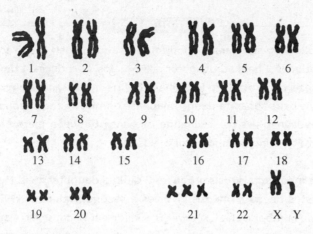

Figure 3.57. Karyotype for a person with Down syndrome, or trisomy 21

ALTERATION OF CHROMOSOME NUMBER

The addition or deletion of an individual chromosome (**aneuploidy**) occurs when homologous pairs fail to separate during meiosis I. In animals, aneuploidy is almost always lethal. Changes in chromosome number by duplication of the entire chromosome set may result in **polyploidy**. Polyploidy is common in plants as the result of hybridization.

INBORN ERRORS OF METABOLISM

Genetic mutations that affect metabolic processes, or **inborn errors of metabolism**, can result in congenital metabolic diseases. Most of these diseases stem from single gene mutations that cause an accumulation of toxic metabolic byproducts. For example, **phenylketonuria** is a disorder resulting from a mutation in the gene for the liver enzyme phenylalanine hydroxylase, which converts the amino acid phenylalanine to the amino acid tyrosine. The mutation creates a dysfunctional enzyme and an accumulation of excessive phenylalanine, which can lead to brain damage and neurological problems. Treatment involves restricting phenylalanine from the diet from birth, so early detection is critical.

Extranuclear Inheritance

The process of meiosis occurs in the nucleus of a eukaryotic cell. **Extranuclear** or **cytoplasmic inheritance** involves the transmission of hereditary material not located in the nucleus. Extranuclear genes occur in the mitochondria and chloroplasts. They may also occur in the cytoplasm in the form of eukaryotic plasmids or viral elements. Since extranuclear organelles and cytoplasm are transmitted by the female parent through the ovum, the transmission of extranuclear genes generally constitutes **maternal inheritance**. Genes found in the organelles are prokaryotic in origin and do not occur on chromosomes. These genes therefore do not replicate by meiosis. Consequently, extranuclear inheritance is also referred to as **nonchromosomal inheritance**.

Which of the following statements about mitosis and meiosis is correct?

(A) Mitosis produces 2 haploid daughter cells; meiosis produces 4 diploid gametes.

(B) DNA synthesis occurs only in interphase before mitosis, not before meiosis.

(C) Homologous pairs separate during anaphase of mitosis and anaphase I of meiosis.

(D) Crossing-over involves the exchange of genes between maternal and paternal chromosomes during prophase I of meiosis.

(D) Answer A is incorrect. Mitosis produces 2 diploid daughter cells. Meiosis produces 4 haploid gametes because meiosis involves a second, reduction division to reduce the chromosome number by half. Answer B is incorrect because DNA synthesis occurs during the S phase of interphase prior to both mitosis and meiosis. However, it does not occur during interkinesis between meiosis I and meiosis II. Answer C is incorrect because homologous pairs do not separate during mitosis. Both parent cells and daughter cells are diploid, with the same number of chromosomes.

GENETICS

The principles of inheritance were first elucidated by the Austrian monk **Gregor Mendel** from his studies of pea plants during the 1860s. However, the significance of his work was not understood until the beginning of the twentieth century, leading to the development of the **chromosomal theory of inheritance**. Mendel's three main observations form the basis of **Mendelian genetics**.

1. **LAW OF SEGREGATION.**
   A. Units of inheritance occur in pairs that segregate during gamete formation.
   B. The inheritance of traits is determined by the mathematical probabilities governing the pairing of these traits during fertilization.
2. **LAW OF INDEPENDENT ASSORTMENT.** Different traits are inherited independently.

Genes

Mendel's units of inheritance are now called genes. A single **gene** is a sequence of DNA that encodes hereditary information and that is located at a specific **locus** (plural: **loci**), or region, of the chromosome. The information encoded by the genes is expressed in the **traits**, or physical characteristics of an organism, by means of the transcription and translation of a polypeptide or protein. Some genes code for RNA. Other genes are not expressed at all. They may be evolutionary remnants that are no longer needed. The physical traits of an organism make up an organism's **phenotype**. The phenotype is influenced by both the genes encoding the trait (the **genotype**) and the environment in which those genes are expressed.

Alleles

Genes occur in homologous pairs in diploid eukaryotic organisms. One gene is inherited from each parent. These genes may be different **alleles**, which are variations of a gene that differ slightly in DNA sequence as a result of mutation or recombination. Maternal and paternal alleles for a single gene occur at the same loci on homologous chromosomes. An organism's genotype is determined by the specific combination of maternal and paternal alleles at one or more loci. Two different alleles will code for slightly different proteins, resulting in differences in the expression of a physical trait in the phenotype. A single gene may have one allele, two alleles, or **multiple alleles** within a population of organisms. However, a single organism can have no more than two different alleles, one from each parent.

Genotype

The genotype of an organism is the combination of alleles inherited from each parent. If a particular gene has two alleles, an organism can have one of three possible genotypes for that gene. Consider two alleles that affect pigmentation, *F* for freckles and *f* for no freckles.

THREE POSSIBLE GENOTYPES FROM TWO ALLELES	
FF	Homozygous dominant
Ff	Heterozygous
ff	Homozygous recessive

Because the order of alleles is not important, *Ff* is the same as *fF*. *FF* and *ff* are **homozygous** because they have the same allele. *Ff* is **heterozygous**. In the case of multiple alleles within a population, there may be more possible genotypes. (See below.)

Dominance

Alleles may exhibit differing levels of dominance: **complete dominance**, **incomplete dominance**, and **codominance**.

COMPLETE DOMINANCE

In complete dominance, a **dominant allele** completely masks the expression of a recessive allele in heterozygous individuals. The recessive phenotype for this trait can be expressed only if the organism carries two recessive alleles. In other words, the organism must have a homozygous recessive genotype. As a result, there are only two possible phenotypes for a single gene exhibiting complete dominance: the dominant phenotype and the recessive phenotype. Table 3.6 shows the genotypes and phenotypes when the allele for freckles (*F*) is dominant to the allele for no freckles (*f*).

> **DOMINANT AND RECESSIVE ALLELES**
>
> Alleles of the same gene may be either dominant or recessive. A dominant gene is always expressed as a trait in the phenotype. A recessive trait may be masked or hidden by the presence of a dominant allele. By convention, the dominant allele of a given gene is usually written as a capital letter. The recessive allele is usually written as the lowercase of the same letter.

Table 3.6 Complete Dominance: Dominant Allele for Freckles (*F*) and Recessive Allele for No Freckles (*f*)

	Genotype	Phenotype
FF	Homozygous dominant	Freckles
Ff	Heterozygous	Freckles
ff	Homozygous recessive	No freckles

INCOMPLETE DOMINANCE

In incomplete dominance, the dominant allele does not completely mask expression of the recessive allele. Three possible phenotypes result, one for each genotype. As shown in Table 3.7, flower color in snapdragons is determined by incomplete dominance. A homozygous dominant plant has red flowers. A homozygous recessive plant has white flowers. In the heterozygous plant, *Rr*, the flower color is an intermediate between dominant red and recessive white. The two colors are blended to result in pink.

Table 3.7 Incomplete Dominance: Dominant Red Allele (*R*) and Recessive White Allele (*r*)

	Genotype	Phenotype
RR	Homozygous dominant	Red flower
Rr	Heterozygous	Pink flower
rr	Homozygous recessive	White flower

CODOMINANCE

In codominance, both alleles are equally expressed, with no blending of traits. Neither allele is dominant or recessive. The gene coding for ABO blood type in humans is an example of both codominance and multiple alleles. This gene codes for proteins incorporated into the plasma membrane of red blood cells. There are three different alleles, *A*, *B*, and *i* (for type O). The *A* and *B* alleles are dominant to the *i* allele. However, *A* and *B* are codominant with each other, as proteins from both genes are expressed in the phenotype. Possible genotypes for a given person are *AA*, *AB*, *BB*, *Ai*, *Bi*, and *ii*. Possible phenotypes are type A, type B, type AB, and type O. (See Table 3.8.)

Table 3.8 Codominance and Multiple Alleles: ABO Genotypes and Phenotypes

Genotype	Phenotype
AA	Type A blood
Ai	Type A blood
BB	Type B blood
Bi	Type B blood
AB	TypeAB blood
ii	Type O blood

Penetrance and Expressivity

The genotype of an organism provides the inherited instructions for a given trait. How that trait is expressed in an organism's phenotype may depend on other genetic or environmental factors. **Penetrance** refers to the likelihood that a physical trait will be expressed. **Expressivity** refers to the degree to which the trait is expressed.

PENETRANCE

Penetrance is the likelihood that a trait specified by a given allele is actually expressed in the phenotype. Penetrance may depend on interactions with other genes, on age, or on environmental factors. An allele with **complete penetrance** is always expressed. However, an allele with **incomplete penetrance** may not be expressed in some individuals who carry the allele. For example, the mutant alleles *BRCA1* and *BRCA2*, which are linked to a genetic form of breast cancer, demonstrate incomplete penetrance. The actual development of cancer in individuals carrying these alleles depends on environmental factors such as diet, smoking, or breast-feeding.

EXPRESSIVITY

Expressivity refers to the degree to which an allele is expressed in the phenotype. Two individuals may have complete penetrance of a trait (100% chance the trait will be expressed) but may differ in the extent to which it appears in the phenotype (expressivity). Differences in expressivity can result in differences in the severity of a genetic disorder among affected individuals who share the same genotype.

Crosses

Different individuals can be mated (crossed) to determine their genotypes and to investigate patterns of inheritance. Crosses frequently are performed between a **wild-type** individual and an individual with a mutant phenotype for a particular trait. Wild-type individuals carry the allele normally found in natural populations. Mutant phenotypes are often, but not always, recessive traits.

SINGLE GENE CROSS

A **single gene cross** involves crossing or mating two individuals and determining the probability of a given genotype or phenotype in the first generation (**F1 generation**) of offspring. If members of the F1 generation are allowed to cross among themselves, their offspring make up the **F2 generation** (second generation). The **genotypic ratio** and **phenotypic ratio** in the offspring are predicted by the mathematical probability of the union of possible gametes from each parent. This probability can be shown in a diagram called a **Punnett square**. Across the top of the square are the alleles that make up the genotype of one parent, and down the left are the alleles of the other parent's genotype. The possible allele combinations in the form of offspring genotypes are written in the interior squares. By convention, the dominant allele with the capital letter is always written first in a genotype of a single trait. Phenotypes are given in parentheses. The Punnett square in Figure 3.58 shows a cross between a red snapdragon and a pink snapdragon and demonstrates that the probability of a red-flowered offspring is 2/4 = 50%.

	R	r
R	RR (red)	Rr (pink)
R	RR (red)	Rr (pink)

Figure 3.58. Punnett square showing a single gene cross exhibiting incomplete dominance

Practice Question

Freckles is a dominant trait. A woman who is homozygous dominant for freckles and a man who is homozygous recessive have children. What are the possible genotypes and phenotypes of the offspring?

Solution: Because freckles is a dominant trait, the allele for freckles is *F*. The allele for the absence of freckles is *f*. Create a Punnett square to show the inheritance of the freckle trait, as in Figure 3.59.

	f	f
F	Ff (freckles)	Ff (freckles)
F	Ff (freckles)	Ff (freckles)

Figure 3.59. Punnett square for a cross between a freckled woman (homozygous dominant) and a non-freckled man

Because each parent is capable of producing only one kind of gamete, the F1 offspring will all have the genotype *Ff*. All offspring will have freckles. The genotypic ratio is therefore 1:1 = 100% *Ff*. The phenotypic ratio is 1:1 = 100% freckled.

Table 3.9 breaks down the relationships in the sample problem. Use this approach to solve more complex problems.

Table 3.9 Genotypes and Phenotypes for Freckled Trait

	Mother	Father
Parental genotypes	*FF*	*ff*
Parental phenotypes	Freckles	No freckles
Possible haploid gamete genotypes	*F* or *F*	*f* or *f*
Possible zygote genotypes	*Ff*	
Possible zygote phenotypes	Freckles	

Practice Question

A freckled man and a freckled woman are both heterozygous for the freckled gene. What is the probability that these parents will produce a child with no freckles?

Genotypes of parents: *Ff* and *Ff*
Possible haploid gametes produced by each parent: *F* or *f*

Solution: Use the Punnett square shown in Figure 3.60 to determine the possible genotypes of the offspring. Then calculate the probability of a child having a phenotype of no freckles.

	F	f
F	FF	Ff
f	Ff	ff

Figure 3.60. A cross of two individuals both heterozygous for freckles

The predicted genotypic ratio of the offspring is:

1/4 *FF* : 1/2 *Ff* : 1/4 *ff* or 1:2:1 *FF*:*Ff*:*ff*

Because freckles is a dominant trait, both *FF* and *Ff* genotypes will have freckles. Therefore, the phenotypic ratio of the offspring is:

3/4 freckles : 1/4 no freckles or 3:1 freckles : no freckles

The probability that these parents will produce a child with no freckles is 1/4.

The **1:2:1 genotypic ratio** and the **3:1 phenotypic ratio** are the standard ratios produced by any cross of two parents who are both heterozygous for a single gene exhibiting complete dominance. This is called a **monohybrid cross**.

DOUBLE GENE CROSS

A **double gene cross** determines the phenotypic and genotypic outcomes for two genes. In a standard Mendelian double gene cross, the two genes are **unlinked**. In other words, they do not occur on the same chromosome pair. As a result, they follow Mendel's law of independent assortment and are inherited independently. The probability of either allele of one gene being passed to a gamete is mathematically independent of the probability of inheritance of the second gene. If both parents are heterozygous for two traits exhibiting complete dominance, the double gene cross is called a **dihybrid cross**.

Practice Question

In pea plants, purple flowers are dominant to white flowers, and tall stems are dominant to dwarf stems. What are the potential genotypic and phenotypic ratios in the offspring of a cross between a plant that is homozygous dominant for both genes with a plant that is homozygous recessive for both genes?

Solution: Gene for flower color: purple allele = *P*, white allele = *p*

Gene for stem length: tall allele = *T*, dwarf allele = *t*

Table 3.10 shows the genotypes and phenotypes of the parents as well as the possible gametes they can produce. Figure 3.61 is a Punnett square of this cross.

Table 3.10 Genotypes and Phenotypes of Homozygous Dominant and Homozygous Recessive Parents in a Double Gene Cross

Parental genotypes	*PPTT*	*pptt*
Parental phenotypes	Purple tall	White dwarf
Haploid gametes (Gametes will contain one copy of *each* gene)	*PT*	*pt*

	PT
pt	PpTt

Figure 3.61. Punnett square double gene cross with parents homozygous for two genes

Genotypic ratio for F1: 1:1 = 100% *PpTt*

Phenotypic ratio for F1: 1:1 = 100% purple tall

All of the offspring of this parental cross are heterozygous, purple, and tall.

Practice Question

If the heterozygous F1 **hybrids** are allowed to interbreed, what will be the expected genotypic and phenotypic ratios in the F2 offspring?

Solution: Each haploid gamete must contain only one copy of each gene, but there must be a copy of each gene in the gamete, e.g., one allele for flower color and one allele for stem height. The possible alleles are *P*, *p*, *T*, and *t*. Use the FOIL method (pairing First, Outer, Inner, Last) to determine the four possible combinations of alleles in the gametes:

(*Pp*)(*Tt*): First = *PT*, Outer = *Pt*, Inner = *pT*, Last = *pt*

Figure 3.62 shows the possible genotypes of the offspring from this cross.

	PT	Pt	pT	pt
PT	PPTT	PPTt	PpTT	PpTt
Pt	PPTt	PPtt	PpTt	Pptt
pT	PpTT	PpTt	ppTT	ppTt
pt	PpTt	Pptt	ppTt	pptt

Figure 3.62. Punnett square for double gene cross with heterozygous parents

Genotypic ratio of F2 offspring:

$$1/16 \; PPTT : 2/16 \; PPTt : 1/16 \; PPtt : 2/16 \; PpTT :$$
$$4/16 \; PpTt : 2/16 \; Pptt : 1/16 \; ppTT : 2/16 \; ppTt : 1/16 \; pptt$$

(also written as a 1:2:1:2:4:2:1:2:1 genotypic ratio)

Phenotypic ratio of offspring: 9/16: 3/16: 3/16: 1/16 or 9:3:3:1 purple tall: purple dwarf: white tall: white dwarf

The **9:3:3:1 ratio** is the standard phenotypic ratio in offspring of a dihybrid cross. 9/16 of the offspring have the dominant phenotype for both genes. 3/16 have a dominant phenotype for one gene and a recessive phenotype for the other. 1/16 have the recessive phenotype for both genes.

> **PUNNETT SQUARE CONVENTIONS**
>
> Alleles of the same gene are written together. The capital letter is written first. The order of genes is the same as shown in the parental genotype.
> Correct: *PpTt*
> Incorrect: *PTpt, pPtT,* or *TtPp*

TESTCROSS

A **testcross** is a cross between an individual with a dominant phenotype but unknown genotype and another individual that is homozygous recessive for the trait. The phenotypic ratios of the offspring will show whether the unknown parent is homozygous dominant or heterozygous.

BACKCROSS

A **backcross** is a cross of an F1 hybrid offspring with either one of the parents (or with an individual of similar genotype to the parent). Backcrossing is used in selective breeding as a means of transferring a novel trait in a hybrid back into the main breeding stock. Individuals carrying the desired trait are backcrossed over multiple generations, resulting in a genetic strain similar to the original parent but carrying the novel allele.

OUTCROSSING AND HYBRID VIABILITY

An **outcross** is a cross between genetically distinct individuals or populations with the purpose of bringing novel genetic traits into a breeding line and increasing the genetic diversity of offspring. The hybrid offspring of an outcross frequently exhibit **hybrid vigor**, or increased viability, as a result of a decrease in homozygous recessive traits.

Sex Determination

In humans and many other animals, females are **homogametic**, with two X chromosomes (XX) forming the homologous pair. Males are **heterogametic**, with a paired X and Y chromosome (XY). Females inherit a copy of an X chromosome from each parent at fertilization. Males inherit an X chromosome from their mothers and a Y chromosome from their fathers. Hence, the father determines the sex of the child. Interestingly, in birds, the male is homogametic.

Sex Linkage

Genes that are located on the X or Y chromosomes are called **sex-linked genes**. The X and Y chromosome differ not only in size and shape but also in the number, type, and location of genes. Most sex-linked genes are **X-linked**. Only a few genes are linked to the small Y chromosome. Both chromosomes contain genes involved in sex determination as well as genes for other traits. The inheritance of X-linked traits differs from Mendelian inheritance patterns because in males the trait is carried only on one chromosome. Because males do not have an extra copy of the gene, they express a recessive trait in the phenotype if they receive a single recessive allele from their mother. Females, in contrast, must inherit a recessive allele from each parent to express the trait. X-linked recessive genetic disorders include red-green color blindness, hemophilia, and male-pattern baldness.

Gene Mapping

The frequency of recombination can be used to map genes on chromosomes. Typically, three-point test crosses are performed between a true-breeding wild-type parent and an individual mutant for three separate genes. The frequency of recombinant offspring is used as a measure of genetic distance. A higher number of recombinant offspring means a greater distance between genes on a chromosome. The maximum distance between genes is 50 LMU (Linkage Map Units), which corresponds to a 50% recombination frequency. This distance corresponds to genes that are unlinked and separated on different chromosomes. Genes with a recombination frequency of less than 50% are linked on the same chromosome, at distances determined by the recombination frequency. Linked genes do not follow independent assortment. Genes with a recombination frequency of 0 are completely linked. These genes are so close together on a chromosome that no recombination occurs, and the genes are inherited as a unit. The frequency of offspring with recombinant genotypes between the three genes will provide a measure of genetic distance between the genes on the chromosome.

POPULATION GENETICS AND HARDY–WEINBERG

A **population** is defined as an interbreeding group of organisms of the same species living in a geographically connected area. Population genetics is the study of the changes in the allele frequencies of a population over time in response to evolutionary pressures, mutation rates, and changes in population size and breeding structure. In order to examine whether a population has undergone genetic changes over time, the population can be compared to a theoretical steady state in which no change is predicted to occur. This theoretical steady state is known as Hardy–Weinberg equilibrium. The Hardy–Weinberg principle of population genetics predicts that within a population, allele frequencies will remain constant over many generations as long as the following conditions exist:

1. Random mating
2. Large population size
3. No mutation
4. No gene flow with other populations
5. No natural selection

Any deviation from Hardy–Weinberg equilibrium in a natural population indicates that the population is experiencing genetic change as a result of one of the above factors.

The sum total of all of the alleles of all genes of all individuals of a population is referred to as the **gene pool**. Under Hardy–Weinberg equilibrium, the frequency of one allele of a given gene is p and the frequency of a second allele at that locus is q. For a gene with one dominant allele (A) and one recessive allele (a), the predicted genotype frequency in each generation if p and q remain constant is

p^2 = frequency of AA

$2pq$ = frequency of Aa

q^2 = frequency of aa

In any population, the sum of the frequencies of each genotype is always 1:

$$p + q = 1 \text{ and } p^2 + 2pq + q^2 = 1$$

Actual allele frequencies in a population may be determined by techniques such as protein gel electrophoresis. These actual frequencies can be compared with the frequencies predicted by the Hardy–Weinberg principle. Any deviation from expected Hardy–Weinberg frequencies suggests that one of the required criteria has been violated and that gene frequencies have changed. Because of this, Hardy–Weinberg calculations can be used as a test of mating structure, gene flow, and natural selection in a population.

EVOLUTION

Evolution is the process of heritable change over time in living things. Evolution occurs over many generations in populations of organisms. A single individual does not evolve. **Microevolution** is short-term evolutionary change. It is measured in the changes in gene frequencies within a population or species over relatively few generations. **Macroevolution** refers to the evolution of new species and higher taxonomic groups over geologic time. Macroevolution results in a pattern of evolutionary relationships that indicates the descent of all living things from a shared common ancestor.

Importance of Variation

Individuals within a population vary. No two organisms are exactly alike. The differences among individuals are caused by genetic differences such as the presence of different alleles in different individuals as well as environmental differences that affect an organism's phenotype during development and over the course of a lifetime. This variation among individuals within a single population results in **within-population variation**. In order for evolution to occur at the population level, heritable within-population variation must occur among individuals.

Populations of organisms also vary. Evolutionary differences between two populations are reflected in the amount of **between-population genetic variation**, measured as differences in the frequencies of alleles in the gene pool. As a result of evolution, populations of organisms become different from one another. Eventually, enough differences accumulate between the populations that individuals in the different populations are no longer able to interbreed, leading to speciation. The greater the between-population variation, the more divergent different populations have become and the more likely they will become different species.

Mechanisms of Evolutionary Change

Evolutionary change can occur randomly, through processes such as mutation. It can also occur nonrandomly, through directional processes such as selection. Processes that alter allele frequencies may either increase or decrease the amount of variation between and within populations. Each of the following processes can lead to evolution.

MUTATION AND RECOMBINATION

Mutation is the ultimate source of all new genetic variation. Point mutations, gene duplications and deletions, and chromosomal translocations and nondisjunctions are all sources of novel genetic traits. Most mutations are neutral, meaning they are neither harmful nor beneficial. Neutral mutations can occur in repetitive sequences of noncoding DNA without affecting the phenotype. For example, single nucleotide polymorphisms (SNPs) are point mutations that are a major source of neutral genetic variation as shown in Figure 3.63. Most SNPs are noncoding. Other mutations, such as those that affect regulatory regions of DNA, can have large effects on the phenotype.

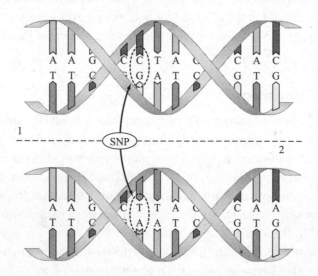

Figure 3.63. A single nucleotide polymorphism (SNP) between DNA molecule 1 and DNA molecule 2 resulting in a C to T substitution mutation (Adapted from: David Hall, on Wikipedia, *http://en.wikipedia.org/wiki/File:Dna-SNP.svg*)

Genetic variation among individuals is also determined by the random **recombination** of alleles that occurs during sexual reproduction as a result of crossing-over, independent assortment, and the recombination of gametes at fertilization. Together, mutation and recombination are the sources of hereditary within-population variation among individuals. At the population level, mutation provides the source of new alleles that alter allele frequencies within a population, leading to between-population differences and evolution.

GENE FLOW

Gene flow is the exchange of genes between two or more distinct populations of the same species. Gene flow results from the migration of individuals or from interbreeding between populations. It leads to increased genetic variation within populations. However, gene flow can cause adjacent populations to become genetically more similar, decreasing variation between populations.

GENETIC LEAKAGE

Leakage is gene flow between species. It can occur when populations of different species come into contact. Leakage can occur only when species are not yet completely reproductively isolated.

GENETIC DRIFT

Genetic drift is the random loss of alleles that occurs in very small populations. Because of the small number of breeding individuals, not every allele is transmitted to the next generation. Alleles are lost as a result of chance, leading to an increase in homozygosity and a decrease in genetic variation among individuals. This decrease in variation can be reversed by gene flow. When gene flow is cut off, genetic drift can lead to rapid evolutionary change in small, isolated populations. The decrease in genetic variation within the population may lead to extinction. At the same time that genetic drift decreases variation among individuals, it increases variation among populations, leading to evolutionary change.

OUTBREEDING

Outbreeding involves crossing individuals from different genetic strains or populations. Typically, the first generation of outbreeding results in **hybrid vigor**, or greater fitness among the F1 hybrids. However, fitness may decline in subsequent generations.

A similar situation can arise in larger populations as a result of **inbreeding** between closely related individuals. Inbreeding lowers the effective population size, resulting in an increase in homozygosity and an increase in the frequency of recessive traits and genetic disorders. This reduction in fitness in inbred populations is **inbreeding depression**. Inbreeding depression is a common occurrence during population **bottlenecks**, or periods of extremely low population size. Inbreeding depression can result in a dramatic loss of genetic diversity that extends through the gene pool of many subsequent generations.

NATURAL SELECTION

Natural selection is the primary mechanism of **nonrandom, directional** evolutionary change. In any population, more individuals are born than can survive and reproduce, leading to **differential survival and reproduction**. The differential survival and reproduction of individuals in a given environment is natural selection. The environment acts as a filter to screen out variants that are more successful. Those with phenotypic traits that aid survival and reproduction in that environment will contribute a higher percentage of genes to the gene pool of subsequent generations. Over many generations, the changes in the frequency of favorable alleles caused by natural selection will result in evolution.

Relative Fitness

Individuals that contribute more offspring to the next generation than others are said to have a higher **relative fitness**. Relative fitness and physical fitness are not the same. Whereas physical fitness may contribute to relative fitness in some circumstances, increased relative fitness is the result of any feature that enhances survival and reproduction. *Survival of the fittest* does not mean survival of the strongest. The fittest individuals are those who succeed in passing their genes to subsequent generations, by whatever means. The fittest individuals are those who are best adapted to their particular environment and way of life. The relative fitness of an individual depends on the environment, and it changes as the environment changes.

For example, in the presence of antibiotics, bacteria possessing a gene for antibiotic resistance will be more successful at survival and reproduction than bacteria lacking the gene. Consequently, the resistant bacteria exhibit higher relative fitness because they are better adapted to that environment. Figure 3.64 shows that the prevalence of antibiotic-resistant individuals in the population increases after selection pressure is applied in the form of an antibiotic. However, expression of the gene for antibiotic resistance is metabolically costly. In an environment where no antibiotic is present, bacteria that lack antibiotic resistance may have a competitive advantage over resistant strains and may show greater fitness, ultimately surviving and reproducing in greater numbers.

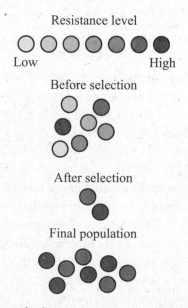

Figure 3.64. Natural selection for antibiotic resistance in bacteria

Adaptation

An **adaptation** is a physical feature or trait that increases an organism's ability to survive and reproduce in a given environment. The term *adaptation* is also used to describe the process whereby an organism adapts to its environment. An adaptation is always the consequence of natural selection. Whether a given trait is adaptive depends entirely on the environment. A trait that is an adaptation in one environment may be useless or even harmful in a different environment. For example, the allele that causes sickle-cell anemia is a deleterious point mutation that causes red blood cells to be deformed, reducing the oxygen-carrying capacity of the blood. However, this same mutation provides protection against malaria. In the presence of malaria, the sickle-cell allele is an adaptation.

If the environment changes, the direction of natural selection will change. Natural selection has no goal. However, natural selection results in increasing adaptation of organisms to their environment over time.

DIRECTIONAL, STABILIZING, AND DISRUPTIVE SELECTION

In any population of organisms, variation in a trait typically exhibits a normal distribution. By definition, most individuals possess the mean value (e.g., size, color) of the trait and increasingly fewer individuals possess traits toward the extreme values. If natural selection favors a particular range of phenotypes, it can result in a shift of the distribution curve toward versions of a trait that bring higher fitness. Natural selection may be directional, stabilizing, or disruptive (see Figure 3.65).

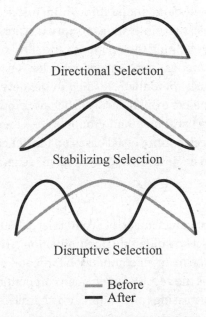

Directional Selection

Stabilizing Selection

Disruptive Selection

— Before
— After

Figure 3.65. The effect of different modes of
natural selection on a normal distribution of variation

Directional Selection

Directional selection shifts the distribution of a trait in one direction, resulting in a change in the mean value of the trait. An example of directional selection is the increase in brain size relative to body size that has occurred during human evolution. Directional selection does not affect the amount of genetic variation within a population.

Stabilizing Selection

Stabilizing selection favors the mean value while selecting against the extremes, decreasing variation. Stabilizing selection favoring a heterozygous phenotype can also result in maintenance of **genetic polymorphism** in the population. The prevalence of the recessive allele for sickle-cell anemia is an example of stabilizing selection and genetic polymorphism. When malaria is present, heterozygous individuals with one normal and one sickle-cell allele have a selective advantage, favoring the persistence of both alleles. Homozygous dominant individuals are susceptible to malaria, whereas homozygous recessive individuals suffer from sickle-cell anemia. In environments where malaria is present, stabilizing selection will favor the heterozygous genotype.

Disruptive Selection

Disruptive selection is selection against the mean, resulting in a **polymorphic species** with more than one phenotypic expression of a trait. Disruptive selection increases variation within a population and may lead to speciation.

KIN SELECTION AND GROUP SELECTION

Natural selection acts at the level of the individual, resulting in evolution at the level of the population. In social species, natural selection has also been shown to act at the level of the extended family via **kin selection**. In kin selection, altruistic individuals who sacrifice their own reproduction by contributing to the reproductive success of family members pass their genes to subsequent generations through **inclusive fitness** by the reproduction of close relatives. For example, when breeding territory is scarce, the offspring of many bird species defer reproduction by helping their parents raise their siblings.

Group selection is a theoretical form of natural selection that would act upon larger groups of unrelated individuals, potentially leading to the development of social behavior. In theory, groups whose members exhibit altruistic behavior toward others could contribute more genes to subsequent generations than groups whose members behave selfishly. The idea of group selection has been controversial based on the difficulty of explaining how genes of altruistic individuals could be passed on to subsequent generations.

SEXUAL SELECTION

Sexual selection is an alternate mechanism of evolutionary change. Unlike natural selection, sexual selection is caused solely by differential reproduction. The change in hereditary traits in a population over time is the result of competition for mates and mating preference. Most commonly, sexual selection is the result of male:male competition for access to females and of females selecting males possessing traits that may be correlated with fitness. Sexual selection may even lead to traits, such as the elaborate tail of the male peacock, that negatively affect an individual's survival by increasing risk of predation or nutritional stress.

Sexual selection can result in **sexual dimorphism**, distinct phenotypic differences between the sexes. Sexual dimorphism is frequently observed in the plumage differences of male and female birds, with the males tending to be brightly colored and the females cryptically colored. Humans also exhibit sexual dimorphism in the difference in body size, muscle mass, and secondary sexual characteristics between males and females. Sexual dimorphism is another form of **polymorphism**, the presence of more than one phenotype within a single species.

Which of the following statements about evolution is correct?

(A) Individuals develop mutations in order to adapt themselves to their environments.

(B) Natural selection is a random process.

(C) Individuals vary, and the traits of individuals who leave more offspring become more prevalent in successive generations.

(D) The strongest individuals have higher relative fitness and will contribute more genes to successive generations.

(C) Of the four statements, only choice C accurately describes evolution by natural selection. Natural selection is the differential survival and, more importantly, reproduction of individuals who possess physical traits that best adapt them to their environment. As a result of differential reproduction, these traits will be passed on to offspring who make up a larger percentage of future generations. Consequently, the prevalence of favorable traits increases in the population.

Answer A can be eliminated for two reasons. First, individuals do not evolve and, consequently, do not adapt. Evolution and adaptation occur at the population level, over many generations, not within the lifetime of a single individual. Second, organisms do not develop mutations in order to survive and adapt. Mutations occur randomly, not for a set purpose. Natural selection acts on mutations and other sources of variation that already exist naturally in a population, resulting in the increased prevalence of favorable traits.

Answer B can be eliminated because natural selection is not random. In fact, it is a highly nonrandom, directional process whereby the environment selects specific traits that enhance survival and reproduction, leading to increasing adaptation.

Answer D can be eliminated because strength and relative fitness are not the same. The strongest individuals may not always be the best at surviving and reproducing. Natural selection may favor those who run rather than fight, those who are small and better able to hide from predators, or those who have genes allowing them to persist in novel environments. Relative fitness depends on both survival and reproduction. Ultimately, individuals who reproduce more than others contribute the most genes to future generations.

Speciation

Speciation involves the formation of one or more new species from an ancestral population. There has been considerable debate as to what constitutes a **species**. Under the **biological species concept**, a species is a group of interbreeding organisms that is reproductively isolated from other such groups. In other words, organisms that may not necessarily resemble one another nevertheless belong to the same species if they can mate with one another and produce viable offspring. Alternatively, individuals that are phenotypically indistinguishable belong to different species if they are unable to interbreed. A limitation of the biological species concept is that it cannot be applied to species that reproduce asexually.

Because the rate of random mutations is fairly constant, the accumulation of neutral mutations in a sequence of DNA can be used as a **molecular clock** to estimate how long ago two species diverged. Some evolutionary change occurs gradually. However, other changes in evolutionary history occur as short bursts of rapid change followed by long periods of stability (**punctuated equilibrium**).

ADAPTIVE RADIATION

Populations that colonize islands or become isolated from other species frequently undergo **adaptive radiation**—the divergence of a single ancestral population into multiple new species. In a novel environment free of competition, the founding population diverges as a result of natural selection and adaptation as individuals exploit new habitats and food supplies. Subpopulations become specialized to fill open **ecological niches**. The Galapagos finches studied by Charles Darwin, seen in Figure 3.66, are a classic example of adaptive radiation leading to specialization. The differences in beak sizes in closely related species of Galapagos finches result from natural selection favoring individuals that can feed on different-sized seeds.

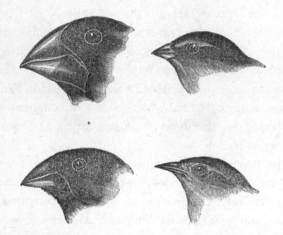

Figure 3.66. Beak adaptations in Galapagos finches (From: Darwin, 1845. *Journal of researches into the natural history and geology of the countries visited during the voyage of H.M.S. Beagle round the world, under the Command of Capt. Fitz Roy, R.N.* 2d edition.)

DIVERGENT AND CONVERGENT EVOLUTION

Most phylogenetic relationships show patterns of **divergent evolution**. In divergent evolution, an ancestral species splits into two or more daughter species that become progressively more dissimilar over time. However, in some cases, organisms will become more similar to one another as a result of similar selection pressures for similar environments or ways of life, a process called **convergent evolution**. Convergent evolution results in similar features in organisms that are not closely related, for example, the wings of birds, bats, and insects or the streamlined body shape of sharks and dolphins. If the organisms involved are closely related members of a single lineage, the independent development of similar traits is termed **parallel evolution**. In convergent and parallel evolution, the common trait was not shared by the common ancestor of the different groups that possess the trait. Similar traits that are not inherited from a common ancestor but instead arise independently

---

ANALOGOUS VERSUS HOMOLOGOUS

The wings of birds and bats are **analogous**. They have a similar structure and function but have a different evolutionary source.

The common bones of the forelimbs of all vertebrates are **homologous**. They may have different structures and functions but evolved from the same structure.

in separate evolutionary lineages are **analogous traits**. In contrast, traits inherited from a common ancestor are **homologous traits**.

HUMAN ANATOMY AND PHYSIOLOGY

Human anatomy is the study of the structure of the organ systems of the body, the specific organs that make up these systems, and the tissues that make up the organs. Human physiology is the study of the functions of these tissues, organs, and organ systems. The human body can be divided into 12 organ systems.

- Nervous system
- Endocrine system
- Circulatory system
- Lymphatic system
- Immune system
- Digestive system
- Urinary system
- Skeletal system
- Muscular system
- Respiratory system
- Integumentary system (skin)
- Reproductive system

Specialized Eukaryotic Cells and Tissues

In humans and other complex multicellular eukaryotes, cells differentiate during embryogenesis into **tissues.** Tissues are groups of cells specialized to perform specific functions. Tissues, in turn, are modified and further specialized depending on their function and location within the organism. Connective tissue, for example, includes such diverse forms as cartilage, bone, and blood, depending on the characteristics of the extracellular matrix. Two or more tissue types may participate to form an **organ**, and organs in turn are combined within an **organ system**.

Animal tissue is divided into four primary tissue types: muscle, nervous, epithelial, and connective.

MUSCLE TISSUE

Muscle tissue makes up skeletal muscle that moves the body. It also lines the walls of organs, dilates and constricts the eye pupils, pumps the blood, and aids in thermoregulation. Muscle cells are elongated and filled with contractile proteins, mainly actin and myosin. These proteins give muscle cells their capacity for **contraction**, the ability of the muscle to shorten to exert force or cause constriction. Muscle cells also exhibit **extensibility** and **elasticity**. Extensibility allows muscle cells to be stretched beyond their resting state. Elasticity is the capacity to return to original size after being stretched. Like nerve cells, muscle cells also demonstrate **excitability** in that they can be stimulated to propagate a nerve impulse.

Muscle tissue is divided into skeletal muscle, cardiac muscle, and smooth muscle. **Skeletal muscle** is **striated**, **voluntary** muscle tissue responsible for locomotion and other movements of the body skeleton. Skeletal muscle also moves the eyes and allows for facial expression. **Cardiac muscle** is **striated, involuntary** muscle tissue found in the walls of the heart.

Cardiac muscle is responsible for the pumping of blood. **Smooth muscle** is **unstriated**, **involuntary** tissue that occurs within the eye and in the lining of blood vessels and hollow organs. Smooth muscle functions in vision and acts to move materials through body passageways. Muscle tissue is discussed in more detail under Muscle Systems.

NERVOUS TISSUE

Nervous tissue includes **neurons** and **glial** (or **neuroglial**) cells. Neurons are specialized cells responsible for conducting electrical impulses in the nervous system. A neuron consists of a cell body, dendritic region, and axon. The **cell body** contains the cell's nucleus. The **dendritic** region receives stimuli. The **axon** transmits signals. Neuroglial cells are support cells that surround neurons and provide nutrients, immune support, and an appropriate external environment for the propagation of impulses. Nervous tissue is discussed in more detail under Nervous System.

EPITHELIAL TISSUE

Epithelial tissues (**epithelia**) surround the exterior of the body and line the walls of body openings, body cavities, and glands. Epithelia protect body surfaces from friction, abrasion, and infection. They cushion, protect, and lubricate body organs. Epithelia absorb, filter, secrete, and excrete substances into and out of the body and body openings. They also detect environmental stimuli. Epithelia can be derived from all three germ layers: endoderm, ectoderm, or mesoderm.

Characteristics of Epithelia

Epithelial tissue may be either **membranous** or **glandular**. Membranous epithelia form sheets of cells that line external and internal surfaces, whereas glandular epithelia form secretory glands. Some secretory glands open via a duct to a **lumen** (hollow opening) or body surface. Others lack an external opening. In general, epithelia have the following five characteristics.

1. **HIGH RATE OF REGENERATION.** Epithelial cells are capable of rapid mitotic division to replace worn or damaged cells.
2. **CELLULARITY.** Epithelial cells are in close contact with adjacent cells and are joined together by specialized contacts. The close relationship of cells is referred to as cellularity, an important characteristic of epithelial tissues. Contacts between cells include tight junctions, desmosomes, and adherens junctions. **Tight junctions** allow sheets of cells to form impenetrable barriers. **Desmosomes** and **adherens junctions** anchor cells to each other and to the underlying surface. Cellularity is important because it allows epithelial tissues to form sheets that regulate the passage of materials across boundaries.
3. **AVASCULARITY.** Although epithelial tissues are innervated by a nerve supply, they are **avascular**, lacking blood vessels. Instead, epithelial tissues rely on the diffusion of nutrients from underlying connective tissue. Multicellular epithelial glands, however, are typically well vascularized due to the penetration of blood vessels within associated connective tissue.
4. **POLARITY.** Epithelial tissues are polarized. They have an **apical surface** that faces out of the body or into the opening, or lumen, of a cavity, duct, or gland. They also have an opposite **basal surface**, where the tissue is attached to underlying cells. These two surfaces are structurally and functionally distinct due to differences in membrane pro-

teins. Tight junctions prevent the migration of membrane proteins between apical and basal surfaces, thus maintaining polarity.

5. **BASEMENT MEMBRANE.** Membranous epithelial tissue is connected to underlying connective tissue by a basement membrane, which is an acellular matrix of glycoproteins and collagen fibers. The upper **basal lamina** is secreted by the basal epithelium. In contrast, the lower **reticular lamina** is secreted by the connective tissue.

CONNECTIVE TISSUE

Connective tissue is the most abundant tissue type in the human body. Also called support cell tissue, it forms bones, tendons, ligaments, blood, fat, the underlying layers of the skin, and the interstitial matrix. The functions of connective tissue include support, protection, locomotion and body movement, transport, insulation, energy storage, and intercellular communication. The specific function of a particular connective tissue depends on the type and location of the tissue. All connective tissue has a common embryonic origin in **mesenchyme**, an embryonic tissue derived primarily from mesoderm. Connective tissue is composed of a variety of cell types embedded in an extracellular, secreted **matrix**.

Extracellular Matrix (ECM)

The extracellular matrix includes a **ground substance** with **fibers** of collagen or elastin proteins. The ground substance may be a liquid as in blood plasma, a gel as in loose connective tissue, or a solid substance as in bone. The ground substance is made of proteins, polysaccharides, and glycoproteins, including **proteoglycans**. These are proteins that carry negatively charged **glycosaminoglycan** (GAG) side chains that trap cations such as Na^+ and attract water molecules by osmosis. The water content and, consequently, the viscosity of the matrix are influenced by the type and concentration of glycosaminoglycans and proteins. Three types of fibers occur in the extracellular matrix.

1. **WHITE FIBERS.** These are made of cross-linked fibrils of **collagen**, the most abundant protein in the body. Collagen fibers provide tensile strength and support to the matrix.
2. **YELLOW FIBERS.** These are composed of the protein **elastin**, which provides flexibility and elasticity. Yellow fibers (also called elastic fibers) are found in the lungs, in blood vessels, in the dermis of the skin, and in other areas that require elasticity.
3. **RETICULAR FIBERS.** These are composed of thin collagen fibers capable of forming a fine, meshlike supportive webbing in soft tissue such as the liver, bone marrow, and lymphatic system.

Other substances in the extracellular matrix include **fibronectin** proteins and **cellular adhesion molecules** (CAMs) such as **integrins.** Fibronectins bind to transmembrane integrins on a cell surface that interact with the intracellular components of the cytoskeleton. Fibonectins also bind to extracellular collagen fibers. In this way, fibronectins and integrins form a link between the cytoskeleton and the extracellular matrix for the transport of cells and materials. This binding also allows for cell-to-ECM and cell-to-cell interactions and for cell signaling. The extracellular matrix plays an essential role in cancer progression. Healthy ECM cells may inhibit cancer. However, abnormal ECM cells may facilitate the spread of cancer.

TIP

-BLASTS VERSUS *-CYTES*

Cells in connective tissue that are actively dividing and secreting extracellular matrix carry the suffix *-blast*. Mature cells that have stopped dividing carry the suffix *-cytes*.

Types of Cells and Tissues

You should be familiar with the common types of connective tissue cells listed in Table 3.11.

Blood is a connective tissue that consists of an abundant, watery matrix containing many specialized cell types. These cells will be discussed in the section "Circulatory, Lymphatic, and Immune Systems."

Connective tissue differentiates from mesenchyme into loose connective tissue, dense connective tissue, cartilage, blood, and bone. Loose connective tissue and dense connective tissue are together considered connective tissue proper. They are characterized by fibroblasts and a relatively soft ground substance.

Table 3.11 Function and Location of Common Connective Tissue Cells

Cell Type	Function/Location
Fibroblasts	Connective tissue proper
Adipocytes	Fat tissue
Chondrocytes	Cartilage
Osteocytes	Bone
White blood cells and macrophages	Immune, extracellular matrix
Mast cells	Histamine release, inflammatory response

Endocrine and Nervous Systems

The endocrine and nervous systems are the primary systems for maintaining **homeostasis**, or a stable internal environment, within the body. Both systems respond to information from the internal and external environment through negative and positive feedback systems that function to maintain the body's internal environment within the narrow limits that support life.

The endocrine and nervous systems depend on **communication**, or transmission of information, to respond to changes in the external and internal environments. Communication within the nervous system occurs by the rapid transmission of electrochemical signals. In contrast, communication within the endocrine system occurs more slowly through the release of chemical messengers into the bloodstream.

THE PANCREAS

The pancreas acts as an endocrine gland by secreting the hormones insulin and glucagon directly into the bloodstream in minute quantities. However, most pancreatic secretions are exocrine secretions.

The Endocrine System

The endocrine system is a set of organs and tissues that produce chemicals called **hormones**. Secreted by specialized cells in **endocrine glands** or in tissues, these hormones are molecules that elicit a response or change in target cells. The target cells may be relatively far away from the source cells. Hormones may be highly specific in the types and locations of target cells, or they may affect many cell types throughout the body.

Endocrine hormones are secreted into the circulatory system. They are released by exocytosis or by diffusion into capillaries that run through the endocrine glands. In contrast to endocrine glands, which are ductless, **ducted (exocrine) glands** secrete their products directly into another organ, not into the circulatory system. Some organs have both endocrine and exocrine functions, such as the pancreas and the testes.

The endocrine system has three main components—the hormones, the receptors on the target cells, and the endocrine glands themselves.

TYPES OF ENDOCRINE HORMONES

Hormones are classified as either **amino acid–based hormones** or **steroid hormones**. Amino acid–based hormones, which are water soluble, may be derivatives of individual amino acids. Instead, they may be polypeptides or proteins. Steroid hormones are lipids derived from cholesterol and are not water soluble. These two types of hormones differ in their solubility in blood and in their method of action on target tissues.

Amino Acid–Based Hormones

Table 3.12 lists several amino acid–based hormones derived from individual amino acids.

Table 3.12 Several Hormones and Neurotransmitters Derived from Amino Acids

Hormone Name	Function	Amino Acid Derivation
Serotonin	Neurotransmitter	Tryptophan
Melatonin	Neurotransmitter	Tryptophan
Histamine	Neurotransmitter	Glutamic acid
Epinephrine (adrenaline)	Adrenal hormone	Tyrosine
Norepinephrine (noradrenaline)	Adrenal hormone	Tyrosine
Thyroxine	Thyroid hormone	Tyrosine

Most amino acid–based hormones are hydrophilic and travel through the blood to bind to extracellular membrane receptors. However, thyroxine is hydrophobic, like the steroid hormones. Consequently, thyroxine must travel through the blood while bound to plasma proteins. It must cross the cell membrane to bind with intracellular receptors.

Most amino acid–based hormones are **peptide hormones** composed of polypeptide chains. Several of these are listed in Table 3.13.

Table 3.13 Several Peptide Hormones

Hormone Name	Function	Additional Information
Calcitonin	Lowers blood calcium levels	Short amino acid chain
Insulin	Decreases blood glucose levels	Long-chain polypeptide
Glucagon	Increases blood glucose levels	Long-chain polypeptide

Steroid Hormones

Examples of steroid hormones include the **sex hormones** and the **adrenocorticoids**. The sex hormones are produced by the gonads and include **estrogen**, **progesterone**, and **testosterone**. The adrenocorticoids are secreted by the adrenal glands. Adrenocorticoids are further divided into **mineralocorticoids** and **glucocorticoids**. The mineralocorticoids are responsible for maintaining sodium and potassium levels. The glucocorticoids regulate blood glucose levels through gluconeogenesis.

Other Chemical Signals

Certain other signaling substances are hormonelike in their functions.

Prostaglandins are lipid-soluble messenger molecules derived from essential fatty acids such as arachidonic acid. Unlike hormones, which are excreted from specialized endocrine glands into the bloodstream, prostaglandins are secreted by tissues throughout the body. Prostaglandins are released into adjacent tissues and are thus local autocrine or paracrine signal molecules (see Cell-Cell Communication) with short-lived effects. Prostaglandins are most notable for generating the inflammation response and for vasodilation. Vasodilation results from the action of prostaglandins on the smooth muscle lining arterioles and arteries.

Growth factors stimulate the growth and development of specific tissues or cells. Growth factors may be either proteins or steroid hormones which, like prostaglandins, have local paracrine or autocrine effects. Growth factors most likely to be tested on the MCAT are erythropoietin (**EPO**) and the vascular endothelial growth factor (**VEGF**). EPO is used to increase the number of erythrocytes in the blood. VEGF promotes growth of new vasculature to supply a tumor. EPO is released in response to vigorous exercise, and VEGF is released by tumors to enhance blood flow to the tumor tissue. The term *growth factor* is sometimes used synonymously with *cytokines*. However, unlike growth factors, cytokines may inhibit cell division or even initiate cell death (apoptosis).

Pheromones are chemical signaling molecules that act outside the body to trigger a physiological response in another individual. Pheromones, in humans, are lipid-soluble molecules excreted with sweat from the exocrine glands of the skin. These compounds are responsible for the unique body odor of an individual. The exact physiological response of humans to pheromones has not been investigated thoroughly. For animals, pheromones are used to signal ovulation, to raise alarms, and to mark a food trail.

MECHANISMS OF ENDOCRINE HORMONE ACTION

Hormones are secreted from the gland in which they are produced and enter the bloodstream to bind with receptors in a **target cell**. One hormone can affect many different target tissues. Some types of hormones bind to plasma membrane receptors. Other types cross the plasma membrane to bind with receptors within the cell.

Plasma Membrane Receptors and Second Messengers

Water-soluble, polar hormones such as peptide hormones travel through the bloodstream to target cells but are unable to cross the plasma membrane. Instead, these hormones exert their action by binding to receptors located on the cell surface. The binding of the receptor and hormone activates intracellular **second messengers** such as **cyclic AMP**. These second messengers then trigger a metabolic cascade, or signal transduction pathway, within the cell.

Intracellular Receptors and Direct Gene Activation

Steroid hormones do not bind to the plasma membrane. Instead, they cross the membrane to bind with receptors within the cell. Because steroid hormones are lipids, they are not water soluble and must bind to carrier proteins to be transported in the blood. Once they reach the cell, steroid hormones are able to diffuse across the nonpolar cell membrane and into the cytosol where they bind with intracellular receptors. The receptor-steroid complex then enters the nucleus and binds directly to DNA to affect gene expression.

Positive and Negative Feedback

Hormones are regulated by **feedback** systems that act to reduce or enhance the effect of the hormone. For example, when blood glucose levels become elevated, the pancreas secretes the hormone insulin. Insulin allows glucose to enter cells, lowering blood sugar. The pancreas senses the decrease in blood glucose and responds by stopping the secretion of insulin. This is an example of **negative feedback** because the effect of the hormone acts to reduce further effects by inhibiting hormone production, thereby keeping body functions within stable limits. Figure 3.67 shows another example of negative feedback.

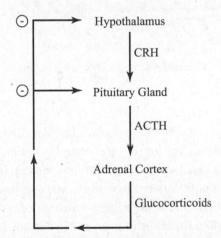

Figure 3.67. Example of negative feedback in the endocrine system

In **positive feedback**, the effect of the hormone causes even more hormone to be released. Humans have just a few examples of **positive feedback**. Some of the significant examples involve childbirth and nursing. During labor, the child presses on and distends the muscles of the cervix, triggering the release of the hormone oxytocin from the pituitary gland. Oxytocin causes muscles in the uterus to contract, leading to more dilation of the cervix, which triggers release of more oxytocin. This positive feedback cycle is finally terminated by the birth of the child.

MAJOR ENDOCRINE GLANDS

Figure 3.68 shows the major organs of the human endocrine system. Although most endocrine organs are found in both males and females, the sex organs differ.

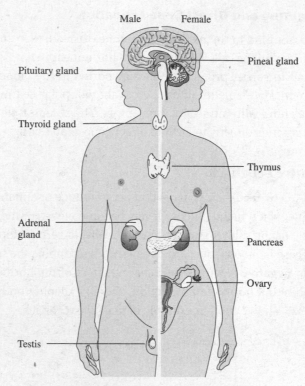

Figure 3.68. Major endocrine glands

Hypothalamus

The hypothalamus is composed of nerve tissue and is considered a part of the brain. The hypothalamus is responsible for integrating the complex communication functions of the endocrine and nervous systems. As part of the nervous system, it plays a crucial role as the "head ganglion" of the autonomic nervous system, sensing internal conditions like temperature and **blood osmolarity**. The hypothalamus provides direct neural links between the conscious regions of the forebrain and the centers of emotional and unconscious control. As such, the hypothalamus directly controls or shares control of diverse functions including body temperature, appetite, water balance and thirst, sexual drive, and emotional responses. In addition to its connections to various parts of the central nervous system, the hypothalamus also has a significant influence on chemical communication and itself acts as an endocrine gland.

> **OSMOLARITY**
>
> The concentration of solutes in blood is usually measured as osmolarity (osmoles per liter). In contrast to a mole, an osmole counts the number of particles of a substance, including ions. One mole of NaCl would yield two osmoles, Na^+ and Cl^-.

All hypothalamus secretions are peptide hormones and include the following:

- **TRH** (thryrotropin-releasing hormone) targets the anterior pituitary to produce TSH (thyroid-stimulating hormone). TRH also stimulates anterior pituitary secretion of prolactin.

- **Dopamine**, in its endocrine role, inhibits the release of prolactin by the anterior pituitary. (Dopamine is also an important brain neurotransmitter),
- **GHRH** (growth hormone–releasing hormone) stimulates release of GH (growth hormone) by the anterior pituitary.
- **Somatostatin** inhibits both GH and TSH release by the anterior pituitary.
- **GnRH** (gonadotropin-releasing hormone) stimulates production of FSH (follicle-stimulating hormone) and LH (luteinizing hormone) by the anterior pituitary.
- **CRH** (corticotropin-releasing hormone) stimulates production of ACTH (adrenocorticotropic hormone) by the anterior pituitary.

The hypothalamic endocrine cells are specialized neurons called **neurosecretory cells**. When nerve impulses are transmitted along the axons of the neurosecretory cells, the impulses trigger the release of hormones rather than of neurotransmitters. There are two sets of neurosecretory cells—parvocellular and magnocellular—that differ in the way that they release hormones and in the region of the hypothalamus that they influence.

Parvocellular neurosecretory cells (*parvo* = "small") store vesicles with several hormones called **releasing factors**. The vesicles are stored in each cell's terminal buds. The releasing factor hormones exit into a capillary bed that is the entry point for the **hypophyseal portal system**. The releasing factors are secreted into hypothalamic capillaries. From there the releasing factors are pumped just a few millimeters to the next capillary bed in the **anterior lobe** of the pituitary gland. The releasing factors either stimulate or inhibit production of anterior pituitary hormones. These include follicle stimulating hormone (FSH), luteinizing hormone (LH), thyroid stimulating hormone (TSH), and others discussed below.

Magnocellular neurosecretory cells extend from the hypothalamus directly into the **posterior pituitary lobe**. Nerve impulses received by the cells trigger the release of the hormones **ADH** (antidiuretic hormone, or vasopressin) and **oxytocin**. ADH and oxytocin are produced by the hypothalamus and subsequently are absorbed by and stored in the posterior pituitary gland until they are secreted.

Pituitary

The pituitary gland is regulated by the hypothalamus through neuroendocrine control. It has two distinct lobes, each releasing different hormones into the bloodstream.

The **posterior pituitary lobe** is really an extension of the hypothalamus. It directly receives two hormones, ADH and oxytocin, which it stores until their secretion is triggered by physiological conditions.

- **ADH** (antidiuretic hormone) is a small peptide hormone that causes kidneys to reabsorb more water from kidney tubules into the bloodstream and to release more concentrated urine. When blood osmolarity increases, sensory neurons in the hypothalamus (**osmoreceptors**) send impulses to the hypothalamic magnocellular neurosecretory cells to release ADH into the posterior pituitary. The ADH is then released by the pituitary into the bloodstream. When ADH reaches the kidneys, it bonds to receptors on the membranes of cells of the collecting ducts. This bonding triggers a release of cAMP (cyclic AMP, a

> **HYPOPHYSEAL PORTAL SYSTEM**
>
> The hypophyseal is one of three portal systems in which blood flows from one capillary bed into another capillary bed instead of directly into venules. The other two are the hepatic and renal portal systems.

second messenger). The release of cAMP increases the permeability of the collecting ducts to water. Water then diffuses from the nephron into the vasa recta (the capillaries surrounding the convoluted tubule and loop of Henle). As the blood becomes more dilute, the hypothalamus releases less ADH, resulting in a reduced rate of water retention. This is a typical example of endocrine regulation via a **negative feedback loop**.

- **Oxytocin** is a small peptide hormone that targets and stimulates the contraction of smooth muscles. Secretion of oxytocin is especially significant in females to promote uterine muscle cell contraction during childbirth and to release milk from mammary glands in lactation.

The **anterior pituitary lobe** produces a wide array of peptide hormones. Some of these are **tropic**. They promote the production of other hormones by other endocrine glands. Others act directly on tissues, without involving other hormones.

The tropic hormones include the following:

- **TSH** (thyroid-stimulating hormone) stimulates thyroid gland production of thyroxine and triiodothyronine.
- **ACTH** (adrenocorticotropin) stimulates the adrenal cortex to produce androgens and corticosteroids.
- **FSH** (follicle-stimulating hormone) in females promotes maturation of an ovarian follicle. In males, it stimulates sperm maturation.
- **LH** (luteinizing hormone) in females triggers ovulation and formation of the corpus luteum. In males, it promotes the production of testosterone.

Two anterior pituitary hormones, GH and prolactin, act directly. Unlike the tropic hormones, these two do not act by stimulating production of other hormones.

- **GH** (growth hormone) stimulates cell growth and reproduction directly. It also stimulates the liver to produce hormones (growth factors) that stimulate bone and cartilage growth.
- **Prolactin** stimulates milk production by the mammary glands.

Thyroid

The thyroid gland is located in two lobes around the trachea, below the larynx and above the sternum. The thyroid produces three hormones. The first two, T_3 and T_4, act as a set. The third hormone is calcitonin.

> **BASAL METABOLIC RATE**
>
> An increased basal metabolic rate means that the chemical reactions of metabolism proceed more quickly and cells consume more oxygen and calories.

Triiodothyronine (T_3) and **thyroxine (T_4)** are both derived from the amino acid tyrosine. They both contain atoms of iodine and act similarly on target cells. T_3 is the more active form. Both regulate basal metabolic rates. They also increase rates of protein synthesis. Finally, T_3 and T_4 are important in growth and nervous system development in children.

Calcitonin lowers blood Ca^{+2} concentrations, resulting in the concurrent uptake and deposition of Ca^{+2} by osteoblasts in bone. Calcitonin functions to decrease excess blood calcium levels, opposing parathyroid hormone, which increases blood calcium levels. Calcitonin levels tend to be higher in young children. However, its function in human physiology is not well understood.

Parathyroids

These four small glands 3–4 mm in diameter are on the dorsal surface of the thyroid gland. Along with the thyroid gland, they regulate blood calcium concentrations.

PTH (**parathyroid hormone**) acts antagonistically to calcitonin. PTH is activated by vitamin D. PTH is secreted when blood Ca^{+2} levels are low. PTH stimulates osteoclast activity, which dissolves bone, mobilizing Ca^{+2} ions. It also enhances kidney reabsorption of Ca^{+2}. PTH stimulates vitamin D activation and release by the kidneys and other tissues.

Pancreas

Most pancreatic tissue is exocrine and produces digestive enzymes and bicarbonate ions that are released into the small intestine via the pancreatic duct. However, in addition, the pancreas is dotted with clusters of cells called islets of Langerhans, which are endocrine tissue.

The hormone **insulin** causes cells (mostly muscle, liver, and adipose) to take up glucose from the bloodstream, lowering blood sugar levels. It also shifts metabolic energy sources from fat to carbohydrates. It promotes cellular uptake of amino acids and consequently protein synthesis. Insulin promotes the uptake of sugar into the liver where it is converted into glycogen. Insulin is secreted by β-cells (beta cells), and its release is regulated by blood sugar concentration. After a meal, when blood glucose rises, β-cells secrete insulin. Insulin binds to receptors on cell surfaces. The hormone-receptor complex initiates a sequence of changes that opens glucose channels so that glucose can diffuse into cells.

Diabetes is the most well known and common disease of the endocrine system. In type I diabetes, insufficient quantities of insulin are produced. In type 2 diabetes, adequate insulin is produced, but problems occur with insulin receptors or with glucose uptake by cells. In either case, high concentrations of carbohydrate accumulate in blood plasma (hyperglycemia). Urine tests show sugar in the urine, indicating diabetes. The high concentrations of sugar in the urine prevent kidneys from reabsorbing water, which leads to dehydration. Because glucose cannot be effectively used as an energy source in diabetics, fat is oxidized at a much higher than normal rate. The result is an accumulation of ketones in the blood. This accumulation can eventually reduce blood pH (ketoacidosis) enough to cause serious complications. If left unmanaged, diabetes can lead to compromised blood flow, muscle weakness, blindness, and a host of other problems.

The hormone **glucagon** is secreted by α-cells (alpha cells) in the islets of Langerhans. Glucagon is antagonistic to insulin. It is secreted in response to low blood sugar. Glucagon causes the liver to convert stored glycogen to glucose. Glucagon also promotes the breakdown of fats and proteins and it stimulates the liver and kidneys to initiate **gluconeogenesis** (glucose synthesis from non-carbohydrates sources). The "hunger" hormones, **gastrin** and **CCK** (cholecystokinin), also stimulate glucagon production.

Somatostatin is secreted by pancreatic δ-cells (delta cells.) Somatostatin production is stimulated by both high blood sugar and high blood amino acid content. It inhibits production of both insulin and glucagon.

Adrenal

The adrenal gland is composed of a **cortex** and a **medulla**. The cortex is derived from the mesoderm and the medulla from the ectoderm. Overall, the adrenal hormones help the body in fight-or-flight situations. They cause vasoconstriction, increased heart rate, increased respiration, and increased blood glucose levels. Adrenal hormones dilate the pupils and also affect the intestines and uterus.

The adrenal cortex is divided into three zones: the **zona glomerulosa** on the outer edge, the **zona fasciculata** intermediately, and the **zona reticularis** bordering the medulla. The cortex produces **corticosteroids**, steroid hormones derived from cholesterol.

The zona glomerulosa produces mineralocorticoids from lipids and cholesterol. Mineralocorticoids function to help retain water, sodium, and chloride. They also increase the urinary loss of phosphorus and potassium by acting on the renal tubules. The most important hormone produced in this zone is **aldosterone**, a mineralocorticoid that regulates the concentration of sodium and potassium in the blood. It is important to recognize that the pituitary gland exerts no control in this zone.

The zona fasciculata and zona reticularis produce glucocorticoids. These hormones are gluconeogenic in nature, regulating blood glucose concentrations. They are regulated by the hormone **ACTH**, produced in the pituitary gland. These hormones convert amino acids into glucose instead of protein and thus increase blood sugar and liver glycogen levels. **Cortisol** is an example of a glucocorticoid that influences carbohydrate, protein, and fat metabolism. Cortisol also affects the permeability of cell membranes, suppresses inflammation, and suppresses the immune system by interfering with the antigen-antibody response.

The zona reticularis produces sex hormones called gonadocorticoids, which include DHEA and estradiol. These hormones have similar functions to the sex hormones produced by the testes and ovaries but are produced in much lower quantities. Because gonadocorticoids are predominantly androgens, they have masculinizing effects and contribute to puberty and sex drive in both males and females. The anterior pituitary exerts a mild control over the production of these hormones.

Problems may sometimes occur with the function of the adrenal cortex. **Addison's disease** is a hypofunction of the adrenal cortex which manifests as chronic adrenal insufficiency. This condition arises from inadequate amounts of steroid hormones. Clinically, the patients exhibit general debility, a weak heart, stomach irritation, and a change in skin color due to deposition of melanin.

Hyperadrenalism syndromes include Conn's syndrome, Cushing's syndrome, and adrenal virilism. **Conn's syndrome** is caused by an overproduction of aldosterone by the zona glomerulosa. **Cushing's syndrome** is the result of excess cortisol produced by the zona fasciculata. **Adrenal virilism** is the premature appearance of secondary sexual characteristics caused by excessive production of androgens in the zona reticularis.

The adrenal medulla is located in the center of the adrenal gland, surrounded by the cortex. The cells of the medulla are modified postganglionic neurons that act as an extension of the sympathetic nervous system. In the medulla, the amino acid tyrosine is converted into a class of hormones called **catecholamines**, which include **epinephrine** and **norepinephrine**. Common synonyms for these hormones are adrenaline and noradrenaline, respectively. These hormones function in the fight-or-flight response. They reduce the blood flow to the internal organs and the skin. They also increase flow to the skeletal muscles, brain, and heart—the organs most directly involved in fighting or fleeing. This redirection of blood flow is effected through vasodilation and vasoconstriction.

Gonads

The testes function as both exocrine and endocrine glands. The primary endocrine hormone of the **testes** is the steroid hormone **testosterone**. The testes secrete testosterone beginning in adolescence in response to luteinizing hormone (LH) secreted by the anterior pituitary. Testosterone is responsible for sexual differentiation in the embryo and for primary and secondary male sexual characteristics. In addition, testosterone augments body hair, muscle strength and mass, and bone density. It also has an effect on the development of the brain.

The **ovaries** are the source of the steroid hormones **estrogen** and **progesterone**. Like testosterone, the production of estrogen is regulated by the anterior pituitary. Progesterone is produced in the corpus luteum after ovulation.

Estrogens are responsible for the development of female secondary sexual characteristics, for the development of the female reproductive tract, and for ovulation. In addition, estrogens affect a wide range of body systems, including bone density, fat deposition, muscle mass, blood clotting, cholesterol levels, fluid balance, and thyroid function. Sharp fluctuations in estrogen levels can have psychological effects, including mood swings and depression.

Progesterone stimulates the walls of the endometrium to prepare for pregnancy. During pregnancy, progesterone suppresses lactation, reduces the potentially harmful maternal immune response, and inhibits the onset of labor. In addition, progesterone has a strengthening effect on myelin, collagen, skin, bones, teeth, ligaments, and thyroid function.

Nervous System: Structure and Function

Whereas communication within the endocrine system occurs slowly through the release of chemical messengers into the bloodstream, communication within the nervous system occurs by the rapid transmission of electrochemical signals. The nervous system receives information from the environment via **sensory receptors**, processes this information, and relays a response to muscles or glands. Figure 3.69 shows the brain, spinal cord, and many nerves in the nervous system. Muscles and glands that carry out a response are called **effectors**. The specialized cells of the nervous system that transmit and process information are **neurons**. Neurons are similar to muscle cells in that they are **excitable**, or capable of responding to stimuli through the generation of electrochemical signals. Like muscle cells, neurons are essentially amitotic and have very little capacity for regeneration.

NEURON STRUCTURE

All neurons have three basic parts, a soma, multiple dendrites, and a single axon. The **soma** (cell body) contains the nucleus and most of the organelles. The multiple dendrites are fingerlike processes extending from the soma that receive information. The single **axon**, or **nerve fiber**, is a long, cellular process that transmits information to other cells. The region between the cell body and the axon is an important area called the **axon hillock**, which acts as a threshold for nerve signals. The dendrites, soma, and axon hillock constitute the **receptive region** of a neuron. The axon is the **conductive region**. If a signal received by the receptive region is strong enough to reach threshold at the axon hillock, the signal will continue (self-propagate) along the axon. Once the signal reaches the end of the axon, the **secretory region**, branches called **axon terminals** transmit information from the neuron to adjacent cells. (See Figure 3.70.)

> **LONG AXONS**
>
> The longest human motor neurons have axons up to 1.5 m long. These neurons go from the spinal cord to the big toes.

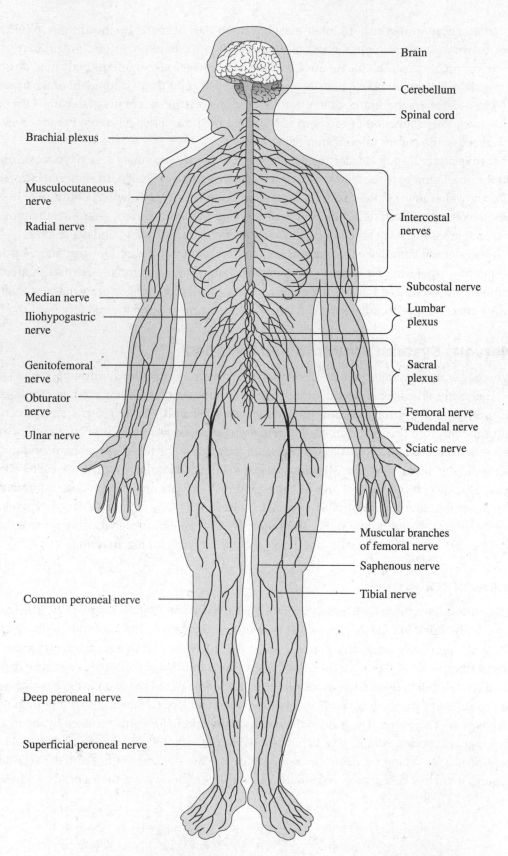

Figure 3.69 Nervous system

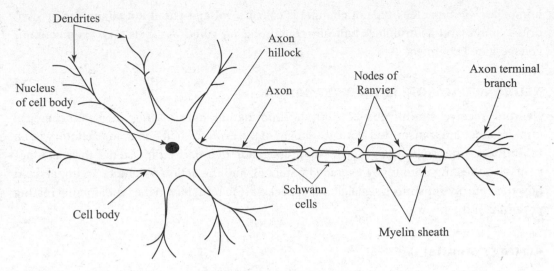

Figure 3.70. Neuron structure

Myelin Sheath

Many vertebrate neurons have axons that are insulated by myelin, a whitish, fatty mixture of lipids and proteins secreted by glial cells. The **myelin sheath** is formed by Schwann cells in the peripheral nervous system and oligodendrocytes in the central nervous system (see Glial Cells below). These support cells wrap around the axon in jelly-roll-like layers that are almost entirely filled with myelin. The myelin sheath insulates the axon against current loss during propagation of the electrochemical signal and speeds up the rate of transmission.

Glial Cells

Neurons carry out the function of transmission; however, the most abundant cells in the nervous system are support cells called **glial cells** (or **neuroglia**). Unlike neurons, glial cells are not excitable. Instead, they function to nourish, support, and protect the neurons and to direct the growth of neurons during development.

Glial cells are specialized for different functions. The most abundant are **astrocytes**, star-shaped support cells that support neurons in the brain and spinal cord (the central nervous system). Other glial cells in the central nervous system include **microglia**, which act as defensive phagocytes, **ependymal cells**, which line fluid-filled brain cavities, and **oligodendrocytes**, which secrete myelin. In the peripheral nerves and ganglia (peripheral nervous system), glial cells include **satellite cells**, which nourish and protect neuron cell bodies, and **Schwann cells**, which myelinate axons and aid in the regeneration of damaged fibers.

Ion Channels

In both neurons and muscle cells, electrochemical signals are initiated by the opening of membrane ion channels. When an ion channel opens, charged ions rush into or out of the cell, resulting in a rapid and reversible change in the difference in charge between the inside and outside of the cell (the membrane potential).

Ion channels are transmembrane proteins that act as gates, allowing ions to pass through the membrane. Some ion channels may be opened by the binding of another molecule, or **ligand**. This type of channel is called a **ligand–gated ion channel**. Other channels are triggered by a change in the electrical potential (voltage across the plasma membrane) in their immediate vicinity. This type of channel is called a **voltage–gated ion channel**. The dendrites, soma, and axon hillock typically contain ligand-gated channels. The axon contains voltage-gated channels.

NEURON FUNCTION: THE NERVE IMPULSE

Neurons receive stimuli and convert the information into a series of electrochemical impulses that are transmitted along the length of the axon to elicit either an **excitatory** or an **inhibitory** response in a target cell. The propagation of a nerve impulse has three components—the resting potential, the graded potential, and the action potential. To understand how the neuron transmits a signal, it is first necessary to understand the fundamental **resting potential** of the neuron.

Resting Potential

TIP

SODIUM-POTASSIUM PUMP

As a mnemonic, think of salt on the outside of a pretzel to remember that the sodium accumulates on the outside of the cell.

The term **resting potential** refers to the difference in electrical charge between the inside and the outside of the cell when the neuron is not actively conducting a nerve impulse. The term *resting* is misleading in that maintaining the resting potential requires energy from ATP to maintain ion gradients. A typical resting potential of a neuron is –70 mV. The negative sign refers to the fact that the inside of the cell is negative relative to the outside.

The resting potential is established by the action of the sodium-potassium (or Na^+-K^+) pump, a protein molecule that is densely distributed throughout the neuron cell membrane. Figure 3.71 shows the sodium-potassium pump. By using energy from the hydrolysis of ATP, the pump forces sodium ions out of the cell and pumps potassium ions into the cytoplasm. For every two K^+ ions pumped into the cell, three Na^+ ions are expelled. This results in a greater number of positive charges outside the cell and thus a relative negative charge inside the cell.

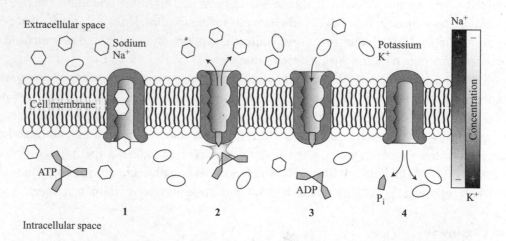

Figure 3.71. Sodium-potassium pump. From left to right, *(1)* three sodium ions inside the cell are drawn into the pump, *(2)* they are expelled, *(3)* two potassium ions from outside the cell are drawn into the pump, and *(4)* they are propelled into the cell.

Initiation of a Signal

A signal begins when sensory information or information from another nerve cell reaches the receptive region. Such external information takes the form of a signal molecule that binds with a ligand–gated ion channel. This binding causes the channel to open, allowing charged ions to enter the cell and altering resting potential. This change in potential in a localized area of the cell is called a **graded potential** because its magnitude depends on the strength of the stimulus. The graded potential may result from the opening of gated sodium channels, in which case, the influx of positive sodium ions will make the interior of the cell less negative and will raise the membrane potential from –70 mV to a number closer to zero. This increase in membrane potential is called a **depolarization**. Graded potentials that depolarize the cell are **excitatory** signals.

Alternatively, a graded potential may result from the opening of potassium or chloride channels, leading to a loss of positive ions or a gain of negative ions within the cell. Either situation leads to a decrease in the membrane potential, which becomes more negative. This type of potential change is a **hyperpolarization**, which is an **inhibitory** signal. Multiple signals reaching the neuron at the same time may include both excitatory and inhibitory stimuli. The overall change in membrane potential is the result of the summation of all the signals reaching the receptive region.

Graded Potential

Graded potentials originate in the receptive region and spread through the cell body toward the axon hillock. The strength of a graded potential weakens with distance. A weak stimulus will result in a weak graded potential that travels only a short distance. However, if the graded potential is large enough, it can alter the resting potential as far as the axon hillock, the "trigger" region of the neuron. For a signal to be transmitted by the neuron, the axon hillock must be depolarized sufficiently to reach a threshold value, typically 10–20 mV above resting potential. In a neuron with a resting potential of –70 mV, the threshold value may be –55 mV. One or more graded potentials that result in a net depolarization of the axon hillock to threshold will initiate a second type of signal, an **action potential**, or **nerve impulse**, in the axon of the neuron.

Action Potential

Action potentials are initiated by the opening of voltage–gated ion channels that occur only in the conductive region of the neuron. These are **sodium channels** and **potassium channels**. The opening of voltage–gated sodium channels leads to depolarization of the neuron, and the opening of voltage–gated potassium channels reverses the depolarization, a process called **repolarization**. Recall that at resting potential the concentration of sodium ions is higher on the outside of the cell, and the concentration of potassium ions is higher on the inside of the cell, creating an electrochemical gradient. If a graded potential raises membrane potential in the vicinity of the axon hillock to threshold (to approximately –55 mV), voltage–gated sodium channels will open, allowing a large influx of Na^+ ions. As a result, the membrane potential can rapidly increase nearly 100 mV, from –70 mV to +30 mV. This is the **depolarization** phase of the action potential.

The area affected by the depolarization is initially small—just the area of the axon adjacent to the axon hillock. However, voltage-gated channels in the axon are placed at close intervals. As a result, adjacent channels down the axon (away from the cell body) are also in a region of increased positive charge and will open, allowing still more positive sodium ions to enter and depolarize the area around it. As a result, each sodium channel down the axon will be triggered sequentially down the entire axon. Because each sodium channel is triggered to open by the opening of adjacent sodium channels in a positive-feedback system, an action potential is self-reinforcing and self-propagating and does not degrade with distance.

Repolarization

The opening of voltage–gated sodium channels is short-lived. Once a voltage–gated ion channel has opened to allow sodium ions to flood the cell, it closes again. The temporary depolarization triggers the opening of a second set of ion channels, the voltage–gated potassium channels located along the axon. The opening of these channels allows K⁺ ions to leave the cell, following their concentration gradient. This exodus of K⁺ results in the second phase of the action potential, **repolarization**. By the time repolarization takes place, the next Na⁺ channel down the axon has already opened, sending the depolarization wave down the axon. The net effect is that each successive area of the axon is first depolarized and then repolarized before returning to the resting potential.

During repolarization, an excess of K⁺ exiting the cell leads to a short period of **hyperpolarization**, in which the cell becomes more negative than the resting potential. This effect is temporary. Within about 2 milliseconds of the depolarization wave reaching one point along the neuron, the sodium and potassium channels have both closed. The sodium-potassium pumps reestablish the resting potential.

In summary, two things happen during an action potential. First, voltage–gated sodium channels open and propagate the nerve impulse. Second, sodium channels close and adjacent potassium channels open and shut to reset the resting membrane potential. Eventually the sodium-potassium pump will restore ionic concentrations in the cell. However, before that becomes necessary, multiple action potentials may be propagated along the same neuron. (See Figure 3.72.)

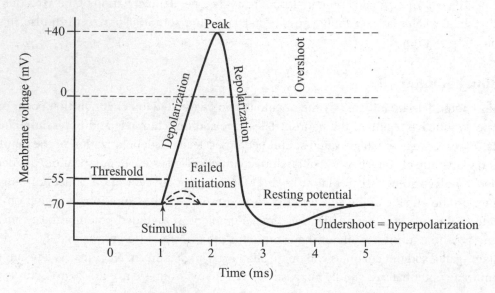

Figure 3.72. Action potential (Adapted from:
http://en.wikipedia.org/wiki/File:Action_potential_vert.png)

The time delay between the opening of Na⁺ channels and the restoration of resting potential is the **refractory period**. Because a membrane cannot be restimulated during the refractory period, an action potential can travel in only one direction along the axon, away from the point of origin along the length of the axon toward the axon terminals.

Nerve Impulse Summary

The nerve impulse is an **all-or-none threshold response**. For an action potential to be generated, the graded potential must depolarize the cell sufficiently to reach threshold. If the stimulus is weak and the resulting depolarization is below threshold, no signal is transmitted. Above the threshold, an action potential is generated and an impulse is transmitted. Once enough Na^+ ions have entered the cell to reach the threshold, any additional sodium triggers the opening of more sodium channels in an unstoppable positive feedback cycle, resulting in an all-or-none response.

In contrast to graded potentials, action potentials always have the same magnitude regardless of the strength of the stimulus. Variation in the strength of the stimulus results in a change in the frequency, not the magnitude, of the nerve impulses. Consider two scenarios. In one, you drop a book onto your foot. In the second, you drop a brick onto your foot. When you drop the brick onto your foot, there will be more nerve impulses per second. However, each impulse will have the same magnitude. A greater frequency of impulses transmitted down the axon is interpreted by the central nervous system as a more powerful signal, such as more intense pain.

SALTATORY CONDUCTION

Myelinated axons speed transmission of nerve impulses because myelin prevents charge leakage—and, consequently, loss of electrochemical potential—across the membrane. However, the myelin sheath surrounding axons is not continuous. Glial cells, such as Schwann cells, are spaced at intervals surrounding gaps called **nodes of Ranvier**. Because voltage–gated sodium channels are concentrated in these gaps, myelinated axons exhibit **saltatory conduction**. *Saltatory* comes from the Latin for "jumping." The action potential "jumps" through the cytoplasm from one node of Ranvier to the next. In contrast, unmyelinated axons have sodium channels along their entire length. Saltatory conduction requires the opening of fewer sodium channels over a smaller membrane surface area, allowing an action potential to propagate more rapidly. The rate of propagation of myelinated axons is approximately 100 times greater than that of unmyelinated axons of the same diameter.

SYNAPSES

Nerve impulses are propagated through the body between neurons or between neurons and effectors, such as muscles or glands. The junction between a neuron and another cell is a **synapse**, as shown in Figure 3.73. Because nerve signals travel in one direction, the nerve cell from which the signal is coming is called the **presynaptic cell**. The cell that receives the signal is called the **postsynaptic cell**. Synapses may be **chemical** or **electrical**.

Chemical synapses are the most common form of synapse. A chemical synapse consists of the axon terminal of the presynaptic neuron, a fluid-filled **synaptic cleft**, and a postsynaptic cell, which may be another neuron or an effector cell. The ends of the axon terminals are modified into bulbous **synaptic knobs** that contain vesicles of chemical **neurotransmitters**. When an action potential arrives at the synaptic knob, voltage–gated calcium channels open in the plasma membrane, triggering vesicles to release neurotransmitter into the synaptic cleft. Neurotransmitter molecules cross the synaptic cleft and bind to postsynaptic membrane receptors, opening ion channels and creating a graded potential in the postsynaptic cell.

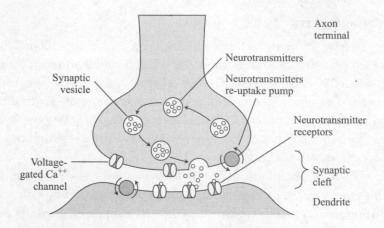

Figure 3.73. Synapse

Depending on the type of receptor and the type of associated ion channel, the binding of neurotransmitter to the postsynaptic cell results in a change in membrane potential that is either depolarizing or hyperpolarizing. Depolarizations result in an **excitatory postsynaptic potential** (**EPSP**) and allow the postsynaptic cell to reach the firing threshold more easily. In contrast, hyperpolarization results in an **inhibitory postsynaptic potential** (**IPSP**). Inhibitory potentials leave the postsynaptic neuron less likely to fire.

Summation of Impulses

Nerve impulses can be transmitted across a synapse to a particular cell through a single transmission. Often, though, the strength of the signal is increased through multiple nerve impulses to the same cell. The process whereby a single cell responds to multiple nerve impulses is called **summation**. Summation can be spatial, temporal, or both.

Spatial summation involves the stimulation of the same postsynaptic cell by more than one axon terminal at the same time. **Temporal summation** involves rapid stimulation of the same postsynaptic cell by several nerve impulses in succession. In both spatial and temporal summation, each firing of an axon terminal releases more neurotransmitter into the synaptic cleft. If both excitatory and inhibitory stimuli are received, the inhibitory stimuli subtract from the effect of the excitatory stimuli, and the cell will be less likely to depolarize sufficiently to reach threshold.

Propagation and Resistance

As a signal propagates from a nerve cell to another cell, no loss occurs in the strength of the signal due to resistance. An action potential will always have the same magnitude even after passing through multiple neurons and synapses.

Neurotransmitter Degradation and Reuptake

Once a neurotransmitter molecule is released into the synaptic cleft, it may be degraded by enzymes, it may diffuse out of the synaptic cleft, or it may be taken up by active transport. An example of enzymatic degradation is the breakdown of acetylcholine into choline and acetic acid by the enzyme cholinesterase. Choline is subsequently transported back into the presynaptic neuron, where it is used in acetylcholine synthesis.

Synaptic Delay

Synaptic delay is the slight delay in signal transmission that occurs at a synapse. Compared with the short amount of time needed for the rapid propagation of an action potential along an axon, slightly more time is needed for information to cross a synapse. Neurotransmitters must be released, cross the synaptic cleft, and bind to receptors, leading to a very slight increase in transmission time.

Synapse Fatigue and Accommodation

If the vesicles at the end of the axon are stimulated to release neurotransmitters over a prolonged period, they may run out of available neurotransmitter. This is called **synapse fatigue**. A fatigued synapse cannot transmit a signal, no matter how much it is stimulated, until neurotransmitter levels are built up again through reuptake or protein synthesis.

If a nerve is subject to a gradually increasing stimulus, it may require increasingly stronger stimulation to initiate a nerve impulse. This is called **accommodation**.

Electrical Synapses

In an electrical synapse, the nerve impulse is transmitted directly from one cell to another via protein channels (**connexons**) located at gap junctions between cells. These protein channels allow multiple cells to be electrically coupled, or synchronized, to fire simultaneously. Unlike chemical synapses, electrical synapses can allow bidirectional as well as unidirectional signal transmission. Because no synaptic delay occurs, transmission is much more rapid than in chemical synapses. However, the signal cannot be amplified across the synapse. Electrical synapses link neurons together in embryonic tissues to coordinate development. In adults, electrical synapses occur in protective reflex arcs and in the retina and cerebral cortex, where rapid transmission is essential.

NEUROTRANSMITTERS

Neurotransmitters are the chemicals released in chemical synapes to trigger responses in the postsynaptic cell. Neurotransmitters include a variety of molecules, including peptides, amino acids, purines, lipids, and even dissolved gases such as carbon monoxide and nitrous oxide. The action of a specific neurotransmitter depends on the type and location of membrane receptors and on the duration of the stimulus. Membrane receptors are specific to a particular neurotransmitter. The same neurotransmitter may elicit either excitatory or inhibitory responses depending on the type of receptor. Neurotransmitters may directly open ion channels. Alternatively, they may signal an intermediary molecule (**second messenger**) that conveys information into the cell. The following describes some of the major neurotransmitters of the central and peripheral nervous systems.

Acetylcholine (ACh)

Acetylcholine is the neurotransmitter of neuromuscular junctions in skeletal muscle. It binds to excitatory receptors to stimulate muscle contraction. Acetylcholine also acts in the brain and the autonomic nervous system.

In neuromuscular junctions, the enzyme acetylcholinesterase breaks down acetylcholine into acetate and choline. Neurotoxins that inhibit the activity of acetylcholinesterase cause tetanus and muscle spasms. Examples include pesticides, strychnine, and the nerve gas sarin. Toxins that block acetylcholine receptors, such as curare, result in paralysis.

In the CNS, acetylcholine is involved in learning and short-term memory. A deficiency of acetylcholine is associated with neurological disorders such as Alzheimer's.

EPINEPHRINE AND NOREPINEPHRINE

Epinephrine (adrenaline) is a derivative of norepinephrine produced by the adrenal medulla.

Dopamine and Norepinephrine

Dopamine and norepinephrine are monoamine neurotransmitters derived from the amino acid tyrosine. In the brain, dopamine is involved in learning, memory and reward systems, motivation, and voluntary movement. Norepinephrine contributes to alertness and arousal. Both molecules are produced in response to stress and contribute to the fight-or-flight response of the sympathetic nervous system.

Dopamine and norepinephrine may also be secreted into the bloodstream to function as hormones. Low dopamine levels are associated with attention deficit disorder (ADD) and Parkinson's disease. High levels are associated with schizophrenia. Drugs that increase dopamine and norepinephrine levels include amphetamines, cocaine, and antidepressants.

Serotonin

Serotonin is another monoamine neurotransmitter that is derived from the amino acid tryptophan. Serotonin acts as a "feel good" neurotransmitter in the brain and spinal cord, where it binds to inhibitory receptors and regulates mood, appetite, sleep, learning, and memory. Approximately 80% of serotonin is produced in the GI tract, where it is involved in peristalsis. Serotonin is also released by the gut into the bloodstream, where it is stored in platelets and functions in blood clotting and vasoconstriction.

Serotonin is removed from the synaptic cleft by monoamine transporter proteins and is degraded by the enzyme monoamine oxidase. Drugs that increase serotonin levels include antidepressants such as monoamine oxidase inhibitors (MAOIs) and selective serotonin reuptake inhibitors (SSRIs), as well as cocaine and amphetamines.

Glutamate

Derived from the amino acid glutamic acid, glutamate is the most abundant neurotransmitter in vertebrates. It is also the primary excitatory neurotransmitter in the brain, where it functions in learning and memory.

GABA (Gamma-Aminobutyric Acid)

The second most abundant neurotransmitter in the brain after glutamate, GABA is derived from glutamate but binds to inhibitory receptors. The effects of alcohol consumption are due to the binding of alcohol to GABA receptors, resulting in inhibition of brain functions involved in motor control, judgment, and decision making.

Endorphins

Endorphins are a group of peptide neurotransmitters that block pain by acting as natural opiates. They are released by the brain and spinal cord in response to pain, exercise, certain foods, and emotion. Endorphins inhibit the release of GABA, increase the production of dopamine, and block the activity of substance P, another peptide neurotransmitter involved in pain sensitivity. The opiate drugs morphine, codeine, and heroin bind to the same receptors.

Adenosine/ATP

In addition to playing critical roles in signal transduction and energy transfer, the purine molecules adenosine and ATP function as neurotransmitters in the brain and sensory pathways. Adenosine binds to inhibitory receptors in the brain, facilitating sleep. ATP is released by sensory neurons in response to injury, initiating a pain response.

Caffeine, another purine, acts as an adenosine antagonist by binding to and blocking adenosine receptors in the brain. Consequently, caffeine acts as a stimulant by reducing the inhibitory effects of adenosine. In addition, caffeine stimulates the sympathetic nervous system, affecting anxiety and alertness. It also increases the production of dopamine involved in pleasure and reward. Figure 3.74 shows the structures of both caffeine and adenosine.

Caffeine   Adenosine

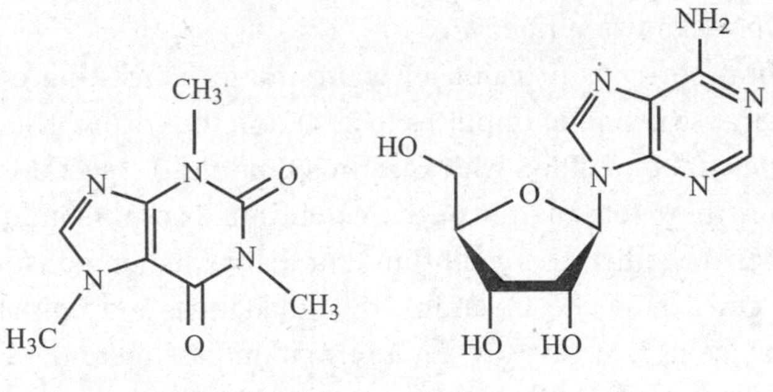

Figure 3.74. Caffeine and adenosine

Nitric Oxide

Nitric oxide is a short-lived dissolved gas that is synthesized as needed and travels out of the presynaptic neuron and across to the postsynaptic neuron by diffusion. It binds with enzymes to produce second messengers such as cyclic GMP. As a neurotransmitter, nitric oxide is involved in learning and memory.

ORGANIZATION OF THE VERTEBRATE NERVOUS SYSTEM

The vertebrate nervous system consists of the **central nervous system** (**CNS**) and the **peripheral nervous system** (**PNS**). The CNS contains the brain and spinal cord. The PNS consists of peripheral nerves and ganglia. Neurons that transmit sensory information toward the brain and spinal cord are sensory (**afferent**) neurons. Neurons that send responses from the central nervous system to muscles and glands (effectors) are motor (**efferent**) neurons. **Interneurons,** or **association neurons**, connect sensory neurons with motor neurons within the central nervous system.

The processing of information in the brain and spinal cord occurs in regions of **gray matter,** which are composed of unmyelinated cell bodies and synapses. **White matter** consists of myelinated axons that function in the transmission of information between brain regions and between the central nervous system and the peripheral nervous system. In the CNS, regions of gray matter are called **nuclei**, and regions of white matter are called **tracts**. In the PNS, axons of multiple neurons are bundled together with blood vessels and wrapped by connective tissue into **nerves**. The majority of nerves, **mixed nerves**, carry both afferent sensory and efferent motor fibers as well as both myelinated and unmyelinated axons. Synapses and collections of cell bodies of the PNS are called **ganglia**.

Central Nervous System (CNS)

The brain and the spinal cord of the central nervous system are responsible for coordination, integration, and processing of sensory information and motor responses. The brain is the primary processing center. The spinal cord relays information between the brain and the body.

The largest portion of the human **brain** consists of the **cerebrum**. The cerebrum is divided into right and left **cerebral hemispheres**, each of which primarily receives information from and exerts control over the opposite side of the body. The outer surface of the cerebral hemispheres, the **cerebral cortex**, is a region of gray matter that is the seat of higher-level functions, including consciousness, reasoning, judgment, sensory processing, and voluntary motor control. The cortex in humans is divided into lobes, as shown in Figure 3.75, and is highly convoluted to maximize surface area.

Below the cerebral cortex is a region of white matter consisting of myelinated tracts responsible for the transmission of impulses to and from the cortex. The cerebrum encloses **ventricles**, or cavities, that are filled with **cerebrospinal fluid**. Several islands of gray matter are found within the white matter of the cerebrum. These include the **diencephalon** and the **basal nuclei**. Together, the cerebrum and diencephalon constitute the **forebrain**. The diencephalon consists of the thalamus, hypothalamus, and epithalamus. The **thalamus** acts as the relay center, or gateway, for information passing to the cerebral cortex. The **hypothalamus** regulates body temperature, hunger, thirst, and sleep, controls the visceral responses of the autonomic nervous system, and acts as the master gland of the endocrine system by secreting hormones that regulate the **anterior pituitary gland**. In the roof of the hypothalamus, the **pineal gland** of the **epithalamus** functions to regulate sleep/wake cycles via secretion of the hormone **melatonin**. Other components of the forebrain include the **amygdala** and **hippocampus**, **basal nuclei**, which along with the hypothalamus forms part of the **limbic system** involved in emotion, visceral response, and memory.

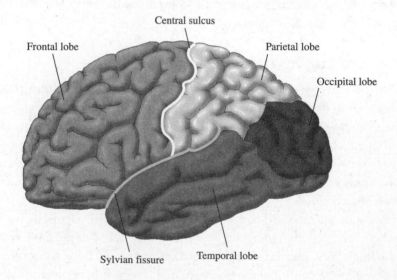

Figure 3.75. Lobes of the brain

Below the cerebrum is the **brainstem**, which consists of the midbrain, pons, and medulla oblongata. The **midbrain** contains auditory and visual reflex centers and functions in maintaining alertness and arousal. In addition, voluntary motor tracts (**pyramidal tracts**) descend from the cerebral cortex through the midbrain and pons to the medulla, where they cross, or **decussate**, over to opposite sides. As a result, voluntary somatic motor response is controlled by brain centers on the opposite side of the body. The **pons** consists primarily of fiber tracts passing to and from the brain, spinal cord, and cerebellum. The **medulla oblongata** is the uppermost extension of the spinal cord. In addition to transferring information, the medulla responds to signals from the hypothalamus to regulate heart rate, blood pressure, respiration, and other autonomic and reflex functions.

The **cerebellum** attaches to the back of the brainstem and forms two highly convoluted lobes of gray and white matter. The cerebellum receives sensory information about body position and movement from the muscles, joints, eyes, and inner ears. It coordinates this input to maintain balance and equilibrium. The cerebellum is also responsible for muscle memory, which is the repetitive, unconscious learning involved in such activities as riding a bicycle or playing the violin.

The **spinal cord** consists of myelinated tracts of white matter surrounding a butterfly-shaped region of gray matter. Afferent neurons of sensory nerves enter the dorsal, or posterior, region of the spinal cord through the **dorsal root**. These neurons synapse with motor neurons or connecting interneurons in the **dorsal horn** of the gray matter. The axons of motor neurons with cell bodies in the **ventral horn** exit the spinal cord through the ventral root. (See Figure 3.76.) Sensory input travels along **ascending tracts** of the spinal cord to the brain. Motor response descends from the brain to the body through **descending tracts**.

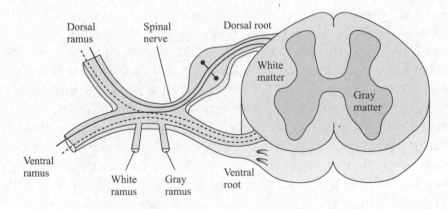

Figure 3.76. Spinal cord and spinal nerve

Peripheral Nervous System

The peripheral nervous system consists of 12 pairs of **cranial nerves** and 31 pairs of **spinal nerves**. The cranial nerves arise from the brain. Cranial nerves may be purely sensory, purely motor, or mixed nerves. The spinal nerves are formed from a fusion of the dorsal and ventral roots on each side of the spinal cord. Spinal nerves are all mixed nerves containing both afferent sensory axons and efferent motor axons. Spinal nerves, in turn, branch to form dorsal and ventral **rami** (branches) of the **peripheral nerves**. **Dorsal rami** innervate the skin and muscles of the back. **Ventral rami** innervate skin, muscles, and viscera of the ventral surface of the body, including the upper and lower limbs. In each of the limb regions, the ventral rami of multiple spinal nerves interconnect to form a **nerve plexus**.

The PNS is divided into the somatic nervous system and the autonomic nervous system. The **somatic nervous system** is involved in voluntary, conscious movement and sensation. It includes both sensory and motor nerve fibers, which innervate the skeletal muscles. The somatic nervous system is also involved in reflex movements.

Reflexes are rapid, involuntary responses to stimuli. Reflexes follow a common neural pathway, or **reflex arc**, through the spinal cord. They bypass higher brain centers to allow a more rapid response. A reflex arc consists of a **sensory receptor**, a **sensory neuron**, an **interneuron**, a **motor neuron**, and an **effector**. During a reflex, sensory receptors activated by a stimulus send information toward the central nervous system along an afferent sensory neuron. This neuron forms a synapse in the gray matter of the spinal cord either directly with a motor neuron (**monosynaptic relfex**) or indirectly via relay interneurons (**polysynaptic reflex**). An efferent response issues from the spinal cord along one or more motor neurons, which in turn activate effectors such as muscles or glands.

Only the simplest of reflexes are monosynaptic. Polysynaptic reflexes allow for feedback control. A polysynaptic reflex can also use several pathways to effect a coordinated response. For example, a polysynaptic reflex can simultaneously cause the contraction of one muscle and the relaxation of an opposing muscle.

The **autonomic nervous system** (visceral nervous system) or **ANS** regulates involuntary, unconscious functions such as breathing, heart rate, digestion, and the body's internal environment in general. The autonomic nervous system receives visceral sensory information from the muscles, joints, and internal organs. The ANS controls visceral motor responses of smooth muscle, cardiac muscle, and glands.

The autonomic nervous system consists of a chain of two neurons that extends from the central nervous system to a visceral effector. The first neuron, the preganglionic neuron, exits the brain or spinal cord, where its cell body is located. The preganglionic neuron synapses with the second, postganglionic neuron in an autonomic ganglion, which is a cluster of postganglionic cell bodies outside the CNS. The postganglionic neuron then sends its axon from the ganglion to a visceral effector, either a muscle or a gland.

The autonomic nervous system is composed of two divisions, the sympathetic nervous system and the parasympathetic nervous system. Figure 3.77 compares both divisions. These divisions have partially antagonistic functions. In general, the sympathetic system can be characterized as the fight-or-flight division. The parasympathetic division is the resting and digesting division.

The fight-or-flight response in the **sympathetic nervous system** involves preparing the body for sudden activity, such as dealing with an external threat or with an exciting situation. Typical sympathetic responses include an increase in heart rate and blood pressure, rapid breathing, and dilated eye pupils. Additional responses include increased blood sugar levels, decreased gut activity, and decreased blood flow to the skin as the body mobilizes energy reserves and diverts blood flow to skeletal muscle and critical organ systems. In addition to the organs of the chest, abdomen, and pelvic cavities, the sympathetic division also innervates the sweat glands and smooth muscle of the skin as well as the smooth muscle that lines all arteries and veins. Innervation of the sweat glands and smooth muscle of the skin results in the cold sweat and goosebumps of the fear response. Innervation of the smooth muscles lining the blood vessels allows for both vasoconstriction and vasodilation.

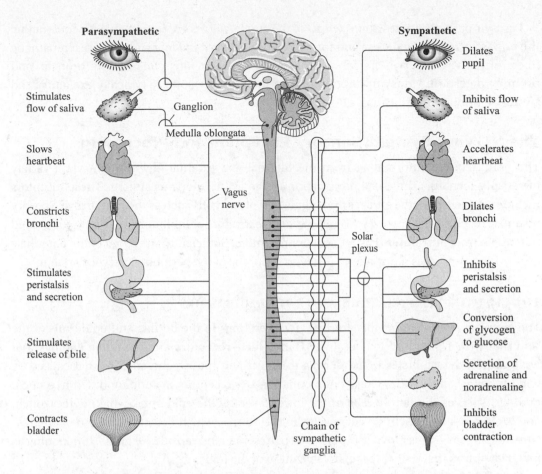

Parasympathetic

Stimulates
flow of saliva

Slows
heartbeat

Constricts
bronchi

Stimulates
peristalsis
and secretion

Stimulates
release of bile

Contracts
bladder

Ganglion

Medulla oblongata

Vagus
nerve

Sympathetic

Dilates
pupil

Inhibits flow
of saliva

Accelerates
heartbeat

Dilates
bronchi

Solar
plexus

Inhibits
peristalsis
and secretion

Conversion
of glycogen
to glucose

Secretion of
adrenaline and
noradrenaline

Inhibits
bladder
contraction

Chain of
sympathetic
ganglia

Figure 3.77. Comparison of the parasympathetic and sympathetic nervous systems
(Courtesy of John W. Kimball, from "Kimball's Biology Pages" at *http://biology-pages.info*.
Used with permission.)

In the sympathetic nervous system, preganglionic fibers arise from the spinal cord in the thoracic (chest) and lumbar (lower back) regions. Short preganglionic fibers exit the spinal cord and immediately synapse with the cell bodies of postganglionic neurons on either side of the vertebral column, forming sympathetic chain ganglia that are linked together vertically. Postganglionic sympathetic fibers generally release norepinephrine. Two important exceptions are the sweat glands and the adrenal medulla, both of which are innervated by sympathetic fibers that release acetylcholine. Norepinephrine and the related hormone epinephrine (adrenaline) bind to **adrenergic receptors** on target effector cells. Acetylcholine binds to **cholinergic receptors**. The response of a tissue or organ to sympathetic stimulation varies depending on the types of receptors present in target cells.

The **parasympathetic nervous system** functions when the body is in a housekeeping mode that conserves energy while allowing body functions such as digestion and excretion to proceed as usual. Parasympathetic fibers exit both ends of the spinal cord in cranial and sacral (pelvic) nerves, giving the parasympathetic division the alternate name of the craniosacral division. The parasympathetic division is distinguished by very long preganglionic axons that travel from the CNS to the vicinity of the target organ or gland before synapsing with the cell bodies of short postganglionic neurons in terminal ganglia. In the parasympathetic nervous system, both pre- and postganglionic neurons release acetylcholine and stimulate cholinergic receptors in target cells.

Parasympathetic fibers within several of the cranial nerves are responsible for constricting the pupils and focusing the eye and for stimulating salivary and tear glands. Parasympathetic fibers of the vagus nerve (cranial nerve X) slow the heart rate, constrict the bronchi, and promote digestion. Parasympathetic fibers in the pelvic region are typically excitatory and stimulate urination, defecation, and sexual arousal.

The Nervous System: Sensory Reception and Processing

The body receives information from the internal and external environment via a variety of sensory receptors that send information to the central nervous system. These receptors include simple free nerve endings and highly complex organs such as the human eye. Sensory response to a stimulus involves the generation of excitatory or inhibitory post-synaptic graded potentials (**receptor potentials**) in sensory receptors. Sufficiently strong receptor potentials trigger nerve impulses along afferent, sensory neurons of the peripheral nervous system.

TOUCH, PAIN, TEMPERATURE, AND PROPRIOCEPTION

The simplest sensory receptors are **free nerve endings** in the dermis and epidermis of the skin that detect pain and temperature. **Hair follicle receptors** are free nerve endings that wrap around hair follicles in the dermis to detect hair movement, such as that caused by wind blowing on the skin. Other cutaneous sensory receptors include modified free nerve endings, such as the **tactile cells** of the lower layers of the epidermis, which detect touch, and **Meissner's** and **Pacinian corpuscles** in the dermis, which detect touch and deep pressure, respectively. Pressure receptors are also present in the capsules of joints, functioning as **proprioceptors** that detect the relative position of the body.

Muscle spindles are proprioceptors that provide information about the degree of muscle stretch. A muscle spindle consists of nerve endings surrounding small muscle fibers (**intrafusal fibers**) in a connective tissue capsule. When the muscle is stretched, as when tension is applied, muscle spindles signal the spinal cord, which reflexively activates motor neurons to contract the muscle. This **stretch reflex** is particularly important in keeping muscles contracted for extended periods to maintain muscle tone and posture. Other proprioceptors include Golgi tendon organs and joint kinesthetic receptors. **Golgi tendon organs** detect excessive stretch in tendons and are responsible for muscle relaxation. **Joint kinesthetic receptors** detect stretch, pressure, and movement in the articular capsules of joints.

OLFACTION AND TASTE

Smell and taste, like hearing and vision, are referred to as special senses because sensory receptors are found in complex, specialized organs. Both smell (**olfaction**) and taste (**gustation**) receptors are **chemoreceptors**, which detect molecules in solution.

Olfaction

Olfactory receptors are located in the mucous membranes lining the nasal conchae of the nasal cavity. These receptors are extensions of the **olfactory nerve** (cranial nerve I). Pseudostratified columnar epithelial supporting cells surround **olfactory receptors cells** to form the **olfactory epithelium**. Olfactory receptor cells are bipolar neurons with modified dendrites that terminate in **olfactory cilia**. These nonmotile cilia line the surface of the olfactory epithelium and are embedded in a mucous layer. Airborne molecules (**odorants**) dissolve into the water-filled mucous layer and bind to receptor proteins on the olfactory cilia. Thousands of different receptor proteins are capable of binding to one or more different odor molecules, allowing for a high level of sensory discrimination.

The bound odorant initiates a metabolic cascade via second messengers. This cascade depolarizes the cell and generates a receptor potential. Axons of olfactory receptor cells pass through the cribiform plate of the ethmoid bone to synapse with second-order neurons in the **olfactory bulb**. A sufficiently strong stimulus triggers action potentials in the second-order neurons. These neurons relay the nerve impulse along the **olfactory tract** to the thalamus and hypothalamus, which direct olfactory input to both the frontal lobe (conscious interpretation) and the limbic system (emotional response and memory).

Taste (Gustation)

Taste receptors are the **taste buds** of the tongue and the linings of the oral cavity. Taste buds on the tongue are found in **papillae**, projections of the mucous membrane on the tongue's surface. Taste buds are flask-shaped bodies containing **gustatory cells**, which are also known as **taste cells**, and basal stem cells embedded in the stratified squamous epithelium of the papillae. The actual chemoreceptive portions of the taste cells are elongated microvilli called **gustatory hairs**. These project outward into the **taste pore**, an opening in the tongue epithelium, where they come into contact with saliva.

Dendrites of sensory neurons wrap around taste cells, each receiving input from multiple receptors within a single taste bud. When the gustatory hairs bind to a food chemical, depolarization of the taste cell leads to the release of neurotransmitter (either serotonin or ATP). If the activation threshold is reached, a nerve impulse is generated in sensory dendrites.

Different taste cells detect different types of chemicals and have different activation thresholds. The five primary taste sensations are sweet, sour, salty, bitter, and umami. **Umami** describes a savory taste that is triggered by the amino acid L-glutamate and certain other molecules. Of the five tastes, the bitter receptors, which detect toxins and spoiled food, are the most sensitive.

Taste input travels along afferent fibers of the facial, glossopharyngeal, and vagus nerves (cranial nerves VII, IX, and X). These nerves go to the medulla of the brainstem, which controls taste reflexes such as salivation and gagging, and then to the thalamus. The thalamus directs input to the **gustatory cortex** in the insula between the frontal and temporal lobes. The gustatory cortex interprets taste sensations and flavor intensity. Taste input, like olfactory input, is also directed through the hypothalamus to the limbic system.

THE EAR

The ear consists of a set of elaborate external and internal structures that capture, amplify, and direct the vibrational energy of sound toward sensory receptor cells. These receptor cells transduce the vibrational stimulus into auditory input. The ear also contains organs of equilibrium responsible for detecting body position and movement.

Ear Structure

The ear is divided into three regions: the external ear, the middle ear, and the inner ear as shown in Figure 3.78. The **external ear** consists of the auricle (pinna) and the external acoustic meatus (external auditory canal). The **auricle** is a concave structure of elastic cartilage and skin. The **external acoustic meatus** penetrates the temporal bone of the skull. The auricle captures sound waves and directs them through the external acoustic meatus toward the tympanic membrane, or eardrum. The **tympanic membrane** is a cone-shaped membrane of connective tissue and epithelial tissue that separates the external ear from the middle ear.

The **middle ear** is a small chamber lined by mucosa that lies between the tympanic membrane and the inner ear. The tympanic membrane attaches to the **ear ossicles**, tiny bones that transmit and amplify sound vibrations. These ossicles include the lateral **malleus** (hammer), a central **incus** (anvil), and a medial **stapes** (stirrup). The medial stapes communicates with the **oval window**, a small opening into the inner ear. Below the oval window is another small opening into the inner ear, the **round window**. The middle ear also contains an opening into the pharynx, the **pharyngotympanic tube (Eustachian tube)**. The pharyngotympanic tube is a flattened, mucosa-lined duct that opens on swallowing or yawning to allow for equalization of air pressure between the middle ear and the body exterior.

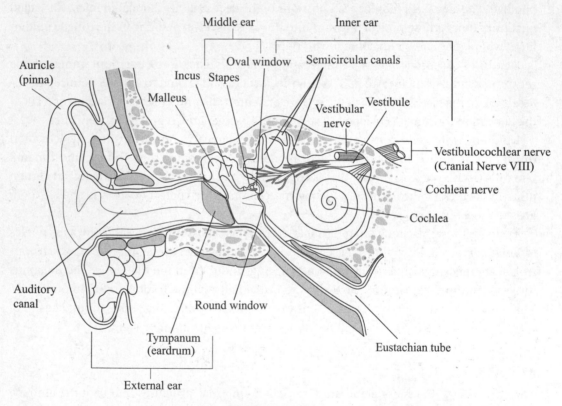

Figure 3.78. Ear

Viral and bacterial infections of the mucosal lining of the upper respiratory tract can also extend into the middle ear via the pharyngotympanic tube, resulting in an ear infection (**otitis media**). Blockage of the pharyngotympanic tube by inflammation, mucus, or pus can lead to pain and hearing impairment as a result of fluid and pressure buildup in the middle ear.

The **inner ear** consists of an interconnected series of fluid-filled, membranous tubes lying within bony chambers embedded within the temporal bone. The bony chambers form three separate structures: the **vestibule** (a central chamber that communicates with the middle ear), the posterior **semicircular canals**, and the anterior **cochlea**. Receptors for equilibrium and motion are found in the first two chambers. The cochlea detects sound. Each chamber is filled with fluid (**perilymph**), which encloses membranous tubes filled with a second fluid, **endolymph**. Perilymph is continuous with cerebrospinal fluid. However, endolymph more closely resembles intracellular fluid.

Structure of the Cochlea

The cochlea (snail shell) is a hollow, spiral-shaped tube through which the membranous labyrinth coils to a dead end. Figure 3.79 shows a cross section of the cochlea. The endolymph-filled interior of the membranous labyrinth forms a central chamber called the **scala media**, or **cochlear duct**. The **organ of Corti**, which is the sense organ for sound, rests on the **basilar membrane** of the cochlear duct. The cochlear duct is bordered on either side by a continuous, perilymph-filled chamber that runs from the vestibule to the apex of the cochlear duct and back down the other side to the round window of the middle ear. The superior portion of the chamber between the vestibule and the apex is the **scala vestibuli**. The inferior portion between the apex and the round window is the **scala tympani**. The floor of the scala vestibuli, the **vestibular membrane**, also forms the roof of the cochlear duct.

Two types of hair cells are found in the cochlea: inner hair cells and outer hair cells. Inner hair cells synapse with nerve terminals to send signals to the brain. However, outer hair cells do not transmit neural signals. Instead, depolarization of outer hair cells triggers the cell to expand and contract at the same frequency of incoming sound, increasing the oscillation and amplifying the signal.

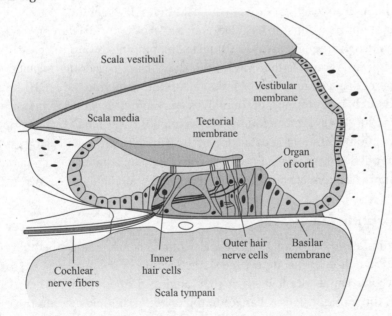

Figure 3.79. Cross section of the cochlea

Sound Transmission and Transduction

Sound waves travel through the external auditory canal to the tympanic membrane, which vibrates in resonance with the frequency and amplitude of the sound. The tympanic membrane transfers sound energy into vibrational energy. The vibration of the tympanic membrane vibrates the ossicles of the middle ear, which act as tiny levers. When the stapes vibrates against the narrow opening of the oval window, the application of force over a small surface area amplifies the signal. The vibration of the stapes against the oval window sets up pressure waves in the fluid perilymph of the inner ear. These waves travel from the vestibule through the scala vestibuli and into the cochlear duct through oscillations of the vestibular membrane. Oscillation of the basilar membrane of the cochlear duct sends the pressure wave through the scala tympani toward the round window, which bulges outward to relieve the pressure.

The organ of Corti in the cochlear duct transduces the vibrational energy of the oscillating fluid into an electrochemical signal which the brain interprets as sound. This organ consists of columnar **hair cells** on the surface of the basilar membrane. The tips of these cells bear elongated, hairlike microvilli (**stereocilia**) that are joined together and embedded in an overlying, gelatinous, **tectorial membrane**. As the pressure wave passes through the cochlear duct, the vertical oscillation of the basilar membrane is translated into a horizontal shearing movement of the stereocilia within the tectorial membrane. The bending of these stereocilia opens ion channels and depolarizes the hair cells. Hair cell receptors release the neurotransmitter glutamate to trigger action potentials within the **cochlear nerve**. The cochlear nerve and the vestibular nerve from the semicircular canals join to form the **vestibulocochlear nerve**, cranial nerve VIII.

Auditory Processing

Auditory input travels from the cochlear nerve to the brainstem, to the auditory reflex centers of the midbrain, and through the thalamus to the **primary auditory cortex** in the temporal lobe. Not all fibers from each ear cross to opposite sides of the brain.

The basilar membrane differs in flexibility and in its sensitivity to different sound frequencies along its length. High-frequency waves vibrate the membrane toward the base of the cochlea. Low-frequency waves travel farther toward the apex before triggering oscillations. The location of maximum displacement of the basilar membrane is interpreted by the central nervous system as the **pitch**, or frequency, of sound. The ear can detect sound frequencies within the wavelengths of 20–20,000 Hz. The **loudness** of a sound is determined by the amplitude of the pressure wave and the amount of deflection of the hair cell stereocilia. A larger pressure wave leads to greater deflection of the hair cells, a larger receptor potential, more neurotransmitter release, and more frequent action potentials, which the brain interprets as a louder sound.

Organs of Equilibrium

Both the vestibule and the semicircular canals contain sense organs of equilibrium. Within the vestibule are hair cells that detect the static position of the head relative to gravity. The three semicircular canals are located at right angles to one another. They detect relative movement in three dimensions. Changes in the direction of fluids within the canals stimulate hair cell receptors to indicate when the body changes direction or when it starts or stops motion. These receptors send their signals via the **vestibular nerve** to the cerebellum and to regions of the brainstem that coordinate balance and equilibrium.

THE EYE

The eye is a specialized sense organ containing receptors cells that detect the wavelength and intensity of light, as shown in Figure 3.80. The eye transduces light energy into action potentials that are relayed to the visual processing centers of the brain to be interpreted as visual images.

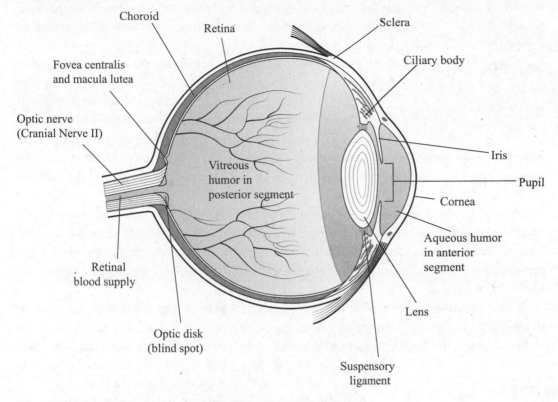

Figure 3.80. Structures of the eye

Eye Structure

The vertebrate eye is a spherical organ consisting of three tissue layers, or tunics, surrounding a fluid-filled interior. The eye is divided into anterior and posterior segments by the lens. The **lens** is a biconvex elastic and transparent structure of epithelial cells and crystalline protein that can change shape to focus light rays onto the light-sensitive cells at the back of the eye. The anterior segment of the eye is filled with a semiliquid **aqueous humor**. The posterior segment contains a gel-like **vitreous humor**.

> **RETINAL IMAGE**
>
> The image projected on the retina is inverted: upside-down and reversed.

The lens is normally flattened for distance vision. Constriction of smooth ciliary muscle relaxes suspensory ligaments, allowing the lens to bulge. The result is **accommodation**, which is the alteration of lens shape necessary for close vision. (See Figure 3.81.)

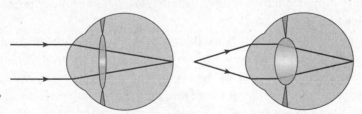

Figure 3.81. Accommodation: The lens flattens for distance vision (*left*) and thickens for close vision (*right*)

The outer layer of the eye, the **fibrous tunic**, forms the **cornea** of the anterior surface of the eye. The cornea is a transparent layer of epithelial and dense connective tissue that protects the eye while allowing light to enter. Along the posterior and lateral exterior surfaces, the fibrous tunic becomes the protective layer of the **sclera**, or white of the eye.

The middle layer, or **vascular tunic**, has a rich capillary supply that nourishes adjacent tissues. Posterior to the lens, the vascular tunic forms the **choroid**, a highly vascular, darkly pigmented layer that absorbs light and acts to prevent reflection within the posterior segment. The vascular tunic also forms the **ciliary muscle, ciliary zonule (suspensory ligament)**, and **ciliary body**. These control the shape of the lens, hold the lens in position, and secrete the aqueous humor of the anterior segment, respectively.

The **iris** is a pigmented band of circular and radial smooth muscle that constricts or dilates to regulate the amount of light passing through a small opening, or **pupil**, into the lens. Because both the focusing of the lens and the constriction or dilation of the iris depend on smooth muscle, these are involuntary processes under control of the autonomic nervous system.

Stimulation of the sympathetic nervous system causes the iris to expand and the pupil to dilate. Parasympathetic stimulation causes the pupil to constrict. Constriction focuses light on the cones at the back of the eye and allows for up close scrutiny in bright light. Dilation reaches more rods along the lateral margins and allows for distance vision and visibility in low light conditions.

The innermost layer, or **nervous tunic**, forms the retina. The **retina** consists of an outer **neural layer** of neurons and light-receptor cells and an underlying **pigmented layer** of epithelial cells. The outermost cells, or **ganglion cells**, have long axons that form the **optic nerve** and connect the retina with the brain. A middle layer contains **bipolar neurons** that synapse with both the ganglion cells and the inner photoreceptor cells, the **rods** and **cones**. The rods and cones are partially embedded in the pigmented layer of the retina.

> ## EYE REFLEXES
>
> The **pupillary reflex** and **accommodation reflex** control the diameter of the pupil and the shape of the lens, respectively.

> ## THE RETINA
>
> Developmentally, the retina is an extension of the optic nerve (cranial nerve II) and hence is part of the central nervous system.

Photoreceptors

The specialized receptor cells of the retina are two types of modified neurons that contain disks of light-absorbing visual pigments. These pigments contain the light-sensitive molecule **retinal**, which is derived from vitamin A. Retinal is bound to different **opsin** proteins to form four different types of pigments. Rods are highly sensitive receptors containing the pigment **rhodopsin**. They are found in high concentrations along the peripheral margins of the retina. Sensory input from rods is most useful in low light or for peripheral vision and is perceived in black and white.

Cones carry one of three different visual pigments to allow for color vision. However, they have a lower sensitivity and consequently are only activated in bright light. Cones occur in highest concentration at the back of the eye in the **fovea centralis**. The high density of cones in the fovea centralis provides for high resolving power and visual acuity when light is focused on this area of the retina.

The Pathway of Light

Light entering the eye must pass through the cornea, aqueous humor, pupil, lens, and vitreous humor before reaching the retina. To reach the photosensitive outer segments of the rods and cones, light must also pass through layers of ganglion cells and unipolar neurons.

Photoreception and Transduction

When rods and cones are exposed to light, the retinal within rhodopsin and the other photopigments undergoes a conformational change and ultimately dissociates from opsin, a process called **bleaching of the pigment**. In the absence of light, these molecules are reassembled. The pigment breakdown initiates an enzymatic cascade that ultimately results in the closure of ion channels and the hyperpolarization of the cell. Hyperpolarization of photoreceptor cells leads to a reduction in the amount of the inhibitory neurotransmitter glutamate released into the synaptic cleft between photoreceptors and bipolar neurons. Bipolar neurons become uninhibited and depolarize, releasing excitatory neurotransmitter onto ganglion cells. The ganglion cells then depolarize and send an action potential through the optic nerve to the brain.

Visual Processing

The paired optic nerves pass through the eye sockets to the **optic chiasma**, where medial fibers cross over to merge with lateral fibers from the opposite eye. Nerve fibers then continue on to the thalamus as **optic tracts**. Because of the crossing of fibers, each optic tract contains complete sensory input from either the right or left visual field. A small number of fibers from the optic tract go to the midbrain, which controls visual reflexes such as the pupillary reflex. From the thalamus, the main **optic radiation** carries visual input to the **primary visual cortex** in the occipital lobe, where the majority of visual processing occurs. The visual cortex is responsible for interpreting contrast and orientation information. The visual cortex also relays visual inputs to other areas of the occipital, temporal, parietal, and frontal lobes, which interpret these inputs as visual images.

The Circulatory System

The circulatory system (cardiovascular system) functions in the transport of nutrients (amino acids, lipoproteins, glucose), gases, hormones, fluids, ions, and wastes around the body. The circulatory system is the avenue through which cells receive fresh nutrients and expel waste. It also helps to fight disease and maintain homeostasis.

The circulatory system has three main components: the heart, the blood vessels, and the blood. The heart and blood vessels work to pump blood through the lungs (**pulmonary circulation**) so the blood can be oxygenated. The oxygenated blood then moves through the rest of the body (**systemic circulation**) before returning as deoxygenated blood back to the heart.

THE FOUR-CHAMBERED HEART

The heart, a fist-sized organ composed of cardiac muscle, powers the circulatory system. In mammals, the heart is organized into four chambers. The two upper chambers are the left and right **atria**. The two lower chambers are the left and right **ventricles**. The thick, vertical wall of muscle separating the left and right sides of the heart is called the **septum**. Figure 3.82 shows the structure of the heart.

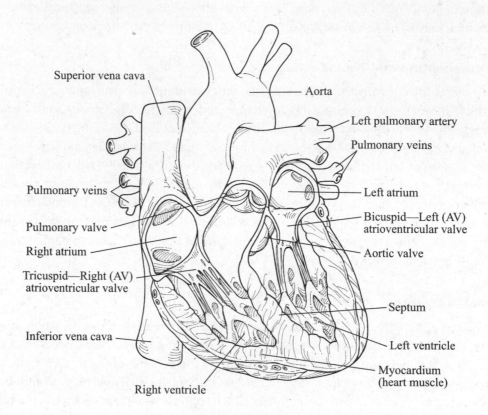

Figure 3.82. Heart

Four valves separate the heart's chambers and prevent backflow of blood. Flow through the heart is directional. The right side of the heart collects deoxygenated blood from the body, channeling it into the **right atrium**. From the right atrium, blood passes through the **right ventricle** to be pumped into the lungs via the **pulmonary arteries**. Blood is oxygenated and returned to the heart through the **pulmonary veins** that enter into the **left atrium**. The blood is then released into the **left ventricle**. This ventricle then contracts its thick muscular wall to generate enough pressure to circulate the blood through the entire body. Blood flow to and from the lungs is the exception to the convention that veins carry deoxygenated blood and arteries carry oxygenated blood. (The other exception is in fetal circulation.) Just remember that *a*rteries carry blood *a*way from the heart, whereas veins carry blood toward the heart.

Two **atrioventricular** (AV) valves separate the atria and ventricles and prevent backflow. The **tricuspid valve** separates the right atrium from the right ventricle. The **mitral** valve separates the left atrium from the left ventricle. Two **semilunar valves**—pulmonary and aortic—prevent blood exiting the ventricles from reentering. The **pulmonary valve** prevents blood that was pumped into the pulmonary arteries from leaking back into the right ventricle. The **aortic valve** does the same for blood pumped into the aorta by the left ventricle.

Contraction of the heart is a two-phase process coordinated by the nervous system. The contraction of the ventricles is called **systole**. This phase begins as the AV valves close to prevent backflow of blood. The sound made by this valve closing is the first heart sound in the heartbeat. In **diastole**, the semilunar valves close and the AV valves open to allow blood from the atria to refill the ventricles. During the diastole, the heart is relaxed. The sound of the semilunar valves closing at the end of systole constitutes the second beat of the heartbeat.

ARTERIAL AND VENOUS SYSTEMS

The human circulatory system is **closed**, which means that it is contained within blood vessels. These blood vessels, which make up the body's **vasculature**, are **arteries**, **arterioles**, **veins**, **venules**, and **capillaries**. Arteries and the smaller arterioles carry blood away from the heart, veins and venules carry blood to the heart, and capillaries penetrate the tissues and connect the arterial and venous blood supply.

Newly oxygenated blood leaves the heart through the biggest artery, the **aorta**. The aorta continually branches to reduce the volume and pressure of the fluid as it passes from the arteries to the smaller arterioles. Then the blood passes to the capillaries, where nutrients and wastes are exchanged with cells. From the tiny, thin-walled capillaries, where blood cells must pass single file, the flow continues through the tissues as capillaries converge to venules and finally the veins. Blood exiting the capillaries enters the venous circulation under low pressure. Ultimately, the blood reenters the heart via the principal veins draining the upper and lower halves of the body, the **superior** and **inferior vena cava**, respectively.

The structural differences between arteries and veins reflect their functional differences. Arteries are thick, strong, and elastic. They have an outer layer of smooth muscle, which offers the resistance necessary to handle and maintain the pressure of the blood pumped from the heart. Veins are thin walled and inelastic, with no smooth muscle. Veins are able to do the work of returning blood to the heart, even in the face of gravity, by using a combination of one-way valves and assistance from the surrounding skeletal muscles. These surrounding muscles can help squeeze blood upward during contraction.

PRESSURE AND FLOW CHARACTERISTICS

During each heartbeat, the pressure the blood exerts on the walls of the blood vessels varies from a maximum (systolic) to minimum (diastolic) as the ventricles contract and relax. Blood is traditionally measured in mmHg (millimeters of mercury) and is written as systolic over diastolic. The pressure provided by the heart drops dramatically in its circuit to accommodate the capillaries, whose walls are only a single cell thick. The interplay between pressures at the capillary level, called **Starling forces**, mediates the proper exchange of nutrients, fluids, and wastes between blood and cells.

CAPILLARY BEDS

Capillaries are by design leaky. As blood moves from the arteriole into the capillary network, its pressure forces fluid, and the accompanying nutrients, into the interstitial space. This **hydrostatic pressure**, the force per unit area that the blood exerts against blood vessel walls, originates from the heart. At the venule end of the capillary bed, hydrostatic pressure has dropped. However, **oncotic** (or **osmotic**) **pressure**, determined by the relatively higher concentrations of solutes in the vessel versus interstitial space, has increased in the capillaries. The key determinant of oncotic pressure in the capillaries is plasma proteins, which are too big to leave the vessels. The osmotic differential generates a pressure and concentration gradient, sucking fluids and wastes from the tissues into the capillaries and the venous circulation.

COMPOSITION OF BLOOD

Blood is a type of connective tissue that consists of blood cells suspended in a liquid plasma matrix. **Plasma** is mostly water; however, it also contains ions (sodium, potassium, calcium, magnesium, chloride, bicarbonate), hormones, glucose, carbon dioxide, and dissolved proteins (albumin, fibrinogen, immunoglobins). Blood cells make up 45% of the blood volume.

The three types of **blood cells** are erythrocytes, leukocytes, and platelets. **Erythrocytes**, commonly referred to as red blood cells, are the most prevalent blood cell. Millions are produced per second from hematopoietic stem cells in the bone marrow. When mature, they are flexible biconcave disks. The only purpose of red blood cells is to transport oxygen. An erythrocyte extrudes its nucleus and most of its organelles, including mitochondria, during development in order to maximize space for oxygen-binding hemoglobin proteins and eliminate oxygen-consuming processes in the cell. Red blood cells, therefore, use anaerobic respiration until their death after about 120 days. At this point, they are removed by the spleen and recycled by macrophages.

Leukocytes, or white blood cells, are cells of the immune system that are also produced in hematopoietic stem cells in the bone marrow. They work to clear the body of infection and foreign materials.

Platelets are small fragments of large cells called megakaryocytes and play an important role in the formation of blood clots. A low platelet concentration in blood can be dangerous because of the possibility of poor clot formation and risk of excessive bleeding (hemorrhage). However, high concentrations can be equally deadly, leading to blood vessel obstructions (thrombosis), stroke, pulmonary embolism, or myocardial infarction (heart attack).

COAGULATION

The inside surface of the body's vasculature is lined with a layer of endothelial cells that normally inhibits platelet activation. Injury to the endothelial layer exposes proteins of the underlying basement membrane to the bloodstream. These proteins, namely collagen and von Willebrand factor, activate platelets. Platelets bind to the exposed collagen and release their contents, activating additional platelets in a positive feedback response. The loose platelet plug must be reinforced with a fibrin mesh to form a stable clot. Fibrin is produced via a complex activation pathway that works to produce prothrombinase, an enzyme that converts prothrombin to thrombin, which in turn cleaves fibrinogen to fibrin.

OXYGEN TRANSPORT

Oxygen bound to hemoglobin is significantly more soluble in blood than free oxygen. So almost all oxygen travels through the body bound to hemoglobin in the bloodstream. This is in contrast to carbon dioxide, which travels through the blood as bicarbonate ion (HCO_3^-), a fact of physiologic importance.

An important property of human blood is its **hematocrit**, which is the proportion of blood volume made up by red blood cells. This percentage is about 48% for men and 38% for women, independent of body size. When blood is centrifuged, the components separate based on their relative densities. Erythrocytes are the densest component and occupy the bottom of the test tube. A thin layer of leukocytes and platelets form on top of the erythrocytes. Plasma, which is the least dense, forms the top layer.

Each erythrocyte is packed with 270 million hemoglobin proteins. Hemoglobin has the capacity to bind an oxygen molecule to each of its four prosthetic heme groups, each with

TIP

SO_2 and PO_2

Don't confuse these with chemical formulas. The S stands for saturation and the P for partial pressure.

a central iron atom. As the first oxygen molecule binds, a conformational shift changes the hemoglobin from its taut state to a relaxed state, which increases hemoglobin's affinity for oxygen. This is called **cooperative binding**. **Cooperative binding** also works in reverse. As the first oxygen is removed from a saturated hemoglobin, the conformational shift increases the ease with which oxygen leaves the protein. This property of hemoglobin results in a sigmoidal dissociation curve that plots the percentage of oxygen saturation of hemoglobin (SO_2) versus the partial pressure of oxygen in the blood (PO_2). For a complete discussion of the oxygen-hemoglobin dissociation curve, see the section "Respiration."

HOMEOSTASIS

Although the primary function of the cardiovascular system is to transport vital gases and nutrients throughout the body, it also serves in **thermoregulation**. When the body becomes overheated, the arterioles can help with cooling by means of **vasodilation**. In vasodilation, the smooth muscle in arteriole walls relaxes and more blood can flow through the arteries that lead to the capillaries close to the skin. Cutaneous veins just below the skin surface also dilate in response to high body temperature. Vasodilation allows the dissipation of heat by convection and conduction. **Vasoconstriction** is essentially the opposite as smooth muscle contracts and blood vessels narrow. This process effectively keeps warm blood away from the skin and conserves heat in cold environments.

Homeostasis in plasma volume is also regulated by the circulatory system. The plasma volume is significant because it affects blood pressure. Volume is generally mediated by blood **osmolality** (concentration of solutes) and hormones. If blood osmolality is high, more fluid will be reabsorbed by capillaries from the tissues and blood volume will increase. ADH and aldosterone are two hormones that increase blood volume. Both hormones act to increase water reabsorption in the kidneys. (These hormones were discussed in "The Endocrine System.")

The Lymphatic System

The **lymphatic system** consists of a network of lymphatic vessels, lymph nodes, and other lymphoid tissues associated with specific organs. The lymphatic system transports the fluid **lymph** throughout the body, ultimately rejoining with the circulatory system through the thoracic duct in the vena cava. The primary functions of the lymphatic system are to circulate fluids and to act as an agent of the immune system.

LYMPH

Lymph is a fluid that is created when blood is forced out of capillaries as interstitial fluid. Lymph is similar in composition to blood plasma. This fluid is absorbed into the lymphatic vessels through lymphatic capillaries called **lacteals**.

Transportation of Lymph

Almost all tissues of the body, except for the central nervous system, drain into the lymphatic system. Unlike blood, lymph does not have a pump to push it through the body. Instead, the lymphatic system relies on the contractions and relaxations of the body's skeletal muscle to push the lymph through the lymphatic vessels. Lymph vessels contain one-way valves that restrict the direction of flow. Lymph ultimately drains into veins at the right lymphatic duct and thoracic duct.

FUNCTIONS OF THE LYMPHATIC SYSTEM

The lymphatic system serves as a pathway for interstitial fluid to be returned to the blood. In addition, lymph helps fight disease primarily by monitoring the body for infection and initiating the humoral immune response. Lymph is a critical component in maintaining homeostasis.

- The lymphatic system is responsible for transporting interstitial fluid from tissues, equalizing the body's fluid distribution, maintaining blood pressure, and preventing edema.
- The lymphatic system absorbs fats and fatty acids from the small intestine through lacteals and transports them to the thoracic duct, where they ultimately rejoin the circulatory system.
- The lymphatic system removes particles and proteins that are too large to pass into the capillaries.
- The lymphatic system transports lymphocytes between the bone marrow and the lymph nodes.
- The lymphatic system transports antigen-presenting cells (APCs) throughout the body as a primary first responder in an immune response.

The role of the lymphatic system in immune response is described in the section "Immune System."

ASSOCIATED ORGANS

The lymphatic system includes a number of organs involved in the immune response. Among these are the **spleen**, **bone marrow**, **thymus**, and **lymph nodes**. In addition to filtering the blood and removing old red blood cells, the spleen synthesizes antibodies and screens out pathogens. The bone marrow produces lymphocytes, a class of white blood cells. These cells mature in the bone marrow as B lymphocytes, or in the thymus as T lymphocytes. The lymph nodes are reservoirs of B and T lymphocytes that target foreign particles and pathogens circulating in the lymph.

Immune System

The immune system is the body's defense against the invasion of disease-causing pathogens, parasites, and foreign or cancerous cells. Immunity can be either **innate** or **adaptive**. Innate immunity is a nonspecific, generalized response to a variety of invaders. An innate immune response is found in a wide variety of organisms, including plants and fungi as well as animals. Adaptive immunity, which is found only in vertebrates, is a highly specific immune response that targets specific pathogens, foreign cells, and malignant cells.

INNATE IMMUNE RESPONSE

The first line of defense in the innate **immune response** system includes the body's physical barriers: the **skin** and **mucous membranes** of the digestive, respiratory, urinary, and reproductive tracts. The skin not only acts as a barrier but also actively secretes acidic and antimicrobial substances such as sweat and sebum. Mucous membranes trap microbes and foreign particles, which are expelled by ciliary action. If these physical barriers are breached, internal innate defenses are activated. The body contains numerous internal defenses.

1. **Nonspecific phagocytes**, such as **neutrophils** and **macrophages**, are specialized white blood cells that engulf foreign or infected cells.
2. **Natural killer (NK) cells** trigger infected cells to commit "suicide" by apoptosis.
3. **Blood proteins**, such as **interferons**, are released by infected cells to activate defensive mechanisms in other cells.
4. **Complement proteins** lyse microorganisms and aid in phagocytosis.
5. The **inflammatory response** increases blood vessel permeability to allow the entry of fluid, phagocytes, and repair cells into an injured or infected area.
6. **Fever**, a bodywide innate response, inhibits microbial reproduction and accelerates repair mechanisms through an increase in body temperature.

ADAPTIVE IMMUNE RESPONSE

The adaptive immune system is a dynamic immune response that mounts an individualized defense against particular pathogens or invaders. The adaptive immune response is designed to remember pathogens in order to destroy them more efficiently and more quickly in subsequent exposures. Unlike innate immunity, which allows a rapid response, adaptive immunity takes time to develop. Adaptive immunity can be **passive**, as when mothers pass antibodies (protective proteins) to their infants across the placenta and through breast milk. Passive immunity is transient, disappearing when the antibodies disappear. With the exception of a few examples of passive immunity, however, most adaptive immunity in humans is **active**. Active immunity is a long-term or even lifetime immunity developed in response to an individual's exposure to specific viruses, bacteria, or other pathogens.

B LYMPHOCYTES AND T LYMPHOCYTES

B lymphocytes (B cells) are distinguished from T lymphocytes (T cells) by the tissue in which they mature and become immunocompetent, or capable of recognizing and binding antigen. B lymphocytes mature in the bone marrow. The "B" stands for bone. T lymphocytes are produced in the marrow but mature in the thymus. The "T" stands for thymus.

WHITE BLOOD CELLS

Both innate and adaptive immunity involve the participation of **leukocytes**, or white blood cells, as part of the **immune response** (see Table 3.14). White blood cells are classified as either **granular leukocytes (granulocytes)** or **agranular (mononuclear) leukocytes**. Granular leukocytes include phagocytic **neutrophils** and **eosinophils**, and the less common **basophils**, which contribute to the inflammatory response. Agranular leukocytes include **monocytes**, which differentiate into phagocytic **macrophages** and **dendritic cells**, and the structurally similar but functionally and developmentally distinct **lymphocytes**. Granular leukocytes and monocytes tend to function in nonspecific, innate responses. Lymphocytes primarily contribute to adaptive immunity. However, the innate and adaptive immune systems are intricately linked. Different types of cells may have roles in both innate and adaptive responses.

Lymphocytes facilitate adaptive immunity through two distinct mechanisms. The first, **humoral immunity**, relies on **antibodies** (blood proteins) produced by cells derived from B lymphocytes. The second, **cell-mediated immunity**, is a cellular defensive mechanism carried out by T lymphocytes to defend against cells that have been infected by fungi or viruses.

Table 3.14 Types of Leukocytes (White Blood Cells) and Their Functions

Type of Leukocyte	Diagram	Main Functions
Neutrophils		Destroy bacteria and fungi
Eosinophils		Destroy larger parasites such as intestinal worms; modulate allergic inflammatory responses
Basophils		Release histamine to trigger inflammatory response

Lymphocytes		• **B cells** (bone marrow cells): humoral immunity; adaptive immune response; release antibodies and assist in the activation of T cells
		• **T cells** (thymus cells): cell-mediated immunity; adaptive immune response
		  – Helper T cells: activate and regulate T cells and B cells, also called T_H or CD4+ cells
		  – Regulatory (suppressor) T cells: return the immune system to normal after infection; prevent autoimmune response
		  – Cytotoxic T cells: destroy tumor-infected or virus-infected cells; also called T_C or CD8+ cells
		  – Natural killer T (NKT) cells: destroy tumor-infected or virus-infected cells
		• **Natural killer (NK) cells:** destroy virus-infected and tumor-infected cells; do not require activation; rapid innate immune response

Monocytes		Migrate from the bloodstream to other tissues and differentiate into tissue-resident macrophages or dendritic cells
Macrophages		Phagocytose (engulf and digest) cellular debris and pathogens; stimulate lymphocytes and other immune cells that respond to the pathogen
Dendritic cells		Antigen-Presenting Cells (APC) that activate T lymphocytes

HUMORAL IMMUNITY

The humoral immune response produces antibodies that circulate in the blood and lymph (the body's "humors") in order to bind to bacteria, viruses, and toxins and target them for destruction.

SELF VERSUS NONSELF

The ability of the immune system to distinguish between the body's own tissues and foreign substances is referred to as **self versus nonself recognition**. Self-recognition is determined by cell surface glycoproteins of the **major histocompatibility complex (MHC)**. Genes of the MHC complex are extraordinarily diverse and result in unique combinations of MHC proteins on the cells of every individual, except for identical twins. Cells display MHC peptides on their cell membranes as self-recognition sites. In infected cells, the MHC peptides attach fragments of foreign antigens, signaling the presence of nonself material and triggering an immune response. Foreign cells introduced in tissue and organ transplants also risk rejection even if MHC proteins are carefully matched between donor and recipient.

Antigens

Antibodies of the humoral response specifically target foreign **antigens**, or substances that the body recognizes as foreign. An antigen is any substance capable of eliciting an immune response. Antigens include macromolecules such as proteins or polysaccharides attached to the outer surfaces of viruses, bacteria, foreign tissue grafts, or pollen grains. A single bacterium may have multiple **antigenic determinants**, or specific binding sites recognized by different antibodies. Antigens may also be smaller molecules, called **haptens**, that attach to body proteins. Haptens can be formed by certain drugs, such as penicillin, as well as by compounds in poison ivy, pet dander, and chemicals such as detergents. Because the combination of hapten and protein is recognized as foreign, these compounds can trigger an immune response.

TIP

ANTIGEN

The word antigen is a contraction of "antibody" and "generating," meaning any substance that generates the production of antibodies.

Antibodies

Antibodies (also referred to as **immunoglobulins** or **Ig**) are proteins with highly specific binding sites to antigens. Each antibody is specific to a particular antigenic determinant.

The basic structure of all antibodies is the same, a Y-shaped molecule built from four polypeptide chains (see Figure 3.83). Two of the chains are light, and two are heavy. The heavy chains at the base of the "Y" form one of five different classes of a **constant (C) region**. However, the tips of antibodies, or **antigen-binding sites (V regions)**, are highly variable and can adapt to a wide range of antigens. The extreme variability and diversity of antibodies results from the shuffling of variable region genes during antibody formation.

Once an antibody binds to an antigen, the antibody contributes to the destruction of the antigen by activating innate defense mechanisms. Antibodies may **neutralize** the virus, toxin, or bacterium by blocking binding sites and preventing the invading organism from attaching to host cells until it can be removed by phagocytes. Antibodies may also cause foreign cells to clump together (**agglutinate**), rendering them harmless, or may cause soluble antigen molecules to **precipitate** out of solution. Several antibodies binding to adjacent receptors on the same cell may bind to (or fix) **complement** proteins, triggering cell **lysis**. Antibody binding may also contribute to **phagocytosis** by signaling phagocytes and providing them with a convenient binding site.

IMMUNOGLOBULINS

The five classes of antibodies are categorized based on their heavy chain constant regions. These classes are IgM, IgA, IgD, IgG, and IgE, or "MADGE." The different antibodies have different roles in the immune response. IgA protects against pathogen entry in mucous membranes. IgG and IgM protect against pathogens in blood and lymph, and both fix and activate complement. The presence of IgM in blood plasma is diagnostic of current infection, and IgG confers passive immunity between mother and fetus. IgD and IgM molecules act as antigen receptors on B cells. IgE binds to mast cells and basophils to trigger histamine release leading to the inflammatory response and, in some cases, allergies.

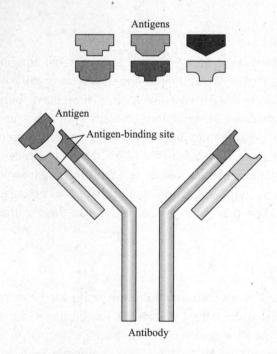

Figure 3.83. Structure of an antibody

B Lymphocyte Response

Antibodies are proteins produced by cellular components of the immune system. B lymphocytes differentiate into antibody-producing cells after being activated by exposure to antigen. B lymphocytes are produced in the bone marrow but migrate into the bloodstream and lymph organs, where they encounter antigen. The antigen binds to a membrane-bound antibody (IgD and IgM) and activates the B lymphocytes, triggering the white blood cells to begin proliferating. An additional agent such as helper T cells usually contributes to B lymphocyte activation.

An activated B lymphocyte proliferates into a **clone** of genetically identical cells. All the descendents of this clone bear the same genes for the production of a single antibody type corresponding to the antigen that initially activated the B lymphocyte. Only those B lymphocytes capable of binding to a specific circulating antigen will proliferate, a process called **clonal selection**.

The clone of B lymphocytes differentiates into two types of cells: **plasma cells** (also known as **effector cells**) and **memory cells**. The plasma cells immediately begin to mass produce antibodies that combat the existing infection. Memory cells do not immediately produce antibodies. However, they stay in the circulatory system for many years, creating **immunological memory**. Memory cells allow for a rapid and more vigorous response to a repeat infection in the future.

The first time that the immune system encounters a specific antigen, the immune response is referred to as a **primary response**. Typically, peak production of antibodies can take from a few days to two weeks. If the same antigen is encountered by memory cells in the future, antibody production begins more quickly and robustly, within a few hours to two days. The rapid response by the memory cells on subsequent exposure is referred to as a **secondary response**.

VACCINES

Vaccines take advantage of the immunological memory created by the humoral response. Vaccination is an artificial means of inducing active immunity. An antigen from a disease-causing organism is deliberately introduced into the bloodstream to initiate a primary immune response. This antigen may be in the form of killed or weakened viruses or viral fragments that are incapable of causing serious disease but that can still activate B lymphocytes. On subsequent exposure to a live virus, memory cells will rapidly initiate a secondary response to prevent infection.

CELL-MEDIATED IMMUNITY

In contrast to humoral immunity, in which antibodies target antigens circulating in blood and lymph, cell-mediated immunity provides a defensive mechanism against infected or abnormal cells within body tissues. In cell-mediated immunity, T lymphocytes destroy the body's own cells that have become infected or cancerous. T cells also destroy foreign cells from tissue grafts, transfusions, or transplants. No antibodies are involved; however, like B cells, T cells must be activated by exposure to an antigen to trigger the immune response.

T cells are produced in bone marrow and then migrate to the thymus to proliferate. In the thymus, T cells also undergo differentiation and acquire secondary characteristics to become specialized for different roles. During childhood, T cells in the thymus undergo a rigorous selection process to eliminate those cells that are incapable of distinguishing self (normal body cells) from nonself (foreign cells or materials that may trigger an antigenic response). Mature T cells then leave the thymus and enter the peripheral circulation, where they make up a majority of the circulating lymphocytes.

T Lymphocyte Response

Although T cells circulate in the blood, they cannot respond to free antigens in the bloodstream. Instead, these lymphocytes must be activated by contact with another cell. These other cells include phagocytic dendritic cells, macrophages, and B lymphocytes, which act as **antigen-presenting cells** (**APCs**). Antigen-presenting cells display fragments of antigen presented on cell-surface MHC proteins.

When T cells encounter and bind to antigen-presenting cells, the lymphocytes must be **costimulated** by additional surface receptors on the APC. If both binding and costimulation occur, the T cell is triggered to undergo clonal selection and proliferation into memory cells and effector cells to mount an immune response against other cells displaying the same antigen. In the process, activated T cells and antigen-presenting cells produce **cytokines**, or cell-signaling molecules, such as **interferons** and **interleukins**. Cytokines set up a positive feedback cycle promoting differentiation and proliferation of T cells. They also enhance innate immune defenses by promoting macrophage activity and inflammation.

Classes of T Cell

The main types of T cells are helper, cytotoxic, regulatory (formerly called suppressor), and natural killer T cells. **Helper (T_H) cells** display CD4+ glycoproteins on their cell surfaces and are consequently also known as **CD4 cells**. T_H cells are critical to the adaptive immune response because they assist in activating both B cells and T cells through the secretion of cytokines such as interleukins.

Cytotoxic (T_C) cells, or **CD8 cells**, display CD8+ glycoproteins. Cytotoxic cells travel through the blood and lymph to encounter virus- or fungal-infected cells as well as cancer cells. When a T_C cell encounters a cell displaying antigen that corresponds to its T cell receptors, the T_C cell binds to the foreign cell and kills it directly. The cytotoxic cell secretes toxins such as **perforins**, which penetrate the cell membrane, and **granzymes**, which degrade cell proteins and induce apoptosis. **Regulatory (T_{reg}) cells** turn off the cell-mediated immune response upon completion in order to prevent **autoimmunity** (the body attacking itself as foreign). **Natural killer T (NKT) cells** combine the functions of T_H and T_C cells. NKT cells are distinct from the natural killer (NK) cells of the innate immune response.

Digestive System

Digestion is the process by which food is **catabolized**, or broken down into smaller components, thus allowing the body to absorb and utilize nutrients. The process of digestion begins when food enters the mouth (**ingestion**). Digestion continues through the esophagus, stomach, and small and large intestines. The liver, gallbladder, and pancreas are involved in digestion. The digestive tract ends at the rectum. (See Figure 3.84.)

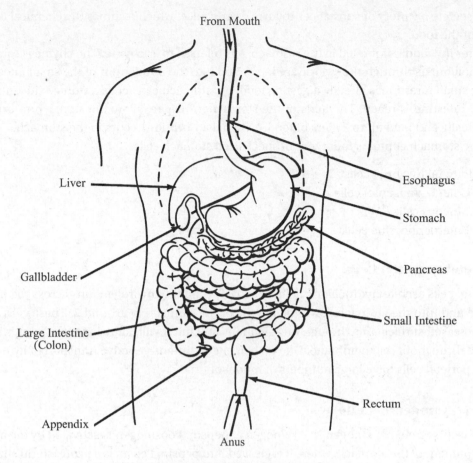

Figure 3.84. The digestive system

INGESTION

Digestion in humans begins in the mouth, where food is mechanically broken down through chewing (**mastication**). Mastication allows the food to be safely swallowed by breaking it into small pieces. Mastication also increases the surface area of the food, allowing the digestive enzymes to be more efficient. Saliva is released from the salivary glands and lubricates the food for its pathway through the digestive system. In addition, saliva contains enzymes that begin the chemical breakdown of food. **Salivary amylase** is an enzyme that catalyzes the hydrolysis of starch into polysaccharides. **Salivary lipase** catalyzes the hydrolysis of lipids into monoglycerides and fatty acids.

Once the food is chewed and swallowed, it enters the pharynx and then the esophagus. The epiglottis moves to cover the trachea, preventing food from entering the lungs. The mass of food, or **bolus**, is moved through the esophagus by **peristalsis**, which is the rhythmic contraction of smooth muscle. The food passes through the gastroesophogeal, or cardiac, sphincter and into the stomach.

THE STOMACH

Once the bolus enters the stomach, the mechanical breakdown of the food continues through the contractions of the muscular stomach wall in a process called **churning**. The epithelial lining of the stomach is folded into pits, forming glands that contain specialized cells. These cells secrete a variety of substances to form gastric juice, which resumes the chemical digestion of the food.

After the food is liquefied in the stomach, it is referred to as **chyme**. The chyme is squirted in small bursts through the pyloric sphincter and into the **duodenum** of the small intestine. If the small intestine is already digesting food, the stomach can act as a storage site until the small intestine is ready. The folds of the stomach, or **rugae**, allow the stomach to expand drastically and hold up to 2 liters of food. Minimal absorption occurs in the stomach.

The stomach contains four types of specialized stomach cells:

1. Parietal (oxyntic) cells
2. Chief (zymogenic) cells
3. Mucous cells
4. Enteroendocrine cells

Parietal (Oxyntic) Cells

Parietal cells secrete hydrochloric acid by actively pumping hydrogen ions across the membrane and into the stomach, lowering the pH of the stomach to around 2. These cells have an increased surface area through invaginations and microvilli, allowing more pumps to be active throughout the membrane. Due to their energy-intensive active transport of hydrogen ions, parietal cells have large numbers of mitochondria.

Chief (Zymogenic) Cells

ZYMOGEN

A *zymogen* is an inactive form of an enzyme. Pepsin is an active enzyme. Pepsinogen is the inactive (zymogen) form.

Chief cells secrete **pepsinogen**, the zymogen of **pepsin**. Pepsinogen is activated by the acidic environment of the stomach, where it is cleaved into pepsin. Pepsin is a **protease**, an enzyme that breaks down proteins.

Mucous Cells

Mucous cells secrete an alkaline mucus, which protects the stomach lining from digestive enzymes and from the acidic environment. Mucous cells line the inside surface of the stomach. An **ulcer** occurs when the acidic gastric juice of the stomach penetrates the epithelial lining of the stomach. Most ulcers are caused by the bacterium *Helicobacter pylori*, which prevents the infected mucous cells from secreting mucus.

Enteroendocrine Cells

Enteroendocrine cells secrete a variety of hormones that affect the secretions from other cells and the motility of food through the stomach.

LIVER

The liver is the largest internal organ in humans. It is involved in numerous biochemical processes, including the production of bile, the regulation of blood glucose levels, and the detoxification of blood.

Production of Bile

The liver produces **bile**. This fluid contains bile salts. Bile **emulsifies** (breaks down) insoluble fats, facilitating their digestion by enzymes. Bile may go through the common hepatic duct directly to the duodenum. Instead, it may travel through the cystic duct to the **gallbladder**, where it can be stored.

Regulation of Glucose Levels

The liver helps to regulate blood glucose levels. It stores glycogen, which can be broken down into glucose (**glycogenolysis**) and released into the blood. The liver can also form glycogen from glucose (**glycogenesis**) and synthesize glucose from noncarbohydrate molecules (**gluconeogenesis**).

If glycogen stores are depleted, the liver oxidizes triglycerides to produce energy and high-energy products that are exported and used by other cells in the body. A consequence of using lipids for an energy source is the production of **ketone bodies**, which are acidic. An excess of ketone bodies, which may occur due to a shortage of insulin in diabetics, lowers the pH of blood and leads to a dangerous state known as **ketoacidosis**. When carbohydrates or proteins are in excess, they are converted into fatty acids and triglycerides through **lipogenesis**. Cholesterol is synthesized and secreted along with bile.

Detoxification of Blood

The liver detoxifies the blood by removing old erythrocytes, which are converted to a component of bile. Many plasma proteins such as clotting factors and **albumin** are synthesized by the liver. Nonessential amino acids are also synthesized by the liver. Ammonia, a toxic by-product of protein degradation, is converted to urea in the liver. The liver also is capable of storing over a year's supply of certain vitamins.

PANCREAS

The **pancreas** is a gland with both endocrine and exocrine components. The **islets of Langerhans** make up the endocrine portion, producing a variety of hormones such as glucagon and insulin.

Exocrine Cells

The exocrine cells of the pancreas produce digestive enzymes, most notably the zymogen proteases **trypsinogen** and **chymotrypsinogen** but also pancreatic lipase and pancreatic amylase. The zymogens and enzymes are secreted in the pancreatic juice through the pancreatic duct and into the small intestine, where the zymogens are activated. In addition, **sodium bicarbonate** ($NaHCO_3$) is produced and secreted in the pancreatic juice. Sodium bicarbonate neutralizes the acidic chyme entering the duodenum from the stomach. Figure 3.85 shows the ducts of the pancreas and liver that are part of the exocrine component.

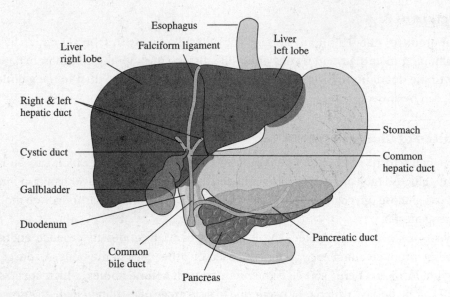

Figure 3.85. The ducts of the liver and pancreas

SMALL INTESTINE

The small intestine is where the final stages of digestion and absorption take place. The small intestine is made up of three parts: the **duodenum**, **jejunum**, and **ileum**. The surface area of the small intestine is dramatically increased due to villi and microvilli. The protruding villi are fingerlike extensions of the intestinal wall. The microvilli are projections coming out of the epithelial cells that line the villi. These microvilli, which cover the villi, are also known as the **brush border** and contain numerous digestive enzymes. The villi and microvilli absorb nutrients from the partially digested fluid that is pushed through the small intestine by peristalsis.

Duodenum

The duodenum is connected to the stomach and is the most active area for digestion. The pancreatic juices mix with the acidic chyme to neutralize the partially digested food and further digest it in the duodenum. Trypsin and chymotrypsin from the pancreas break apart proteins into smaller polypeptides, which are further degraded into amino acids along the brush border. Lipids are emulsified by the bile salts. Pancreatic lipase entirely degrades the lipids into fatty acids and monoglycerides. These products are absorbed by the epithelial cells and combine with proteins to form lipoproteins called **chylomicrons**. Chylomicrons are released via exocytosis into the lacteals of the lymph system and eventually enter the circulatory system through the thoracic duct, where they transport the nonpolar lipids through the bloodstream. Carbohydrates in the small intestine are broken into smaller polysaccharides by pancreatic amylase. These polysaccharides are further broken down at the brush border and in the epithelial cells into monosaccharides before being passed into the blood stream. Other carbohydrates remain undigested throughout the small intestine.

LIPOPROTEINS AND BLOOD CHOLESTEROL

Chylomicrons are the largest lipoproteins involved in lipid transport. Other lipoproteins include high-density lipoproteins (HDL) and low-density lipoproteins (LDL). High dietary fat intake can result in high blood cholesterol in the form of elevated LDL levels, which can lead to cardiovascular disease. In contrast, cholesterol carried by high-density lipoprotein is frequently termed "good cholesterol" because of a correlation with cardiovascular health.

Jejunum and Ileum

Absorption of water and nutrients takes place throughout the small intestine. However, the majority of absorption occurs in the jejunum and ileum. The pH of the fluid is slightly alkaline when it reaches the end of the small intestine.

LARGE INTESTINE

The processed food from the ileum is passed to the large intestine, which is made up of the colon, cecum, appendix, and rectum. One major job of the large intestine is the absorption of water and electrolytes from the food. However, specialized digestion also takes place. Certain undigested substances, such as complex saccharides, are broken down by the **gut flora**. The huge population of bacteria in the gut flora is mostly symbiotic or commensal, not parasitic. These microorganisms enable humans to absorb additional nutrients broken down by the specialized enzymes of the microorganisms. Some intestinal microorgansims synthesize vitamins. One type of bacteria in the gut is *Escherichia coli*. Most *E. coli* strains are commensal, although pathogenic strains in contaminated food have caused disease outbreaks and food poisoning.

The bacteria in the large intestine ferment some of the nutrients, producing gas as a by-product. The large intestine also forms **feces**, which contain the remaining indigestible food mixed with other waste products from the body, such as erythrocytes. The **rectum** is located at the end of the large intestine and stores the feces until the feces are ready to be excreted. Excretion of feces is controlled by the anal sphincter.

ENDOCRINE AND NERVOUS SYSTEM CONTROL

The digestive system is tightly regulated by the endocrine and nervous systems. Hormone-secreting (enteroendocrine) cells within the digestive system make up the largest endocrine system in the body, the **enteric endocrine system**. These cells are dispersed in and among other secretory cells in the organs and epithelia; however, because they are endocrine cells, the hormones they produce are secreted into the bloodstream and affect target tissues throughout the body. Because they are embedded in the epithelia, enteric endocrine cells are able to monitor and receive feedback from the lumen through their apical border, allowing for regulatory control. For example, the hormone secretin is produced by endocrine cells within epithelial cells of the small intestine in response to the presence of acid in food arriving from the stomach. Secretin triggers release of bicarbonate-rich solutions from the pancreas, neutralizing the stomach acid. When acid levels drop, secretin levels drop. Table 3.15 describes major digestive hormones and their functions.

The digestive system is also under the control of the autonomic nervous system, which exerts sympathetic and parasympathetic control over peristalsis, secretion, and absorption. The gut is under the control of the **enteric nervous system**, a separate division of the autonomic nervous system formed by nerve plexi in the lining of the esophagus, stomach, and intestine. The enteric nervous system can function independently of the central nervous system. The intestine is the largest producer and reservoir of the neurotransmitter serotonin in the body. The digestive system plays a critical role in the absorption of amino acid precursors necessary for the synthesis of amino-acid based neurotransmitters and hormones and in the absorption and processing of cholesterol for steroid hormone synthesis.

Table 3.15 Hormones of the Enteric Endocrine System

Location	Hormone	Stimulus	Function
Stomach	**Ghrelin**	Fasting	"Hunger hormone" through action on hypothalamus; stimulates release of growth hormone from the anterior pituitary
Stomach	**Gastrin**	Food (amino acids, peptides) in the stomach lumen	Gastric acid secretion
Small Intestine	**Cholecystokinin**	Food (amino acids, fatty acids) in the small intestine	Secretion of bile and pancreatic enzymes
Small Intestine	**Secretin**	Gastric acid in small intestine	Secretion of bicarbonate from pancreas and liver to neutralize stomach acid
Small intestine	**Gastric Inhibitory Polypeptide**	Fat and glucose in small intestine	Inhibits gastric motility and acid secretion; enhances the release of insulin from the pancreas
Pancreas (B cells)	**Insulin**	High blood glucose levels	Reduces glucose levels by stimulating tissues to uptake glucose and stimulating liver to convert glucose to glycogen
Pancreas (A cells)	**Glucagon**	Low blood glucose levels	Increases glucose levels by stimulating glycogen breakdown and gluconeogenesis in liver
Pancreas (D cells)	**Somatostatin**		Inhibits the release of other pancreatic hormones; inhibits release of growth hormone by pituitary

The Urinary System

The urinary system is also called the excretory system (see Figure 3.86). The **kidneys** are the primary organ of the urinary system, although many other organs play roles in excretion. The kidneys are attached to the **urinary bladder** via **ureters**. The bladder empties its contents to the outside of the body via the **urethra**. Elimination is under the control of a muscular sphincter in the urethra.

The main function of the urinary system is to remove nitrogenous waste, such as ammonia and urea. However, the urinary system also plays a key role in **homeostasis**. By controlling water and electrolyte retention, the urinary system is able to control both the blood pressure and pH of the blood.

KIDNEY

A kidney consists of two regions: the outer **renal cortex** and the inner **renal medulla**. The renal medulla is made up of **renal pyramids**. The pyramids are cone-shaped tissues formed by **nephrons**, the basic filtering units of the kidney.

The renal cortex is responsible for **ultrafiltration**, in which small molecules are pushed out of the capillaries due to a high pressure gradient. The renal medulla plays a critical role in **osmoregulation**, or maintaining the proper amount of water and salt in the blood.

NEPHRON

The functional unit of a kidney is a **nephron** (see Figures 3.87 and 3.88). A nephron is composed of a renal corpuscle and a renal tubule.

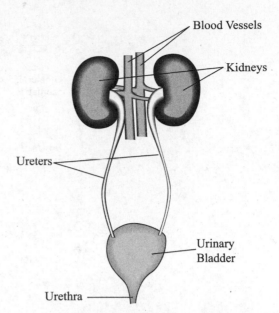

Figure 3.86. Urinary system

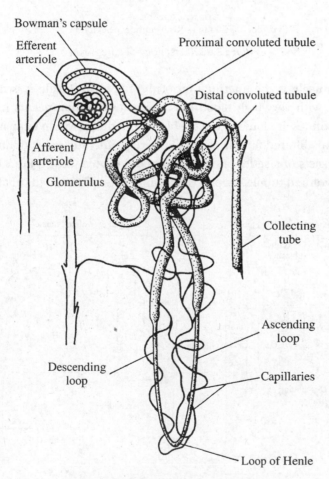

Figure 3.87. Anatomy of a nephron

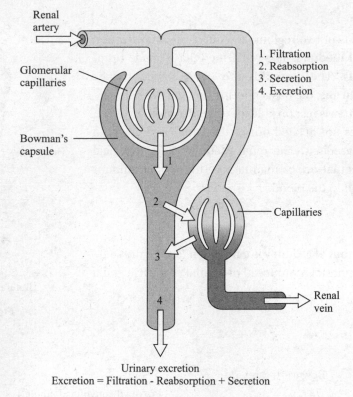

1. Filtration
2. Reabsorption
3. Secretion
4. Excretion

Renal artery

Glomerular capillaries

Bowman's capsule

Capillaries

Renal vein

Urinary excretion
Excretion = Filtration - Reabsorption + Secretion

Figure 3.88. Physiology of a nephron

The **renal corpuscle** is the filtering unit of the nephron. Inside it is the **glomerulus**, a capillary network with very high blood pressure. Ultrafiltration occurs in the glomerulus. Water and small solutes are forced from the blood into the **Bowman's capsule**, a cup-shaped collecting area. This filtered fluid is called **glomerular filtrate** and is drained into the renal tubule, which consists of a series of ducts. The **renal tubule** (see Figure 3.89) is made up of the proximal convoluted tubule, loop of Henle, and distal convoluted tubule.

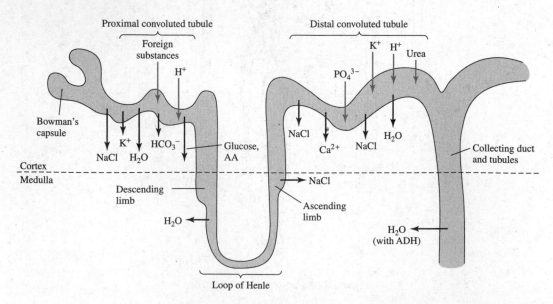

Figure 3.89. Physiology of the renal tubule and collecting duct

Proximal Convoluted Tubule

Most of the reabsorption of water and nutrients in the glomular filtrate occurs in the **proximal convoluted tubule**. Glucose, amino acids, ions (such as K^+, Na^+, and Cl^-), and water are reabsorbed through facilitated diffusion and secondary active transport, powered by the sodium concentration gradient. Foreign substances, such as drugs, are secreted. The glomerular filtrate pH is regulated by the proximal convoluted tubule through the exchange of bicarbonate and hydrogen ions.

Loop of Henle

The filtrate flows from the proximal convoluted tubule into the **loop of Henle**. The lower part of the loop is the only part of the renal tubule that is in the renal medulla. The rest of the renal tubule is located in the renal cortex. The first part of the loop of Henle is known as the **descending limb**. It is permeable to water but mostly impermeable to sodium. Because the interstitial fluid is hypertonic, water passively flows out of the filtrate in the descending limb. The latter part of the loop of Henle, the **ascending limb**, is impermeable to water. Sodium pumps actively pump sodium out of the filtrate and into the interstitial fluid, causing the interstitial fluid to become increasingly hypertonic.

Distal Convoluted Tubule

After the loop of Henle, the filtrate enters the **distal convoluted tubule.** This portion of the renal tubule relies on active transport for much of the reabsorption that occurs and is heavily controlled by the endocrine system. In particular, **parathyroid hormone** causes more calcium to be reabsorbed while increasing the secretion of phosphate. **Aldosterone** causes more sodium to be reabsorbed while increasing the secretion of potassium. Like the proximal convoluted tubule, drugs and toxic substances are also secreted here.

Collection of Urine

After passing through the distal convoluted tubule, the filtrate flows into a collecting duct. Numerous renal tubules connect to a common collecting duct. The permeability of the duct to water is controlled by **antidiuretic hormone (ADH)**. The presence of ADH significantly increases the permeability of the collecting duct to water, causing water to flow out of the filtrate and increasing the concentration of urine. This is known as a **countercurrent system**. The water flows out of the substrate due to the hypertonic conditions in the medulla created by the sodium pumps of the loop of Henle. Caffeine and alcohol inhibit ADH, increasing water loss through urine.

Urine from each kidney is emptied through a **ureter** and collected in the bladder. The bladder is an elastic muscular organ that stores urine until it is ready to be expelled. At that point, the urine passes through the involuntary **inner urethral sphincter** and voluntary **outer urethral sphincter**, into the **urethra**, and finally out of the body.

Regulation of Blood Pressure

The kidneys are responsible for regulating blood pressure through the **renin-angiotensin system**. This system is controlled in part by the **juxtaglomerular apparatus**, a structure inside the kidney that can sense stretching, indirectly measuring blood pressure. Decreased stretching indicates decreased blood pressure. Low blood pressure triggers the release of the enzyme **renin,** which increases the production of **angiotensin I**. Angiotensin I is then converted to **angiotensin II**. This hormone acts as a vasoconstrictor to increase blood pressure and causes the release of aldosterone to increase the reabsorption of sodium and water into the blood. (See Figure 3.90.)

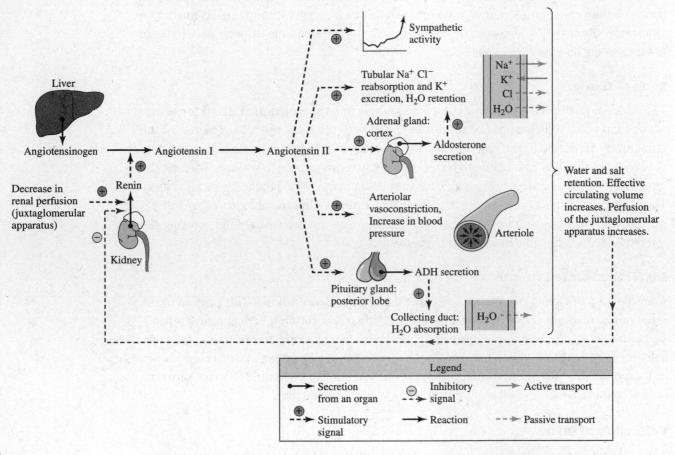

Figure 3.90. Diagram of the renin-angiotensin system

The Skeletal System

The skeletal system consists of the bones, cartilage, and joints of the body. The skeletal system has many functions:

- Provide structural support
- Provide physical protection to organs and body cavities
- Act as levers for muscular action
- Provide cavities for blood formation (hematopoesis)
- Store calcium and phosphate
- Store fat (as bone marrow)
- Act as a reservoir of other minerals and growth factors

BONE TISSUE

The skeletal system is composed of three types of connective tissue: compact bone, spongy bone, and cartilage. Compact and spongy bone are both types of **osseous tissue**. The cells of osseous tissue include osteoclasts, osteoblasts, and osteocytes. **Osteoclasts** are bone-resorbing cells that break down old bone to allow for bone growth and remodeling. **Osteoblasts** are bone-forming cells. Osteoblasts actively secrete the organic matrix, or **osteoid**, composed of a proteoglycan ground substance and abundant collagen fibers. The **osteoid** becomes hardened by the addition of calcium phosphate, which crystallizes into **hydroxyapatite** crystals. The osteoid also contains fibers of collagen protein to provide a degree of elasticity. A mature osteoblast that is no longer secreting osteoid becomes a mature **osteocyte** surrounded by the mineral bone matrix.

CARTILAGE

Cartilage is a form of connective tissue that provides firm, compressive support while retaining some elasticity. Cartilage lacks nerves and blood vessels. Instead, it is nourished by an external membrane called the perichondrium. The embryonic skeleton is entirely composed of hyaline cartilage. In an adult, cartilage persists in the joints, rib cage, larynx, trachea, nose, ears, and epiglottis. Cartilage also acts as cushioning pads between the vertebrae and between pelvic bones in adults.

TYPES OF BONE

Bones are organs composed of osseous tissue with associated connective, vascular, and nervous tissue. Table 3.16 lists the different types of bones.

Table 3.16 Types of Bones

Type	Examples
Long bones	Long bones of the appendages, such as the femur and humerus
Short bones	Carpal bones of the wrist, tarsal bones of the ankles
Flat bones	Skull, ribs, scapulae, and sternum
Irregular bones	Vertebrae Os coxae of the pelvis
Sesamoid bones	Rounded or irregular bones within the tendons, such as the patella of the knee

BONE GROWTH AND REMODELING

Osteogenesis, or **ossification**, is the process of bone growth. There are two mechanisms of ossification, both of which involve the replacement of an existing tissue by bone. The first mechanism, **intramembranous ossification**, involves the formation of bone (**dermal bone**) from a fibrous connective tissue membrane. During embryonic development, dermal bones that form by intramembranous ossification include the mandible, or lower jaw, and the roofing bones of the skull. The second mechanism, **endochondral ossification**, replaces cartilage with bone to produce the remainder of the adult skeleton. Both types of ossification occur by the activity of osteoblasts that secrete new organic matrix that is later hardened by the addition of calcium and phosphate crystals. Both mechanisms of ossification contribute to the healing of bone fractures.

Bone also undergoes continuous **remodeling**. Existing bone is broken down by the process of **osteolysis**, or **resorption**. Osteoclasts secrete digestive enzymes that break down bone matrix to release stored calcium and phosphate. As old bone is broken down, new bone is generated by the activity of both osteoclasts and osteoblasts. Bone remodeling and the storage or release of calcium is regulated by calcitonin, which promotes the storage of calcium in bone, parathyroid hormone, which triggers calcium release to the bloodstream, and vitamin D, which interacts with parathyroid hormone to promote calcium absorption and release. Calcitonin and parathyroid hormone are produced in the thyroid and parathyroid glands. However, vitamin D may be obtained through dietary sources or, in humans and some other mammals, may be derived from cholesterol on exposure of the skin to ultraviolet light. Vitamin D must subsequently be activated in the liver and kidneys to the biologically active form, calcitriol. On average, bone remodeling leads to the replacement of 10% of adult bone mass every year.

> ### BONE LOSS
>
> The rate of bone formation or bone loss is determined by the ratio of the activity of osteoblasts versus osteoclasts. Bone formation occurs at a slightly lower rate than bone resorption. This results in a gradual decrease in bone density with age that may lead to osteoporosis. Medications developed to treat osteoporosis target the activity of osteoclasts.

SKELETAL STRUCTURE

The human skeleton (Figure 3.91) is an internal framework, or **endoskeleton**, of 206 bones and associated cartilage. The endoskeleton provides support and protection, as does the exoskeleton of arthropods and other invertebrates. A protein exoskeleton, however, limits the body size of the organism. The mineralized endoskeleton of vertebrates overcomes this disadvantage. The endoskeleton also provides attachment points for muscle.

The skeleton consists of both **axial** and **appendicular** skeletal components. The axial skeleton includes the skull, vertebral column, and rib cage. The appendicular skeleton consists of the limbs and limb girdles. Bones articulate with one another and with associated cartilages through a variety of **joints**.

Joint Structure

Joints occur at points of **articulation**, or contact, between bones. Joints are classified structurally as either fibrous joints, cartilaginous joints, or synovial joints. Table 3.17 lists the different types of joints and describes their differences.

Table 3.17 Types of Joints

Type	Details and Examples
Fibrous joints	Highly immovable joints formed by fibrous connective tissue Example: The sutures between the flat bones of the skull
Cartilaginous joints	Rigid, mostly immobile joints with cartilage providing firm, cushioning support between bones Examples: The joints between the ribs and sternum; the joints between the vertebrae
Synovial joints	Freely movable joints that consist of a fluid-filled cavity surrounded by a synovial membrane and fibrous joint capsule. Most joints of the body are synovial. Examples: Knee, elbow, and shoulder joints

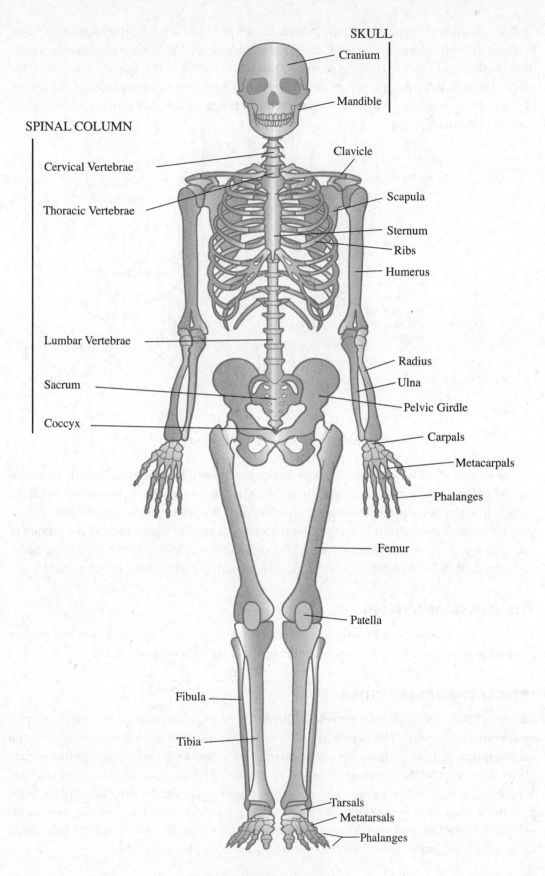

SKULL
— Cranium
— Mandible

SPINAL COLUMN

Cervical Vertebrae

Thoracic Vertebrae

Clavicle

Scapula

Sternum

Ribs

Humerus

Lumbar Vertebrae

Radius

Sacrum

Ulna

Pelvic Girdle

Coccyx

Carpals

Metacarpals

Phalanges

Femur

Patella

Fibula

Tibia

Tarsals
Metatarsals
Phalanges

Figure 3.91. Human skeleton

The structure of a typical **synovial joint** is shown in Figure 3.92. A **joint capsule** of dense irregular (fibrous) connective tissue surrounds the joint and provides resistance to multidirectional tensile force. The inner layer of the joint capsule is a synovial membrane that secretes **synovial fluid**, a viscous lubricating substance. Within the joint capsule, the articulating surfaces are lined with hyaline **articular cartilage**, which provides a smooth, glassy surface to reduce friction.

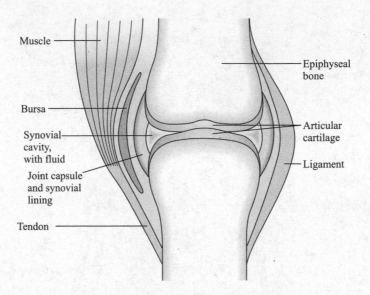

Figure 3.92. Structure of the synovial joint

The joint is stabilized by ligaments and muscle tendons. **Ligaments** are cords of dense, regular connective tissue that connect bone to bone. Muscle **tendons** cross joints to attach muscle to bone. **Bursae** are fluid-filled capsules found between ligaments and bone. Bursae provide cushioning support in areas of high friction. Sesamoid bones such as the **patella** of the knee may also form within tendons where they cross over joints. In the knee joint, fibrocartilage pads called **menisci** provide additional support and resistance to compression.

The Muscular System

The muscular system functions to provide structural support and mobility, line and protect internal organs, and aid in thermoregulation and in circulation of body fluids.

MUSCLE TISSUE STRUCTURE

Muscle tissue is composed of **muscle fibers**, elongate fused cells that originate from embryonic mesoderm. The equivalent of the plasma membrane in a muscle fiber is the **sarcolemma**, and the cytoplasm is **sarcoplasm**. Muscle fibers are packed with rodlike organelles called **myofibrils** that run the length of the fiber and are specialized for contraction. Myofibrils, in turn, are composed of protein **myofilaments**, primarily **thin filaments** of **actin** and **thick filaments** of **myosin**. Muscle tissue is well-vascularized to provide oxygen for aerobic respiration, and muscle cells contain abundant mitochondria. Adult muscle tissue undergoes very limited cell division and has little capacity for regeneration.

Muscle tissue is either **striated** or **smooth**. Striated muscle contains striations—transverse bands of alternating dark and light regions visible under a light microscope. These bands are formed by the distribution of contractile proteins in **sarcomeres**, the fundamental units of contraction. The end-to-end arrangement of sarcomeres in a myofibril is responsible for striations. In smooth muscle, striations are absent because contractile proteins are not arranged in sarcomeres.

Muscle tissue also can be characterized as either **voluntary** or **involuntary**. Voluntary muscle is under conscious control. Involuntary muscle is under unconscious regulation by the autonomic nervous system, by tissue pacemakers, and by local hormonal and chemical signals.

Figure 3.93 shows the three types of muscle tissue: skeletal muscle, cardiac muscle, and smooth muscle. **Skeletal muscle** is typically attached to the skeleton and functions in voluntary movement. Both **cardiac muscle** and **smooth muscle** are involuntary. Cardiac muscle is found in the heart. Smooth muscle is found in the skin, eyes, and the walls of hollow organs.

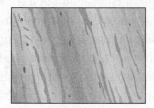
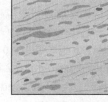
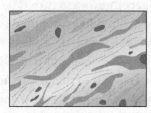

Skeletal muscle   Smooth muscle   Cardiac muscle

Figure 3.93. Three types of muscle tissue (Source: SEER Training Modules, *Muscle Tissue*. U.S. National Institutes of Health, National Cancer Institute. Accessed March 2011. ‹*http://training.seer.cancer.gov/*›)

Skeletal Muscle

Skeletal muscle tissue is **striated** and **voluntary**. It consists of **elongated**, **multinucleated**, **unbranched** cells reaching up to 30 cm in length. Skeletal muscle tissue combines with connective tissue, blood vessels, and nerves into **muscles**, which are the organs of the muscular system. Skeletal muscles function in body movement, including movement of the limbs, movement of the eyes, and movement of the skin for facial expression. Skeletal muscles also maintain body posture.

Most skeletal muscles attach on either side of a body joint, acting to move and stabilize the joint. The point of attachment that remains fixed is termed the **origin**. The point of attachment that moves as a result of muscle contraction is the **insertion**. Because muscle can only contract, not extend, pairs of muscles act in opposition to one another. One acts as a prime mover, or **agonist**. Another acts as an **antagonist** to exert pull in the opposite direction.

A single skeletal muscle consists of thousands of individual muscle fibers, or cells, each enclosed in a sheath of connective tissue (see Figure 3.94). Multiple muscle fibers are bundled together into **fascicles** wrapped by another connective tissue layer. Groups of muscle fascicles are bundled together to form an entire muscle. An outer sheath of connective tissue surrounds the muscle. This outer sheath is continuous with the dense connective tissue of cordlike **tendons** and sheetlike **aponeuroses** (layers of flat tendon), which transmit force from muscle to bone and from muscle to muscle.

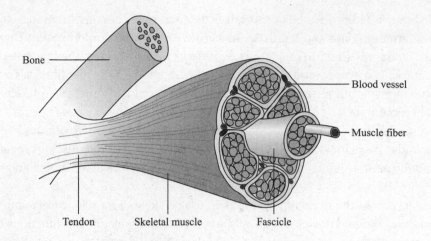

Figure 3.94. Structure of a skeletal muscle

Sarcomere structure. The sarcomere is the fundamental unit of contraction in a skeletal muscle fiber. In a sarcomere, dark A bands are formed from transverse bands of **myosin thick filaments**, which partially overlap **actin thin filaments**. The A band is bisected by a lighter H zone, in the center of which is an M line of protein that anchors the thick filaments. Light I bands consist of thin filaments attached to perpendicular Z lines. A single sarcomere extends from one Z line to the next and is composed of a dark A band bordered by half of a light I band on either side. (See Figure 3.95.)

REMEMBERING THE BANDS

Use mnemonics to remember dark and light bands:

d = A = rk = A band

L - I = ght = I band

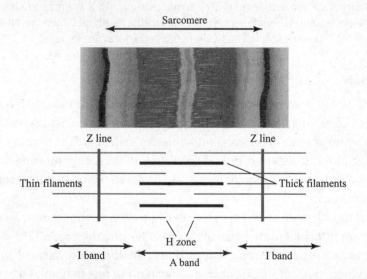

Figure 3.95. Sarcomere, showing bands.
During contraction, Z lines are pulled closer together.

Thick filaments consist of myosin chains that bear globular heads with binding sites for actin. Myosin chains are wound around an **elastic (titin) filament** that acts as a central core running between the M line and opposite Z lines. Elastic filaments align thick filaments and aid in elastic recoil of the sarcomere after contraction. (See Figure 3.96.)

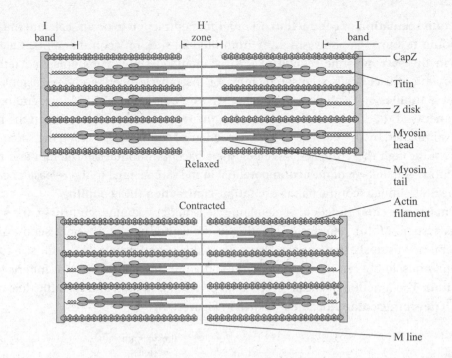

Figure 3.96. Relaxation and contraction of sarcomere
(Adapted from David Richfield on *http://en.wikipedia.org/wiki/Sarcomere.*)

Thin filaments are composed of two chains of actin that twist about each other like strings of pearls. Actin thin filaments extend from the point of attachment at the Z line toward the thick filaments, overlapping with thick filaments at the outer edge of the A band. Additional strands of the regulatory protein **tropomyosin** are also entwined with the actin strands. A second regulatory protein, **troponin**, forms a complex that binds to tropomyosin. In a relaxed muscle, tropomyosin blocks access to the myosin binding sites on the actin filaments. For contraction to occur, calcium must bind to the troponin complex, which changes in conformation and pulls tropomyosin away from actin binding sites. Myosin heads then bind to exposed binding sites on actin and initiate contraction.

Sliding filament model. According to the sliding filament model, contraction occurs when myosin heads bind to actin filaments and pull them toward the H zone, shortening the sarcomeres. The myosin heads are the motors that drive contraction. Prior to binding actin, myosin heads must be activated into a cocked position by the hydrolysis of ATP. The binding of myosin heads to actin forms **cross-bridges**. On binding, a myosin head swivels or rachets into a new position, pulling along the actin strand and returning the myosin head to a low energy state. ATP is required to release actin-myosin cross-bridges and recock the myosin heads to continue the cycle. During contraction, cross-bridges are formed, broken, and reformed as myosin heads on each thick filament rachet along the thin filament. The contraction of a muscle is the result of the combined effect of the contraction of individual sarcomeres arranged in series within the muscle fibers.

> **RIGOR MORTIS**
>
> The prolonged contraction of muscles after death is caused by the failure of membrane ion pumps, which leads to an influx of calcium into muscle cells. This triggers cross-bridge formation. As no ATP is available to break the cross-bridges, muscles remain contracted until proteins eventually degrade.

Calcium regulation of contraction. In order for contraction to occur, calcium must bind to troponin to move tropomyosin away from binding sites on actin filaments. Calcium is stored in the **sarcoplasmic reticulum (SR)**, a modified smooth endoplasmic reticulum of embryonic muscle cells. The sarcolemma of the muscle fiber sends extensions called **transverse tubules** or **T tubules** to encircle each sarcomere. The T tubules extend between enlargements of the sarcoplasmic reticulum in the region of each Z disk. When the muscle fiber is stimulated by the nervous system, an action potential travels along the sarcolemma and down through the T tubules, signaling the adjacent SR to release calcium and initiate contraction. The linkage of the action potential in the sarcolemma to the release of calcium from the SR to initiate contraction is **excitation-contraction (EC) coupling**.

The neuromuscular junction. Skeletal muscle is under voluntary control by the somatic nervous system. **Motor neurons** originating in the central nervous system send axons via peripheral nerves to skeletal muscle. Nerve fibers divide and penetrate the muscle to reach individual muscle fibers. One motor neuron and all of the muscle fibers it innervates is a **motor unit**. The junction of one axon terminal of a motor neuron and an individual muscle fiber is a **neuromuscular junction** as shown in Figure 3.97.

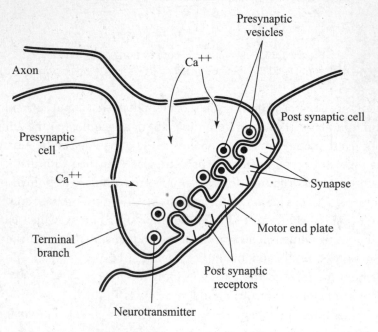

Figure 3.97. Neuromuscular junction

The axon terminal and **the motor end plate**, or adjacent membrane of the muscle fiber, are separated by a narrow fluid- and protein-filled gap called the **synaptic cleft**. The axon terminal is filled with **synaptic vesicles** containing the neurotransmitter **acetylcholine (ACh)**.

When the motor neuron is depolarized by an action potential, Ca^{2+} ions flood into the axon terminal and trigger the exocytosis of ACh from synaptic vesicles. Acetylcholine diffuses across the synaptic cleft and binds to ACh receptors located on folds of the sarcolemma at the motor end plate. These receptors are **ligand–gated ion channels** that open upon binding ACh, allowing Na^+ to enter and K^+ to exit through the sarcolemma. As more sodium ions cross the membrane than potassium ions, the muscle fiber is locally depolarized, resulting in a change in **end plate potential**. Once the end plate potential reaches a threshold value, adjacent **voltage–gated ion channels** open and an action potential is propagated along the sarcolemma and down into the T tubules, triggering contraction. Contraction is terminated as acetylcholine in the synaptic cleft is broken down by the enzyme **acetylcholinesterase**. This results in termination of the signal and restoration of the resting membrane potential at the motor end plate.

Nervous system regulation of contraction. The nervous system regulates the degree of muscle contraction by varying the frequency and the strength of the stimulus. Stimulus frequency affects the force of contraction generated by individual muscle fibers. Stimulus strength determines the number and type of motor units that participate in contraction. Both stimulus frequency and strength affect the force of contraction of the muscle as a whole.

1. All-or-none response
2. Graded response
3. Stimulus strengh (recruitment of motor units)
4. Isotonic versus isometric contraction

In an **all-or-none response**, a single action potential stimulating all the fibers of a single motor unit results in a **muscle twitch**. A muscle twitch consists of three stages. The first stage is a **latent period** between the propagation of the action potential and the release of calcium from the SR. During the second stage, a **period of contraction** occurs when actin and myosin are actively forming cross-bridges. The third stage is a **period of relaxation** when calcium concentrations decline as calcium is taken up by the sarcoplasmic reticulum. Depending on the type of muscle fiber, muscle twitches may be fast and of short duration, or they may be slow and prolonged. However, in all cases, a muscle twitch is an all-or-none response. Once the action potential threshold is reached within the sarcolemma of a muscle fiber, the fiber fully contracts.

In contrast to the all-or-none response of individual muscle fibers, an entire muscle is capable of a **graded response**. An entire muscle exhibits a range in the degree of contraction that varies from delicate movements to heavy lifting. This graded response can be achieved by altering the stimulus frequency. A single action potential results in a single muscle twitch. However, if the nerve stimulus is repeated before the first contraction terminates, the separate contractions combine in a process of **wave summation** (**temporal summation**.)

Wave summation occurs because each stimulus increases the concentration of intracellular calcium. At a low frequency of nerve stimulation, each stimulus arrives before the muscle has completely relaxed. The resulting **temporal summation** results in **incomplete tetanus**, which is a partial but sustained contraction. Note that muscle tetanus is a normal physiological event in muscle contraction that should not be confused with the disease of the same name.

At a higher frequency, when the stimulus is applied so rapidly that no relaxation occurs between muscle twitches, the muscle will achieve **complete tetanus**. This is a smooth, sustained contraction generating maximal muscle tension. Most muscle contraction involves incomplete tetanus, as complete tetanus occurs only as a result of extreme stimulation. After any prolonged tetanus a muscle may begin to **fatigue**, losing the ability to contract despite nervous stimulation.

The strength of muscle contraction can also be controlled by **strength of the stimulus** from the nervous system. A stronger stimulus leads to a greater depolarization of the muscle fibers. The stimulus strength determines the number and type of individual motor units that are activated by the somatic nervous system (the **recruitment of motor units**). At low levels of stimulus, the first motor units to be activated are small-diameter, highly excitable fibers with a low response threshold. At higher stimulus levels, larger-diameter, less excitable motor units are recruited. The greater the number of motor units stimulated to contract, the stronger the contraction of the entire muscle.

The amount of movement in a skeletal muscle depends not only upon the force of contraction but also upon the amount of load or force opposing contraction. In an **isotonic contraction**, the muscle shortens and moves the load. In an **isometric contraction**, the load is greater than the force generated by the muscle and the muscle cannot shorten. Instead, the muscle exerts **tension** against the load. Isotonic contractions result in body movement. Isometric contractions triggered by stretch receptors and spinal reflexes help determine **muscle tone**, the state of partial skeletal muscle contraction needed to maintain body posture and stabilize joints.

Energy for contraction. At low to moderate levels of activity or during aerobic exercise, muscle contraction is a highly aerobic process. Muscle contraction depends on abundant mitochondria and a continuous supply of oxygen to generate ATP through **aerobic respiration**. Initially, blood glucose is the primary energy source. During sustained exercise, cellular respiration utilizes glycogen stores and free fatty acids that are converted to glucose through the process of gluconeogenesis.

In the absence of oxygen, muscle cells have a specialized backup system for rapidly generating ATP. Muscle cells maintain stores of **creatine phosphate**, a molecule capable of reversible phosphorylation of ADP to ATP in a reaction catalyzed by creatine kinase enzymes.

$$\text{Creatine kinase}$$
$$\text{Creatine phosphate} + \text{ADP} \leftrightarrow \text{Creatine} + \text{ATP}$$

The creatine phosphate system acts as a reserve of stored phosphate that can be used to regenerate ATP for several seconds at the onset of intense muscle activity.

When sudden exertion must proceed longer than a few seconds, muscles utilize **anaerobic glycolysis** and **lactic acid fermentation** to generate ATP until the heart rate and respiratory rate increase sufficiently to increase the oxygen supply. During anaerobic respiration, glycolysis provides the source of ATP. In order to regenerate NAD^+ required for the oxidation of glucose, the pyruvic acid produced by glycolysis is converted to lactic acid. Lactic acid eventually diffuses out of the muscles and is transported by the bloodstream to the liver. The liver can convert the lactic acid to blood glucose. Alternatively, lactic acid can be used as an energy source by the skeletal muscles, liver, kidneys, and heart. Lactic acid leads to an **oxygen deficit**, which must be repaid after exercise, when lactic acid is converted in the presence of oxygen back to pyruvic acid.

Types of skeletal muscle fibers. Skeletal muscle fibers are categorized into three types based on the color of the fiber and the type of contraction:

1. Slow oxidative fibers (Type I)
2. Fast oxidative fibers (Type IIa)
3. Fast glycolytic fibers (Type IIb)

Each motor unit contains only one type of fiber. However, a muscle may have a mix of fiber types. The type of muscle fiber in a motor unit affects the speed and duration of contraction.

Slow oxidative fibers (Type I) are slow twitch red fibers. These are slow to contract but are capable of extended contraction without fatigue. They utilize aerobic pathways and fatty acids as an energy source. They contain abundant mitochondria and **myoglobin** (red-pigmented oxygen-storage molecules) and are well vascularized. Muscles that contain many Type I fibers are used in endurance exercise and in maintaining posture.

Fast oxidative fibers (Type IIa) are intermediate red fibers with abundant myoglobin, mitochondria, and capillaries. They utilize aerobic, glycolytic, and anaerobic pathways. Fast oxidative fibers contract more quickly but fatigue more readily than Type I fibers. Type IIa fibers can function for extended periods of anaerobic activity such as middle distance running.

Fast glycolytic fibers (Type IIb) are fast twitch white fibers with little myoglobin and few mitochondria and capillaries. They contain large amounts of stored glycogen. Type IIb fibers generate ATP very rapidly through glycolytic and anaerobic pathways but fatigue rapidly. They are used for short bursts of intense activity.

Cardiac Muscle

Cardiac muscle is **involuntary**, **striated** muscle that forms the walls of the heart and pumps blood through the body. Cardiac cells are **uninucleate**, **branching** cells joined by **intercalated disks** visible as dark, tranverse lines under a light microscope. Intercalated disks are formed by intercellular connections including desmosomes and gap junctions. Desmosomes, which are also called macula adherens, bind adjacent cells together. Gap junctions allow for the rapid intercellular transmission of action potentials necessary for cardiac cells to contract simultaneously. Involuntary contraction of cardiac muscle is initiated by the sinoatrial node pacemaker of the heart but can be regulated by parasympathetic and sympathetic innervation. Although striated muscle does not readily regenerate, recent evidence suggests that cardiac cells undergo a limited amount of cell division in adults.

Smooth Muscle

Smooth muscle is **involuntary**, **nonstriated** muscle that lines the hollow organs of the body, including the stomach, intestines, bladder, uterus, blood vessels, and bronchioles, where it moves materials through passageways. Smooth muscle also occurs in the arrector pili muscles of the skin and in the ciliary body and iris of the eye. In smooth muscle, **spindle-shaped cells** are arranged in sheets, typically in two layers—one longitudinal and one circular. Contraction of the longitudinal layer results in shortening of the muscle. Contraction of the circular layer results in elongation of the muscle and constriction of the lumen, or hollow cavity, within the organ. Relaxation of smooth muscle dilates the lumen of the vessel.

Smooth muscle tissue is unstriated because it lacks sarcomeres. Instead, thin and thick filaments occur in a spiral arrangement within the cell. T tubules and an enlarged sarcoplasmic reticulum are absent. Most of the calcium necessary to trigger muscle contraction comes from the extracellular space. There is no troponin complex. Instead, calcium binds to the protein **calmodulin**, triggering phosphorylation of myosin to initiate contraction.

Smooth muscle contraction is typically slow and sustained. It occurs simultaneously in all fibers. However, multiunit smooth muscle capable of rapid contraction occurs in the iris of the eye, the trachea, and the linings of large blood vessels. Involuntary contraction of smooth muscle may be triggered by the autonomic nervous system, by hormones, by local signals, or by tissue pacemakers. For example, the hormone oxytocin triggers uterine contractions, the local release of histamine triggers bronchoconstriction, and tissue pacemakers trigger peristalsis.

Innervation of Involuntary Muscle

Cardiac and smooth muscle may receive both sympathetic and parasympathetic innervation from the autonomic nervous system. Sympathetic control leads to increased heart rate, vasoconstriction in the blood vessels of the skin and abdomen, vasodilation of blood vessels serving skeletal muscle, dilation of the bronchi, stimulation of the sweat glands, and dilation of the iris. On the other hand, parasympathetic control results in decreased heart rate, peripheral vasodilation, bronchoconstriction, peristalsis, salivation, and pupillary constriction.

Function of Muscles in Thermoregulation

Muscle can convert the chemical energy of ATP to the mechanical energy of contraction at approximately 40% efficiency. The remaining energy is lost as heat. This excess heat is used by the body for thermoregulation. When body temperature is low, the **shivering reflex** may initiate involuntary contractions of the skeletal muscle around critical organ systems to generate heat.

Function of Muscles in Peripheral Circulation

Muscle contraction assists the circulatory system in returning blood and lymph to the heart. Circulation is also affected by **muscle tone**, the low level of contraction maintained in relaxed muscle by reflexive contraction of individual muscle fibers. Venous return depends highly on muscle tone and muscular activity, as does the movement of lymph out of the tissues and through lymph nodes.

The Respiratory System

The respiratory system is designed as an air-blood interface for the exchange of oxygen and carbon dioxide in the body. Figure 3.98 shows the respiratory tract. The lungs dispose of carbon dioxide from the body while bringing oxygen into the blood for transport throughout the body. Respiration is accomplished by simple diffusion. Oxygen and carbon dioxide move from an area of high partial pressure (or concentration) to an area of low partial pressure. The respiratory tract has special mechanisms for conditioning the air taken in from the environment and for protecting itself against disease organisms and contamination.

PROTECTING THE RESPIRATORY TRACT

As air enters the nose, it passes through the nasal cavity, the pharynx, the larynx, the trachea, the bronchi, and the bronchioles, ending up in the alveoli. The air contains particles, including bacteria and debris. In the nose and upper respiratory tract, these particles are filtered out by hairs and mucous material in the nose and in the **mucociliary tract**. The air is also made warmer and more humid. The mucus in these areas is constantly pushed upward by small cilia, eventually reaching the nose and throat. At that point, the mucus is eliminated through the nose, by swallowing, or by expectoration.

The alveoli lack cilia and mucus. Contamination in the alveoli is controlled by macrophages and leukocytes that debride the area and clear contaminants via the lymphatic system.

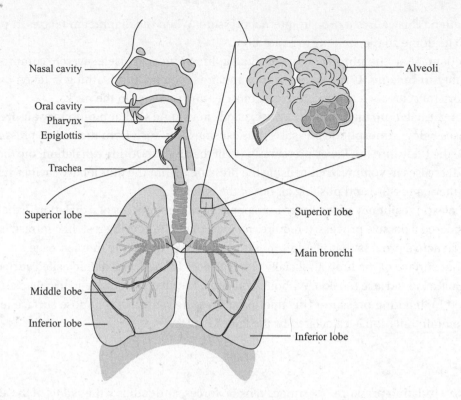

Figure 3.98. The respiratory tract

In addition, the autonomic nervous system helps protect the respiratory tract. The autonomic system innervates the smooth muscles lining the **bronchioles** (terminal portions of the airways). Parasympathetic stimulation causes **bronchoconstriction**, such as in an asthma attack, to protect the alveoli from harmful contaminants. Sympathetic stimulation causes relaxation of these same bronchioles.

FUNCTIONS OF RESPIRATION

Respiration involves the following:

1. Ventilation of the lungs
2. Gas exchange between the lungs and blood
3. Transport of gases in the blood
4. Gas exchange between the blood and interstitial fluids of the body

Ventilation of the Lungs

Normal spontaneous breathing is under the control of motor neurons, especially the **phrenic nerve** to the diaphragm. Intercostal nerves innervate the external and internal intercostal muscles, which elevate the ribcage. Conscious control of breathing originates in the cerebral cortex and travels through the pons and medulla of the brain. However, for the most part, breathing is involuntary and is regulated through the respiratory center located in the medulla.

The diaphragm is the primary muscle involved in breathing. It is innervated by the phrenic nerve. The impulse for inspiration is produced in the **medulla oblongata**. In its relaxed state, the diaphragm is dome shaped. The signal to inhale causes the diaphragm to contract and thus flatten. This causes a drop in internal pressure. When the diaphragm relaxes, it pushes up into its dome shape, helping to expel air.

Any damage to the phrenic nerve or the diaphragm muscle itself severely compromises the ability to breathe. If the diaphragm is impaired, control of breathing is taken over by accessory muscles such as the intercostal muscles and scalenes in the neck.

During inhalation, the thoracic cavity expands in volume so that **pulmonary air pressure** decreases below atmospheric pressure, thus causing air to rush from the higher-pressure air outside the body into the lower-pressure space of the alveoli. During exhalation, the thoracic cavity decreases in volume, thus causing the pressure within the pulmonary cavity to exceed atmospheric pressure and pushing air out of the lungs.

The **elastic resiliency** of the lungs is responsible for the process of exhalation. Exhalation is considered a passive process. It requires no muscular effort during rest. In contrast, inhalation is an active process that requires muscular effort to expand the thoracic cage.

The inner surface of the lung (especially in the alveoli) is lined with a fluid called **surfactant**, which has a low surface tension. Without surfactant, the alveoli would tend to collapse unless opposed by inflating pressure. The amount of pressure required to oppose surface tension and maintain inflation is calculated by the law of Laplace:

$$p = \frac{2T}{r}$$

where p = inflation pressure, T = surface tension forces, and radius = the radius of the alveoli.

Because the lungs are lined by a liquid (constant surface tension), as the radius decreases (deflation), the distending pressure increases. Smaller alveoli require a greater distending force than larger alveoli due to the smaller radius.

The inability to produce surfactant is a key problem in hyaline membrane disease. Infants with this deficiency may die of respiratory distress because their lungs collapse with each breath.

The **transpulmonary pressure** is the pressure that keeps the lungs inflated. Transpulmonary pressure is defined as the pressure differential ($P_{pul} - P_{ip}$) between the **intrapulmonary** (**alveolar**) **pressure** (P_{pul}) in the alveoli and the **intrapleural pressure** (P_{ip}) of the pleural cavity. The transpulmonary pressure is always positive, and the intrapulmonary pressure is close to atmospheric pressure at rest, moving between slightly positive and slightly negative at each breath. Both the thoracic wall and the lung surface of the pleural cavity are lined by serous membranes, and the space between is filled with serous fluid. The intrapleural pressure is always negative and is less than intrapulmonary pressure because the outward pull of the thorax resists the inward pull of the lungs, which tend to collapse because of the surface tension of fluid within the alveoli. On inspiration, the thorax expands outward and the diaphragm pulls downward, expanding the volume of the thoracic cavity. The intrapleural pressure becomes more negative. Because the thin layer of serous fluid acts as an adhesive between lungs and thorax, the lungs also expand, decreasing intrapulmonary pressure relative to atmospheric pressure, and sucking air into the alveoli. On expiration, the elastic recoil of the lungs and thorax decreases the volume of the lungs, and air is expelled.

The volume of air that is moved into and out of the lungs at each normal breath is the **tidal volume (TV)**. The maximum amounts of air that can be forcibly inhaled and exhaled are the **inspiratory reserve volume (IRV)** and the **expiratory reserve volume (ERV)**, respectively. After forcible expiration, there is still an amount of residual air in the lungs, the **residual volume (RV)**. The total amount of exchangeable air in the lungs is the **vital capacity (VC)**. Vital capacity is the sum of TV, IRV, and ERV. The total amount of air in the lungs, the **total lung capacity** (**TLC**), is the vital capacity plus the residual volume. For normal adult males, total lung capacity is approximately 6000 mL, and vital capacity is 4800 mL.

Not all inspired air contributes to gas exchange in the alveoli. The volume of air that fills up respiratory passages outside the alveoli is **anatomical dead space**. The actual volume of air that is involved in alveolar ventilation in each inspiration is the tidal volume minus the anatomical dead space. If tidal volume is 450 mL, and anatomical dead space is 150 mL, the volume of air involved in gas exchange is 300 mL. If alveoli cease to function due to blockage or collapse, the alveolar dead space is added to the anatomical dead space to calculate the total volume of air that does not contribute to gas exchange, the **total dead space**.

The **alveolar ventilation rate** (**AVR**) measures the ventilation rate of the lungs. The alveolar ventilation rate is calculated as:

$$AVR = frequency \times (TV - dead\ space)$$
$$(mL/min)(breaths/min)(mL/breath)$$

The alveolar ventilation rate of a person with TV is 450 mL, dead space is 150 mL, and the alveolar ventilation rate of a person who is breathing 12 times per minute is 12 breaths per minute times 300 mL per breath, or 3600 mL per minute.

Gas Exchange

Gas exchange through simple diffusion occurs in the **alveoli** of the lungs, which provide an enormous surface area with an extremely thin capillary barrier. The alveolus is the only area for gas exchange. Other areas, including the tracheobronchial tree, function as anatomic dead space that simply facilitates movement of air but not diffusion of gases. The oxygen passes from the alveolar air spaces (**respiratory zone**) to the blood in the capillaries surrounding the alveoli. The diffusion of oxygen from the alveoli into the blood follows a specific pathway.

ALVEOLAR PATHWAY

1. Alveolar air
2. Surfactant (lowers surface tension)
3. Alveolar epithelium (simple squamous epithelium)
4. Fused basal laminae of alveolar epithelium and capillary endothelium
5. Capillary endothelium (simple squamous epithelium)
6. Blood plasma
7. Erythrocytes (red blood cells)

Oxygen molecules bind to hemoglobin in the red blood cells. Hemoglobin contains four iron atoms, each of which can bind to one O_2 molecule. In a process known as **cooperativity**, the binding of an O_2 molecule to an iron atom increases the rate at which other O_2 molecules will bind. The same accelerating effect happens when an O_2 molecule is released, leading to rapid unloading of O_2.

Several factors determine the extent to which the blood will be saturated with oxygen. These include the oxygen tension (partial pressure in mm Hg), the pressure of CO_2, the pH, concentration of 2,3-diphosphoglycerate (DPG), and the temperature. In the lungs, these factors are ideally maximized for maximum saturation. However, as the blood circulates through the body, conditions reverse and favor decreased saturation. As a result, oxygen will tend to leave the blood and become available for tissues in the body. The balance between these conditions governs the transport of oxygen and carbon dioxide from the lungs to other tissues. This balance is described in the oxygen dissociation curve (Figure 3.99).

Transport of Gases

In the blood, the oxygen is transported in the form of oxyhemoglobin. Normal hemoglobin values are 14 g/100 mL for women and 16 g/100 mL for men (with an average of 15 g/100 mL). Each gram of hemoglobin can combine with 1.39 mL of oxygen. The volume of dissolved oxygen in fully oxygenated blood (the **oxygen capacity** of blood) can be calculated as: .

$$(15 \text{ g Hb}/100 \text{ mL blood}) \text{ H } (1.39 \text{ mL O}_2/\text{g Hb}) = 21 \text{ mL O}_2/100 \text{ mL blood}$$

Gas Exchange Between Blood and Body Fluids

Figure 3.99 shows several factors that affect the affinity of hemoglobin for oxygen: pH, temperature, and DPG concentration. These factors determine how much oxygen can bind to hemoglobin.

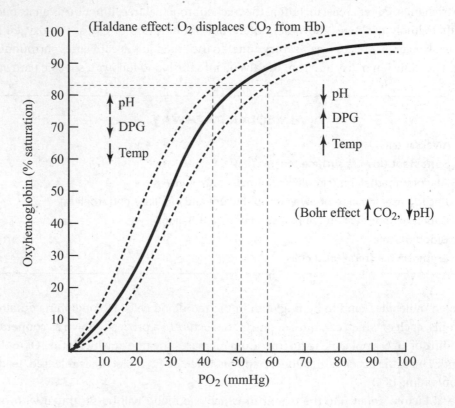

Figure 3.99. Oxygen-hemoglobin dissociation curve

These factors affect the sigmoid-shaped curve on the oxygen dissociation curve, which shows the percent of oxygen saturation versus the partial pressure of oxygen (PO_2). A decrease in pH, an increase in temperature, or an increase in DPG will facilitate the release of oxygen in the tissue capillaries. This is plotted as a shift of the curve to the right.

In the lungs, the partial pressure of oxygen is around 110 mm Hg. On the oxygen dissociation curve, this would indicate a maximized saturation of about 97%. As blood moves through the body, it may pass tissues that are actively metabolizing, such as muscles that are contracting. In these tissues, the oxygen pressure is more typically in the range of 40 mm Hg. Based on the curve, the saturation of oxygen in the blood would drop to about 82%. This means that oxygen would be released from the blood into the metabolizing tissues. Active metabolism in tissues typically results in an increase in temperature and carbon dioxide concentration that causes oxygen to leave hemoglobin.

Carbon dioxide must also be transported through the bloodstream from the tissues to the lungs, where it is expelled. Carbon dioxide is nonpolar and does not readily dissolve in the blood, although approximately 5% of blood CO_2 is dissolved in plasma. Hemoglobin can carry carbon dioxide, but at a very low binding affinity. Most carbon dioxide is transported in the form of bicarbonate ions, HCO^{3-}. CO_2 combines with water to form bicarbonate with the help of the catalyst carbonic anhydrase:

$$CO_2 + H_2O \leftrightarrow H_2CO_3 \leftrightarrow H^+ + HCO^{3-}$$

Bicarbonate is an extremely important buffer for blood, which needs to remain at a pH of 7.4 for optimal functioning. Consider how changes in the surrounding fluid's pH would shift the oxygen-hemoglobin dissociation curve. An increase in carbon dioxide concentration shifts the curve to the right. According to Le Châtelier's principle, in the equilibrium above, an increase in carbon dioxide would cause an increase in the concentration of H^+. This increase would decrease the pH. A decrease in pH would shift the oxygen-hemoglobin dissociation curve to the right. In contrast, an increase in pH would shift the curve to the left. The **Bohr effect** states as much; increasing the concentration of protons and/or carbon dioxide and increasing pH will reduce the oxygen affinity of hemoglobin.

NERVOUS SYSTEM CONTROL OF RESPIRATION

Respiration is under both voluntary and involuntary control by the central nervous system. The brainstem provides involuntary control by the autonomic nervous system, but this can be overridden to an extent by voluntary input from the cerebral cortex. Blood levels of oxygen and carbon dioxide and pH are monitored by chemoreceptors in the medulla, the aorta, and the carotid arteries. Autonomic nervous system response is carried out by glossopharyngeal and vagus cranial nerves. Strenuous exercise results in lower blood pH, triggering an increase in respiration rate. Respiration rate is also affected by temperature and emotional state.

Integumentary (Skin) System

The integumentary system is composed of the skin and associated nerves, capillaries, fatty deposits, glands, hairs, and sensory organs. The skin is the largest organ in the body. It acts as a tough but flexible waterproofing layer that protects the body from abrasion, dessication, injury, UV damage, and infection. The skin also synthesizes vitamin D. It contributes to the maintenance of homeostasis by regulating body temperature and excreting wastes, salts, and water.

STRUCTURE

The skin consists of two layers: an outer **epidermis** of epithelial tissue and an inner **dermis** of connective tissue. Below the dermis is the **hypodermis**, a subcutaneous fat layer that is not considered part of the skin. The skin is also called the **cutaneous membrane**. Figure 3.100 illustrates the layers of the skin.

Epidermis

The epidermis is the body's outermost defense against injury, infection, and water loss. It is composed of stratified squamous epithelial tissue that forms 4 to 5 avascular layers. The most abundant cells are **keratinocytes**. These cells produce intermediate filaments of **keratin**, a fibrous structural protein that contributes to the durability and toughness of the skin. Keratinocytes divide continuously by mitosis in the deepest cell layer of the epidermis adjacent to the underlying connective tissue of the dermis.

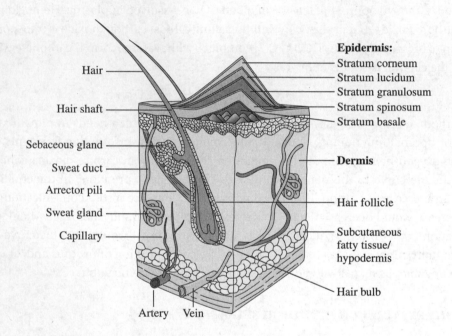

Figure 3.100. Layers of the skin

As new cells are generated, older cells are pushed upward. The older cells become tightly bound together by desmosomes, fill with keratin and waterproofing glycolipids, and begin to die as they move farther away from the dermal blood supply. The outermost layer of the epidermis is composed of dead, keratin-filled cells that continuously slough off and are replaced by underlying layers. Replacement of the entire epidermis occurs approximately once a month. **Calluses** are thickenings of the epidermis that form protective pads in areas exposed to excessive friction.

Other cell types found in the lower layers of the epidermis include **melanocytes**, **Langerhan's cells**, and **tactile (Merkel's) cells**. Melanocytes produce the pigment **melanin**, which shields the DNA in dividing keratinocytes from UV damage. Variation in the amount of melanin produced results in variation in skin color. Langerhan's cells (dendritic cells) are macrophages that function in immune response. Tactile (Merkel's) cells are sensory receptors that respond to touch.

Dermis

The dermis is a thick layer of loose and dense connective tissue that underlies and nourishes the epidermis. Unlike the epidermis, the dermis contains an abundant blood supply. It supports nerve fibers, glands, sensory receptors, smooth muscle, and the growing portions of accessory structures such as hair and nails. The network of **collagen** and **elastin** fibers in the extracellular matrix of the dermis gives the skin its tensile strength and elasticity.

Hypodermis

The hypodermis consists of a layer of adipose tissue underlying the dermis. Although the hypodermis is not structurally part of the skin, it contributes to the skin's ability to regulate body temperature by providing insulation against heat loss.

Accessory Structures

Hair and **nails** are epidermally derived structures that consist primarily of the protein keratin. Nails are flattened, corneous (hornlike) structures on the dorsal surface of the tips of fingers and toes in primates, structurally similar to the claws and hooves of other vertebrates. Hairs are shafts of keratin produced in the dermis within hair follicles, pockets of epithelial cells surrounded by a connective tissue sheath. Hair growth proceeds from the base of the follicle toward the surface.

A small, smooth muscle called the arrector pili attaches to the base of each hair. Sympathetic nervous system stimulation of the arrector pili causes the muscle to contract and raise the hair in response to cold temperature or strong emotion, increasing the thermal boundary layer and causing goosebumps. Hair follicles are usually associated with an oil-producing sebaceous gland.

Two classes of exocrine glands are found in the dermis. **Sebaceous glands** found in association with hair follicles secrete **sebum**, a waxy substance containing lipids, antibacterial compounds, and cellular debris. Sebum coats, protects, and lubricates the skin.

Sudoriferous glands, or **sweat glands**, secrete sweat, which is a solution of water, salt, and urea. Sweat glands originate in the dermis and carry their secretions through ducts that penetrate the epidermis. Sweat cools the body by evaporation. Excessive sweating can cause dehydration and electrolyte imbalance. Specialized sweat glands in the skin of the armpits, nipples, and genital region secrete fats and proteins as well as sweat to nourish the bacteria responsible for body odor. The activity of sweat glands is under the control of the sympathetic nervous system.

SPECIFIC FUNCTIONS OF THE SKIN

Physical Protection

The tough keratinized outer layer of the skin protects against abrasion and provides a barrier against infection by disease organisms. Melanocytes in the epidermis protect the body against ultraviolet radiation. The relative impermeability of the skin protects against water loss.

Thermoregulation

The skin assists in the regulation of body temperature through vasoconstriction or vasodilation of capillary networks in the dermis, a process under the control of the sympathetic nervous system. Blood may be shunted toward or away from cutaneous blood vessels to regulate radiant heat loss. In addition, the production of sweat results in evaporative cooling. The subcutaneous fat layer of the hypodermis provides thermal insulation, as does the erection of hair on the surface to create a thermal boundary layer.

Osmoregulation and Excretion

Sweating results in the excretion of water and salt, allowing the skin to regulate water and ion balance. The skin also aids in waste removal by excreting urea, drug residues, and metabolites.

Sensory Reception

Sensory reception is a primary function of the skin. In addition to tactile cells (the touch receptors at the boundary between the dermis and epidermis), the skin also contains temperature, pain, and touch receptors (**Meissner's corpuscles**) in the dermis. **Pacinian corpuscles** in the lower dermis act as pressure receptors. Hairs can also participate in sensory reception because of free nerve endings associated with the hair follicle.

Vitamin D Synthesis

Upon exposure to UVB radiation, the skin synthesizes vitamin D precursors from a form of cholesterol. These precursors are converted to vitamin D by the liver, kidneys, and macrophages of the immune system. Vitamin D is necessary for bone growth and calcium metabolism. It also contributes to immune function.

Reproductive System

Reproduction of humans and other terrestrial vertebrates occurs via **internal fertilization**. Both males and females have **external** and **internal genitalia**, structures designed for the transmission of sperm from the male to an ovum located in reproductive organs inside the female. Internal genitalia include the **gonads**, reproductive and endocrine organs responsible for the production of gametes and sex hormones. In males, the gonads are **testes**. In females, they are **ovaries**. Male and female gonads and genitalia are homologous structures that have the same embryonic origin.

Germ cells within the gonads undergo meiosis to produce gametes for sexual reproduction. (See "Meiosis and Genetic Variability," beginning on page 404.) Germ cells differ from somatic cells in that they are the only cells in the body capable of undergoing meiosis as well as mitosis. The process of meiosis in males is termed **spermatogenesis** because it results in the production of **spermatozoa**, or sperm, which are the male gametes. In females, meiosis is **oogenesis**. It results in the production of **ova**, or female gametes. Ova are much larger than sperm. They contribute cytoplasm, mitochondria, and other organelles to the resulting embryo. Meiosis is discussed in greater detail in the section "Meiosis and Genetic Variability."

MALE REPRODUCTIVE SYSTEM

The male reproductive system is composed of external genitalia, gonads, accessory glands, and a system of ducts that convey sperm out of the body (see Figure 3.101). The male genital, or **penis**, is the copulatory organ responsible for transmitting sperm to the female during

sexual intercourse. The penis is an external organ located in the pelvic region. During sexual arousal, the penis becomes erect as a result of increased blood flow to specialized tissues located within the shaft. The erect penis is inserted into the vagina of the female and ejaculates sperm into the female reproductive tract. Below the penis is the **scrotum**, an external pocket of skin that encloses the paired testes. Testes develop in the abdominal cavity but descend into the scrotum before birth. By remaining outside the body wall, the scrotum maintains a lower temperature necessary for sperm development. The penis and scrotum together constitute the male external genitalia.

Sperm originate in the coiled **seminiferous tubules** of the testes, where they are stimulated to develop by the androgen hormone **testosterone** at the onset of puberty. Testosterone is secreted in the testes by **Leydig cells** located between the seminiferous tubules. Other cells, **Sertoli cells**, act as nurse cells that nurture and protect the developing sperm.

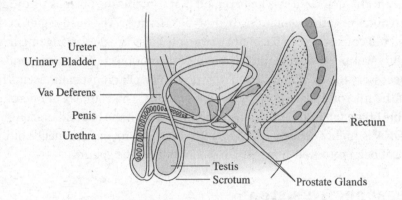

Figure 3.101. The male reproductive system

Sperm pass from the seminiferous tubules into the **epididymis**, an accessory structure of coiled ducts on the outside of the testis, where they mature and become motile. Sperm remain stored in the epididymis until ejaculation, when they are propelled by contraction of smooth muscle into the **vas deferens**, a muscular duct that travels into the abdominal cavity through the **inguinal canal** as part of the **spermatic cord**. The paired vasa deferentia from each testis travel around and below the bladder to join into a common **ejaculatory duct,** which travels into the **prostate gland** to merge with the **urethra**. In the process, sperm cells are mixed with seminal fluid and secretions from the **seminal vesicles**, prostate gland, and **bulbourethral glands** to form **semen**, the ejaculatory fluid. Semen contains alkaline secretions to neutralize the acidity of the female reproductive tract. It also contains sugars, enzymes, prostaglandins, and nutrients to nourish, activate, and protect the sperm. Semen exits the body through the urethra, which forms a common outlet for both the reproductive and urinary tracts.

Spermatogenesis

The male germ cells of the testes are called **spermatogonia**. They are located in the outer margin of the seminiferous tubules. These germ cells divide continuously by mitosis, replicating as new spermatogonia until adolescence. At adolescence, stimulation of the testes by the pituitary gonadotropins FSH and LH increases the activity of testosterone, leading spermatogonia to differentiate mitotically into **primary spermatocytes**. Primary spermatocytes move through support cells toward the lumen of the tubule and undergo meiosis I to form haploid **secondary spermatocytes**. Each of these then undergoes meiosis II to form four **spermatids**. Spermatids are subsequently modified into **spermatozoa** (sperm) before being released into the lumen of the seminiferous tubule for export to the epididymis. Sperm production is continuous from puberty through old age. Millions of sperm are released during each ejaculation, and new sperm are constantly being formed.

Sperm Morphology

Spermatozoa are characterized by a **head region** that contains the nucleus surrounded by the **acrosome**, an outer covering containing hydrolytic enzymes. The head region connects to a **midpiece** and **tail** consisting of a flagellum of microtubules in a 9+2 arrangement, with mitochondria tightly wound about the microtubules of the midpiece. The mitochondria provide the energy necessary for the propulsion of the sperm. Flagellar movement occurs by the sliding action of the microtubules linked by dynein proteins. The complex of microtubules and motor proteins of the tail is also called the **axoneme**. Within the haploid nucleus of the head region, the DNA is highly condensed. Most of the cytoplasm and organelles of the original spermatid have been removed to maximize the motility of the sperm.

FEMALE REPRODUCTIVE SYSTEM

The female reproductive system must not only function in gamete production but must also provide a suitable environment for fertilization and fetal development. The female external genitalia consists of the **vulva**. It is located in the **perineum**, the superficial region of the pelvic floor between the anus and the pubic symphysis. The vulva includes the **mons pubis**, the **clitoris**, the **labia majora**, and the **labia minora**. The mons pubis is a rounded region of fatty deposits that supports the growth of pubic hair beginning in puberty. The clitoris is a projection of erectile tissue homologous to the penis in the male. It is located just anterior to the external opening of the urethra, which in females is not part of the reproductive tract. The labia are folds of skin and adipose tissue that enclose the clitoris, urethra, and the opening to the **vagina**, or birth canal. The vagina receives the penis during sexual intercourse and acts as a passageway for sperm, for menstrual fluid, and for an infant during delivery.

As shown in Figure 3.102, the vagina terminates within the pelvic cavity at the **cervix**, the constricted opening of the **uterus**. The uterus is a thick-walled, elastic pouch of smooth muscle that functions to nourish and protect a developing fetus. The uterus also undergoes strong muscular contractions to propel an infant through the birth canal during childbirth. The lining of the uterus, or **endometrium**, responds to hormonal control. It becomes thickened and vascularized each month in preparation for the implantation of a fertilized ovum. In the absence of fertilization, the endometrium is shed via the process of **menstruation**.

Ova begin forming in the paired ovaries, which are located on either side of the uterus. The ovaries communicate with the uterus via the **fallopian tubes** (**oviducts** or **uterine tubes**). An immature oocyte released from the ovary is swept off the surface of the ovary by fingerlike projections (**fimbriae**) of the fallopian tube. The immature oocyte is then conveyed toward the lumen of the uterus by the movement of cilia and the contraction of smooth muscle.

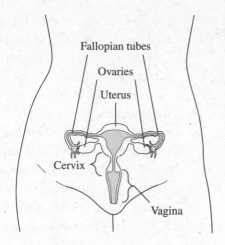

Figure 3.102. The female reproductive system

Fertilization typically occurs within the fallopian tubes. After several days, the embryo implants in the endometrium of the uterus. After implantation, the embryo undergoes development and is nourished by the **placenta**, a highly vascularized structure formed by the union of maternal and fetal tissues and blood supply.

Oogenesis and the Reproductive Cycle

The **oogonia**, or female germ cells, undergo the first stages of meiosis while a female infant is still in the mother's uterus. However, daughter cells remain arrested in prophase I as **primary oocytes**. A human female is born with more than 1 million primary oocytes, of which 250,000 may remain by the onset of puberty. Fewer than 500 will be released as functional gametes during a woman's reproductive lifetime of approximately 40 years.

> ### ECTOPIC PREGNANCY
>
> An **ectopic pregnancy** occurs when an embryo develops outside of the uterus. Ectopic pregnancies may occur if an embryo implants within the fallopian tube or in the abdominal cavity. Ectopic pregnancies cannot be sustained due to the inability of the fallopian tube or body cavity to nourish and contain a developing fetus. The resulting miscarriage can result in hemorrhage.

Oocytes are located in the outer cortex of the ovary in small, pouchlike **ovarian follicles**. Each month starting at puberty, several follicles at a time are stimulated by FSH and LH to begin the **ovarian cycle** and resume **oogenesis**. Of these, only one will become a **mature follicle** and release a functional gamete during the process of **ovulation**.

In contrast to spermatogenesis, the cytoplasmic divisions in oogenesis are unequal. The daughter cells produced by the two divisions of meiosis are three small **polar bodies** and only one gamete, a **secondary oocyte** that is arrested at metaphase II. As a result, the female gamete is much larger than the male and contributes virtually all of the cytoplasm and organelles to the embryo. Oogenesis also differs from spermatogenesis in that typically only one viable ovum is produced per month between puberty and menopause. A woman produces far fewer gametes over her reproductive lifetime than a man, but the energy invested in each gamete is much greater.

In the ovary, the developing follicle enlarges and produces the estrogen **estradiol**. In high concentrations, estradiol stimulates the anterior pituitary to produce a rapid increase in LH via positive feedback, triggering ovulation, which is the rupture of the mature follicle and the release of a secondary oocyte for fertilization. Ovulation occurs approximately 14 days after the onset of the ovarian cycle. Only if the oocyte is fertilized by a sperm will the egg complete meiosis II.

After ovulation, the ruptured follicle becomes a **corpus luteum** (yellow body). It secretes **progesterone** and some estrogen, stimulating the growth of uterine lining (**endometrium**) in preparation for implantation of a fertilized embryo as part of the **uterine** or **menstrual cycle**. Progesterone and estradiol also inhibit the production of FSH and LH. If the oocyte is not fertilized, the corpus luteum degenerates, progesterone levels fall, and **menstruation** ensues. Menstruation is the shedding of the uterine endometrium. The resulting increase in FSH and LH initates a new ovarian and menstrual cycle. A complete reproductive cycle lasts approximately 28 days.

Hormonal Regulation

The monthly cycle of ovulation and menstruation is under the control of regulatory hormones produced by the brain and the ovaries. At the beginning of the cycle, the hypothalamus secretes gonadotropin releasing hormone (GnRH) to trigger the anterior pituitary to release luteinizing hormone (LH) and follicle stimulating hormone (FSH). These gonadotropin hormones promote development of a mature follicle and ovulation. At the same time, gonadotropins stimulate the ovaries to produce the steroid hormones estradiol and progesterone, which thicken the uterine lining in preparation for implantation. High levels of estradiol and progesterone produced by the ovaries inhibit gonadotropin secretion, causing FSH and LH levels to drop, preventing maturation of additional follicles. In the absence of fertilization, the degeneration of the corpus luteum in the ovary causes estradiol levels to drop, triggering menstruation. Low levels of estradiol remove inhibition on gonadotropin secretion by the pituitary, and the ovulatory cycle begins again (see Figure 3.103).

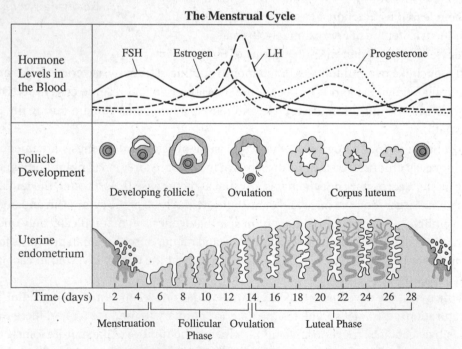

The Menstrual Cycle

Figure 3.103. The female reproductive cycle

FERTILIZATION, IMPLANTATION, AND DEVELOPMENT

Sperm can survive for up to 5 days in the female reproductive tract. However, the secondary oocyte is viable for only 12–24 hours after ovulation. During sexual intercourse, tens of millions of sperm are transferred to the female reproductive tract. Only a few of these will survive the journey through the acid uterine environment and arrive at the correct location within one of the fallopian tubes.

In order to fertilize an oocyte, sperm must first undergo a process called **capacitation**, which may take several hours. Capacitation involves the weakening of the acrosomal membrane (around the head of the sperm) through interaction with uterine secretions to allow the release of hydrolytic enzymes that enable the sperm to penetrate the outer layers of the ovulated secondary oocyte. These layers include the corona radiata and the zona pellucida. The outer **corona radiata** is composed of follicular cells. The **zona pellucida** is a clear extracellular matrix of glycoprotein. It contains a receptor that binds to the head of the sperm and initiates the release of acrosomal enzymes.

The enzymes secreted by many different sperm break down the zona pellucida, finally exposing the plasma membrane of the secondary oocyte. The first sperm to penetrate the zona pellucida binds to sperm receptors on the surface of the plasma membrane. The sperm and oocyte membranes fuse, and the sperm head and the flagellum are incorporated into the oocyte. The entry of the sperm into the oocyte triggers the release of Ca^{2+} ions from the endoplasmic reticulum. This initiates a signal transduction pathway that triggers the **cortical reaction**: cortical granules secrete enzymes by exocytosis into the zona pellucida to prevent the entry of additional sperm. The release of calcium ions also activates the egg to begin embryonic development.

Fertilization

Once the sperm nucleus has penetrated the plasma membrane, the oocyte nucleus completes meiosis II to form two daughter cells. One is a nonfunctional polar body. The other is the functional **ovum**, or completed haploid daughter cell. Fertilization does not technically occur until the chromosomes of the sperm and ovum combine. At this point, the fertilized ovum becomes a diploid **zygote**, which immediately undergoes DNA replication to prepare for mitosis and embryonic development.

FRATERNAL VERSUS IDENTICAL TWINS

If more than one oocyte is released at ovulation, both oocytes can be fertilized by separate sperm and result in **fraternal twins**. Fraternal twins are genetically equivalent to full siblings born separately and are not identical. Fertility drugs can stimulate the maturation of more than one ovarian follicle at a time and lead to the release of multiple oocytes, resulting in fraternal twins and similar **multiple births**.

Identical twins are the result of a single fertilized ovum that divides into two embryos. The resulting twins share identical DNA since they originated from the same cell.

Implantation

The zygote completes its first cell division within 36 hours. It continues to divide as it travels down the fallopian tube, reaching the **blastocyst** stage of development by the time it arrives in the uterus. Approximately 6 or 7 days after ovulation, the blastocyst undergoes **implantation** into the wall of the endometrium, where it erodes uterine capillaries and becomes surrounded and nourished by the maternal blood supply. If implantation is successful, the blastocyst secretes **human chorionic gonadotropin (hCG)**. This hormone stimulates the corpus luteum to continue to produce progesterone and estrogen to maintain the uterine lining and prevent menstruation and ovulation.

DETECTING PREGNANCY

Pregnancy tests can detect the presence of hCG secreted by the developing embryo in maternal blood or urine as early as one week after fertilization.

Placentation

In the beginning of pregnancy, fetal and maternal blood vessels and membranes intertwine to form an organ called the **placenta**. Extensions of fetal extraembryonic membrane called **chorionic villi** interact with blood vessels in the endometrium to form a placental disk of tissue and blood vessels attached to the uterine wall. Another fetal membrane, the **allantois**, forms the **umbilical cord**, which connects the embryo to the placenta. Although the maternal and fetal blood supplies have no direct contact, the placenta allows for the transfer of nutrients and oxygen from the mother and for the removal of nitrogenous waste and carbon dioxide from the fetus. Maternal antibodies are also capable of crossing the placental barrier.

The placenta is fully developed by the end of the first three months of pregnancy. As the placenta is developing, it takes over the function of secreting progesterone and estrogen from the corpus luteum, which degenerates as hCG levels drop. Increasing levels of progesterone and estrogen maintain the pregnancy and stimulate development of mammary glands for milk production (**lactation**).

Development and Birth

The average duration of a normal human pregnancy is 9 months, or 40 weeks from the first day of a woman's last menstrual period, divided into 3 trimesters of 3 months each. During the first 9 weeks, the **zygote** undergoes development from a single cell to a multicellular **embryo** with developing limbs and organ systems. After 9 weeks, the embryo becomes a **fetus**. A fetus born before 37 weeks is considered preterm and is less likely to survive. Birth is preceded by the onset of **labor**, or uterine contractions that dilate the cervix to allow for the passage of the baby. The baby is delivered through the vagina (birth canal). A newborn infant remains attached via the umbilical cord to the placenta. During the last stage of labor, the placenta separates from the uterine wall and is delivered separately.

DEVELOPMENTAL BIOLOGY

After fertilization, the development of a fertilized ovum into an embryo is **embryogenesis**. Embryogenesis involves mitotic cell division and cellular differentiation.

Embryogenesis

Embryogenesis, or **morphogenesis**, involves several steps. These are cleavage, blastula formation, gastrulation, neurulation, and organogenesis.

CLEAVAGE AND BLASTULA FORMATION

Immediately following fertilization, the zygote begins preparations to divide by mitosis, a process known as **cleavage**. The dividing cells spend very little time in the G1 and G2 stages of interphase, progressing rapidly through each S phase to the next phase of mitosis. Little cell growth occurs between divisions. The zygote divides into progressively smaller cells called **blastomeres**. By the 16–32 cell stage, the embryo has become a **morula**, a solid ball of blastomeres; see Figure 3.104. After approximately 7 cell divisions, the cells undergo **compaction**. The blastomeres flatten and adhere closely via tight junctions and gap junctions between cells. Compaction results in the formation of the **blastula**, a hollow ball of more than 100 cells surrounding a fluid-filled cavity called the **blastocoel**. The process of blastula formation is **blastulation**.

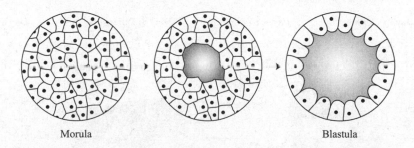

Morula   Blastula

Figure 3.104. Blastulation

Meroblastic versus Holoblastic Cleavage

In certain species that provide **yolk** to nourish the embryo, cleavage is **meroblastic,** or incomplete. It results in unequal distribution of yolk toward the **vegetal pole** of the developing embryo. The opposite **animal pole** contains the blastocoel and the rapidly dividing blastomeres, which will continue to form the embryo. In mammals, cleavage is complete or **holoblastic**, resulting in an embryo that divides symmetrically during cleavage.

Blastocyst Formation in Mammals

In mammals, compaction results in the formation of a **blastocyst**, which is analogous to the blastula in other species. The blastocyst consists of an outer layer of cells called the **trophoblast**, a fluid-filled **blastocyst cavity**, and an **inner cell mass**. The inner cell mass, located at the **embryonic pole**, will develop into the embryo proper and extraembryonic membranes.

    The inner cell mass divides into two layers, the **hypoblast** and **epiblast**. They form a pear-shaped, bilaminar **embryonic disk**. The hypoblast cells are located on the surface of the inner cell mass facing the blastocoel or blastomeric cavity. Expansion of hypoblast around the cavity transforms the blastocoel into the **yolk sac**, or **umbilical cavity**. Adjacent epiblast cells lie between the hypoblast and the trophoblast. Development of a fluid-filled space between the trophoblast and the epiblast forms the incipient **amniotic cavity,** which will enclose and cushion the embryo. Figure 3.105 shows the various stages of human embryogenesis.

The trophoblast also divides, forming an outer **syncytioblast** and an inner **cytotrophoblast**. The syncytioblast is a multinucleate syncitium that functions to invade the uterine lining during implantation, secreting enzymes that erode maternal capillaries and causing the embryo to be bathed in maternal blood. Both the syncytioblast and the cytotrophoblast, combined with **extraembryonic mesoderm** derived from the epiblast, form the **chorioic villi** of the **chorion**. The chorion combines with maternal tissues and blood vessels to form the **placenta**.

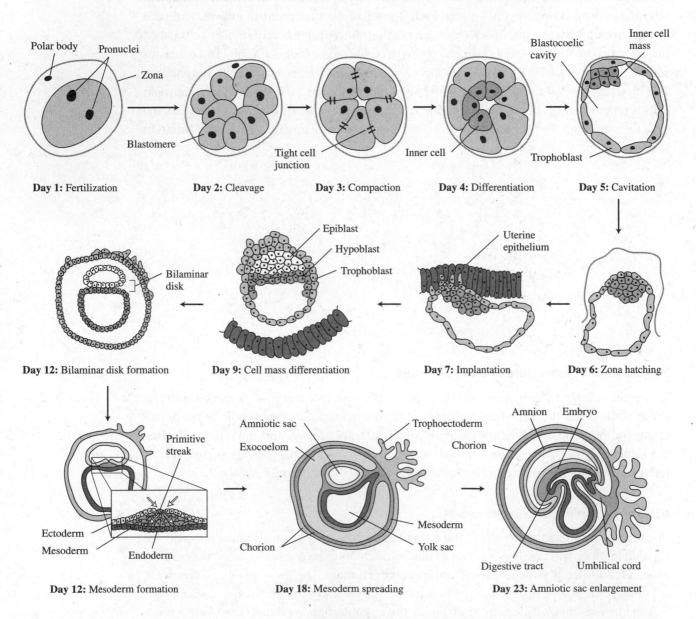

Figure 3.105. Human embryogenesis

GASTRULATION

Gastrulation is the process in which the three primary **germ layers** are formed—the **ectoderm**, **mesoderm**, and **endoderm**—along with an **archenteron**, or primitive digestive tract. The process of **gastrulation** varies among organisms. However, it generally involves some of the cells from the outer layer (ectoderm) of the blastula folding in to create a new layer as shown in Figure 3.106. A blastula that has undergone gastrulation is called a **gastrula**.

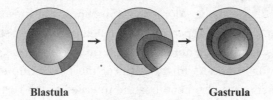

Blastula   Gastrula

Figure 3.106. Gastrulation

Cell movements are made possible by a loss of cell-cell adhesion in the outer layers of the embryo, allowing cells or cell layers to slide past one another. During gastrulation, the archenteron forms when the outer layer of the embryo invaginates at the **blastopore** and pushes inward toward the blastocoel. Ultimately, this pocket will displace the blastocoel and form the gut, a hollow digestive tube lined by endoderm that extends through the embryo. The outer layer of the gastrula becomes the ectoderm. The mesoderm forms a middle layer from individual migratory **mesenchyme cells** that move throughout the embryo.

During gastrulation in mammals and birds, epiblast cells move toward the posterior center line of the embryonic disk. They form a thickened line called the **primitive streak**, creating the anterior/posterior axis of the embryo and resulting in bilateral symmetry. Cells along the primitive streak **ingress** or push inward and downward toward the hypoblast, forming a **primitive groove** equivalent to the blastopore. Cells reaching the bottom layer of the primitive groove displace hypoblast cells and become the endoderm, which will surround the developing gut. Cells remaining on the surface become the ectoderm. A third layer of epiblast cells move laterally between the other two layers to form the mesoderm. Some of these mesodermal cells become mesenchymal (stem cells). Although hypoblast cells do not contribute to the embryo, they aid in determining the location of the primitive streak and form part of the yolk sac or umbilical cord.

NEURULATION AND ORGANOGENESIS

In vertebrates and other chordates, the first step of **organogenesis**, or organ development, is the formation of the **notochord**. This is a rigid rod derived from dorsal mesoderm that forms above the archenteron or below the primitive groove along the longitudinal axis of the embryo. Once the notochord is formed, **neurulation** begins. Neurulation is development of the **neural tube**, which becomes the central nervous system.

During neurulation, cell-signaling interactions between the mesoderm of the notochord and overlying ectoderm induce the ectoderm to thicken and form the **neural plate**. This neural plate then folds upward and inward along each side to form **neural folds** down the midline of the embryo. The neural folds close together from anterior to posterior to form a hollow neural tube, which will become the **dorsal hollow nerve cord**, which lies dorsal to the notochord. An anterior enlargement of the nerve cord becomes the brain, and the posterior extension becomes the spinal cord.

In vertebrates, the formation of the neural tube is accompanied by the pinching off or delamination of **neural crest cells** from the ectoderm of the neural tube as part of an **epithelial** to **mesenchyme transition**. Neural crest cells migrate throughout the body and become a variety of structures, including portions of the jaw, teeth, ear ossicles, heart valves, and nervous system.

Along the notochord, the mesoderm condenses into repeated, segmented units called **somites**. Mesenchymal cells from the somites surround the notochord to form the vertebrae, which largely replace the notochord except for remnants in the form of the cartilaginous intervertebral disks. Mesenchyme from the somites also becomes the muscles of the vertebral column and rib cage. On either side of the vertebral column, the **coelom**, or body cavity, forms within lateral mesoderm. In vertebrates, the coelom will become the **ventral body cavity**, which houses the heart, lungs, and abdominal viscera. See Figure 3.107.

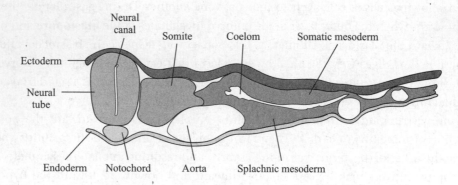

Figure 3.107. Cross section of vertebrate embryo after neurulation, showing germ layers, neural tube, notochord, somites, and coelom

MAJOR STRUCTURES FROM PRIMARY GERM LAYERS

The germ layers ultimately differentiate into tissues and organs of the adult as shown in Figure 3.108 and Table 3.18.

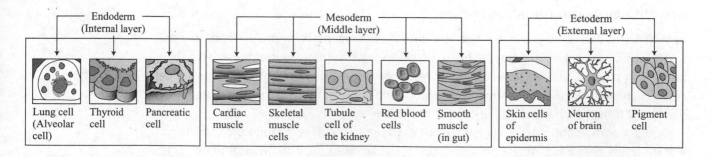

Figure 3.108. Major structures derived from the primary germ layers

Table 3.18 Embryologic Origin of Major Body Tissues and Organs

Ectoderm (Outer Layer)	Mesoderm (Body cavity)	Endoderm (Lining of Archenteron)
Integumentary system and mucous membranes: Outer epithelial layer of skin, mouth, pharynx, and anus	Muscular system: Skeletal, cardiac, and smooth muscle	Respiratory system: Epithelial lining of trachea, bronchi, alveoli
Epithelial-derived structures: Hair follicles, sweat and mammary glands, cornea and lens of eye	Bones and connective tissue: Cartilage, tendons, ligaments, loose connective tissue, the dermis of the skin, blood	Digestive system: Epithelial lining of esophagus, stomach, intestines

Associated digestive and endocrine glands: Liver, pancreas; lining of thymus, thyroid, and parathyroid |
Nervous system: Brain, spinal cord, peripheral nerves and ganglia, epidermal sensory receptors, pineal and pituitary glands	Circulatory, lymphatic, reproductive, and urinary systems: Blood vessels, spleen, reproductive organs, kidneys, smooth muscle of bladder	Epithelial lining of urethra, bladder, and reproductive systems
Adrenal medulla	Adrenal cortex	
Neural crest cells: Ectodermally derived stem cells		

Developmental Mechanisms

In multicellular organisms, cell specialization occurs as a single-celled zygote divides to become an intricate system of diverse cell types and cooperative tissues. The zygote begins as **totipotent**. In other words, it is able to differentiate to become any cell type. As the zygote begins cleavage, the embryonic cells lose their totipotency after the 16-cell stage. The inner cell mass can no longer form extraembryonic membranes. These cells are now **pluripotent**, which means they are able to develop into any of the three germ layer tissues. Cells that are pluripotent are also known as **stem cells**.

As embryonic cells continue mitosis, they eventually reach a **determined** state, after which their fate cannot be changed even if the cells are transplanted or provided with appropriate signals. **Differentiation** is the process by which cells continue to develop toward their ultimate cell type. Differentiation determines the

REGENERATIVE CAPACITY OF STEM CELLS

Stem cells can exist in both embryonic and adult tissues. Some organisms, such as salamanders, earthworms, planaria, and some lizards, have the ability to regrow body parts after loss or damage. The ability to activate stem cells to regenerate tissues in adult organisms is an area of active biomedical research.

cell's size, metabolic activity, morphology, membrane potential, and responsiveness to signals. As cells differentiate, their DNA does not change. Instead, genes are turned on and off in a specific developmental sequence as regulatory genes alter gene expression and protein synthesis. Gene expression is primarily mediated by **cell-to-cell communication** (**cell signaling**).

In cell-to-cell communication, the various cells of the developing organism influence each other. Ligands from one cell may bind with receptors on another cell, thus conveying information that will determine how genes are expressed in the second cell. The process of one cell influencing the developmental fate of other cells is called **induction**.

Apoptosis, or programmed cell death, is also a developmental mechanism. The classic example is the programmed death of cells between the fingers and toes in the developing human embryo, allowing the digits to separate.

Senescence and Aging

Cellular senescence is the cessation of mitotic division accompanied by phenotypic changes related to gene expression. Senescent cells can remain metabolically active. Senescence occurs during embryonic development and in response to various stressors. Recent evidence suggests it also plays a role in tissue repair, wound healing, tumor suppression, and organismal aging. **Organismal senescence**, or **aging**, is the senescence of the entire organism, characterized by a progressive decline in physiological function and increased susceptibility to degenerative diseases. Aging is a complex process modulated by genetic as well as environmental factors. The process of aging can differ among individuals and among different types of organisms. Ultimately, aging leads to death through failure of the body's homeostatic mechanisms. The biology of aging is an area of active research.

TEST QUESTION

During development of the gastrointestinal tract, endoderm develops into the epithelial lining and mesoderm develops into smooth muscle. In the absence of mesoderm, the epithelial lining will fail to form. The relationship between endoderm and mesoderm during organ development is an example of:

(A) differentiation.

(B) induction.

(C) pluripotency.

(D) gastrulation.

(B) Induction occurs because the mesodermal cells influence the developmental fate of the ectodermal cells through cell-to-cell signaling.

Answer A is incorrect because differentiation refers to the process of cell specialization, whereas induction and cell signaling are the mechanisms that lead to differentiation. In the absence of induction, no differentiation will occur. Answer C is incorrect because pluripotency refers to the ability of cells to remain unspecialized and to retain the ability to differentiate into any of the three germ layers. In this case, both mesoderm and ectoderm are undergoing differentiation and, therefore, loss of pluripotency. Answer D is incorrect because gastrulation refers to the development of the germ layers in the embryonic gastrula before organogenesis. However, induction is also important during gastrulation.

SUMMARY

Biology constitutes the largest part of the MCAT. Carefully review the topics in this chapter. You should understand cell biology and the differences between eukaryotic and prokaryotic cells. Review metabolic reactions of cells with a particular focus on the role of enzymes. In the area of microbiology, review fungi, bacteria, and viruses. Be sure to understand DNA and protein synthesis. You will need to know the structure and function of DNA and RNA, the mechanism of DNA replication, and the transcription and translation of DNA and RNA into protein. Be familiar with the mechanisms of generating recombinant DNA and understand its uses.

Eukaryotic cell replication is an important topic on the MCAT. Be familiar with the cell cycle, mitosis, and cytokinesis, including the role of apoptosis and the relationship of the cell cycle to cancer. Review meiosis and the concept of genetic variability, including sexual and asexual reproduction and chromosomal mutations. It is important that you understand the fundamental concepts of genetics, including Mendelian and sex-linked crosses and pedigree analysis. Review population genetics and the Hardy-Weinberg equilibrium. Be sure you are clear on the concepts of evolution, including the role of random variation, nonrandom natural selection, and geographic isolation in the generation of new species.

The MCAT tests all aspects of human anatomy and physiology. Review specialized eukaryotic cells and tissues and then move on to the specific systems of the body. Be sure to review the nervous and endocrine systems, the circulatory, lymphatic, and immune systems, the digestive system, the excretory system, the skeletal and muscle systems, the respiratory system, the skin (integumentary) system, and the reproductive system. Finally, make sure you understand the developmental mechanisms of developmental biology.

It is helpful to go through the biology review chapter several times in full. You should also examine any questions that you miss in your practice tests and then use the chapter to review the concepts that caused you to miss the question.

> **DIRECTIONS:** This Biology test contains four passages. Each passage is followed by a series of questions. Read the passage, and then choose the one answer that is best. Some questions are not based on a passage or each other. If you are not sure of an answer, eliminate the answer choices that you think are wrong and choose one of the remaining answers.

PASSAGE I

Anaphylaxis is an acute, life-threatening allergic reaction affecting multiple organ systems. Rapid onset of an anaphylactic reaction can occur as a result of exposure to insect stings, medications such as penicillin, and dietary allergens such as nuts and shellfish. Anaphylaxis results in a systemic inflammatory response of connective tissue and mucous membranes. In susceptible individuals, an initial exposure to a potential antigen sensitizes B lymphocytes, resulting in the production of IgE antibodies. For B cells to produce IgE instead of other classes of immunoglobulins, B cells must interact with CD4$^+$ T helper cells that have been activated by exposure to antigen-presenting cells to secrete the cytokine interleukin-4 (IL-4). Large numbers of IgE antibodies bind to Fc receptors on mast cells and basophils.

On subsequent exposure, binding of multiple antigens to antigen-specific IgE causes cross-linking of Fc receptors. This triggers a signal cascade that results in degranulation and release of histamine and other inflammatory mediators, including leukotrienes, fatty molecules that make up the slow-reacting substance of anaphylaxis (SRS-A). Histamine causes vasodilation of postcapillary venules. It also increases the permeability of blood vessels, allowing fluid and leukocytes to leak into tissues. Leukotrienes in SRS-A are potent smooth muscle contractors that cause prolonged bronchoconstriction.

In a severe anaphylactic reaction, vasodilation, loss of blood volume, and bronchoconstriction can result in lowered blood pressure, shock, and death by cardiovascular collapse and asphyxiation. The treatment for anaphylaxis is intramuscular injection of epinephrine, which activates the fight-or-flight response to increase heart rate, constrict blood vessels, and dilate bronchi. In addition, antihistamines, bronchodilators, and IV fluids may be administered.

1. Mast cells and basophils are triggered to release histamine by binding of:
    (A) IgE to Fc receptors.
    (B) cytokine to B lymphocytes.
    (C) antigen to IgE-Fc receptor complexes.
    (D) antigen to B lymphocytes.

2. According to the passage, which of the following contribute to asphyxiation due to anaphylaxis?
    (A) Vasodilation of pulmonary venules, leading to decreased blood pO_2
    (B) Excessive fluid in pulmonary capillaries, leading to decreased alveolar pO_2
    (C) Smooth muscle constriction in alveoli, leading to decreased alveolar pO_2
    (D) Smooth muscle constriction in bronchioles, leading to decreased blood pO_2

3. Basophils are found in:
    (A) pulmonary capillaries.
    (B) pulmonary epithelia.
    (C) loose connective tissue of the dermis.
    (D) microvascular endothelium.

4. Epinephrine is a hormone that activates:
    (A) cholinergic receptors of the parasympathetic nervous system.
    (B) cholinergic receptors of the sympathetic nervous system.
    (C) adrenergic receptors of the parasympathetic nervous system.
    (D) adrenergic receptors of the sympathetic nervous system.

5. All of the following would correctly explain why an initial exposure to a potential antigen would NOT be likely to result in a future anaphylaxis EXCEPT:
    (A) an absence of Fc receptors.
    (B) failure of CD4$^+$ T helper cells to activate IL-4.
    (C) failure of CD4$^+$ T helper cells to interact with B lymphocytes.
    (D) failure of B lymphocytes to interact with cells that have been exposed to antigen-presenting cells.

PASSAGE II

Bacteria may be classified phenotypically as either gram-positive or gram-negative based on the color that they turn when Gram's stain is applied. A few bacteria are gram-indeterminate. These do not respond to Gram's stain. These categories of gram-positive and gram-negative correspond to certain physical and chemical differences in the cell walls of the bacteria. Gram-positive bacteria include *Staphylococcus, Streptococcus, Clostridium,* and *Listeria.* Gram-negative bacteria include *Neisseria, Campylobacter,* and *Francisella.*

Both gram-negative and gram-positive bacteria may occur in various shapes, which are often reflected in their nomenclature. *Staphylococcus,* for example, have the round or dotlike shape signified by the ending *-coccus* (plural *-cocci*).

The genus *Clostridium,* which consists of obligate anaerobes, includes *C. botulinum, C. perfringens, C. tetanus,* and *C. difficile.* These bacteria are responsible for botulism, gas gangrene, tetanus, and pseudomembranous colitis, respectively. Spore-forming bacteria such as *Clostridium* form spores in order to maintain viability and remain protected in unfavorable environments. Once conditions are more favorable, the spores germinate into the active, disease-causing bacteria.

C. botulinum produces the botulinum toxin. The toxin causes paralysis of affected muscles, typically the respiratory muscles. Botulism is most commonly caused by eating improperly canned or preserved food. Children less than 1 year of age are particularly susceptible to botulism infection when fed raw honey, possibly because they lack sufficient intestinal flora to competitively inhibit *C. botulinum* in the small intestine and possibly because their stomach acid is not as strong as that of adults.

6. Tetanus bacteria are bacilli. It can be concluded that tetanus bacteria are:
   - (A) rod-shaped and turn dark blue/violet when the Gram stain is applied.
   - (B) round and turn pinkish red when the Gram stain is applied.
   - (C) rod-shaped and do not change color when the Gram stain is applied.
   - (D) round and turn blue-violet when the Gram stain is applied.

7. Which of the following best explains the main cause of botulism as it is stated in the passage?
   - (A) The botulism bacteria outcompete the beneficial bacteria in the small intestine.
   - (B) Canned food is typically low in oxygen.
   - (C) The respiratory muscles of infants are smaller and less developed than those of adults.
   - (D) Preserved and canned foods, if old, can become exposed to the air.

8. Assuming that the botulinum toxin acts at the neuromuscular junctions of muscles, which of the following would be consistent with the toxin's action?
   - (A) Stimulating the breakdown of acetylcholine
   - (B) Stimulating the release of norepinephrine
   - (C) Inhibiting the breakdown of norepinephrine
   - (D) Stimulating the release of acetylcholine

9. Botulinum toxin is one of the most potent toxins known. The word *potent* in this example most likely means that:
    (A) an infection by *C. botulinum* will be of long duration.
    (B) once the infection takes hold, the immune system is not able to overcome it.
    (C) a small amount of metabolic by-product of the bacteria can cause significant pathology.
    (D) toxins produced by the bacteria are difficult to destroy in the environment.

The following questions do not refer to a descriptive passage and are not related to each other.

10. Short interfering RNA (siRNA) is currently being tested as a novel biochemical therapeutic agent. After being introduced into cells, siRNA functions as a gene silencer, acting between the transcription and translation stage of protein production. Given this information, it is most likely that short interfering RNA:
    (A) stimulates the 7-methylguanosine capping of mRNA and its polyadenylation.
    (B) combines with tRNA and prevents it from incorporating amino acids.
    (C) combines with the coding strand of DNA and prevents its unwinding.
    (D) combines with mRNA and induces its breakdown.

11. Parthenogenesis is a form of reproduction in which females produce offspring without fertilization from a male. Parthenogenetic offspring may be produced by meiosis, followed by the fusion of gametes of a single female, a process called automixis. Automictic offspring would be:
    (A) diploid and genetically identical to mother and to each other.
    (B) diploid and genetically distinct from mother and from each other.
    (C) haploid and genetically identical to mother and to each other.
    (D) haploid and genetically distinct from mother and from each other.

12. The puncturing of the pleural cavity results in a condition called pneumothorax. This condition would result in collapse of the alveoli due to:
    (A) equalization of intrapleural pressure with intrapulmonary pressure.
    (B) equalization of intrapulmonary pressure with atmospheric pressure.
    (C) an intrapulmonary pressure greater than intrapleural pressure.
    (D) an intrapleural pressure less than atmospheric pressure.

PASSAGE III

Body mass index (BMI) is a statistical tool in current use to identify individuals at risk for weight-related health problems. Body mass index uses a person's height and weight to provide an estimate of total body fat, assuming an average body composition within a given population. The formula for calculating the body mass index is:

$$BMI = kg/m^2$$

Although body mass increases as the cube of linear dimensions, BMI is scaled to vary inversely with the square of height. Consequently, BMI is least accurate at height extremes.

In the United States, BMI statistics are based on a predominantly Caucasian population. A healthy adult BMI is considered to be in the range of 18–25. Individuals with a BMI below 18 are considered underweight. Individuals with BMI over 25 are considered overweight. Those with BMI over 30 are considered obese. Use of BMI to assess adiposity is widespread, despite the fact that it fails to account for variation in body fat percentage due to differences in bone density and muscle mass.

The prevalence of obesity as assessed by BMI has been increasing in the United States, particularly in children. Obesity is correlated with a number of health conditions. These include high blood pressure, high cholesterol level, insulin resistance and type 2 diabetes, heart disease, stroke, respiratory problems, gallbladder disease, and several forms of cancer.

13. In which of the following examples would BMI underestimate the percentage of body fat?

   I.   A long-distance runner
   II. An elderly person with osteoporosis
   III. A person of average height with short legs relative to torso length
   IV. An unusually tall person with long legs relative to torso length

   (A) I and III only
   (B) I and IV only
   (C) II and III only
   (D) II and IV only

14. If BMI accurately estimates body fat, a person with a BMI over 30 may exhibit:
   (A) high levels of high-density lipoprotein.
   (B) elevated blood glucose levels.
   (C) decreased cardiac output.
   (D) decreased vascular resistance.

15. Excess cholesterol is removed from blood by the:
   (A) pancreas.
   (B) spleen.
   (C) liver.
   (D) kidneys.

16. Gallbladder disease could potentially have what affect on an individual?
    (A) Insufficient lipid absorption by microvilli in the duodenum
    (B) Difficulty with carbohydrate digestion in the small intestine due to a deficiency of amylase
    (C) Buildup of uric acid in the blood
    (D) Inability of the liver to convert glycogen to glucose

17. An average value for normal blood pressure is considered to be 120/80. The number 120 mm Hg is the:
    (A) blood pressure in the pulmonary circuit.
    (B) pressure in the left ventricle prior to contraction.
    (C) arterial pressure when the heart is relaxed.
    (D) arterial pressure when the ventricles are contracting.

18. Compared with a person with average body fat, a person with a high percentage of body fat may have difficulty with thermoregulation because:
    (A) a high surface area to volume ratio leads to a higher percentage of superficial capillaries.
    (B) a low surface area to volume ratio leads to greater retention of body heat.
    (C) sweat glands do not penetrate adipose tissue.
    (D) a higher percentage of body fat results in a higher metabolic rate.

19. High blood pressure would initially affect the kidneys by:
    (A) increasing the volume of filtrate produced by the glomerulus.
    (B) decreasing the collection of water and solutes within Bowman's capsule.
    (C) decreasing the amount of water reabsorbed by the loop of Henle.
    (D) increasing the amount of filtrate secreted by peritubular capillaries.

The following questions do not refer to a descriptive passage and are not related to each other.

20. All of the following cells primarily function through exocytosis EXCEPT:
    (A) fibroblasts.
    (B) osteoblasts.
    (C) chondrocytes.
    (D) phagocytes.

21. Posttranslational modification in the eukaryotic cell may be carried out by which of the following?
    (A) Ribosome
    (B) Mitochondria
    (C) Endoplasmic reticulum
    (D) Nucleus

22. In the condition myasthenia gravis, antibodies to the acetylcholine receptor cause muscle weakness. Which of the following may represent a potential therapeutic agent?
    (A) A substance that inhibits release of acetylcholine
    (B) An acetylcholinesterase stimulator
    (C) An acetylcholinesterase inhibitor
    (D) A substance that stimulates receptor endocytosis

23. Which of the following represents the correct order of embryonic development starting from conception?
    (A) zygote → morula → gastrula → embryo → fetus
    (B) zygote → morula → gastrula → fetus → embryo
    (C) gamete → zygote → gastrula → embryo → fetus
    (D) zygote → gastrula → morula → embryo → fetus

PASSAGE IV

One of the most common lethal genetic diseases is cystic fibrosis, which is caused by a defect in the CFTR gene on chromosome 7. In healthy individuals, it encodes a transmembrane protein that facilitates ion transfer across cell membranes. The mutated gene product cannot effectively transport chloride ions into cells, leading to an increased extracellular concentration of chloride ions. Cystic fibrosis exhibits an autosomal recessive mode of inheritance.

One of the complications of cystic fibrosis is a malfunction of exocrine glands (such as the pancreas) because of the increased viscosity of mucus and other secretions that may block the ducts. The result is pancreatic insufficiency and malabsorption. A similar problem occurs in the sinorespiratory tract, causing breathing difficulties, lung collapse, and even pneumonia.

Other genetic conditions such as Huntington's chorea and myotonic dystrophy are caused by an increased number of trinucleotide repeats in certain genes. These repeats often increase in number in each human generation. As a result, more severe manifestations of the disease often occur at an earlier age, a phenomenon termed **anticipation**. Myotonic dystrophy is characterized by cataracts, testicular atrophy, baldness, and an inability for muscles to relax once they have contracted. Huntington's chorea is characterized by involuntary movements, incontinence, and muscle rigidity and is often fatal.

An example of a genetic disorder caused by a sex chromosome mutation is Turner syndrome. Most commonly, it is caused by a missing X chromosome, leading to an XO genotype. Affected individuals are phenotypically female. Common features include a short, webbed neck, nonfunctional ovaries, incomplete female genital development, and absence of menstruation.

24. Which of the following may be expected to show manifestations of cystic fibrosis?
    (A) Kidney stones from concentrated urine
    (B) Low blood flow from viscous blood
    (C) Sinus infections from viscous secretions
    (D) Joint immobility from viscous cartilage

25. Which of the following may represent a potential reason for the increased frequency of pneumonia seen in cystic fibrosis?
    (A) Obstruction and infection of airways
    (B) Immune dysfunction causing susceptibility to infections
    (C) Increasing antibiotic resistance of bacteria
    (D) Excess intracellular chloride

26. Which of the following could be used as a diagnostic test for cystic fibrosis?
    (A) Low mucus viscosity
    (B) Low sweat chloride
    (C) Low sweat sodium
    (D) Elevated tear chloride

27. From the information in the passage, what can be concluded regarding the inheritance patterns of cystic fibrosis?
    (A) Both genes of the homologous pair need to have a mutation for the disease phenotype to be expressed.
    (B) Only one gene of the homologous pair needs to have a mutation for the disease phenotype to be expressed.
    (C) The Y chromosome needs to be affected for the disease phenotype to be expressed.
    (D) The X chromosome needs to be affected for the disease phenotype to be expressed.

28. Which of the following is true about the phenomenon of anticipation over successive generations?
    (A) Earlier age of occurrence of genetic mutations
    (B) Greater ability to predict the disease
    (C) Longer waiting period before the disease manifests
    (D) More severe symptoms

29. Which of the following may describe a person with myotonic dystrophy?
    (A) A person with salty skin and repeated coughing
    (B) A person with stiff muscles and repeated arm movements
    (C) A female with short stature, a shieldlike chest, and a webbed neck
    (D) A person with the inability to release the grip after a handshake

30. Consider a case in which, during the fertilization of an ovum, the sperm lacks a Y chromosome as a result of chromosomal nondisjunction. The resulting individual would most likely exhibit Turner syndrome in which of the following ways?
    (A) The individual would have nonfunctioning testes and an underdeveloped penis.
    (B) The individual would have nonfunctioning testes and underdeveloped penis and might exhibit minimal breast growth.
    (C) The individual would have nonfunctioning ovaries and an underdeveloped penis.
    (D) The individual would have nonfunctioning ovaries and underdeveloped female genitalia.

The following questions do not refer to a descriptive passage and are not related to each other.

31. Leber's hereditary optic neuropathy (LHON) is an irreversible condition that causes early-onset blindness. It is inherited by mutations carried in mitochondrial DNA. Which of the following can be concluded about LHON?
    (A) An LHON patient's mother was also probably affected.
    (B) An LHON patient's father was also probably affected.
    (C) Only an LHON patient's sons will be affected.
    (D) Only an LHON patient's daughters will be affected.

32. A virus that uses DNA to encode genetic information is treated with a drug that blocks the enzyme reverse transcriptase. This drug will:
    (A) block transcription of viral DNA into host RNA.
    (B) block transcription of viral RNA into protein.
    (C) enhance transcription of viral RNA into host DNA.
    (D) have no effect on viral transcription.

33. Anticancer drugs damage DNA in rapidly dividing cells. All of the following would be expected NOT to suffer such damage from anticancer drugs EXCEPT:
    (A) the cerebral cortex.
    (B) skeletal muscle.
    (C) intestinal epithelia.
    (D) cardiac cells.

34. A pulmonary embolism is a blood clot that passes from the venous systemic circulation to the lungs. Blockage of blood flow to a lung results in hyperventilation, leading to reduction in PCO_2. In addition, a pulmonary embolism is likely to result in:
    (A) blockage of pulmonary veins, leading to decreased PO_2
    (B) blockage of pulmonary veins, leading to increased alveolar O_2
    (C) blockage of pulmonary arteries, leading to decreased SO_2
    (D) blockage of pulmonary arteries, leading to decreased blood pH

ANSWER KEY

1. C	**6.** A	**11.** B	**16.** A	**21.** C	**26.** D	**31.** A
2. D	**7.** B	**12.** A	**17.** D	**22.** C	**27.** A	**32.** D
3. A	**8.** A	**13.** D	**18.** B	**23.** A	**28.** D	**33.** C
4. D	**9.** C	**14.** B	**19.** A	**24.** C	**29.** D	**34.** C
5. B	**10.** D	**15.** C	**20.** D	**25.** A	**30.** D	

ANSWERS EXPLAINED

1. **(C)** Histamine release is triggered by a second exposure to antigen that binds to IgE on Fc receptors of mast cells and basophils.

2. **(D)** Smooth muscle constriction in bronchioles blocks airways, leading to lowered blood pO_2.

3. **(A)** Basophils are leukocytes found in blood.

4. **(D)** Epinephrine (adrenaline) acts on alpha- and beta-adrenergic receptors, triggering the fight-or-flight response of the sympathetic nervous system.

5. **(B)** The passage states that antigen-presenting cells activate the $CD4^+$ T cells, leading them to produce IL-4. $CD4^+$ T cells do not activate IL-4.

6. **(A)** Bacilli are rod shaped, as opposed to cocci, which are round or dot shaped. Choices B and D can be eliminated. Tetanus bacteria are identified in the passage as *Clostridium* and gram-positive. Because both gram-positive and gram-negative bacteria are described as turning colors under Gram staining, choice C can be eliminated. Therefore, it is help-ful, but not necessary, to know that gram-positive bacteria stain dark blue-violet.

7. **(B)** The passage states that the main cause of botulism is improperly canned or preserved foods and that *Clostridium botulinum* is an obligate anaerobe, meaning it can grow only in the absence of oxygen, eliminating choice D. Choice A refers to infant botulism, which is not the main cause, and the answer does not explain botulism in adults. Choice C also refers to infant botulism, and the cause it cites is not supported by the passage.

8. **(A)** The passage states that the toxin causes paralysis, so it must act by preventing nerve signals from propagating. Acetylcholine is the neurotransmitter for skeletal muscle synapses. Norepinephrine is the neurotransmitter for autonomic synapses. Either the release of acetylcholine must be inhibited or the breakdown of it must be stimulated.

9. **(C)** The question refers to the toxin produced by *C. botulinum*, not to the bacterial infec-tion itself. Answers A and B are out. Potency refers to the action of the substance on the body, eliminating choice D.

10. **(D)** The question says that siRNA acts between the stages of transcription (producing mRNA from DNA) and translation (mRNA attaching to a ribosome and tRNA bringing amino acids). Thus options B and C are wrong. Choice A refers to normal posttranscrip-tional mRNA processing, which would actually help gene expression.

11. **(B)** The offspring produced will be diploid because the fusion of two haploid ova will result in a complete set of homologous chromosomes. The offspring will differ genetically from the mother and potentially from each other as a result of crossing over during meiosis.

12. **(A)** The pressure that keeps the lungs inflated is the transpulmonary pressure, or the difference between the negative intrapleural pressure (P_{ip}) of the pleural cavity and the intrapulmonary pressure (P_{pul}) of the alveoli, which is approximately atmospheric pressure. If a lung is punctured, the negative intrapleural pressure increases to atmospheric pressure, or to the equivalent of P_{pul}. Since $P_{pul} = P_{ip}$, transpulmonary pressure goes to zero, and the lung collapses from surface tension and elastic recoil of the alveoli.

13. **(D)** An elderly person with osteoporosis would have relatively less weight in bone than an average person. The resulting low BMI would be an underestimate of body fat because the value assumes average bone density. A tall person with long legs has more height than an average person with the same amount of body fat in the torso, resulting in an artificially low BMI because of the inverse relationship between height and BMI. Individuals I and III would both have a BMI that overestimates body fat for their weight and stature. A long-distance runner would have a high BMI that doesn't accurately reflect body fat because of the higher than average contribution of muscle mass to weight. A person with short legs relative to torso length would have an above average weight for his or her height because of the greater than average contribution of the torso, and its associated organs, to total weight.

14. **(B)** Insulin resistance and type 2 diabetes lead to elevated blood glucose levels. Choice A is incorrect because high cholesterol levels are associated with increased levels of low-density lipoprotein (LDL) in the blood, not HDL. Choices C and D can be eliminated because both would increase, not decrease, in individuals with excessive body fat.

15. **(C)** The liver removes cholesterol from the blood and converts it to bile salts for excretion.

16. **(A)** Insufficient production of bile or blockage of the bile duct by gallstones would prevent the emulsification of fats in the small intestine and thereby reduce absorption by microvilli.

17. **(D)** The number 120 refers to the systolic blood pressure, the pressure detected in the brachial artery when ventricles are contracting.

18. **(B)** A person with more body fat would have a lower, not higher, surface area to volume ratio because of the increase in abdominal mass. Consequently, that person would retain more body heat due to relatively lower surface area for evaporative cooling and fewer superficial capillaries relative to body mass. Choice C can be eliminated because sweat glands are in the dermis and epidermis of the skin, above the fat layer of the hypodermis. Choice D can be eliminated because body fat lowers metabolic rate relative to muscle.

19. **(A)** Filtrate leaves the capillaries of the glomerulus under high pressure. An increase in blood pressure increases the amount of filtrate produced. The Bowman's capsule would collect more filtrate. Water is not reabsorbed by the loop of Henle. Secretion of filtrate is the role of the glomerulus, not of the peritubular capillaries.

20. **(D)** All the other cells are responsible for secreting substances necessary for their respective tissues. Fibroblasts secrete extracellular matrices and collagen. Osteoblasts secrete osteoid matrix for bone formation. Chondrocytes secrete cartilaginous matrix for cartilage formation. Phagocytes—white blood cells—primarily use endocytosis (taking materials into the cell) because their role is to take in foreign particles.

21. **(C)** Posttranslational modification in eukaryotic cells is the modification of a translated protein or polypeptide within the endoplasmic reticulum, Golgi body, or cytoplasm.

22. **(C)** The therapeutic agent should either increase the number of receptors or cause the acetylcholine that is normally in the synapse to stay there longer. Acetylcholinesterase breaks down acetylcholine. So an acetylcholinesterase inhibitor allows more acetylcholine to function. Receptor endocytosis would decrease the number of available receptors.

23. **(A)** The morula develops before the blastula and gastrula. Choice C is incorrect because the gamete appears before conception.

24. **(C)** Both the paranasal sinuses and the respiratory tract form a functional continuum from the nose down to the lungs, and both produce mucus in healthy individuals. The other answer choices are not considered secretions from glands, which are affected in cystic fibrosis. Also, the passage does not mention the other answer options but does state that problems occur in the sinorespiratory tract.

25. **(A)** The passage mentions that a similar problem occurs in the lungs as is described in the pancreas. High extracellular chloride results in thick, viscid secretions that block the ducts and prevent normal secretion.

26. **(D)** The passage mentions that chloride ions are not transported into the cell, leading to a higher concentration in extracellular secretions. All the other choices mention low concentrations.

27. **(A)** The condition is described as autosomal recessive. Choice B refers to dominant conditions. Answers C and D refer to abnormalities of the sex chromosomes, not of autosomes.

28. **(D)** The passage states that the disease appears earlier and has more severe symptoms. Choice A is incorrect because the genetic mutations themselves are present at conception. Choices B and C are incorrect because anticipation does not refer to prediction or to a waiting period.

29. **(D)** The passage states that affected individuals have trouble with releasing muscles from their contracted state. Choice A refers to a person with cystic fibrosis, choice B to someone with Huntington's chorea (excessive movement), and choice C to a person with Turner syndrome.

30. **(D)** Without a Y chromosome, the individual's genotype would be XO, exactly the same as the Turner syndrome individuals described in the passage.

31. **(A)** The condition can be passed down only from the mother (and not the father) as it is encoded in mitochondrial DNA. An affected mother will pass the mutation to all her children, regardless of sex, because mitochondrial DNA is inherited from the mother.

32. **(D)** Reverse transcriptase is an enzyme found in retroviruses that converts viral RNA to viral DNA within the host cell. It would have no effect on a DNA virus.

33. **(C)** A characteristic of epithelial tissue is rapid regeneration via mitotic cell division. Adult neurons and muscle cells are highly specialized and are essentially incapable of cell division.

34. **(C)** Blood flows from the systemic circulation to the heart and then from the heart to the lungs via pulmonary arteries, not veins. Choice C is correct because a reduction in the surface area of contact between the alveoli and blood capillaries leads to a decrease in the amount of oxygen diffusing into the blood and consequently a decrease in the oxygen saturation of hemoglobin. Choice D is incorrect because hyperventilation leads to lower PCO_2 levels, increased alkalinity, and a higher blood pH.

For online practice, go to
http://barronsbooks.com/tp/mcat

Organic Chemistry

4

→ **ORGANIC COMPOUND FUNCTIONAL GROUPS**

→ **THE COVALENT BOND**

→ **MOLECULAR STRUCTURE AND SPECTRA**

→ **SEPARATION AND PURIFICATION**

→ **HYDROCARBONS**

→ **OXYGEN FUNCTIONAL GROUP COMPOUNDS**

→ **AMINES**

Each biological sciences section of the MCAT contains approximately 12 to 20 questions on organic chemistry. Most are in conjunction with a passage. A few are independent questions.

This chapter reviews the basic principles of organic chemistry and covers the topics on the MCAT topic outline published by AMCAS. To master the MCAT Organic Chemistry, study this review, do the exercises in the chapter, and work on as many MCAT practice tests as possible.

ORGANIC COMPOUND FUNCTIONAL GROUPS

A functional group is defined as a characteristic group of atoms in an organic compound that has a predictable chemical reactivity. Memorize the functional groups listed in Table 4.1 and be able to identify them in complex molecules. MCAT problems often present large organic compound structures that contain many different combinations of functional groups. The key to understanding how these large and often strange-looking molecules behave is to identify their functional groups and remember how the functional groups interact with other organic compounds and standard reaction reagents.

Table 4.1 Organic Compound Functional Groups

Hydrocarbon Functional Groups*

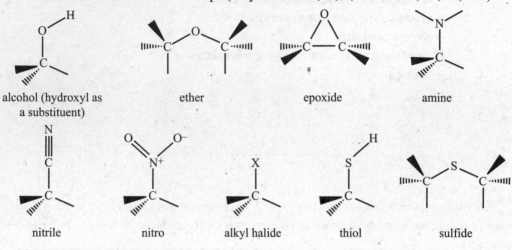

alkene   alkyne   aryl (phenyl as a substituent)

* By definition, alkane hydrocarbons contain no functional groups.

Heteroatom Functional Groups (may contain O, N, S, and X = F, Cl, Br, or I)

alcohol (hydroxyl as a substituent)   ether   epoxide   amine

nitrile   nitro   alkyl halide   thiol   sulfide

Carbonyl (C=O) Containing Functional Groups

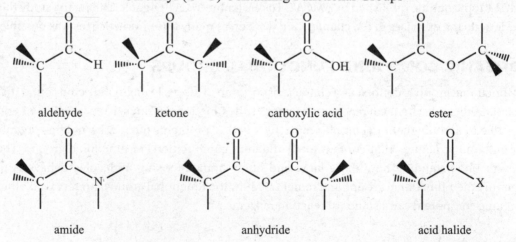

aldehyde   ketone   carboxylic acid   ester

amide   anhydride   acid halide

THE COVALENT BOND

Organic chemistry is the study of carbon-containing compounds. Of the various types of bonds formed by these compounds, by far the most important are **covalent** bonds. In most cases, carbon atoms are bonded to each other or to the elements H, O, N, X (where X = F, Cl, Br, and I), S, and P (these non-carbon atoms are also occasionally bonded to each other). Some organic compounds include ionic bonds, but these are not nearly as common. The shape (structure) of organic molecules is usually defined by the carbon-carbon covalent bond, making it the most important bonding scheme in organic chemistry.

Sigma (σ) and Pi (π) Covalent Bonds

The **valence bond** theory qualitatively predicts the length and strength of covalent bonds in molecular compounds. This theory is also useful in predicting the three-dimensional shapes of molecules. This model for bonding (originally postulated by the chemist Linus Pauling) is based on three elements:

> ### TWO KINDS OF BONDING
>
> **Covalent bonding:** the sharing of two or more valence electrons between atoms.
> **Ionic bonding:** the transfer of one or more valence electrons between atoms. This transfer creates oppositely charged ions (positively charged **cations** and negatively charged **anions**) that are attracted to each other. Their "sticking together" creates an ionic bond.

- Overlap of atomic orbitals containing unpaired valence electrons
- Localization of valence electrons in the orbital overlap region between atoms (the bonding region)
- The formation of hybrid orbitals from atomic orbitals to optimize orbital overlap between bonding atoms.

S AND P ORBITALS

The s and p orbitals are the key to understanding organic bond formation. The s orbital is shaped like a sphere and can hold two valence electrons of opposite spins. The p orbitals exist in sets of three (usually referred to as the p_x, p_y, and p_z orbitals) and can hold a total of six valence electrons. These orbitals are shaped like a figure eight.

An s atomic orbital   A p atomic orbital

Figure 4.1. The shapes and geometries of p and s atomic orbitals

ORBITAL HYBRIDIZATION

In some molecules, atomic orbitals containing unpaired valence electrons overlap to form covalent bonds. However, in most cases, the geometry of the atomic orbitals is not correct for optimum overlap (that is, the greatest area of overlap to give the strongest, shortest bond). Usually, in order to optimize orbital overlap, **orbital hybridization** takes place. The most common types of orbital hybridization are:

- The combination of an s and a p atomic orbital to give two sp hybrid orbitals
- The combination of an s and two p atomic orbitals to give three sp^2 hybrid orbitals
- The combination of an s and three p atomic orbitals to give four sp^3 hybrid orbitals

Note that in the orbital hybridization process, the number of atomic orbitals combined is always equal to the number of hybrid orbitals formed. Figure 4.2 shows the approximate shapes of the sp^3, sp^2, and sp hybrid orbitals. Although the hybrid orbitals have similar shapes, they are different in size.

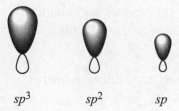

$$sp^3 \qquad sp^2 \qquad sp$$

Figure 4.2. The shapes and relative sizes of the sp^3, sp^2, and sp hybrid orbitals

The hybrid orbitals shown in Figure 4.2 are common in covalent bonding and result in three main molecular shapes. A **linear** shape (bond angle of 180°) results when two sp hybrid orbitals are back to back (large orbital lobe oriented away from the atom). With three sp^2 hybrid orbitals on an atom, the most stable arrangement is **trigonal planar** (bond angles of 120°). With four sp^3 hybrid orbitals, the lowest energy arrangement is a **tetrahedral geometry** (bond angles of 109.5°).

The three hybrid orbital bonding geometries shown in Figure 4.3 are by far the most common in organic compounds.

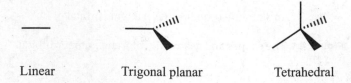

Linear   Trigonal planar   Tetrahedral

Figure 4.3. The most common molecular geometries for bonding atoms in organic compounds

Carbon atoms always use hybrid orbitals when forming bonds, as do certain other elements, including oxygen and nitrogen. In organic compounds, hydrogen and halogen atoms almost always form single bonds. Thus, their bonding orbitals are not hybridized during the bonding process. They use their unhybridized *s* and *p* atomic orbitals and unpaired electrons to bond. Some MCAT organic chemistry questions ask you to predict the kind of hybrid orbitals the central atom in a molecule uses to form bonds and the resulting molecular shape.

Figure 4.4 shows how the central carbon atom in methane (CH_4) mixes an *s* and three *p* atomic orbitals to produce four hybrid sp^3 orbitals. Each of the four sp^3 hybrid orbitals, centered on the carbon atom, is used to make a covalent bond with the *s* atomic orbital from each of the four hydrogen atoms in the molecular formula. The resulting molecule has a tetrahedral shape with 109.5° bond angles. The drawing on the left shows the approximate regions of bond orbital overlap in the methane molecule (between the carbon sp^3 orbitals on the central carbon atom and the four hydrogen *s* atomic orbitals). The graphic on the right shows a standard 3-D line structure drawing of methane.

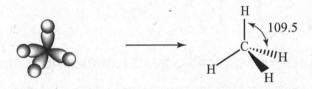

Figure 4.4. Central carbon atom in methane

SIGMA AND PI BONDS

Orbital overlap between both *p* atomic and hybrid orbitals can occur in two distinct orientations. The most common is **end-to-end overlap** between two *p* atomic orbitals, a *p* atomic orbital and a hybrid orbital, or two hybrid orbitals. Bonds that result from this kind of orbital overlap are referred to as *sigma* (σ) bonds and form the bonding skeleton of organic compounds (called the sigma skeleton). The second kind of overlap is **side-to-side overlap**, usually between two *p* atomic orbitals. Bonds that result from this type of orbital overlap are called *pi* (π) bonds and only occur in conjunction with the formation of σ bonds. Figure 4.5 shows pictorial examples of these two kinds of orbital overlaps and the resulting bond types.

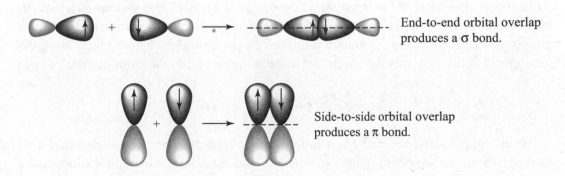

End-to-end orbital overlap produces a σ bond.

Side-to-side orbital overlap produces a π bond.

Figure 4.5. The formation of σ and π bonds by end-to-end and side-to-side orbital overlap

Structural Formulas

There are several common methods for showing the structure of an organic compound molecule on a two-dimensional surface (such as a piece of paper, blackboard, or a computer screen).

LEWIS STRUCTURE

A complete representation showing all atoms and bonds in the molecule is called a Lewis structure. Shown in Structure 1—referred to as (1)—is the Lewis structure for the alkyl compound normal hexane (C_6H_{14}).

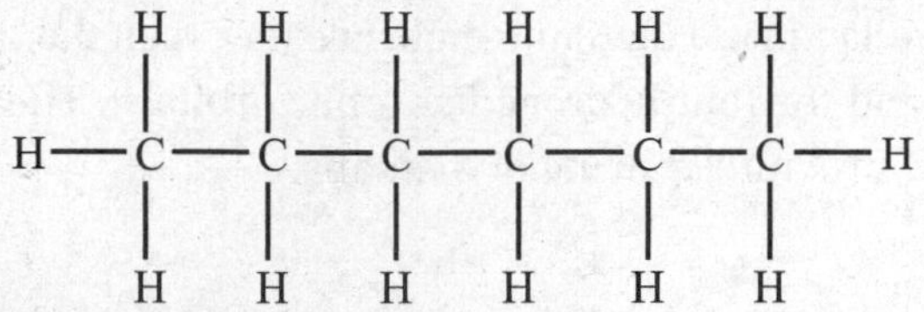

(1)

> ### BE ABLE TO DRAW AND READ LEWIS STRUCTURES
>
> Know how to draw and read 2-dimensional Lewis structures. If necessary, practice them using examples from a general chemistry text. Many MCAT chemistry questions require you to be good at this.

CONDENSED STRUCTURE

Another more abbreviated form referred to as *condensed* shows all the atoms in the structure, but only some or none of the bonds. The rest of the molecular structure implies the presence of the missing bonds. Structure 2 shows the condensed structure for normal hexane.

$$CH_3CH_2CH_2CH_2CH_2CH_3 \quad (2)$$

LEWIS SKELETAL STRUCTURE

Yet another even more abbreviated form in common use is the Lewis **skeletal** structure. In this case only the covalent bond skeleton is shown. The presence of the carbon and hydrogen atoms associated with the compound is implied by the bonding scheme. Again, using the example of normal hexane, the skeletal structure is shown in the following diagram:

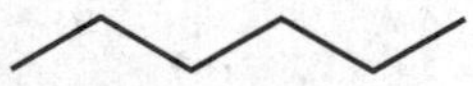

(3)

When using skeletal structures to represent compounds, all noncarbon atoms other than hydrogen must be explicitly shown. It is best to also show all nonbonding electron pairs ("loan pairs"). This chapter will mainly use skeletal structures to represent molecules.

The following diagrams are some relatively simple examples of Lewis skeletal structures. The molecular formula is shown first, followed by the skeletal structure. Draw a complete Lewis formula to the right of each example. Check that your Lewis formula contains exactly the same number and types of atoms as indicated in the molecular and skeletal formulas. Answers to most of the practice questions are given at the end of the Organic Chemistry chapter.

1. Molecular formula: $C_6H_{11}N_1O_1$

    Skeletal structure:

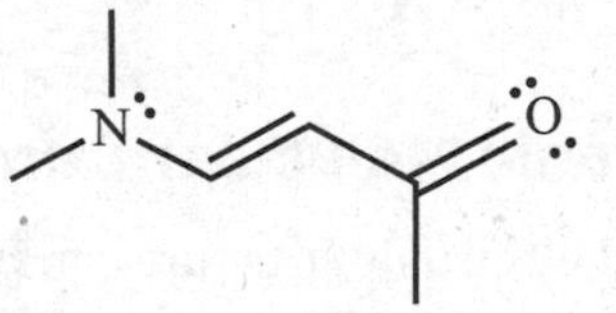

(4)

2. Molecular formula: $C_8H_{11}F_1O_1$

    Skeletal structure:

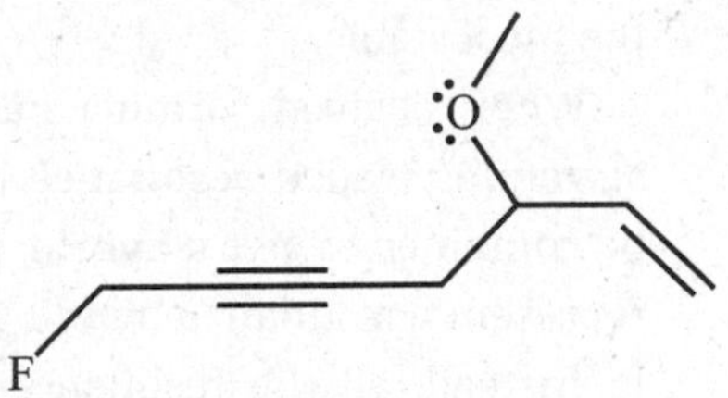

(5)

3. Molecular formula: $C_9H_{10}O_3$

    Skeletal formula:

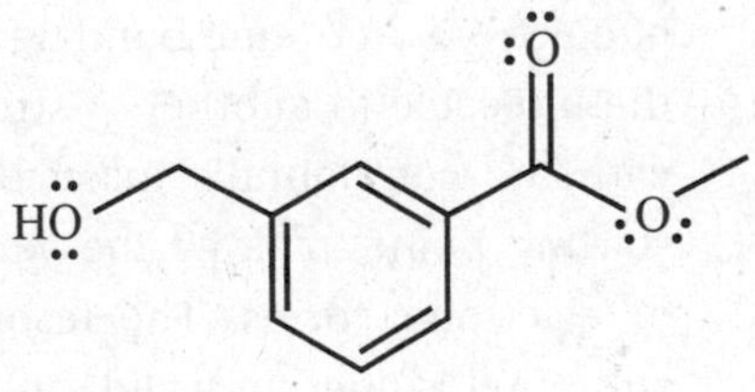

(6)

Multiple Bonds in Organic Compound Molecules

Many organic molecular compounds contain multiple covalent bonding interactions, commonly called simply **multiple bonds**. A simplified bonding symbology is used to easily represent multiple bonds, which are actually combinations of σ and π bonds. A single line between bonding atoms implies a single σ bond. Two lines between bonding atoms implies a double bond consisting of a σ and a π bond. Three lines between atoms refer to a triple bond consisting of a single σ and two π bonds. The carbon-carbon bonds in the following compounds ethane, ethene (commonly called ethylene), and ethyne (commonly called acetylene) illustrate the use of this symbology. Triple bonds are shorter and stronger than double bonds. Double bonds are shorter and stronger than single bonds. In general, the shorter the bonding interaction between two atoms, the more energy it takes to break the bond.

Table 4.2 Comparison of Multiple-Bond Characteristics

$$H_3C \longrightarrow CH_3 \qquad H_2C =\!\!= CH_2 \qquad HC \equiv\!\!\equiv CH$$

one σ bond	one σ bond and one π bond	one σ bond and two π bonds
(C–C single bond)	(C–C double bond)	(C–C triple bond)
Length: 154 pm*	Length: 134 pm	Length: 121 pm
Energy: 356 kJ/mol	Energy: 598 kJ/mol	Energy: 813 kJ/mol

*1 pm = 10^{-12} m

[Data from Cotton, F. A., Wilkinson, G. and Gaus, P. L. *Basic Inorganic Chemistry*, 3rd ed. New York: Wiley, 1995; p. 12.]

Resonance Forms of Organic Molecular Compounds

In many cases, more than one valid electronic structure can be drawn for a given molecular formula. Any possible electronic structure for a molecular formula is correct, assuming it has not broken any basic rules (such as the octet rule), but it may not be the best. The best structure is defined as the electron arrangement that gives the molecule the lowest possible potential energy. In other words, it is the structure that is the most stable.

When a given formula has several valid electronic structures (called **resonance** forms), the structures can be combined to give a **hybrid**. It is usually not possible to represent a resonance hybrid very accurately by drawing it. Instead, all the resonance forms that contribute to the hybrid must be shown. The process of drawing resonance forms of molecules is referred to as **electron pushing**. Curved arrows are used to show the movement of electrons from one bonding or nonbonding region in the molecule to another. A structural isomer consistent with the compound's molecular formula is used as a starting point to draw the various possible resonance or electronic forms. The resonance forms of a single structural isomer are valid only for that isomer and are not to be confused with those of other possible structural isomers of the compound.

> ### THE OCTET RULE
>
> The octet rule comes from Lewis bonding theory.
>
> **Period 2 elements can have only up to eight valence electrons around their nuclei and no more.** The low energy orbitals of these elements (the 2s and 2p) can hold up to eight electrons. Once filled, there are no other accessible orbitals to hold electrons.
>
> **Period 1 elements, such as hydrogen, can have no more than two valence electrons around their nuclei** because only the 1s orbital can be occupied.
>
> **Period 3 and higher elements can have eight or more valence electrons around their nuclei and do not follow the octet rule.**

(7)

In Structure 7, a pair of bonding π electrons is being moved from between the carbon–oxygen bond to the more electronegative oxygen atom. Double-headed arrows are used to show the transition from one resonance form to another. A double-headed arrow should only be used when drawing resonance forms of a molecule. As with all representations of molecular structures based on Lewis theory, only the valence electrons associated with the molecule are considered in the resonance scheme.

There are some basic guidelines for drawing resonance forms:

- Only lone pair electrons and π bonding electrons may be moved.
- Under no circumstances can σ bonds be broken. The σ skeleton of the molecule must remain intact.
- The "octet rule" as defined by Lewis bonding theory cannot be violated, though sulfur and phosphorus can form expanded octets.
- When given a neutral skeletal structure, start by creating charge separation between two bonding atoms by moving a pair of π bonding electrons between two atoms to the more electronegative atom. This will usually work if a π bond is present in the molecule. The result will be two atoms bonded to each other with equal and opposite formal charges. (See Structure 7 in the earlier example.)
- If the given skeletal structure is a cation, push electron density (a lone pair of electrons or a pair of π bonding electrons) toward the positive charge. (Do not break the octet rule.)
- If the given skeletal structure is an anion, push electron density (a lone pair of electrons or a pair of π bonding electrons) away from the negative charge. (Again, do not break the octet rule.)

FORMAL CHARGE CALCULATIONS

Often, one or two of the resonance forms will contribute more character to the hybrid and some forms may contribute very little. The more stable the form, the more it contributes. The best skeletal structure is the resonance form that contributes the most to the hybrid. **Formal charge calculations** can be used to determine the best resonance form of the skeletal structure for a given molecular formula. The following equation can be used to calculate the formal charge of any atom in a skeletal structure.

$$\text{Formal Charge}_{\text{Atom}} = \text{Element's Group \#} - (\text{\# of bonds} + \text{\# of unshared electrons})$$

Note: The species' total charge (usually zero unless it's an ion) must be the same as the sum of the formal charges of all the atoms in the molecule or ion. The element's group # can be found on the periodic table.

The following example illustrates the process of drawing the important resonance forms and determining which is the most stable (lowest in energy) for simple organic molecular compounds.

GUIDELINES FOR FORMAL CHARGES ON ATOMS

- Charges closest to zero are preferred.
- The absolute value of nonzero charges should be as small as possible.
- Negative charges should be on the most electronegative atoms.

Practice Exercise 2

Given the following skeletal Lewis formula (Structure 8), draw the important resonance forms. Which one is the lowest energy form?

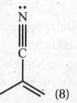

(8)

Approach: The compound molecule is neutral, so begin by pushing a pair of bonding π electrons between the C–N triple bond onto the more electronegative N atom. This gives a new resonance form with charge separation. Next, look for other lone pairs or π electron pairs that can be moved without breaking the octet rule.

Solution: Shown below are the only three important resonance forms. Note the use of curved arrows to show electron movement.

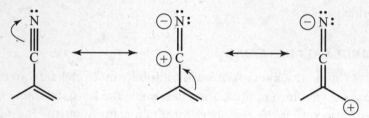

Figure 4.6. Three correct forms

The first resonance form is the most important (lowest in energy) because its C and N atoms all have zero formal charges. Given a neutral molecule, this will usually be the case.

Practice Exercise 3

Draw the important resonance forms of the organic molecules in Structures 9, 10, and 11, based on their skeletal Lewis formulas. (Answers appear at the end of this section.)

1.

(9)

2.

(10)

3.

(11)

Valence Shell Electron Pair Repulsion (VSEPR) Molecular Shape Theory

An alternate method for predicting the shapes of simple organic compounds is to use VSEPR theory. This approach uses a much-simplified explanation for molecular shapes and has advantages when there is limited time to look at the details of bond formation using an orbital overlap approach (for example, valence bond theory).

This method of predicting shapes involves electron pair repulsion between bonds in molecules. When a molecule has two bonds to a central atom, the geometry when the bonds are farthest apart from each other is a linear shape (180°). This geometry minimizes electron–electron repulsion between the two bonding regions of the molecule and provides the greatest distance possible between the two covalent bonds.

When a molecule has three bonds to a central atom, the predicted geometry is trigonal planar with bond angles of 120°—again, as far apart as the bonds can get from each other. Four bonds to a central atom give a tetrahedral shape (bond angles of 109.5°), and so on.

> ### THE MOST COMMON SHAPES FOR ORGANIC COMPOUND BONDING CENTERS
>
> - linear
> - trigonal planar
> - tetrahedral

VSEPR theory can be used to predict the type of hybridization that occurs in complex organic compound bonding centers and is the simplest approach for answering many MCAT questions.

Use the following method to assign the bonding hybridization for carbon, oxygen, and nitrogen atoms in organic compounds:

1. Draw a valid Lewis skeletal structure (2-D representation) of the compound. Be sure not to break the octet rule.
2. Count the number of *electron groups* around each of the bonding centers in the molecule (e.g., each C, N, and O atom bonding center). An electron group is a single bond, a double bond, a triple bond, a nonbonding lone electron pair, or less commonly a single unpaired nonbonding electron. Each of these electron configurations is counted as one and only one electron group. (They all count the same!)
3. Assign the bonding atom's hybridization based on the number of electron groups surrounding it. Bonding atoms with two electron groups are *sp* hybridized, atoms with three electron groups are sp^2 hybridized, and atoms with four electron groups are sp^3.

The following exercise illustrates the use of this procedure.

Practice Exercise 4

Assign the bonding hybridization to each of the C, O, and N atoms in the skeletal formula in Structure 12.

$$(12)$$

Approach: Using the above procedure, count the electron groups around each of the C, O, and N atoms and assign the hybridization.

Solution:

$$(13)$$

Practice Exercise 5

Assign the correct orbital hybridization to all the C, O, and N atoms in the compounds represented by Structures 14, 15, and 16. (Answers appear at the end of this section.)

1.

$$(14)$$

2.

$$(15)$$

3.

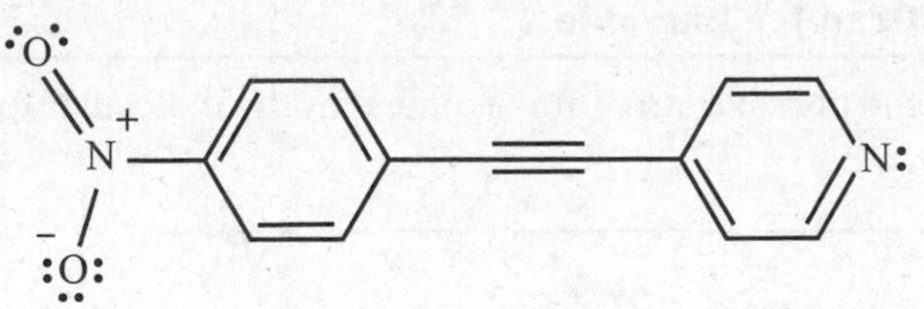

(16)

Organic Molecular Compounds and Chemical Isomerism

Chemical **isomers** are compounds that differ in certain ways but have the same molecular formula. They fall into three basic categories.

1. **STRUCTURAL ISOMERS.** Also known as **constitutional** isomers, structural isomers have the same molecular formulas but differ in the way atoms in the molecule are bonded to each other.

2. **STEREOISOMERS.** Stereoisomers have the same molecular formula and connectivity but differ in the way their atoms are arranged in space. Stereoisomers cannot be interconverted by σ (single) bond rotation.

3. **CONFORMERS.** Also known as **conformational** isomers, conformers have the same molecular formula and connectivity, but temporarily differ due to rotation about σ bonds in the molecule. Conformational isomers are actually the same compound because different conformations can be interconverted by σ bond rotation to produce identical conformers. The most common examples of this type of isomerism are based on alkane (single bond saturated hydrocarbons) molecules. Conformers of alkanes are discussed in the **Hydrocarbons** section of this chapter.

MCAT questions on chemical isomers are quite common. Be sure to understand all three types of isomerism.

STRUCTURAL ISOMERS

Most molecules can form structural isomers, even if they have relatively simple molecular formulas. Because of this, be careful not to assume that a simple molecule does not have isomers. In general, the greater the number of atoms in a compound, the more structural isomers that formula can represent. This is seen most easily with alkanes but holds true for almost any category of organic compound. Structures 17, 18, and 19 depict the possible structural isomers for the molecular formula C_2H_4O. The use of skeletal Lewis structures is usually the fastest way to determine and depict all the structural isomers for a given molecular formula.

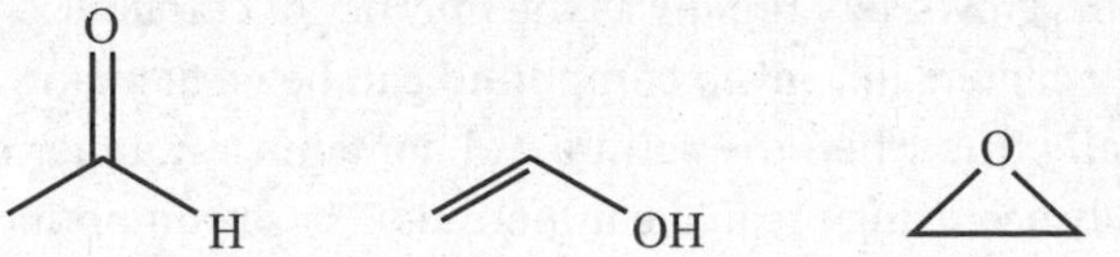

(17, 18, 19)

Draw, using skeletal structures, all the possible structural isomers for the molecular formula C_3H_8O. (Hint: There are three.)

STEREOISOMERS

Sterioisomers of organic compounds fall into two categories:

1. **Enantiomers** are compounds that are nonsuperimposable mirror images of each other. This type of stereoisomer always comes in pairs that are sometime referred to as the left and right-handed isomers of the compound.
2. **Diastereomers** are compounds that are non-mirror image stereoisomers of each other. This category includes all forms of stereoisomerism except enantiomers.

In order for a compound to exist as an enantiomer, it must be chiral. The Greek term *chiral* literally means handedness, as in a right and a left version of something. Human hands are often used to explain the concept of **chirality** as it relates to nonsuperimposable mirror image isomers. Right and left hands reflect into each other but cannot be fully superimposed on each other. This same property is also exhibited by enantiomers. They have handedness and are mirror images of each other, but they cannot be superimposed.

It is not necessary to have a detailed understanding of the concept of chirality to answer MCAT questions. Chiral compounds can be easily identified using one simple rule: They must contain at least one **chirality center**. A chirality center is a carbon atom that is sp^3 hybridized and has four different atoms or groups of atoms attached to it. Figure 4.7 shows a pair of enantiomers. They are nonsuperimposable mirror images of each other and both contain a single chirality center, designated by an asterisk. Identify the chirality center in each of the isomers.

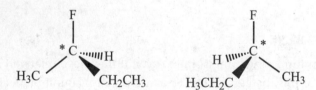

Figure 4.7. A pair of enantiomers containing one chirality center

Chiral molecules often contain more than one chirality center. The number of stereoisomers possible for a given compound is 2^n, where n is the number of chirality centers. If the compound has one chirality center, it will have two stereoisomers. Compounds with two centers may exhibit up to four stereoisomers and those with three can have up to eight. The number of possible isomers grows very rapidly as the number of chirality centers increases.

Finding all the chirality centers in a given compound can be challenging and takes some practice. This is particularly true when the compound contains a number of carbon rings, as found in many naturally occurring organic compounds. These compounds are often isolated from plants and animals and contain many rings and many chirality centers. Figure 4.8 shows a cholesterol molecule. Each of the chirality centers is identified with an asterisk. Notice that the molecule has eight chirality centers, so it can exhibit up to 256 stereoisomers. Past MCAT questions have tested this concept. Practice identifying chirality centers in other complex molecules, such as ones given in organic chemistry textbooks.

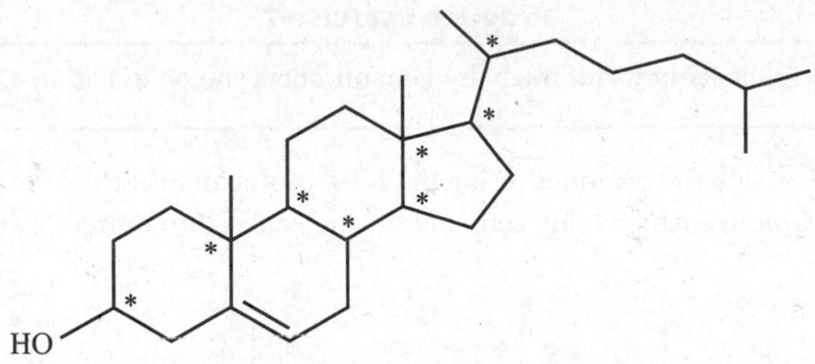

Figure 4.8. A cholesterol molecule

Because large numbers of stereoisomers are possible for compounds with even a few chirality centers, it is necessary to use a special nomenclature system to clearly indicate which isomer is being referred to. This procedure involves assigning the absolute configuration of the chirality center(s) using an *R* or *S* prefix (usually included in the compound's name). Each of the four groups bonded to the chiral carbon in the chirality center is assigned a priority (1, 2, 3, or 4). The lowest priority group (4) is positioned behind the chiral carbon, leaving the remaining higher priority groups (1, 2, and 3) in a trigonal planar configuration. If the groups' priorities around the chiral carbon are 1 to 2 to 3 (highest to lowest priority) in a clockwise direction, the center is designated *R*. If the groups' priorities around the chiral carbon are counterclockwise, the center is designated *S*.

The prioritization process for the groups attached to the chiral carbon in the chirality center uses the Cahn-Ingold-Prelog (C-I-P) protocol. This protocol compares the atomic numbers of the atoms bonded directly to the chiral carbon in the chirality center. The atom with the highest atomic number is assigned the highest priority (1). The atom with the next highest atomic number is second priority (2), and so on, until all four atoms attached to chirality center carbon are given priorities. If two or more of the attachments are groups of atoms (e.g., an organic functional group), the atomic numbers of the atoms in the groups bonded first to the chirality center carbon are compared and given priorities as above. If two or more of the atoms bonded to the chiral carbon are the same, the atomic numbers in the atoms in the attached groups are compared. The one with the higher atomic number is assigned the higher priority. If the atoms at this level are the same, movement is to the next atoms in the groups, and so on, until a difference is found. The atom at this point with the higher atomic number gets the higher priority. The following example shows how to assign the *R* and *S* configuration to chirality centers using the C-I-P system.

> **HOW TO FIND CHIRALITY CENTERS**
>
> ■ Look for the four different groups attached to each of the carbons at the center of the chirality centers.
> ■ When the chirality center is in a ring, follow all the bonds away from the chiral carbon.
> ■ Look for differences between the attachments. Remember that skeletal structures don't show hydrogen atoms. You may want to draw them in.

Designate the chirality centers for the pair of enantiomers shown in Figure 4.7 as *R* or *S*.

Approach: First, assign the priorities (using the C-I-P protocol) to each of the groups bonded to the chiral carbon in each chirality center of the molecules (Structures 20 and 21).

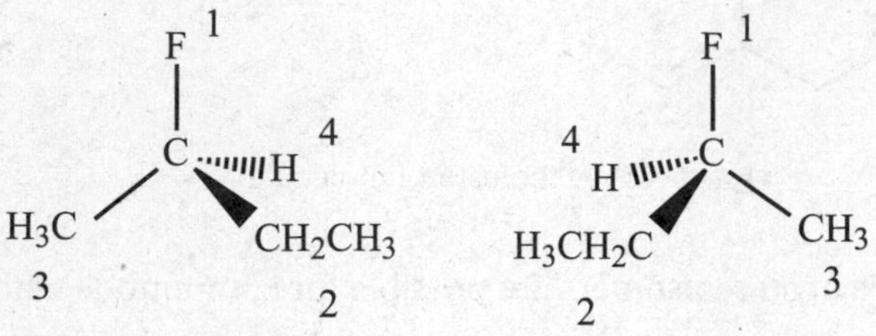

(20, 21)

Next, conceptually turn each of the molecules so that the lowest priority group (in this case it is an H atom for both structures) is hidden behind the carbon at the center of the chirality center. This will leave the remaining three groups in a planar configuration around the chirality center's chiral carbon (Structures 22 and 23).

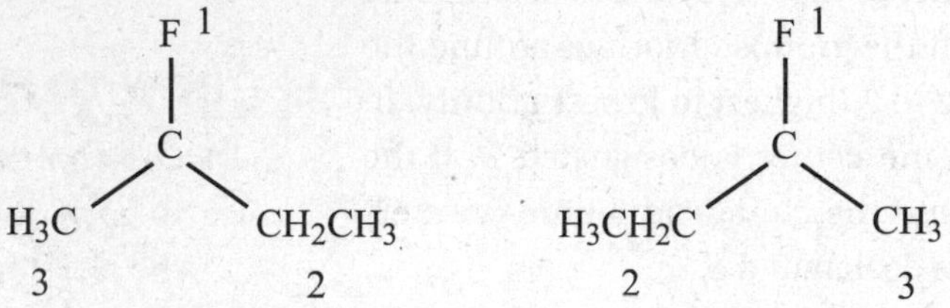

(22, 23)

Finally, observe the direction (clockwise or counterclockwise) when going from the highest priority group to the lowest priority group around the chirality center, as in Structures 22 and 23.

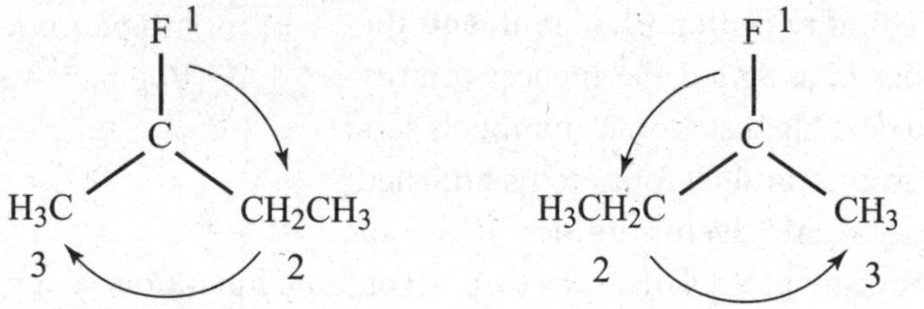

Clockwise (*R*)   Counterclockwise (*S*)   (24, 25)

In Structures 24 and 25, the direction of the priorities (highest to lowest) for the molecule on the left is clockwise. Its chirality center is designated *R*. The direction for the molecule on the right is counterclockwise, so its chirality center is designated *S*.

(26, 27)

TIP

MIRROR IMAGE ENANTIOMERS

The *R* enantiomer is the mirror image of the *S* enantiomer. When they are placed directly opposite each other, as in the example, the isomers reflect into each other.

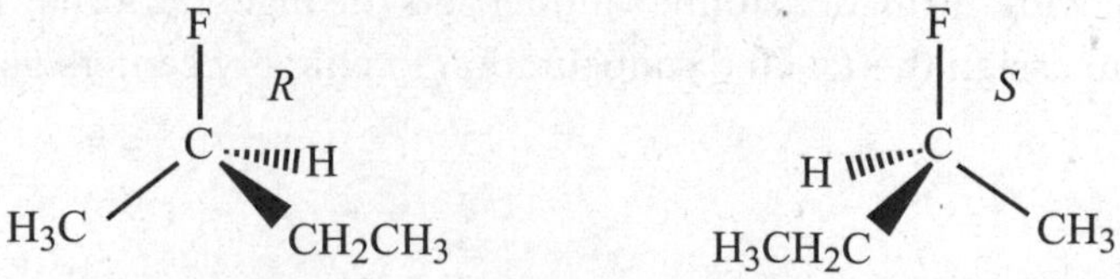

Practice this procedure so you can correctly assign the *R* and *S* designations to chirality centers. The example provided in Structures 26 and 27 is relatively simple partly because of the way the two stereoisomers are drawn. Note that the lowest priority group (the hydrogen atom) was already positioned so that it was behind the chirality center carbon. Stereoisomer molecules will not always be drawn this way. Sometimes the molecule will be drawn with the lowest priority group in front of the chirality center carbon or to the side. In these cases, you will have to conceptually rotate the molecule until the lowest priority group is behind the chirality center carbon, leaving the higher priority groups in front. This takes practice.

In Practice Exercise 8, test your skill in assigning *R* and *S* configurations to chirality centers using the above process.

Practice Exercise 8

Designate the chirality centers in molecule Structures 28, 29, and 30 as *R* or *S*.

Note that there may be more than one chirality center present in a given molecule.

1.

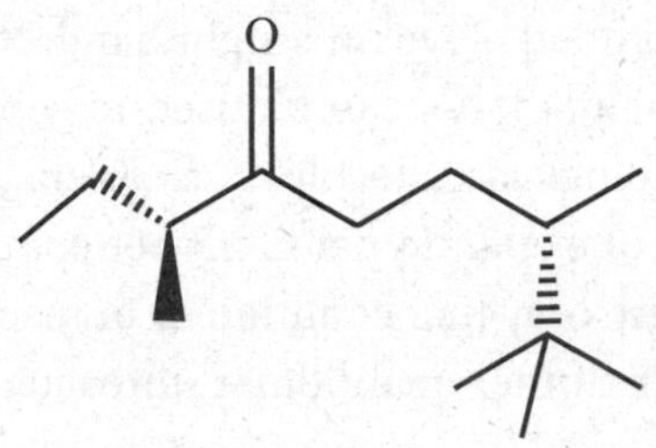

(28)

2.

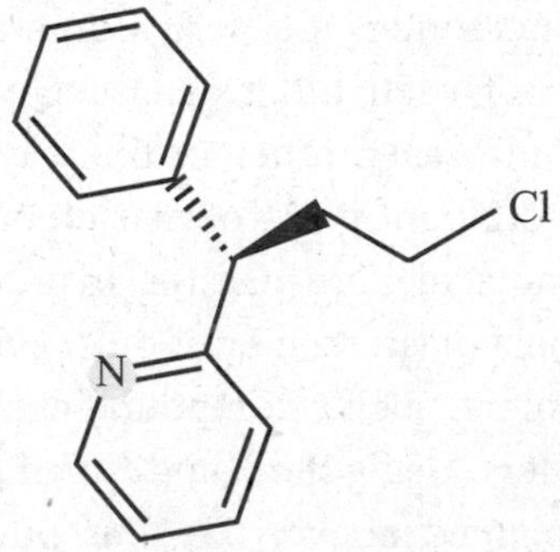

(29)

3.

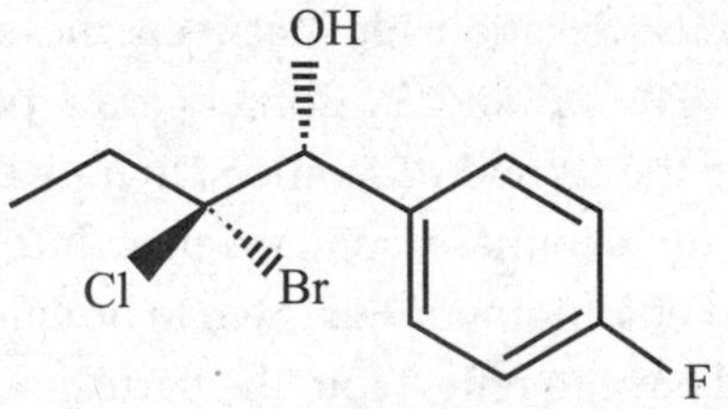

(30)

TIP

HYDROGEN ATOMS IN SKELETAL STRUCTURES

The molecules in this exercise are depicted with skeletal structures, which by convention do not show hydrogens. Don't forget they are still there!

To see the chirality centers more clearly, try drawing in some or all of the hydrogen atoms.

The physical and chemical properties of enantiomers are exactly the same, with two exceptions:

1. When plane-polarized light is passed through a solution of a pure enantiomer, it will rotate the light in a specific direction and a specific number of degrees. A solution of the other enantiomer in the pair (the mirror image) will rotate the same light the same number of degrees but in the opposite direction. This phenomenon is known as **optical activity** and is a property of any pure chiral stereoisomer. Stereoisomers that rotate light to the right (clockwise) are referred to as **dextrorotatory** (often labeled in the compound's name as **d** or **+**) and those that rotate light to the left (counterclockwise) are called **levorotatory** (**l** or **−**).

TIP

R AND S VERSUS (+) AND (−)

Important note! There is no relationship between the *R* and *S* configuration designations and the optical rotation designations of (+) and (−).

When equal amounts of two enantiomers are made into a solution and plane-polarized light is passed through the sample, there is no optical rotation. In other words, the sample is optically inactive. A sample with equal amounts of two enantiomers is called a **racemic mixture** or a **racemate** and is always optically inactive.

2. Another difference between paired enantiomers is in their interaction with other chiral media. The members of a pair of enantiomers often exhibit different reaction rates from each other with other chiral molecules. This again has to do with the handedness of the enantiomer. One pure enantiomer may geometrically fit together better with another chiral molecule and thus produce a reaction transition state that is of lower energy. The other pure enantiomer may not have the right geometry to easily interact with this same chiral molecule. The rate of the reaction between the chiral molecule and the better-fitting enantiomer will be faster and in some cases, much faster.

This situation is similar to trying to put a left-handed glove on a right hand. It may go on but it will never fit well. The property of handedness can be used to separate mixtures of enantiomers from each other. Large biological molecules such as enzymes, which are chiral, usually have a preference for only one enantiomer (it fits better in their active site) and will use only that enantiomer in reactions it catalyzes, leaving the other enantiomer unreacted and unchanged.

USING ENZYMES TO SEPARATE ENANTIOMERS

Enzymes are complex chiral biological molecules that increase the speed of (catalyze) reactions in all living organisms. Organic chemists have isolated many kinds of enzymes from plants and animals. These enzymes are now regularly used to catalyze reactions in the laboratory and industry.

One of the main laboratory uses for these enzymes is the separation of mixtures of enantiomers. This is particularly important in the pharmaceutical industry.

As stated earlier, diastereomers are stereoisomers that are not mirror images of each other. These types of isomers do not reflect into each other in the way that enantiomers do. Many different types of diastereomeric relationships between molecules are possible. In order for a chiral compound to be a diastereomer, it must contain at least two chirality centers. Such a compound can exist as up to four stereoisomers. Using the *R* and *S* configuration nomenclature explained above, the four possible isomers are *RR*, *SS*, *SR*, and *RS*.

The stereochemical relationship between these isomers is as follows. The *RR* and *SS* isomers are a pair of enantiomers, as are the *SR* and *RS* isomers. In both cases, the two chirality centers in these isomers reflect into each other. Note that the *RR* and *SR* isomers are not a pair of enantiomers. For them to be enantiomers, the two chirality centers of one molecule would have to reflect into the corresponding two chirality centers of the other molecule. Because these two stereoisomers are not mirror images of each other, they are diastereomers. Figure 4.9 shows two compounds that contain two chirality centers each and exhibit this type of isomerism.

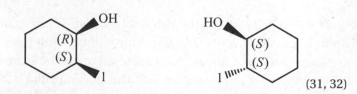

Figure 4.9. Two nonsuperimposable stereoisomers that are diastereomers

As can be seen by the chirality center configurations assigned to these two molecules (left molecule *R, S* and the right molecule *S, S*) they are stereoisomers of each other but not mirror images.

There is a special kind of chiral diastereomer that is called a **meso compound**. A meso compound, like all chiral diastereomers, must contain at least two chirality centers, but it also must have a plane of symmetry that allows one side of the molecule to reflect into the opposite side. This kind of molecule is a mirror image of itself. One side of the molecule reflects exactly into the other side. As a result, it is optically inactive.

There is another type of diastereomer that is not a chiral compound and instead of having two chirality centers has two sp^2 hybridized carbon atoms adjacent to each other. This kind of organic compound is called an **alkene** and contains one or more carbon–carbon double bonds. As described earlier in this section, carbon–carbon double bonds in organic molecules consist of one σ bond and one π bond. Free rotation is possible around carbon–carbon single (σ) bonds, but not carbon–carbon double bonds. Because of the side-to-side overlap of the *p* atomic orbitals that form the π part of the double bond, rotation is very restricted. Rotation about a carbon–carbon double bond requires enough energy to break the π part of the bond and does not happen under ambient conditions. Because of the rigid nature of the carbon–carbon double bond, groups attached to either side of the bond are fixed in space and cannot interact with each other. This property of the double bond leads to what are called cis/trans stereoisomers. Figure 4.10 shows a pair of cis/trans isomers.

trans-1,2-dibromoethene   *cis*-1,2-dibromoethene   (33, 34)

Figure 4.10. The cis and trans isomers of 1,2-dibromoethane

If two atoms of the same type are on opposite sides of the double bond, the isomer is assigned the **trans configuration** (molecule on the left). If two atoms of the same type are on the same side of the double bond, the isomer is assigned the **cis configuration** (molecule on the right). As with the *R* and *S* designations for chirality centers, cis and trans designations appear as prefixes in the compound names.

Why are cis and trans isomers considered diastereomers? Note that the only difference between the left and right molecule shown above is the way the atoms are arranged in space. The connectivity is the same and so are their molecular formulas. Thus cis and trans isomers are stereoisomers. However, the two molecules are not nonsuperimposable mirror images of each other. If the two molecules are not enantiomers and are non-mirror image stereoisomers of each other, they must be diastereomers.

There is another type of nomenclature that is used to distinguish these alkene stereoisomers from each other. The designations are similar to cis and trans; they are the **E and Z isomers**.

The E and Z designation is most commonly used when there are no like groups attached to the double bond. It can be used to indicate the stereochemistry of any alkene. As with the *R* and *S* designations, the procedure for assigning E or Z to a specific stereoisomer involves the use of the C-I-P prioritization rules. The following example shows how to specify the E and Z configurations of alkene stereoisomers.

E AND Z

E is from the German word *entgegen*, which means "opposite." For a mnemonic, think of it as "ecross" (across).

Z is from the German word *zusammen*, which means "together." For a mnemonic, think of it as "zide by zide" (side by side).

Practice Exercise 9

Designate the alkene stereoisomer in Structure 35 as E or Z.

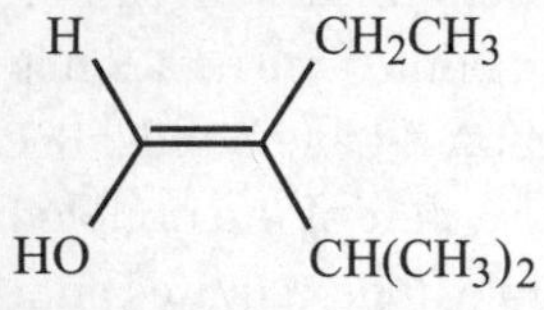
H
CH2CH3
HO
CH(CH3)2

(35)

Approach: Divide the given molecule into two parts by cutting the horizontal double bond in half. Structure 36 shows the left side of the molecule after being segmented.

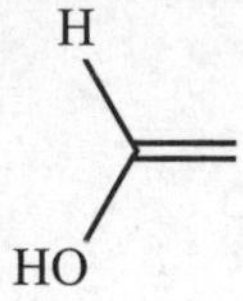
H
HO

(36)

Next, use the C-I-P rules to prioritize the groups as either first (1) or second (2). In this case, the two atoms attached directly to the double bond are oxygen and hydrogen. Because oxygen has the higher atomic number, it gets first priority and hydrogen second. See the result in Structure 37.

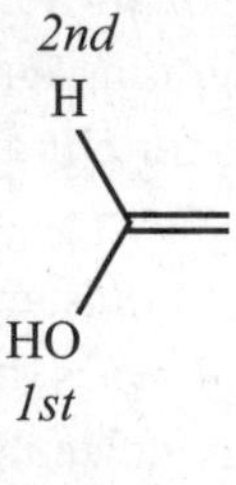
2nd
H
HO
1st

(37)

The groups attached to the right side of the molecule (Structure 38) are prioritized in exactly the same way.

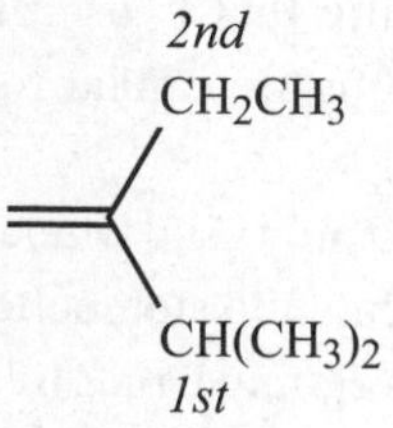
2nd
CH2CH3
CH(CH3)2
1st

(38)

Now put the molecule back together, as shown in Structure 39.

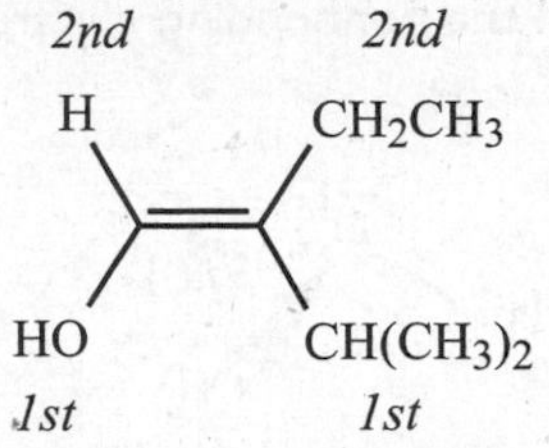

(39)

If the two first-priority groups attached to the double bond are on the same side, the isomer is designated as Z and if they are on opposite sides, the isomer is designated as E. In this case, they are on the same side, so the stereo-isomer is Z, as shown in Figure 4.11.

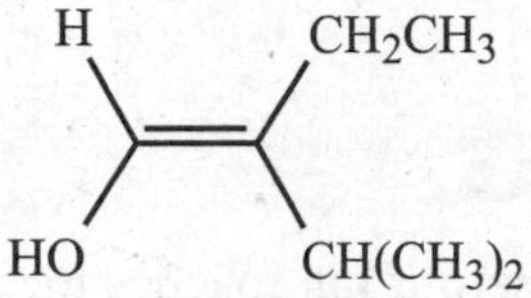

(40)

Figure 4.11. Z isomer

WHAT'S NOT IN THE DIAGRAM

Remember that skeletal structures of molecules don't show hydrogens.

In this case, for simplicity, nonbonding electron pairs are also not shown. See Structures 41, 42, and 43.

Practice assigning E and Z designations to alkene stereoisomers in the following exercise.

Practice Exercise 10

Designate the following alkene stereoisomers as E or Z.

1.

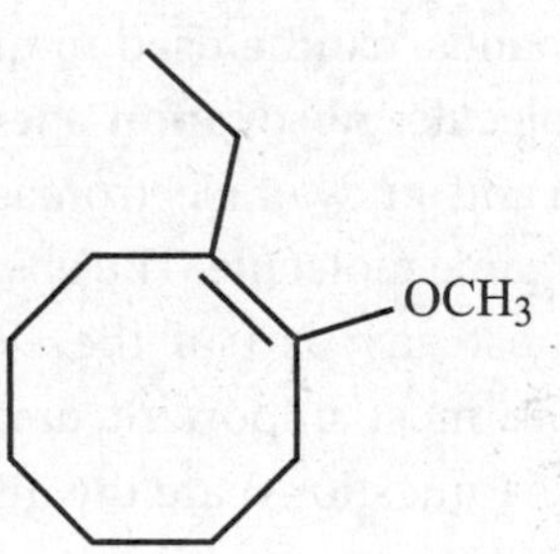

(41)

2.

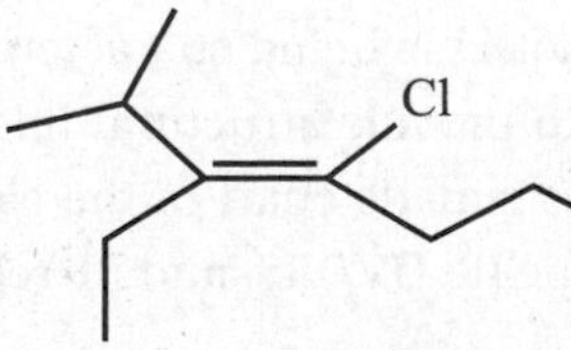

(42)

3.

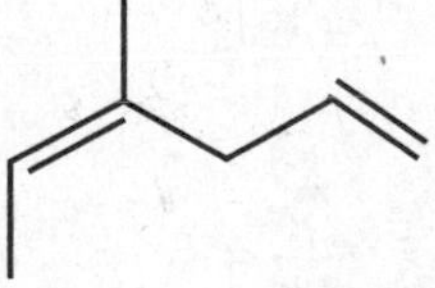

(43)

In what type of hybrid orbital will the nonbonding electron pair on the oxygen atom in the trimethyloxonium ion be found?

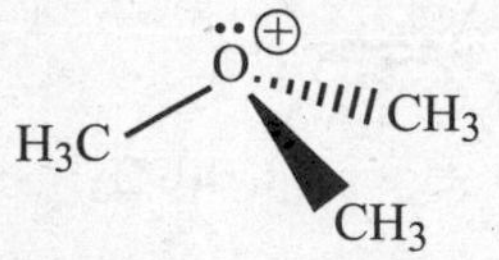

(A) sp^3

(B) sp^2

(C) sp

(D) p

(A) There are four electron groups around the oxygen.

MOLECULAR STRUCTURE AND SPECTRA

In the history of the study of organic compounds, numerous approaches for the characterization of molecular structures have been developed. When chemists isolate or synthesize an organic compound, they must have a reliable method for assigning a structure to the compound and, eventually, an IUPAC name. This is particularly important for safety, research, and legal reasons (for example, the patent application process) if the compound has never been previously isolated or synthesized.

The most powerful and efficient methods currently in use to characterize the structure of organic molecules involve absorption and emission spectroscopic and spectrometric techniques. These tools are quite sophisticated and, in the right hands, can be used to quickly and confidently assign a structure to a complex organic molecule. **Absorption spectroscopy** involves the detection and study of electromagnetic radiation absorbed by an organic molecule. The absorbed radiation can be from almost any part of the electromagnetic spectrum, but the most important areas for organic chemistry (and MCAT questions) are the infrared (IR), ultraviolet/visible (UV/VIS), and radio frequency (RF) regions. In **emission spectroscopy**, electromagnetic radiation emitted by the molecule being characterized is detected and interpreted to provide structural information. Figure 4.12 shows a schematic chart of the electromagnetic spectrum. Note the IR, UV/VIS, and RF regions.

WHAT IS IUPAC?

IUPAC stands for the *International Union of Pure and Applied Chemistry*. Among other things, this union of chemists has developed and sanctioned a systematic method of nomenclature for chemical compounds. This method of naming compounds is the recognized international standard.

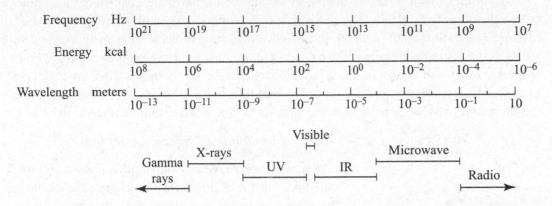

Figure 4.12. The electromagnetic spectrum

Past MCAT exams have often contained questions related to spectroscopic characterization concepts. You may be given a spectrum and have to choose the answer with the correct substance or you may be given a substance and have to choose the correct spectrum.

Absorption Spectroscopy

The most important types of radiation absorption for characterizing organic compounds are in the IR and UV/VIS ranges. The most important of these techniques, IR spectroscopy, will be reviewed first, followed by an overview of UV/VIS spectroscopy.

IR ABSORPTION SPECTROSCOPY

The data obtained from IR spectra is usually used to identify the **functional groups** associated with the compound being studied. This can immediately tell chemists if they are working with an alcohol, ketone, amine, or other common molecule. If the spectrum is more complex, it may indicate the presence of several different functional groups. Typically, radiation from the middle of the infrared spectrum is employed in IR spectroscopy. The energies of photons within this region correspond to energy differences between vibrational states in covalently bonded molecules. For this reason, IR spectroscopy is also called **vibrational spectroscopy**.

In accordance with quantum theory, these vibrational states are quantized; thus, molecules will only absorb infrared photons with specific energies. When IR radiation is absorbed, the molecule will vibrate (with its atoms moving relative to each other as if attached by springs) at a faster rate. There are two types of vibrational modes: **stretches**, in which bond lengths change, and **bends**, in which bond angles change. Furthermore, there are two types of stretches—**symmetric** and **asymmetric**—and four types of bends—**rocking, scissoring, wagging, and twisting**. See the following website for animated examples of each:

http://www.shu.ac.uk/schools/sci/chem/tutorials/molspec/irspec1.htm

FUNCTIONAL GROUPS

A **functional group** is an atom or group of atoms with specific chemical and physical properties. The functional group is often the reactive portion of the molecule.

There are about 25 most common functional groups in organic compounds. Compounds often contain more than one. At the beginning of this chapter is a table of the functional groups you should know.

Not all possible vibrational modes absorb infrared radiation, however. Only those that change the dipole of the molecule during movement are "IR-active." Those modes that do not—for example, the symmetric stretch of $O=C=O$ along the axis of the molecule—are IR-inactive. Additional modes may be created when vibrations interact with each other, or couple, to form combination modes.

An IR spectrum is plotted as percent transmittance versus frequency, but instead of using reciprocal time (that is, s^{-1}), frequency is given in reciprocal wavelengths or **wave numbers** (cm^{-1}). The relationships between wave number, wavelength (λ), and frequency (ν) for electromagnetic radiation are as follows:

wave number (in cm^{-1}) = $1/\lambda$ (in cm) = ν (in s^{-1})$/c$, where $c = 3.00 \times 10^{10}$ cm/s

The typical wave number range used in IR spectroscopy is 4000–400 cm^{-1} (corresponding to a wavelength range of 2.5×10^{-4} to 2.5×10^{-3} cm or 2.5–25 µm) and is usually plotted from highest to lowest frequency (thus the highest energy vibrations are to the left and the lowest are to the right). Figure 4.13 is the IR spectrum for formaldehyde, $H_2C=O$, and provides a good example of some of the most common types of bond vibrations found in the spectra of organic molecules. Note the stretching vibrations in the region above 1400 cm^{-1} and the bending vibrations at wave numbers below 1400 cm^{-1}.

Because each vibrational state is further split into rotational and translational states, each absorption occurs over a range of frequencies rather than at just one. This causes both broadening of the absorption signal, which appears as a band rather than a peak, and the appearance of additional "structure" in the spectrum in the form of shoulder and side bands usually near more intense bands.

The intensity of bands is affected by three principal factors: concentration of the compound (which equally affects the intensity of all absorptions), **bond polarity** (the more polar, the stronger the absorption), and the level of asymmetry in the molecule. In general, the more asymmetry between the bonds, the stronger the absorption band will be, as predicted by quantum mechanics.

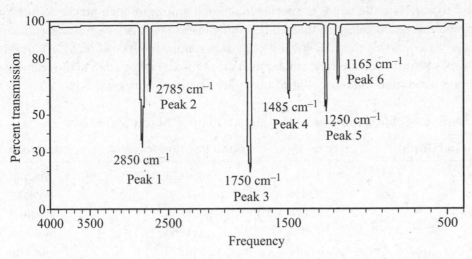

Figure 4.13. The IR absorption spectrum for formaldehyde. The peaks are as follows:

Peak 1	CH_2	2850 cm^{-1}	Asym stretch
Peak 2	CH_2	2785 cm^{-1}	Sym stretch
Peak 3	C=O	1750 cm^{-1}	Stretch
Peak 4	CH_2	1485 cm^{-1}	Scissor
Peak 5	CH_2	1250 cm^{-1}	Rock
Peak 6	CH_2	1165 cm^{-1}	Wag

The frequencies of specific IR bands are affected by any factor that affects vibrational energy. Stretching modes, which require more energy to excite, occur at higher energies, and thus higher frequencies, than do bending modes. Also, the shorter and thus stronger the bonds involved in a vibration, the higher the energy, and thus frequency, of the absorption. Vibrational modes involving triple bonds are at higher frequencies than those involving double bonds, which are, in turn, at higher frequencies than modes involving single bonds. Another important factor involves **inductive effects**. Electron-withdrawing and conjugated substituents typically weaken adjacent bonds and thus lower their absorption frequencies. Additionally, the presence of hydrogen bonding must be considered, as it tends to broaden absorption bands for O–H and N–H stretches, especially in solutions or liquids in which fast hydrogen exchange is possible.

In general, O–H, N–H, and C–H stretches are found between 3700 and 2700 cm^{-1}, multiple bond stretches (in roughly the order C≡N, C≡C, C=O, C=C, aromatic) between 2300 and 1400 cm^{-1}, and single bond stretches between 1600 and 1300 cm^{-1} for N–O and between 1300 and 900 cm^{-1} for C–O, C–N, and C–C. In fact, the 4000 to 1300 cm^{-1} range is called the *functional group region* because bands within it are often well separated and relatively strong. Because of this,

> **IR SPECTROSCOPY ON THE MCAT**
>
> A detailed understanding of the factors that affect absorption band shape, strength, and position is not necessary for the MCAT.
>
> The most important thing to remember is the general position (in cm^{-1}) of the absorption bands for the most common kinds of bonds and functional groups.

it is easy to correlate the bands to specific functional groups, though precise identification of a compound based solely on the bands is difficult. Table 4.3 shows the absorption band positions (in cm^{-1}) for the functional groups most often referenced in MCAT questions. Study Table 4.3 until you are very familiar with the approximate position of the referenced IR absorption bands and the functional groups to which they correspond.

Table 4.3 Important Functional Group IR Absorption Bands

Functional Group	Bond Type	Band Position (cm^{-1})	Intensity
Alkanes	C–H	3000–2850	Strong
	C–C	~1200	Weak
Alkenes	=C–H	3095–3010	Medium
	C=C	~1650	Medium
Alkynes	≡C–H	~3300	Medium
	C≡C	2260–2100	Medium
Aromatics	Ar–H	3100–2900	Weak
	C–C	1625–1425	Medium
Aldehydes	H–C=O	~2810, 2710	Medium
	C=O	1740–1690	Strong
Ketones	C=O	1750–1680	Strong
Carboxylic Acids	O–H	3000–2500	Strong, Broad
	C=O	1780–1710	Strong
Alcohols	O–H	3600–3200	Strong, Broad
Amines	N–H	3500–3200	Medium
Ethers	C–O	1150–1050	Strong

Most bending frequencies are found in the range of 1400 cm^{-1} to 600 cm^{-1}. Unfortunately, this overlaps significantly with the stretching frequencies for single bonds and also with the frequencies for many of the combination vibrational modes mentioned above, quite often making this region of the spectrum too crowded and complicated to interpret. However, a band-for-band match within this frequency range between the IR spectra of a known compound and a sample of an unknown compound is strong proof that the two compounds are identical. Therefore, this range is called the **fingerprint region** (from about 1500 to 500 cm^{-1}).

Quantitative analysis using IR spectroscopy is more difficult than with other analytical methods because of deviations from Beer's law, which requires a linear relationship between absorbance and concentration. Deviations can be due to imperfections in mirror movement within the interferometer, relatively narrow absorption bands, the difficulty in providing consistent or measurable path lengths, and the relatively low sensitivity of IR detectors as compared to detectors used in other methods.

Some MCAT exam questions require you to identify common functional groups in organic molecules directly from the IR spectra of compounds. Figures 4.14 through 4.20 show example spectra of simple compounds containing many of the common functional groups likely to be encountered on the MCAT. Careful study of these examples will help you recognize and internalize the band patterns for functional groups commonly seen on the MCAT.

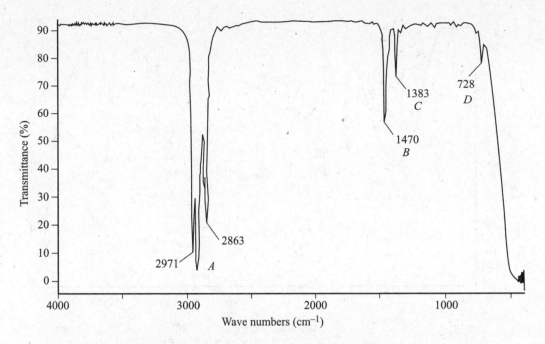

Figure 4.14. The IR absorption spectrum of the alkane octane. Point *A* is a C–H stretch, *B* is C–H scissoring, *C* is C–H methyl rock, *D* is long-chain methyl rock. Note the key bands common to ***alkanes*** (C–H stretch bands).

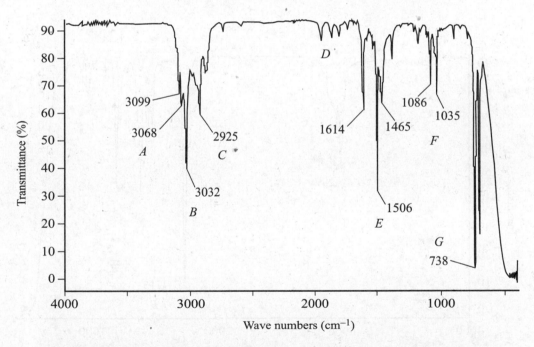

Figure 4.15. The IR absorption spectrum of the aromatic compound toluene. Aromatic C–H stretches are left of 3000 and alkyl C–H stretches are right of 3000. Points *A* and *B* are aromatic C–H stretches. *C* is an alkyl C–H stretch. *D* represents overtones. *E* is C–C stretches in the aromatic ring. *F* is in-plane C–H bending. *G* is out-of-plane (oop) C–H bending. Note the key bands common to ***aromatic*** compounds (aromatic C–H stretches).

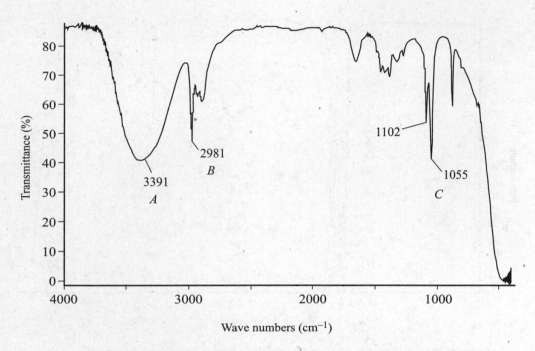

Figure 4.16. The IR absorption spectrum of the alcohol ethanol. Point **A** is an O–H stretch. **B** is a C–H stretch. **C** is a C–O stretch. Note the key bands common to **alcohols** (broad O–H stretch and C–O stretch).

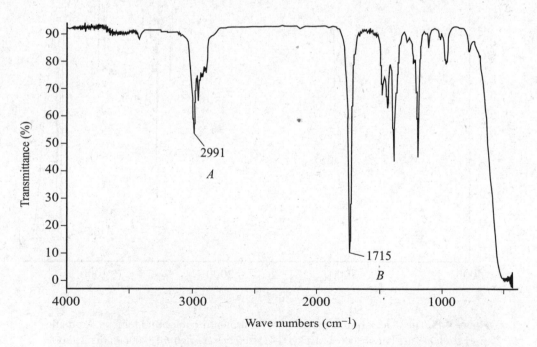

Figure 4.17. The IR absorption spectrum of the ketone 2-butanone. Point *A* is a C–H stretch. *B* is a C=O stretch. Note the key band common to **ketones** (C=O stretch).

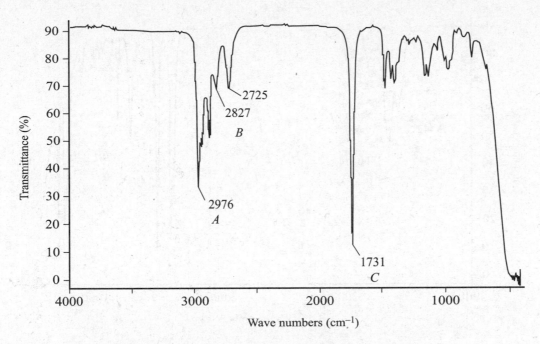

Figure 4.18. The IR absorption spectrum of the aldehyde butyraldehyde. Point *A* is an alkyl C–H stretch. *B* represents aldehyde C–H stretches. *C* is a C=O stretch. Note the key bands common to **aldehydes** (C–H stretch and C=O stretch).

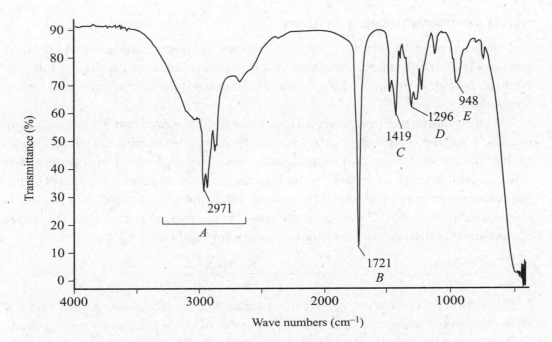

Figure 4.19. The IR absorption spectrum of the carboxylic acid hexanoic acid. Note the key bands common to **carboxylic acids** (very broad O–H stretch and C=O stretch). Point *A* represents O–H and C–H stretches. *B* is a C=O stretch. *C* is an O–H bend. *D* is a C–O stretch. *E* is an O–H bend.

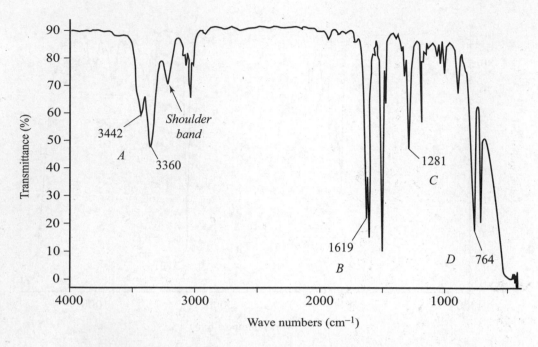

Figure 4.20. The IR absorption spectrum of the amine aniline. Point *A* represents N–H stretches (primary amines). *B* is an N–H bend (primary amines). *C* is a C–N stretch. *D* is an N–H wag (primary and secondary amines). Note the key bands common to a primary *amine* (N–H stretches—two present and C–N stretch). Notice that only one N–H stretch appears for a secondary amine and none appears for a tertiary amine, but the C–N stretch will be present for all.

UV/VIS ABSORPTION SPECTROSCOPY

The applications of UV/VIS absorption spectroscopy are quite specialized and for MCAT purposes require only a brief discussion. This type of absorption spectroscopy is used primarily to provide information about the degree of unsaturation and conjugation in organic compounds.

The terms **saturated** and **unsaturated** refer to the hydrogen atom content of organic compounds. Saturated compounds contain the maximum possible number of hydrogen atoms in their molecules. Unsaturated compounds contain fewer hydrogen atoms because they contain multiple bonds, rings, or other functional groups that reduce their potential hydrogen content. Any combination of multiple bonds, rings, and functional groups is possible in unsaturated compounds. The majority of organic compounds are unsaturated. The **degree of unsaturation (DU)** can be calculated using the following formula:

$$DU = \frac{2C+2+N-(H+X)}{2}$$

In this formula, C is the number of carbon atoms, N is the number of nitrogen atoms, H is the number of hydrogen atoms, and X is the number of halogen atoms in the compound.

If the molecular formula of a compound is known, its DU can be calculated (using the above formula) and used to estimate the number of possible multiple bonds and rings it contains. This information can be very valuable in ultimately determining its complete atomic structure.

In unsaturated compounds **conjugation** refers to a specific arrangement of double bonds in the molecule. A compound is conjugated when its double bonds alternate with single bonds. Examples of **isolated** and **conjugated** double bonds are shown in Structures 44 and 45.

Isolated Double Bonds   Conjugated Double Bonds   (44, 45)

The wavelength (represented by the Greek letter λ) of the radiation in the UV/VIS part of the spectrum is commonly given in **nanometers (nm)**. The range most important for molecular structure information is relatively narrow, falling roughly between 200 nm and 500 nm. This range starts in the near ultraviolet region and overlaps into the violet/blue region of the visible part of the spectrum. The majority of unsaturated compounds absorb radiation in the 200 to 400 nm range, but a few absorb longer wavelength radiation in the visible region.

When an organic molecule is irradiated with electromagnetic energy, the radiation, depending on its wavelength, may be absorbed or it may pass though the compound. IR radiation absorbed by molecules causes their covalent bonds to vibrate (resulting in stretching and bending), but the energy of UV/VIS radiation is much higher and leads to a change in the molecule's electron configuration. In organic compounds containing double bonds, absorption of UV/VIS radiation energy results in the promotion of electrons from **bonding** molecular orbitals (ψ, referred to as ground state) to higher energy **antibonding** molecular orbitals (ψ^*, referred to as excited state) in the compound. The energy absorbed during this transition (which is called a $\pi \rightarrow \pi^*$ transition) is measured and interpreted in order to provide structural information about the molecule being irradiated.

Other kinds of electron transitions can occur when radiation is absorbed if certain functional groups are present in the molecule. For example if a carbon–oxygen double bond (called a carbonyl group) is present, an $n \rightarrow \pi^*$ (where n refers to a nonbonding molecular orbital) transition is observed. This transition involves the promotion of an electron from a ground state nonbonding molecular orbital to an excited state antibonding molecular orbital and requires less energy than a $\pi \rightarrow \pi^*$ transition.

TIP

A NANOMETER

$1 \text{ nm} = 10^{-9} \text{ meters}$

MOLECULAR ORBITAL THEORY

This is one of many theories for explaining atom bonding in molecular compounds. When atomic orbitals are combined linearly (a mathematical operation), two kinds of molecular orbitals are usually produced— bonding and antibonding. A nonbonding orbital is also possible.

Bonding MOs are lower in energy than the orbitals they were derived from and help stabilize the bonding interaction.

Antibonding MOs are higher in energy than the atomic orbitals from which they were formed. They destabilize the bonding interaction.

Nonbonding MOs neither stabilize nor destabilize the bonding interaction.

Graphs of spectra. UV/VIS spectra of organic compounds are usually recorded by irradiating samples with continually increasing wavelengths of radiation (from higher to lower energy). When the energy of the radiation is sufficient to promote an electron to a higher energy level, energy is absorbed and the absorption is observed as a positive peak (rather than a negative band as in IR spectroscopy) in the spectrum. Spectra are displayed with the wavelength in nanometers at the bottom of the graph and relative absorption (which is unitless) along the left vertical axis. Figure 4.21 shows as an example the UV/VIS absorption spectrum of the compound isoprene.

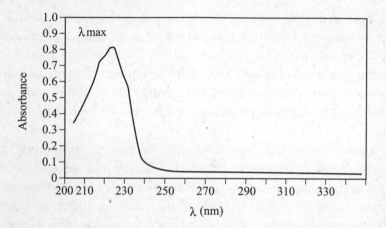

Figure 4.21. The UV/VIS absorption spectrum of isoprene. Max = 222 nm

Unlike IR spectra, UV/VIS spectra generally have very few features. As seen in Figure 4.21, there is often only a single broad absorption peak, referred to as λ **max**. Spectra of other more complex molecules may show additional absorption peaks because of additional electron transitions. This can be seen in the UV/VIS absorption spectrum of a conjugated ketone (below).

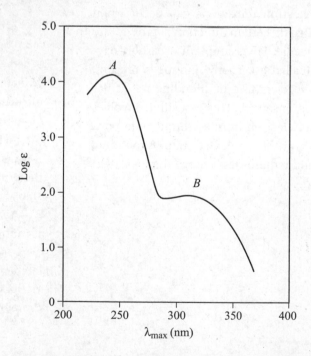

Figure 4.22. The UV/VIS absorption spectrum of a conjugated ketone.
[Source: *http://www.cem.msu.edu/~reusch/VirtualText/Spectrpy/UV-Vis/spectrum.htm*]

Note the two absorptions peaks (*A* and *B*) resulting from two different electron transitions, $\pi \to \pi^*$ and $n \to \pi^*$. Also note that this spectrum has been plotted using the log of the molar absorptivity (ε) for the vertical axis. This is an alternative to using absorption (A) and can make some spectra easier to interpret.

The degree of conjugation in an organic compound can be estimated from its UV/VIS spectrum. In general, the longer the conjugated double bond system in the molecule, the lower the energy required for a $\pi \to \pi^*$ transition and thus the longer the wavelength of the energy absorbed.

Most λ max absorption peaks are found between 200 and 400 nm, but when the conjugation system is really long, as for example in the compound β-carotene (with 11 conjugated double bonds and a λ max of 455 nm), the λ max absorption may fall in the visible part of the electromagnetic spectrum. Compounds with this characteristic UV/VIS spectrum appear colored to the human eye. The general rule is that for every conjugated double bond, the absorption energy wavelength is increased by approximately 30 to 40 nm. Additional isolated double bonds generally do not increase the absorption wavelength. The addition of alkyl groups (for example, methyl, ethyl, propyl) to the conjugation system of the molecule adds about 5 nm to the wavelength's absorption.

Mass Spectrometry

Mass spectrometry (MS) uses high-energy electrons (often in the form of a beam) to eject electrons from and break bonds in molecules. The technique is destructive and usually results in a significant level of molecular fragmentation. Electron beam bombardment literally causes the exposed molecule to fall into pieces. Even though the molecule being studied absorbs energy during the fragmentation process, neither the energy absorbed nor emitted is measured or studied. Mass spectrometry is not considered to be a spectroscopic technique. Instead, it focuses on the detection of positively charged species resulting from the molecular degradation process.

The most important molecular characterization clues obtained from mass spectrometry are:

■ An estimate of the molecule's mass (its molecular weight in atomic mass units)

■ The molecule's **fragmentation pattern**, which is usually unique and can sometimes be matched to a database of known MS fragmentation patterns. If a high confidence match is obtained with a compound in the database, the compounds are either identical or very similar.

In many cases, just the opportunity to obtain an estimate of the molecule's molecular weight is reason enough to conduct a mass spectrometry experiment. The molecular weight, along with **elemental analysis** data, will usually allow the researcher to determine the molecule's molecular formula—an invaluable starting point for assigning its molecular structure.

The first species formed during electron bombardment is a radical-cation (a positively charged ion with an odd number of electrons) and results from the ejection of a single electron from the analysis molecule. This radical-cation is referred to as the **molecular ion** and is represented by M^+. Because the loss of a single electron from a molecule has essentially no effect on its mass, the M^+ represents the molecular weight of the original compound. The M^+ is inherently unstable and, once formed, begins to spontaneously decompose into various fragments. Some of the fragments are cations or radical cations, which are sorted by mass using a strong magnetic field present inside the MS instrument. The magnetic field deflects the flight paths of positively charged species as a function of their mass. The paths of heavier ions are deflected less than light ones. Because of shorter flight paths, heavier ions reach the instrument's detector before lighter ones. Neutral fragments, such as radicals or molecules, do not interact with the magnetic field and are not detected by the instrument.

MS spectra are plotted with the amount of each cation (**relative intensity**) detected on the vertical axis versus their masses (from lowest to highest) on the horizontal axis. More specifically, the cations' masses are represented by their **mass-to-charge ratio (m/z)**. The charges of the detected cation fragments are almost always +1, so their m/z ratio (mass/1) is an accurate measure of their true masses. Figure 4.23 shows a typical MS spectrum for the compound hexane.

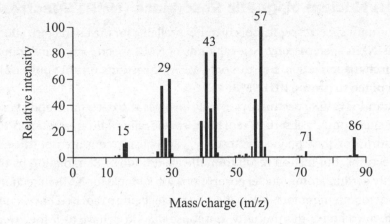

Figure 4.23. The mass spectrum of the alkane hexane
(Source: *http://www.chem.arizona.edu/massspec/*)

To prepare for MCAT questions on this topic, be familiar with three important features of most MS spectra, shown in Figure 4.23. First look for the **base peak.** This is the tallest peak (highest relative intensity) in the spectrum, and it represents the most stable cation fragment. This peak is automatically scaled to 100 and all the other spectrum peaks representing ions in lower abundance are smaller.

Next find the molecular ion peak (the **M peak**), which is usually the first significant peak (to the right of the others) with the largest m/z in the spectrum. This peak represents the molecular weight of the compound. In the case of the example spectrum in Figure 4.23, the hexane's molecular weight is 86 amus. Because all organic compounds contain carbon, about 99 percent of which is the carbon-12 isotope, there is usually a much smaller peak in front of the M peak, called the **M + 1 peak** (this peak is one m/z unit higher than the M peak) which results from the presence of a small amount of carbon-13 isotope in the sample.

Other peaks with an m/z greater than the M + 1 peak are also sometimes present in the spectrum. These are often due to the presence of various halogen isotopes (such as ^{37}Cl and ^{81}Br) in the sample molecules.

The third feature to look for is the pattern of ion peaks shown in the spectrum. These peaks represent the fragmentation pattern of the molecular ion and are usually unique to the molecule being analyzed. Although an exact interpretation of the peak pattern is not usually possible, it can provide clues as to the types of functional groups present in the sample's molecules. For example, if the M peak in a particular MS spectrum has an m/z of 113 and another nearby peak (to the left of the M peak) has an m/z of 78, it can be concluded with confidence that a chlorine atom (35 amus) was lost from the molecular ion and a chloro group must be present in the sample compound molecules.

> ### ESTIMATING M⁺
>
> A mass spectrometer detects the masses of individual molecules. Because of this, the whole-number atomic masses of the most common individual isotopes must be used to estimate the mass of the **M⁺**. For example, the compound in Figure 4.23, hexane, has a whole-number mass of 86 [(6 C × 12 amu) + (14 H × 1 amu) = 86 amu].

Proton (¹H) Nuclear Magnetic Resonance (NMR) Spectroscopy

The most important spectroscopic tool currently available for the characterization of organic compounds is NMR spectroscopy. Several kinds of NMR spectroscopy are commonly used for molecular characterization, but the only MCAT questions on this powerful technique have been confined to **proton (¹H) NMR**.

As with IR and UV/VIS spectroscopy, NMR involves the detection (and presentation in the form of a spectrum) of absorbed radiation, specifically **radio frequency (RF)** radiation. Unlike other forms of absorption spectroscopy, NMR absorptions are not caused by energy changes of electrons, but instead result from the absorption of RF radiation by the nuclei of the atoms. Only certain atomic nuclei absorptions are suitable for NMR detection.

The primary requirement for NMR is that the nuclei being irradiated have a **nuclear spin**. Not all atomic nuclei have this property, but those that do behave as if they were spinning about an axis. Because all nuclei are positively charged, those that spin create their own minute magnetic fields, which can interact with external magnetic fields. The nuclei of both hydrogen and carbon-13 atoms have spin. This makes the use of this technique very valuable for the study of organic compounds because to some extent they always contain these two elements.

Because the nucleus of the atom is all that is studied in this procedure, hydrogen atoms can be referred to simply as protons and the absorption technique is called proton (¹H) NMR. In the absence of an external magnetic field, the spins of protons are randomly oriented, but when exposed to a strong external field, they each become aligned with it. Because each proton has its own magnetic field, there are two possible alignment orientations with the external field, either with it (parallel to it) or against it (antiparallel to it.) Figure 4.24 shows what this orientation process might look like when protons with randomly oriented spins are exposed to an external magnetic field.

The energies of the two possible orientations are not the same. Protons that are antiparallel to the external field are slightly higher in energy than those that are parallel. When a lower energy proton in the parallel state absorbs exactly the right amount of energy, supplied by RF radiation, it can be promoted into the higher energy antiparallel state. When this occurs, the proton is said to have **spin-flipped** and is in **resonance** with the applied RF radiation.

This phenomenon is the basis for nuclear magnetic resonance spectroscopy. The energy absorbed is detected and represented as a peak in an NMR spectrum. The higher the strength of the applied magnetic field, the higher the frequency of the RF radiation required to flip the proton from the parallel spin state to the antiparallel spin state.

> ### TESLA AND GAUSS
>
> 1 tesla (T) = 1×10^4 gauss (G).
>
> Both of these units are commonly used to measure the strength of magnetic fields.

To obtain an NMR spectrum of a compound, the sample is placed inside the field of a superconducting magnet (ranging in strength from about 4.7 to 21.6 tesla) and irradiated with RF radiation of various frequencies (ranging from ~200 to 920 MHz depending on the strength of the instrument's magnetic field). The energy absorbed by the various nuclei generally appears as sharp peaks in the spectrum.

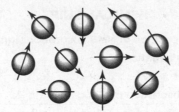

Randomly oriented
spinning protons

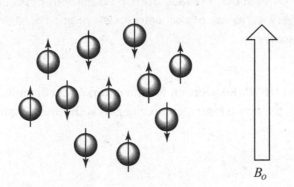

Spinning protons
aligned *with* and *against*
an external magnetic
field (B_o)

B_o

TIP

HYDROGEN AND PROTONS

In discussions related to ^{1}H NMR spectroscopy, the terms *hydrogens* and *protons* are used interchangeably.

Figure 4.24. The alignment of protons with randomly
oriented spins by an applied external magnetic field (B_0)

On the graph of the NMR spectrum, the vertical axis represents the relative intensity of the RF absorption peaks and the horizontal axis shows the position of the absorption peaks. Peak positions (referred to as **chemical shift**) are plotted from high frequency (called **downfield**) on the left to low frequency (called **upfield**) on the right. NMR absorption peak positions are measured relative to a standard reference signal produced by **tetramethylsilane (TMS)** that is added to the analysis sample before the experiment. The TMS absorption signal is arbitrarily assigned at 0 parts per million (ppm). Most NMR absorption signals are well downfield from the reference TMS signal. Figure 4.25 shows the basic layout of a ^{1}H NMR spectrum.

^{1}H NMR Spectrum Orientation

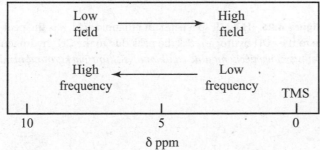

Figure 4.25. The basic format of a ^{1}H NMR spectrum

A typical ^{1}H NMR spectrum for the compound ethanoic acid (commonly referred to as acetic acid, the active ingredient in vinegar) is shown in Figure 4.26.

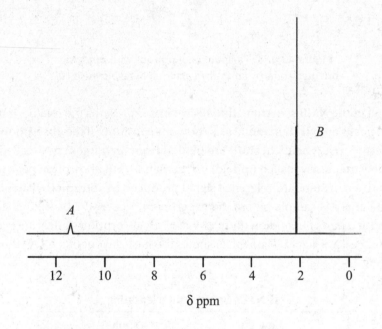

δ ppm

Figure 4.26. ^{1}H NMR spectrum for ethanoic acid: *A* is the peak due to the –OH hydrogen, *B* is the peak due to the CH$_3$ hydrogens. (Source: *http://www.chemguide.co.uk/analysis/nmr/background.html#top*)

The spectrum shows only two absorption peaks at approximately 2.1 ppm and 11.4 ppm. The upfield peak (2.1 ppm) is due to energy absorbed by three protons attached to a carbon and the downfield peak arises from a proton attached to oxygen. Why do these absorptions appear in such different locations in the spectrum and what basic compound characterization information does NMR spectroscopy provide?

NMR spectroscopic data provides the key information needed to map out the carbon-hydrogen skeleton of an organic compound. This carbon-hydrogen connectivity, along with a little additional information (such as a molecular formula and possible functional groups present) is key to assigning a compound a complete structural formula. There are four key pieces of information that an NMR spectrum can provide.

1. **THE NUMBER OF ABSORPTION SIGNALS (PEAKS) IN THE SPECTRUM.** The number of peaks that are observed in a ^{1}H NMR spectrum tells the analyst the number of different magnetic environments that the compound's protons (hydrogens) are experiencing. In other words, the number of peaks seen in the spectrum indicates the number of magnetically nonequivalent protons in the molecule. If all the proton environments are the same, then only one peak is observed, but this is relatively rare. In most cases protons attached to different atoms in the compound have different magnetic characteristics. The example spectrum shown in Figure 4.26 shows two peaks, which indicates that two different "kinds" of protons are present in the ethanoic acid molecule.

2. **THE POSITION (CHEMICAL SHIFTS) OF THE PEAKS IN THE SPECTRUM.** **Shielded** and **deshielded** are terms used to categorize the different magnetic environments of protons. Shielded protons tend to have higher electron density around them and feel the external magnetic field of the spectrometer relatively less. These protons are usually, but not always, bonded to lower electronegativity atoms, such as carbon, or are a significant distance from other more electronegative atoms, such as oxygen, nitrogen, or halogens, in the compound. Peaks associated with shielded protons are usually found upfield (closer to the TMS peak) at lower absorption frequencies. Deshielded protons have lower electron density around them and feel the external magnetic field of the spectrometer relatively more. They are usually either bonded directly to a significantly higher electronegative atom or near one in the molecule being analyzed. The signals from these protons appear downfield (farther away from the TMS peak) at high absorption frequencies.

Just by looking at a proton's chemical shift, it is possible to determine which type of atom it is either bonded to or very near in the compound's structure. For example, as Figure 4.26 shows, the absorption peak for a hydrogen attached to a highly electronegative oxygen atom in ethanoic acid is significantly farther down field (11.4 ppm) relative to the hydrogens attached to a much less electronegative carbon atom (2.1 ppm). The chemical shifts of protons in NMR spectra can provide valuable information about the structural connectivity and possible functional groups present in the molecule. Figure 4.27 shows the relative chemical shift ranges for protons associated with the functional groups most commonly seen on the MCAT.

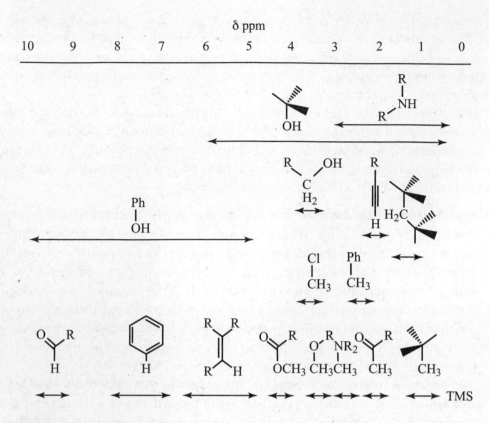

Figure 4.27. The relative chemical shifts of protons in ^1H NMR Spectra. Note: Protons attached to alkene and phenyl functional groups are significantly less shielded (farther down field) than protons attached to most other types of atoms. This is because of proton's interaction with the π bonding system in these functional groups.

3. THE SPLITTING PATTERNS OF THE ABSORPTION SIGNALS. When a carbon with hydrogen substituents is bonded to one or more carbons with hydrogen substituents, the absorption signals of the neighboring hydrogens are split into **groups of peaks**. The splitting is caused by the nonequivalent neighboring hydrogens' magnetic fields interacting with each other. If a hydrogen (or group of hydrogens) has no immediate neighbors, as can be seen in the spectrum of ethanoic acid (Figure 4.26) its absorption signal remains unsplit and it appears as a single peak or **singlet**. The hydrogens' magnetic fields in ethanoic acid are too far apart to "feel" each other.

In general, the number of peaks an absorption signal is split into is equal to the number of its neighboring hydrogens plus one peak. This is called the ***n* + 1 splitting rule**, where ***n*** is the number of immediate neighboring hydrogen atoms that the absorption signal interacts with. This splitting pattern leads to groups of peaks that are referred to as **doublets** (one neighboring hydrogen), **triplets** (two neighboring hydrogens), **quartets** (three neighboring hydrogens), **pentets** (four neighboring hydrogens), and **sextets** (five neighboring hydrogens). When a signal is split into more than six peaks it is referred to as a **multiplet**. Figure 4.28, the ^1H NMR spectrum of ethyl acetate, shows an example of the peak splitting phenomenon.

Notice the peak groups (from left to right)—a quartet, a singlet, and a triplet. The annotated structural formula of ethyl acetate (Structure 46) shows how the molecule's protons interact with each other to produce this splitting pattern.

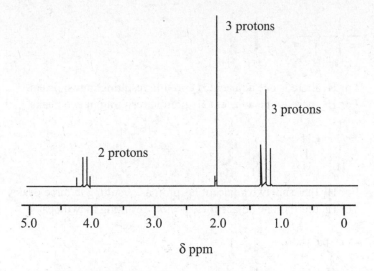

Figure 4.28. ^{1}H NMR spectrum for ethyl acetate. Note: The numbers next to each peak group indicate the number of protons associated with each absorption signal in the spectrum.

(46)

Point *A* is CH_3 next to carbon without attached hydrogens (a singlet). Point *B* is CH_3 next to carbon with two hydrogens attached (a triplet). Point *C* is a CH_2 next to carbon with three attached hydrogens (a quartet).

As can be seen from the ethyl acetate example, the splitting patterns observed in NMR spectra can provide valuable information about the connectivity of the carbon skeleton and the number of hydrogens attached to each of the skeleton carbons. There are certain splitting patterns that are seen repeatedly in ^{1}H NMR spectra. The ones most commonly seen in spectra encountered on the MCAT are shown in Figure 4.29. The reviewer should become familiar with these patterns and the structural information they provide.

There is an important exception to the splitting phenomenon. Generally, when protons are attached to atoms that are significantly more electronegative than carbon, such as oxygen or nitrogen, their absorption signals are not split. These proton signals appear as ***singlets*** even if they are next to a carbon with hydrogen. The reason these protons signals are not split is rather complex. Being aware of this exception is important for the MCAT, but a complete understanding of the mechanism is not.

4. THE RELATIVE SIZE OF THE PROTON ABSORPTION PEAKS. The relative areas under the absorption peaks in a ^{1}H NMR spectrum provide data about the relative ratios of the different kinds of protons present in the compound being analyzed. The area under each peak is measured in the form of an integral line (also called an integral trace) which is computer generated. The integral line is superimposed on top of the NMR spectrum and crosses over all the peak groups in steps from left to right.

A. 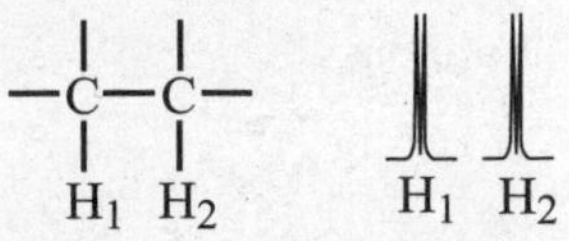 $-\overset{|}{\underset{H_1}{C}}-\overset{|}{\underset{H_2}{C}}-$

For H_1 there is one adjacent H_2 proton, resulting in two peaks.
For H_2 there is one adjacent H_1 proton, resulting in two peaks.

B. 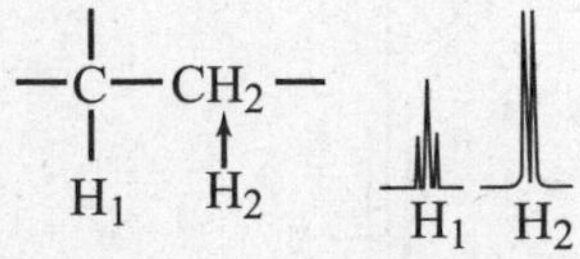 $-\overset{|}{\underset{H_1}{C}}-\underset{\underset{H_2}{\uparrow}}{CH_2}-$

For H_1 there are two adjacent H_2 protons, resulting in three peaks.
For H_2 there is one adjacent H_1 proton, resulting in two peaks.

C. 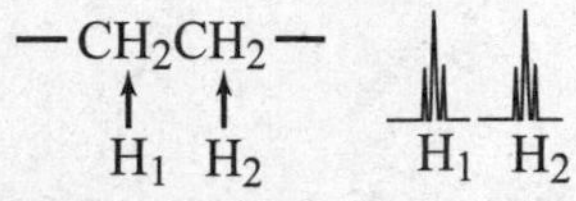 $-\underset{\underset{H_1}{\uparrow}}{CH_2}\underset{\underset{H_2}{\uparrow}}{CH_2}-$

For H_1 there are two adjacent H_2 protons, resulting in three peaks.
For H_2 there are two adjacent H_1 protons, resulting in three peaks.

D. 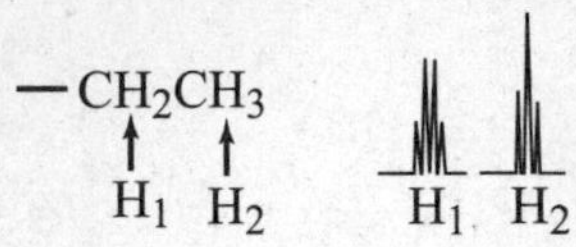 $-\underset{\underset{H_1}{\uparrow}}{CH_2}\underset{\underset{H_2}{\uparrow}}{CH_3}$

For H_1 there are three adjacent H_2 protons, resulting in four peaks.
For H_2 there are two adjacent H_1 protons, resulting in three peaks.

E. 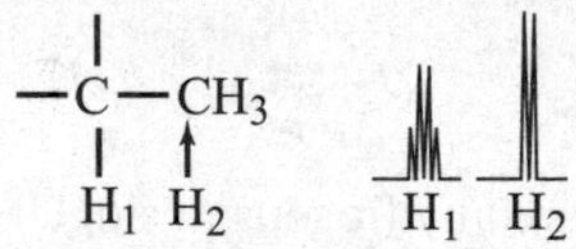 $-\overset{|}{\underset{H_1}{C}}-\underset{\underset{H_2}{\uparrow}}{CH_3}$

For H_1 there are three adjacent H_2 protons, resulting in four peaks.
For H_2 there is one adjacent H_1 proton, resulting in two peaks.

Two peaks = doublet, three peaks = triplet, four peaks = quartet

Figure 4.29. ^{1}H NMR spectra splitting patterns commonly seen on the MCAT

The height and number of peaks in a peak group correspond to the number of protons with the same approximate chemical shift. The heights of the steps of the integral trace are proportional to the area under the peak groups. Figure 4.30 shows an example ^{1}H NMR spectrum, of the compound propanoic acid, that includes the integrator trace. The spectrum shows three different peak groups, indicating that three different kinds of protons are present in the compound.

The relative heights of the integrator line steps associated with each peak group in the figure show that the ratios of the different kinds of protons (from left to right) in propanoic acid are 1:2:3. In this particular case, this ratio represents the actual number of different kinds of protons in the molecule: the –COOH group (1 proton), the –CH$_2$ group (2 protons), and the –CH$_3$ group (3 protons). This is often, but not always, the case. Sometimes the integral areas only provide the relative number of different kinds of protons in a compound.

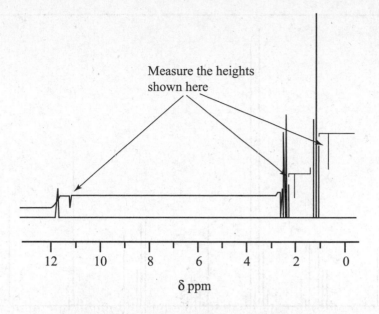

Figure 4.30. ¹H NMR spectrum of propanoic acid, CH_3CH_2COOH, showing the integrator trace.

Practice Exercise 11

Assign a structural formula to an unknown compound. The spectral data (an IR spectrum, an MS spectrum, and a ¹H NMR spectrum) and molecular formula associated with an unknown compound are given below.

Unknown Compound's Molecular Formula: $C_5H_{10}O_2$

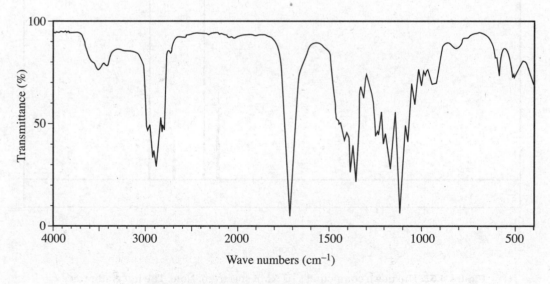

Figure 4.31. Unknown compound's IR spectrum

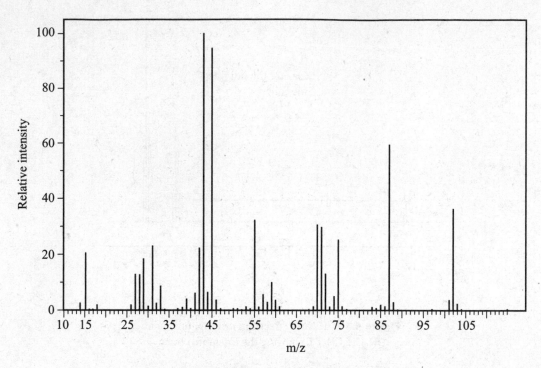

Figure 4.32. Unknown compound's MS spectrum

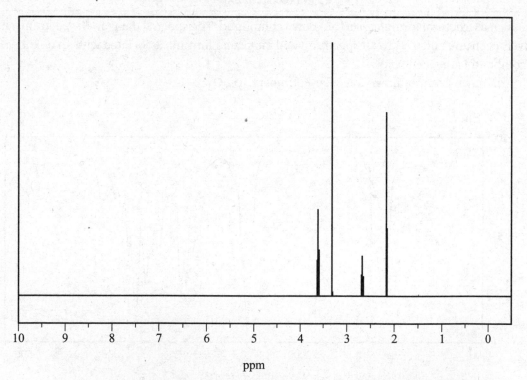

Figure 4.33. Unknown compound's ¹H NMR spectrum. Note: The integrator trace
is not shown on this spectrum. Try to estimate the number of hydrogens associated
with the absorptions using the relative sizes of each peak group (total of four groups).
This may take some trial and error to get right.

Using the above information, propose the best possible structural formula for the
unknown compound.

SEPARATION AND PURIFICATION TECHNIQUES

Before a compound can be fully characterized, used in a synthesis scheme, tested in a product or clinical trial, or patented, it must meet certain purity standards. Depending on the application, these standards may require an extremely pure substance (>99.9%) or something only relatively pure (~90%). Organic chemists spend considerable time perfecting purification processes, procedures that separate the desired compound from the rest of the matrix.

The most common separation processes are:

- Extraction
- Distillation (several kinds)
- Chromatography (many kinds)
- Recrystallization
- Electrophoresis
- Sublimation
- Centrifugation
- Filtration (several kinds)
- Decanting

For the MCAT, you should have a very basic understanding of all of these techniques, but you should be particularly familiar with **extraction**, **distillation**, **chromatography**, **recrystallization**, and **filtration**.

Extraction

Extraction is the selective partitioning of a desired substance into a phase from which it can be easily removed. The process separates the substance from other components in the matrix and thus to some extent purifies it. There are several possible phase combinations for an extraction process (solid–liquid, liquid–liquid, gas–liquid, and others.) The most common procedure is **liquid–liquid** extraction.

The most critical factor in a liquid–liquid extraction is the selection of the two liquid phases. In most cases one liquid will be water and the other some low boiling, relatively nonpolar organic solvent. It is most important that the two liquids be **immiscible**. They must form separate layers, like oil and water, in the extraction vessel and cannot dissolve into each other.

Other important criteria for liquids used in an extraction are:

- Neither liquid can react in a chemically irreversible way with the desired solute (the compound the chemist is trying to isolate).
- The extracting liquid added to the compound solution must have a higher affinity for the solute than the solvent it is dissolved in. The higher the affinity (referred to as the **partition coefficient**) of the extracting liquid the better.
- Once the solute has been partitioned into the higher affinity liquid (the extracting solvent), it must be relatively easy to remove that liquid (for example, by evaporation).

Liquid–liquid extractions are carried out using a special piece of laboratory glassware called a **separatory funnel**. These specially shaped funnels have a ground glass/Teflon stopcock and ground glass/Teflon stopper. Figure 4.34 shows an example.

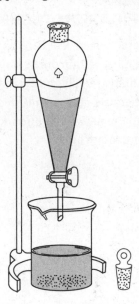

Figure 4.34. Standard separatory funnel supported on a ring stand.
Note: The shaded organic phase is being drained into a beaker leaving the colorless aqueous phase in the funnel. The ground glass stopper is used to seal the funnel while the contents are being shaken.

The use of a separatory funnel for extractions is straightforward. Place the compound solution in the funnel and then add an extracting solvent, making sure the two liquids form separate layers. Next, the funnel is sealed with a stopper (see Figure 4.34) and shaken to allow the two liquid phases to commingle. After shaking, the liquid phases are allowed to separate. Finally, the extracting liquid, which now hopefully contains the desired compound, is drained from the funnel and saved.

MISCIBILITY

Miscible: The two liquids are soluble in each other and form a single phase, like water and alcohol.

Immiscible: The two liquids are insoluble in each other and form two phases, like oil and water.

Depending on the organic solvent used, the aqueous phase may be on the top (organic phase is more dense) or on the bottom (organic phase is less dense). More than one extraction with the extracting solvent is usually performed to make sure all the solute (desired compound) has been removed from the original solution. The extraction volumes are combined, and the solvent is usually evaporated, leaving the isolated compound.

Liquid–liquid extraction is often used to separate weak organic acids and bases from a reaction matrix. This takes advantage of the fact that both of these classes of compounds can often be converted to water-soluble salts.

Figure 4.35 shows a flow chart of a procedure used to separate a carboxylic acid (in this case benzoic acid) from a neutral compound (naphthalene) by extracting (shaking in a separatory funnel) the organic phase (diethyl ether) with a dilute aqueous solution of sodium hydroxide.

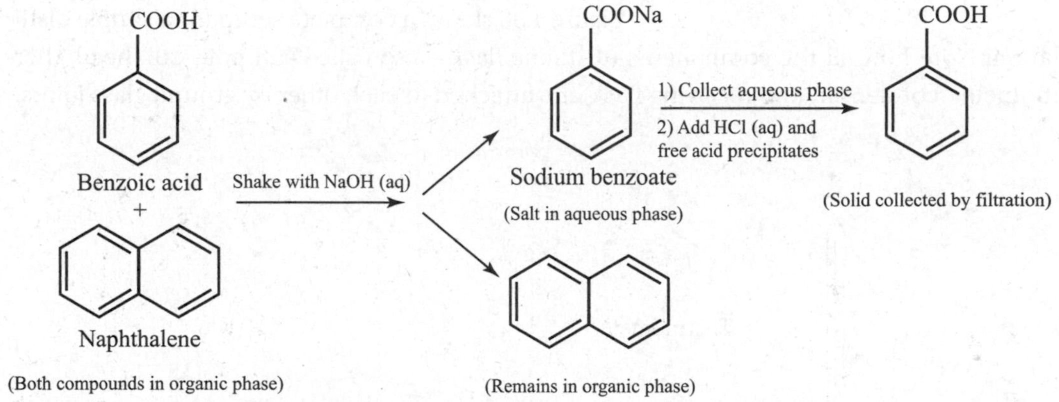

Figure 4.35. Separation of benzoic acid from naphthalene by aqueous sodium hydroxide extraction

As seen in the figure, benzoic acid reacts with aqueous sodium hydroxide (while being shaken in a separatory funnel) and is converted into the water-soluble salt, sodium benzoate. This salt migrates into the aqueous phase. The neutral naphthalene is unchanged and remains in the organic phase. The aqueous phase containing the sodium benzoate is collected and acidified to give a precipitate of the free benzoic acid, which is collected by filtration. A very similar scheme can be used to separate a weak organic base, such as an amine, from a neutral compound, except that the amine is shaken with an aqueous solution of an acid (such as hydrochloric acid). The amine reacts with the acid to form a soluble salt, which, as in the above example, migrates into the aqueous phase. The free amine is isolated by adding base to the collected aqueous phase.

An organic acid and organic base can also be separated from each other using the above principles. For practice, devise a scheme for carrying out such a separation. Questions involving this kind of separation have appeared on the MCAT.

Distillation

When separation of two or more **miscible** liquids is required, **distillation** is usually used. Distillation involves preferentially vaporizing a liquid (or liquids) with a high vapor pressure and then condensing the vapor back to a liquid so that it can be collected. Liquids with low boiling points vaporize at lower temperatures than those with high boiling points. The larger the difference between the liquids' boiling points, the easier the separation by this procedure. Depending on the difference between the volatility of the liquids, different forms of distillation are used.

SIMPLE DISTILLATION

This technique is used to separate relatively low boiling (<150°C) liquids that have large differences in boiling points. There should be at least a 30°C difference in boiling points for simple distillation to be successful. This procedure can also be used to separate a liquid from nonvolatile impurities, such as soluble salts and high molecular weight solutes.

Figure 4.36 shows a complete setup for a simple distillation. Note how all the components (distilling flask—also called still pot—still head, thermometer, condenser, and receiving flask) are attached to each other by ground glass joints.

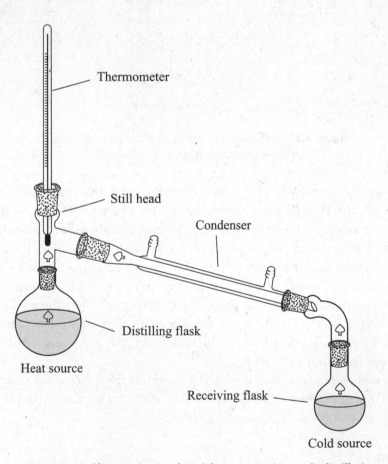

Figure 4.36. Glassware setup for a laboratory scale simple distillation

The liquids to be separated are placed in the distilling flask and heated. When the lower boiling liquid's boiling point is reached, its vapors begin to travel though the still head until they reach the condenser (which is usually cooled by tap water) where the cold surface recondenses the vapor into a liquid. The liquid flows down the angled condenser by gravity, eventually dripping into the receiving flask (usually cooled in an ice bath). As long as the boiling temperature of the liquid, as verified by the thermometer, remains relatively constant, it can be assumed that the liquid being collected is pure.

VACUUM DISTILLATION

This procedure is very similar to simple distillation but is used for separation of liquids that boil above 150°C. At ambient temperatures, such liquids would have to be heated to high temperatures before they would begin to vaporize. In many cases they are heat sensitive and instead of vaporizing, they would decompose before they begin to boil. If the pressure is lowered by a vacuum source, the liquids' vapor pressures increase and they boil at lower temperatures. The lower the pressure, the lower the temperature at which they boil. Lower boiling points can prevent heat-induced decomposition. This type of distillation, like simple distillation, requires a boiling point difference of at least 30°C.

The only difference in the glassware setup for this type of still is the addition of a side-arm connector to the adaptor between the condenser and the receiving flask (see Figure 4.36). Figure 4.37 shows an example of this type of vacuum adaptor.

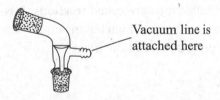

Vacuum line is attached here

Figure 4.37. Vacuum adaptor for low pressure distillations

FRACTIONAL DISTILLATIONS

This type of distillation can separate liquids whose boiling points are closer together than 30°C. Sophisticated setups can separate liquids that boil as close to each other as a couple of degrees. For this procedure, the basic still setup remains the same, except that a **fractionating column** is placed between the still head and the distilling flask. This setup is designed to force the vapor mixture from the distilling flask to condense and revaporize over and over again as it rises through the fractionating column. Each condensing-revaporizing cycle results in a slight enrichment in the proportion of the lower boiling liquid in the vapor phase. By the time the vapor mixture reaches the top of the column, it is composed almost exclusively of the lower boiling component. Figure 4.38 shows an example of a fractionating column used for fractional distillations.

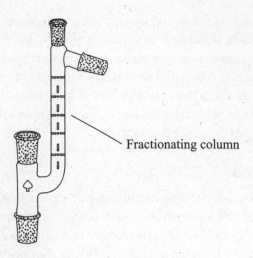

Figure 4.38. A fractionating column used for fractional distillations

There are a number of different kinds of fractionating columns. The one shown in the figure above has small glass protrusions that extend from the wall of the column into the interior. These tiny glass "fingers" serve as condensing sites as the vapor mixture rises through the column. Other fractionating columns are simple glass tubes that have been filled with high surface area materials such as copper wool, glass beads, or even coarse glass wool. The compounds being separated are collected using a different receiving flask for each compound. These different collections are called **fractions**. It is also possible to perform a **fractional vacuum** distillation to separate high boiling liquids whose boiling points are close to each other, although the procedure is a little tricky.

Chromatography

The most advanced methodology currently available for separating mixtures of substances is a large set of techniques collectively referred to as **chromatography**. This separation process is used daily in laboratory and industrial settings around the world. There are hundreds, if not thousands, of different kinds of chromatography, with entire journals devoted to the use and development of new methods.

For the MCAT, you should be familiar with two phases present in all chromotography—the **stationary phase** and the **mobile phase**. The general process for chromotography involves first introducing the sample (usually a mixture of compounds) to a stationary phase. The stationary phase is a medium of some type (for example, paper, silica gel, or a viscous oil) for which the components of the sample mixture have an affinity, meaning that to some degree the components all stick to the medium. The sample mixture clinging to the stationary phase is then exposed to a mobile phase, usually a liquid or a gas. The mobile phase moves through the stationary phase, carrying the sample components with it.

> **"GRAPH OF COLORS"**
>
> **Chromatography** literally means "graph of colors" because its earliest use by German chemists was to isolate plant pigments.

This process is called **elution**. Depending on the affinity of each component for the stationary phase (how "hard" they stick together), the component moves at a different rate as the mobile phase carries it along. The lower the component's affinity for the stationary phase, the more quickly it moves as it is carried by the mobile phase. The higher the component's affinity, the more slowly it moves. The key separation mechanism that allows the process to work is that all the components of the sample mixture have slightly different affinities for the stationary phase. Thus, over time, as the mobile phase moves through the stationary phase, the mixture components are separated because they move at different rates.

Based on the desired applications, there are generally two categories of chromatography:

1. Those that are used for **analytical** purposes
2. Those that are used for **preparative** purposes

The analytical methods are used to provide data about the sample mixture, such as the number and relative amounts of its components and the identity of the components. Preparative methods are used to separate and actually isolate components (in some cases on an industrial scale) from the sample mixture so that their properties can be further studied.

ANALYTICAL CHROMATOGRAPHY

Thin-layer chromatography (TLC) is one of the most commonly used types of analytical chromatography. It can also be adapted for preparative uses, but it is generally limited to producing small laboratory scale samples. This description will focus on its analytical application.

The stationary phase of TLC is, as the name implies, a thin layer of medium that is coated onto a glass, plastic, or metal plate. The most commonly used media are silica gel and alumina. These are highly polar materials and result in a "polar phase" TLC plate. The more polar an analite, the more strongly it interacts with the polar phase on the plate and the more slowly it moves with the system's mobile phase. There are other media that are also used to prepare nonpolar or "reverse phase" TLC plates, but these are not as common. The mobile phase for this technique is a solvent system, usually a mixture of two or more slightly polar and nonpolar organic solvents.

The sample mixture (usually in solution phase) is placed near the bottom of the TLC plate (called the **origin**) as a small curricular spot, using a very thin glass capillary tube. See Figure 4.39 for an example of a TLC plate with sample spots.

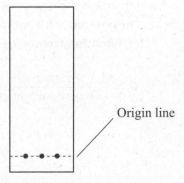

Figure 4.39. TLC plate with sample spots on origin line

The plate is allowed to dry and is then placed in a sealed elution chamber containing a small amount of the solvent system (a few millimeters in the bottom of the container). As soon as the plate (the stationary phase) makes contact with the solvent (the mobile phase) at the bottom of the chamber, it begins to move up the plate by capillary action. A faint line that is formed by the moving solvent is referred to as the **solvent front**. As the solvent moves up the plate, the sample mixture components begin to separate (based on their affinity for the plate medium) into individual spots. Figure 4.40 shows a simulated "time-lapse" view of this process.

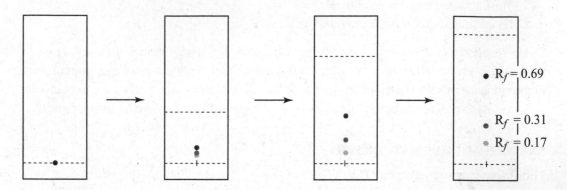

Figure 4.40. A simulated time-lapse view of the solvent front moving up a TLC plate. Note: The lower dotted line represents the sample origin line and the upper dotted line the solvent front. Observe how the solvent front moves up the plate and the sample component spots get more separated over time.

When the solvent front nears the top of the TLC plate, the plate is removed from the elution chamber, the position of the front marked (a pencil should be used), and the solvent allowed to evaporate. There are a number of ways to visualize the component spots. Sometimes they absorb light in the visible part of the spectrum and they appear colored to the human eye, making them easy to see. More often they absorb in the UV region. To visualize these spots, the plate is irradiated with UV radiation from a "black light," which makes them glow violet or blue-violet.

The position of the component spots can be quantified using **retention factor** (R_f) calculations where:

$$R_f = \frac{\text{Distance spot moved from the origin}}{\text{Distance solvent front moved from the origin}}$$

TLC PLATES

The typical TLC plate is between 10 and 15 cm long, and it can take 15 to 20 minutes for the solvent front to reach near the top of the plate. Theoretically, the longer the plate, the greater the possible separation between the components spots. However, there are practical considerations that limit the length of TLC plates.

Distances used to calculate R_f's are usually measured in centimeters; thus, these length units cancel in the calculation and R_f's are unitless. It should be noted that R_f values are always less than or equal to one ($R_f \leq 1$) because the distance the spot moved must be less than the distance of the solvent front. There are tabulated R_f values for specific compounds in reference books that can be compared to those calculated for lab experiments. This may allow the identification of some sample components, but the comparison is only valid if the reference R_f's and the experiment R_f's were obtained under identical experimental conditions. The TLC plate to the far right in Figure 4.40 above shows the R_f's (from bottom to top of plate R_f's = 0.17, 0.31, and 0.69) for the component spots for the simulated sample mixture elution.

Other common types of analytical chromatography include **paper chromatography** and **gas–liquid chromatography (GLC)**.

Paper chromatography is very similar to but less effective than TLC. Instead of a medium coated plate, a strip of porous paper is used for the stationary phase. A solvent system moves up the paper by capillary action separating the components of the sample as in TLC.

Gas–liquid chromatography (GLC) is a more sophisticated and sensitive procedure that involves the use of an instrument called a **gas chromatogram (GC)**. In this case, the stationary phase is often a viscous silicon oil that coats the inside of a long very thin glass column, which is housed inside the gas chromatogram instrument. The temperature of the column is carefully controlled by computer-defined settings. The column can be heated to a constant temperature or the temperature can be varied.

The mobile phase for this process, unlike in the other techniques described above, is a gas. The gas, often helium or nitrogen, flows through the column at various rates, depending on the desired experiment conditions. The sample mixture is introduced into the column (the stationary phase) either neat or in solution with a heated syringe. Only very small samples (microgram levels are enough) are needed for good analytical results. As the gas flows through the heated column, it forces the vaporized sample mixture into contact with the oil coating on the interior of the column. Different components of the mixture have different affinities for the oil coating (as well as different boiling points) and move though the column at different rates, resulting in separation. As the mixture components exit the column, they are detected by various types of sensors, depending on the instrument setup.

Once detected, the components appear as peaks of varying heights on a computer screen. The chromatogram gives information about not only the number of components in the mixture, but the relative amount of each as well. A significant limitation of this type of chromatography is that the sample components must be fairly volatile to make it through the instrument column. High molecular weight compounds cannot generally be analyzed by this procedure because they decompose prior to vaporizing. Figure 4.41 shows a schematic diagram of a very basic instrument used for GLC experiments.

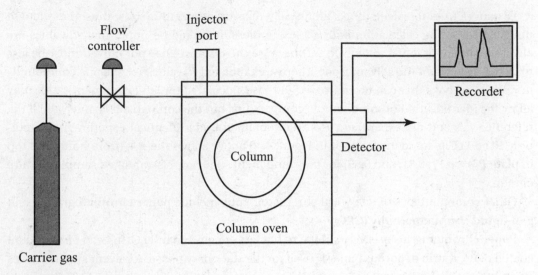

Figure 4.41. Schematic diagram of a simple gas chromatograph used for GLC experiments

PREPARATIVE CHROMATOGRAPHY

Most forms of preparative chromatography involve the use of media-packed columns. As with other forms of chromatography, there are many kinds of media that can serve as the stationary phase, but the most commonly used for organic compounds are silica gel and alumina. As with TLC, these media produce a very polar stationary phase.

In its simplest form, a long glass or quartz column is packed with medium. The column has one open end and a stopcock valve with a fritted glass filter (to retain the medium) at the other end. Figure 4.42 shows an example of such a column.

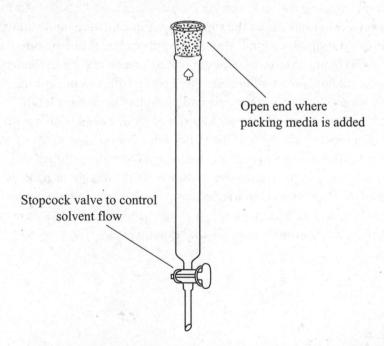

Open end where
packing media is added

Stopcock valve to control
solvent flow

Figure 4.42. Glass/Quartz column used for holding packing media

The packing process can be done either dry or wet (the column is first filled with a solvent and then the medium is added). A few centimeters of sand are usually added to the top of the media column to stabilize it. Following packing, the stopcock is opened and a solvent system (the mobile phase) is carefully added to the top of the column until it is freely flowing out the open valve at the bottom. Once a few volumes of solvent have flowed through the column, the solvent level is allowed to drop until it is just below the sand layer at the top of the column. The stopcock is then closed. The column cannot be allowed to run dry, because this can cause the tightly packed medium to "crack" and create fissures, degrading the column's separation ability.

The last step of the setup is to introduce the sample mixture to be separated onto the sand layer at the top of the column. This must be done carefully in order to avoid disturbing the packed medium. Typically, if the sample is a liquid, it is placed on the sand neat. If it is a solid, a very concentrated solution can be used. Once the sample has settled a centimeter or so into the sand, the stopcock is opened and small amounts of the solvent system are carefully added until the column is full. Some columns have a glass bulb that can be attached to the top of the column so that it can hold large volumes of solvent. Otherwise, the user must continually add new solvent, not letting the level drop below the sand.

The separation process occurs as the solvent system (the mobile phase) flows through the tightly packed media (the stationary phase) carrying the sample mixture. It is sometimes possible to see bands of different colors form, corresponding to different components of the mixture. To be able to see colored bands, as with colored spots for TLC, is the exception. If a quartz column is employed, it will allow UV radiation to pass. Violet glowing bands can be seen if the lab is darkened and the column is illuminated with a powerful black light. As the component bands reach the bottom of the column, they flow out and are collected as **solution fractions** (sample components dissolved in the mobile phase). After all the desired fractions are collected, the solvent is evaporated from each one to yield a pure sample of each component. Pure multi-gram or larger quantities of each component can be obtained this way.

An automated type of packed column chromatography similar to GLC called **high performance liquid chromatography (HPLC)** can also be used to obtain fairly large quantities of hard-to-purify compounds. It uses pre-packed medium columns with very high separation ability housed inside a temperature-controlled instrument connected to a computer. The mobile phase, just as with simple column chromatography, is a solvent system that is pumped through the stationary phase column media at very high pressures.

The various mixture components are detected as they leave the column and collected as solutions fractions, just as with simple column chromatography.

Recrystallization and Filtration

An easy and effective way to purify solid organic compounds is to **recrystallize** them. This separation process relies on the fact that as the temperature of a solvent increases, the solubility of a solute increases. Likewise, as the temperature of a solvent decreases, the solubility of a solute decreases.

Purification by recrystallization involves taking an impure (or crude) solid compound, dispersing it in a cold or room temperature solvent contained in a beaker, and then heating the mixture until a solution is formed. The hot solution is then sometimes poured through filter paper (referred to as a **hot filtration**) to remove any insoluble impurities. The resulting clear solution can be further heated if necessary to make sure it remains completely homogeneous. Next, the beaker is covered and insulated and the hot solution allowed to very slowly cool to room temperature.

HPLC

High performance liquid chromotography was once referred to as high pressure liquid chromatography, but the term is no longer common.

TEMPERATURE AND SOLUBILITY

Higher temperature generally means higher solubility. There are a few exceptions to this rule, particularly among ionic compounds, but it almost always holds true for organic compounds.

As the solution cools, the solubility of the compound being purified decreases and at some point, assuming too much solvent was not used, it begins to fall out of solution as pure crystals. In general, the slower the solution cools, the larger the resulting crystals. Large crystals of the compound are desirable because they are easier to collect and often higher in purity. In most cases, the impurities, which were a minor portion of the original crude compound, remain in solution. Thus the compound is purified by selective solubility—with the compound less soluble and the impurities more soluble. Choosing the correct recrystallizing solvent is critical for achieving this balance. In order to maximize the recovery of the "recrystallized" compound, the mixture is usually cooled below room temperature using an ice bath or other cooling source. This further reduces the solubility of the compound, which facilitates additional crystal formation.

Once crystallization is deemed complete, the crystals are typically collected by either **gravity** or **vacuum filtration**. Figure 4.43 shows what the cooled, recrystallized compound might look like before filtration.

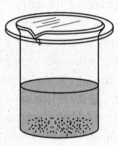

Figure 4.43. Recrystallized compound ready for collection

Note that the beaker is covered with a watch glass to provide insulation, which facilitates slower cooling of the solution. Observe the newly formed crystals on the bottom of the beaker.

As indicated earlier, the most important factor in achieving a good recrystallization result is solvent selection. The balance between the compound's solubility in the hot solvent and its solubility at lower temperatures has to be just right. Often, as in chromatography separations, a solvent system composed of two or more solvents is used. The most common systems involve dissolving the compound to be purified in a fairly polar solvent first and then adding small amounts of a nonpolar solvent until the compound just begins to come out of solution. This tipping point is apparent when the mixture begins to become slightly cloudy. Next the mixture is heated until completely clear and a slow cooling process started. The reverse system, in which the dissolving solvent is nonpolar and small amounts of a polar solvent are added, is also common.

The second most important factor is deciding how much of the solvent system to use. Usually less is better. Too much solvent prevents crystals from forming. Reheating the mixture and boiling off some of the excess solvent can correct this, but this wastes solvent and can be hazardous if the solvent is flammable. A better approach is to use less solvent and more heat (without boiling) and add a little more solvent as needed to completely dissolve the crude compound.

Pure compound crystals formed during recrystallization are typically collected by filtration. If they are not extremely fine, vacuum filtration is the best choice. This approach uses a Buchner funnel and filtration flask. There are a number of different designs for this equipment but the setup must have a side-arm connector that can be attached to a vacuum source—thus the term vacuum filtration. Figure 4.44 shows an all-glass vacuum filtration system.

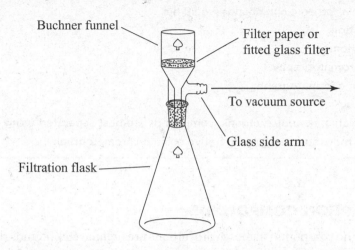

Figure 4.44. Laboratory glassware setup for vacuum filtration

The compound crystals are suspended in the recrystallization solvent and poured into the Buchner funnel and vacuum applied. As the pressure in the filtration flask is lowered by the vacuum source, solvent (the **filtrate**) is pulled through the porous Buchner funnel (some require filter paper and other designs have a fitted glass filter), leaving behind the solid crystals. The crystals are usually washed with pure cold solvent to remove any surface impurities. Here again, it is almost always better to be conservative with the amount of solvent used to wash the crystals. Too much solvent will often dissolve some of the desired compound, lowering the yield.

If the crystals are very small, like a fine powder, the pores of the filter may become clogged when vacuum is applied. In this situation, it is best to use **gravity filtration**, which uses larger pieces of filter paper that are less prone to becoming clogged. The folded or fluted filter paper is inserted into a regular glass funnel. As the name implies, the solvent slowly flows through the filter paper by gravity into a receiving flask, leaving the crystals behind. Figure 4.45 shows the glassware for this simple setup. As with vacuum filtration, the collected compound crystals should be washed with cold solvent and allowed to dry as the final step.

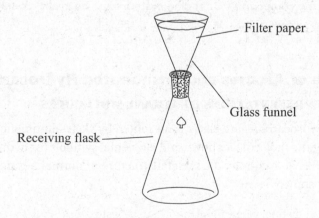

Figure 4.45. Glassware setup for gravity filtration

The most appropriate method for separating a large quantity of a mixture of nonvolatile, nonpolar organic compounds would be:

(A) distillation.

(B) extraction.

(C) gas chromatography.

(D) column chromatography.

(D) Nonvolatile, nonpolar, organic compounds are best separated using chromatography and more specifically preparative column chromatography.

HYDROCARBON COMPOUNDS

As implied by the compound name, hydrocarbons are organic compounds that contain only the elements hydrogen and carbon.

The MCAT focuses on knowledge and concepts related to one particular hydrocarbon, **alkanes**. Alkanes have the general molecular formula $C_N H_{2N+2}$, where N is a positive whole number integer. Alkanes are called **saturated** hydrocarbons because they contain the maximum number of hydrogen atoms possible for their molecular structures.

Compounds consisting of only hydrogen and carbon that contain less than the maximum numbers of allowable hydrogen atoms are referred to as **unsaturated** hydrocarbons. There are three categories of unsaturated hydrocarbons:

1. **Alkenes:** general formula of $C_N H_{2N}$
2. **Alkynes:** general formula of $C_N H_{2N-2}$
3. **Aromatic:** compounds.

AROMATIC COMPOUNDS AND HÜCKEL'S RULE

The term *aromatic* originally referred literally to the fragrance of some organic compounds. Today it describes a special group of compounds that follow **Hückel's rule**. To be aromatic it must possess **$4n + 2\pi$ electrons** (where n is a positive integer). Also, the compound's π bonding system must be **cyclic, conjugated,** and in a planar conformation.

Nomenclature of Alkanes and Unsaturated Hydrocarbons

STRUCTURAL REPRESENTATIONS OF ALKANE MOLECULES

The structures of hydrocarbons are easily represented by skeletal nomenclature. Only the σ bonding skeleton of the molecule is shown and elemental symbols for hydrogen and carbons atoms are omitted. As an example, the skeletal structure of normal hexane (Structure 47), a common alkane, is shown below.

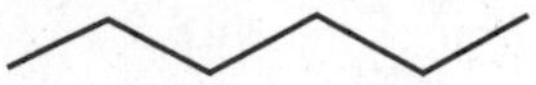

(47)

ABBREVIATED IUPAC RULES FOR NAMING ALKANES

A detailed understanding of the nomenclature of organic compounds is not necessary for most MCAT questions. If you are asked to recognize the name of a compound, it will most probably be an alkane. You should be familiar with the specific naming rules, then, for alkanes.

To understand the naming rules, we can divide alkanes into two categories: **normal** or open chain structures and **cyclic** structures.

The most important factor in correctly naming **normal** (open chain) **alkanes** is identifying the longest and most branched carbon chain (the principal chain) in the compound's structure. This provides the base name for the compound, using a Greek prefix (in most cases) indicating the number of carbon atoms in the principal chain followed by the letters "**ane**" for alkane. The principal chain prefixes for up to ten carbons are as follows: meth-, eth-, prop-, but-, pent-, hex-, hept-, oct-, non-, and dec-. The first four can be remembered by the mnemonic "***mom eats peanut butter***" (**m**eth-, **e**th-, **p**rop-, and **b**ut-).

Small carbon branches (called alkyl substituents) attached to the principal chain are named and numbered so as to give the lowest set of attachment numbers possible. When writing the final compound name, substituents attached to the principal chain are listed in alphabetical order in front of the base name with their respective attachment numbers shown first. A list of the most common alkyl substituents along with their structures is shown in Table 4.4.

Table 4.4 Common Alkyl Substituents and Their Structures

Methyl	Ethyl	Propyl
$-CH_3$	$-CH_2CH_3$	$-CH_2CH_2CH_3$

n-Butyl	Isopropyl	Isobutyl
$-CH_2CH_2CH_2CH_3$	$-CHCH_3$ $\mid$ CH_3	$-CH_2CHCH_3$ $\mid$ CH_3

sec-Butyl	*tert*-Butyl
$-CHCH_2CH_3$ $\mid$ CH_3	CH_3 $\mid$ $-CCH_3$ $\mid$ CH_3

When naming **cyclic alkanes** (those that have a closed-ring structure) there are two additional considerations. First the prefix *cyclo-* must be added to the compound's principal chain name, as in *cyclohexane* for a cyclic six-membered ring. Second, depending on how the compound's structure is represented, the stereochemistry of the substance may need to be indicated in the name. The term "stereochemistry" refers to the three-dimensional arrangement of two or more substituents attached to the ring. In this review, only the case in which there are two substituents will be considered. When drawing cyclic structures, a solid shaded wedge-shaped bond indicates that the substituent is attached to the top side of a ring. A dashed or dotted bond indicates that the substituent is on the bottom side of a ring. When two substituents are on the same side of the ring, their stereochemistry is referred to as *cis*. When two substituents are on opposite sides of the ring (top and bottom) they are referred to as *trans*.

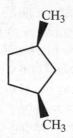

cis-1, 3-dimethylcyclopentane

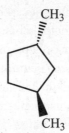

trans-1, 3-dimethylcyclopentane   (48, 49)

To indicate the specific stereochemistry for a cyclic alkane, the prefix *cis*- or *trans*- is placed at the very beginning of the full name. Structures 48 and 49 and their associated names provide examples of the use of cis and trans nomenclature for cyclic alkanes.

A summary of the IUPAC rules for naming alkanes is shown below.

IUPAC NOMENCLATURE FOR ALKANES

(Summary of Rules)

1. Find the longest chain in the compound.[a,b]
2. Name each substituent group that is attached to the principal chain.
3. Alphabetize the substituent groups (methyl, ethyl, propyl, and so on).[c]
4. Number the principal chain from the end that gives the smallest number at the first point of difference.
5. Name the principal chain using the Greek prefix that corresponds to the number of carbons it contains and assign numbers to each substituent.

[a]If two chains are of the same length, choose the most branched as the principal.

[b]If the compound is cyclic, add the prefix *cyclo*- to the parent chain name. If stereochemistry is indicated, use the terms *cis* and *trans*.

[c]Note: The prefixes *sec*- and *tert*- are not used in alphabetization.

It should also be noted that chirality centers may be present in hydrocarbon molecules. If the stereochemistry of these centers is shown in the structural formula (usually with wedge- and dash-shaped bonds), the absolute configuration is also shown in the name. The chirality center designation (*R* or *S*—see the section on the Covalent Bond for the details on determining chirality center assignments) is written first, followed by the number of the carbon in the principal chain. This information usually follows cis/trans designations for cyclic compounds, although the cis/trans designation is often omitted from the name when the compound's stereochemistry is specified.

Practice Exercise 12

By far the best plan for becoming skilled at naming organic compounds is lots of practice. Use the summary of IUPAC rules to name the following alkane structural formulas (50, 51, and 52).

1)   2)   3)   (50, 51, 52)

It is unlikely that you will need to understand names of complicated **unsaturated hydrocarbons**. There are, however, a few points you should know.

The **alkene** functional group is a carbon–carbon double bond. Note the change in suffix from *-ane* to *-ene* for these compounds. The principal chain from which the alkene molecule's name is derived must be the longest chain that contains the double bond. One or more double bonds may be present in an alkene and Greek prefixes are used to show the number of double bonds (*diene* means two double bonds, *triene* means three, *tetraene* means four, and so on). If the stereochemistry around the double bond is shown in the structural formula, the specific designation must be shown in the name (cis/trans or E/Z. See the section on the Covalent Bond for details). Study the following alkene structure (53) and its associated name as an example.

(Z)-5-ethyl-6-methyloct-2-ene　　(53)

The **alkyne** functional group is a carbon–carbon triple bond. Note the change in suffix from *-ane* to *-yne* for these compounds. Alkynes are named in almost exactly the same way as alkenes. The base name of the molecule comes from the longest chain that contains the triple bond. Multiple triple bonds are indicated, as with alkenes, by using Greek prefixes. Because the carbons in the triple bonds are *sp* hybridized, these functional groups do not exhibit any stereochemistry. This makes the naming process for alkynes less complicated. See the following alkyne structure and associated name as an example.

2,3-dimethyloct-4-yne　　(54)

Aromatic compounds (which may not be in the strict sense true hydrocarbons because they often contain atoms other than hydrogen and carbon) contain the **phenyl** (sometimes also referred to as benzene) functional group, which consists of a six-membered carbon ring with three alternating carbon–carbon double bonds (remember the phenyl ring's hydrogens are not shown). There are many IUPAC accepted common names for mono-substituted aromatic compounds. Be familiar with the names and structures (55, 56, 57, 58, and 59) of the following substances:

benzene　　toluene　　benzoic acid　　aniline　　phenol　　(55, 56, 57, 58, 59)

It is also worth the time to become familiar with a few heterocyclic and polycyclic aromatic compounds. The reviewer should be able to recognize the names and structures of the following compounds (60, 61, and 62):

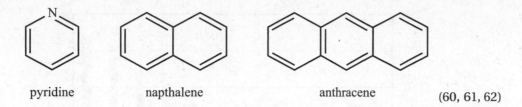

pyridine   napthalene   anthracene   (60, 61, 62)

The process for naming **disubstituted** aromatic compounds uses a simple terminology to indicate the relative positions of the two groups on the phenyl ring. If the groups attached to phenyl ring carbons are next to each other, the configuration is called *ortho* (abbreviated in names as "*o*"). If they are attached to ring carbons with one unsubstituted carbon in between, the configuration is referred to as *meta* (abbreviated as "*m*") and if the groups are attached to ring carbons straight across from each other, the substitution pattern is called *para* (abbreviated as "*p*"). The following constitutional isomers (Structures 63, 64, 65) of dichlorobenzene illustrate this naming process.

o-dichlorobenzene   *m*-dichlorobenzene   *p*-dichlorobenzene   (63, 64, 65)

Aromatic compounds with more than two substituents are named using a numbering system similar to that for cycloalkanes to indicate where substituents are on the benzene ring. Although not particularly difficult to learn, it is unlikely that you will be required to answer questions on the MCAT that use this naming procedure.

Properties and Uses of Alkanes

Most alkanes (as well as other hydrocarbons) are derived from petroleum through a procedure referred to as "cracking" or refining, which involves a form of distillation. This process yields both straight chained (normal) and branched alkanes.

The melting and boiling points of normal alkanes show a very regular increase in temperature as the number of carbons in their chains increase. This trend is directly associated with a rise in the dispersion forces (the weakest of the intermolecular forces) between the molecules as their molar masses increase. Greater numbers of electrons in the larger alkanes are more easily polarized, leading to stronger attractive forces and higher boiling points. See Figure 4.46 for a graphical representation of this trend.

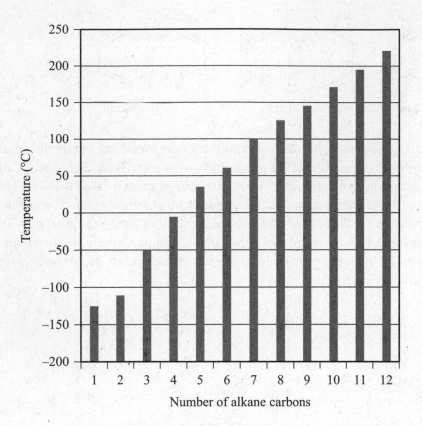

Figure 4.46. Alkane boiling points

Because the elements hydrogen and carbon, which make up alkanes, have relatively similar electronegativities, the magnitudes of dipole moments in their covalent bonds are low. This makes the molecules very nonpolar—one of the alkanes' most unusual properties. The alkane carbon chains are "coated" with nonpolar hydrogen atoms, which make them hydrophobic. This along with their relatively low densities generally prevents them from mixing with water; instead, hydrocarbon molecules agglomerate and float on top as oily films.

The most common uses of alkanes are as fuels, solvents, and precursors for the synthesis of more complex molecules. The only current source of the complex array of hydrocarbons used in today's society is petroleum.

The physical properties of unsaturated hydrocarbons follow pretty much the same trends as alkanes except they tend to be slightly more polar due to the polarizability of the π portion of their multiple bonds. More specifically, trans alkenes tend to be less polar than cis alkenes because they are generally more symmetric. Aromatic hydrocarbons can be considerably more polar if they contain highly electronegative atoms (e.g., oxygen, nitrogen, and halogen atoms).

As with most organic compounds, alkanes can exist in different isomeric forms. Isomers have the same molecular formulas but differ in the way their atoms are bonded to each other (constitutional isomers) or are arranged in space (stereoisomers). Any alkane with a molecular formula having four or more carbon atoms can exhibit constitutional isomerism. Both normal butane and isobutane have the same molecular formula but different molecular structures. The structures (in skeletal format) of these two alkanes are shown below (Structures 66 and 67). As the number of carbons in alkanes increases, the number of possible constitutional isomers grows rapidly. For an alkane with 20 carbons, there are 366,319 possible constitutional isomers.

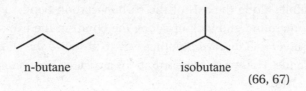

n-butane   isobutane

(66, 67)

Another related topic often studied in conjunction with simple alkanes is **conformational analysis**, a kind of temporary structural isomerism. Because the σ bonds in the skeletons of alkanes have the freedom of rotation, there are many different ways that the various parts of a molecule can move relative to each other. The simple two-carbon alkane ethane can be used to illustrate this point. Figure 4.47 shows two different conformational structures of ethane (these representations are sometimes called saw-horse forms).

Eclipsed   Staggered

Figure 4.47. The most important conformations of ethane

Note that the structure on the left has all the hydrogen–carbon bonds on each of the two ethane carbons aligned relative to each other. This conformation of ethane is call **eclipsed**. In the structure on the right, the position of the carbon in the background (the one toward the top of the figure) has moved relative to the same carbon in the structure on the left. This change was made by allowing a 180° rotation about the σ carbon–carbon bond in the molecule and results in a new conformation called **staggered**. These two **conformers** of ethane have different stabilities (energies) and because of **torsional strain** in the eclipsed form, the staggered form is lower in energy. There are obviously other possible conformations of ethane depending on the degree of rotation about its carbon–carbon bond, but the two that differ most in energy, and thus are the most important, are staggered and eclipsed.

THREE KINDS OF STRAIN

There are three different kinds of strain associated with the various conformers of organic compounds.

Torsional strain is caused by electron-electron repulsion between eclipsed bonds.

Steric strain occurs when two groups of atoms are too close to each other and try to occupy the same space.

Angle or **ring** strain is discussed in detail under the topic of cyclic alkanes later in this section.

If one looks carefully along the axis of the carbon–carbon bonds (align one's eye with the carbon in the foreground and look up along the bond) in the two structures shown in Figure 4.47, the observer will discover another way to visualize the staggered and eclipsed conformations of ethane. These new representations are called **Newman projections** and are shown in the Figure 4.48.

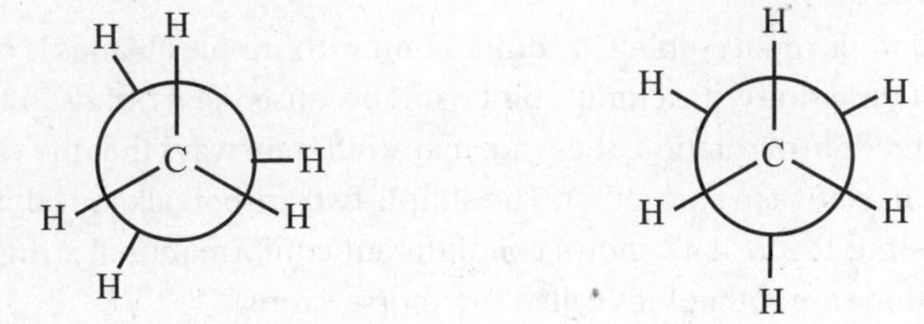

Eclipsed   Staggered

Figure 4.48. The eclipsed and staggered Newman projections of ethane

The conformations of normal butane, another simple alkane, are often studied. As with ethane, its conformers are best represented with Newman projections. If one looks along the bond axis of carbons 2 and 3 in the butane structural formula in Figure 4.49 (left eclipsed sawhorse form) the eclipsed Newman projection (on the right) can be visualized.

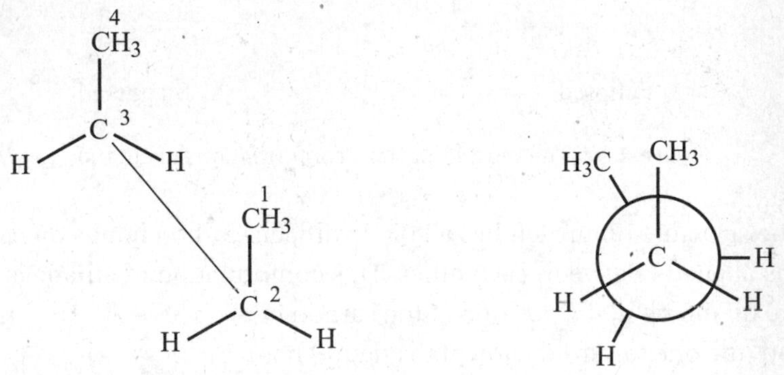

Eclipsed   Eclipsed

Figure 4.49. An eclipsed conformation of butane
(sawhorse on the left and Newman on the right)

Figure 4.50 shows all the important conformations of butane using Newman projections along with their relative energies. Each of the conformations is successively generated (going from left to right) by fixing the position of the butane molecule's second carbon (see Figure 4.49) and allowing carbon three to rotate about the C_2–C_3 bond axis. Each new conformation is generated by a C_2–C_3 bond rotation of 60°. As might be expected from the ethane example, Figure 4.50 clearly illustrates how the various staggered conformations (bottom of the figure) of butane are lower in energy than the less stable eclipsed forms (top of the figure).

Cycloalkanes, alkanes with closed ring molecular structures, are generally less stable than their open chain counterparts. Their lower stability is associated with a property called **ring strain**. Forcing the carbon atoms in an open chain structure into a closed ring causes this kind of molecular strain. The carbon atoms of all alkanes have optimum bond angles of

109.5° (those of a tetrahedron) and when forced into small rings, these angles are significantly distorted. This causes an inherent increase in the energy of the molecule and thus instability (atomic orbital overlap is reduced by the nonoptimum angles, which makes the bonds weaker). Figure 4.51 shows a graph of relative ring strain as a function of ring size.

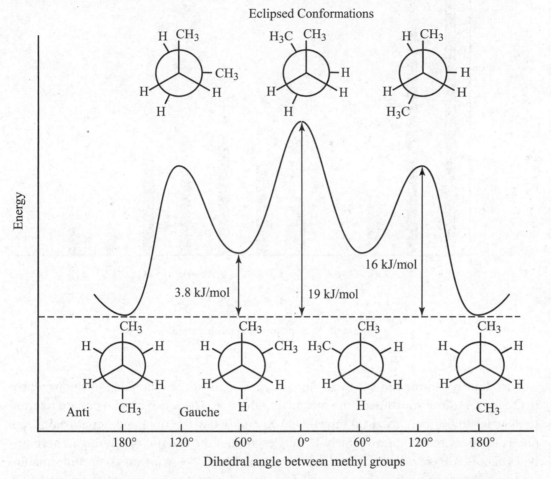

Figure 4.50. The relative energies of the conformations of butane

TIP

DIHEDRAL ANGLE

The dihedral angle on the *x*-axis of the graph in Figure 4.50 refers to the angle between the two terminal methyl groups of butane in the Newman projections.

The graph shows that small rings are particularly strained and large rings (those with 12 or greater carbons) are significantly less strained. It also shows an interesting and important anomaly associated with six-membered cycloalkane rings. They exhibit essentially no ring strain and are just as stable as the open chain form. At first this may seem puzzling, but this circumstance is due to an exceptionally stable conformation that six-membered rings can assume. The ring is not flat but assumes a more stable puckered shape. This low energy conformation is referred to as the **chair** conformer. The chair conformation of cyclohexane has been studied extensively and there is a standard way to represent this conformer on a two-dimensional surface. Begin by drawing two parallel lines and then connect them with two zigzag lines in a closed box. Shown below (Structure 68) is the standard representation for the chair conformation of cyclohexane.

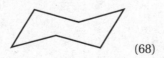

(68)

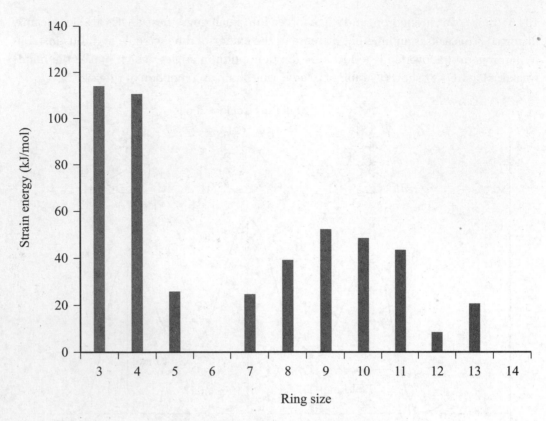

Figure 4.51. Cycloalkane ring strain energies

The chair conformation has two different types of substituent bonding positions where hydrogens or other substituents are attached to the ring. These two bond types are referred to as **axial** (these bonds extend directly above and below the ring) and **equatorial** (these bonds are oriented at approximately 45° angles around the equator of the ring). These two types of bonds occur on each carbon in the six-membered ring, so for any chair conformation there are always six axial and six equatorial bonds. The chair conformation on the left, below (Structure 69) shows only the axial bonds, and the one on the right (Structure 70), only the equatorial bonds, so they can easily be distinguished from each other.

TIP

AXIAL AND EQUATORIAL BONDS

These can also be referred to as axial and equatorial positions.

(69, 70)

Structure 71 shows both the axial and equatorial bonds present on the cyclohexane ring with hydrogens attached—the complete structure (molecular formula C_6H_{12}).

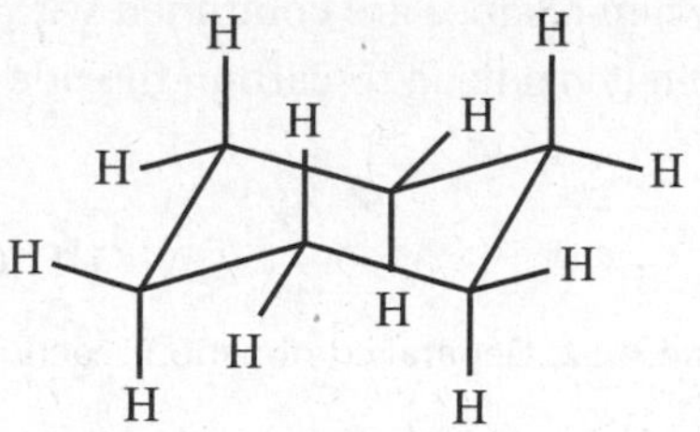

(71)

Just like open chain alkanes, cyclohexane can have substituents other than hydrogen attached to the ring. In general, these larger substituents (more bulky than hydrogen) are more stable in the equatorial position than in the axial. The equatorial position provides more room and thus a less crowded conformation with lower energy. Structures 72 and 73 show a methyl substituent in the axial and equatorial positions, respectively. The equatorial methyl is clearly further removed from the rest of the ring and less crowded.

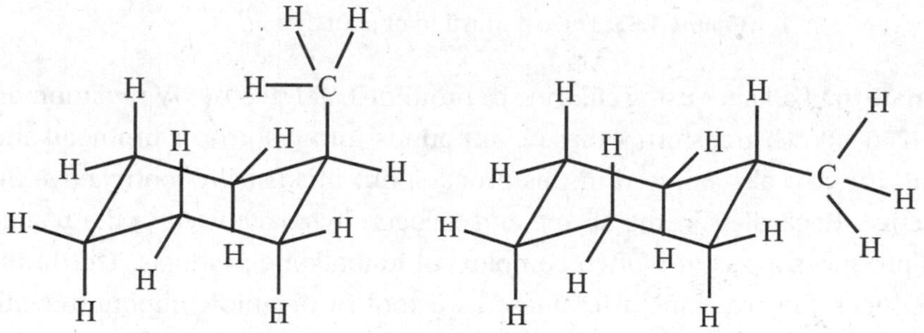

(72, 73)

Hydrocarbon Chemical Reactions

ALKANE REACTIONS

Simple alkanes used as starting materials for other processes are not synthesized directly, but usually obtained by the **pyrolysis** of larger, more complex alkanes obtained from petroleum. Alkanes are relatively inert compounds and do not undergo chemical changes easily. As a result of their limited reactivity, many low boiling alkanes such as pentane, hexane, heptane, and octane make excellent solvents (media) for conducting synthetic organic reactions. There are few synthetically useful reactions that use alkanes as starting materials, but their **combustion** reactions are of immense commercial importance. One other alkane reaction commonly studied in organic chemistry courses is **halogenation**. This reaction has appeared on the MCAT exam.

GENERALIZED REACTION SCHEMES

The schemes shown in this review are often unbalanced and may leave out certain reactant counter ions, side product molecules, solvents, and detailed reaction conditions. In general, the reaction schemes shown here show you only what you need to know for the MCAT.

Alkane combustion occurs when alkanes are combined with sufficient oxygen under the right conditions and are completely oxidized to carbon dioxide and water products (Figure 4.52).

$$C_NH_{2N+2} + O_{2\,(g)} \rightarrow NCO_{2\,(g)} + (N+1)H_2O_{(g)} + \Delta$$

Figure 4.52. General combustion reaction for alkanes

This reaction is extremely exothermic. As a result, large amounts of heat (Δ) are released. This makes alkanes excellent fuels for heating living spaces and cooking. They are also ideal for use in the internal combustion engines. The process requires a high temperature, such as a flame or spark, for its initiation and the mechanism is a very complex and poorly understood free-radical chain reaction. An example reaction, the combustion of pentane, follows (Figure 4.53).

$$C_5H_{12\,(l)} + 8\,O_{2\,(g)} \xrightarrow{\Delta} 5\,CO_{2\,(g)} + 6\,H_2O_{(g)}$$

Figure 4.53. The combustion of pentane

The **halogenation** of alkanes using chlorine or bromine catalyzed by UV radiation or high temperatures (250–400°C) transforms these compounds into chloro- or bromoalkanes. In some cases fluorine can also be used in this process, but it is usually too reactive. Iodine is often unreactive. Regardless of the alkane and halogen reactants used in the reaction, it almost always produces a mixture (often complex) of **haloalkane** products. This limitation significantly reduces the reaction's usefulness as a tool in organic compound synthesis. The general reaction for this process is shown in Figure 4.54, where X is Cl or Br and rarely F or I.

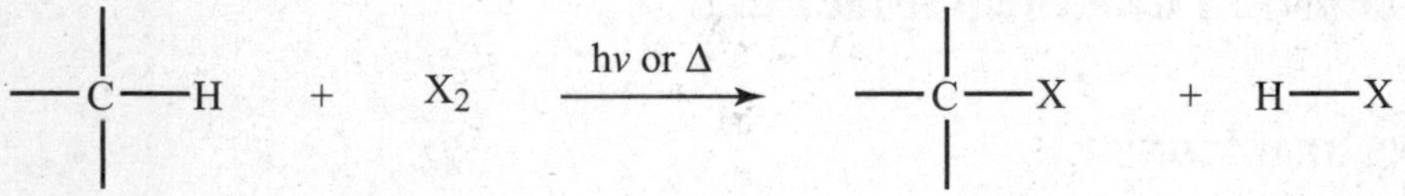

Figure 4.54. Free radical halogenation of alkanes

The halogenation of alkanes is one of the most studied reactions in organic chemistry and has provided much insight into the particulars of free-radical reaction mechanisms. As can be seen from the general reaction above, halogen atoms in this process replace hydrogen atoms (a substitution process). Depending on the position of a hydrogen atom in the alkane structure, its reactivity toward substitution by halogen atoms varies considerably, with some hydrogens being very reactive and others less so. This spectrum of hydrogen atom reactivities toward replacement by halogen atoms leads to the mixtures of haloalkane products cited above.

UNSATURATED HYDROCARBON REACTIONS

The reactions (both to prepare and derivatise) of unsaturated hydrocarbons are much more numerous, varied, and complex than those for alkanes. Focus on recognizing the reaction patterns (elimination, addition, substitution, reduction, oxidation, and so on) common to these compounds. It is not particularly helpful just to memorize reactions. Grouping reactions into the above patterns (also called mechanisms) can help cut down on the number of flash cards you may need to keep them straight.

Alkenes are most commonly prepared by **elimination reactions**. Two elimination reactions studied in organic chemistry courses are **dehydration of alcohols** and **dehydrohalogenation of alkyl halides**. The product of both of these reactions is an alkene. Figure 4.55 shows the general reaction schemes for these processes.

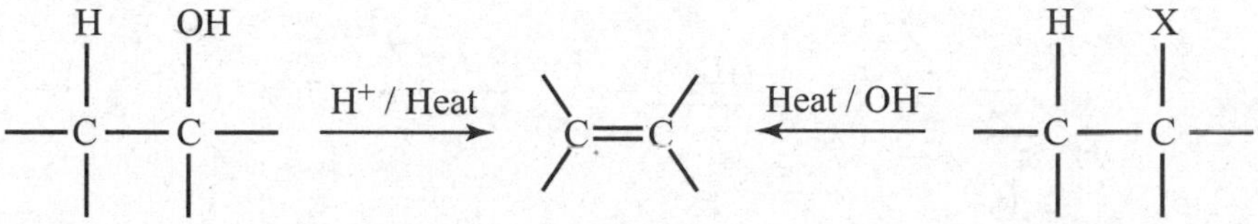

Figure 4.55. Elimination reactions commonly used to prepare alkenes

There are two commonly accepted mechanisms for alkene-forming elimination reactions:

1. **Monomolecular Elimination (E1)** and
2. **Bimolecular Elimination (E2)**

E1 reactions exhibit first-order kinetics and consist of a two-step process. The first step, which is rate determining and therefore slow, involves the formation of an intermediate **carbocation** (R–C+) resulting from the loss of a leaving group (usually a water molecule or a halogen anion). In the second step, which is fast, the loss of a proton (usually under acidic conditions) adjacent to the carbocation leads to the alkene product. Elimination reactions of this type are not usually very synthetically useful because they often produce mixtures of alkenes and substitution products. Figure 4.56 shows the steps of this process.

RECOGNIZE REACTION PATTERNS

Recognizing common reaction patterns helps you mentally organize and remember the large number of chemical reactions in organic chemistry. Be sure to review the specific patterns of elimination, addition, substitution, reduction, and oxidation.

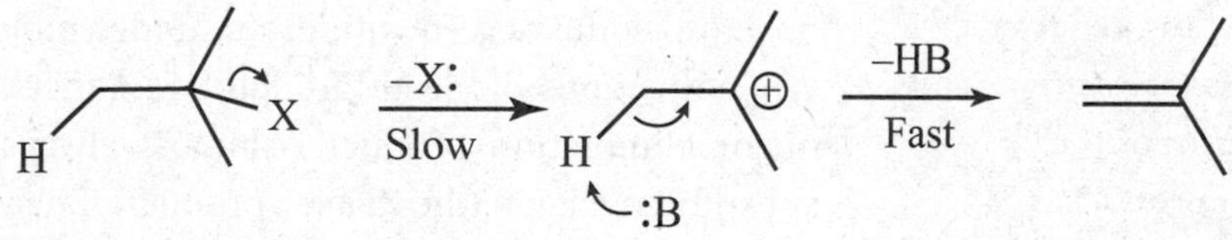

Figure 4.56. The E1 reaction mechanism where X is a leaving group and :B is a base

E2 reactions exhibit second order kinetics and occur in a single step. In this process, a proton is abstracted (removed) from a carbon next to a carbon with a **leaving group** (as with E1 reactions, usually a water molecule or a halogen anion). As the proton is abstracted by a strong base, the remaining electron pair moves between the adjacent carbon, and the leaving group departs with a pair of electrons. An *anti*-periplaner bond geometry (almost coplanar) between the reactive proton and leaving group stabilizes the transition state of this process and can significantly increase the reaction's rate. The net outcome of this concerted process is the formation of a double bond—an alkene product. Because this reaction

REACTION MECHANISMS ON THE MCAT

MCAT questions often present you with laboratory **kinetic data, reaction conditions,** and **product ratios** and then require you to use this data to draw conclusions about **reaction mechanisms.** These questions can take a lot of time because they require not only basic chemistry knowledge but also critical analysis of the data to reach a logical conclusion about a mechanism.

proceeds without the formation of an intermediate carbocation, there is less chance of a product mixture forming. Depending on the starting compound's structure, though, a mixture of alkenes can possibly result. From a stereochemical perspective, trans products, due to their lower energy, are favored over cis products. Figure 4.57 shows the E2 mechanism.

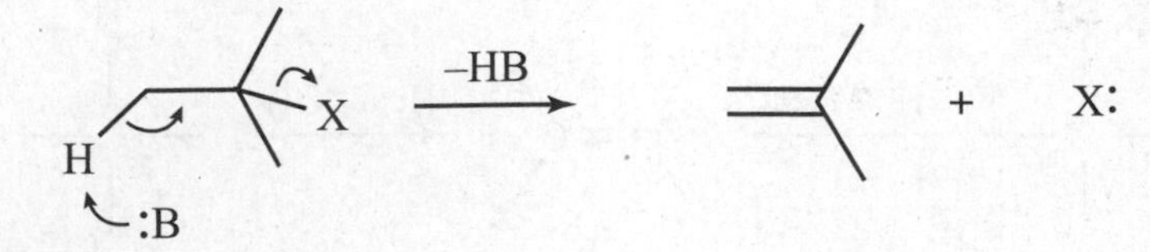

Figure 4.57. The E2 reaction mechanism where X is a leaving group and :B is a base

Reactions with *heat* and *basic conditions* proceed almost exclusively through E2 (usually desirable). If there is more than one β carbon with a reactive proton next to the leaving group of the substrate, a mixture of alkenes usually results. The process is regioselective. In most cases, the more substituted, lower-energy alkene will predominate; this is known as "Zaitsev's rule." This outcome is illustrated by the real reaction example shown in Figure 4.58.

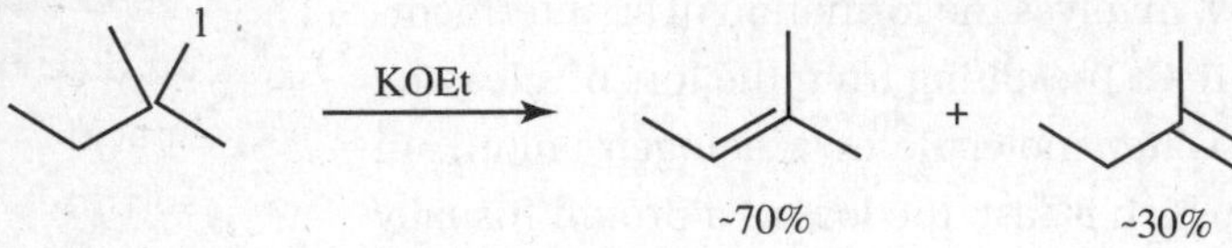

Figure 4.58. An elimination reaction that produces a mixture of E2 products

REACTION WEBS

In most reaction web diagrams, the reactants and products have been generalized to represent the most common form of the reaction. Usually only the main product is shown. There are often additional products that are not shown because they are minor or not essential to understanding the reaction outcome.

In general, *heat* and *acidic conditions* (such as the dehydration of alcohols) will produce an E1 product often mixed to some degree with other, undesirable products. When reactions proceed through an E1 mechanism, the major elimination product is almost always the more substituted alkene (the Zaitsev product). Be familiar with both of these elimination reaction mechanisms.

Alkenes can undergo many different **addition reactions** that result in many types of new compounds. The π portion of the alkene double bond can act as a nucleophile (a species attracted to the nucleus of an atom) that is attracting electrophiles. The electrophiles use the π electrons to form σ bonds and thus "add" to the alkene functional group. This makes alkenes a versatile starting point for the synthesis of more complex and valuable substances. Figure 4.59 shows an addition reaction web, which includes common examples.

Alcohols can be prepared by either reaction 1 (Figure 4.59) [oxymercuration–mercury acetate ($Hg(OAc)_2$) followed by sodium borohydride ($NaBH_4$) reduction] or reaction 6 [borane (BH_3) followed by basic hydrogen peroxide (H_2O_2)]. Reaction 1 results in **Markovnikov addition** of water and reaction 6 **non-Markovnikov syn addition** of water. The two methods are complementary.

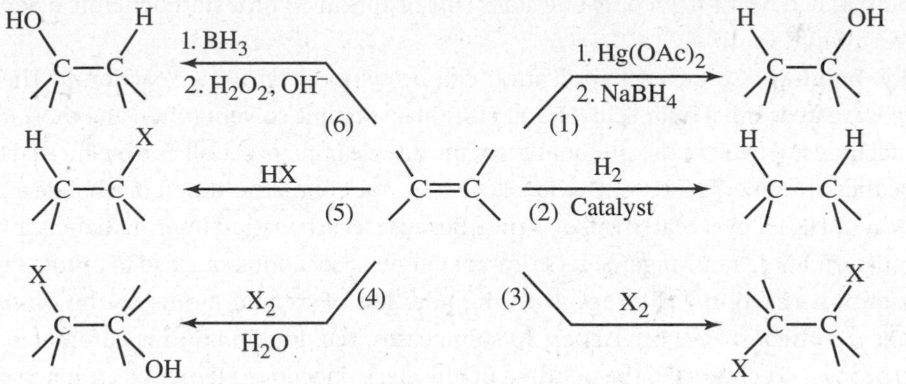

Figure 4.59. Alkene addition reaction web

MARKOVNIKOV'S RULE

Vladimir Markovnikov was a Russian chemist who discovered a predictable pattern for addition reactions involving carbocation intermediates. "Mark's" rule refers to the addition of a reactant (e.g., halide anion, hydroxyl anion, etc.) to the more substituted carbon in the double bond of an alkene. Different reaction conditions allow a chemist to add reactants in either Mark or non-Mark orientation to an alkene double bond.

In reaction 2, the addition of H_2 is catalyzed by a supported transition metal (e.g., Pt, Pd, Ni, Rh, etc.) in a syn stereochemical fashion. The product is an alkane.

Reactions 3 [addition of a halogen (X_2, where X = Cl or Br) to give a *1,2-dihalide*] and 4 (addition of aqueous halogen to give a *1,2-halohydrin*) proceed by the same mechanism, the first step of which is the formation of a **halonium ion** intermediate (Structure 76).

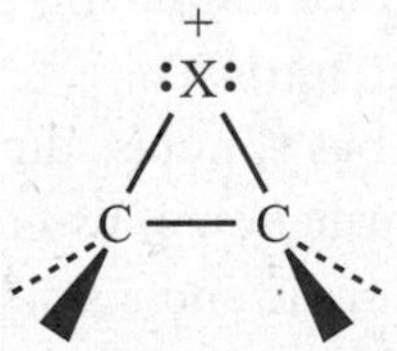

(76)

It can be seen from the halonium ion's structure that one side of the carbon–carbon bond is blocked by a halogen cation (X+); thus nucleophilic (a species that's attracted to the nucleus of a carbon) addition of either X– (reaction 3) or H_2O

ADDITION REACTION STEREOCHEMISTRY TERMS

Syn: In the **syn** process, the addition reactants add to the same side of a double or triple bond. Structure 74 shows a generalized **syn** addition product where *X* and *Y* are the addition reactants.

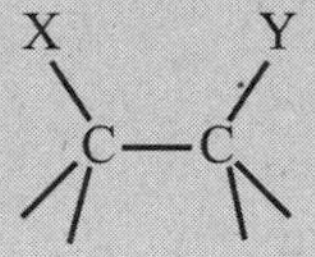

(74)

Anti: In the **anti** process, the addition reactants add to the opposite sides of a double or triple bond. Structure 75 shows a generalized **anti** addition product where *X* and *Y* are the addition reactants.

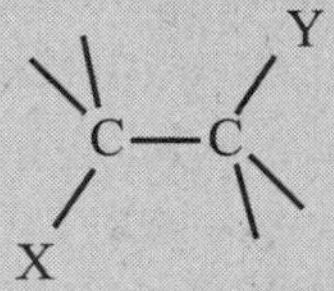

(75)

Don't confuse the terms **syn** and **anti**, which refer to reaction mechanism processes, with cis and trans, which refer to a pair of alkene stereoisomers and more specifically a pair of diastereomers.

(reaction 4) can occur from only one side. This results in an **anti** stereochemical addition for both reactions.

Alkyl halides (also called haloalkanes) can be synthesized using reaction 5. The starting alkene is treated with a **halo acid** (HCl or HBr) in an organic solvent (often an ether). The reaction mechanism involves the protonation of the double bond of the alkene by the acid to form a carbocation intermediate (C+). This is followed by nucleophilic addition of a halide anion (X–). Addition of HX follows Markovnikov's rule. Because a carbocation intermediate is involved in the transformation, rearrangements to lower energy carbocations can lead to product mixtures.

Oxidation reactions often result in the addition of oxygen atoms to the double bond carbons (sp^2 hybridized) of alkenes. In some cases, the double bond is completely cleaved in the process. Technically, the bonding of any electronegative element's atoms to carbon is considered to be oxidation. However, many of the reactions shown in the alkene web (Figure 4.59) are not generally classified this way. Figure 4.60 shows those reactions that are commonly considered to be alkene oxidations.

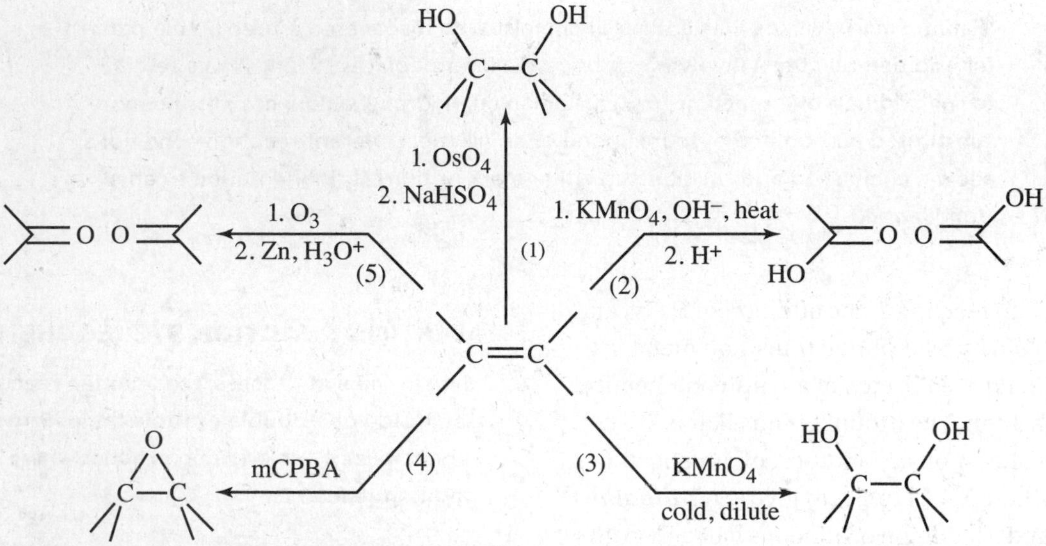

Figure 4.60. Alkene oxidation reaction web

As shown in reaction 1 in Figure 4.60, an alkene can first be treated with osmium tetroxide (OsO_4) to produce a cyclic osmate, which is then cleaved by addition of aqueous sodium bisulfite ($NaHSO_4$). The reaction proceeds by **syn** addition to produce a **diol**. This procedure has some drawbacks related to the expense and toxicity of osmium tetroxide.

In reaction 2 of Figure 4.60, treatment of an alkene with hot, basic, potassium permanganate ($KMnO_4$) results in cleavage of the double bond and the formation of two **carboxylic acid** fragments. If the alkene is symmetric, the fragments are the same and a single carboxylic acid product is produced. If the alkene is asymmetric, two different carboxylic acids are formed, which may be difficult to separate.

Reaction 3 is similar to reaction 1 except that the oxidative conditions are much milder and the product produced is a diol with a **syn** addition orientation.

Epoxides (also called oxiranes) are produced when alkenes are reacted with peroxycarboxylic acids. In reaction 4, *m*-chloroperoxybenzoic acid (MCPBA) is used to effect such an oxidation. Another commonly used reagent is peroxyacetic acid (PAA).

Ozonolysis of an alkene is shown in reaction 5. This oxidative process results in the formation of carbonyl compounds—either **ketones** or **aldehydes**, depending on the alkene's structure. First, the alkene is reacted with ozone to form a molozonide that isomerizes to an ozonide intermediate that is immediately reduced with acidic zinc to the carbonyl-containing product.

The **Diels–Alder reaction** (a name reaction) is an unusual addition process that proceeds by neither a polar nor radical mechanism. It is a particularly useful reaction for synthesizing organic compounds that contain rings. The reaction is classified as a cycloaddition and involves reacting a **conjugated diene** with an **alkene** (called a **dieneophile**). These species combine in a cyclic transition state and produce a ring through the simultaneous formation of two carbon–carbon bonds. The mechanism of this process is termed **pericyclic** because the reaction product is produced in a single concerted step by the cyclic redistribution of bonding electrons.

The diene in the reaction must be able to assume a conformation that allows both of its double bonds to align on the same side of their connecting sigma bond (see Structures 77 and 78, which show the aligned and unaligned forms). This conformation is sometimes referred to as the *s*-cis form. If the diene has large terminal substituents, the *s*-cis conformation can be unstable (high energy) and its lower energy *s*-trans form may predominate. Such dienes react slowly or not at all with the dieneophile.

s-cis form
- reactive

s-trans form
- unreactive

(77, 78)

For the reaction to proceed at a reasonable rate, the dieneophile must have an electron-withdrawing group or groups attached to its double bond carbons. The withdrawing species are usually some kind of carbonyl containing functional group (for example, aldehyde, ketone, ester, carboxylic acid, etc.) although other polarized groups can also work.

Another aspect of the Diels-Alder reaction is that it forms a *predominant* product when stereoisomer formation is possible. Thus the reaction is considered to be *stereoselective*. Figure 4.61 shows a generalized scheme for the Diels-Alder reaction for the formation of a six-membered ring.

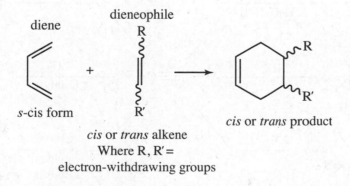

Figure 4.61. A generalized Diels–Alder reaction

The generalized reaction in Figure 4.61 shows the formation of a six-membered ring. Rings of other sizes, commonly five-membered rings and bicyclic compounds, can also be synthesized by this process.

There are only a few practical ways to **synthesize alkynes**, and even the available methods require harsh conditions and often produce low yields. One approach is dehydrohalogenation of **vicinal** (side-by-side) dihalides. Figure 4.62 shows this elimination reaction.

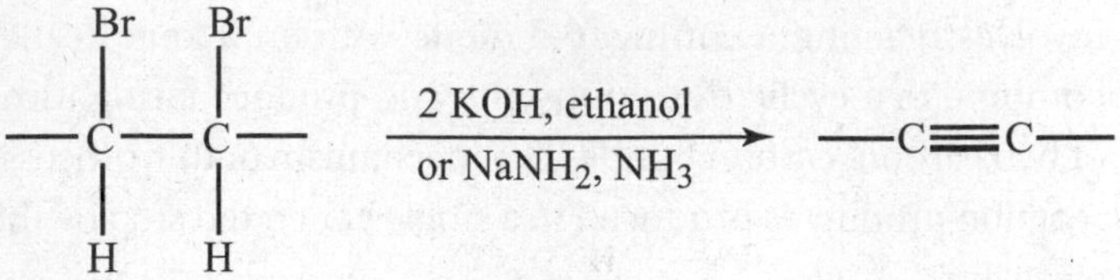

Figure 4.62. Preparation of an alkyne by dehydrohalogenation

ACIDIC PROTONS

Protons attached to *sp*-hybridized carbons in a triple bond (H–C≡C–) are slightly acidic (pK_a ~ 25). The resulting acetylide anion is stabilized by the high *s* orbital character (50%) of the carbon carrying the negative charge (⁻C≡C–).

It is better to start with a simple alkyne and further derivatise it. Using a very strong base such as sodium amide (NaNH$_2$), terminal alkynes can be deprotonated to produce salts of an acetylide anion.

The salt of the acetylide anion is not generally isolated but rather immediately reacted with a primary alkyl halide (RCH$_2$–X, where X = Cl, Br, and I) to produce an internal alkyne. If acetylene (H–C≡C–H) is used to prepare the acetylide ion, it can be alkylated to produce a terminal alkyne. This process is one of the important methods available for forming carbon–carbon bonds. Figure 4.63 shows the general reaction scheme for this procedure.

Figure 4.63. The synthesis of an internal alkyne by acetylide ion alkylation

As with alkenes, alkynes undergo a number of different addition reactions to produce new categories of organic compounds. Figure 4.64 shows an addition reaction web that includes the most common examples.

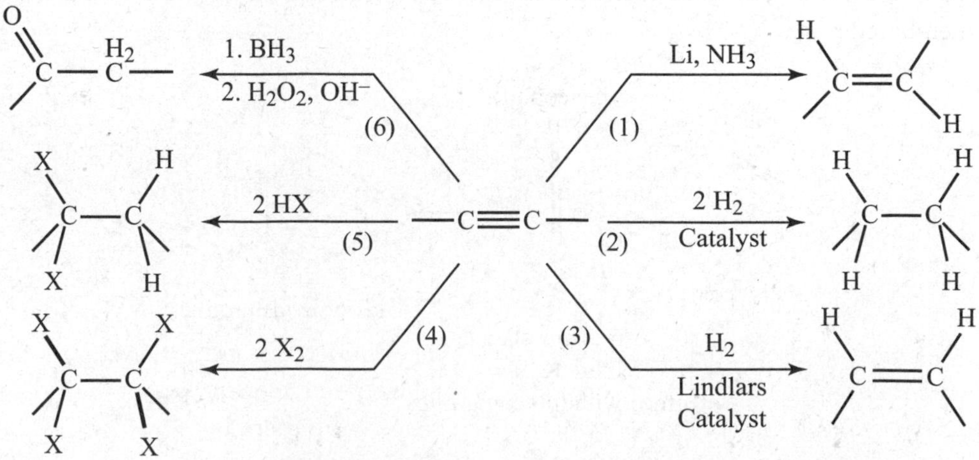

Figure 4.64. Alkyne addition reaction web

Note that, in the figure, reductive addition to produce alkanes and alkenes can be accomplished using reactions 1, 2, and 3. Reaction of an alkyne with excess H_2 and a standard transition metal catalyst (Pt, Pd, Ni, Rh, etc.) produces an alkane by **syn** addition. A *trans*-alkene is produced by treating an alkyne with Li metal in liquid ammonia (NH_3) and a *cis*-alkene by reaction of an alkyne with one equivalent of H_2 and **Lindlar's catalyst**.

Alkyl halides are produced from alkynes by reactions 4 and 5. Alkynes reacted with excess halogen (X_2, where X = Cl, Br, and I) result in tetrahalides (reaction 4). Those reacted with excess haloacid (HCl or HBr) in an organic solvent produce **geminal** (attached to the same carbon atom) **dihalides** (reaction 5).

As with alkenes, hydroboration/oxidation of alkynes produces **carbonyl compounds**. Terminal alkynes produce aldehydes, and internal alkynes give ketones. Reaction conditions for the two processes are slightly different, but to convert an internal alkyne to a ketone, the oxidation conditions (step 2 in the process) must be basic.

Strong oxidizing agents such as potassium permanganate/base or ozone produce **oxidation reactions** that lead to the cleavage of alkyne triple bonds and the formation of carboxylic acids. These reactions, except for the starting alkyne, are almost identical to reactions 1 and 4 in Figure 4.60 (alkene oxidation reaction web). The processes may require more heat and time to completely cleave the very strong triple bond, and product yields are often lower.

Reactions of the benzene ring. In contrast to the previously discussed unsaturated hydrocarbons, the most important reactions of simple aromatic compounds are not addition reactions, but substitution reactions. The double bonds in the benzene (or phenyl) ring are unreactive toward addition except under very special conditions. Instead, because of the ring's high π electron density, the ring acts as an electron donor and thus attracts and reacts with electron-deficient species (electrophiles). Figure 4.65 shows a substitution reaction web for benzene that includes the most common examples.

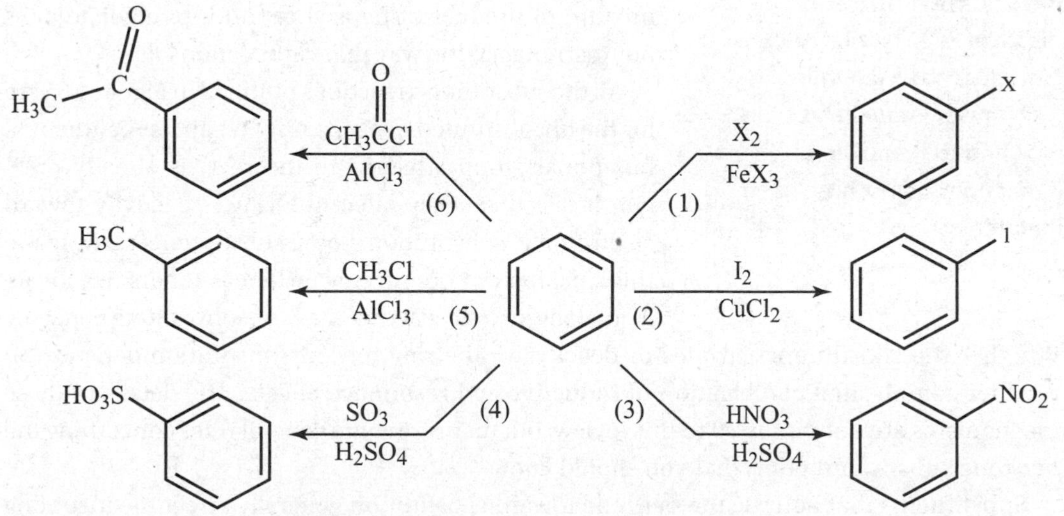

TIP

LINDLAR'S CATALYST

Lindlar's catalyst is a "poisoned" Pd metal catalyst that is less active than the standard version.

Figure 4.65. Benzene substitution reaction web

As can be seen from the above figure, many different functional groups can be attached to the benzene ring using substitution reactions. **Halogenated benzene** compounds can be prepared by using reactions 1 and 2, where X in reaction 1 is either Cl or Br. Note that these reactions require the addition of a co-reactant (FeX_3 and $CuCl_2$) to allow the reaction to proceed at a practical rate. Otherwise they are too slow. These co-reactants act as catalysts and significantly improve these reactions' rates and product yields. Specifically, they interact with the halogen and make it a better electrophile by polarizing it so that it behaves like X+.

Reaction 3, the nitration of benzene, is a classic organic chemistry reaction. **Nitrobenzene** (or another nitrated aromatic compound) is used as a precursor for the preparation of many other important chemicals, explosives, and pharmaceutical agents. Sulfuric acid (H_2SO_4) and nitric acid (HNO_3) react to produce the nitrating agent, the **nitronium ion** (NO_2^+) in this reaction.

Sulfonation of benzene is shown in reaction 4. This is a historically important reaction, because **aromatic sulfonic acids** were once used to prepare dyes and sulfa drugs. Here sulfur trioxide (SO_3) and sulfuric acid (the mixture is referred to as fuming sulfuric acid) react to form HSO_3^+, which is the sulfonating electrophile.

Reaction 5 is a name reaction, **Friedel–Crafts alkylation**, and is a very important method for synthesizing alkyl benzenes. In the example shown, aluminum trichloride ($AlCl_3$) catalyzes the formation of CH_3^+ (a carbocation, another strong electrophile) from chloromethane, which goes on to react with the electron rich benzene ring. Almost any alkyl halide can be used in this reaction, making it very versatile. If there is already another functional group attached to the benzene ring, in many cases the reaction fails. Another limitation involves the formation of a carbocation (R–C+) intermediate. Carbocations, depending on their structures, can rearrange to form new, more stable (lower energy) carbocations. When this can happen, the reaction produces what can be a hard-to-separate mixture of alkyl benzenes.

The last reaction, 6, shown in Figure 4.65 is called **Friedel–Crafts acylation** (as opposed to alkylation). In this variation of the alkylation reaction, the electrophile is R–$^+$C=O, an acyl cation which, like the carbocations in reaction 5, react with the benzene ring to form an acyl benzene. As with alkylation, almost any carboxylic acid chloride will work in this reaction and it has the advantage of not giving a mixture of products. The acyl cation intermediate does not rearrange in the way that carbocations do.

All the substitution reactions outlined in Figure 4.65 are for the unsubstituted benzene ring. When a substituent (a functional group attached to the ring) is already present, it can drastically affect the ring's reactivity toward electrophilic substitution. Some substituents activate the ring, making it more reactive, whereas others deactivate it, making it less reactive than unsubstituted benzene.

NAME REACTIONS

Many reactions in organic chemistry are named after their discoverers. For example, the alkylation reaction described in Figure 4.65 is named after chemists Friedel and Crafts. Some students find that knowing the names of these reactions helps in remembering the reactions.

Whether the substituent activates or deactivates the ring toward substitution depends on a rather complicated combination of **inductive** and **resonance** effects. The details of these mechanisms are not discussed in this review, but there are some general rules concerning the **benzene substituent effect** that you should know.

Substituents that activate the benzene toward substitution generally direct the incoming electrophile to the *ortho* and *para* ring positions relative to the group already present. Functional groups that fall into this category include:

- –R, –OR, –OH, –OC=OR, –NHC=OR, –NH_2, and NR_2 (where R is an alkyl group)

Substituents that deactivate the benzene ring always direct the incoming electrophile to the *meta* ring position relative to the group already present. Functional groups in this category include:

■ –C=OOH, –C=OOR, –C=OR, –C=OH, –NO$_2$, and –SO$_3$H (where R is an alkyl group)

EXCEPTIONS

Unfortunately, as is usually the case, there is an exception to these hard-and-fast rules. Halogen ring substituents (–F, –Cl, –Br, and –I) are **deactivating**, but direct the electrophile to *ortho/para* ring positions.

The following exercise illustrates the use of the above substituent effect rules.

Practice Exercise 13

Given the following acylation reaction of phenol (Structure 79) predict the major product(s).

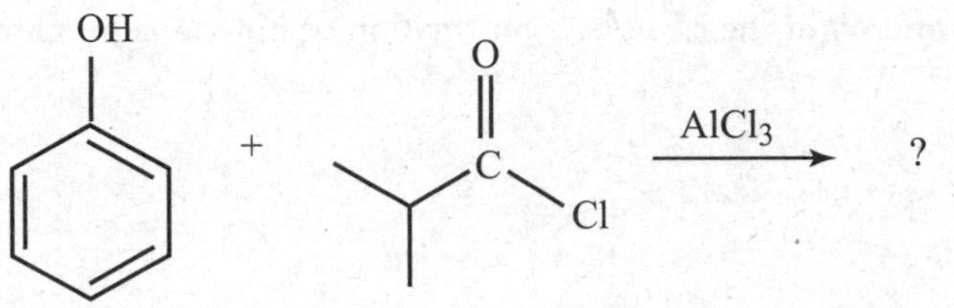

(79, 80)

Solution: The ⁻OH group of phenol is an activating, *ortho/para* director. Thus there are two major products (Structures 81 and 82):

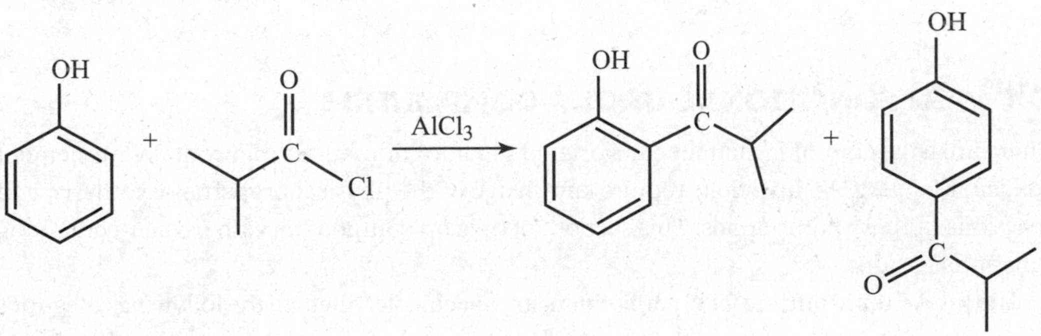

(81, 82)

Practice Exercise 14

Given the following nitration reaction of bromobenzene (Structure 83) predict the major product(s).

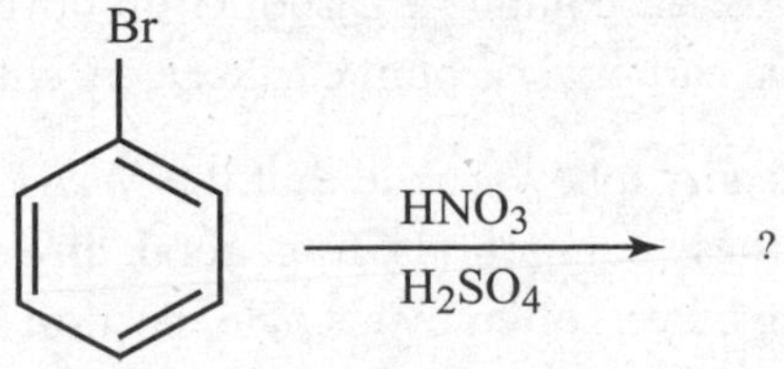

(83)

Even though the benzene ring is normally unreactive toward addition, there is one important addition reaction you should know—the addition of hydrogen to the double bonds of the benzene ring. This process requires elevated temperature/pressure and a powerful hydrogenation catalyst (finely divided rhodium metal supported on carbon—Rh/C—is often used). This reaction, shown in Figure 4.66, reduces the benzene ring to cyclohexane.

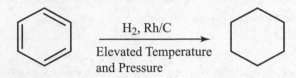

Figure 4.66. Metal (Rh) catalyzed addition of hydrogen gas (H_2) to benzene

---

TEST QUESTION

The relatively high energy of the gauche conformation of butane is primarily associated with:

(A) angle strain

(B) torsional strain

(C) steric strain

(D) orbital strain

(C) The most important strain energy associated with this conformation of butane is the result of a steric interaction between two methyl groups.

OXYGEN FUNCTIONAL GROUP COMPOUNDS

There are a number of important categories of organic compounds that contain the element oxygen. Many MCAT questions require knowledge of the physical properties, synthesis, and reactions of these compounds. This section focuses on compounds with oxygen-containing functional groups.

The MCAT topic outline for organic chemistry specifically refers to the following categories of oxygen-containing compounds (functional group name and associated general formula of each follows):

TIP

ETHER

The ether functional group, which also contains oxygen, is not included in the MCAT topic outline.

- **Alcohols:** contain a hydroxyl group
- **Aldehydes:** contain a carbonyl group
- **Ketones:** contain a carbonyl group
- **Carboxylic Acids:** contain a hydroxyl group bonded to a carbonyl carbon
- **Carboxylic Acid Derivatives:** all contain a carbonyl group along with various other **hetero atoms** bonded to the carbonyl carbon (e.g., oxygen, chlorine, and nitrogen)

A general review of each category follows. Note that the MCAT seems to be particularly fond of questions that involve these compounds. In general, any one of these compounds can be converted into any of the others, often by a single reaction step. The many chemical reactions of these compounds can be hard to remember because they can seem so similar. Look for general reaction patterns and prepare a unique set of flashcards for reactions associated with each functional group.

Alcohols and Phenols

Alcohols and **phenols** (aromatic alcohols) are defined by their **hydroxyl** functional groups. More specifically, alcohols have hydroxyl groups bonded to sp^3 carbons and phenols to sp^2 carbons of phenyl (benzene) rings. They can all be thought of as derivatives of the water molecule, in which one of the hydrogens has been replaced with carbon. Figure 4.67, below, shows generalized structural examples of these two types of compounds.

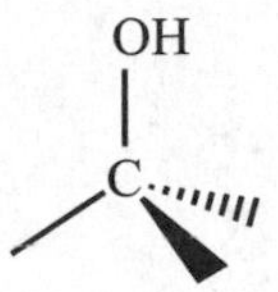

An Alcohol 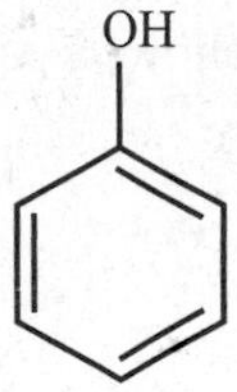   A Phenol

Figure 4.67. Generalized structures of an alcohol and a phenol

NOMENCLATURE

Alcohols are named using IUPAC rules, by replacing the -*e* suffix of alkane with the suffix -*ol*. For example, methane becomes methanol and ethane becomes ethanol. For more complex alcohols, identify the longest carbon chain (principal chain) containing the carbon with the hydroxyl group, and its position in the chain must be given the lowest possible number. Small **alkyl groups** on the principal chain must be named and numbered. The root name of the alcohol is derived from the principal chain. The following structure (84) illustrates the naming process (which is very similar to the naming of hydrocarbons).

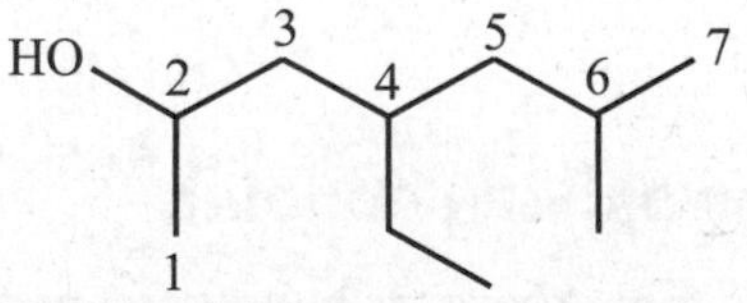

4-ethyl-6-methyl-2-heptanol   (84)

Notice that the longest continuous chain (principal chain) with an attached hydroxyl group is seven-carbons (numbered chain); thus the root name for this compound is heptanol. The carbon with the attached hydroxyl group is given the lowest number (2), which defines the numbers for the ethyl (4) and methyl (6) substituents, which are listed in the name in alphabetical order.

Alcohols that are commonly used in industry or in domestic settings, and have a very long history, are often named using the word alcohol as the root—non-IUPAC nomenclature. Examples are methyl and ethyl alcohol. Also the term *diol* is commonly used to refer to compounds that have two hydroxyl groups (often directly adjacent to each other). Phenols are named in the same way as substituted benzene compounds. The root name for this class of compounds is always phenol. For example, *m*-chlorophenol has a chloro group attached to the phenol ring in the *meta* position.

PROPERTIES AND USES

Because of the presence of the highly electronegative oxygen atom in alcohols, the hydroxyl functional group is very polarized. It is, in fact, so polarized that, like water, alcohols are capable of forming **hydrogen bonds** with themselves, other alcohols, carboxylic acids, amines, and water. Alcohols with up to four or five carbons are so polar that they are miscible with water, unlike the majority of organic compounds. When the alkyl part of alcohol molecules is larger than 5 carbons, they no longer dissolve in water and behave more like hydrocarbons. Figure 4.68 shows a generalized scheme for hydrogen bonding between two alcohol molecules.

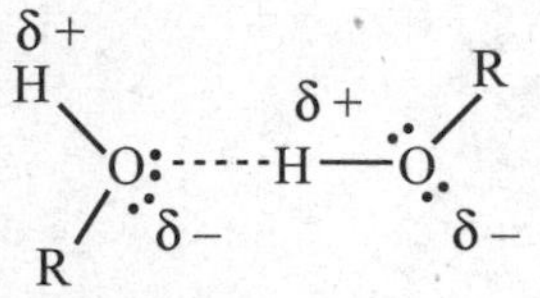

Figure 4.68. A hydrogen bond interaction between two highly polarized alcohol molecules

Hydrogens attached to the oxygens of hydroxyl groups in alcohols have another special property in addition to being capable of hydrogen bonding. They are more acidic than the hydrogens attached to many other functional groups, with pK_a's ranging from ~15.5 (approximately the pK_a of water) to 18.0 for alcohols with many branched alkyl groups. Simple alkyl group branches attached to a carbon are electron donating, an inductive effect. If a carbon with a hydroxyl group has several alkyl groups attached to it, the electron-donating effect will destabilize the anion (referred to as an **alkoxide**) formed when the hydroxyl proton is lost. This makes the protons of hydroxyl groups in highly branched alcohols less acidic. Figure 4.69 shows the destabilizing electron-donating effect of alkyl groups (denoted as *R* in the figure) on an alkoxide anion.

HYDROGEN BONDING

The intermolecular attractive force known as **hydrogen bonding** can occur only between molecules in which a hydrogen atom is attached to a highly electronegative atom. These atoms include oxygen, nitrogen, and fluorine. This kind of bonding is possible in these cases because the hydrogen's single electron is essentially stripped away from its nucleus when attached to a highly electronegative atom. The remaining almost "bare" proton carries a highly positive charge and is very electrophilic. Hydrogen bonding is one of the strongest intermolecular forces (forces between molecules) and extremely important in many organic and biological reaction processes.

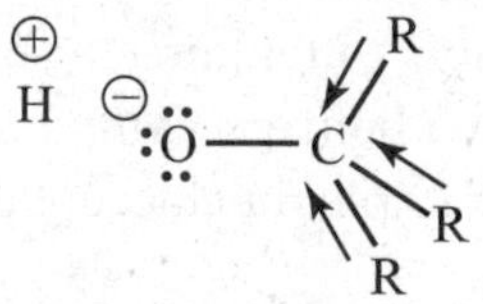

Figure 4.69. Destabilization of an alkoxide anion by alkyl group electron donation

Note that the arrows in the diagram imply electron flow toward the oxygen anion from the R groups (where R is any alkyl group—in this case there are three alkyl groups attached to the carbon bearing the negatively charged oxygen atom). The oxygen anion is destabilized by the presence of alkyl groups and thus the species is less likely to lose its hydroxyl proton (the group is shown in its ionized state).

REVIEW OF ACIDITY

The term **acid** refers to a species that can *donate protons* (H^+ *ions*). There are several factors that determine how acidic a compound is. These include what kind of atom the hydrogen is attached to (*the element effect*), if there are electron donating or withdrawing atoms or groups in the compound (*the inductive effect*), if other resonance forms of the compound can spread out the charge and stabilize an anion resulting from the loss of a proton (*the resonance effect*), and what kind of orbital hybridization the atom bearing the acidic proton has (*the orbital effect*). Often several of these effects may be at play at the same time in a compound. In such a situation they can be additive, making a hydrogen either very acidic or very non-acidic, or they may counter each other, resulting in a less dramatic effect on acidity. The relative acidity of hydrogens can be quantified by using pK_a's (a base ten log scale of the deprotonation/protonation equilibrium constant K_a).

The lower the pK_a of a given hydrogen, the more acidic, or easily ionized, it is.

Methanol and ethanol are two of the most important of all industrial chemicals and are used widely as solvents, in drug formulation and synthesis, in polymer synthesis, as gasoline additives, and in foods and beverages. Ethanol is the active ingredient in all alcoholic beverages.

REACTIONS

There are several commonly used methods for synthesizing *alcohols* and *phenols*. Alkenes can be converted to alcohols using **addition reactions**. This has been described above in the Hydrocarbon Compounds section.

Another technique is the use of **substitution reactions**. These reactions are classified by their mechanisms in a way analogous to the elimination reactions (E1 and E2) covered under Hydrocarbons. The most important for the synthesis of alcohols is **bimolecular nucleophilic substitution (S_N2)**. These reactions are effective for the preparation of alcohols from primary (1°) and secondary (2°) alkyl halides when reacted with a hydroxide base (e.g., sodium or potassium hydroxide). Highly branched alkyl halides usually give elimination products and produce low alcohol yields. Figure 4.70 shows the generalized mechanism for these reactions.

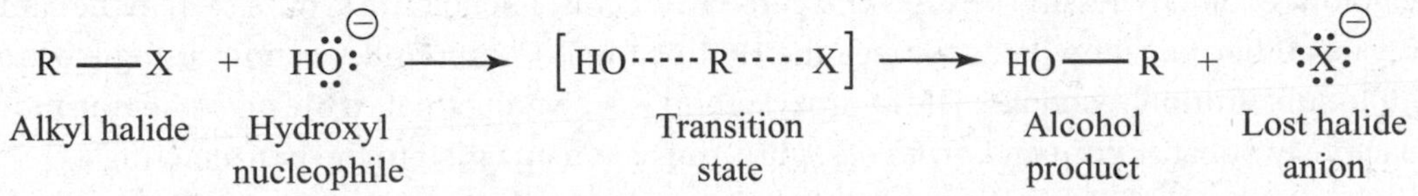

Figure 4.70. The S_N2 reaction mechanism where R–X is a 1° or 2° alkyl halide

As can be seen in the figure, the term *bimolecular substitution* comes from the fact that two separate reactants (the substrate and the nucleophile) must come together to form the transition state, which then leads to the loss of a halide anion and to the alcohol product. These reactions exhibit **second order kinetics,** which supports the bimolecular mechanism. Factors that affect the rate and yield of these reactions include the identity of the "leaving" halide atom (generally bromine and iodine are the best halogen leaving atoms), the reaction solvent (polar aprotic solvents that cannot hydrogen bond are best), and the structure of the alkyl halide substrate (1° are better than 2°. Usually 3° do not work).

Unimolecular nucleophilic substitution (S_N1) can also produce alcohol products, but they often result in mixtures. When branched alkyl halide substrates are reacted with hydroxide bases in polar protic solvents, elimination products, namely alkenes, usually dominate. Few or no alcohol products are produced.

Figure 4.71 shows the general two-step mechanism for this process.

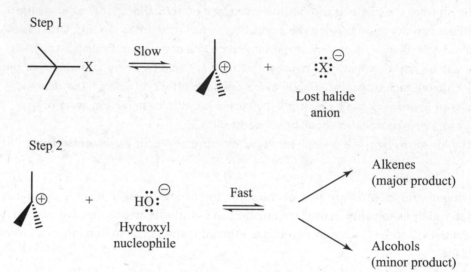

Figure 4.71. The S_N1 reaction mechanism

The first step of the mechanism involves the spontaneous loss of a halide anion (X–) and formation of an intermediate carbocation. Because this step is slow, it determines the rate of the reaction and as such these processes exhibit first order kinetics. In the second step, which is fast, the carbocation intermediate reacts with a hydroxide anion to form either alkenes (if the anion acts as a base and abstracts a proton from the carbocation) or alcohols (if the anion acts as a nucleophile and attacks the carbocation directly). As indicated earlier, this process is usually not a good way to prepare alcohols, but both of these substitution mechanisms regularly show up in MCAT exam passages and you should be familiar with them.

Other common methods for synthesizing alcohols are the reduction of carbonyl compounds and the reaction of carbonyl compounds with organometallic reagents, both of which are types of addition reactions. These processes are discussed later in this section under the reactions of aldehydes and ketones and carboxylic acids. Phenols are synthesized in the same ways as other benzene derivates (see the Hydrocarbon Compounds section) using electrophilic substitution reactions. The hydroxyl group is activating (makes the benzene ring more reactive to substitution) and *ortho/para* directing when attached to the benzene ring.

The **reactions** of alcohols are quite varied with some of the most important falling into the category of oxidation. This is also an important reaction category for hydrocarbons. Recall that the elimination of water (H_2O) from alcohols can be used to prepare alkenes, another common hydrocarbon. Figure 4.72 shows a generalized reaction web for some of the most important reactions of alcohols.

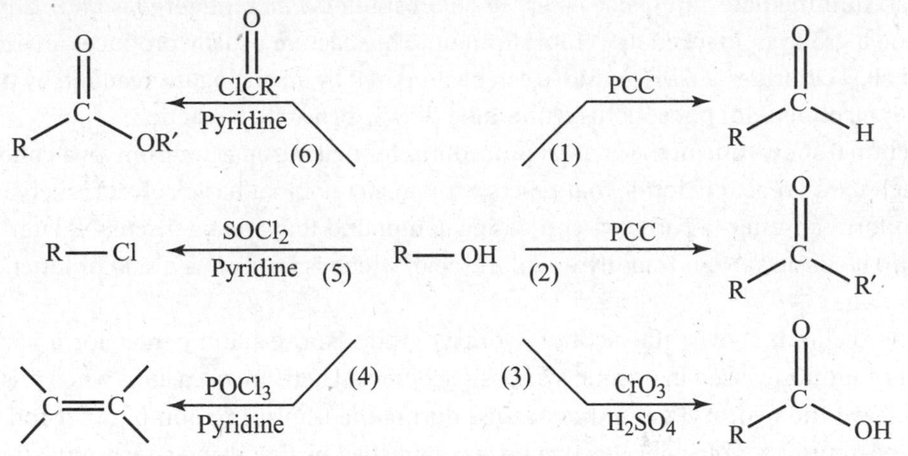

Figure 4.72. Alcohol reaction web

If a 1° alcohol is treated with the mild oxidizing agent pyridinium chlorochromate (PCC, see reaction 1), it is transformed into an aldehyde. The same process (reaction 2) produces ketones from 2° alcohols. Because of valence considerations, 3° alcohols cannot be directly oxidized.

Reaction 3 in the figure shows the use of a stronger oxidizer (chromium trioxide) in sulfuric acid. This reaction produces **carboxylic acids** from 1° alcohols. These harsh conditions often produce low yields of the acids. This reaction gives **ketones** from 2° alcohols.

There are several ways to dehydrate alcohols to prepare *alkenes*. Reactions using strong aqueous acid and heat can sometimes be used, but this approach, because of the formation of an intermediate carbocation, often produces mixtures of alkenes. A better and milder approach uses phosphorus oxychloride ($POCl_3$) in the basic solvent pyridine (see reaction 4). This reaction proceeds by an S_N2 mechanism and thus avoids the problematic formation of carbocations.

Alcohols can be transformed into **alkyl halides** using S_N2 reactions. As with the formation of alcohols from alkyl halides (the reverse process discussed earlier in this section) 1° alcohols are better than 2°, and 3° usually do not work. The limitation in all these reactions is that the hydroxide anion (^-OH) is a very poor leaving group. This problem can be overcome by transforming it into a much better leaving group using the reagent *p*-toluenesulfonyl chloride (commonly referred to as tosyl chloride). Figure 4.73 shows the generalized reaction of an alcohol with this compound followed by reaction with a nucleophile—in this case a halide anion (X–).

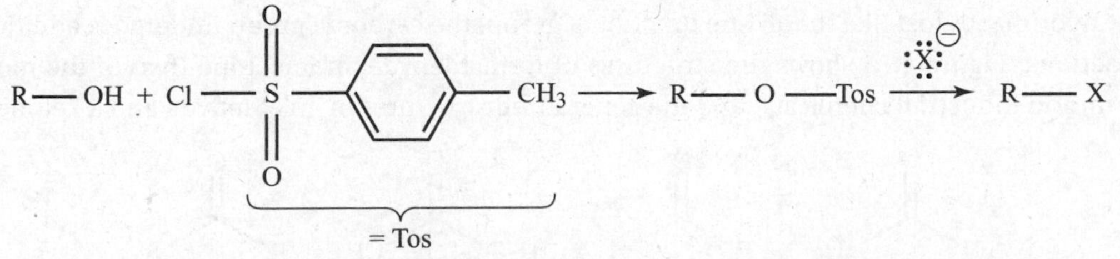

Figure 4.73. Preparation of an alkyl halide from an alcohol using tosyl chloride.
Note: The alcohol must be 1° or 2° and X may be Cl, Br, or I. The R-O-Tos intermediate shown is commonly referred to as a tosylate.

Reaction 5 in Figure 4.72 shows another reagent, thionyl chloride ($SOCl_2$), which is valuable for the specific preparation of **alkyl chlorides** from 1° and 2° alcohols. This reaction forms an intermediate "inorganic ester" (a chlorosulfite), which undergoes an S_N2 process when the R group is attacked by a chloride anion. The reaction usually produces an excellent yield of alkyl chlorides. **Alkyl bromides** can be prepared by an analogous reaction by treating 1° and 2° alcohols with phosphorus tribromide (PBr_3), also an S_N2 reaction.

Reaction 6 shows one of the general procedures for making an ester from an alcohol. This approach uses an acid chloride that reacts with an alcohol in a basic solvent, such as pyridine, to form an ester (a carbonyl-containing compound that will be discussed later in this review). The basic solvent traps hydrochloric acid, which is formed as a side product during the reaction.

As the diagram shows, the alcohol hydroxyl group is a reaction center for a variety of reagents commonly used in organic synthesis schemes. There are occasions when it is desirable to leave the hydroxyl group unchanged during the transformation of other functional groups present in a molecule. This can be accomplished by first using a technique that protects the hydroxyl group—that is, a reaction that changes the hydroxyl group into an unreactive species that can later be reversed when other reactions have been completed. The net process leaves the hydroxyl group unchanged. One of the most common methods of alcohol protection is reaction with chlorotrimethylsilane. This process produces a trimethylsilyl (TMS) ether, which is inert to oxidizing agents, reducing agents, and organometallic addition reagents. Figure 4.74 shows the generalized protect/de-protect reactions of an alcohol using chloro-TMS (protection) and acid (de-protection).

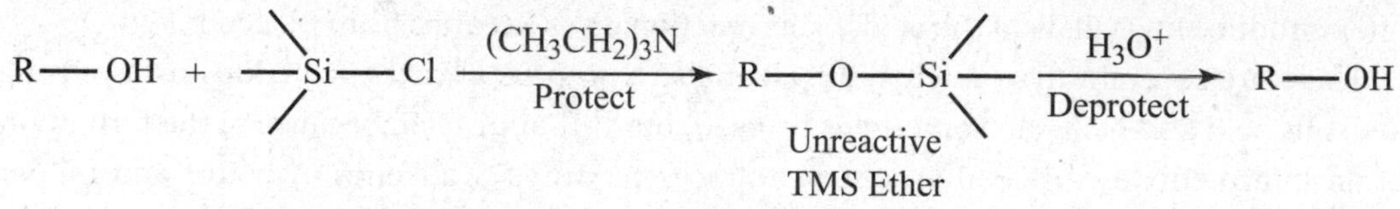

Figure 4.74. The protection/de-protection of an alcohol hydroxyl group

The TMS protecting group can be easily removed by reacting the TMS ether with aqueous acid, as shown in the above figure. Note that the alcohol is regenerated in this step (the TMS ether is converted into a TMS alcohol—TMS–OH by-product).

Aldehydes and Ketones

Aldehydes and **ketones** belong to the family of carbonyl-containing compounds. The carbonyl group consists of a carbon–oxygen double bond (C=O). Both aldehydes and ketones contain the carbonyl group. They are some of the most numerous naturally occurring organic compounds. Both the carbon and the oxygen atoms in the carbonyl double bond are also sp^2 hybridized. Just like the alkene functional group, the carbonyl group undergoes addition reactions. Figure 4.75 shows the structures of formaldehyde and acetone (two of the most common industrial chemicals) and the generalized structures of an aldehyde and a ketone.

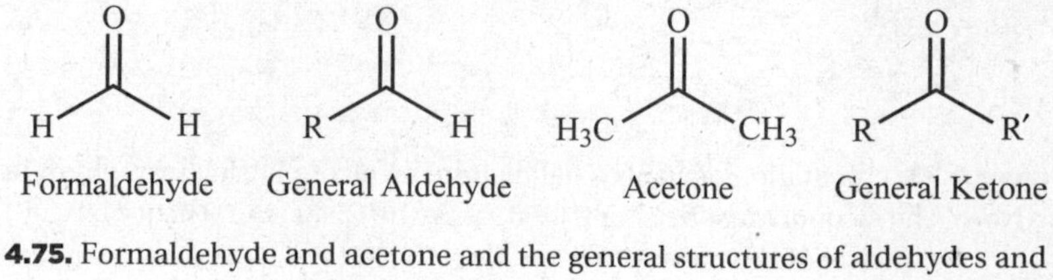

Figure 4.75. Formaldehyde and acetone and the general structures of aldehydes and ketones

NOMENCLATURE

Aldehydes are named using IUPAC rules by replacing the *-e* suffix of alkane with the suffix *-al*. For example, methane becomes methanal and ethane becomes ethanal. The common name for the simplest aldehyde, formaldehyde, is accepted by IUPAC. For compounds with longer carbon chains, the aldehyde group is always designated the number one carbon (it has to be terminal) and the rest of the chain numbered from there on with substituents receiving these numbers depending on where they are attached. The following structure (85) provides an example.

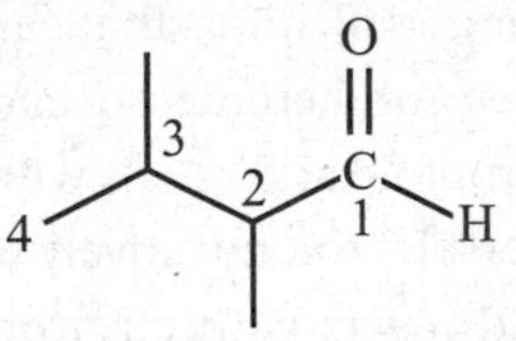

2,3-dimethylbutanal (85)

The longest chain containing the aldehyde group is four carbons, and thus the root name of the compound is butanal (the compound also has two attached methyl substituents at positions 2 and 3 along the chain). When it is necessary to refer to the aldehyde group as a substituent, the prefix *formyl-* is used.

Ketones are named using IUPAC rules by replacing the *-e* suffix of alkane with the suffix *-one*. For example, propane (the smallest carbon chain that can be a ketone) becomes propanone and butane becomes butanone. The principal chain is the longest chain that contains the ketone group and is numbered from the end nearest the carbonyl carbon. The following structure (86) provides an example.

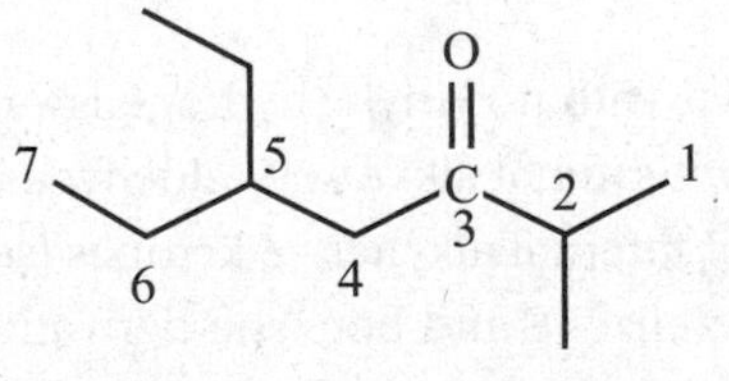

5-ethyl-2-methyl-3-heptanone (86)

The longest chain containing the ketone group is seven carbons and thus the root name of the compound is heptanone, with the carbonyl group in the 3 position (the compound also has an ethyl and a methyl group attached to the principal chain in the 2 and 5 positions respectively). When it is necessary to refer to the ketone group as a substituent, the prefix *oxo-* is used.

PROPERTIES AND USES

The carbon–oxygen double bond (the carbonyl group), to a major extent, defines the physical and chemical properties of aldehydes and ketones. The carbonyl group, because it contains oxygen, is highly polarized. Most of the group's electron density resides at the oxygen end (which carries a partial negative charge) with the carbon end being electron deficient with a partial positive charge. The generalized carbonyl structure (87) shown below illustrates this property.

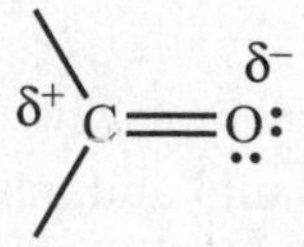

$$\delta^+ \overset{\diagdown}{\diagup}C = \overset{\delta^-}{\underset{\cdot\cdot}{O}}:$$

(87)

As a result of the polarized carbonyl group, aldehydes and ketones have elevated boiling points relative to similar alkanes and alkenes. This is because of the dipole–dipole intermolecular attractive forces between these molecules. They are not capable of true hydrogen bonding, but the partially negatively charged oxygen in the carbonyl can act as a hydrogen acceptor with molecules such as water and alcohols that can hydrogen bond.

The carbonyl group gives aldehydes and ketones special chemical properties. The positively charged carbon acts as an electrophile and reacts with the same kinds of nucleophiles already covered in this review. Conversely, the negatively charged oxygen has, as might be expected, nucleophilic properties and reacts with electrophiles. Another property of carbonyls is that the hydrogens on carbons directly adjacent to the carbonyl carbon (called the α *position*) are slightly acidic (pK_a ~ 17–19) and can be removed by a strong base. This phenomenon is important in the synthesis of more complex carbonyl-group-containing compounds and will be discussed later in this review. Aldehydes and ketones are widely used for a vast range of purposes, including over-the-counter drugs and home building materials.

SYNTHESIS AND REACTIONS

Review the following methods for preparing aldehydes and ketones.

- Oxidation of primary alcohols → aldehydes (see page 615)
- Oxidation of secondary alcohols → ketones (see page 615)
- Oxidative cleavage of alkenes with at least one vinylic hydrogen → aldehydes (see page 604)
- Oxidative cleavage of alkenes with no vinylic hydrogens → ketones (see page 604)
- Hydroboration/oxidation of terminal alkynes → aldehydes (see page 606)
- Hydroboration/oxidation of internal alkynes → ketones (see page 606)
- Friedel-Crafts acylation of benzene and benzene derivatives → aromatic ketones (see page 607)

Another valuable technique for the synthesis of aldehydes on a laboratory scale is the **partial reduction of esters** by treatment with the reagent diisobutylaluminum hydride (DIBAH). Figure 4.76 provides a generalized example of this synthetic process.

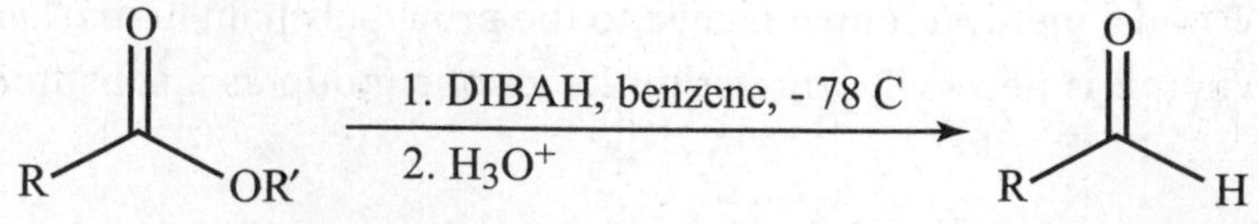

Figure 4.76. A method for the preparation of aldehydes from esters

The most important reactions of aldehydes and ketones fall into three categories:

1. Nucleophilic addition (which includes reduction reactions)
2. Enolate ion reactions
3. Oxidation

Nucleophilic addition involves the attack of the partially positive carbon (an electron deficient reaction center, or electrophile) in the carbonyl group by a myriad of neutral and negatively charged nucleophiles. These reactions produce many new, valuable functional groups that can be retained in the molecule or transformed to other groups. The general mechanistic scheme for this large group of processes is shown in Figure 4.77 below.

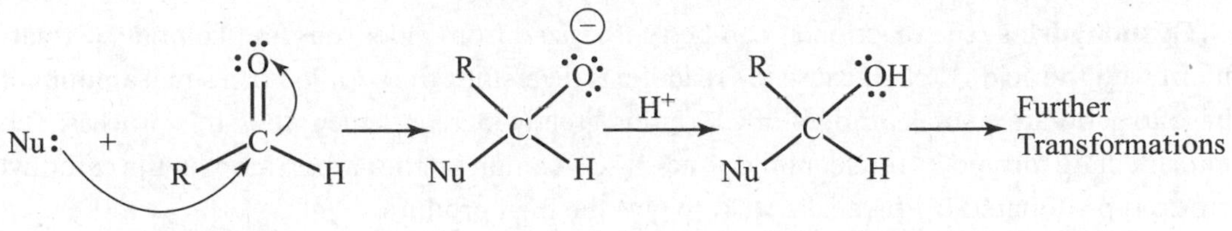

Figure 4.77. Nucleophilic addition to the carbonyl functional group

The nucleophile shown in Figure 4.77 is neutral, but it can also have a formal negative charge. In many cases, the hydroxyl group, shown in the third species (left to right) of the figure is lost (often as water) and only the functional group associated with nucleophile remains. This species then often undergoes further changes, which produce the target product. The starting compound shown in the scheme is an aldehyde, but exactly the same process takes place with ketones.

Figure 4.78 shows a nucleophilic addition reaction web that includes many of the most important examples of this reaction type. Note that the molecule at the center of the reaction web is generalized and can represent either an aldehyde or a ketone.

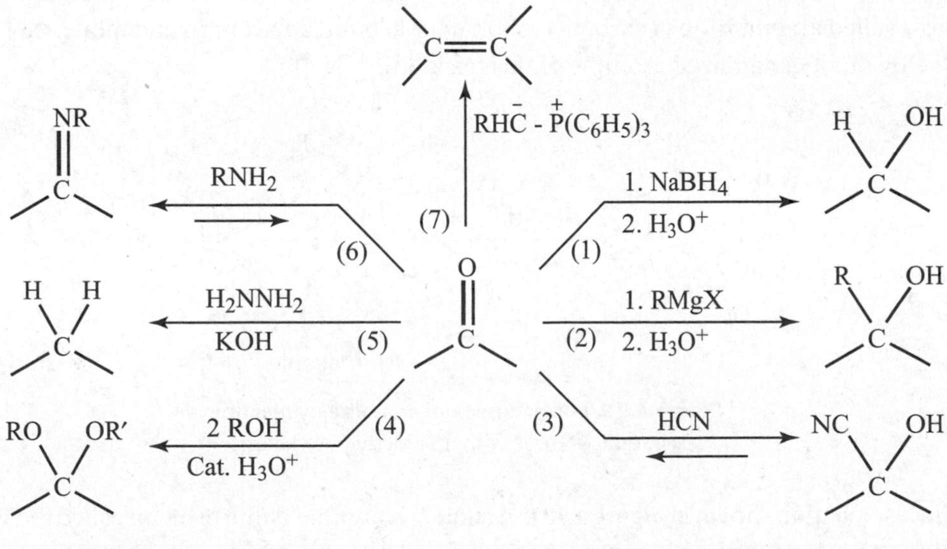

> **WHY ALDEHYDES ARE MORE REACTIVE THAN KETONES**
>
> - Aldehydes have less steric hindrance at the carbon of the carbonyl group.
> - Their carbonyl groups are more polarized than those of ketones. This makes the carbon in the carbonyl group more positive and thus more attractive to nucleophiles.

Figure 4.78. Nucleophilic addition reaction web for aldehydes and ketones

In reaction 1, the use of a hydride donor (in this case, sodium borohydride, $NaBH_4$, with a proton source) leads to the formation of alcohols from aldehydes and ketones. Another commonly used reducing agent for this process is lithium aluminum hydride ($LiAlH_4$) followed by the addition of water, another proton source.

More complex alcohols can be produced from aldehydes and ketones (see reaction 2) by reaction with a Grignard reagent (RMgX, where X is usually Cl or Br). This reaction begins with the positively charged Mg ion complexing with the partly negatively charged carbonyl oxygen. This further polarizes the carbonyl bond and makes its carbon more susceptible to attack by the R:$^-$ nucleophile of the Grignard reagent. Aqueous acid is added in the second step to protonate the intermediate and give an alcohol.

Cyanohydrins (see reaction 3) can be synthesized from aldehydes and ketones by treatment with the acid HCN. Because the reaction is reversible, the addition of a small amount of base to generate a small amount of CN$^-$ anion greatly increases the rate of this process. The intermediate formed by nucleophilic attack by CN$^-$ anion on the carbon atom in the carbonyl group is protonated by the acidic HCN to give the final product.

When two equivalents of an alcohol in the presence of a catalytic amount of acid (the process is reversible) are reacted with an aldehyde or ketone, an **acetal** (see reaction 4) is produced. The nucleophilic addition of the first equivalent of alcohol initially produces a hydroxy ether called a **hemiacetal**. The mechanism involves an initial protonation of the carbonyl oxygen and two subsequent nucleophilic attacks by alcohol molecules on its carbon. Loss of water and a proton leads to the formation of the acetal.

Reaction 5 is called the **Wolff–Kishner** reaction. It is a convenient method for changing carbonyl groups into a CH_2. In this process the carbonyl is first reacted with hydrazine, H_2NNH_2, to form a hydrazone intermediate, which, when heated, loses nitrogen gas (N_2) to form an alkane. The protons needed to form the CH_2 group come from the reaction solvent, which is usually dimethyl sulfoxide (DMSO).

Nucleophilic addition of primary (1°) amines, shown in reaction 6, to ketones and aldehydes yields products that are called **imines**. This reaction process proceeds much as the others outlined in Figure 4.78, with the amine nitrogen attacking the partially positively charged carbon of the carbonyl, followed by the loss of water and a proton from the tetrahedral intermediate. If a secondary amine is used in this process, a slightly different compound is formed, called an **enamine** (a carbon–carbon double bond adjacent to an amine; see Figure 4.79 below for a generalized example of this reaction).

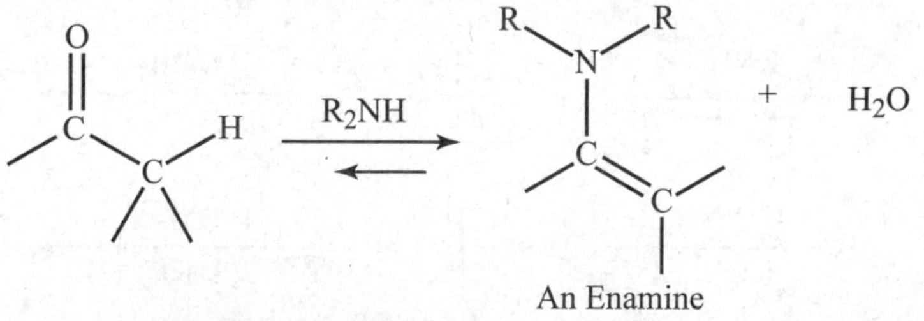

Figure 4.79. Formation of an enamine by reacting a secondary amine with an aldehyde or ketone

The last reaction shown in Figure 4.78 (reaction 7) is another name reaction called the **Wittig** reaction. It is used to form alkenes by coupling the carbonyl carbon in aldehydes or ketones to another carbon provided by a phosphorus-containing reactant called an **ylide** [$R_2C=P(C_6H_5)_3$ is the generalized formula for a commonly used ylide]. Nucleophilic attack at the carbon of the carbonyl by the ylide carbon produces a metastable four-membered ring intermediate consisting of two joined carbons, an oxygen from the carbonyl, and the phosphorus atom of the ylide. This species spontaneously decomposes to give the alkene and triphenylphosphine oxide [$O{=}P(C_6H_5)_3$]. This reaction produces only a single alkene structural isomer, and the carbon–carbon double bond is always where the carbonyl group was in the aldehyde or ketone.

Enolate ion reactions. Remember that the hydrogens on either side of the carbonyl groups of aldehydes and ketones (as well as some other carbonyl containing functional groups) are slightly acidic. It is, in fact, possible for one of these hydrogens to be transferred to the oxygen atom of the carbonyl group, resulting in another isomer called an **enol**. For aldehydes and ketones with α carbons bearing hydrogen, when the keto and enol forms are at equilibrium, the keto form dominates, but there is still a tiny amount of the enol form (about 0.0000001%). These two isomers, which differ only in the placement of a single proton, are called **tautomers**.

> **ENOLIZATION**
>
> The two tautomers associated with aldehydes and ketones are called the **keto** and the **enol** forms. The process of converting between these is called **enolization**. The equilibrium between the two strongly favors the keto form. The enolization equilibrium of aldehydes and ketones is seen in Structure 88:
>
> 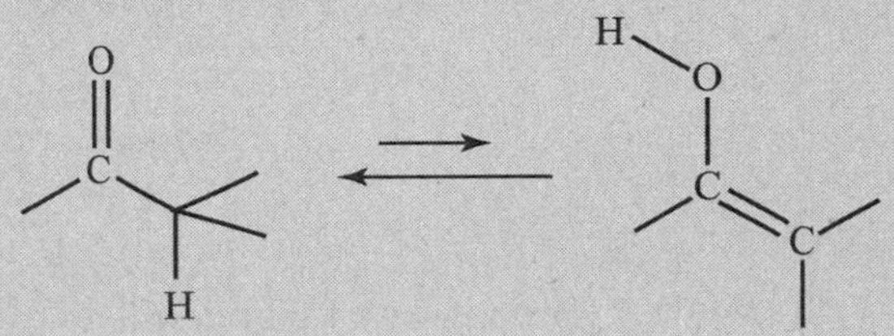
>
> (88)

Because the hydrogens in the α positions to the carbonyl group are acidic, they can be removed by using strong base. When these carbons are deprotonated, the resulting carbanions (fully negatively charged carbon atoms) are called **enolates**. These resonance stabilized carbanions can, like any negatively charged species, act like nucleophiles and add to electron-deficient sites in reactions. **Enolate** ions participate in a number of types of nucleophilic addition reactions.

One classic enolate reaction of aldehydes and ketones is the **aldol** (*ald* from aldehyde and *ol* from alcohol) **condensation**. In this reaction, the enolate ion formed by abstraction of a proton by base from the α carbon of an aldehyde or ketone goes on to attack the carbon of the carbonyl of another aldehyde or ketone molecule. The product of the reaction is called an **aldol** and contains both a carbonyl group and an alcohol group β to the carbonyl. The generalized process of forming an aldol is shown below in Figure 4.80. Because this reaction is an equilibrium-driven process, the yield of many condensate reactions is low, with aldehydes generally giving higher yields. The aldol product of the condensation reaction can be dehydrated (caused to lose water) by heating. This leads to the formation of an α, β unsaturated aldehyde or ketone.

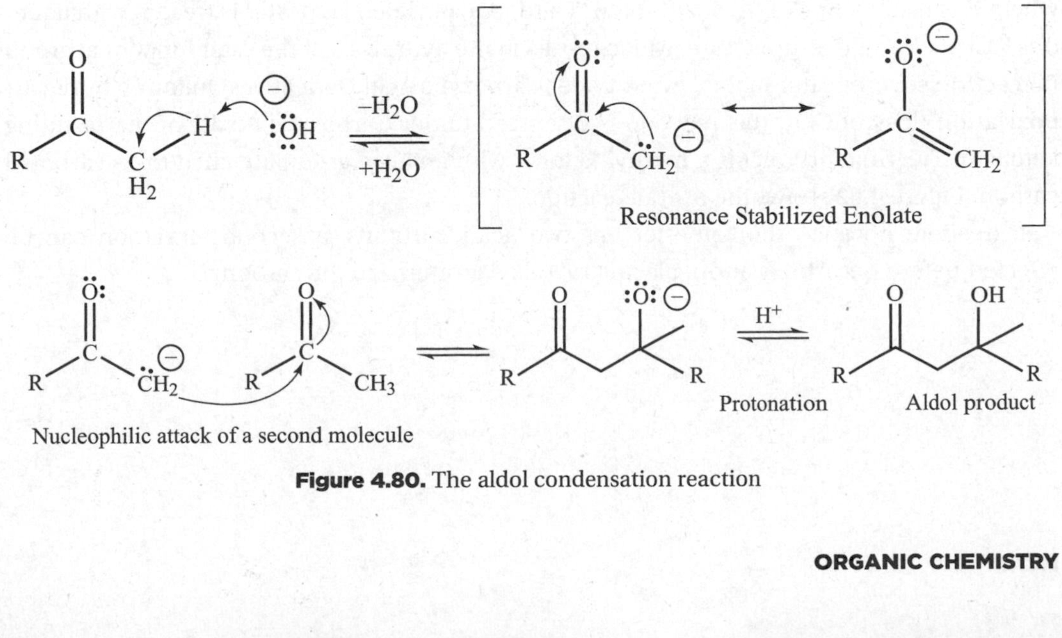

Figure 4.80. The aldol condensation reaction

A variation of the aldol condensation reaction is the direct alkylation of ketones. In order to completely convert the ketone reactant to an enolate, a strong hindered base is necessary. Lithium diisopropylamide (LDA) is commonly used to form the enolate, which then reacts with an alkyl substrate with a good leaving group (usually an alkyl halide) in an aprotic solvent giving the alkylated product (see Figure 4.81 for an example of this reaction). This is clearly an S_N2 reaction. Aldehyde substrates almost always give poor yields of the alkylated products because they tend to condense with themselves (see the aldol condensation reaction in Figure 4.80) instead of reacting with the alkyl halide.

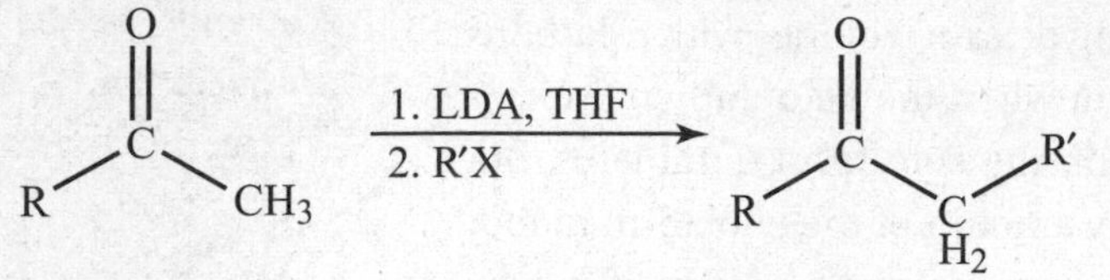

Figure 4.81. Direct alkylation of ketone α carbons.
Note that X is usually iodine in this reaction.

Carbons with hydrogens α to two carbonyl groups are particularly acidic (pK_a ~ 9), mostly because of resonance stabilization. Upon deprotonation by a base, the resulting enolate can spread out its negative charge over both carbonyls. Structure 89 shows the charge delocalization process.

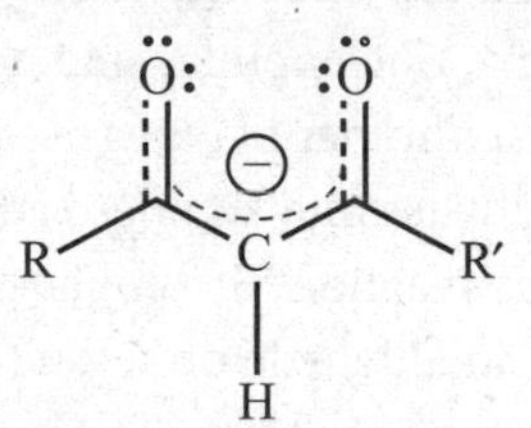

(89)

Several alkalation reactions take advantage of the high acidity of these special protons, because a simple base such as sodium hydroxide (NaOH) can be used to form enolate ions. The most important of these alkylation processes uses a ketoester commonly called ethyl acetoacetate (see Figure 4.82) and is referred to as the **acetoacetic ester synthesis**. This reaction process consists of three basic steps. First is the formation of an enolate by reaction of base with ethyl acetoacetate. Second, the enolate is reacted with a primary alkyl halide (RX, where X is usually Br or I) in S_N2 fashion. Third, the alkylated ketoester is treated with aqueous HCl at elevated temperature, which results in the hydrolysis of the ester functional group (a reaction covered later in this review under Carboxylic Acid Derivatives) followed by decarboxylation (loss of CO_2; this reaction is discussed under Carboxylic Acids) of the resulting ketoacid. The final product is a **methyl ketone**, with an alkyl group attached to its carbonyl carbon. Figure 4.82 shows the overall reaction.

If desired, because the ketoester has two acidic protons, a second alkylation can be effected before decarboxylation, placing *two* alkyl groups α to the carbonyl.

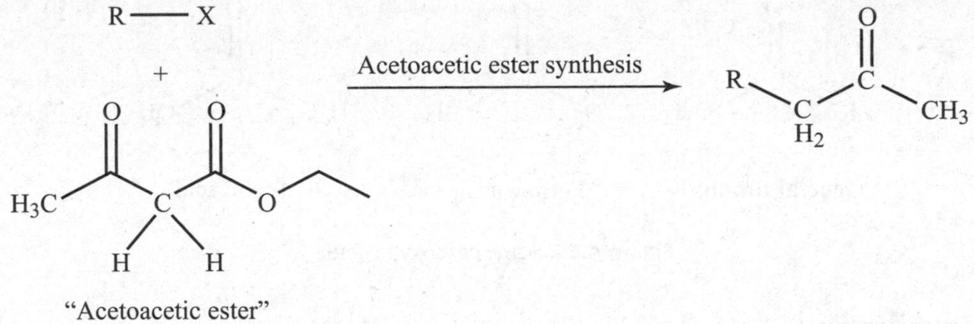

Figure 4.82. The acetoacetic ester synthesis used for the alkylation of ketones

Enolate anions produced from methyl ketones can react with halogens. As a result, the hydrogens α to their carbonyls are replaced with halogen atoms (usually Br or I). If an excess amount of the halogen is used, all the hydrogens are replaced and a **haloform** (HCX_3) product is produced, which is a good leaving group. The starting methyl ketone is converted into a carboxylate salt. This transformation, known as the **haloform reaction**, is shown in Figure 4.83.

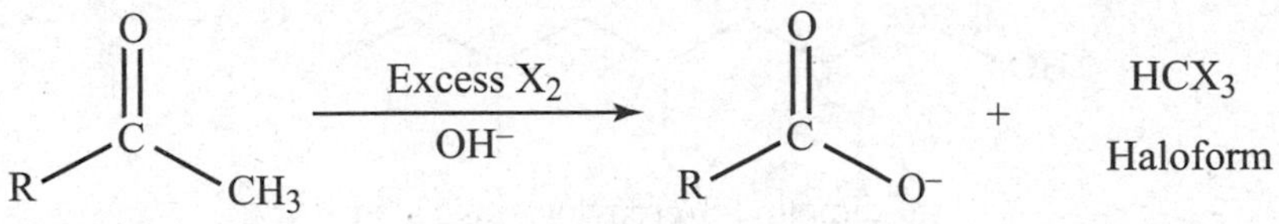

Figure 4.83. The haloform reaction—reaction of a methyl ketone with excess X_2

Oxidation. Although not a particularly useful reaction, it is possible to oxidize aldehydes to **carboxylic acids** using a number of reagents. Figure 4.84 provides a generalized example of this process.

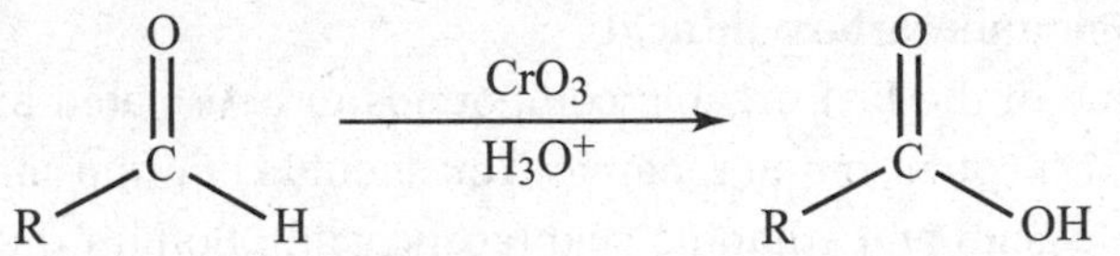

Figure 4.84. Oxidation of aldehydes to carboxylic acids

> **HALOFORM REACTIONS WITH IODINE**
>
> When iodine (I_2) is used in a haloform reaction, the process produces iodoform (HCI_3), which is a yellow precipitate that can be used to confirm the presence of a methyl ketone. Other kinds of ketones don't give a positive **iodoform test**.

Carboxylic Acids

Other members of the carbonyl-containing family of compounds are carboxylic acids. The molecules of these substances all contain a **carboxyl functional** group. The atomic architecture of this group consists of a hydroxyl group attached to the carbon of a carbonyl group. These compounds are often referred to as "organic acids" and are one of the most important and numerous classes of naturally occurring organic molecules. Figure 4.85 shows a generalized structural formula for a carboxylic acid and two of the simplest varieties, formic acid and acetic acid.

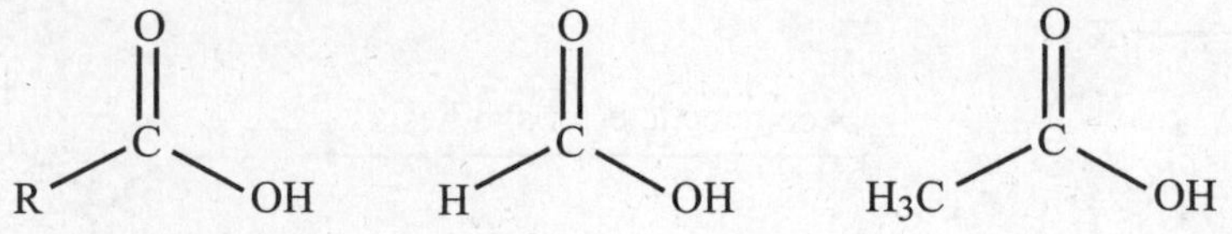

Figure 4.85. Some carboxylic acids

NOMENCLATURE

There are two accepted forms of IUPAC nomenclature for carboxylic acids. The most commonly used involves replacing the -*e* suffix of the corresponding alkane with -*oic* **acid**. As with aldehydes, the carboxyl group is always terminal, so it is designated number 1 in the principal chain (the longest continuous carbon chain containing the carboxyl group) of the molecule. The following example (structure 89) shows the IUPAC naming process for these compounds.

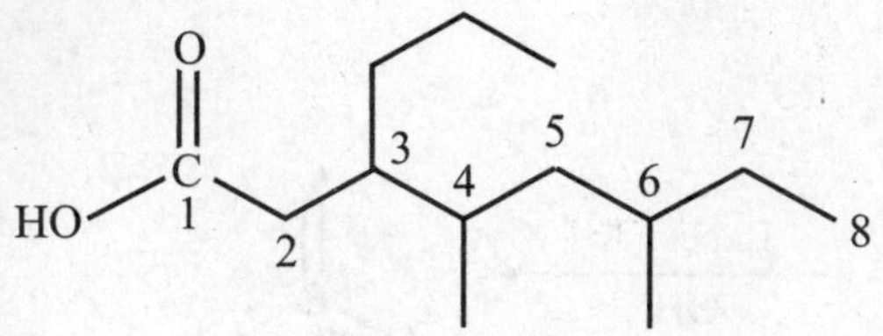

4,6-dimethyl-3-propyloctanoic acid

(89)

The principal chain in the compound contains eight carbons, so the root name for the compound is **octanoic acid**. The number assignments of the other substituents, two methyl groups at carbons 4 and 6 and a propyl group at carbon 3, are defined by the carboxyl group at carbon number 1 in the principal chain.

Another approach is used if a compound has a carboxyl group bonded to a carbon ring. In this case the suffix -*carboxylic* **acid** is used. For example, a cyclopentane ring with a carboxyl group attached would be called **cyclopentanecarboxylic acid**.

Because carboxylic acids were some of the first organic compounds to be isolated and characterized, they have many IUPAC accepted common names. You should know the common name for methanoic acid (formic acid) and ethanoic acid (acetic acid). Both of these acids are shown in Figure 4.85.

PROPERTIES AND USES

As with alcohols, carboxylic acids are capable of hydrogen bonding, and as such have significantly higher boiling points than their corresponding alkanes. Most of these acids can also exist as hydrogen bonded cyclic **dimers**, which is a particularly strong intermolecular interaction. This property makes the boiling points of carboxylic acids even higher than those of alcohols. Figure 4.86 shows how this interaction can occur between two acid molecules.

As might be expected, because of their hydrogen bonding abilities many of the smaller acids (less than six carbons) are water soluble.

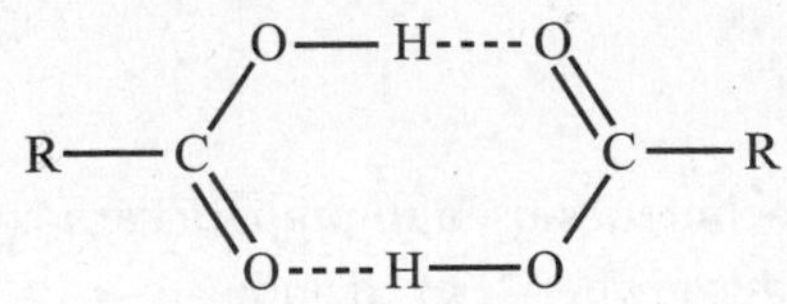

Figure 4.86. Generalized carboxylic acid hydrogen bonded dimer

The defining property of carboxylic acids, as their name implies, is their high acidity. Their acidic properties are largely due to the resonance stabilization of the carboxylate anion that is formed when its hydroxyl proton is lost. Figure 4.87 shows how the negative charge of the ion is delocalized over both oxygens of the carboxyl group.

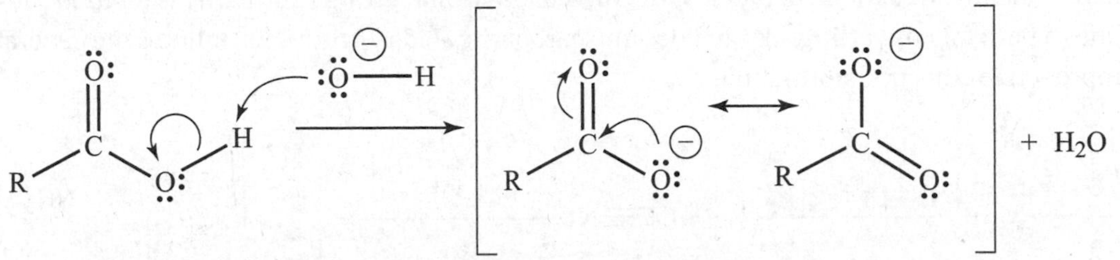

Figure 4.87. Delocalization of the carboxylate anion of a carboxylic acid

As the above figure illustrates, the carboxyl proton readily reacts with hydroxide bases to form water and the carboxylate anion. This is similar to enolate formation. The pK_a's of carboxylic acids that have small attached alkyl groups have a tight range of ~4.7–4.9 (for example acetic acid's $pK_a = 4.75$). The carboxylate can be further stabilized by electron-withdrawing groups attached at the α carbon position, resulting in a corresponding increase in acidity. For example, triflouroacetic acid (F_3CCOOH: note the three added, highly electronegative fluorine atoms) has a $pK_a = 0.20$.

Reaction of carboxylic acids with hydroxide bases (e.g., NaOH or KOH) produces metal carboxylate salts (see Figure 4.87; the metal cation is not shown) that are quite soluble in water because of their ionic character. This behavior can be used to purify acids by using a basic aqueous solution (the base reacts with the acid to form a salt) to extract them from an organic phase, followed by acidification of the aqueous extract. The crude "free acid" often precipitates from the acidic solution and can then be collected by filtration for further purification. As with other carbonyl-containing compounds, the hydrogens α to the carbonyl of carboxylic acids are also acidic and notably more acidic (pK_a~ 10) in β-dicarboxylic acids (also called 1,3-dicarboxylic acids). Abstraction of a proton from the carbon between the two carboxyl groups of these compounds produces an anion that is stabilized not only by resonance, but also by the electron-withdrawing effects of both carboxyl groups. 1,3-ketoacids, organic compounds that contain both a carboxyl group and a ketone group, exhibit similar α hydrogen acidic behavior.

Benzoic acid ($pK_a = 4.2$), a benzene ring with one attached carboxyl group, is the simplest aromatic carboxylic acid. Deactivating groups attached to its aromatic ring, because of their electron withdrawing properties, tend to increase benzoic acid's acidity. Activating groups (which are electron-donating) make it less acidic.

SYNTHESIS AND REACTIONS

Synthesis

Many of the most common techniques used to prepare carboxylic acids have already been covered in earlier sections of this review. They include

- Oxidation of alcohols → carboxylic acids (see page 615)
- Oxidation of aldehydes → carboxylic acids (see page 623)
- Oxidative cleavage of alkenes → carboxylic acids (see page 604)
- Oxidative cleavage of alkynes → carboxylic acids (see page 606)

Nitrile hydrolysis. Two additional processes can also be used to synthesize carboxylic acids. One involves the **hydrolysis of the nitrile functional group** ($^-C\equiv N$). This method provides a path for converting alkyl halides into carboxylic acids. Figure 4.88 outlines the general approach for this transformation.

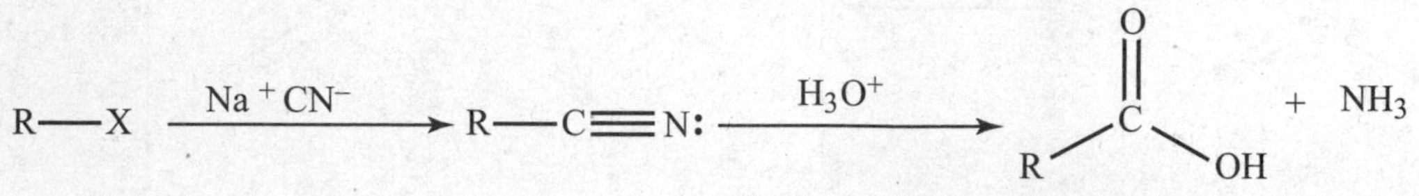

Figure 4.88. Preparation of carboxylic acids from alkyl halides

As can be seen in the figure, an alkyl halide can be readily converted into a nitrile by S_N2 reaction with a nucleophilic cyanide anion (CN^-, in this case provided by the sodium cyanide salt). The resulting nitrile is then hydrolyzed by treatment with aqueous acid. A by-product of the reaction is ammonia gas. This procedure, because it involves an S_N2 reaction to make the nitrile, works best for primary alkyl halides, although some secondary substrates also give good yields. It is not a good method for converting tertiary alkyl halides to acids because of competing elimination reactions.

Another approach that invoves the carboxylation of **Grignard reagents** can be used for tertiary alkyl halides. Figure 4.89 shows the general process for this reaction, which uses carbon dioxide gas as the carboxyl source.

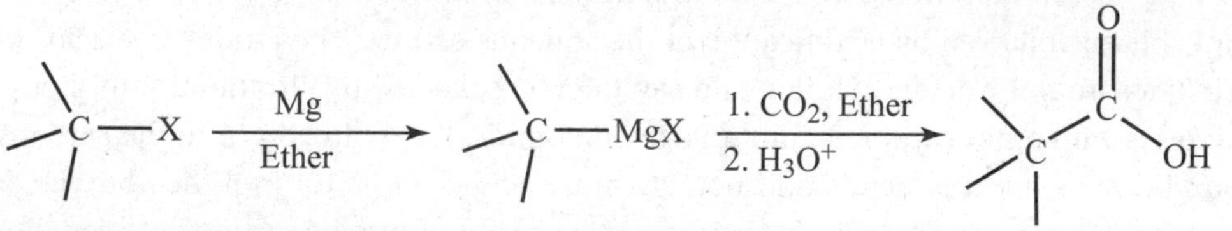

Figure 4.89. Conversion of tertiary alkyl halides to carboxylic acids

REDUCING AGENTS

Reducing agents contribute the nucleophilic hydride anion (H:–), which attacks the partially positively charged carbon of the carbonyl group in, for example, a carboxylic acid. The overall result is the addition of hydrogen atoms to the reacting substrate's active site.

Like any carbonyl-containing compound, carboxylic acids under certain conditions may undergo nucleophilic substitution. Few of the substitution reactions already covered for aldehydes and ketones are applicable to carboxylic acids because the hydroxyl of the acid's carboxyl is a poor leaving group. With a few exceptions, the hydroxyl group must be converted into a better leaving group before reactions of this type are practical.

Reactions

A couple of reactions that are directly applicable to carboxylic acids follow. One is **reduction**, using lithium aluminum hydride ($LiAlH_4$) or borane (BH_3), of carboxylic acids to primary alcohols. Because of the high oxidation state of the acid, it can be difficult to get this reaction to go to completion. Running it at elevated temperature in an aprotic solvent improves yields. (See Figure 4.90 for a generalized example of the reaction.) In step one of the transformation, the acid is reduced to an alkoxide anion (RCH_2O^-) through the loss of water, which is protonated in the second step by aqueous acid to give the alcohol. The use of BH_3 in this reaction improves the rate and it is a more selective reducing reagent.

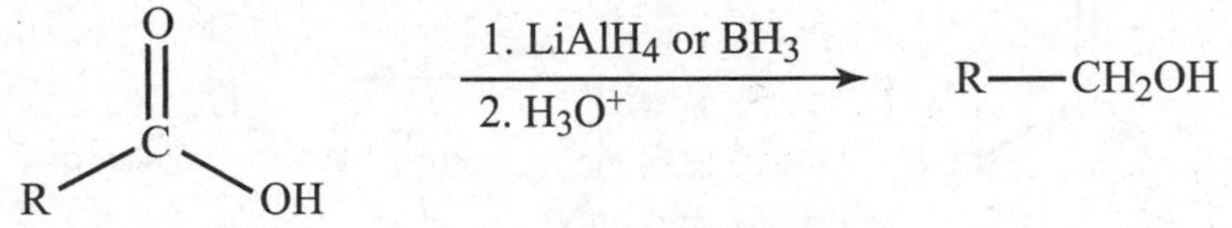

Figure 4.90. Reduction of a carboxylic acid to a primary alcohol

Decarboxylation of carboxylic acids (a type of elimination reaction) was already mentioned in the discussion of the acetoacetic ester synthesis. This is not a general reaction of carboxylic acids but is unique to 1,3-dicarbonyl compounds (those compounds that contain two carbonyl functional groups, one of which is a carboxylic acid, separated by one carbon atom—often a β-keto acid). Upon heating, these types of carboxylic acids lose their carboxyl groups as carbon dioxide (CO_2) gas. The mechanism of this process involves a cyclic conformation, and this accounts for the need for a second carbonyl group β to the carbonyl group of the acid. Figure 4.91 shows the decarboxylation reaction mechanism.

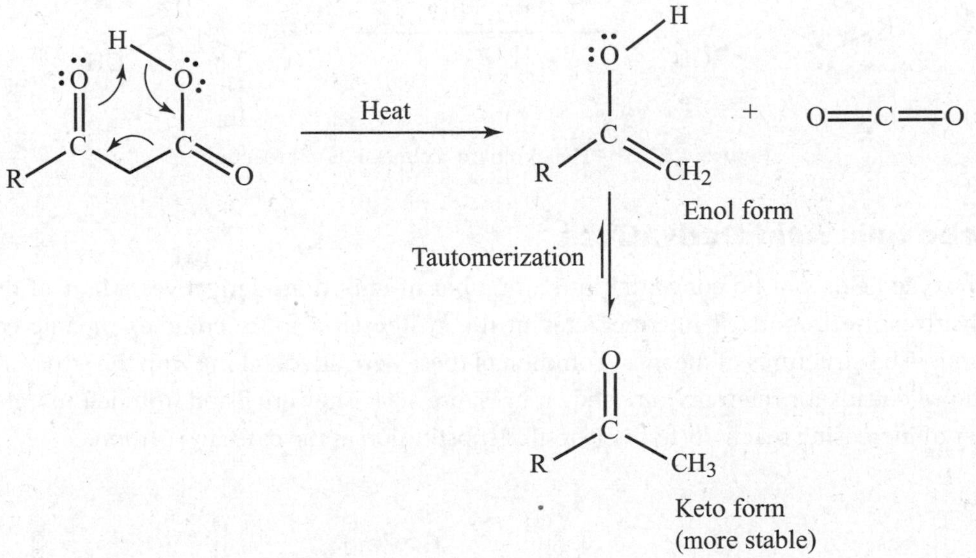

Figure 4.91. The decarboxylation mechanism of a β-keto acid

Esterification is another important reaction of carboxylic acids. There are a number of methods used to prepare esters from acids and they all involve reaction with an alcohol. One of these procedures was shown earlier in Figure 4.72, the alcohol reaction web reaction. This process involves first converting a carboxylic acid into an acid chloride (a very reactive carbonyl compound, which will be discussed later in this section under Derivatives of Carboxylic Acids), which is then reacted with an alcohol to produce an ester.

Fischer esterification refers to the formation of esters by heating carboxylic acids in an alcohol solvent with a catalytic amount of acid (only a few drops are needed). This reaction gives good yields, but is effectively limited to producing methyl, ethyl, propyl, and butyl esters because their corresponding alcohols must be used as solvents in the process. It would be possible to use more complex higher-boiling alcohols in the reaction, but the large quantity required would be expensive and separating the excess alcohol from the ester product difficult. (See Figure 4.92 for the generalized Fischer esterification reaction.)

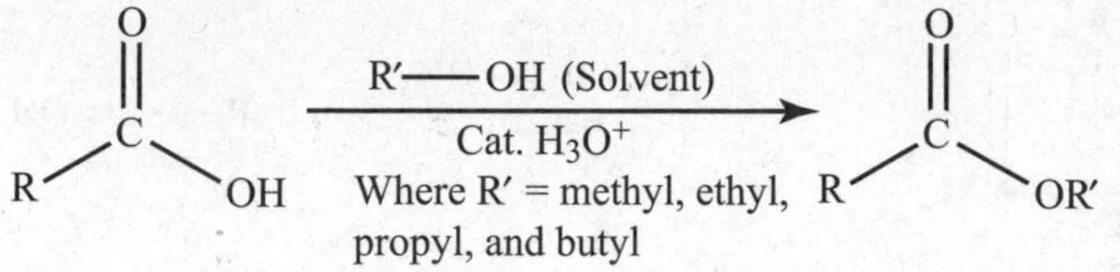

Figure 4.92. The Fischer esterification reaction

The hydrogens on carbons α to the carbonyl group of carboxylic acids are slightly acidic and can theoretically be abstracted by strong base. Unfortunately, these types of carboxylic acids do not enolize sufficiently for them to be effective nucleophiles, so they do not generally undergo the same enolate nucleophile reactions observed with aldehydes and ketones. There is, however, a way to brominate the α carbon of carboxylic acids. This is known as the **Hell–Volhard–Zelinskii (HVZ) reaction**. Figure 4.93 provides an example of this reaction.

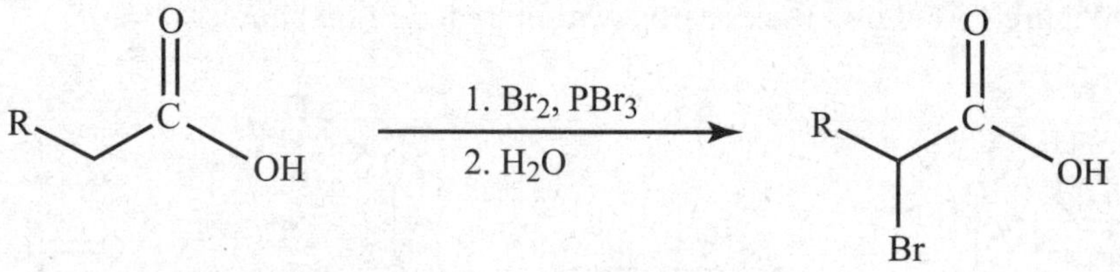

Figure 4.93. The Hell–Volhard–Zelinskii (HVZ) reaction

Carboxylic Acid Derivatives

Carboxylic acids can be converted into a number of important derivatives. Many of these derivatives are important intermediates in the synthesis of more complex organic compounds. The structures of the most common of these derivatives (along with the structure of carboxylic acids for reference) are shown in Figure 4.94. They are listed from left to right in order of increasing reactivity to nucleophilic substitution at the carbonyl carbon.

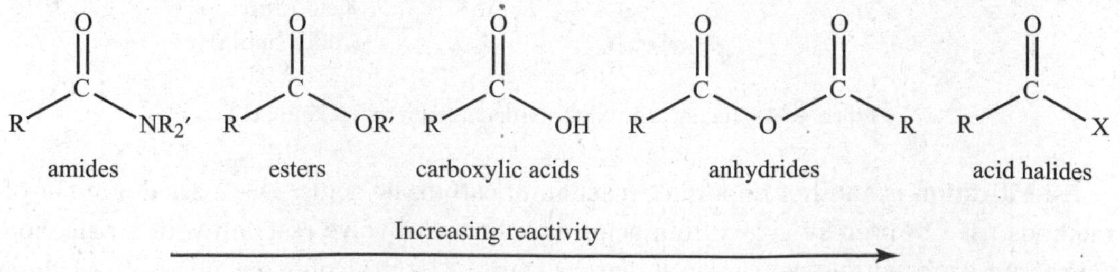

Figure 4.94. Common carboxylic acid derivatives

All carboxylic acid derivatives can undergo nucleophilic attack at the carbonyl carbon, depending on the reaction conditions. The order of reactivity outlined in Figure 4.94 can be explained by the tendency of the group attached to the carbonyl carbon (shown on the right side of each structure in the figure) to leave. The better the leaving group, the more reactive the compound to nucleophilic substitution. As a leaving group is lost, it typically becomes an anion. The lower the pK_a of the leaving group's conjugate acid, the more stable its anion will be. For example, the conjugate acid of an acid chloride's leaving group, the chloride anion, is HCl, which is extremely acidic ($pK_a \sim -7$). The chloride anion leaving group is quite stable without its proton. Thus acid chlorides are very reactive toward nucleophilic substitution reactions. The pK_a of an amide's leaving group, which is an amine, is about 40, which makes the anion (NR_2^-) very unstable. It is a poor leaving group because of its basic character. Amides are the least reactive toward nucleophilic substitution.

The generalized mechanism for nucleophilic substitution reactions of carboxylic acid derivatives is shown in Figure 4.95. This process starts out with nucleophilic attack at the carbonyl carbon (where Z is the carboxylic acid derivative's leaving group) and results in a new carbonyl-containing product.

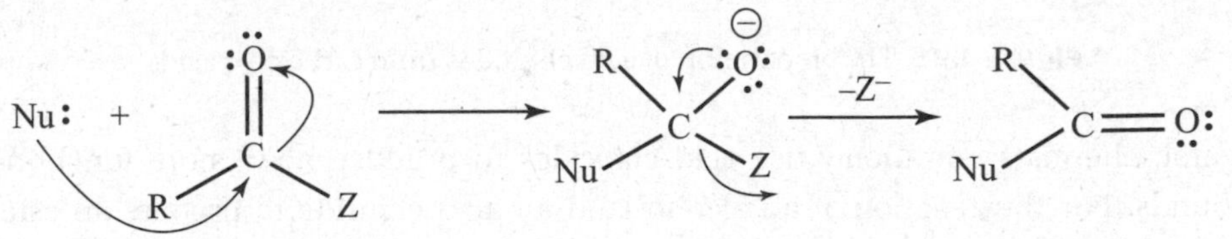

Figure 4.95. The generalized nucleophilic substitution mechanism for carboxylic acid derivatives

Note the loss of Z, the leaving group of the carboxylic acid derivative. As with other similar mechanisms, the nucleophile (Nu:) may be neutral or negatively charged, but it must have an available lone electron pair.

ACID HALIDES

Acid halides (also called acyl halides) are named under the IUPAC system by changing the -*ic* acid suffix of the parent carboxylic acid to -*yl* **halide**. The most common type of acid halide on the MCAT is an **acid chloride**.

The following example (Structure 90) shows the IUPAC naming process for an acid chloride.

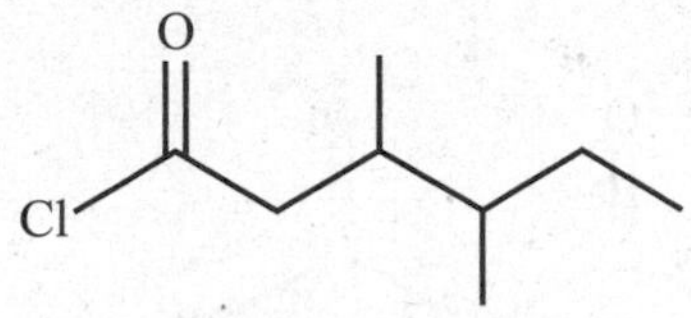

> **SUBSTITUTION REACTIONS UNDER ACIDIC CONDITIONS**
>
> In some substitution reactions run under acidic conditions, the protonation of the oxygen carbonyl makes the carbonyl carbon more susceptible to nucleophilic attack. These conditions make the reaction rates of less reactive derivatives, such as amides, faster.

3,4-dimethylhexanoyl chloride

(90)

TIP

ACID BROMIDES AND IODIDES

Acid bromides and iodides exist, but are rarely referred to in general organic chemistry studies.

Properties and Uses

Acid halides are very reactive and highly susceptible to hydrolysis. They must be protected from contact with sources of water such as humid air. The primary use of these substances is as intermediates in the synthesis of more complex organic compounds.

Synthesis and Reactions

The standard way to synthesize acid chlorides is the treatment of a carboxylic acid with the reagent thionyl chloride ($SOCl_2$). The reaction is usually run in a basic solvent such as pyridine, which captures HCl, a by-product of the process (see Figure 4.96). The reaction proceeds by an S_N2 type mechanism. Other types of acid halides can be synthesized by similar procedures.

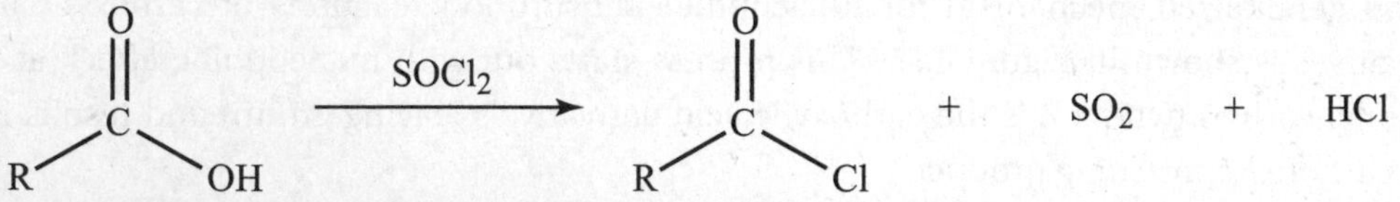

Figure 4.96. The preparation of acid chlorides from carboxylic acids

Organic chemists commonly use acid chlorides to produce new, more functionalized compounds. For the reaction of an alcohol and an acid chloride to prepare an ester, see Figure 4.72. This is often the most efficient way to produce an ester, and the reaction yields are high.

Another important reaction involving an acid chloride is Friedel–Crafts Acylation, which is used to make **alkyl aryl ketones**. For a generalized example of this transformation see Figure 4.65. This procedure involves the generation of an **acylium ion** by reaction of an acid chloride with a Lewis acid such as $AlCl_3$. The acylium cation reacts with the substrate through an electrophilic aromatic substitution mechanism.

Figure 4.97 shows a reaction web that includes three additional reactions that involve acid chlorides.

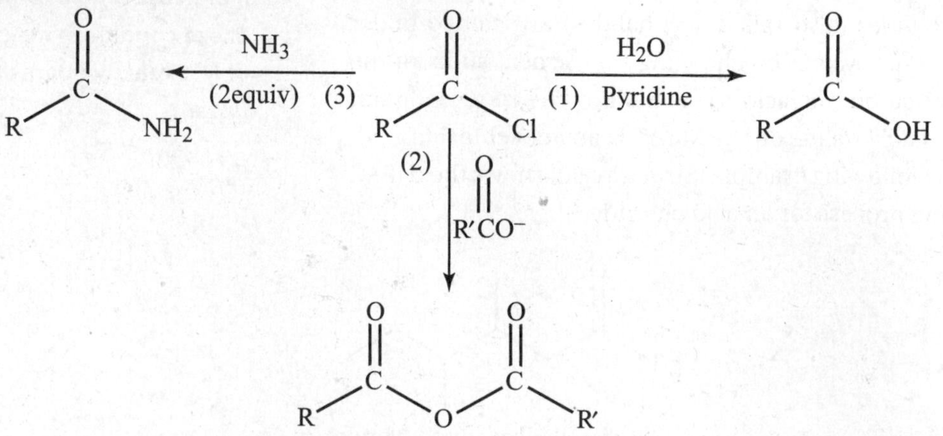

Figure 4.97. Acid chloride reaction web

Reaction 1 in Figure 4.97 shows the hydrolysis of an acid chloride to produce a carboxylic acid. The basic solvent pyridine reacts with HCl evolved in process to form a **pyridinium hydrochloride salt** (not shown).

Anhyrdrides are formed when an acid chloride is reacted with a **carboxylate salt** (see reaction 2. Only the carboxylate anion is shown). The carboxylate anion acts as a nucleophile, attacking the acid chloride carbonyl carbon. The chloro group leaves as an anion as the anhydride product is formed.

A variety of **amides** can be synthesized by reacting acid chlorides with ammonia (NH_3; see reaction 3) or primary and secondary amines. Two equivalents of the basic nitrogen reactant must be used. One equivalent acts as a nucleophile, attacking the acid chloride carbonyl carbon. The other acts as a base and reacts with the HCl by-product produced in the reaction to form an ammonium chloride salt (the salt is not shown in the reaction diagram). Primary, secondary, and tertiary amides can be prepared using this approach.

ANHYDRIDES

Anhydrides come in two forms, symmetrical and mixed. **Symmetric anhydrides** are named using the IUPAC system by replacing the *acid* suffix of the parent carboxylic acid with the term *anhydride*. **Mixed anhydrides**, which are produced from two different carboxylic acids, are named by alphabetizing the names of both acids and replacing the suffix *acid* with *anhydride*. The following structures (91 and 92) illustrate both of these IUPAC naming rules.

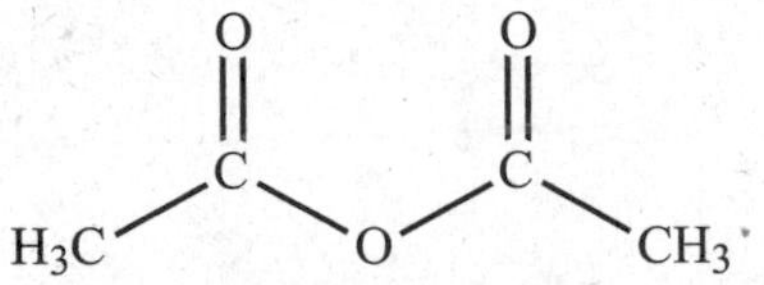

acetic anhydride   (91) 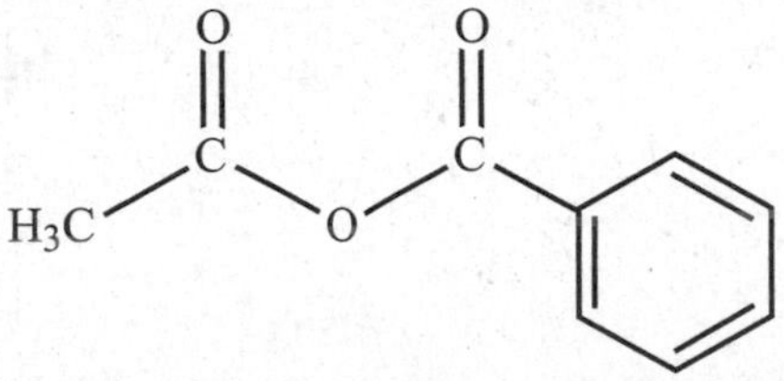   acetic benzoic anhydride   (92)

Properties and Uses

Similar to acid chlorides, although less reactive, anhydrides are easily hydrolyzed when they are exposed to water and must be stored in a cool, dry environment. Anhydrides, particularly acetic anhydride, are commonly used reagents for the acylation of alcohols and amines. These reactions are used in the pharmaceutical industry. Polymers containing many anhydride functional groups (called polyanhydrides) can be used to make biodegradable plastics.

Synthesis and Reactions

As was shown earlier (see Figure 4.97, reaction 2), both symmetric and mixed anhydrides can be synthesized by reacting an acid chloride with a carboxylate salt. This is probably the most common method to prepare a mixed anhydride.

A number of cyclic anhydrides (such as phthalic and succinic anhydride, both common names) can be produced by simply heating the corresponding dicarboxylic acids to a high temperature, which results in the loss of water (a dehydration process). Under these conditions, five-membered anhydride rings form. Figure 4.98 shows an example of this reaction. In this example, succinic acid (common name) is converted to succinic anhydride (common name).

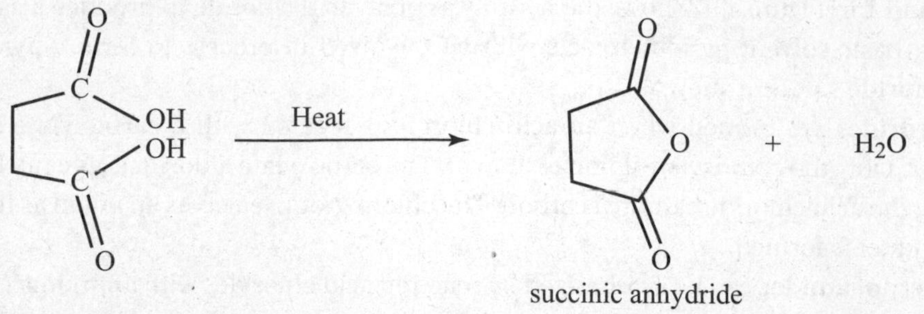

Figure 4.98. The thermal synthesis of a cyclic anhydride (succinic anhydride)

The important reactions for anhydrides are similar to those for acid halides. Figure 4.99 shows a reaction web that includes some reactions that involve anhydrides (note the similarity to Figure 4.97).

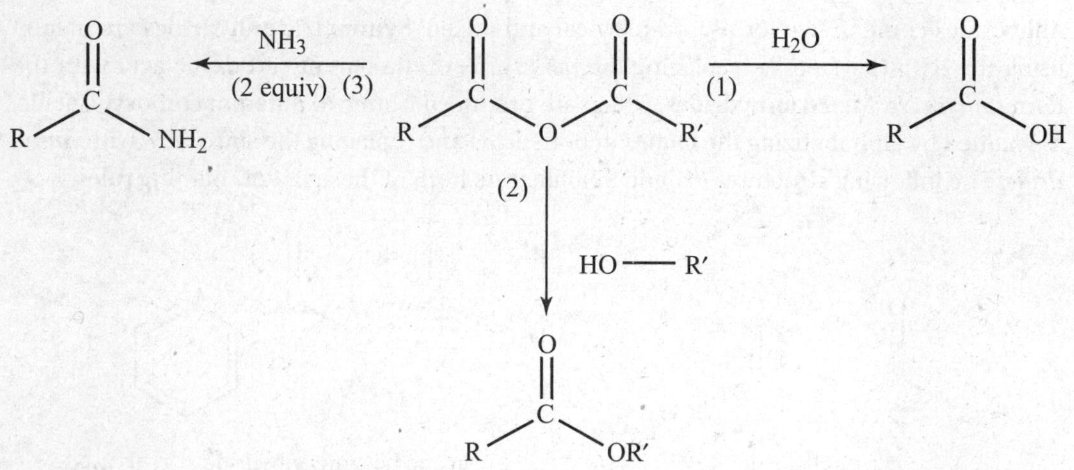

Figure 4.99. Reaction web for anhydrides

Reaction 1 shows the hydrolysis of an anhydride to produce a carboxylic acid. If the anhydride is symmetric, two moles of the same acid will be produced. If a mixed anhydride is used, a 1:1 mixture of the two parent carboxylic acids will result. Because separating the mixture can be difficult, this is generally not a good way to make a carboxylic acid.

In reaction 2, an anhydride is reacted with an alcohol to prepare an ester. This is yet another approach to synthesizing an ester but can have drawbacks because one mole of a carboxylic acid by-product (not shown in the figure) is produced in the process. Separating the acid from the ester may not be easy.

As with acid chlorides, amides can be prepared (see reaction 3) by treating an anhydride with two moles of ammonia or with a primary or secondary amine. Just as with acid chlorides, two moles of the nucleophile are required because one mole of ammonium carboxylate salt is produced as a by-product (not shown in the figure).

Anhydrides can also be used in place of acid chlorides for Friedel–Crafts Acylation reactions.

ESTERS

For IUPAC naming purposes, esters are thought of as being derived from the dehydration product of an alcohol reacting with a carboxylic acid. The part contributed to the ester from the alcohol comes first in the name and is often just an alkyl group. The part contributed from the carboxylic acid appears second in the name and is referred to as an acyl group (RCO⁻). This group is named by changing the *-ic* acid suffix of the carboxylic acid to the suffix *-ate*. For example, an ester produced by combining ethanol and acetic acid would be named *ethyl* (from the ethanol) *acetate* (from the acetic acid). Structure 93 shows another example of this naming procedure.

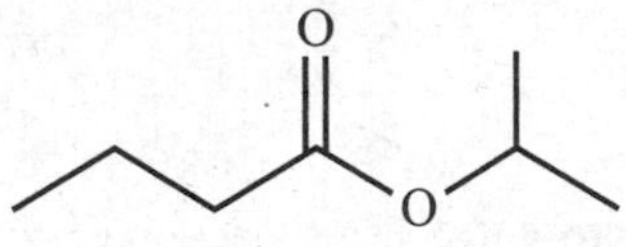

isopropyl butyrate　　　(93)

Properties and Uses

Esters, like other carboxylic acid derivatives, can undergo hydrolysis reactions, but they are much less reactive with water than acid halides and anhydrides. Under normal ambient conditions esters are fairly stable and the low boiling ones such as **ethyl acetate** can be used as solvents for a variety of applications. These solvents are fairly polar due to the oxygen atoms in their structures. There are many naturally occurring esters that have very pleasant odors. These are often found in the flowers and fruits of plants.

Synthesis and Reactions

A number of methods for making esters have already been discussed in this review. Esters can be prepared by:

- Reaction of an acid chloride and an alcohol (Figure 4.72, reaction 6)
- Reaction of an anhydride and an alcohol (Figure 4.99, reaction 2)
- The Fischer esterification process (Figure 4.92)

All of these methods, as well as other less known procedures, have their merits and drawbacks depending on the specific synthetic application. Many factors must be considered before selecting the most appropriate technique.

The most common reactions involving esters are hydrolysis, transforming them into amides, and a process called **transesterification**, which makes a new ester from a starting ester substrate. Figure 4.100 shows generalized examples of all these reactions.

Hydrolysis of esters can be carried out under either acidic (see above figure, reaction 1) or basic conditions. The acidic process is acid-catalyzed and only a few drops of added acid are needed, but as indicated above, it is a reversible equilibrium process. The first step of the reaction mechanism is the protonation of the carbonyl's

> **EQUILIBRIA**
>
> According to Le Châtelier's principle, when a reaction's equilibrium is disturbed, the reaction will adjust its equilibrium position. Adding a reactant shifts the reaction's equilibrium to the right (product side). Removing a reaction product also shifts the process to the right.

oxygen. One way to force the reaction toward the product side and completion is to remove the alcohol product as it produced. Another approach, which is usually easier, but may have other limitations, is to use a large excess of water, which is the nucleophile in the reaction.

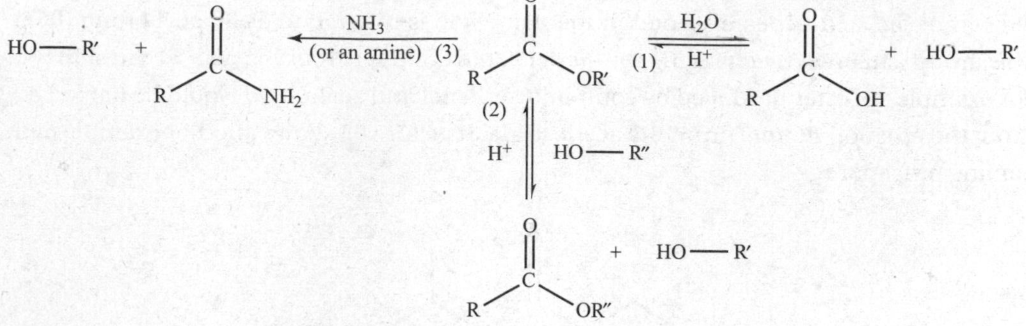

Figure 4.100. Ester reaction web

When ester hydrolysis is conducted under basic conditions, it is not base-catalyzed, and a full equivalent of base is required. The reaction product is a **carboxylate salt**. This approach is historically very old and is referred to as **saponification**. It has been used for thousands of years in soap-making processes to hydrolyze triacylglycerols (the primary components of animal fats) to produce **fatty acid salts** and **glycerol** (1,2,3-propanetriol). Fatty acid salts produced this way have long aliphatic carbon chains attached to the polar carboxylic acid group. (See Structure 94 below. Note that the metal counter-ion from the base, also commonly called lye, isn't shown.) These substances possess both polar and nonpolar properties in the same molecule, which makes them ideal for cleaning applications.

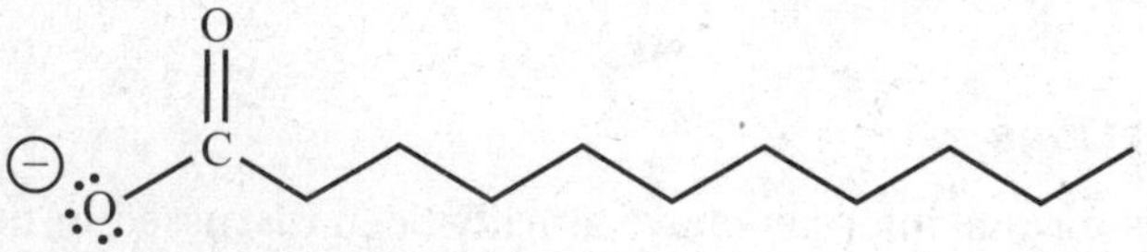

(94)

Acid-catalyzed transesterification (see reaction 2 in Figure 4.100) involves the use of alcohols as nucleophiles to attack an ester substrate's carbonyl carbon. This results in the loss of the ester's alkoxy group and the addition of a new one provided by the alcohol nucleophile. The starting ester is transformed into a new ester. Like acid-catalyzed hydrolysis of esters, this reaction is a reversible equilibrium process, and an excess of the alcohol nucleophile must be used for the reaction to be successful.

As with other carboxylic acid derivatives, esters can be transformed into amides (reaction 3 in Figure 4.100). By using ammonia or primary or tertiary amines as the nucleophile, many different kinds of amides can be produced. The alkoxy leaving group of the ester produces a full equivalent of alcohol if the reaction is taken to completion. Because esters are not particularly reactive, elevated temperatures are usually required to increase this reaction's rate.

Other reactions involving esters already discussed in this section include the transformation of an ester to an aldehyde (see Figure 4.76) and the Acetoacetic Ester Synthesis used for the alkylation of ketones (see Figure 4.82).

AMIDES

Amides are analogous to esters in that they contain two groups—an amine group and an acyl group. Primary amides are named by replacing the *-ic acid* suffix of the carboxylic acid contributing the acyl group with the suffix -*amide* (other suffixes such as -*oic* acid and -*ylic* acid are treated the same way). With secondary and tertiary amides, alkyl groups attached to the amide nitrogen atom must be named. If there is more than one group and they are the same, the prefix *di-* is used. If they are different, the names of the groups appear in alphabetical order at the beginning of the complete IUPAC name. All groups attached to the amide nitrogen atom are given an *N-* prefix, which precedes the name of the alkyl group. Structure 95 shows an example of this naming process that uses all the rules.

N-ethyl-*N*-methylbutyramide   (95)

Properties and uses

Amides are not easily hydrolyzed because the resulting amine anion is not a good leaving group. It is a relatively strong base compared to the other leaving groups discussed in this section. This is an important factor when considering their properties and uses. Primary and secondary amides are quite polar and are capable of intermolecular hydrogen bonding. As such, they have higher melting and boiling points than other comparable carboxylic acid derivatives and they are often water soluble due to their hydrogen bonding properties. Many natural products contain amide functional groups. Proteins are polyamides.

Synthesis and Reactions

A number of methods for making amides have already been covered in this review. Amides can be prepared by:

■ Reaction of an acid chloride with NH_3 or an amine (primary or secondary) (see Figure 4.97, reaction 3, page 630)
■ Reaction of an anhydride with NH_3 or an amine (primary or secondary) (see Figure 4.99, reaction 3, page 632)
■ Reaction of an ester with NH_3 or an amine (primary or secondary) (see Figure 4.100, reaction 3, page 634)

Important reactions of amides include **hydrolysis** and a name reaction called the **Hofmann rearrangement**.

As with esters, amides can undergo **hydrolysis** under either acidic or basic conditions, but the processes must be considerably more strenuous than with esters. Under acid conditions, the first step of the reaction mechanism involves protonation of the oxygen atom of the amide carbonyl carbon with water acting as a nucleophile (as with ester hydrolysis, a large excess of water must be used). The amine-leaving group in this reaction ends up in the form of a protonated ammonium salt. Under basic conditions the final products are a free amine and a carboxylate salt (the last step of the reaction mechanism is actually an acid-base reaction), again similar to basic ester hydrolysis (see Figure 4.101).

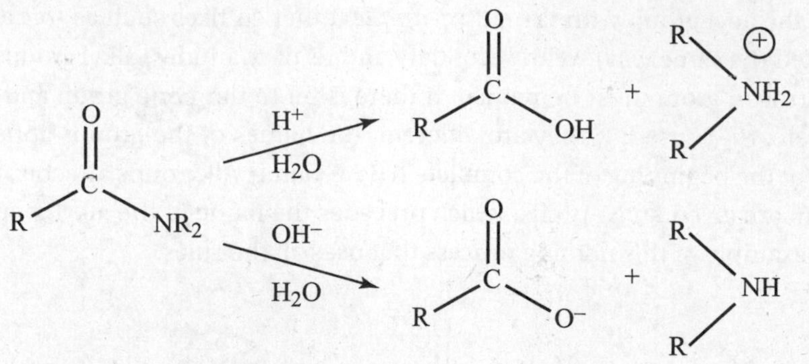

Figure 4.101. Amide hydrolysis reactions

The **Hofmann rearrangement** transforms primary amides into **primary amines**. The reaction results in the formation of an **isocyanate** (R–N=C=O) intermediate, which is hydrolyzed to give an amine product, with loss of the original carbonyl carbon as carbon dioxide. See Figure 4.102 for a generalized example of this reaction.

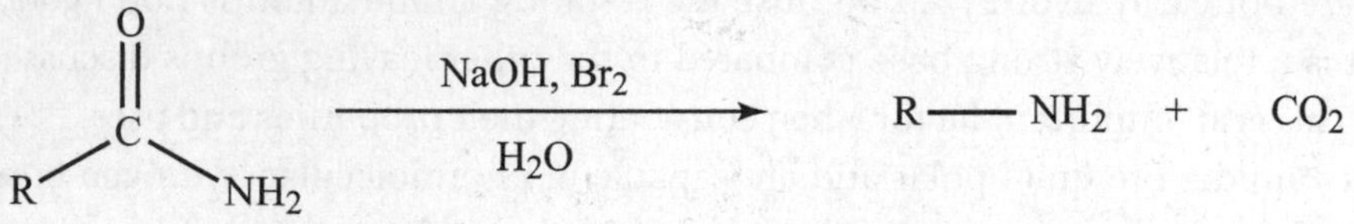

Figure 4.102. The Hofmann rearrangement reaction

The base reagent deprotonates the primary amide nitrogen, which then becomes brominated by nucleophilic substitution. A second deprotonation of the bromoamide results in a bromoamide anion. The R-group attached to the amide carbonyl carbon then migrates over to bromoamide anion nitrogen, which leads to the formation of an isocyanate.

TEST QUESTION

When an aldehyde is reacted with hydrogen cyanide a "cyanohydrin" is formed. This process is best termed:

(A) electrophilic addition.

(B) electrophilic substitution.

(C) nucleophilic addition.

(D) nucleophilic substitution.

(C) Hydrogen cyanide is a good nucleophile and adds to the carbonyl carbon of aldehydes and ketone.

AMINES

Several types of nitrogen-containing organic compounds have been discussed earlier in this review. Most of these were covered in the Oxygen-Containing Functional Groups section. These nitrogen-containing compounds included cyanohydrins, imines, enamines, nitriles, isocyanates, and amides. The preparation of nitrobenzene was discussed in the Hydrocarbon Compounds section.

The **amines** are another, and even more important, nitrogen-containing functional group. Amines have the general formula NR_3 where R can be a hydrogen, alkyl group, or aryl group. All amines can be thought of as derivatives of ammonia (NH_3). Figure 4.103 shows the general 3-D structure of an amine and example amine compounds triethylamine (a commonly used solvent) and aniline (an arylamine).

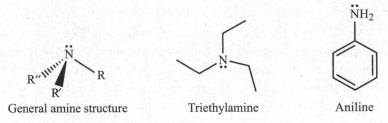

General amine structure   Triethylamine   Aniline

Figure 4.103. General amine structure and examples

As can be seen above, substituents are attached to the sp^3 hybridized nitrogen (resulting in a tetrahedral geometry about the nitrogen) by single covalent bonds. In their neutral form, amine nitrogens always have an associated lone valence electron pair. This feature of the amine structure plays an important part in the functional group's chemical properties. Amines are classified by the number of alkyl and/or aryl groups (Rs) attached to their nitrogen atoms: a **primary amine** has one R attached (RNH_2:); a **secondary amine** has two (R_2NH:), and a **tertiary amine** three (R_3N:). Note in Figure 4.103 that triethylamine is a tertiary alkyl amine and aniline (common name) is a primary aryl amine.

Nomenclature

There are several ways to name amines using the IUPAC system. For amines with simple alkane groups attached to the nitrogen atom, the final *-e* of the alkane name is changed to the suffix *-amine*. For example, an amine group with an isopropane attached to its nitrogen would be called **isopropanamine**. One with cyclohexane bonded to the nitrogen would be named **cyclohexanamine**.

> ### QUATERNARY AMMONIUM SALT
>
> A fourth group can also be bonded to the nitrogen using its lone electron pair. In this case the nitrogen atom must carry a formal positive charge (R_4N^+) and the species is called a **quaternary ammonium salt** (the counter ion is not shown in the formula).

Alternatively, the suffix *-amine* can simply be added to the alkyl substituent's name. For example, an amine with one isopropyl group attached to its nitrogen can be named **isopropylamine**. Secondary and tertiary amines in which the alkyl groups are the same are named by adding the standard prefixes *di-* or *tri-* to the alkyl group name. See the compound triethylamine in Figure 4.103. If an amine functional group is a lower priority substituent attached to a compound structure with higher priority substituents, such as a carboxylic acid or alcohol functional group, the prefix *amino-* is added to the beginning of the name. Structure 96 shows an example of this naming approach.

4-aminohexanoic acid   (96)

Aryl amines are usually named as derivative of aniline (see Figure 4.103), the simplest aromatic amine.

HETEROCYCLIC AMINES

When the nitrogen of an amine functional group is found inside a ring structure, the compound is called a **heterocyclic amine**. Each type of heterocyclic ring system has its own principal (parent) name. Most of these ring systems have common names such as **pyrrole** (a five-membered aromatic ring containing a nitrogen) and **pyridine** (a six-membered aromatic ring containing a nitrogen). The details of the IUPAC system for naming these amines is beyond the scope of this review and it is very unlikely that the test taker will encounter an MCAT question where this knowledge is required.

Properties and Uses

Simple amines have an approximately tetrahedral shape with a lone electron pair associated with the nitrogen atom. Because nitrogen is fairly electronegative (~3.0) amines are capable of forming hydrogen bonds. These bonds are not as strong as those formed by alcohols, carboxylic acid, and water, because oxygen is more electronegative (~3.5). As such ammonia and low molecular weight amines have boiling points that are higher than the corresponding alkanes, but lower than similar alcohols. Like alcohols, and because they can hydrogen bond, amines having fewer than five or six carbon atoms in their structures are usually soluble in water. Tertiary amines, because they cannot hydrogen bond, generally have lower boiling points and are not water soluble.

The most important chemical property of amines is that they can act as weak bases and are sometimes referred to as organic bases. Figure 4.104 shows how the lone pair of an amine can accept a proton from a proton donor (an acid).

DEFINITIONS OF BASES

The **Brønsted–Lowry** definition of a base is that it is a proton-accepting species. Amines use their nitrogen lone pairs to form a bond with a proton, also known as a **hydrogen cation**. Neutral species that accept protons via a lone pair are called **Lewis bases**.

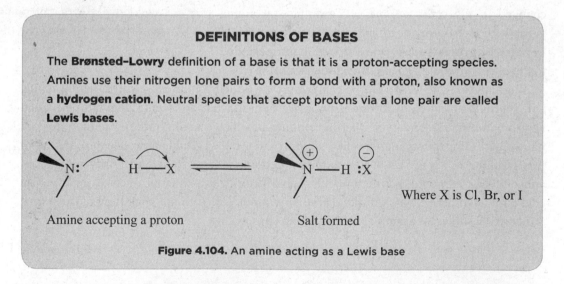

Where X is Cl, Br, or I

Amine accepting a proton   Salt formed

Figure 4.104. An amine acting as a Lewis base

The result of the process shown above is the formation of a quaternary ammonium salt, described earlier in this section. Amines are more basic than oxygen-containing organic compounds (even though the oxygen-containing compounds usually have multiple lone electron pairs) and water because the nitrogen with the lone pair is less electronegative. This makes the lone pairs that are attached to the nitrogens in amines more accessible for bonding with protons, because these lone pairs are not held as tightly as lone pairs that are attached to oxygen. This simple point explains why amines are more basic than most other organic compounds. It also explains why amines are often good nucleophiles.

In general, because alkyl groups are electron donating, alkyl amines (pK_a ~ 40–41) are stronger bases than unsubstituted ammonia (pK_a ~ 36). The effect of pushing electron density toward the nitrogen atom of the amine is that it is more willing to share its lone pair with a proton and is thus more basic. It also makes the nitrogen less willing to give up a proton, for the same reason.

Aryl amines are less basic than alkyl amines because the lone pair of the nitrogen can be delocalized on the aromatic ring of these compounds, thus making it less available for bonding. Figure 4.105 shows this process for the aryl amine aniline (pK_a ~ 25).

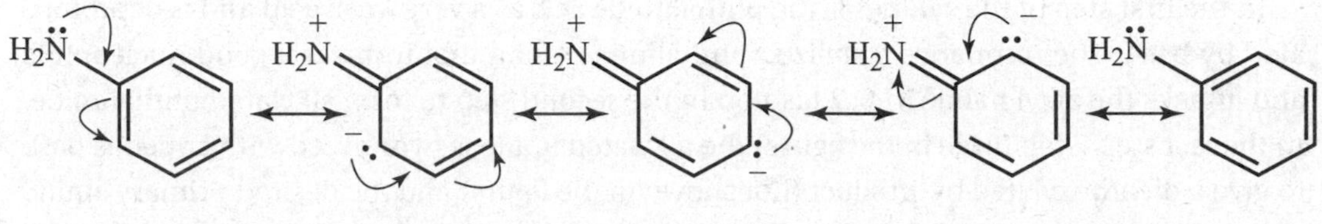

Figure 4.105. Delocalization of the nitrogen lone pair of aniline on the benzene ring

As might be expected, electron-donating groups attached to the aromatic ring of aryl amines make the aryl amines more basic, and electron-withdrawing groups make aryl amines less basic.

Amines are used extensively in industry to prepare pharmaceuticals, pesticides, and fertilizers. A number of different kinds of **diamines** (these contain two amine functional groups) can be polymerized with various carboxylic acid derivatives to prepare **polyamides**, commonly known as **nylons**. Many different kinds of amines occur in nature, some of which are very biologically active. Examples include: atropine, nicotine, caffeine, coniine, adrenaline, mescaline, and morphine.

Synthesis and Reactions

SYNTHESIS

There are many methods for preparing amines. Some amine synthesis reactions were previously discussed in the Oxygen-Containing Functional Groups section of this review. These involved the general hydrolysis of amides to given amines (see Figure 4.101) and the transformation of primary amides to primary amines, known as the Hofmann rearrangement (see Figure 4.102).

Amines are often good nucleophiles, but standard S_N2 reaction processes (for example, reaction of ammonia with a primary alkyl halide) to make more alkylate amines usually produce mixtures. Mixtures occur if ammonia, primary amines, or secondary amines are used because the reaction cannot be stopped after only one or two substitutions. For each proton present on the amine nucleophile, a substitution is possible. Tertiary amine substrates produce quaternary ammonium salt products. If a primary amine is desired and the necessary amide substrate is available, the Hofmann rearrangement can be used, but if this is not the case, a process called the **Gabriel synthesis** can be used. This innovative approach uses what is effectively a blocked primary amine precursor, phthalimide, which prevents the multiple substitution reaction issues associated with regular S_N2 techniques. A generalized example of the Gabriel synthesis is shown in Figure 4.106 below.

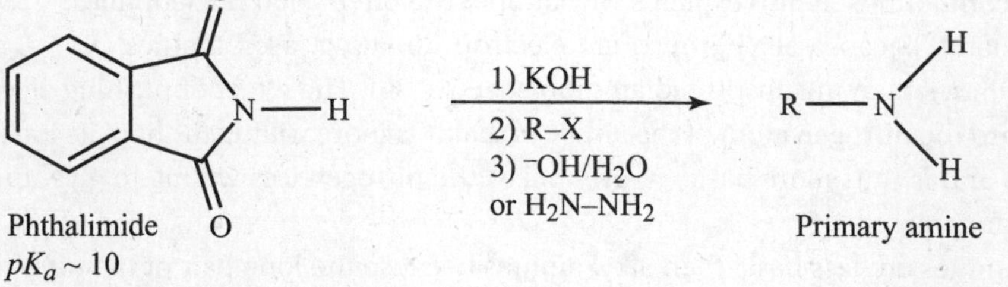

Figure 4.106. The Gabriel synthesis used to prepare primary amines

In the first step of the synthesis, the phthalimide acts as a very weak acid and is deprotonated by base. The resonance stabilized phthalimide anion that forms is a good nucleophile and attacks the alkyl halide in S_N2 fashion in the second step to form alkylated phthalimide. In the last step (step three in the figure) the alkylated imide is hydrolyzed with aqueous base to give a dicarboxylated by-product (not shown in the figure) and the desired primary amine product. Alternatively hydrazine can be used in the last step to remove the blocking group.

It is also possible to reduce other nitrogen-containing functional groups in order to produce amines. There are many methods for doing this. One of the most important of these is the reduction of **imines**. This technique is referred to as **Reductive Amination** and is quite versatile because almost any aldehyde or ketone can be converted to an imine and then reduced to an amine. Figure 4.107 shows a generalized approach to this transformation.

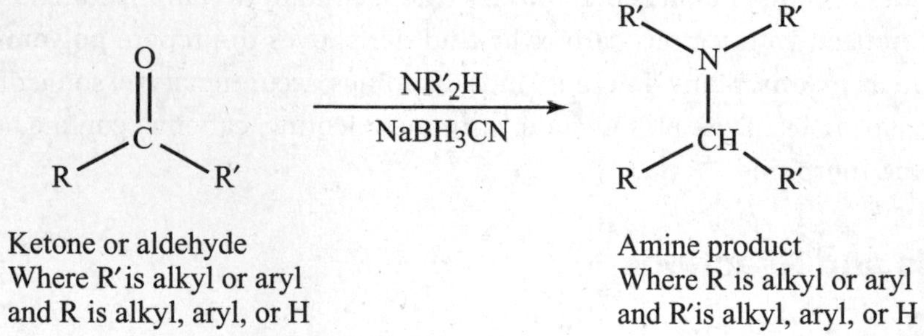

Figure 4.107. The preparation of primary, secondary, and tertiary amines by reductive amination

As can be seen in the figure, this method can be used to synthesize primary (when ammonia is used), secondary (when a primary amine is used), and tertiary (when a secondary amine is used) amines. Note that one alkyl group bonded to the nitrogen of the amine product comes from the carbonyl compound. The remainder of the structure comes from ammonia or the amine reactant. The reagent sodium cyanoborohydride ($NaBH_3CN$) is usually used for the reduction step (the imine is not isolated) although many other reducing agents will work (e.g., H_2/Ni).

Other function groups that are often reduced to amines include **nitro** groups (Figure 4.108), **nitriles** (Figure 4.109), and **amides** (Figure 4.110).

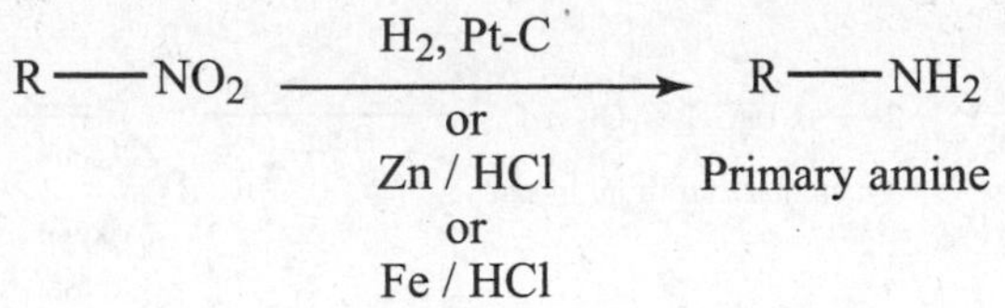

$$R\!-\!NO_2 \xrightarrow[\substack{\text{or} \\ Zn/HCl \\ \text{or} \\ Fe/HCl}]{H_2,\ Pt\text{-}C} R\!-\!NH_2$$

Primary amine

Figure 4.108. The reduction of nitro compounds to prepare primary amines

$$R\!-\!C\!\equiv\!N \xrightarrow[\text{2. }H_2O]{\text{1.}LiAlH_4} R\!-\!CH_2NH_2$$

Primary amine

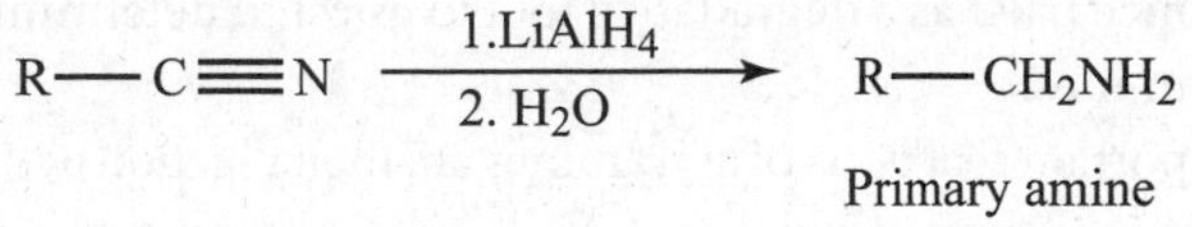

Figure 4.109. The reduction of nitrile compounds to prepare primary amines

Amide
Where R is alkyl or aryl
and R′ is alkyl, aryl, or H

Amine product
Where R is alkyl or aryl
and R′ is alkyl, aryl, or H

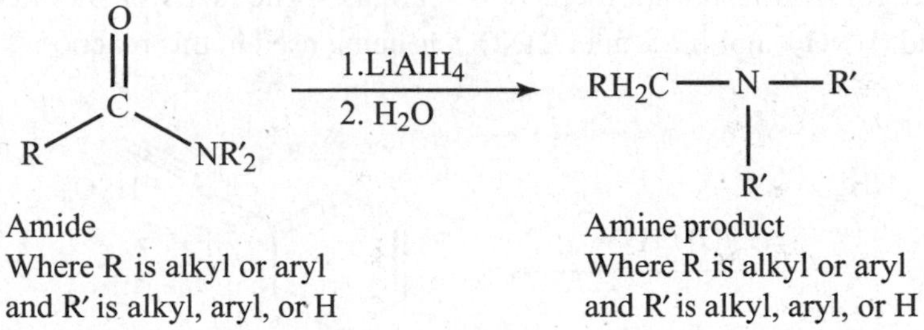

Figure 4.110. The reduction of amides to prepare primary, secondary, and tertiary amines

REACTIONS

The reactions of amines, particularly aryl amines, are some of the most important synthetic tools in organic chemistry. The synthesis of amides from amines has already been covered in the Oxygen-Containing Functional Groups section of this review. Amides can be made by:

- Reaction of ammonia or an amine with an acid chloride (see Figure 4.97, reaction 3, page 630)
- Reaction of ammonia or an amine with an anhydride (see Figure 4.99, reaction 3, page 632)
- Reaction of ammonia or an amine with an ester (see Figure 4.100, reaction 3, page 634).

The alkylation of tertiary amines, discussed earlier in this section, works well to make quaternary ammonium salts, but this S_N2 process is not a suitable reaction for other kinds of amines.

Amines can be converted into alkenes by a process called the **Hofmann Elimination** (also referred to as **exhaustive methylation**). In this procedure, to make the NH_2^- anion a better leaving group, the amine substrate is first reacted with excess iodomethane to produce a quaternary ammonium salt. This reaction is followed by heating the salt with silver oxide (Ag_2O), which acts as a base to effect an elimination that occurs by a concerted E2 mechanism. This step gives an alkene, water, and a trimethylamine by-product. Figure 4.111 shows this two-step process for a primary amine substrate.

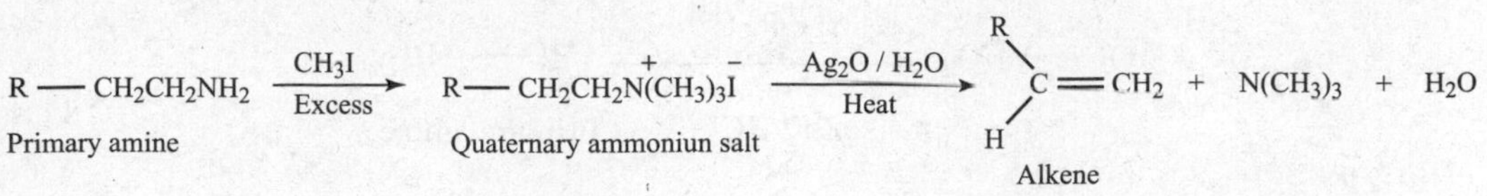

R—CH₂CH₂NH₂ $\xrightarrow[\text{Excess}]{\text{CH}_3\text{I}}$ R—CH₂CH₂N(CH₃)₃I $\xrightarrow[\text{Heat}]{\text{Ag}_2\text{O / H}_2\text{O}}$ (alkene structure) + N(CH₃)₃ + H₂O

Primary amine · · · · · · · · · · · · Quaternary ammoniun salt · Alkene

Figure 4.111. The Hofmann elimination reaction process for a primary amine

The Hofmann elimination reaction is not used much any more but is historically important because it was once used as a degradative tool to assist in determining the structures of naturally occurring amines.

By far the most important reactions of aryl amines are their reaction with nitrous acid (which is generated *in situ*) to form arenediazonium salts. This reaction, referred to as the **Sandmeyer reaction**, is compatible with many different kinds of ring-substituted anilines. Alkyldiazonium salts can also be prepared but they are dangerously explosive and generally cannot be isolated (see Figure 4.112 for the diazotization reaction of aniline). The reviewer should carefully note that *nitrous* acid (HNO_2), not *nitric* acid (HNO_3), is being used in this reaction.

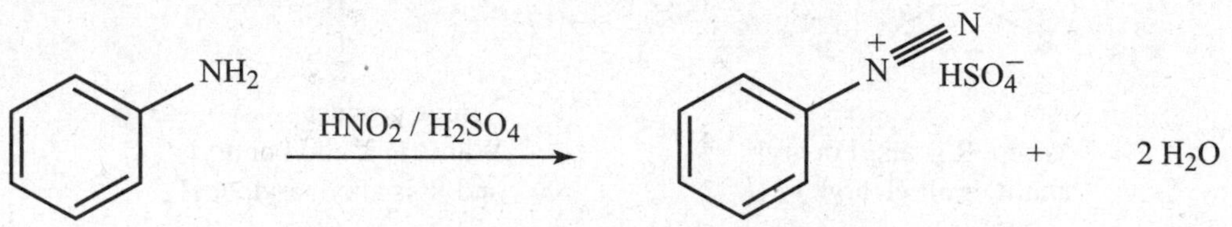

Figure 4.112. The diazotization of aniline

The diazonio group (–N⁺≡N) can be replaced by nucleophiles to make numerous substituted aromatic compounds, which is why this reaction pathway is so important. Figure 4.113 shows the generalized reaction for the substitution of the diazonio group with a nucleophile (note the loss of the diazonio group as nitrogen).

THE MOST IMPORTANT PATHWAY FOR AROMATIC SUBSTITUTION

The overall pathway of nitration of the aromatic ring → reduction of the nitro group to an amine → diazotization of the amine group → and substitution by an appropriate nucleophile is probably the most important method of aromatic substitution.

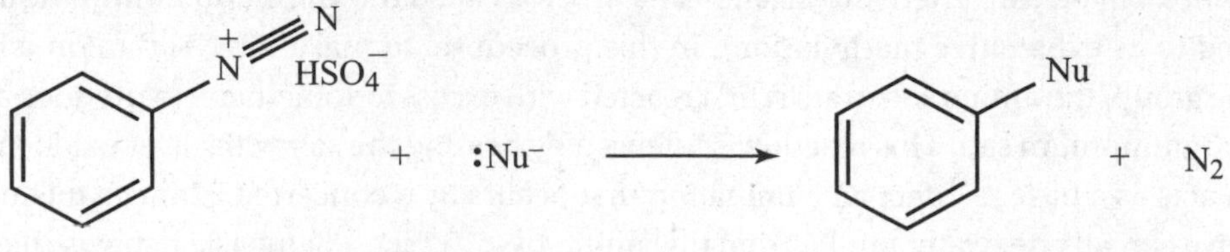

Figure 4.113. Nucleophilic replacement of the diazonio group of an arenediazonium salt

Figure 4.114 shows a generalized arenediazonium salt nucleophilic substitution reaction web.

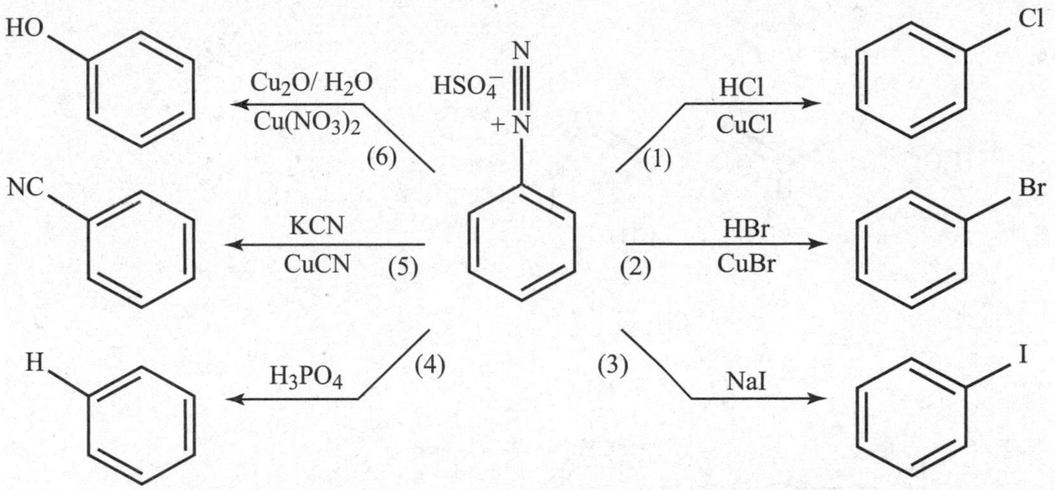

Figure 4.114. A nucleophilic substitution reaction web for arenediazonium salts

AROMATIC AZO COMPOUNDS

Arenediazonium salts can be coupled to form **aromatic azo compounds** (Ar–N=N–Ar'). These compounds are sometimes brightly colored because of their extended conjugated π electron systems. Historically, they have been used extensively as dyes.

TEST QUESTION

A method for preparing primary amines from primary amides, which involves an isocyanate intermediate, is an example of:

(A) the Gabriel synthesis.

(B) reductive amination.

(C) the Hofmann rearrangement.

(D) the Curtius rearrangement.

(C) This process is an important name reaction.

ANSWERS TO PRACTICE QUESTIONS
Practice Exercise 1. Lewis Formulas

1.

2.

3.

Practice Exercise 2. Resonance Forms

The solution is given in the chapter.

Practice Exercise 3. Resonance Forms

1.

2.

3.

Practice Exercise 4. Bonding Hybridization

The solution is given in the chapter.

Practice Exercise 5. Bonding Hybridization

1.

2.

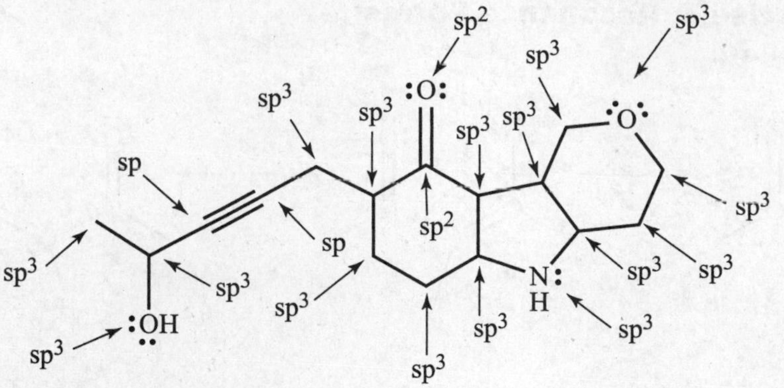

3.

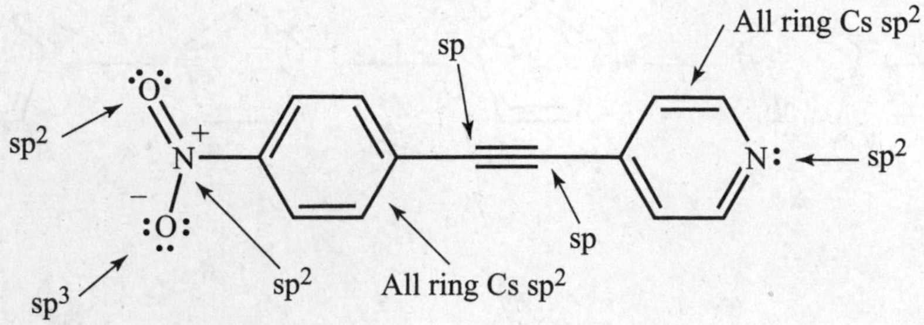

Practice Exercise 6. Structural Isomers for C$_3$H$_8$O

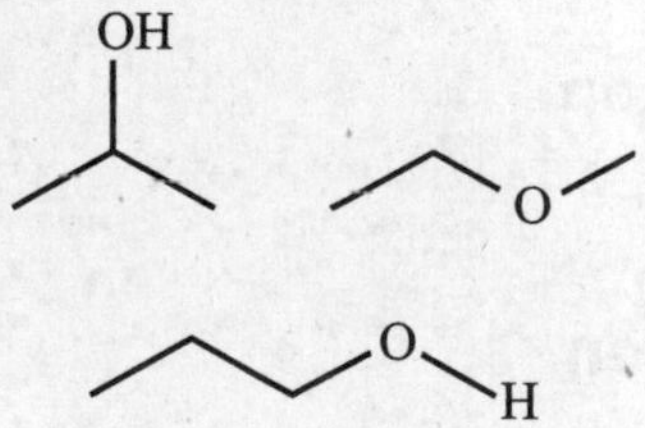

Practice Exercise 7. Designating Chirality Centers

The solution is given in the chapter.

Practice Exercise 8. Designating Chirality Centers

1.

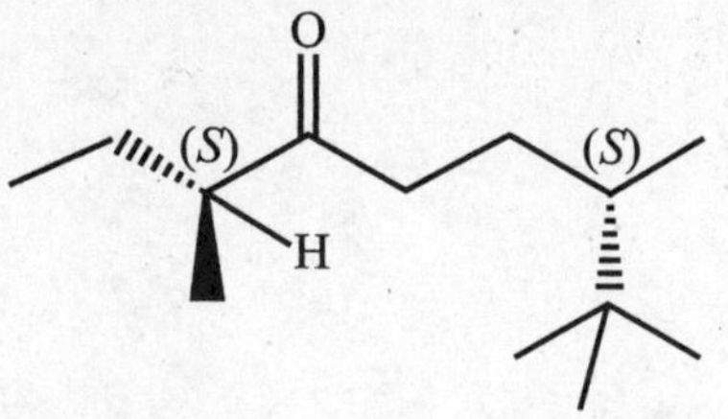

2.

3.

Practice Exercise 9. Designating Alkene Stereochemistry

The solution is given in the chapter.

Practice Exercise 10. Designating Alkene Stereochemistry

1.

2.

3.

Practice Exercise 11. Using Spectroscopic Data to Assign a Structure

The IR spectrum indicates that ketone and ether functional groups may be present.

Some isomers that are consistent with this data and the given formula ($C_5H_{10}O_2$) are:

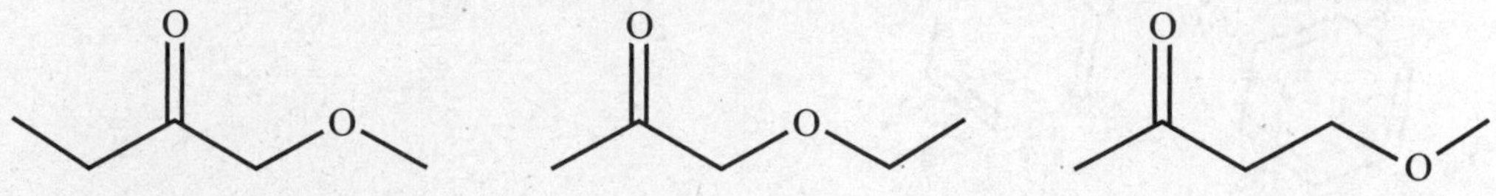

Of these, the isomer that is most consistent with the ^{1}H NMR spectrum data is:

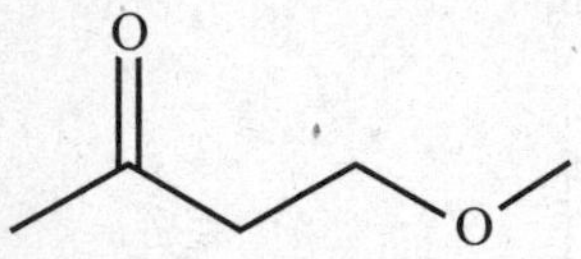

Practice Exercise 12. Naming Alkanes

1.

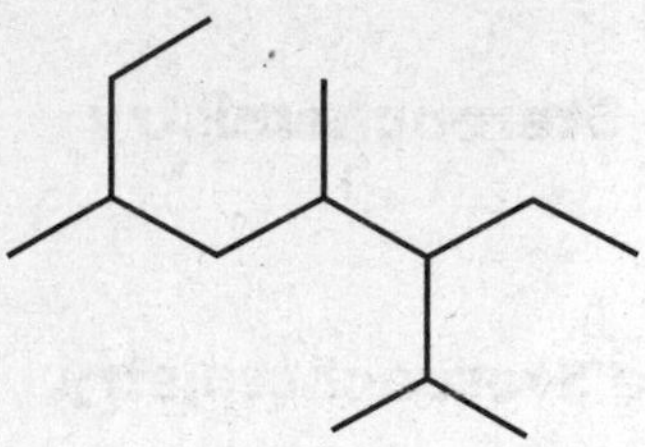

3-ethyl-2,4,6-trimethyloctane

2.

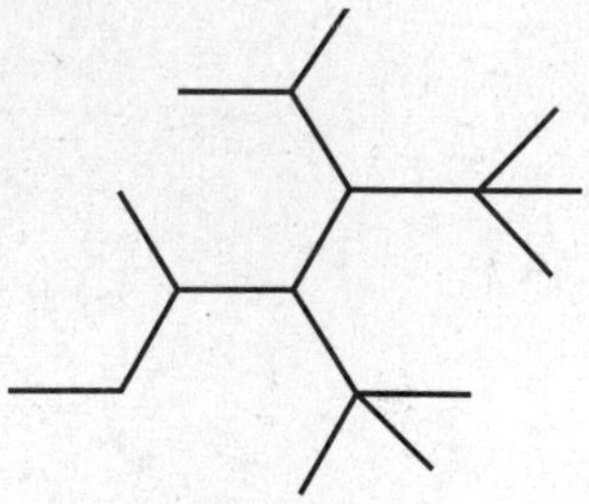

4-(*tert*-butyl)-3-isopropyl-2,2,5-trimethylheptane

3.

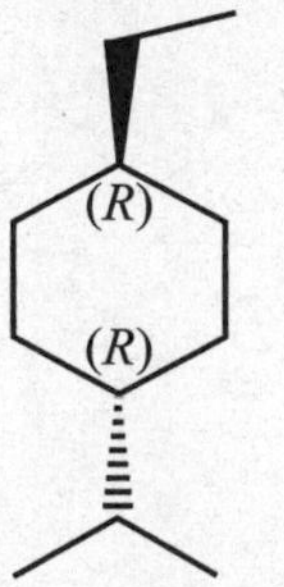

(trans)-1-ethyl-4-isopropylcyclohexane

Practice Exercise 13. Electrophilic Aromatic Substitution

The solution is given in the chapter.

Practice Exercise 14. Electrophilic Aromatic Substitution

Bromine is a deactivating *ortho/para* director; thus the products of the reaction are:

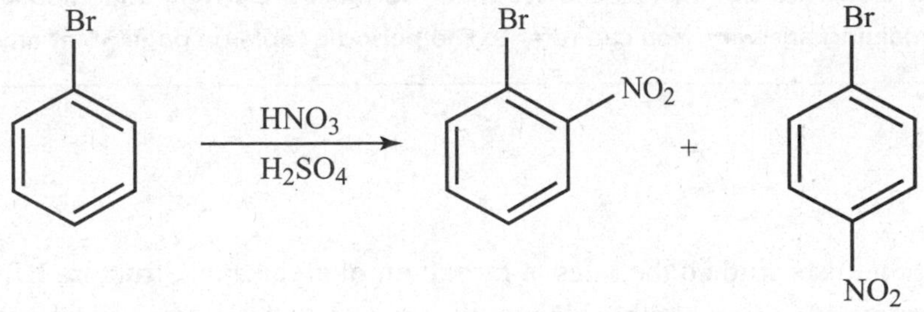

SUMMARY

This chapter has covered eight major topics in organic chemistry that are important for the MCAT. It is helpful to go through the chapter in full several times. Also, as you continue to practice MCAT questions, come back to the chapter and use it to review any concepts that you missed in your practice questions.

Review covalent bonds, starting with sigma and pi bonds and including structural formulas, multiple bonds in organic compound molecules, resonance forms, valence shell electron pair repulsion (VSEPR), molecular shape theory, and chemical isomerism. As you study molecular structure and spectra, be sure to review absorption spectroscopy, mass spectrometry, and proton nuclear magnetic resonance (NMR) spectroscopy.

Separation and purification is an important topic. Review extraction, distillation, chromatography, and recrystallization and filtration. The MCAT will test knowledge of hydrocarbons. Review and understand the nomenclature of alkanes, along with their properties and uses. Understand hydrocarbon chemical reactions.

Review the oxygen functional group compounds. Be sure to specifically review alcohols and phenols, aldehydes and ketones, and carboxylic acids and their derivatives. Review amines, beginning with their nomenclature, and be sure to understand their properties and uses, synthesis, and how they react.

Finally, review the biological molecules. These include carbohydrates, amino acids and proteins, lipids, and phosphorus compounds (phospholipids). Remember that the MCAT is often more concerned with your understanding of concepts than with a simple memorization of facts. If you do not feel that you understand a concept well, take the time to review it again in this chapter.

PASSAGE I

A team of chemists studied the rates of formation of an alkene (Structure **III**) produced from the reaction of sodium methoxide and the cis and trans isomers of 1-bromo-4-(*tert*-butyl)cyclohexane (Structures **I** and **II**). It was proposed that the reaction occurred by a bimolecular elimination (E2) mechanism (see Scheme **I**).

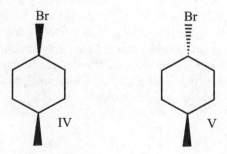

Scheme **I**

Both the cis and trans isomers produced the same product (Structure **III**), but researchers were surprised to find that the *cis* isomer formed the alkene at a much faster rate than the trans isomer. When the *tert*-butyl group of the substrate 1-bromo-4-(*tert*-butyl)cyclohexane was replaced by a methyl group, Structures **IV** and **V**, the reaction rates for the formation of the alkene were about the same for both isomers.

Based on these experiments, it was concluded that the *tert*-butyl group associated with reactants I and II must be responsible for the difference in reaction rates.

1. What are the absolute stereochemical designations for the chirality centers in compound I?
    (A) *R* and *R*
    (B) *S* and *S*
    (C) *R* and *S*
    (D) The molecule does not contain any chirality centers.

2. What is the role of the sodium methoxide in these reactions?
    (A) Abstraction of a proton from the cyclohexane carbon with the bromine substituent.
    (B) Nucleophilic attack of the cyclohexane carbon with the bromine substituent.
    (C) Nucleophilic attack of the cyclohexane carbon with the *tert*-butyl substituent.
    (D) Abstraction of a proton from the carbon α to the bromine substituent.

3. The correct IUPAC name for the alkene (Compound **III**) formed in these reactions is:
    (A) (*S*)-4-(*tert*-butyl)cyclo-1-hexene.
    (B) (*S,Z*)-4-(*tert*-butyl)cyclo-1-hexene.
    (C) (*R*)-4-(*tert*-butyl)cyclo-1-hexene.
    (D) (*R,E*)-4-(*tert*-butyl)cyclo-1-hexene.

4. In the lowest energy conformation of Compound **II**, the bromine and *tert*-butyl substituents on the cyclohexane ring would be:
    (A) bromine axial, *tert*-butyl equatorial.
    (B) bromine equatorial, *tert*-butyl axial.
    (C) both axial.
    (D) both equatorial.

5. The difference in the reaction rates of Compounds **I** and **II** was attributed to the *tert*-butyl substituent. What factor associated with this substituent would most likely affect an E2 reaction rate?
    (A) Cyclohexane ring strain
    (B) Deactivation of the cyclohexane ring to nucleophilic attack
    (C) Steric forces that affect the cyclohexane ring conformation
    (D) Torsional strain

The following questions do not refer to a descriptive passage and are not related to each other.

6. Which of the following solvents would best facilitate an S_N2 substitution reaction?
    (A) Water
    (B) Hexane
    (C) Dimethylformamide
    (D) Ethanol

7. The stereochemical relationship between the two compounds shown below can best be described as:

(A) stereochemically identical.
(B) a pair of enantiomers.
(C) a pair of meso compounds.
(D) a pair of diastereomers.

PASSAGE II

The synthesis of a class of compounds containing the pyrrolizidine bicyclic ring system is of interest to drug researchers because this ring architecture occurs in a number of alkaloids. Investigation of several approaches to synthesize the simplest of these compounds, Structure **I**, led chemists to a process that resulted in a mixture of two isomers of 3-hydroxypropylpyrrolidine (Compounds **IVa** and **b** in a 4:1 mixture). One of these isomers, Compound **IVa**, can be converted into the desired product pyrrolizidine (Structure **I**).

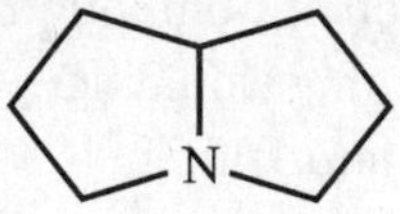

Pyrrolizidine (I)

The procedure used to prepare Compounds **IVa** and **IVb** is shown in Scheme I.

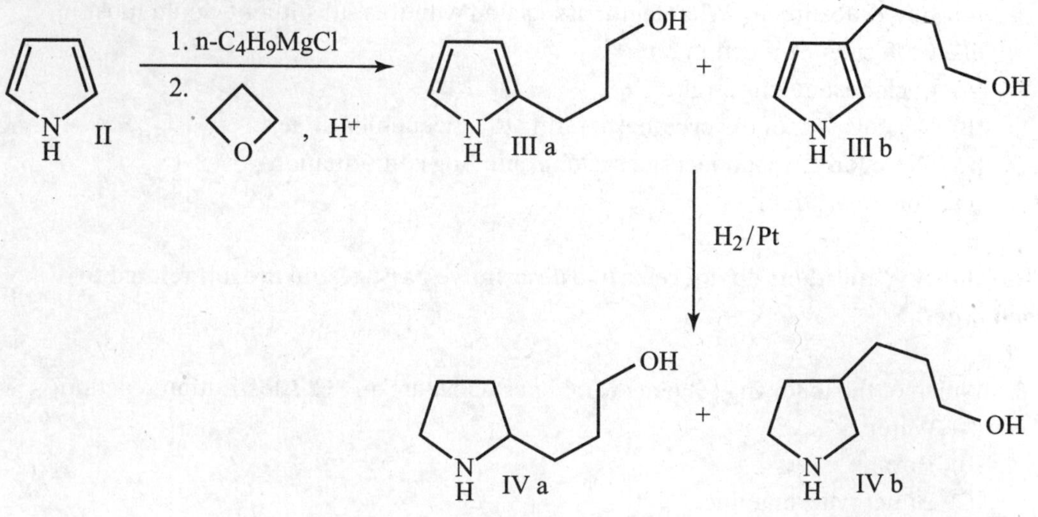

Scheme I

Only Compound **IVa** was converted into pyrrolizidine (**I**) using the one-step method shown in Scheme **II**.

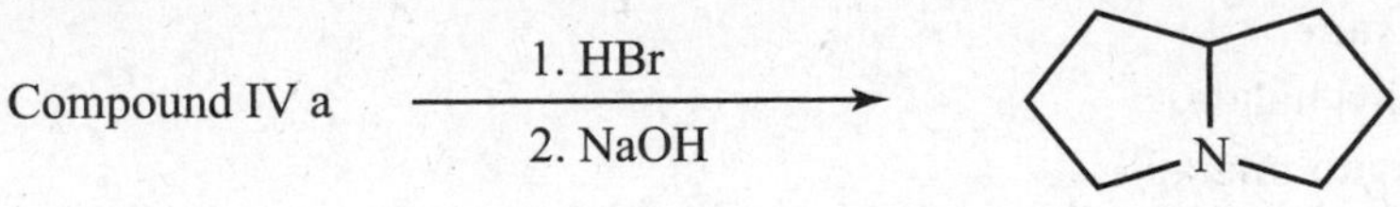

Compound IV a $\xrightarrow[\text{2. NaOH}]{\text{1. HBr}}$

Pyrrolizidine (I)

Scheme II

8. Compound **I** is best described as:
   (A) a primary amine.
   (B) a tertiary amine.
   (C) an aromatic amine.
   (D) an amide.

9. The relationship between Compounds **IIIa** and **IIIb** is that:
   (A) they are stereoisomers.
   (B) they are mirror images.
   (C) they are constitutional isomers.
   (D) they are anomers.

10. What is the first step of the cyclization mechanism shown in scheme II?
    (A) Protonation of the hydroxyl group by HBr
    (B) Bromination of the amine group in the five-membered ring
    (C) Protonation of the amine group in the five-membered ring to form a hydrobromide salt
    (D) Substitution of the hydroxyl group by bromine from attack by bromide anion

11. If Compound **IVb** were cyclized in the same manner as Compound **IVa**, the product would be:
    (A)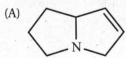

    (B)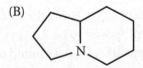

    (C)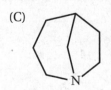

    (D)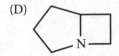

12. The reagent used in the first step of Scheme **I** is:
    (A) an alkene.
    (B) an alkane.
    (C) an alkyl halide.
    (D) an organometallic.

PASSAGE III

The oxidation of pyrrole by hydrogen peroxide produces a crystalline product with the molecular formula $C_8H_{10}N_2O$ and a melting point of 136°C (see Scheme **I**).

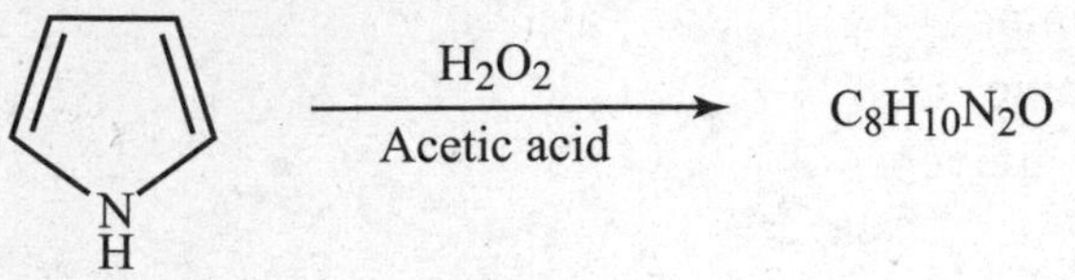

Scheme I

When first synthesized in the early 1920s, chemists assigned this compound the following structure (Structure **I**):

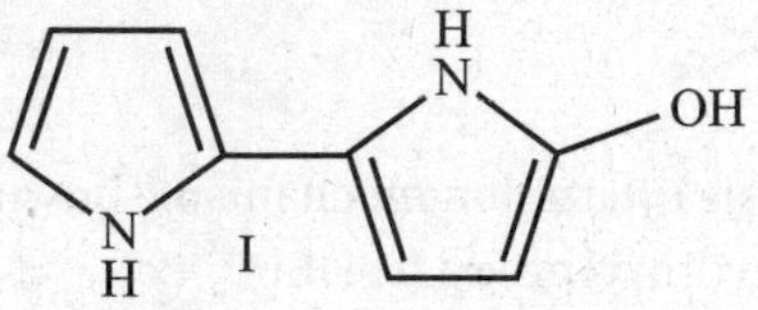

Structure **I** was generally accepted until the mid 1960s when a study provided spectroscopic evidence (from IR, UV/VIS, and proton NMR spectral data) that a different structure (Structure **II**) must instead be correct.

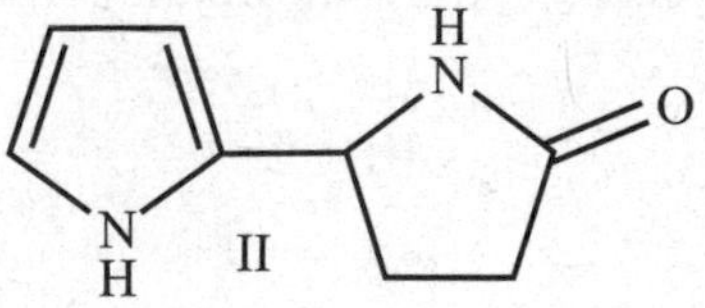

Structure **II** was later independently synthesized (melting point 136°C). Using the reaction in Scheme **II**, it was converted into Compound **III**, which was proposed to be 2,2′-pyrrolypyrrolidine. The characterization data associated with Compound **III** were later found to be identical to the well-known 2,2′-pyrrolypyrrolidine, thus confirming the researchers' earlier assumption.

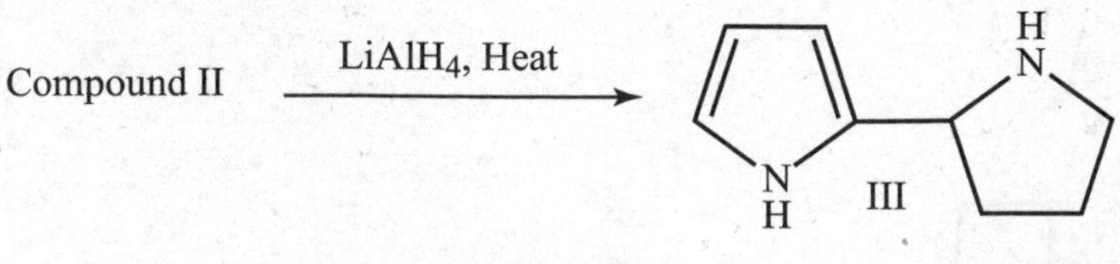

Scheme II

13. The pK_a of the ammonium ion of pyrrole (see Scheme I) is ~0.40. The pK_a of the ammonium ion of pyridine is ~5.3. Which of the following is true?
    (A) Pyrrole is a weaker acid than pyridine.
    (B) Pyrrole is a stronger base than pyridine.
    (C) Pyrrole is a weaker base than pyridine.
    (D) Both pyrrole and pyridine are weak acids.

14. Compound **II** shows IR absorption bands at ~3430 cm^{-1} (weak) and ~1690 cm^{-1} (strong, sharp). These bands are associated with:
    (A) amine and hydroxyl functional groups.
    (B) amine and carbonyl functional groups.
    (C) hydroxyl and carbonyl functional groups.
    (D) hydroxyl and amine functional groups.

15. The reaction of Compound **II** with LiAlH$_4$ to produce Compound **III** can best be described as:
    (A) an oxidation.
    (B) a reduction.
    (C) a dehydrogenation.
    (D) a decarboxylation.

16. Compound **II** contains the following functional group structure:

    What is the name of this functional group?
    (A) Amide
    (B) Amine
    (C) Lactone
    (D) Lactam

17. Given the available data, what is clearly inconsistent with the assignment of Structure **I** as the oxidation product of pyrrole?
    (A) Structure **I** is an unstable enol compound.
    (B) Structure **I** wouldn't show IR absorption bands for amine functional groups.
    (C) The melting point of Structure **I**
    (D) The molar mass of Structure **I**

The following question does not refer to a descriptive passage.

18. Given the following data (see Table 1 below), which amino acid has the highest isoelectric point (pI)?

Table 1. pK_a Values for Ionizable Groups of α-Amino Acids

Amino Acid	α-COOH	α-NH$_3^+$
Alanine	2.35	9.87
Glutamine	2.17	9.13
Leucine	2.33	9.74
Valine	2.29	9.72

(A) Alanine
(B) Glutamine
(C) Leucine
(D) Valine

ANSWER KEY

1. D	**4.** D	**7.** D	**10.** C	**13.** C	**16.** D
2. D	**5.** C	**8.** B	**11.** C	**14.** B	**17.** D
3. B	**6.** C	**9.** C	**12.** D	**15.** B	**18.** A

ANSWERS EXPLAINED

1. **(D)** Due to symmetry, there are no chirality centers in this compound.

2. **(D)** Abstraction of a proton α to the bromine substituent by the methoxide anion allows the elimination of the leaving group, bromine, and the formation of a double bond.

3. **(B)** Structure **III** has *one chirality center* and *one double bond.* Using the *R* and *S* designations for chirality centers and the E/Z rules for assigning stereochemistry to alkenes, the chirality center is *S* and the double bond is *Z.* Only answer B specifies these assignments.

4. **(D)** *Trans*-1,4-disubstituted cyclohexanes must have both substituents in either the *axial* or *equatorial* position. Of these two possible conformations, the case where both substituents are in the *equatorial* position is the lower energy one.

5. **(C)** The large *tert*-butyl group effectively locks the cyclohexane ring of Compounds **I** and **II** (cis and trans isomers) into a specific chair conformation. The conformation of the *cis* reactant allows an anti-periplanar elimination, which is geometrically very favorable and fast. The trans reactant conformation does not.

6. **(C)** S_N2 reactions are best conducted in polar aprotic solvents. The only polar aprotic solvent listed is dimethylformamide (DMF).

7. **(D)** The structures shown are alkene cis/trans isomers. These non-mirror image stereoisomers are referred to as diastereomers.

8. **(B)** The nitrogen in Compound **I** has three alkyl group attachments associated with the ring system, so it is a tertiary amine.

9. **(C)** Compounds **IIIa** and **IIIb** have the same molecular formulas but different atomic connectivity, so they are constitutional isomers.

10. **(C)** HBr is a very strong acid and will immediately react with the basic amine group in Compound **IVa** to form a hydrobromide salt.

11. **(C)** When Compound **IVb** is cyclized, it forms a *bridged* polycyclic structure (only answer C shows this category of ring system).

12. **(D)** The reactant in step 1 of Scheme **I** is a *Grignard reagent* and contains a metal (magnesium) and organic ligands.

13. **(C)** The ammonium ion of an amine is the protonated, or acidic, form of the compound. The lower the pK_a of a compound, the stronger an acid it is. In this case, pyrrole is a weaker base than pyridine because its protonated form is a stronger acid.

14. **(B)** Recall that a weak absorption around 3400 cm^{-1} indicates the presence of an *amine* functional group, and a strong sharp absorption band from about 1800–1650 cm^{-1} indicates the presence of a *carbonyl* group.

15. **(B)** In this reaction, hydrogen atoms are added to one of the pyrrole rings in the compound. The addition of hydrogen atoms to carbon atoms is defined as *reduction* in organic chemistry. Also, lithium aluminum hydride is a reducing agent.

16. **(D)** The cyclic form of an amide functional group is called a *lactam*.

17. **(D)** The molar mass of Structure **I** (148.2 g/mol) doesn't match the molar mass of the molecular formula, $C_8H_{10}N_2O$ (150.2 g/mol), determined for the oxidation reaction shown in Scheme **I**.

18. **(A)** The *isoelectric point* (*pI*) of an amino acid is the pH at which it exists primarily in neutral form. The value of the *pI* can be estimated for neutral amino acids by calculating the average of the α-COOH and α-NH$_3^+$ pK_a's.

For online practice, go to
http://barronsbooks.com/tp/mcat

Biochemistry

5

→ **AMINO ACIDS AND PROTEINS**

→ **CARBOHYDRATES**

→ **LIPIDS**

→ **PRINCIPLES OF BIOENERGETICS**

→ **METABOLISM**

Biochemistry topics account for 25 percent of the questions on both the Biological and Biochemical Foundations of Biological Systems and the Chemical and Physical Foundations of Biological Systems sections of the MCAT.

INTRODUCTION

Biochemistry shares many elements with biology, organic chemistry, and general chemistry. This chapter expands on the concepts found in the chapters for these three areas and reviews the topics that are critical to biochemistry.

COMPOUNDS

Amino Acids and Proteins

All **amino acids** contain two functional groups and, as the name implies, one is an amine group (discussed in the Amines section of this review) and the other a carboxylic acid group (discussed in the *oxygen functional group compounds* section of this review). Many amino acids occur naturally, and many others that do not occur in nature have been synthesized. Amino acids can be joined together by amide or, more specifically, **peptide bonds** to produce polyamides (more commonly referred to as **polypeptides**), which are **proteins**. Proteins are one of the most numerous and important biomolecules found in nature. They perform, among other roles, structural, catalytic, transport, and regulatory functions in living systems.

AMINO ACIDS

Naturally occurring amino acids are often referred to as α-**amino acids** because their amino functional group (NH_2) is bound to the α carbon. The other two substituents at the α carbon are usually a hydrogen atom and a variable group, often referred to as an **R-group**. All naturally occurring amino acids, with the exception of one, have a chirality center at the α carbon. Only one enantiomer of these compounds is produced in nature, so all natural amino acids (again with the exception of one) are optically active. As with monosaccharides, the absolute stereochemistry of amino acids is assigned using **D** and **L** prefixes. All naturally occurring optically active amino acids are **L** enantiomers. With few exceptions, these are the only amino acid stereoisomers found in natural proteins. Figure 5.1 shows the generalized structure of an L-α-amino acid.

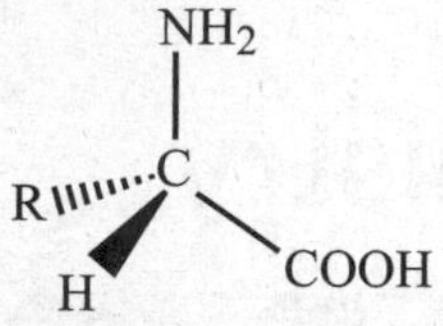

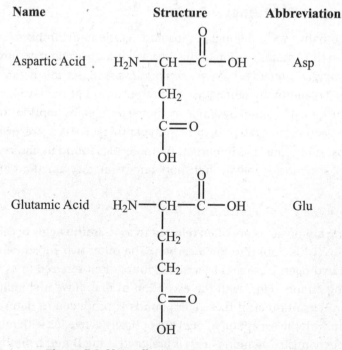

L-α-amino acid

Figure 5.1. The generalized structure of a naturally occurring amino acid

CHIRALITY AND ENANTIOMERS

The concepts of chirality and enantiomers are defined in Chapter 4 Organic Chemistry.

Until recently D-amino acids were considered rare in nature. It is now known that they do occur in significant concentrations and have a critical impact on a number of biological processes. For example, D-serine functions as a neurotransmitter and is a co-agonist for the NMDA receptor. As a result, it may be an important factor in the study of disorders involving the NMDAR. These include ischemia, schizophrenia, and degenerative disorders of the nervous system.

The 20 amino acids found in nature are commonly classified by the chemical characteristics of their *R-groups*. These compounds fall into three categories:

- Acidic amino acids
- Neutral amino acids
- Basic amino acids

The structures, common names, and three-letter name abbreviations of these naturally occurring compounds are shown in Figures 5.2, 5.3, and 5.4. (No structural stereochemistry is shown in the figures.)

Name	Structure	Abbreviation
Aspartic Acid	$H_2N-CH-C-OH$ (with C=O above, CH_2, C=O, OH below)	Asp
Glutamic Acid	$H_2N-CH-C-OH$ (with C=O above, CH_2, CH_2, C=O, OH below)	Glu

Figure 5.2. Naturally occurring acidic amino acids

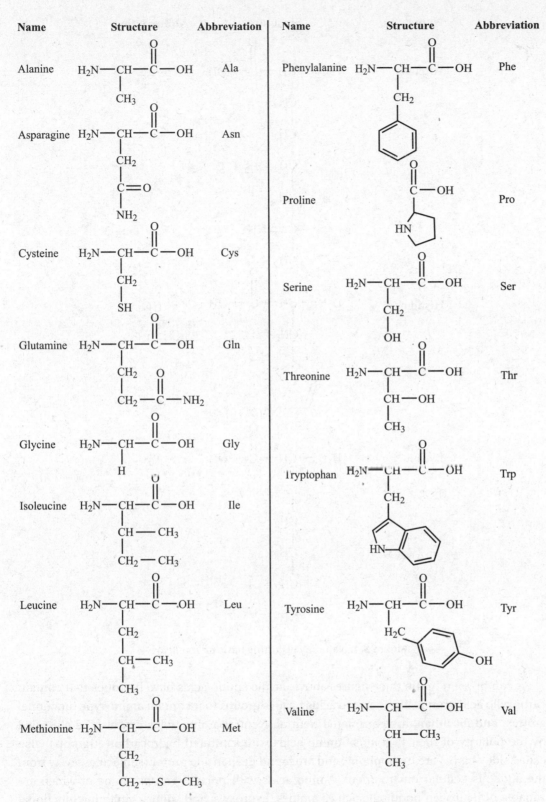

Figure 5.3. Naturally occurring neutral amino acids

Name	Structure	Abbreviation

Arginine

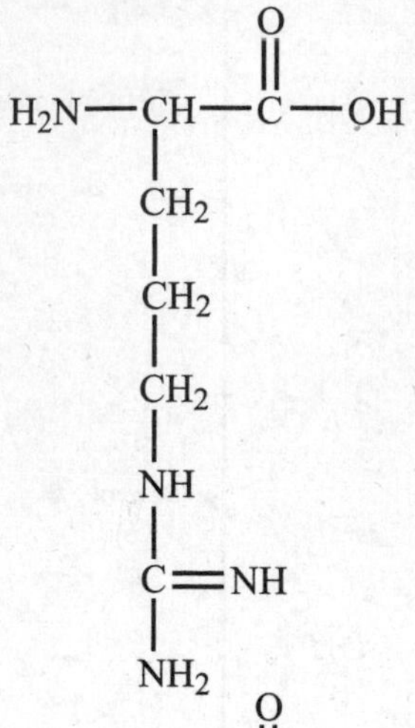

$$H_2N-CH-\overset{\overset{\displaystyle O}{\|}}{C}-OH$$

with side chain:
CH$_2$
CH$_2$
CH$_2$
NH
C$=$NH
NH$_2$

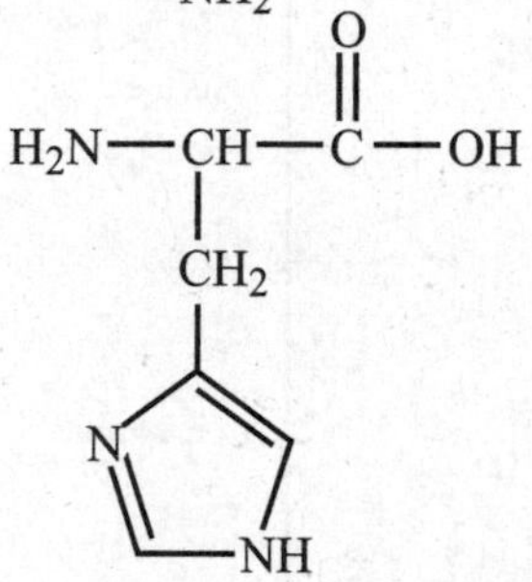

Arg

Histidine

$$H_2N-CH-\overset{\overset{\displaystyle O}{\|}}{C}-OH$$

His

Lysine

$$H_2N-CH-\overset{\overset{\displaystyle O}{\|}}{C}-OH$$

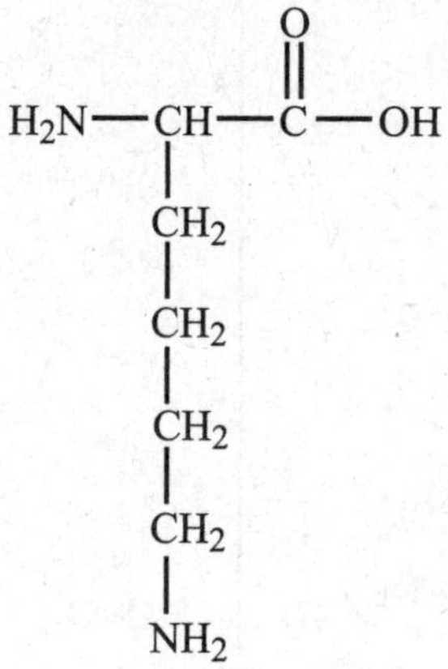

Lys

Figure 5.4. Naturally occurring basic amino acids

As can be seen in the three figures above, acidic amino acids have R-groups that contain carboxylic acid groups, basic amino acids have R-groups that contain amine type functional groups, and all others are considered neutral. Neutral amino acids can also be classified by the polarity of their R-groups. Amino acids with saturated hydrocarbon R-groups (also called side chains) are hydrophobic and are found deep inside protein molecules, away from the aqueous cellular environment. Amino acids with polar R-groups (some of which are capable of hydrogen bonding) such as amides, hydroxyls, and sulfur-containing functional groups are usually found on the surface of proteins, where they come into contact with water and/or other hydrophilic molecules.

Synthesis of Amino Acids

Many plants and bacteria can synthesize the entire complement of amino acids de novo, whereas mammals can synthesize only about half of them. In humans, substrates for amino acid synthesis are drawn from glycolysis, the citric acid cycle, or the pentose phosphate pathway and nine of the 20 can be made from common intermediates. A tenth, tyrosine can only be synthesized from one of the essential amino acids, phenylalanine, while the remainder must be obtained from the diet. As amino acids are important for research, human supplements, and animal feed additives, they are industrially produced in great quantities by a variety of means. Techniques include substrate modification of appropriate precursors by enzymes, harvesting as products of fermentation, or in some cases by de novo synthesis. The Strecker synthesis and Gabriel synthesis are two means by which synthesis of a variety of amino acids can be achieved. The Gabriel synthesis uses phthalidimide to transform an alkyl halide into a primary amine. The Strecker synthesis converts an aldehyde or ketone to an amino acid.

Acid–Base Behavior of Amino Acids

Because amino acids contain both a basic (amine group) and an acidic (carboxylic acid) functional group, these compounds can undergo an intramolecular acid–base reaction in which a proton is transferred. The resulting species, which is an intramolecular salt (contains a positively charged ammonium ion and negatively charged carboxylate ion) is called a **zwitterion**. Figure 5.5 shows the intramolecular proton transfer process. Under neutral conditions amino acids exit primarily as zwitterions. This property makes them very polar and explains their high melting points and water solubility.

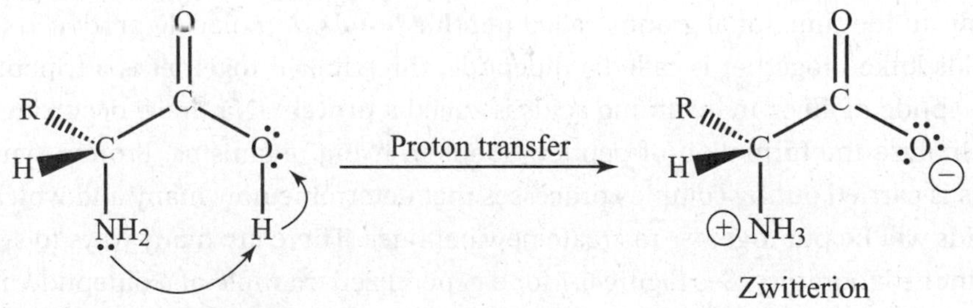

Figure 5.5. Amino acid proton transfer resulting in a zwitterion

The neutral zwitterion salt, which exists at pH ~7, is changed into a cation at low pH, where excess protons are available. At pHs above 7 where excess hydroxide anions are present it is converted into an anion. Figure 5.6 shows the different charge form for neutral amino acids (not acidic or basic R-groups) at different aqueous solution pHs.

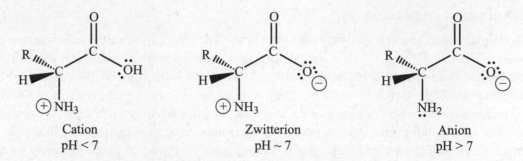

Figure 5.6. The effects of pH on the formal charge of an amino acid

The pK_a's of amino acid carboxyl groups range from about 2.0 to 2.6 and the pK_a's of the protonated form of their amine groups (ammonium ions) are from ~9.0 to 10.3.

Isoelectric Point

The isoelectric point (pI) of an amino acid is the pH at which it exists mostly as a zwitterion. The pI for neutral amino acids can be estimated by taking the average of the pK_a values for the carboxyl group (—COOH) and the protonated α-amine group (α-NH_3^+). The pIs of amino acids vary from one another, a property that is exploited in some methods of separation. Proteins also have pIs corresponding to overall charge neutrality and can be separated by a method known as isoelectric focusing.

PEPTIDES

Just as saccharide units can be linked together by glycosidic bonds, amino acids can be linked together by amide functional groups called **peptide bonds**. A molecule produced from two amino acids linked together is called a dipeptide, three linked together is a tripeptide, and so on. A peptide of 40 or more amino acids is called a **protein**. Naturally occurring enzyme systems catalyze the formation of peptide bonds in living organisms. Protein synthesis in living cells is carried out by complex processes that determine how many and which type of amino acids will be put together to create new peptides. There are many ways to synthesize peptides in the laboratory. See Figure 5.7 for a generalized example of a dipeptide molecule. This peptide is shown in its neutral form, which would predominate at a pH of 7. The end with the free protonated amine (shown on the left side) is called the N-terminal residue, and the end with the free carboxylate anion (shown on the right side) is the C-terminal residue.

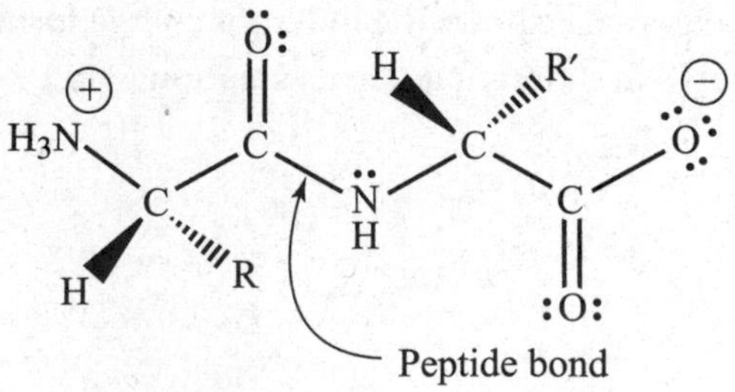

Figure 5.7. A generalized dipeptide

Just as with generic amide bonds, peptide bonds can be hydrolyzed. In living organisms, specialized enzymes facilitate this reaction under ambient conditions. Peptide bonds, which are resonance stabilized, are very strong, and vigorous conditions are required to break them. Figure 5.8 shows the laboratory hydrolysis reaction of a generalized dipeptide. Note that the charges shown on the amino acid hydrolysis products are for a neutralized solution.

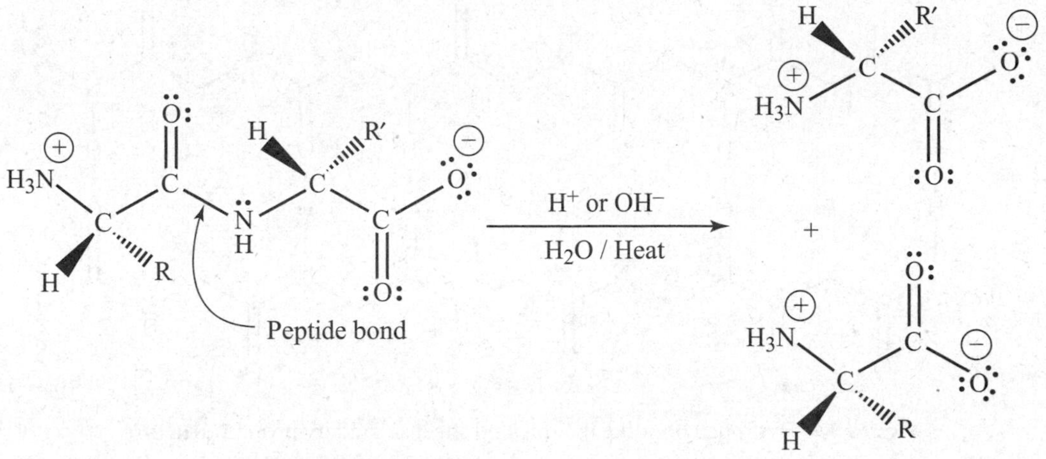

Figure 5.8. Hydrolysis of a dipeptide

PROTEINS

Proteins (polypeptides) consist of many amino acid units (referred to as residues) linked together by peptide bonds. A protein molecule may contain as few as 40 amino acids or as many as tens of thousands. Proteins are often structurally complex, and whether the protein is primarily structural (for example collagen) or primarily functional, the overall shape of the molecule is of paramount importance. Individual polypeptides may be covalently bonded to others, incorporated into helixes or sheets through hydrogen bonding, folded in complicated ways due to a number of intra- and intermolecular interactions, and so on. A hierarchy has been developed to organize and describe the many structural aspects of proteins. The elements of this hierarchy are described below.

Primary and Secondary Structures

PRIMARY PROTEIN STRUCTURE. The amide bond and the polypeptide's specific amino acid sequence are the key elements that define **primary** protein structure. Rotation about the amide bond is restricted due to resonance, but the other σ bonds in the protein backbone are free to rotate. This allows polypeptides to twist and fold based on the particular amino acid residues present.

SECONDARY PROTEIN STRUCTURE. Hydrogen bonding between neighboring amino acids in peptide molecules is the most important factor in determining **secondary** protein structure. Two common secondary structural features arise from these interactions: (1) **the β-pleated sheet** and (2) **the α-helix**.

1. **The β-pleated sheet** involves extended parallel peptide chains held together by intra-molecular hydrogen bonds. The bonds are in the plane of the sheet and between the carbonyl oxygen atoms on one chain and the amine hydrogen atoms on another. The R-groups of the amino acids extend above and below the plane of the sheet. Figure 5.9 shows a schematic of this structural arrangement.

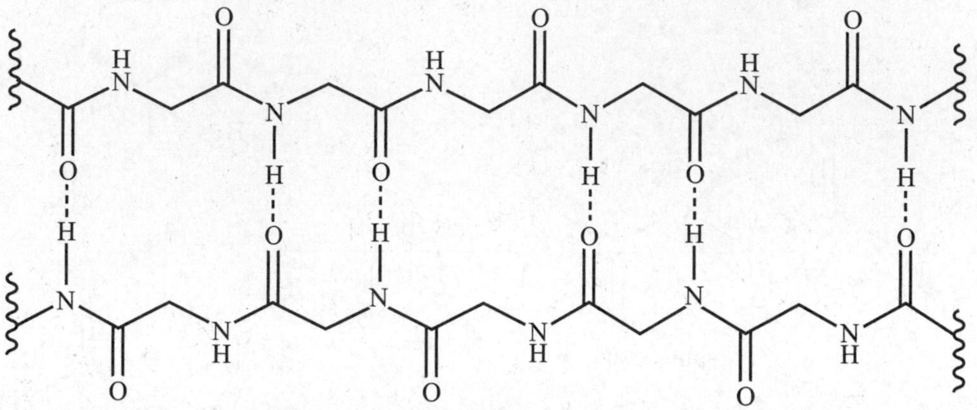

Figure 5.9. Hydrogen bonding in β-pleated sheet secondary protein structure

2. **The α-helix** forms when a peptide chain coils clockwise into a spiral about a central axis. Each turn of the helix is 3.6 amino acid residues in length, and as with the β-pleated sheet, the spiral is stabilized by intramolecular hydrogen bonding. The R-groups of the amino acids in the helix extend outward from the central axis. Some amino acid residues are not flexible enough to exist in an α-helix structure. As a result, proteins containing these residues cannot adopt a helical shape.

Three-Dimensional (Tertiary and Quaternary) Structures

Protein structures above secondary are three-dimensional. Those structures are reviewed in this section, along with enzyme and protein function.

TERTIARY PROTEIN STRUCTURE. Whereas secondary structures are related to localized areas in the polypeptide, the **tertiary** structure is concerned with the overall 3-D shape of the entire protein molecule. Proteins are placed into two categories based on their tertiary structure: (1) long strands or sheets called **fibrous** proteins and (2) heavily folded spherical shapes called **globular** proteins.

The R-groups attached to the amino acids that make up the protein polymer have an important effect on tertiary structure. R-groups can be polar (including hydrogen bonding) or nonpolar, acidic or basic, rigid or flexible, and so on. Based on the combination of these properties, the protein chain folds into a conformation that makes it more stable. Each of the R-group interactions lowers the free energy of the protein molecule, leading to its optimized 3-D conformation. Covalent bonding between cysteine thiol groups (–S–H) also plays a role in stabilizing tertiary structure. Reactions between thiol functional groups form disulfide bonds (–S–S–) inside of and between peptide chains.

QUATERNARY PROTEIN STRUCTURE. The combination of two or more polypeptides results in a **protein complex**. The relative relationship between the folded protein chains in the complex is called **quaternary** structure. The relationship of the peptide molecules to each other is always key to the function of the protein complex. The protein hemoglobin is composed of four separate peptide molecules (two α and two β subunits) packed into a well-defined 3-D shape. It can only function as an oxygen binder (carrier) if all four subunits are present and in the right relationship to each other.

Conformational Stability

Detailed examination of protein stability (defined as the tendency for a protein to assume a particular conformation and remain in that shape) reveals several opposing tendencies: one of these is the formation of a solvation layer in which a highly ordered shell of water molecules surrounds hydrophobic components of the protein. This high degree of enforced order potentially robs the water in the solution of entropy. Some of these losses can be countered, however. Just as when added to water, phospholipids spontaneously assemble into balls so that the hydrophobic hydrocarbon chains are in the interior of the ball away from water, globular proteins will fold in such a way as to tuck the hydrophobic side chains deep into the interior of the molecule. Folding the protein leads to a loss of entropy versus its unfolded state, but this is more than repaid by the reduction of entropy losses in the water. Ionic and hydrogen bonding between polar compounds is also important in maintaining stability. This is especially so when polar groups are forced into the interior of the protein by virtue of their proximity to nonpolar regions. Without other ions with which to form salt bridges (anion-cation pairs) or with which to hydrogen bond, these polar side chains can be a very destabilizing influence. Paired with the right counterion, however, such interior bonds are extremely important in stabilizing the conformation.

Denaturing Protein

The function of almost any protein can be affected or completely destroyed by denaturing it. In fact, even modest changes in environmental pH or temperature can cause significant loss of function. There are several ways to disrupt secondary and tertiary structure while leaving the primary structure intact. The simplest of these is the application of heat, which adds enough energy to break the noncovalent bonds that maintain the three-dimensional shape. The fact that subsequent cooling does not restore function indicates that the effect of heat is permanent. Some other methods of denaturation include the addition of alcohols, which disrupt hydrogen bonding; exposure to acids and bases or high ionic strength solutions, which disrupt both hydrogen bonding and salt bridges; and the use of reducing agents, which break disulfide bonds. Detergents and organic solvents cause denaturation through disruption of hydrophobic interactions within the core of highly folded proteins.

> **ALCOHOL AS A DISINFECTANT**
>
> The disinfectant property of alcohol is due in part to alcohol's ability to disrupt hydrogen bonding.

In denaturation, the loss of the native conformation and the associated loss of function are usually, but not always, permanent. In some cases, the denaturation can be reversed. The tendency for proteins to fold into the lowest energy state can result in a denatured protein recovering its original conformation. In such cases, all of the information needed to assume the correct three-dimensional structure is contained within the primary sequence.

Molecular chaperones are proteins with the specific function of protecting other proteins from denaturation, protecting newly formed proteins from aggregation, and assisting in proper folding. The HSP70 (heat shock protein) family is one of the better studied and is named for the occurrence of these proteins during periods of heat stress. Because proteins have hydrophobic segments that potentially can interact with similar segments on other proteins or within the protein itself, there is the potential for segments to "stick together," which would result in large aggregates that are nonfunctional. By combining with these hydrophobic regions, HSPs protect newly synthesized proteins or newly heat denatured proteins and buy time for the proper folding to occur. They can also maintain a partially unfolded state until a protein has been moved across a cellular membrane, at which time the protein may be degraded or activated.

In other cases, the chaperones actually assist in the folding process. It is now believed that some form of either protection against misfolding or assistance in proper folding is a common requirement and that age-related decline in this function or genetic errors causing dysfunction of these mechanisms are the cause of many diseases. Particularly notable are a group of diverse diseases classified as amyloidoses. These are named after and characterized by the accumulation of insoluble protein aggregates that are connected via regions of beta-pleated sheets before folding or repair can occur.

Protein Function

ENZYME FUNCTION. As noted above, functional roles played by proteins include catalytic, transport, storage, defensive, and regulatory functions. It is impossible to overstate the importance of proteins as enzymes in catalyzing the chemical reactions that support life. The relatively tame conditions under which life exists is insufficiently energetic (too cool, too dilute) to propagate at anywhere near enough speed or sufficient specificity all of the various chemical reactions on which life depends. For life to exist, nature needed enzymes, and with very few exceptions (some RNA has catalytic activity), all enzymes are proteins. Enzymes act on substrates (the chemicals being combined or modified) and speed up the reaction by a factor of several orders of magnitude. A typical enzyme is made up of two or more subunits (has quaternary structure), is much larger than the chemical substrates on which it acts (though the active site itself is typically quite small in comparison with the entire molecule), and is subject to regulation—either by simply increasing/decreasing the amount of enzyme present or through interactions with regulatory substances.

NONENZYMATIC PROTEIN FUNCTION. In addition to their critical role in catalyzing chemical reactions, other functional proteins perform a diverse set of activities that can be broadly categorized as follows. (All are described in Chapter 3, Biology, with the exception of motor functions, which are reviewed in the box on the next page.)

Proteins that perform motor functions are examples of **molecular motors**, molecules that convert energy into mechanical work. Motor functions operate across a range of scales from a subcellular level up to a skeletal level. For example, at the subcellular level, proteins are responsible for the movement of materials within the cytoplasm and for chromosomal segregation during cell division. At the cellular level, proteins facilitate bulk movement across the cell membrane (endo- and exocytosis). At a more macroscopic level proteins are responsible for propulsion by way of cilia and flagella and for contraction of muscle tissues such as smooth, skeletal, and cardiac muscle.

> **CATEGORIES OF NONENZYMATIC PROTEIN FUNCTION**
>
> **IMMUNOLOGIC**—For example, antibodies are proteins that defend against an almost infinite variety of potentially harmful agents.
>
> **SIGNALING/COMMUNICATION**—For example, hormones, growth factors, and their respective receptors provide for signaling between cells with uncanny specificity. Also, as ion channels, proteins allow for the property of excitability.
>
> **TRANSPORT**—For example, transporters carry many materials with limited water solubility, such as fat and oxygen. Also, membrane transporters permit precise regulation of the intracellular environment.
>
> **STORAGE**—For example, myoglobin stores oxygen in the muscle cell.
>
> **MOTOR FUNCTIONS**—For example, actin and myosin are proteins responsible for skeletal motor movement.

All of these motor processes can be subdivided into two broad categories: those motors based on the polymeric proteins actin and myosin and those based on microtubules. Both types covert chemical energy in the form of ATP into mechanical energy with moderate to very high efficiency.

Separation Techniques for Proteins

There are a number of protein separation techniques, several of which are discussed in Chapter 4, Organic Chemistry. The most important laboratory technique in biochemistry is **electrophoresis**. Electrophoresis is commonly used for protein separation as well as for the separation of other macromolecules, such as nucleic acids. The technique is based on differences in charge and/or size among the molecules to be separated, which are subjected to a strong electric field within some type of porous media. This separates the sample into a series of bands that can then be either stained in order to visualize them or collected for further study.

Of the many varieties of electrophoresis, one widely used for analyzing protein is referred to as gel electrophoresis. This technique employs gels that can be made into molecular sieves of different size ranges. The proteins are either run in their native form so that separation occurs based on tertiary (or quaternary) structure or they may first be deliberately denatured using heat, detergent, and reducing agents (to break disulfide bonds). This process converts the proteins from their native shape into linear molecules while coating the protein with excess charge, so that most proteins will sort according to molecular weight (SDS-PAGE). A powerful variation of this technique (2-D electrophoresis) first separates the sample by isoelectric point (isoelectric focusing) using a gel that has a pH gradient built into it. Under these conditions, the protein will migrate until it reaches the pH where it is neutral and is no longer attracted by the electric field. Adding SDS-PAGE electrophoresis (the second dimension of separation) at this point allows mixtures of potentially many thousands of proteins to be individually resolved.

Carbohydrates

Carbohydrates, or "hydrates of carbon," are the largest group of biomolecules found in nature. They have the general formula $C_N(H_2O)_N$ and are hydroxylated analogs of saturated hydrocarbons (alkanes). Many of the hydrogen atoms of their alkane analogs have been replaced with either –OH groups or oxygen atoms. These –OH groups or oxygen atoms are usually bonded to carbon atoms.

Carbohydrates fall into four categories.

1. **Monosaccharides** are the simplest carbohydrate structures and consist of a single saccharide unit (sometimes called simple sugars).
2. **Disaccharides** are molecules containing two saccharide units bonded together.
3. **Oligosaccharides** are short macromolecular chains of saccharide units.
4. **Polysaccharides** are long macromolecular chains of hundreds or even thousands of saccharide units (sometimes called sugar polymers).

MONOSACCHARIDES

Simple sugars are classified by the number of carbon atoms in their backbones, usually 3 to 7, and the type of carbonyl functional group present, an aldehyde or a ketone. Different names are used to specify the number of carbons in the sugar backbone:

- 3-carbon sugars are called **trioses**.
- 4-carbon sugars are **tetroses**.
- 5-carbon sugars are **pentoses**.
- 6-carbon sugars are **hexoses**.
- 7-carbon sugars are **heptoses**.

If the functional group in the monosaccharide backbone is an aldehyde, the sugar is referred to as an **aldose**. If the functional group present is a ketone, the sugar is referred to as a **ketose**. The generalized structure of a monosaccharide is shown in Figure 5.10. The simplest common monosaccharide is a triose (three-carbons) aldose (aldehyde) and has the common name **glyceraldehyde**.

Carbonyl group at carbon 1 or 2 (aldehyde at C 1 or ketone at C 2)

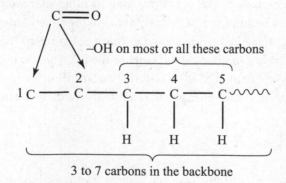

Figure 5.10. General structure of a monosaccharide molecule

The general physical properties of monosaccharides include

- The ability to form hydrogen bonds, which makes them very polar;
- Water solubility, even though they are generally insoluble in organic solvents;
- A High melting point because of strong intermolecular interactions;
- A sweet taste, even though their relative sweetness varies greatly.

All monosaccharide molecules contain one or more chirality centers and, as such, exhibit stereoisomerism.

In addition to the general structure shown above, there are a number of ways to represent the molecular structures, including stereochemistry, of these compounds. The most common method to show both the stereochemistry and connective structure of sugar molecules is to use **Fischer projections**. In these 2-D representations, chirality centers in the backbone of the sugar are shown as bonds crossing each other at right angles to form a cross. The chiral (or achiral—both are often present) carbons in the backbone are omitted for clarity. The projection is usually positioned so that the sugar backbone (which is drawn as a series of crosses) is oriented vertically, parallel with sides of the medium it is presented on (a piece of paper, black board, computer screen, and so on). Figure 5.11 shows the Fischer projections of glyceraldehyde and some other common monosaccharides.

Review stereochemistry of organic compounds in the Covalent Bond section of this chapter.

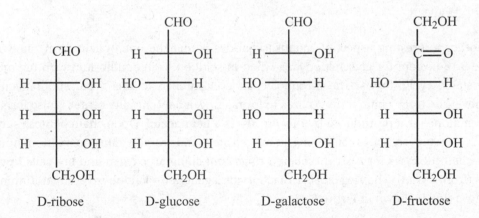

Figure 5.11. The Fischer projections of some common monosaccharides

Note the "D" reference in front of each of the sugar names in Figure 5.11. This is a stereochemical designation used for carbohydrates, which was developed before the adoption of the **R** and **S** system. This older approach is in common use today for sugars and can be illustrated using the Fischer projections of the two stereoisomers of glyceraldehyde (R and S forms—see structures 1 and 2 below). In this system, the two enantiomers of glyceraldehyde, which has one chirality center, are designated as D and L.

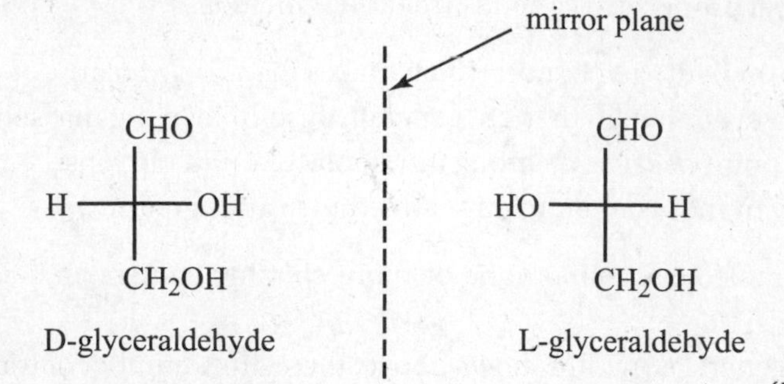

D-glyceraldehyde   L-glyceraldehyde

$$(1, 2)$$

The D and L designations indicated for glyceraldehyde can be applied to all sugar Fischer projections. If the hydroxy group bonded to the carbon of the last chirality center in the sugar backbone (always shown at the bottom of the projection) is on the right (as in D-glyceraldehyde) the sugar is designated D. If the hydroxy group is on the left (as in L-glyceraldehyde) the sugar is designated L. Using this set of rules, it can clearly be seen that all the monosaccharides shown in the Fischer projection figure are "D" sugars (in every case the hydroxy group on the last chiral carbon in the backbone is on the right).

> ## EPIMERS
>
> A pair of D or L sugar stereoisomers differing in structure by only one chirality center are referred to as **epimers**. A pair of epimers usually has a diasteromeric relationship. Both members of the pair must have the same D/L designation, and both must have a single complementary chirality center of opposite configurations.

Another interesting aspect of monosaccharides is that the open chain form, shown in Figure 5.12 (except for glyceraldehyde), when in solution, is in equilibrium with the much more stable cyclic forms. The intramolecular cyclization reactions occur spontaneously. Whenever the open chain form cyclizes to form a ring, a new chirality center is also formed. The functional group produced by this process is a **hemiacetal**. Open chain pentose sugars form five-membered rings containing an oxygen atom and are called **furanoses** (from furan). Open chain **hexoses** form six-membered rings containing an oxygen and are called **pyranoses** (from pyran). The ring closure reaction for a generalized aldohexose sugar forming a pyranose ring is shown in Figure 5.12.

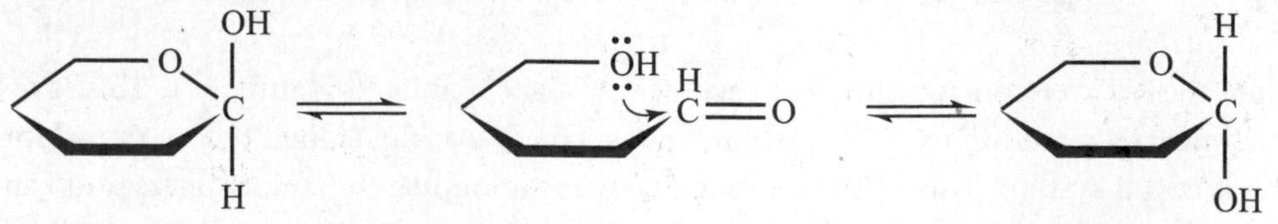

Figure 5.12. Ring closure reaction of a generalized aldohexose monosaccharide

It can be seen from the figure that two rings, which are **epimers** of each other, form when the ring closure occurs to form a hemiacetal. More specifically these cyclic sugar isomers are referred to as **anomers**. Anomers are cyclic monosaccharide stereoisomers that differ in the position of the hydroxy group associated with their hemiacetal functional groups. As a specific example, Figure 5.13 shows the two anomers of the very common aldohexose, D-glucose.

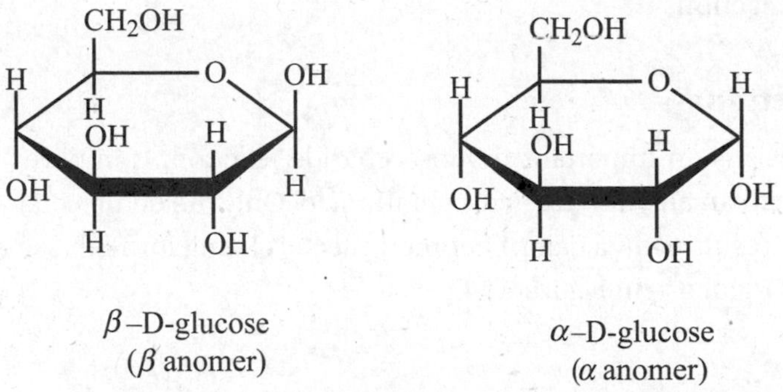

β–D-glucose
(β anomer)

α–D-glucose
(α anomer)

Figure 5.13. The α and β anomers of D-glucose

Observe that when the two hydroxy groups adjacent to the oxygen atom are together on the same side of the pyranose ring (*cis*), the anomer is designated β, and when the two hydroxy groups are on opposite sides of the ring (*trans*), the anomer is designated α. This is true for any cyclic monosaccharide. Each of the above anomers can be isolated and crystallized. If one of these pure anomers is placed in solution, only a trace of the open chain compound of D-glucose will form, and at equilibrium the α and β anomers predominate and exist in an ~2:1 ratio. The α anomer is favored because its trans configuration makes it less sterically hindered and thus lower in energy. A process that results in the spontaneous formation of a mixture of the α and β anomers of any monosaccharide is called **mutarotation**.

Other monosaccharides, such as aldopentoses and ketohexoses, form furanose rings instead of pyranose rings. This process occurs in exactly the same way as seen in Figure 5.13, but a five-membered ring is the result.

HAWORTH PROJECTIONS

The anomers in Figure 5.13 are represented by **Haworth projections**. These projections involve taking a similar Fischer projection and turning it in space so that it is lying on its right side, and then closing it into a ring. When converting a Fischer projection into a Haworth projection, any group on the right side of the Fischer projection will be on the bottom of the Haworth projection. Any group on the left side will be on the top.

In addition to the **intramolecular interactions** of monosaccharides previously described, monosaccharides also undergo **intermolecular interactions**. Because in solution they exist in both open and cyclic forms, the functional groups available for reaction are the hemiacetal, hydroxy, and carbonyl. Reactions discussed in this review include:

- The formation of acetals at the anomeric carbon, known as a **glycoside** in sugar chemistry
- **Esterification** of the hydroxyl groups
- **Oxidation** reactions

Glycoside Reactions

Glycoside synthesis is an important monosaccharide reaction. It involves treatment of the sugar molecule with an alcohol and hydrochloric acid. Only the hemiacetal –OH reacts under these conditions, resulting in a pair of anomeric acetals being formed (see an example reaction involving α-D-glucose in Figure 5.14).

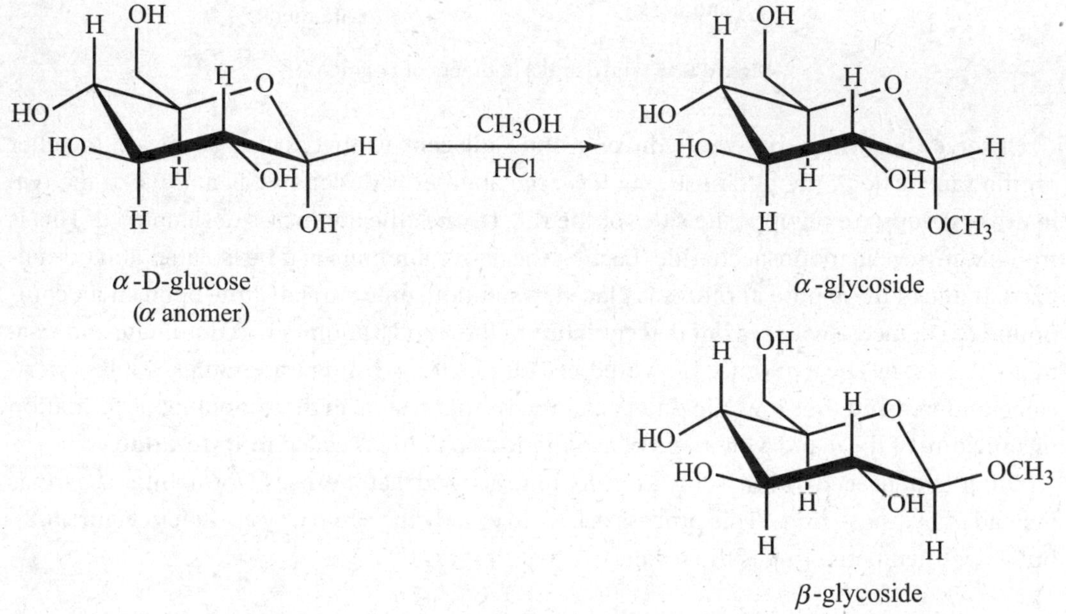

Figure 5.14. Reaction of α-D-glucose to form anomeric glycosides

Note in the above example that both the α- and β-glycosides form. Unlike their hemiacetal analogs, glycosides are stable in water and do not mutarotate. Because glycosides are acetals, they hydrolyze in acidic aqueous solution. The products of this reaction are (1) cyclic hemiacetals and (2) a molecule of alcohol. A mixture of two hemiacetal anomers is formed when a pure glycoside is hydrolyzed.

Esterification

Because monosaccharides have hydroxy groups, they can participate in esterification reactions just like other alcohols. Numerous ways to prepare esters have already been discussed in this review, but a common method used for sugars involves reacting them with acetic anhydride and in a basic solvent. Figure 5.15 shows this process (note the **chair** conformation of these pyranose compounds—yet another way to represent monosaccharides). Acetyl chloride can also be used in this reaction.

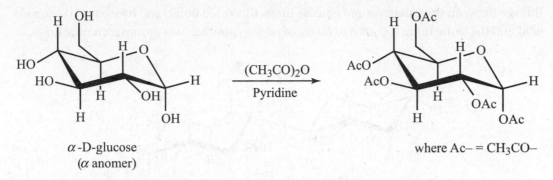

α-D-glucose
(α anomer)

where Ac– = CH₃CO–

Figure 5.15. Esterification of glucose with acetic anhydride

Oxidation

Because the cyclic forms of monosaccharides spend a short time in their acyclic forms in solution, reactions associated with aldehyde and ketone functional groups are possible. For example, aldehydes are easily oxidized by various agents to carboxylic acids. See Figure 5.16 for an example of this reaction. Note that the open-chain form of the sugar is participating in the reaction.

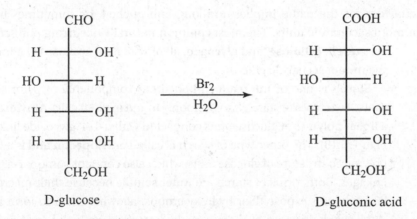

D-glucose

D-gluconic acid

Figure 5.16. Oxidation of D-glucose to D-gluconic acid

The use of bromine and water gives a good yield of the acid product (see Figure 5.16). The aldehyde group of many sugars can be oxidized by the various "spot test" reagents such as **Tollens's**, **Benedict's**, and **Fehling's**, but none of these reactions gives a high yield of the acid.

DISACCHARIDES

Disaccharides contain two monosaccharide units. The three most commonly occurring disaccharides are **maltose**, **lactose**, and **sucrose**. Sometimes the two units are the same monosaccharide (as in the sugar maltose, which contains two glucose molecules) and sometimes they are different (as in the sugar lactose, which contains one galactose and one glucose molecule). Sucrose contains one glucose unit and one fructose unit. The two monosaccharide units in a disaccharide are most commonly bonded between the carbon-1 of the first unit and the carbon-4′ of the second unit by a glycoside linkage (other linkages also occur—sucrose has a 1-2′ glycoside linkage). The first unit's anomeric carbon (C-1) can have either an α or β orientation. Figure 5.17 shows the structure of lactose, which has a β-1-4′ glycoside linkage between the galactose and glucose units. Glycoside bonds will hydrolyze in aqueous acid and the same thing happens to disaccharides to produce two monosaccharide units.

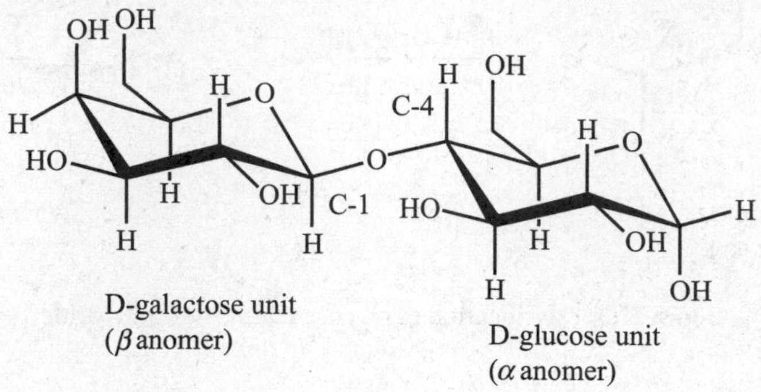

Figure 5.17. The molecular structure of the disaccharide lactose

OLIGO- AND POLYSACCHARIDES

Oligosaccharides contain at least three and usually less than ten monosaccharide units. The units can be all the same, or a number of different types of monosaccharide molecules may be present.

Polysaccharides, as the name implies, are long unbranched, or sometimes branched, polymers of monosaccharide units. The most common naturally occurring polysaccharides are **starch**, **cellulose**, and **glycogen**, all of which are exclusively composed of the monosaccharide glucose.

> **PRIMES**
>
> Primes (') are used in linkage designations to indicate the saccharide unit that does not contain the glycoside (acetal) functional group.

Starch is one of the main carbohydrate components of plant seeds and roots. Two types of starch are commonly found in plant cells. **Amylose** starch is a linear polymer of glucose units connected with α-1-4′ glycoside linkages (see Figure 5.18). The other type of starch is called **amylopectin** and is a branched polymeric structure of glucose units, which also contains some α-1-4′ glycoside linkages. Both forms of starch are water soluble because their macromolecular structures expose their hydroxy groups, allowing them to form hydrogen bonds. The α-1-4′ glycoside linkages of these carbohydrates can be hydrolyzed by enzymes present in most plant-eating vertebrates. In other words, they are digestible.

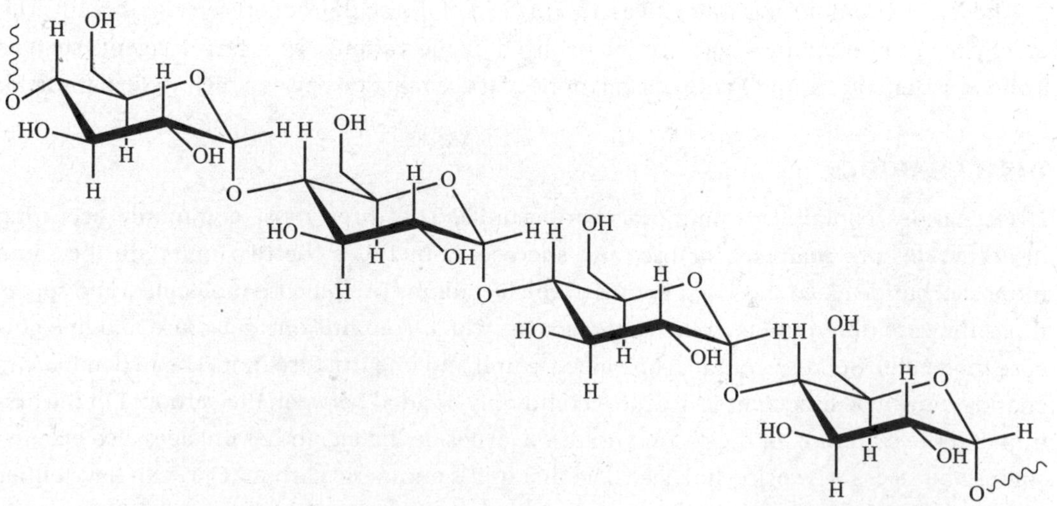

Figure 5.18. A structural representation of an amylose starch molecule

Cellulose is even more common than starch and is found in the cell walls of all plants. This polysaccharide is a linear polymer of glucose units bonded together with β-1-4′ glycoside linkages (see Figure 5.19). Through hydrogen bonding, these long carbohydrate polymers form extensive **3-D networks**. These strong interpolymer bonds make cellulose insoluble in water. Vertebrates, including humans, do not have enzymes that can hydrolyze β-1-4′ glycoside linkages, making cellulose indigestible. Herbivores rely on symbiotic microorganisms to digest cellulose.

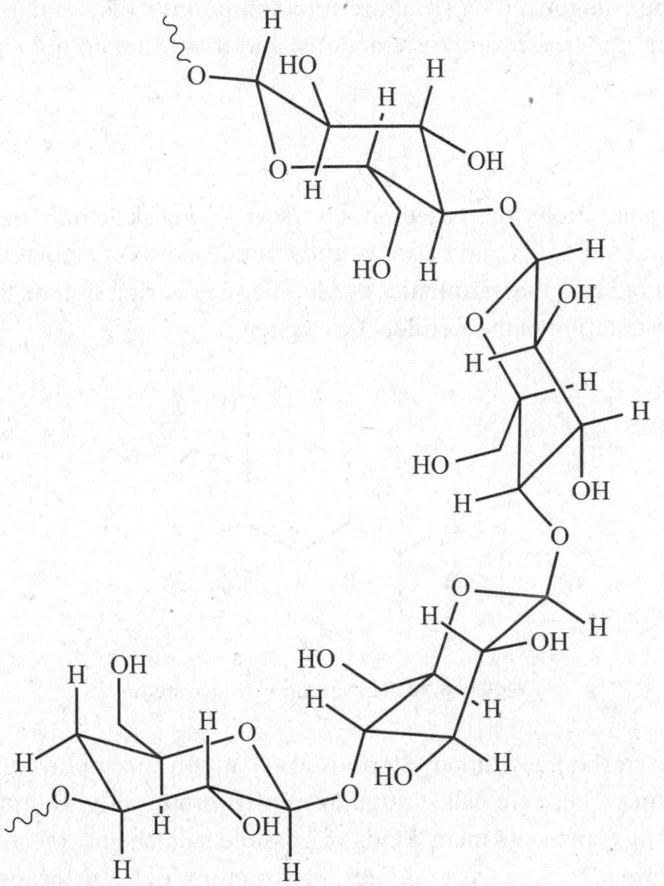

Figure 5.19. A structural representation of a single cellulose polysaccharide unit

The highly branched polymer **glycogen** is used to store polysaccharides in animals, usually in liver or muscle tissue. Its α-*glycoside linkages* are easily and quickly hydrolyzed to produce glucose when an animal needs a quick burst of energy.

Lipids

Lipids are a collection of naturally occurring bioorganic molecules that are defined not by their specific chemical structures, but by their nonpolar properties. All of these substances are in general hydrophobic and can be isolated from living organisms by extraction with nonpolar solvents. Some of the common biomolecules included in this category are oils, fats, waxes, hormones, some types of vitamins, and complex cellular components. The MCAT subject outline specifically refers to the following types of lipid molecules:

- Steroids
- Terpenes
- Triacylglycerols and free fatty acids
- Phospholipids
- Waxes

Lipids can also be categorized by structure into compounds that contain ester functional groups, which can undergo hydrolysis reactions, and those that do not contain ester functional groups.

STEROIDS

Steroids are nonpolar molecules based on a tetracyclic ring skeleton. The four rings in the skeleton are designated A, B, C, and D. A, B, and C are fused six-membered rings, and D is a fused five-membered ring that terminates the six-membered ring system. See Figure 5.20 for a structural representation of the steroidal ring system.

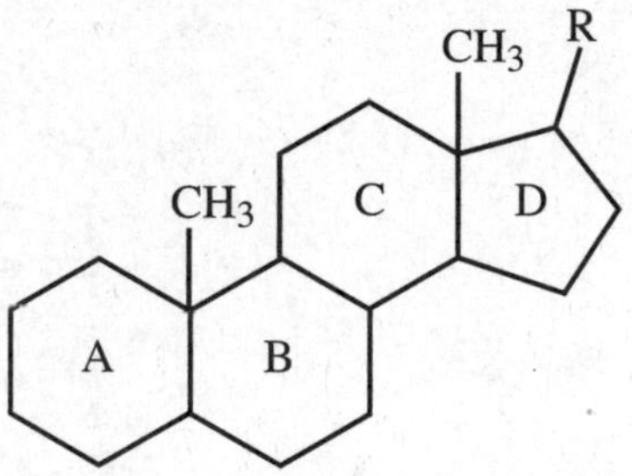

Figure 5.20. The steroidal ring system

As can be seen in the figure, many steroids also contain two methyl groups at the indicated ring junctions. These are called **angular methyl groups**. The R-group shown off the five-membered ring represents many kinds of possible side chains. Most steroids function as hormones. Figure 5.21 shows as examples the structures of **testosterone** and **estradiol** (a form of estrogen.) Note the presence of an aromatic ring in this structure.

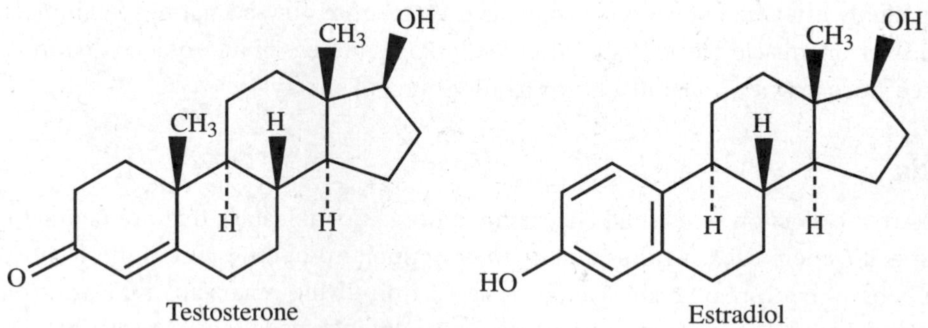

Figure 5.21. Two steroid hormones

Another well-known steroid is **cholesterol**. Cholesterol is a waxy steroid metabolite found in all cell membranes of animals and can be produced biosynthetically. It is important because it is a precursor for the synthesis of a range of compounds including the steroid hormones, vitamin D, and bile. It is also found in the membranes of animal cells where it adds strength, reduces permeability, and participates in endocytosis. Elevated levels of some lipoproteins (proteins responsible for transport of lipids in the body) have a significant role in the development of atherosclerosis.

TERPENES

Chemically, the nonpolar extract of most plant oils consists mostly of a mixture of lipids called **terpenes**. Literally tens of thousands of terpenes have been isolated and characterized from plants, and even though their structures are quite diverse, they are all considered to be related to each other. The structural feature that is key to this relationship is the **isoprene unit**. All terpenes, despite their structural differences, arise from the head-to-tail bonding of two or more isoprene units. Carbon-1 is referred to as the **head**, and carbon-4 the **tail** of the isoprene unit (see structure 3 below).

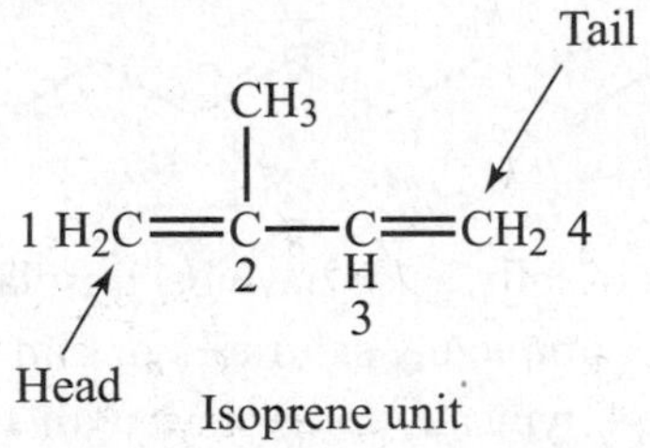

$$\text{Tail}$$
$$\text{CH}_3$$
$$1 \; \text{H}_2\text{C}=\underset{2}{\text{C}}-\underset{\underset{3}{\text{H}}}{\text{C}}=\text{CH}_2 \; 4$$

Head   Isoprene unit

(3)

Terpenes are classified by the number of isoprene units in their structures. Monoterpenes contain two isoprene units. Two examples of these compounds are shown in Figure 5.22.

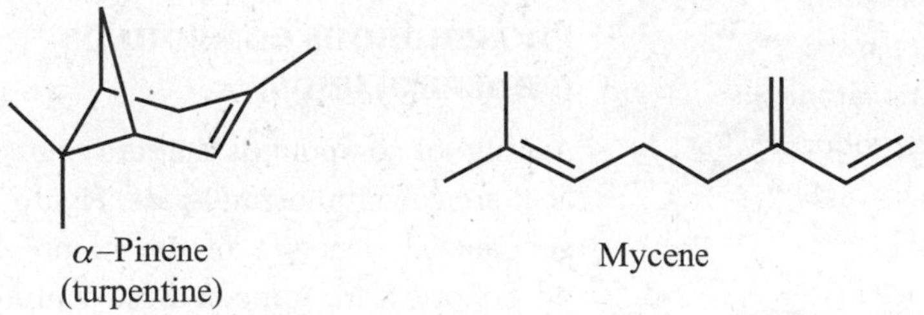

α–Pinene
(turpentine)

Mycene

Figure 5.22. The monoterpenes α-pinene and mycene

More complex terpenes that contain a number of isoprene units and often contain oxygen atoms are found in both plants and animals and are part of a number of biological synthesis pathways. For example, in invertebrates, terpenes function as hormones.

TRIACYLGLYCEROLS AND FREE FATTY ACIDS

Naturally occurring **fats** and **oils** are chemically very similar. Both of these substances are **triacylglycerols**, which are triesters of glycerol (a triol) and various carboxylic acids. Depending on the source of the fat or oil (plant or animal), the structure of the carboxylic acid portion of the triester molecule can vary considerably. Most commonly, the acids have long saturated or unsaturated carbon chains attached α to their carbonyl groups. Structure 4 shows a generalized example of a triacylglycerol molecule (where R, R′, and R″ represent nonpolar hydrocarbon chains of various lengths). This structure can represent either a fat or an oil.

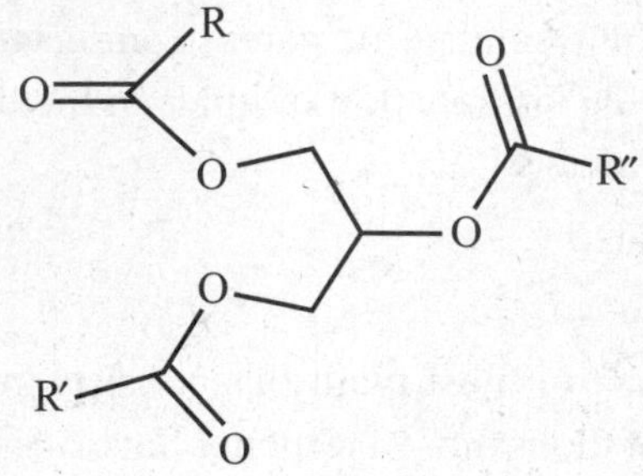

(4)

Triacylglycerols, like all esters, can be hydrolyzed to give glycerol and free carboxylic acids. The free acids produced by the hydrolysis process are commonly called **fatty acids**. Structure 5 below represents the saturated fatty acid commonly named **lauric acid**.

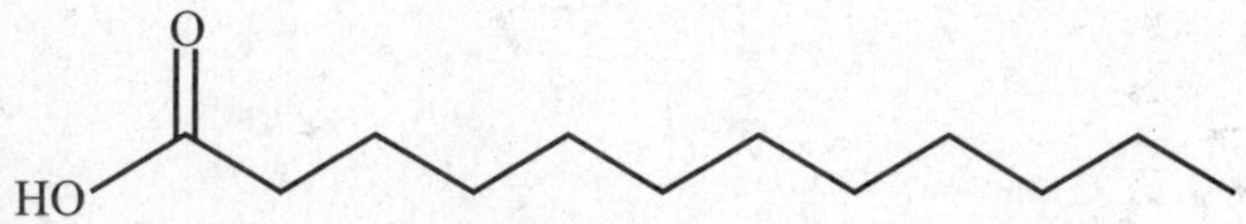

(5)

More than 100 different kinds of fatty acids have been isolated and characterized. Their hydrocarbon side chains can be completely saturated or can contain one or more alkene bonds. These hydrocarbon groups typically range in length from 12 to 20 carbon atoms. The presence of double bonds, almost always the *cis* isomer, in the hydrocarbon chains of fatty acids, considerably lowers their melting points.

SOAP

The process of hydrolyzing fat using a strongly basic aqueous solution and heat is called *saponification*. This process results in the formation of metal salts of aliphatic fatty acids. Isolating and purifying these salts produces what is commonly called *soap*.

PHOSPHOROUS COMPOUNDS (PHOSPHOLIPIDS)

A group of compounds that are esters of phosphoric acid are called **phospholipids**. Figure 5.23 shows the generalized structure of the mono- and diester of phosphoric acid. Some of these compounds, **glycerophospholipids**, are very similar to the triacylglycerols (fats and oils) discussed above. They have a **glycerol backbone** with two fatty acid carboxylic acid esters, but the third ester linkage is a phosphoric acid diester. One side of the phosphate group is linked to the glycerol backbone and the other to an amino alcohol called **ethanolamine**. The charged phosphorus group that replaces one of the fatty acid tails makes this end of the molecule polar. When added to water, the phospholipids spontaneously assemble into micelles or into bilayers for the same reason that the predominantly hydrophobic segments of a protein get buried into the interior of the molecule. It is this spontaneous formation of phospholipids into lipid bilayers that forms the basic plan for the membranes of all cells.

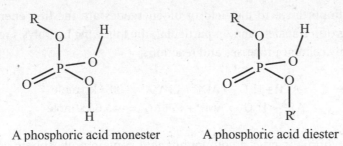

A phosphoric acid monester   A phosphoric acid diester

Figure 5.23. Esters of phosphoric acid

Another large class of phospholipids is the **sphingomyelins**, which are found extensively in nerve and brain tissue. These compounds are amide/esters of a **dihydroxyamine** (common name **sphingosine**).

Finally, one other class of lipids are the waxes, which are found most commonly in plants but also are found in some bacteria, insects, and higher animals. Sebum, the oily substance secreted onto human hair and skin consists of waxes.

PROCESSES

The first part of this chapter reviewed biochemical compounds. The second part now will review biochemical processes involving these compounds.

Principles of Bioenergetics

As the term implies, bioenergetics is a detailed energy accounting of all the biochemical processes occurring within a living system. This important topic within biochemistry uses thermodynamic concepts such as heat, work, enthalpy, entropy, and Gibbs free energy, which are reviewed in Chapter 1, General Chemistry. Of central importance is the concept of Gibbs standard free energy change, denoted by the symbol $\Delta G°$.

The equation $\Delta G° = \Delta H - T\Delta S$ (recall that H is enthalpy, S is entropy, and T is temperature) relates the fundamental quantities involved. It is **standardized** when all reactants and products of a reversible reaction are at 1 molal concentration, while temperature is assumed to be 25C°. Because most biochemical reactions occur at close to a neutral pH of 7, this additional condition is often imposed and reflected by the use of the prime symbol in $\Delta G°'$. Units of free energy change are most often expressed in kJ/mole.

It is possible to add and subtract the various $\Delta G°$ for each of the participants in a reaction. This allows the computation of the overall predicted free energy change and concentrations at equilibria as $\Delta G° = -RT\ln(K_{eq})$. When the overall free energy change is negative, the reaction is spontaneous and able to perform work. If positive, the reaction is not spontaneous and requires the input of energy to proceed. The energy is typically in the form of ATP.

Free energies predict only that a reaction can occur and say nothing about the rate at which the reaction will occur. Almost all reactions of biological interest are enzyme-dependent. As a result, the reaction rate is dependent not only on the concentrations of the reactants but also on the concentration and speed of the enzymes involved. Conditions within the cell or cellular organelle where the reaction is taking place invariably are different from standard conditions. For this reason, the $\Delta G°'$ should be thought of as only an estimate. Instead, it is the actual ΔG under specific physiological conditions that determines whether a reaction is spontaneous, and may be significantly different than the estimate based on standard conditions.

Of particular importance to the field of bioenergetics are the free energies associated with phosphate group transfers and, in particular, the following hydrolysis reactions of ATP, which power many cellular processes and reactions:

$$ATP + H_2O \rightarrow ADP + Pi \; \Delta G^\circ = -30.5 \text{ kJ/mole}$$
$$ATP + H_2O \rightarrow AMP + PPi \; \Delta G^\circ = -45.6 \text{ kJ/mole}$$

ATP is but one of many crucial compounds that contain a phosphate group. Phospho-enolpyruvate, creatine phosphate, acetyl phosphate, and the many phosphorylated sugars are such examples and are often ranked according to their free energy of hydrolysis. ATP occupies an intermediate position among these, meaning that it can readily accept phosphoryl groups from compounds with higher phosphate transfer potential (such as phosphoenolpyruvate or PEP). It can also readily donate phosphoryl groups to those with lower potential. For example, this allows rapid regeneration of ATP in skeletal muscle from pools of creatine phosphate, and it allows ATP to phosphorylate sugars as the first step in a variety of pathways.

It is not the breaking of the phosphate bond itself that drives these diverse chemical reactions. Breaking bonds requires energy. Instead, it is the rearrangement and formation of new bonds with lower sums of energies and entropy that account for the difference. ATP is not "hydrolyzed" in a single step that simply liberates heat. With few exceptions, the hydrolysis occurs in two steps. The first step activates either the substrate or enzyme. In the second step, the phosphate-containing compound is displaced.

The use of phosphate group transfers provides a mechanism by which the energy of ATP hydrolysis can be captured and linked to make many reactions possible. One example is the "activation" via phosphorylation of sugars, nucleosides, and amino acids as a first step in the synthesis of polypeptides, nucleic acids, and polysaccharides. In order to function, enzymes are often dependent on the binding energy of the covalently bound phosphate (alternatively PPi, or AMP) to either the enzyme itself or the substrate. An additional benefit of the phosphorylation strategy in living systems is that phosphorylated compounds such as sugars, because they are polar, are much less permeant. For this reason, they can be trapped within the cell (or in a cellular subcompartment) in higher concentrations than otherwise would be possible.

Electrochemistry is another important area of bioenergetics. Electrochemistry is reviewed in Chapter 1, General Chemistry. Briefly, electrochemistry deals with chemical reactions in terms of electron flow. One chemical is oxidized (loses electrons), while the other is reduced (gains electrons), and the tendency to gain or lose electrons is expressed as a voltage. By pairing and balancing half-cell reactions into the overall reaction, one can calculate the tendency for a reaction to go in one direction or the other in a manner analogous to that of free energies.

The importance of electrochemistry can be appreciated by considering a process crucial to life—the formation of ATP in mitochondria. The overall process can be viewed as a flow of electrons from relatively reduced compounds, such as carbohydrates (which are oxidized in the process) to oxygen (which is reduced during the formation of water). The transfer of these electrons occurs over the many steps involved in glycolysis, the citric acid cycle, and ultimately the respiratory chain located within mitochondria. Although there are hundreds of different intermediates involved in a variety of catabolic pathways, nature here is very conservative, relying on the same handful of electron carriers that can be found in various locations within the cell. Some of these carriers are soluble coenzymes, and some are physically associated with one another in large mitochondrial membrane bound complexes. NAD^+, nicotinamide adenine dinucleotide, and its analog, $NADP^+$, are both very mobile and soluble nucleotides that participate as in a wide variety of redox reactions and are based on the vitamin niacin. NAD^+ primarily participates in reactions catalyzed by a dehydrogenase and results in the loss of hydrogen (oxidation of substrate). The now reduced version, NADH, can be used as a reducing agent in a coupled reaction, or alternatively, can transfer its electron to mitochondrial NAD^+, which can be subsequently oxidized to produce ATP. $NADP^+$ by contrast primarily participates in anabolic reactions, where it functions as a reducing agent.

Another pair of coenzymes used in oxidative-reduction reactions are FAD and FMN, which are found in close association with enzymes known as flavoproteins. They are both derived from the vitamin riboflavin. Besides being in tight association (sometimes even covalently bound) with a specific enzyme (versus flitting from one enzyme to another, as does NAD^+) these coenzymes can participate in either one or two electrons transfers. Because of the affiliation with a variety of different flavoproteins, they have differing redox potentials. Flavoproteins function in a diverse set of metabolic roles. One example is the beta oxidation of fats and the citric acid cycle. In this process the electrons accepted during the conversion of succinate to fumarate are ultimately used to generate ATP in the respiratory chain.

Metabolism

The section below reviews metabolism, including principles of metabolic regulation, the metabolism of fatty acids and proteins, glycolysis, gluconeogenesis, the pentose phosphate pathway, and hormonal regulation of metabolism.

PRINCIPLES OF METABOLIC REGULATION

The term *metabolism* refers to all the chemical and physical processes necessary to sustain life and has two main aspects: catabolism and anabolism. **Catabolism** results in the breakdown (decomposition) of large chemicals into smaller ones. Energy is released and then stored in the form of ATP. **Anabolism** is the opposite. Anabolism builds (synthesizes) large molecules from simpler ones, such as building proteins from amino acids, and this synthesis requires energy. Anabolic steroids are so named because they promote anabolic reactions such as building muscles.

Homeostasis

Whatever their size or complexity, all organisms face a great challenge, that of maintaining **homeostasis**—the state in which internal biochemical conditions are in balance—in the face of an ever-changing environment. As large imbalances in internal conditions can result in disease or death of the organism, it is a subject of great interest how organisms manage this feat. Homeostasis requires controlling the concentration of thousands of chemicals within often narrow limits and, even more challenging, having the ability to alter the concentrations of some chemicals to meet a temporary demand or change of environmental conditions while maintaining near-constant concentrations of many others. Homeostasis is made even more challenging by the fact that many of these substrates share several intersecting pathways that form a highly complicated web of metabolic activity. The following are general principles that guide the processes of homeostasis.

- Use common metabolites to partition pathways into separate compartments within the cell—cytoplasm, endoplasmic reticulum, mitochondria, and so on.
- Control synthetic pathways so that surplus is avoided.
- Avoid futile cycles where destruction and synthesis of a substrate occur simultaneously.
- Use fuels most suited for the immediate circumstances.

A much better understanding of how these principles are incorporated by organisms now exists as a result of major advances in genetic engineering and molecular biology.

Homeostasis requires two related yet distinct concepts: **metabolic regulation**, which operates on short time scales at the molecular level to maintain a dynamic steady state, and **metabolic control**, which acts over larger time scales to increase or decrease the output of a particular pathway in response to changing conditions. Exactly how this is accomplished is dependent on the particular pathway involved. Some commonly employed strategies include:

- Regulation of enzyme's catalytic activity via substrate, product, and cofactor levels as well as through allosteric interactions, covalent modification (often phosphorylation/dephosphorylation), and interactions with other regulatory proteins
- Regulation of the amount of enzyme present via regulation of transcription and subsequent translation of the enzyme
- Sequestration of enzymes and the regulation of transporter activity

Two additional facts are useful for understanding metabolic regulation. First, whereas many enzymes operate at near equilibrium conditions (where the actual $\Delta G'$ is less than 6 kJ/mole), others operate far from equilibrium. It is these latter that are often subject to the greatest regulation, as they can function as one-way valves. Second, contrary to older models that supposed that regulation involved tight control over a single step in a metabolic pathway, we now know that control is much more diffuse and that several different enzymes in a cascade may be under independent control at different levels.

Regulation of Gluconeogenesis and Glycolysis

The regulation of gluconeogenesis and glycolysis provides a helpful example of the principles of metabolic regulation. The specifics of gluconeogenesis appear later in this chapter: to summarize, under conditions of intense exercise or starvation, the level of blood glucose must be maintained by the liver to meet the demands of glucose-dependent tissues such as the brain. New glucose can be synthesized from pyruvate and other materials in several steps that are the reverse of glycolysis. Three of the steps in glycolysis are far from equilibrium and function as one-way valves and, thus, cannot be run in reverse. Because of this, the synthesis of glucose requires different enzymes than those used in glycolysis. Below are descriptions of these three reactions.

REACTION 1: HEXOKINASE/GLUCOSE-6-PHOSPHOTASE. Here we see that by using different isozymes in different tissues, coordination of resource utilization is achieved. In muscle, hexokinase activity is inhibited by product formation putting a natural brake on the process. The form of hexokinase in the liver is different in several important respects. First, it has a much lower affinity, Km, for glucose than its counterparts, which serves to prevent phosphorylation of glucose that is in short supply and needed by other organs. Second, it is not inhibited by accumulation of its product. This allows glucose utilization to continue unimpeded so that it may be diverted for other purposes such as glycogen synthesis or through the pentose phosphate pathway. Finally, when glucose is scarce and fructose more abundant, liver hexokinase is "hidden" within the nucleus, where it has no access to cytoplasmic stores.

Additionally both hexokinase and the competing glucose-6-phophotase levels are subject to transcriptional regulation that is reciprocal, meaning that low energy states characterized by small ATP/AMP ratios lead to an increase in gluconeogenesis while simultaneously suppressing glycolysis.

REACTION 2: PHOSPHOFRUCTOKINASE-1 (PFK-1) and the corresponding "reverse" enzyme **FRUCTOSE 1,6 BISPHOSPHOTASE (FBPase-1).** PFK-1 and FBPase-1 are subject to several types of regulation, including hormonal. These include:

1. Allosteric effects of ATP, ADP, and AMP on PFK-1, which are further modulated by citrate levels and other indicators that catabolic needs are being met by burning other fuels;
2. Allosteric inhibition of AMP on FBPase-1;
3. The effect of glucagon and insulin, which promote gluconeogenesis and glycolysis, respectively.

This latter effect is delivered via fructose 2,6-bisphosphate levels, which shut down PFK-1 activity while promoting FBPase-1 activity. Interestingly, the levels of fructose 2,6-bisphophate are controlled by a separate protein that can catalyze the formation or disappearance of F2,6-B depending on its state of phosphorylation. This in turn is regulated by glucagon and insulin signals, the former acting through cAMP-dependent protein kinase, while insulin activates the dephosphorylating enzyme, phosphoprotein phosphatase. Finally, yet another effect on fructose 2,6-bisphosphate levels is mediated by a product of the pentose phosphate pathway, which increases glycolysis in the liver as a prelude to increased fatty acid synthesis when carbohydrate levels are high.

REACTION 3: PYRUVATE KINASE. The last step of glycolysis (and first step of gluconeogenesis) is also highly regulated by multiple actions at different levels. Like hexokinase, pyruvate kinase exists in several tissue specific forms (isozymes), which are all inhibited by abundant energy supplies but differentially influenced by glucagon. The liver isozyme is inactivated by glucagon via phosphorylation, which serves to spare glucose needed elsewhere in the body while increased levels of cAMP brought about by epinephrine stimulation have the expected stimulatory effect on catabolic processes in muscle.

Meanwhile, the reaction that starts gluconeogenesis uses the substrate pyruvate, to which the enzyme pyruvate carboxylase adds a carboxyl group, making oxaloacetic acid (OAA). This enzyme is under the influence of multiple factors, including substrate availability itself. Pyruvate is at an important branch point. When energy levels are low, the cell favors further oxidation via the citric acid cycle. When energy levels are adequate, rising levels of acetyl-CoA inhibit further production and stimulate gluconeogenesis via positive allosteric effects on pyruvate carboxylase. The subsequent step, that of converting OAA to phosphoenolpyruvate (PEP), is also under hormonal regulation. Namely, high glucagon levels stimulate transcription of more of the gene encoding for it, while slowing the breakdown of the newly transcribed mRNA. Insulin on the other hand sets into motion a sequence of events across a variety of tissues. This sequence involves protein kinases and culminates in anabolic effects such as increased fat production and cellular growth, while reducing production of enzymes needed for gluconeogenesis.

Regulation of Glycogen Metabolism

Glycogen is a large, highly branched polysaccharide that is a form of energy storage in animals and is found in a variety of tissues, chiefly muscle and liver. The regulation of its synthesis and breakdown further illustrates the principles of metabolic regulation and control. Here we review additional examples of

1. Allosteric interactions;
2. Hormonal control, including an enzymatic cascade in response to the catabolic hormones epinephrine and glucagon;
3. The use of isozymes to differentiate responses between liver and muscle;
4. The role of other second messengers in coordinating energy use and storage.

The formation of glycogen involves four enzymes and the use of sugar nucleotides to

1. Catalyze the formation of alpha 1-4 glycosidic linkages between the glucose monomers and
2. Provide periodic branch points so that the overall shape is roughly spherical. The use of sugar-nucleotides such as UDP-glucose serves to make the initial step irreversible and committed to glycogen synthesis. The process involves a commonly employed tactic that uses the free energy of pyrophosphate breakdown (in parentheses) to drive the reaction far to the right of equilibrium.

$$\text{glucose-1 phosphate} + UTP \rightarrow \text{UDP-glucose} + PPi \ (PPi \rightarrow 2Pi)$$

The second step requires the enzyme glycogen synthetase, which forms the glycosidic linkage, thereby lengthening the glycogen by one sugar residue. Periodic branch points are later introduced by a branching enzyme, while the initial seed for the glycogen polymer is catalyzed by the enzyme glycogenin. Glycogenin assembles the first seven linkages before turning over the task of additional lengthening to glycogen synthase. It is noteworthy that the enzymes for production, degradation, and regulation of these processes are found in the glycogen granules themselves associated in a large complex.

Glycogenolysis is in many ways the reverse of these reactions and as might be expected employs a different set of enzymes. One of these enzymes is only found in the endoplasmic reticulum (ER) of liver. It converts the phosphorylated sugar, G6-P, to glucose that can then be passed on to other tissues.

Important sites of overall regulation between the synthesis and degradation of glycogen include the enzymes glycogen synthase and its counterpart, glycogen phosphorylase. Both of these exist in active and inactive forms that can be rapidly interconverted by protein kinases. The respective protein kinases are in turn activated by glucagon (or epinephrine in muscle) and insulin. In the first case, adenylate cyclase is activated by one of the catabolic hormones. This in turn generates cAMP and activates protein kinase A, which in turn activates phosphorylase b. Finally, phosphorylase b converts glycogen phosphorylase B (inactive) into the active form, glycogen phosphorylase A. Such an avalanche of events where the output of a hormonal signal activates another enzyme that in turn activates a third enzyme and so forth, is referred to as an **enzymatic cascade**. An enzymatic cascade allows signals in the body to be greatly amplified. Once glucose levels begin to rise, the process is shut off through an allosteric effect on phosphorylase B. This makes phosphorylase B susceptible to dephosphorylation thus inactivating it. Insulin enhances the inhibition.

Glycogen synthase is subject to a similar set of controls but instead it is activated by dephosphorylation. This takes place via the enzyme phosphorylase A phosphatase 1 (PP1). PP1 also inactivates phosphorylase in a form of reciprocal control. Glycogen synthase is inactivated by a number of protein kinases, the most important of which is glycogen synthase kinase 3 (GSK-3). Thus, insulin exerts its anabolic effect by both blocking GSK-3 (through an inositol second messenger that leads to activation of protein kinase) and activating PP1. In addition there are several allosteric and covalent regulatory effects on PP1itself. These include positive allosteric regulation by G6-P such that PP1 acts as a glucose 6-phosphate sensor. At the same time, its catabolic counterpart glycogen phosphorylase acts as a glucose sensor.

Metabolic Control Analysis

An increasingly sophisticated array of biochemical techniques has been brought to bear on the analysis of metabolic control, a highly mathematical subdiscipline of biochemistry that seeks to quantify exact relations between variables within a metabolic pathway and the total flux through that pathway. One example is the effect that individual enzymes have on the overall output of the pathway. For instance, deeply rooted in the history of biochemistry is the notion that the speed through a single rate-limiting step (bottleneck) is what controlled overall output of the pathway. This turns out to be seldom if ever the case, and instead control is parsed out between several enzymes in the pathway.

The extent to which a particular enzyme is a factor in overall flux is reflected in what is referred to as a **flux control coefficient**, C. In a simple chain reaction pathway, this coefficient varies between 0 (no influence) and a theoretical maximum of 1. At a value of 1, the total flux is governed by a single enzyme as in the example of the rate limiting step notion. In pathways that branch, it is even possible to have a negative impact of flux by siphoning intermediates away from the pathway under study. In this case it has a negative coefficient. In all cases, the sum of the control coefficients equals one.

A second parameter of interest is that of the **enzyme elasticity coefficient**, ε. This coefficient characterizes the response of an enzyme to a change in the concentration of substrate, product, or other regulating substance. This is relatively simple to determine experimentally when the purified enzyme is available. The determination relies on quantitative techniques that use a variety of plot types. Simple Michaelis-Menton kinetics, which plot velocity as a function of substrate concentration, reveal a hyperbolic-shaped function when no cooperativity is present. The elasticity coefficient in this case varies between 1 at low concentrations (reflecting high sensitivity to a change in [s]) and zero when the velocity is near maximum and minimally influenced by changes in [s].

Finally the overall change in flux through a pathway in response to the effect on a single enzyme by another agent such as a hormone can be assessed by calculating a third parameter, **the response coefficient**, R. This coefficient is simply the product of the control coefficient for that enzyme and the enzyme elasticity when measured with respect to the outside agent. In other words, the overall flux sensitivity is just a particular enzyme's sensitivity to the hormone multiplied times the relative importance of that step in the overall sequence. Unless that particular step exerts significant impact on overall control, acceleration or deceleration of that particular step will be of little consequence.

METABOLISM OF FATTY ACIDS

Fatty acids and their digestion, mobilization, and transport were described earlier in this book. This section reviews the fatty acid oxidation, ketones, anabolism of fats, and metabolism of proteins.

Oxidation of Fatty Acids

Fats are an important dietary source of essential nutrients and are found in all living things. As they contain twice as many calories per gram as either carbohydrates or proteins, they are a highly efficient form of energy storage, and as much as 60% of the available energy can be reclaimed during their breakdown. The breakdown of fat (primarily in the form of triacylglycerol) begins with an attack on the lipid droplet itself. These droplets are found mainly in adipocytes but occur in a variety of tissues, including liver and skeletal muscle. Fat droplets are now known to be a much richer and sophisticated structure than previously thought. They are now considered an organelle, complete with phospholipid monolayer embedded with various proteins, including protective perilipins. They have a dynamic interplay with other cellular organelles. Under hormonal signaling, utilization of fat begins with the breakdown of triacylglycerols into (1) three free fatty acids (FFA) and (2) the glycerol backbone. The glycerol backbone is degraded via glycolysis. Free fatty acids are then transported bound to albumin to the destination tissues, such as skeletal muscle or heart. In the destination tissues, they are taken up and transported to the mitochondria, where they are consumed. Long chain fatty acids (C > 14), however, must first undergo a transformation involving three reactions before they can be moved into the mitochondrion by a transport mechanism known as the carnitine shuttle. The first reaction involves activation of the fatty acid by combining it with CoA. This reaction burns ATP and is a commitment to further oxidation, versus that of being recycled in a synthetic step such as the formation of membrane phospholipids:

$$\text{Fatty acid} + \text{CoA} + \text{ATP} \rightarrow \text{Fatty acid-CoA} + \text{AMP} + 2\,\text{Pi}$$

Now activated, the fatty acid-CoA can exchange the CoA with carnitine in the outer membrane and be ferried across the membrane, where it can then release the carnitine in exchange for another CoA, again on the inner membrane. In effect this swaps CoAs from one pool with CoAs from another.

In the case of those FFAs that are both saturated and have an even number of carbons, oxidation is relatively straightforward. Two carbon segments are clipped one at a time in the form of Acetyl-CoA, which is then oxidized in the citric acid cycle. Clipping the two carbon acetyl groups requires that the fatty acid be first modified by the combined action of three enzymes. This process

1. Adds a double bond;
2. Subjects the double bond to hydration forming a beta hydroxyl-acyl CoA;
3. Oxidizes the beta hydroxyl bond to the ketone (hence the description of the process as beta oxidation).

The product, a beta-ketoacyl-CoA, then is shortened via attack at the alpha-carbon-releasing acetyl-S-CoA while replacing the CoA-SH at the end of the FFA so that the cycle can be repeated. This occurs until only an acetyl-CoA remains. Note that two electron carriers participate in the dehydrogenation (FAD) and oxidation (NAD$^+$), both of which can then donate the electrons to the respiratory chain, generating ATP in the process.

Net reaction for the 16 carbon FFA:

$$Palmitoyl\text{-}CoA + 7Co\text{-}A + 7FAD + 7NAD^+ \rightarrow 8 \text{ acetyl-Co-A} + 7FADH_2 + 7NADH + 7H^+$$

Transfer of the electrons and oxidative phosphorylation results in 28 ATP on top of those derived from the oxidations of the 8 acetyl CoA. Each of those contributes an additional 10ATP/acetyl CoA, bringing the total to 108, or about three times the amount in a glucose molecule, despite weighing only 1.5 times as much.

In the event that either the fatty acid has an odd number of carbons or possesses double bonds, additional enzymes are needed. If the FFA is unsaturated, reactions occur as above until the naturally occurring *cis* double bond interferes with further degradation. At that point, an additional enzyme converts the bond to the trans form. If the FFA is polyunsaturated, yet another enzyme is required, but the overall stoichiometry is unaffected. If the FFA possesses an odd number of carbons, the final cleavage leaves a propionate-CoA as one of the products, instead of two acetyl-CoA. The propionate is ultimately converted to succinyl-CoA via addition of a carbon and subsequent rearrangement involving three enzymes and the use of two cofactors, biotin and B_{12}. It should be mentioned that beta oxidation is not confined to mitochondria. It also occurs within perixosomes, which appear to specialize in the catabolism of very long and/or branched FFAs. The absence or dysfunction of perixosomes can cause serious disease. It should also be mentioned that another form of oxidation, omega oxidation, is carried out in the ER and attacks the carbon from the opposite end (omega), producing double-ended fatty acids that can be combined with acetyl CoA and oxidized by the beta pathway in the mitochondria.

Ketone Bodies

An important feature of fat catabolism is the production of ketone bodies, which are produced in the liver and exported to other tissues during times of need. This is particularly important in the brain, which has a limited ability to burn fat directly. The chemicals themselves—acetone, acetoacetate, and beta-hydroxybutyrate—are soluble and do not coalesce into "bodies" of any type as the name implies. They simply represent a temporary form of transport so that acetyl CoA can get from the liver to where energy is needed.

After about two days of low carbohydrate intake, the predominant form of catabolism in many tissues including the brain becomes ketone based and the increased concentration of these products in the blood is referred to as ketosis. In contrast with a serious derangement of metabolism referred to as diabetic ketoacidosis (DKA), ketosis is associated with a relatively mild elevation of ketones. In addition to supplying needed calories to many tissues, these ketones may be beneficial in some cases of epilepsy and for those seeking to lose weight (e.g., Atkins, South Beach diets). In the case of DKA, depletion of citric acid cycle intermediates result in the overproduction of acetyl CoA and in turn, very high levels of ketones in the blood, which can lead to a life threatening acidosis.

The production of ketones begins with the condensation of acetyl CoA to form acetoacetyl CoA, which is then converted to acetoacetate. From acetoacetate, either acetone or beta hydroxybutyrate is formed. Acetone is both toxic and volatile, and in higher concentrations leads to an unmistakable breath odor similar to that of nail polish remover.

Anabolism of Fats

This topic is complex owing to the many structures and roles in which lipids play a key part, ranging from the basic cellular boundaries of all living things to the central role in energy storage, heat insulation, the storage of fat soluble vitamins, and finally the signaling agents such as prostaglandins, steroid hormones, and the second messenger system using diacylglycerol. One striking characteristic of fat metabolism—and which is an important theme in regulation—is that the body partitions catabolism and anabolism into separate compartments. Besides occurring in the cytoplasm, anabolism relies on an entirely different set of enzymes (unlike glycolysis/gluconeogenesis, which share seven enzymes). As the basis for synthesis, the cell utilizes the three carbon acetylated compound, malonyl-CoA, not acetyl CoA. In fact, the commitment to synthesis begins with an ATP-dependent reaction that transfers a carboxyl group to acetyl-CoA to form malonyl-CoA. In the case of simple saturated FFAs, the remainder of the synthesis occurs on a remarkable and large enzyme complex. This complex catalyses seven separate reactions that result in a transfer of two carbons per cycle (the third carbon of malonyl-CoA is released as CO_2 during transfer and provides energy to the process) and can be summarized as

$$7\text{Malonyl-CoA} + \text{Acetyl-CoA} + 14\text{H}^+ + 14\text{NADPH} \rightarrow$$
$$\text{Palmitic acid} + 7CO_{23} + 8\text{CoA} + 14\text{NADP}^+ + 7H_2O$$

Note that the electron carrier is NADPH, which is typically used as an electron donor in anabolic reactions.

In the event that unsaturated fatty acids are needed, mammals are limited to desaturation at the carbonyl end or at the $\Delta 9$ position. This explains the need for us to consume essential fatty acids, which add a greater variety of double bonds, especially at the $\Delta 9,12$ positions in the case of linoleic acid, and at $\Delta 9,12,15$ positions in linolenic acid. Linoleic acids provide the carbon skeleton for the synthesis of eicosanoids, which are a group of very important signal molecules including prostaglandins, thromboxanes, and leukotrienes. Once fatty acids have been formed, the body can use them to synthesize triacylglycerols (energy storage), phospholipids, and sphingolipids (membrane components). The fatty acids can also be used as membrane components capable of acting as second messengers (eiconasoids, sphingomyelin, phosphatidylinisotol, and diacylglycerol).

Some aspects of regulation, such as the partitioning of anabolism in the cytoplasm and catabolism within the mitochondrion, have been discussed above. Additional aspects of regulation include hormone signaling. Epinephrine and glucagon provide the initial signal to mobilize FFAs from lipid droplets, while simultaneously inhibiting synthesis. Other signals include suppression of the carnitine shuttle by malonyl-CoA (thus avoiding a futile cycle) and the relative amounts of citrate (stimulates synthesis) and palmitoyl-CoA (suppresses synthesis).

SYNTHESIS OF CHOLESTEROL AND OTHER STEROIDS. A second and essential group of lipids that the body is capable of synthesizing is cholesterol and its many derivatives. These derivatives include a number of steroid hormones, bile, and vitamin D. Cholesterol itself is an essential component of plasma membranes, where it can represent a significant portion of the total membrane lipids (30% in red blood cells). It has important effects on the physical properties of the membrane, including stiffening it and making it less permeable. Cholesterol is also found in high concentrations in myelin and is involved in a number of other transmembrane transport and signaling activities. Because of the link between high cholesterol levels and the development of cardiovascular disease, the metabolism of cholesterol has been extensively studied. Dietary restriction of cholesterol when combined with exercise can have a beneficial impact on blood levels, but several classes of medication including the "statins" have been shown to have a greater effect on reducing levels and slowing the progression of atherosclerosis, particularly in high-risk patients.

The synthesis of cholesterol begins in much the same way as ketone bodies with a pair of condensation reactions that successively unite 3 acetyl-CoA molecules into the six-carbon compound HMG-CoA. The next reaction, which occurs in smooth ER, is rate limiting, is highly regulated, and is the target of the statin drugs. It requires the enzyme HMG-CoA reductase and the use of two NADPH electron donors to form mevalonate. From mevalonate and the expenditure of three ATP, a decarboxylase converts the activated mevalonate into the five-carbon activated isoprene, Δ^3-isopentenyl pyrophosphate.

This compound and an isomer of it next participate in a head to tail condensation that forms the ten-carbon geranyl-PP1 to which another Δ^3-isopentynl pyrophosphate is added, forming the 15-carbon farnesyl-PP1. Two of these combine in a head-to-head condensation to form the 30-carbon squalene (synthesized by squalene synthase and requiring another NADPH). The net cost for squalene synthesis is 18 ATP (3 for each of the 6 isoprenes) and 13 NADPH.

Squalene is next converted to the 2,3-epoxide by the enzyme squalene monooxygenase in preparation for a cascade of reactions that causes the four rings to close (Figure 5.24).

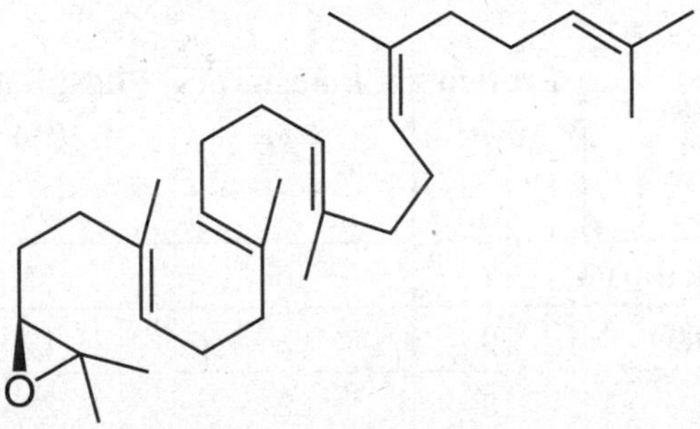

Figure 5.24. 2,3 squalene epoxide, showing the cascade of ring closures

This reaction is the result of strain in the epoxide ring, which is attacked by a proton. This causes the A ring to close, followed by zipping up of the B, C, and D rings (along with movement of methyl groups). The end product of this process is lanosterol. Lanosterol is then converted in a sequence of reactions to cholesterol. Figure 5.25 summarizes the steps in the synthesis of cholesterol.

Cholesterol has a variety of possible destinations and fates. For example, cholesterol produced in the liver can be used to form bile acids, which act as detergents. By emulsifying fat droplets within the small intestine, bile facilitates the enzymatic attack by lipase. Much of the cholesterol destined to be exported to other tissues is first esterified, making it even more insoluble in water. To transport cholesterol, the body uses carrier proteins (**apoproteins**). When combined with various lipids, these proteins are called lipoproteins. Lipoproteins come in a variety of sizes (and densities) and have different duties. The apoproteins themselves are divided into five classes—Apo-A through Apo-E—and each is associated with one or more types of lipoproteins. (See Table 5.1.)

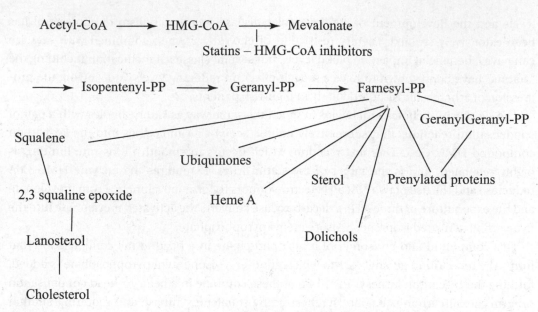

Figure 5.25. A summary of cholesterol synthesis

Table 5.1 Composition of Lipoproteins

Density (g/mL)	Class	Protein (%)	Cholesterol (%)	Phospholipid (%)	Triacylglycerol and Cholesterol Ester (%)
<0.950	Chylomicrons	<2	8	7	84
0.950–1.006	VLDL	10	22	18	50
1.006–1.019	IDL	18	29	22	31
1.019–1.063	LDL	25	50	21	8
>1.063	HDL	33	30	29	4

As shown in Table 5.1, chylomicrons function to transport dietary triacylglycerols taken from chyme through the lacteals and general lymphatic channels before entering the circulation, where they are transported to adipose or tissues in need. VLDLs (very low-density lipoproteins) transport both excess fatty acids and TAGs (converted from carbohydrates) from the liver to (1) adipose tissue for storage and (2) cardiac muscle for oxidation. As TAGs are removed from VLDLs, their density increases and are then referred to as IDLs (intermediate density lipoproteins) and LDLs (low-density lipoproteins).

LDLs transport cholesterol to peripheral tissues, where the LDL binds to specific LDL receptors. The cholesterol and other LDL components are either stored in droplets or used in membranes. Because of their role in the formation of atheromas (inflammatory cholesterol containing lesions on arterial walls), this type of cholesterol is sometimes referred to as bad cholesterol. By contrast, high-density lipopoteins are made up of much more protein and less fat, and they are referred to as good cholesterol because they generally transport cholesterol away from the periphery and back to the liver.

Cholesterol is the precursor from which the steroid hormones are synthesized. To review, sex hormones, mineralcorticoids such as aldosterone, and glucocorticoids are all cholesterol based and synthesized in the gonads or adrenal cortex. Most of these molecules are quite similar to one another and differ from cholesterol in that most or all of the eight carbons linked to C17 on the D ring have been cleaved. The various steroids are produced by the action of mixed function oxidases (also known as monooxygenases). These reactions differ from other oxidative reactions insofar as one of the two oxygen atoms of the participating molecule O_2 is reduced in the formation of water, and the other oxygen atom appears in the product. The hydrogen is provided by NADPH but is donated through the action of an intermediate cytochrome P-450 enzyme.

Cytochrome P-450s are critical in the synthesis of many lipids (including cholesterol itself) and are also essential to the breakdown by the liver of many substances, including toxins found in food as well as in many medications. Finally, it should be noted that cholesterol and its derivatives are not the only important biomolecules that are synthesized from Δ^3-isopentenyl pyrophosphate. The class of molecules referred to as isoprenoids (resembling isoprene) include the other fat soluble vitamins A, E, and K, the quinone electron carriers found in mitochondria (ubiquinone), and chloroplasts (plastiquinone) to name a few examples. The pathways for some of these substances are shown in Figure 5.25.

METABOLISM OF PROTEINS

The synthesis of proteins from amino acids, as well as the digestion of proteins, is reviewed in Chapter 3, Biology. It should be recalled that in addition to being the building blocks of proteins, amino acids serve a variety of other functions, including as signaling molecules (hormones, neurotransmitters), as a substrate for the synthesis of porphyrins, and as the precursors for nucleotides, while some nonstandard amino acids play a central role in the urea cycle.

Here we examine the catabolism of amino acids and discuss the problem of ammonia excretion. Dietary protein can account for a significant fraction of our caloric requirements and the intake of the average American is clearly in excess of the approximately two ounces needed to maintain good health. As there is no storage form for excess amino acids, the body has no choice but to oxidize any surplus. A problem faced by any land-based organism is that oxidation involves removal of the amino group, and a potential by product of the process is ammonia. Organisms have evolved cunning mechanisms to deal with this issue, which by and large ends in the hepatocyte with the production of urea. Urea is a relatively nontoxic and highly soluble compound that can be excreted by the kidneys, where it serves another critically important purpose: concentrating urine and reclaiming water. (Other nitrogen waste comes from metabolism of the nitrogenous bases. Nitrogen found in pyrimidine bases is also converted to urea; the nitrogen from purines ends up as the less soluble uric acid, which can reach high enough concentrations to crystallize out of solution into needlelike crystals during episodes of gout.

Ammonia is produced in a number of tissues. In small amounts it presents no threat, but these tissues are incapable of eliminating ammonia themselves and so must find a way to transport it to the liver, where it can be converted to urea. The most common method is to use amino acids as ammonia transporters. In vigorously exercising skeletal muscle, pyruvate is produced in abundance and can be aminated through the addition of an amino group. This is done by the enzyme alanine aminotransferase (ALT). This process forms alanine, which along with lactate (see Cori cycle) can then be shipped to the liver. In tissues other than skeletal muscle, a second amino group is used to convert glutamate to glutamine, which the liver converts back to glutamate in preparation for disposal.

The overall theme is to funnel the ammonia potentially being produced into the amino group of glutamine. Glutamine is a single intermediate that can be efficiently disposed of by the liver through oxidative deamination. This process is called trans-deamination. It consists of first using transaminases to swap amino groups. The groups are swapped from the amino acid intended for oxidation to a common acceptor (glutamate). Trans-deamination spares the body the metabolic burden of having many redundant pathways specific to each amino acid. Once in the liver, glutamate and glutamine become ammonia donors along with aspartate to form urea in an array of reactions split between the cytosol and mitochondria. Although the overall process is endergonic, requiring four high-energy phosphate bonds per urea molecule produced, much of this energy is offset through the formation of fumarate. Fumarate can generate NADH through conversion to OAA. The sharing of intermediaries between the urea cycle and citric acid provides flexibility in overall metabolic processing of amino acids and other compounds.

$$\text{Net reaction: } 2NH_4^+ + HCO_3^- + 3ATP + H_2O \rightarrow \text{urea} + 2ADP + 4Pi + AMP + 2H^+$$

Amino acids can be characterized by their potential to become either glucose (via gluconeogenesis) or ketones (via acetyl CoA). The former are more common. Only two—leucine and lysine—are purely ketogenic. Five of the amino acids can end up as either ketones or glucose, depending on need.

GLUCONEOGENESIS AND THE PENTOSE PHOSPHATE PATHWAY

Gluconeogenesis (GNG)

Gluconeogenesis literally means the creation of new sugar (glucose) from non-carbohydrate substrates. Normally as sugar reserves are depleted, the body breaks down glycogen that has been formed earlier during times of energy abundance. In the absence of such sugar stores, however, the liver (and kidney to a lesser extent) start to produce new sugar from "scratch" using a variety of materials, including pyruvate, lactate, amino acids, glycerol, and any of the numerous TCA cycle intermediates. Although the making of new sugar in this manner costs the organism energy in the form of high-energy phosphate bonds (ATP and GTP), there are many circumstances in which the body must do so. These include taking care of the brain and nervous tissues, which normally rely on glucose exclusively, or extending the duration of anaerobic exercise (Cori cycle). The kidneys, testes, and erythrocytes likewise depend on glucose. GNG is of more than academic interest: greater understanding of the process and its regulation may lead to improved treatment of diabetes, help to combat the cachexia of cancer, and assist in devising better, more individualized weight loss plans.

Summary of Reactions and the Differences Between GNG and Glycolysis

GNG:

$$2 \text{ pyruvate} + 4 \text{ ATP} + 2 \text{ GTP} + 2 \text{ NADH} + 6 \text{ H}_2\text{O} + 2 \text{ H}^+ =$$
$$\text{glucose} + 4 \text{ ADP} + 2 \text{ GDP} + \text{NAD}^+ + 6 \text{ Pi}$$

Glycolysis:

$$\text{glucose} + 2 \text{ ADP} + 2 \text{ Pi} + 2 \text{ NAD}^+ = 2 \text{ pyruvate} + 2 \text{ ATP} + 2 \text{ NADH} + 2 \text{ H}_2\text{O}$$

By adding the reactions above, the net cost of GNG can be determined. The production of a single glucose from two pyruvate molecules requires the expenditure of 4 ATP and 2 GTP. Two of these ATP can be subsequently recovered by breaking down the glucose, leaving a net expense of 4 high-energy phosphate bonds.

Although it is advantageous for the body to be able to either break down glucose or reassemble it from its byproducts—depending on the needs of the moment—it also invites potential chaos. In the extreme case, the two reactions could form an endless loop, splitting and subsequently reforming glucose at a cost of 4 ATP/GTP per loop. This is called a **futile cycle**.

The body has a mechanism for avoiding a futile cycle and for controlling the overall net effect of the two processes (GNG and glycolysis). This is made possible through enzymatic regulation. To understand this regulation, it is necessary to consider that 6 of the 10 steps of GNG are exactly the same as for glycolysis, using the same enzymes, only run in reverse. These 6 occur at conditions close to equilibrium, allowing them to be run in either direction. Because the steps are so easily reversible, the enzymes involved are not helpful for regulating the direction of the reaction. The remaining steps of glycolysis cannot be run in reverse without a significant energy input. To reverse these steps, GNG uses a different pathway, employing different enzymes than those of glycolysis. This serves two purposes: First, it provides a way around the steps that would be energetically infeasible. Second, it provides a mechanism for preventing futile cycling through a process of **reciprocal regulation**. Reciprocal regulation refers to a state in which the conditions that activate one pathway (e.g., glycolysis) inhibit the other (e.g., GNG). By this means, it is impossible for both pathways to run at the same time, which would result in a futile cycle. This is similar to the relationship between insulin and glucagon. Reciprocal regulation could not be achieved if all of the reactions of glycolysis could be run in reverse. A simplified summary of some of the regulation is shown below, including the factors that activate or inhibit the processes. These are the reactions that are different (not simply reversed) in GNG than in glycolysis.

Abbreviations	
PEP = phosphoenolpyruvate	F6BP = fructose 6 phosphate
PYR= pyruvate	F1,6BP = fructose 1,6 bisphosphate
OAA = oxaloacetic acid	G6P = glucose 6 phosphate

Reaction 1

Glycolysis:

$$F6BP \rightarrow F1,6BP \text{ via enzyme phosphofructokinase}$$

Activated by low ATP and inhibited by high ATP

GNG:

$$F1,6BP \rightarrow F6BP \text{ via fructose 1,6 bisphostase}$$

Inhibited by AMP

Reaction 2

Glycolysis:

$$PEP \rightarrow pyruvate$$

Inhibited when the enzyme pyruvate kinase (liver only) is phosphorylated; this happens in response to epinephrine.

GNG:

$$pyruvate \rightarrow OAA \rightarrow PEP$$

Second reaction increased by phosphorylation via increased transcription of gene for the enzyme PEP carboxykinase. Insulin inhibits transcription of this gene (hormonal control).

Reaction 3

Glycolysis:

$$glucose \rightarrow G6P$$

Catalyzed by enzyme hexokinase, which is inhibited by product build-up.

GNG:

$$G6P \rightarrow glucose + phosphate$$

Glucose-6-phosphatase catalyzes the reverse reaction and is the last step in GNG.

Pentose Phosphate Pathway (PPP)

This cytosolic pathway provides an important alternative to the usual fate of glucose-6-P, that of complete oxidation. In complete oxidation (via glycolysis and the citric acid cycle) approximately 30 to 38 ATP are produced. In PPP, the cell trades all of the potential ATP energy for the opportunity to generate NADPH, an important anabolic cofactor used in the synthesis of fatty acids. PPP also allows the cell to generate ribose-5-P, an important nucleotide precursor. Predictably, those cells where the pentose phosphate pathway is most active are (1) those engaged in large amounts of lipid synthesis (gonads, adrenal cortex) and (2) those with a high turnover rate (many types of epithelium) that have a high demand for nucleic acid synthesis. Other tissues that benefit from this pathway are those exposed to high levels of oxidative stress, which can be partly countered by high levels of NADPH and glutathione, a potent antioxidant. In either case, the potential energy from glycolysis is swapped for increased reducing power.

The PPP is divided into two phases: the oxidative phase, which converts glucose 6-P to ribose 5-P (the pentose phosphate) generating NADPH, and the non-oxidative (reductive) phase. The latter series of reactions involves a number of different phosphorylated carbohydrates of various lengths that can be used to regenerate the glucose 6-P by way of gluconeogenesis, and which when done repeatedly, leads to the net reaction:

$$1 \text{ glucose 6-P} + 12 \text{ NADP}^+ \rightarrow 6 \text{ CO}_2 + 12 \text{ NADPH} + 10 \text{ H}^+$$

Alternatively, the many intermediates and products of the non-oxidative phase can be (1) used to synthesize a variety of compounds, including aromatic amino acids, or (2) oxidized for ATP, depending on the cell's particular needs at the time. In those cells with a high demand for ribose 5-P, the non-oxidative phase, which is energetically neutral, can be run in reverse. This produces three ribose-5-P from two fructose-6-P and one glyceraldehyde-3-P. The commitment step of the oxidative phase of the PPP is noteworthy for its dependence on the enzyme glucose 6-P dehydrogenase. The deficiency of this enzyme is a relatively common genetic disorder, affecting perhaps 7% of the world's population. It can lead to an increased fragility of erythrocyte membrane and hemolytic anemia. However, it has the curious property shared with sickle cell anemia of providing its victims with protection against malaria. Regulation of how much of the available glucose 6-P is used in the PPP versus glycolysis depends to a large extent on the relative abundance of the electron acceptor NADP$^+$ required for the first step reaction. NADP$^+$ has a positive allosteric effect on G6PD, so the reaction naturally slows as NADP$^+$ is converted to NADPH, causing an increased flux of glucose through the glycolytic pathway.

HORMONAL REGULATION AND INTEGRATION OF METABOLISM

This section reviews the mechanisms of neuroendocrine control and coordination of metabolic activities, examines the collective, tissue-specific effects of the major hormones, and concludes with a review of some of the many factors thought to control body mass. These factors, when dysfunctional, may help to explain the factors that underlie obesity.

Neuroendocrine Function

The nervous and endocrine systems operate together and can rightfully be considered a single system of coordination and control by which overall organismal homeostasis is achieved. Primary goals of such a system are the maintenance of long-term fluid, electrolyte, and calorie balance in the face of widely changing environmental conditions. Because of the diverse and specialized functions and properties of the different tissues and organs, such a task can only be accomplished through the sensing and communication of data at many levels. Generally, although the two systems (endocrine and nervous) have highly overlapping functions, important differences include the time scale over which the two systems operate and the specificity of the information flow. The nervous system tends to be more rapid in detecting changes, in its response, and in signaling this information to very specific locations.

Both systems use signal molecules that depend on a high degree of receptor specificity (very low dissociation constants). The free energy of hormone binding to receptors changes the transformational state of the receptor resulting in a signal to the cell interior. There may also be changes in sensitivity to future messages of the same sort via up and down regulation. However, the results may also reverberate forward to related tissues and also be fed back to the original messenger. The molecular messengers, principally hormones and neurotransmitters, share many mechanistic features and may even be the same chemicals. This is the case with epinephrine and norepinephrine. These hormones function in the event of emergency in both the autonomic nervous system, through conventional neurotransmission, and the endocrine system. The adrenal cortex converts specific electrical signals into a call for all hands on deck via the same chemicals, only now blood-borne and thus felt potentially by every cell in the body.

The mechanisms by which both the nervous and endocrine systems engage their targets are also the same and are described in greater detail in Chapter 3, Biology. To briefly review, receptor-ligand interaction results in one or more of the following events within the target cell:

1. A second messenger system is activated with resulting allosteric modification of enzyme activity.
2. A receptor tyrosine kinase is activated, resulting in phosphorylation of other proteins.
3. Receptor-G protein interactions increase cGMP.
4. Mechanical effects transmit through the membrane onto components of the cell's cytoskeleton.
5. Changes take place in transmembrane voltage secondary to permeability changes in the membrane (ion channels opening and closing).
6. Regulatory effects take place at the level of transcription and are usually mediated by lipid-soluble hormones.

With some exceptions, the hormones that mediate these effects are generally classified as protein/polypeptide versus steroid-based hormones. The sphere of influence of a hormone can be endocrine, paracrine, and/or autocrine. Hormones can bind to membrane-bound receptors or to receptors inside the cell. The mechanisms of action of these different types are quite different, as are the time scales of effects. For example, hormones that bind to membrane-bound receptors act more quickly but have less-persistent effects compared to hormones that bind within the cell, act more slowly, and have longer lasting effects. Peptide hormones tend to be more like nervous system signals. They bind to membrane-bound receptors and have effects that are produced almost immediately via changes in levels of enzymatic processes. In contrast, most steroid and other water-insoluble messengers (there are some exceptions that bind to the membrane) bind within the cell and act principally on DNA, altering the level of transcriptional activity of genes.

The eicosanoids hormones (prostaglandins, thromboxanes, and leukotrienes) are an increasingly important topic in medicine and pharmaceutical sciences, as these arachidonic acid-based substances mediate many aspects of inflammation. They depart from many of the generalizations made about hormones as they are fat soluble, yet act through a diverse array of membrane-bound receptors/second messenger systems and are produced by many cells whose effects are local (paracrine). The classic steroid hormones (sex hormones, glucocorticoids, and mineralocorticoids) are joined by the retinoids, vitamin D, and the thyroid hormones as hormones that bind to nuclear receptors and effect transcription.

Finally, the hierarchical organization of the endocrine system provides opportunity for levels of nested control loops as well as an opportunity to interface with the nervous system. In this hierarchy, activity of many glands is controlled by the pituitary, which in turn is regulated by the hypothalamus.

Tissue-Specific Metabolism

This section summarizes differences in metabolism between major tissues in the body and then reviews the effects of the control systems and interactions between them.

In addition to countless other functions, the liver has the important job of maintaining fuel homeostasis for the other tissues of the body, the needs of which vary considerably. For instance, the heart preferentially oxidizes fatty acids, the brain is dependent on glucose, and skeletal muscle uses a combination of its own glycogen, fat, sugar, and protein. Within the liver, glucose 6-P and acetyl-CoA are metabolic branch points for several interconnecting pathways that determine overall production levels of many key substances. Glucose 6-P has a variety of fates available to it: export to other tissues as glucose, formation of glycogen for energy storage, the synthesis of various lipids, the production of ATP locally (via glycolysis and the citric acid cycle), or the formation of reducing power (NADPH) via the pentose phosphate pathway. Amino acids, meanwhile, are necessary for several biosynthetic pathways, such as being incorporated into proteins or made into sugar for export via gluconeogenesis. Additional amino acids can, through conversion to pyruvate and acetyl CoA, be made into fats, glycogen, or any of the fates described above for glucose 6-P. Fats either received from dietary sources or synthesized within the liver have several important fates: export either as FFAs bound to albumin, as triacylglycerols (TAGs) or cholesterol bound to lipoproteins, or as soluble ketone bodies. Alternatively, fats can be used locally for the production of bile salts or simply stored locally, which in turn permits the storage of several fat-soluble vitamins.

Adipose tissue is of two types: the white form (WAT) and the brown form (BAT). White is by far the predominant form and is found throughout the body, where it serves as insulation and an efficient form of energy storage. Recall that within adipocytes, fat is found in the form of large droplets that literally fill the cell, and the fat is constantly being synthesized during periods of surplus caloric input. During times of energy need, TAGs are hydrolyzed into FFAs, which can then be used by the heart and skeletal muscles for energy. In humans, BAT is most important in early infancy as a means of regulating body temperature. Infants, due to their large surface area to volume ratio, are at particular risk for hypothermia and use BAT for generating body heat, in part because infants are not able to produce the shiver reflex. This takes place through an interesting process whereby oxidation and phosphorylation (ATP formation) are deliberately uncoupled so as to produce heat directly from the oxidation of fats. BAT may be a misnomer as it now appears that it may more closely resemble muscle than ordinary WAT and can serve throughout life as an adaptation to cold climates.

Muscles of all types convert ATP into contractile force in one of the rare cases in which ATP is hydrolyzed directly and the energy is converted to a conformational change. Because cardiac and different skeletal muscle have such different work profiles, the metabolic demands are considerably different. The heart, which must work continuously, utilizes the energy-rich fatty acids to a much greater extent. On the other extreme, vigorously exercising skeletal muscle quickly outstrips the capacity of the blood to supply oxygen or glucose and converts glycogen to lactate through fermentation of glucose. The lactate is sent to the liver, where glucose is regenerated during the oxygen debt phase in the Cori cycle. Muscle fibers not geared for the explosive fast-twitch work rely on a mixed diet, depending on the level of activity. Both cardiac and skeletal muscles can use ketone bodies.

The brain and other nervous tissues are very metabolically "high-maintenance" and require a constant supply of glucose from the blood in order to function. Early symptoms of hypoglycemia (low blood sugar) often include confusion, which can quickly progress to coma, convulsions, and death unless treated. These high-energy needs stem from the dependence of large sodium and potassium gradients, which must be maintained through the Na-K ATPase transporter. Because the brain has minimal glycogen stores and has a barrier (the blood-brain barrier) that prevents fats from being utilized, it is at the mercy of glucose resources supplied by the liver and is one reason why glucose in the blood is so tightly regulated. It can, however, adapt to extended periods of fasting/starvation by using ketone bodies (principally beta hydroxyl butyrate) but switching to this fuel requires an adjustment period of some 48 hours.

Hormonal Regulation of Fuel Metabolism

There are four hormones that are critical to long- and short-term metabolic homeostasis: insulin, epinephrine (and norepinephrine), glucagon, and cortisol. The effects of each vary, and each is tissue specific (for simplicity glucagon is assumed to affect only the liver). Only insulin (growth hormone is not considered here) is anabolic, whereas the effects of the others are considered to be catabolic. Three tissues appear to be most sensitive to the effects of insulin: these are adipose tissue, the liver, and skeletal muscle. Indeed without insulin, blood sugars increase to toxic levels, resulting in widespread metabolic dysfunction and death. In the intact organism, insulin has a number of important effects. It increases the uptake of glucose in muscle, fat, and liver. It increases the synthesis of glycogen in muscle and liver. It increases lipid synthesis within the liver and fat. Because of reciprocal inhibition, it also prevents glycogen breakdown and other catabolic activities that would cause futile cycling. Release of insulin from beta pancreatic cells is driven by glucose levels via ATP formation. When ATP levels are high, ATP-gated K^+ channels close, leading to depolarization and calcium-triggered exocytosis (secretion).

The primary catabolic hormones, epinephrine and glucagon, have opposite effects. In the liver, glucagon stimulates both the breakdown of glycogen and the formation of new glucose (gluconeogenesis). Fatty acids are mobilized and ketones produced. Glycolysis is reduced within the liver in order to spare it for other tissues. In short, this is a concerted effort by the liver to make glucose available for the brain and other tissues. Norepinephrine, the primary sympathetic nervous system neurotransmitter, has similar effects. When blood sugar begins to drop or some other emergency is sensed by the brain, norepinephrine is released by the sympathetic nervous system, which innervates critical tissues directly, as well as innervating the adrenal medulla. The adrenal medulla serves as an extension of the sympathetic nervous system by secreting epinephrine into the blood so that the distress signal is felt throughout the body. Muscle and adipose tissue respond in a catabolic fashion by breaking down FFAs and increasing glycolysis. The liver responds as it does to glucagon by mobilizing energy stores and *decreasing* glycolysis so as to increase glucose production for export. Furthermore, epinephrine stimulates glucagon release while inhibiting insulin secretion, which further coordinates the effects.

Cortisol, the other major stress hormone, has mixed effects. In the short term, most of the effects have positive adaptive value and support maintenance of glucose and glycogen supplies. However, these effects can come at the expense of muscle mass and protein loss in other tissues. Over time, these effects are definitely detrimental, as seen in Cushing's disease, where there is generalized muscle wasting, thinning of skin and bone, and loss of immune function.

Obesity and Regulation of Body Mass

Obesity is a major health concern, as there are significant links between greater BMI (body mass index) and the risk of diseases such as diabetes mellitus, heart disease, and cancer. Diabetes mellitus exists in two forms: type I, which most often appears in childhood or adolescence and is associated with an autoimmune process that destroys the cells in the pancreas responsible for insulin production (beta cells), and type II, which appears later in life and is associated with insulin resistance. Type II is becoming epidemic among some populations and is appearing at increasingly earlier ages. A better understanding of the connection between obesity and diabetes, along with the development of strategies for prevention and better pharmacologic management is now a major priority of medical research.

Some significant progress in such an understanding has been made in the past few decades. Although it might seem that weight control should be as simple as decreasing calorie intake and increasing calorie expenditure, the story turns out to be not that simple. For example, shifts in the overall efficiency of metabolism and the control of appetite are quite complex. One significant finding is that adipose tissue secretes hormones known as adipokines, which have effects on metabolism and eating behavior that are reliably linked in genetic experiments. Although it has long been known that experimental manipulation of the hypothalamus can lead to abnormal feeding behavior, it has been found that an increase in one of these adipokines, leptin, causes both a decrease in appetite and an increase in metabolic expenditures, including expression of the protein thermogenin. Thermogenin makes inner mitochondrial membranes porous, effectively forming a short circuit in oxidative phosphorylation, so that burning of fat produces heat and not ATP (much as it occurs in BAT). Appetite-controlling neuropeptides have been discovered in the hypothalamus and include one that stimulates appetite (neuropeptide Y) and one that depresses appetite (melanocyte stimulating hormone or MSH). The effect of leptin is to reduce appetite by increasing MSH.

However intriguing, it seems unlikely that evolutionary pressures have resulted in robust mechanisms to prevent obesity when most organisms struggle to find and consume enough food, and indeed experiments to decrease body mass by increasing leptin levels have been disappointing. A more likely explanation is that leptin is but one of several interrelated signals that serve to maintain warmer body temperatures when fuel is plentiful and encourages increased exploration and activity. During leaner times, decreased leptin results in lower body temperatures and energy conservation. It makes sense that leptin has strong effects on the hypothalamus. In addition to controlling behavioral responses such as feeding, the hypothalamus exerts a strong influence on specific endocrine processes and the overall metabolic state. It is the thermoregulatory center. It drives the sympathetic nervous system. And by way of the hypothalamic hormones (releasing factors), it controls thyroid hormone, glucocorticoid, and reproductive hormone levels. The response to reduced leptin levels makes perfect economic sense in response to starvation: thyroid hormone (basal metabolism) and reproductive hormone levels drop, whereas both short- and longer-term stress hormones (epinephrine and cortisol) are raised.

AMPK (5′ AMP-activated protein kinase) inhibits fatty acid synthesis and promotes fat oxidation in both muscle and liver. AMPK rises in response to leptin and another adipokine, adiponectin. Adiponectin is another protein hormone with many leptin-like effects. These effects are mediated through AMPK and are catabolic while at the same increasing insulin sensitivity. Other important effects of adiponectin, particularly from a medical perspective, include reducing atherosclerosis. It may be that the effect of leptin, adiponectin, and insulin together act to maintain body mass and adipose levels within narrow windows. In any event, their discovery has led to the development of new pharmacologic strategies in the treatment of diabetes, along with the finding that in humans with diabetes type II, adiponectin levels are reduced.

Other pathways involved in the maintenance of body mass and eating behaviors include ghrelin, which is secreted by the stomach. Ghrelin stimulates appetite when the stomach is empty via receptors in the hypothalamus and growth hormone secretion by the pituitary. It has effects on the appetite opposite to both leptin and insulin. That is, it increases appetite but operates on a short time scale. There is a medical condition associated with high levels of ghrelin that leads to uncontrollable eating, and some bariatric procedures may have a beneficial effect by reducing post prandial levels sooner so that satiety is reached before over-consumption of food. Finally, a group of transcription factors known as PPARs (peroxisome proliferator-activated receptors) have various effects that include control of differentiation by fibroblasts into adipocytes, lipid synthesis, and beta oxidation of fats and production of ketone bodies. Some current medications are agonists of different classes of PPAR, which help to control diabetes and hyperlipidemias. Active research into development of drugs that increase one class of PPARs, PPARδ, may offer a potential breakthrough in control of obesity.

SUMMARY

This chapter began with a review of compounds that are critical to biochemistry. These included amino acids and peptides, followed by proteins. For proteins, the primary and secondary structures were reviewed. Then three-dimensional protein structure was discussed, including tertiary and quaternary structures, enzymes and protein function, and electrophoresis.

The next compounds reviewed were carbohydrates, including monosaccharides, disaccharides, and oligo- and polysaccharides. Finally, the compound section reviewed lipids, including steroids, terpenes, triglycerols and free fatty acids, and phosphorous compounds.

The second part of the chapter reviewed processes important to the study of biochemistry. The principles of bioenergetics were reviewed. Then the chapter covered the various aspects of metabolism, starting with principles of metabolic regulation, including homeostasis, the regulation of glycolysis and glyconeogenesis, the regulation of glycogen metabolism, and metabolic control analysis.

Next the chapter reviewed gluconeogenesis and the pentose pathway. The final topic of review was hormonal regulation and integration of metabolism.

PASSAGE I

Three of the important metalloproteins to which oxygen binds in the human body are myoglobin (Mb), the fetal form of hemoglobin (HbF), and the adult form of hemoglobin (HbA). The percent saturation of oxygen correlates to the partial pressure of oxygen. This is shown in Figure 1.

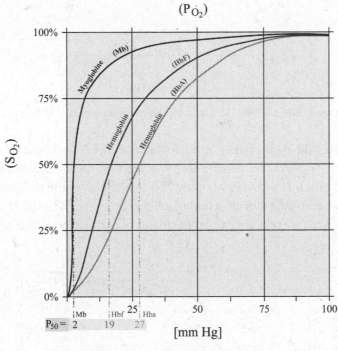

Figure 1.

The oxygen partial pressures corresponding to 50% occupancy by oxygen (P_{50}) are also listed for the three proteins. Myoglobin is monomeric and displays a hyperbolic binding curve avidly binding to oxygen even at very low substrate concentrations, whereas both forms of hemoglobin are tetrameric, consisting of four subunits, each of which can bind to an oxygen.

The binding of oxygen molecules is dependent on occupancy. This is shown by the fact that the dissociation curves for hemoglobin are sigmoidal in shape. This is an example of cooperativity, which is common among oligomeric protein complexes. Cooperativity is an allosteric effect in which events at one region of the molecule influence distant sites in other regions of the molecule. Allosteric modulation can be either positive, as seen here, or negative.

Figure 2 is a family of similarly obtained curves for HbA demonstrating the effects of changing temperature, pH, and DPG (2,3-diphosphoglycerate) concentrations. Increasing H^+ causes a rightward shift of adult hemoglobin, an example of the Bohr effect. Increasing DPG causes a similar reduction in affinity. Neither effect appears to alter cooperativity.

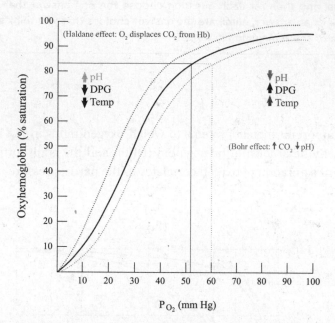

Figure 2. Effect of pH, DPG, and temperature on hemoglobin curves

Figure 3 compares the dissociation of hemoglobin samples obtained from normal individuals, those with the sickle cell trait, and those with the sickle cell disease as part of a preliminary investigation aimed at developing new medicines for the treatment of sickle cell anemia. Sickling, whereby the defective hemoglobin precipitates, damaging cell membranes and making the red blood cells inflexible, begins to occur as blood saturation levels drop below 60%.

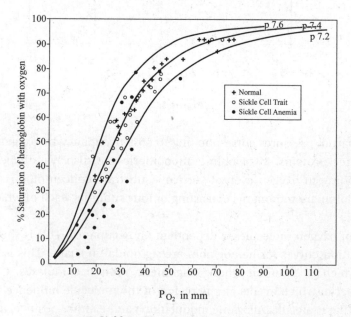

Figure 3. Sickle cell trait and disease versus control

1. Oxygen saturation is routinely measured in patients using pulse oximetry. Oxygen partial pressure required for 80% saturation in a newborn whose hemoglobin is of the HbF type would be closest to:
   (A) 25 mm Hg.
   (B) 35 mm Hg.
   (C) 46 mm Hg.
   (D) 98 mm Hg.

2. The P_{50} (half-occupancy) of the three protein molecules in Figure 1 is affected by all of the following factors EXCEPT:
   (A) positive allosteric modulation.
   (B) negative allosteric modulation.
   (C) partial pressure of oxygen.
   (D) cooperativity.

3. In an effort to mitigate against the effects of desaturation (lowered O_2 levels) in sickle cell anemia, which of the following treatments, assuming that each would be feasible and without negative side effects, would be most effective for a patient whose saturation level was dropping and approaching 60%?
   (A) Lowering the body temperature while reducing levels of DPG
   (B) Decreasing the affinity of sickle cell hemoglobin for oxygen while increasing cooperativity
   (C) Decreasing the H^+ level while transfusing with fetal hemoglobin
   (D) Decreasing pH while increasing DPG levels

4. The Bohr effect is shown in Figure 2 as the rightmost curve is displaced rightward relative to the normal curve (in the middle). This effect is mediated by either CO_2 or H^+, which both bind reversibly at sites other than the heme prosthetic group. The Bohr effect is technically considered a:
   (A) positive allosteric effect.
   (B) negative allosteric effect.
   (C) covalent modification of hemoglobin.
   (D) none of the above.

5. Consider a runner whose leg muscles are producing large amounts of both carbon dioxide and protons. Ventilation is adequate so that the carbon dioxide levels and pH in the lungs are normal. What would be predicted about oxygen delivery to the runner's leg muscles?
   (A) No significant change
   (B) A significant decrease due to the decreased affinity of hemoglobin for oxygen
   (C) A significant increase due to the decreased affinity of hemoglobin for oxygen
   (D) Without additional data, cannot be determined

6. Figure 2 describes both the Bohr effect and the Haldane effect. The relationship between the two can best be described as:
   (A) independent phenomena describing two different processes.
   (B) a competitive relationship between oxygen and carbon dioxide for different sites on the same hemoglobin molecule.
   (C) dual positive allosteric effects in a reciprocal relationship.
   (D) mixed allosteric effects; one is positive while the other is negative.

ANSWER KEY

1. B   **2.** C   **3.** A   **4.** B   **5.** C   **6.** B

ANSWERS EXPLAINED

1. **(B)** Choice B is correct. Finding 80% on the y-axis and following it over to the line representing HbF shows that the x-coordinate is a little to the left of the mark midway between 25 and 50, which would represent 37.5. Even though the value of the x-coordinate is an approximation, it must be larger than 25, so choice A is out. Choice C is out because an x-value of 50 corresponds to a y-value that is clearly above the midpoint between 75 and 100 (87.5). Choice D results from mistakenly finding 80 on the x-axis instead of the y-axis.

2. **(C)** Choice C is correct. Choice A, positive allosteric modulation, includes cooperativity (choice D), which refers to the phenomenon in which the binding of oxygen at one site increases the affinity of another site for oxygen. As a result, the saturation of the molecule for any given partial pressure of oxygen changes, affecting the point at which the molecule is 50% saturated (P_{50}). Choice B refers to an effect in which binding at one site *reduces* the affinity at other sites. However, this still changes P_{50}, even though it does so in the opposite direction from choice A. Partial pressure of oxygen does not change the P_{50} for a curve. It is one of the measures used to determine the P_{50}.

3. **(A)** Choice A is correct. To prevent saturation from dropping below 60% at a given partial pressure of oxygen, the curve must be shifted to the left. Both lowering temperature and reducing DPG shift the curve to the left. Choice A is the only choice for which both of the interventions shift the curve to the left. Choice B is incorrect because decreasing affinity lowers the oxygen level, even though increasing cooperativity increases it. Choice C is incorrect because decreasing the H^+ shifts the curve to the right regardless of the effect of fetal hemoglobin. Choice D is incorrect because both factors shift the curve to the right.

4. **(B)** Choice B is correct because the affinity for oxygen is reduced by CO_2, the allosteric modulator. Choice A is incorrect because it describes a situation in which the binding of the allosteric modulator (CO_2) increases the affinity of hemoglobin for oxygen. Choice C is incorrect because it describes the situation for carbon monoxide and nitric oxide, neither of which is mentioned. Choice D is incorrect because choice B is correct.

5. **(C)** Choice C is correct because, although a negative allosteric effect, the impact on transport is positive as the local changes in exercising muscle facilitates unloading at the tissues. Choice A is incorrect because there is a significant shift in affinity as revealed

by the differences in the three curves. Choice B is incorrect because the amount of oxygen unloaded is clearly greater under conditions causing the Bohr effect. Choice D is incorrect because there is enough information.

6. **(B)** Choice B is correct because binding by either oxygen or CO_2 inhibits the other process. Choice A is incorrect as the two can be viewed as reciprocal effects of the same phenomenon, B. Choices C and D are incorrect because these are both negative allosteric effects.

For online practice, go to
http://barronsbooks.com/tp/mcat

PART 2
Social Sciences

Psychology

6

→ **SENSORY PROCESSING**

→ **COGNITION AND LANGUAGE**

→ **PSYCHO-BIO CONSTRUCTS OF BEHAVIOR**

→ **SOCIAL CONSTRUCTS OF BEHAVIOR**

→ **LEARNING, ATTITUDE, AND BEHAVIOR**

→ **THE NOTION OF SELF AND IDENTITY FORMATION**

→ **ATTITUDES AND BELIEFS THAT AFFECT SOCIAL INTERACTIONS**

→ **ACTIONS AND PROCESSES UNDERLYING SOCIAL INTERACTIONS**

Psychology is one of the components of the Psychological, Sociological, and Biological Foundations of Behavior section of the MCAT. About 60% of the questions in this section will be drawn from psychology. The psychology topics on the test are based on concepts taught in an introductory college-level psychology course.

INTRODUCTION

The study of human psychology begins with the simple sensory perceptions that form the basis of experience and then expands into the realm of cognitive development—attention, cognition, consciousness, memory, and language. Out of this rich realm of cognitive ability comes the personality—the basis of human behavior. Psychology studies both the proper functioning of the human mind and the disorders that affect the psyche. Finally, psychology studies how individual humans interact with each other—both functionally and dysfunctionally—in the context of society.

PERCEPTION AND COGNITION

Perception of the world through the senses is the foundation of human experience. Cognitive abilities—attention, cognition, consciousness, memory, and language—are founded in direct sensory experience.

Sensory Processing

Sensory processing refers to the reception of information through the senses and the organization of the information by the nervous system. **Sensation**, at its most basic level, is the process of receiving information from the environment through the **sensory receptors** of the various **sensory organs**. The sensory organs, including the eyes, ears, nose, tongue, and skin, receive information from the environment. The sensory receptors translate that information into signals that are sent to the nervous system and provide information about the environment.

FOUNDATIONAL CONCEPTS

The basic concepts of sensory threshold, sensory adaptation, and signal detection theory are helpful in understanding sensory processing.

Sensory Threshold

If a stimulus from the environment is too mild, it may not be perceived by the individual. The absolute sensory threshold of a stimulus is the smallest magnitude of a stimulus that an individual accurately recognizes and is able to report 50% of the time. The difference threshold is the smallest detectable difference (the just noticeable difference, or jnd) between a baseline stimulus and a second stimulus.

Webber's law states that the magnitude of the just noticeable difference (jnd) from a baseline stimulus changes depending on how large the baseline stimulus is. Specifically, the jnd is directly proportional to the size of the baseline stimulus. Whereas a person might be able to detect a two-degree temperature change at a low baseline temperature, the same person would only be able to detect a four-degree change from a starting temperature that was twice as high.

Psychophysics

Psychophysics is the study of the interaction between physical stimuli and the sensations perceived by the brain. To put it another way, psychophysics studies the way that the brain recognizes and detects physical stimuli from a person's environment. Webber's signal detection theory (1830s) laid the foundation for the development of psychophysics (1860s). Psychophysics measures the **absolute threshold**, which is defined as the smallest stimulus that an individual is able to identify; **discrimination threshold**, which is the ability to detect a difference between two stimuli; and **scaling**, which is a measure of the strength of the stimuli. An example of absolute threshold is the quietest volume setting on a radio at which a listener can still detect the sound of the radio. The numbers on the radio dial that signify a lower or a higher volume are an example of scaling. The starting and ending points on the dial represent levels at which an individual can identify a change in volume. This scenario exemplifies measurement of the discrimination threshold.

Psychophysics uses the **method of limits**, **method of adjustment**, and **method of constant stimuli** to identify the **difference threshold**—the smallest amount by which a stimulus can vary such that a person can detect the change. When using the method of limits to identify an individual's difference threshold, a scientist presents the subject with stimuli of increasing or decreasing strength to detect when the subject is able to differentiate between the stimuli. The method of adjustment is an interactive method of identifying the difference threshold. When using this strategy, the scientist designs the experiment in a way that allows the test subject to control the strength of the stimuli. The subject increases or decreases the stimuli in order to identify the difference threshold. The interactive component differentiates the method of adjustment from the method of limits. The method of constant stimuli measures an individual's difference threshold by presenting stimuli of various strengths as a way of identifying the upper and lower thresholds of **just noticeable difference**. An example of the method of constant stimuli in a medical care setting is an auditory test. The technician administers a series of beeps at varying volumes and frequencies to determine an individual's hearing scores. The method of constant stimuli is considered a more effective strategy to use than the method of limits or the method of adjustment because it prevents the subject from anticipating the next stimulus and therefore increases the accuracy when measuring thresholds.

Sensory Adaptation

Sensory adaptation refers to the fact that under continued or extreme stimulation, the sensory receptors undergo physiological changes that result in a change in the degree of sensitivity. Typically, sensory adaptation occurs when there is strong stimulation and results in lessened sensitivity. When exposed to loud sounds, the amount of sound transmitted to the inner ear is reduced. In bright light, the pupil contracts to admit less light. After being in cold water for a short period, a person begins to perceive the water as less cold. Sensory adaptation can also occur in the absence of stimulation, typically resulting in increased sensitivity. For example, in the dark, the eye becomes more sensitive to light. An important conclusion from both Webber's law and sensory adaptation is that an individual's experience of sensation is relative.

Signal Detection Theory

Signal detection theory examines the degree to which environmental factors—such as auditory noise, visual distraction, olfactory distraction, or any other sensory interference—make it difficult for a person to correctly identify the presence or absence of a specific **target** stimulus. Consider a person trying to determine whether a particular phone is ringing in a room in which there are many other sounds, such as voices, machine noise, and other phones ringing. The extraneous noise makes it more difficult to correctly identify whether or not the target phone has rung. Signal detection theory uses experimental means to quantify how accurate a person's responses are. There are four possible responses—a **correct rejection** (correctly reporting that the phone did not ring), a **miss** (failing to report that the phone did actually ring), a **hit** (correctly reporting that the phone did ring), or a **false alarm** (reporting that the phone rang when it did not).

THE PRIMARY SENSES

Although many senses contribute to our perception of the world, humans rely primarily on vision and hearing.

Vision

To interpret the raw visual stimuli from the eyes requires complex processing in the visual centers of the brain. Distinct brain cells called **feature detectors** allow the brain to detect and recognize specific kinds of visual stimuli, including shapes and movement. The **parallel processing theory** explains that the brain processes sensory input, including visual stimuli, in multiple ways at one time. For example, a person can register color, shapes, and movement at the same time, rather than as individual tasks, which increases the efficiency of visual processing.

Vision plays a unique role in a person's ability to navigate through the world. It is the basis for physical mobility and contributes to success in interpersonal relationships, commerce, independence, and communication through the use of visual symbols (the ability to read). The loss of vision may have biological, psychological, and social effects on a person. People who lose their vision quickly might experience Charles Bonnet syndrome, in which the brain fills in for missing visual information by providing hallucinatory images. Sleep deprivation can also occur, as changes in daylight no longer regulate the sleep schedule. These biological changes can bring about anxiety or depression. Both congenital and acquired blindness can result in limitations in opportunities for employment, relationships, and social activities and can restrict mobility and independence.

Hearing

Although the ability to hear helps people avoid dangerous situations, the primary importance of hearing in humans is in spoken language, which for most people is the key to communication, social relationships, employment, and entertainment. Helen Keller said that deafness cuts one off from people, whereas blindness cuts one off from things. Unlike loss of vision, an impairment or loss of hearing does not affect mobility or the ability to fit into society visually (hair styles, fashion, ways of moving.) Hearing loss has been described as an invisible handicap.

If severe hearing loss occurs in early childhood, the learning of spoken language can be impaired, along with the development of certain cognitive skills, and the learning of social conventions. These negative effects of hearing loss can be nearly completely avoided if the child is exposed to fluent adult native users of a manual-visual ("sign") language and has regular contact with other children who use the same language. Although people with a serious hearing loss from early childhood may always have limited social opportunities with hearing people, they can have a high-quality social life with other users of their manual-visual language, in much the same way as an immigrant who does not speak English.

There are systems of manual codes that represent elements of a spoken language, such as fingerspelling or signed English, but many researchers believe that such codes lack important aspects of natural language, whether spoken or manual. As in all language learning, it is important that children have role models of adult users who have sophisticated, natural language skills.

When hearing loss occurs in late childhood or adulthood, the primary effect is loss of social connection because of the difficulty of spoken communication and the depression and isolation that might follow. Use of assistive technologies, such as hearing aids and devices for writing messages, can help the person adjust, as can learning to advocate for oneself. This can include being able to explain one's limitations and abilities to others and asking others to adjust their communication behavior, such as speaking more loudly, facing the person with a hearing loss, or writing or gesturing when necessary.

Practice Question

Two individuals are walking down a noisy street together. The individual on the left is speaking. The individual on the right drops behind the individual on the left, circles behind her companion, and repositions herself on the left side. After repositioning herself she says, "There that's better." What can be surmised from this interaction?

Solution: We can surmise that the individual on the right who repositioned herself to the left has unilateral hearing loss in the left ear. She adapted herself to the environment, a noisy street, by repositioning herself so that she could clearly hear the other person speaking.

OTHER SENSES

In addition to vision and hearing, the other senses contributing to perception in humans are the somatosensory system, taste, smell, kinesthetic sense, and vestibular sense.

The **somatosensory system** refers to the senses that register sensations and stimuli of the body. The body has several modalities that register these stimuli, such as touch (physical contact), temperature, proprioception (position and movement of the body, which is conveyed through the activation of neural stimuli in the joints and muscles), pain, tickling, and itching. The body relies upon its **kinesthetic sense** to identify body positioning, proprioception, and movement.

Pain is primarily an aspect of the somatosensory system. It is both a physical and emotional experience. It has been demonstrated that people have a shorter memory for physical pain than for emotional pain. Further, researchers have found that some emotional pain can be relieved in the same way that physical pain is relieved—with an analgesic. In addition, physical pain can often be relieved through the use of a **placebo**, a substance with no actual physical effect but which the patient believes can have an effect. The term **placebo effect** is used to describe the perceived outcomes that occur as a result of suggestions or expectations when a group of test subjects is given a medication that is demonstrated to not have an impact on the individual who takes the medication. The **gate theory of pain** suggests that pain signals can be blocked by other stimuli introduced into the nervous system, such as massage or temperature.

Taste and smell are senses that in modern times are only marginally necessary for survival, mobility, or communication but without which the quality of life can be diminished. People who lose the ability to taste or smell food can experience severe depression.

The body's **vestibular system** is responsible for balance and orientation. It works in conjunction with the body's proprioceptive senses to notify individuals of where they are at spacially in the world and how they are moving. It also helps to maintain their sense of orientation and interaction with gravity. People who experience strong disequilibrium in their vestibular system may experience motion sickness. Those who lose partial functioning of their vestibular system due to a tumor or other illness may require physical therapy to relearn how to process environmental stimuli effectively.

Practice Question

A craniotomy patient has recently been moved from ICU to a recovery room. He requests additional pain medication and is told that he must wait an additional 3 hours before receiving more pain medication. He begins stroking a rough washcloth to distract himself from the pain. What theory of pain management does this represent?

Solution: The patient is exemplifying the gate theory of pain—stimulating his other senses to block the pain signals.

PERCEPTION

Perception is defined as the interpretation of the information that is received from the senses. Information received from the sense organs must be organized, identified, and interpreted by the brain.

A fundamental aspect of perception is **perceptual constancy**. Consider the sound of a siren as it approaches. The actual frequency and loudness of the sound change continually, but the brain interprets the sound as a single constant "object"—a siren. Similarly, if one observes a person riding on a merry-go-round, the angle of the person's profile and the person's position in space change continually relative to the observer's position, but the brain creates the interpretation of a constant object.

In humans, the perception of visual information is more highly developed than perception of other senses. The three most important aspects of visual perception are form, depth, and motion.

The ability to perceive form is an aspect of **visual constancy**, also known as **form constancy**. The perception of form is based on seeing visual outlines as constituting an object. The constancy of the form is maintained regardless of the fact that it may take on a different shape, size, or even be present in a different environment than the last time that it was seen.

Depth perception allows us to determine how far away an object is. There are two types of environmental cues that indicate depth—**monocular** and **binocular**. Monocular clues are those that can be seen with one eye, such as the size of an object, linear perspective, and detail. Binocular clues require both eyes and make use of the slight difference between the image from each eye to interpret depth.

Motion is also perceived through an understanding of environmental clues. To distinguish whether an external object is moving or one's body is moving involves relying upon both visual and vestibular sensory systems. The vestibular system communicates information about balance and body position. The visual system registers movement of an object relative to the background surrounding the object. Visual processing has a bias toward assuming that a background is stationary. As a result, an optical illusion can be created by moving a background and leaving the object stationary.

There are several perspectives on how perceptual processing occurs. **Gestalt theory** suggests that the brain organizes bits of information into larger patterns and that we perceive the world through these patterns. Psychologists distinguish between bottom-up and top-down processing. Bottom-up processing focuses on using small bits of information to develop a larger picture. In top-down processing, the individuals incorporate their experiences, knowledge, and expectations to interpret lower-level bits of information. It is typically assumed that both types of processing occur in perception.

COGNITION

The primary elements of cognition include attention, consciousness, memory, language, intelligence, and problem solving.

Cognition and Language

Sensory information and perception form the basis for the higher-level activities of cognition, including the complex functioning of language. This discussion of cognition includes attention, the processes of cognition, consciousness, memory, and language.

ATTENTION

Attention is a state of focused awareness on a given set of stimuli. **Selective attention** is the process of filtering out extraneous stimuli to direct attention onto the object of interest. **Divided attention** is placing attention onto more than one object simultaneously such that the attention to each object is diminished.

COGNITION

Cognition refers to the ability to take in, process, store, and retrieve information and to think and learn as needed.

Information-Processing Model

The information-processing model is used to explain how human beings receive, process, organize, store, retrieve, and respond to information they receive from their environment. The mind is thought to receive information in much the same way as a computer. **Sensory registers** are the input devices—such as eyes, ears, nose, skin, tongue—that receive the information from the environment. Information from sensory registers is converted to neurological information, which is communicated to the **short-term memory**. In the short-term memory, the information is sorted, processed, discarded, used, or transferred to the **long-term memory**. After information is processed, there may be a response. This response is referred to as the **output**. Output may be a behavior or action. It may be a verbal or a nonverbal response.

Cognitive Development

Cognitive development passes through predictable childhood and adolescent stages, as outlined by Swiss psychologist Jean Piaget. In addition to predictable stages for childhood development, certain changes in cognition can also occur in late adulthood, including both loss of abilities and gaining of new abilities. Cognitive development is influenced by heredity, environment, and culture.

> ### OBJECT PERMANENCE
>
> Peekaboo—a game that adults play with infants—teaches and practices object permanence.

PIAGET'S STAGES OF COGNITIVE DEVELOPMENT. Piaget outlined predictable patterns in early childhood and adolescent cognitive development. He believed that all individuals learn and develop cognitively in a linear manner and must pass through one stage of development (at approximately the same ages) by achieving certain tasks, before moving on to the next stage of development. Piaget described the learning process using the terms schema, adaptation, assimilation, accommodation, and disequilibrium.

A **schema** is a cognitive framework that includes an individual's ability to think and to organize thoughts. **Adaptation** refers to the learning of skills that are necessary for an individual to cognitively assess and process the environment and make the changes necessary for survival. **Assimilation** refers to the processing of new information and integration of it into their existing schema, so that it can be retrieved later when needed. **Accommodation** refers to adjustments to a schema in the face of new information that cannot be assimilated based on the old schema. A situation that cannot be assimilated based on an existing schema results in a state of **disequilibrium**.

Piaget's stages of development are described below.

STAGE 1: THE SENSORIMOTOR PERIOD (APPROXIMATELY 0–2 YEARS). Between birth and 2 years old, the infant learns that it has senses and receives information from those senses that give it information about its world. An infant displays goal-directed behavior, not just automatic responses to stimulus. Finally, an infant develops **object permanence**, the knowledge that an object continues to exist even if it is unseen. Object permanence is important because it allows an individual to begin problem solving through visualization.

STAGE 2: THE PREOPERATIONAL THOUGHT PERIOD (APPROXIMATELY 2-7 YEARS). In this stage, the child is able to think in symbols that represent objects or people when they are not physically present. The child does not yet think logically. Piaget posited that there are three barriers to the development of logical thought that are characteristic of the preoperational stage—egocentrism, centration, and irreversibility. **Egocentrism** is the inability to see a situation from another person's point of view. The child is unaware of the needs, thoughts, and perspectives of others. **Centration** is a child's focus on only one aspect of an object or situation to the exclusion of all others. A frequently used example is when a row of blocks is laid out and then the blocks are moved closer together. A child who is asked whether there are now more, fewer, or the same number of blocks will say there are fewer because the child is focusing only on the length of the row. **Irreversibility** refers to a child's inability to understand that actions, such as moving blocks, can be undone and returned to the original state.

The three developmental tasks that a child must learn in the preoperational stage are classification, seriation, and conservation. **Classification** is the ability to sort, identify, and distinguish items based upon similarities or differences. A child who can separate the toy cars from the toy dinosaurs is able to classify. **Seriation** describes a child's ability to organize objects according to a given characteristic such as size, length, weight, or volume. **Conservation** refers to a child's ability to understand that the amount/size/volume of an object can remain unchanged although it may change in shape or appearance. The classic example of this is pouring a specific amount of liquid from a wider container into a narrower but taller container. The child without conservation believes that the narrower container holds more liquid because it is taller.

STAGE 3: THE PERIOD OF CONCRETE OPERATIONS (APPROXIMATELY 7-11/12 YEARS). During the concrete operational period children begin developing concrete logical thinking. They are capable of more complex thoughts, understand the reversibility of actions, can view a situation from multiple perspectives, and improve their use of symbols, which allows the development of math and language skills and enhances memory. Children at this stage are capable of concrete, but not abstract, thought.

> **PREOPERATIONAL STAGE**
>
> The three developmental tasks of the preoperational stage are classification, seriation, and conservation.

STAGE 4: THE PERIOD OF FORMAL OPERATIONS (APPROXIMATELY 11/12-16 YEARS). During the period of formal operations adolescents develop the capacity for abstract thought, more advanced classification skills, inferential reasoning, and higher-order reasoning. They begin to analyze the world in new ways as their ability to engage in abstract thought expands. They no longer rely on the concrete to understand the world around them.

> **SOCIOCULTURAL DEVELOPMENT**
>
> Vygotsy referred to the adult who guides a child's learning and knowledge as the More Knowledgeable Other.

THE IMPORTANCE OF PIAGET'S THEORIES. Piaget's theories were groundbreaking in the field of cognitive development and changed the way that people understood children. His theories were applied to education, promoting the idea of readiness to learn based upon the developmental stages. Later researchers have suggested that the stages of development may not be as black and white as Piaget suggested. For example, many adults have difficulty completing some of the tasks proposed for the formal operational stage of development.

THE ROLE OF CULTURE, HEREDITY, AND ENVIRONMENT IN COGNITIVE DEVELOPMENT. Culture and environment play an important role in cognitive development. This concept was developed by Lev Vygotsky in his theory of sociocultural development. Vygotsky stated that cognitive development occurs when a child is guided by an adult. The culture in which children are raised influences their development, problem solving, values, and abilities. From a more global perspective, some societies send children to school, and others keep children in close contact with adults for a large part of the day. A society that sends children to school imparts cultural knowledge and contributes to cognitive development in a formalized environment. In a culture in which children are kept in contact with adults for a large part of the day, knowledge is transmitted in a less formal way, through learning from elders and absorbing culturally relevant knowledge and skills through contact with the adults.

The role of heredity vis-à-vis environment in cognitive development has long been debated. Studies of twins show that genetics account for about half of an individual's cognitive development.

COGNITIVE CHANGES IN LATE ADULTHOOD. After the age of 60, people begin to experience diminished ability to process information in the following domains: verbal meaning, spatial orientation, inductive reasoning, number ability, and word fluency. In addition, they typically develop a decline in sensory acuity, with the result that an input must be stronger to be noticed.

Memory also declines with age. This is true for both short-term and long-term memory. Short-term memory holds information that is being consciously used for integrative reasoning, calculations, or inferential thought. In a healthy person, information can be held in short-term memory for 20 to 30 seconds. Declines in short-term memory can result in information being lost from short-term memory more quickly, a reduction in the amount of information that can be held, and a reduction in the efficiency of processing. People with short-term memory deficiency might easily forget what the immediate task was that they were trying to do. Long-term memory can hold information indefinitely and is the storehouse of a lifetime of memories. With long-term memory loss it is more difficult to recall details from the past.

There are four generalizations that researchers have made about memory and cognition as it relates to aging. First, mental processes slow with age. Second, the elderly demonstrate declines in memory. Third, the elderly are less likely to use memory strategies and techniques to support an increased level of functioning. Often they do not see their declines as impairments. Finally, memory problems in the golden years often do not have as negative an impact on quality of life as many people fear.

Some types of memory do not decline with age. Procedural memory—how to do things—does not typically decline, nor does the capacity to remember emotional events. Some types of memory, including semantic knowledge (such as vocabulary) continue to improve.

Biological Factors that Affect Cognition

Cognitive development in a child is affected by biological factors such as the level of functioning of the senses, intelligence, genetics, nutrition, environmental toxins, injury, and maturation of the nervous system in general. Because sensation is the foundation of cognition, if the primary sense organs do not function in a healthy way, as in impaired vision or hearing, cognitive development may be slowed or impaired. General intelligence has a positive correlation to cognitive development. Cognitive development is affected by the level of neurological and motor maturation. Children who are below the norms in these areas may also show delays in cognitive development. Pathological physical conditions or injuries can potentially affect cognition if they result in damage to the brain.

Genetic factors that influence cognitive development include chromosomal abnormalities, such as Down's syndrome (an extra copy of chromosome 23) and single gene mutations, such as in phenylketonuria. Cognitive disorders such as autism, dementia, attention deficit disorder (ADD), and dyslexia are strongly influenced by both genetic and environmental factors.

Poor nutrition can disrupt cognitive development. For example, iodine deficiency is one of the main causes of preventable intellectual disability in the world and can reduce IQ by 10 to 15 points. Deficiencies of micronutrients have been implicated in differences in intelligence among different populations.

Environmental toxins, such as lead, impair cognitive development. Drugs taken during pregnancy or while breastfeeding can harm neurological development. Alcohol, when present in the blood during pregnancy, can cause fetal alcohol syndrome, which includes reduced IQ and other physiological abnormalities.

Problem Solving and Decision Making

Problem solving refers to the mental processes used to identify, analyze, and solve a problem. The problem-solving process requires identifying that there is a problem, fitting the problem into a conceptual framework (including labeling and describing it), identifying existing knowledge that is relevant to the problem, and understanding the various aspects of the problem.

The methods by which problems are solved involve a combination of learned tools and novel insight, or intuition. On one extreme, a problem might be suddenly solved by an unexpected insight. Insight might happen because the current problem is similar to a previous one but the connection is so remote that the process is unconscious. A **trial-and-error approach** uses learned strategies but incorporates intuitive insights into how to apply the strategies in novel ways for the current problem. At the other extreme, a mechanical, problem-solving **algorithm** can be applied. An algorithm is a specific set of steps that can be depended on to lead to a successful result. Using a recipe is an example of following an algorithm. An algorithm involves virtually no novelty or insight.

OBSTACLES TO PROBLEM SOLVING. Problem solving can fail through applying a valid strategy incorrectly or through applying an invalid or ineffective strategy. Even a valid problem-solving strategy can fail if it incorrectly assumes that a current problem is similar to a previous one. Some problem-solving methods, such as applying an algorithm, might result in a solution but in a way that is less efficient than another method.

A **heuristic** is similar to an algorithm in that it involves following a specific procedure but a heuristic is often an overly simplified general rule of thumb. If it works, it might save time, but it is too general to work frequently. Yelling "Quiet!" whenever your dog barks is an example of a heuristic. It runs the danger of failing to solve the real problem if the dog needs to go outside or is warning you about an intruder or a fire.

People use many different types of heuristics for problem solving. Examples include availability, representative, anchoring and adjustment, affect, cognitive laziness, attribute substitution, and fast and frugal.

The **availability heuristic** occurs when an individual overestimates the likelihood that an event will occur based on how quickly and easily an idea or association can be recalled. An example is a college student's fear of dying in a campus shooting. The likelihood of that event occurring is much less than the ease with which the idea is recalled.

A **representative heuristic** attempts to predict something about an unknown situation based on information about a situation that is assumed to be similar. The problem with this is that one similarity between two situations does not necessarily mean that the situations are similar in all ways. One example is assuming that all college students are intelligent because a person knows several college students who are intelligent. Another example is assuming that it will not rain tomorrow because it has already rained for three days or assuming that it will rain tomorrow for that same reason. Both are unwarranted assumptions about an unknown based on information assumed to be representative.

The **anchoring and adjustment heuristic** is used to create an estimate from the foundation of an already-known quantity. This path of reasoning can lead to inaccurate estimates. Consider the sales manager who is asked to create a sales projection for the upcoming year based upon the prior year's sales. If the sales manager is able to create an accurate estimate of sales growth, he or she will produce an accurate projection. However, if the sales manager is not attentive to market indicators that are warning of an economic downturn, the use of anchoring and adjustment could lead to an inaccurate projection.

Emotions are used when applying the **affect heuristic** to a decision-making process. *Affect* refers to the emotions that are triggered by the words used in a particular description. An individual who responds to the emotionally charged words in an advertisement is displaying the affect heuristic in his or her decision making. People would rather eat the "freshest, juiciest hamburger in town" than a "ground beef patty" even though the products are the same.

Cognitive laziness suggests that an individual will use a variety of techniques to reduce the effort involved in the decision-making process. **Attribute substitution** occurs when an individual intuitively and unconsciously substitutes a heuristic attribute to simplify the decision-making process.

False assumptions or **irrelevant information** can sabotage problem solving. When a problem is complex, there is a tendency to focus on one or two aspects of the problem, but these aspects may be irrelevant.

Certain nonrational processes can interfere with effective problem solving. Although much of effective problem solving occurs outside of rational thought—such as in intuition—factors that block rational thought can lead to ineffective solutions. Problem solving is frequently influenced by **biases**. Biases are automatic preferences for a specific action. For example, a certain person, when forced to decide between two equally appealing choices on a menu, might always choose the cheaper of the two. Such a bias is often unconscious and may distort problem solving by overriding rational input. Similarly, if the current problem causes a strong emotional reaction, or if the anticipation of the solution causes a strong emotional reaction, the emotions can override information that the rational mind tries to provide.

Certain rigid attitudes can obstruct effective problem solving. In some people, a fixed mental set results in relying on the same strategies for any problem. **Functional fixedness** is a similar hindrance to problem solving, in which a person can only conceive of using an object in one "standard" way and is unable to think flexibly about other ways that the object can be used to solve the problem. **Belief perseverance** is the refusal to abandon a belief in the face of evidence against it. With belief perseverance people are unreasonably overconfident in their beliefs.

A gardener is attempting to plant seeds in a garden but is unable to find the garden shovel. Instead, the gardener goes to the kitchen, takes a large spoon, returns to the garden, and uses the spoon to dig the holes needed to plant the seeds. The gardener demonstrates cognitive flexibility, which is the opposite of which problem-solving obstacle?

(A) Belief perseverance

(B) Biases

(C) Functional fixedness

(D) False assumptions

(C) The gardener did not fall victim to functional fixedness. Although a spoon is traditionally used to serve food, the gardener found an alternative use for that object as a garden shovel, which demonstrates cognitive flexibility.

PROBLEM-SOLVING THEORIES. Various branches of psychology view problem solving from their own perspectives. Cognitive theorists examine problems using the **problem space theory**. The problem space is considered to be the current state of affairs, the desired state of affairs, and all possible options in between that could lead toward achieving the desired state of affairs. Behaviorists observe that people use **the law of effect**, meaning that they engage in problem solving after a period of trial and error, having found what does and does not work, and that people repeat that behavior even in situations where it may not be as useful. The gestalt approach to problem solving views problem solving as requiring people to restructure the way they think of the problem, moving toward a productive process that will produce a flash of insight.

Intelligence

Intelligence is influenced by both heredity and the environment. Intelligence can be defined as the ability to learn from experience, to be flexible/adaptable in new situations, to grasp and interpret new or absent concepts, and to use that understanding to shape one's surroundings. The degree and types of intelligence vary widely among human beings.

THEORIES OF INTELLIGENCE. There are two theoretical approaches to understanding intelligence—the theories of general intelligence and multiple intelligences. The **theory of general intelligence** posits that individuals have an overall intelligence that pervades their functioning in all domains. In other words, a person who is smart will be smart in all areas. In theory, the person would be equally gifted in both math and English. Researchers validated this theory when they found that individuals who score high in one domain of functioning are more likely to score high across several domains of functioning. One criticism of the theory of general intelligence is that it does not account for human diversity.

The theory of **multiple intelligences** suggests that a person may have one or several areas in which he or she demonstrates a high level of functioning but this does not necessarily predict a high level of functioning in other domains. In other words, a person can demonstrate high intelligence in language but struggle with mathematical reasoning skills.

MULTIPLE DEFINITIONS OF INTELLIGENCE. Intelligence can be defined as the ability to learn from experience, be flexible/adaptable in new situations, grasp and interpret new or abstract concepts, and use that understanding to shape one's surroundings. Historically, certain aspects of intelligence have been measured and evaluated through an intellectual quotient test (IQ test). Such tests rely on a relatively narrow definition of what constitutes intelligence.

> ### MULTIPLE INTELLIGENCES
>
> Intelligence is not limited to verbal or mathematical skills. Intelligence can be based on musical ability, visual/spatial skill, language, logic/math, physical skills, interpersonal skills, intrapersonal skills, naturalistic intelligence, existential intelligence, and moral sense.

Howard Gardner proposed the theory of multiple intelligences. He initially identified eight sensory modalities: musical/rhythmic, visual/spatial, linguistic, logical/mathematical, bodily/kinesthetic, interpersonal, intrapersonal, and naturalistic. He later added existential modalities. Gardner posited that each person has a certain level of intelligence (mastery) within each domain, and the level of the person's intelligence might vary significantly from domain to domain. For example, an individual might have high bodily/kinesthetic intelligence, such as an Olympic athlete, while exhibiting only average intelligence in other areas, such as logical/mathematical reasoning or linguistic performance. The person might even have below average intelligence in some domains.

L. L. Thurstone developed the theory of primary mental abilities, which is another multiple intelligences theory. In contrast to Gardner, Thurstone divided intelligences into the following categories: word fluency, spacial reasoning, verbal comprehension, perceptual speed, numerical ability, inductive reasoning, and memory.

Another theorist, Robert Sternberg, proposed the **triarchic theory of intelligence**. He hypothesized that intelligence is a characteristic that leads to real-world success and has three underlying aspects that contribute to all applications of intelligence: analytical/problem-solving intelligence, creative intelligence, and practical intelligence. He was interested in how people integrate these three intelligences in practical situations. He noted that although different cultures may define intelligence in distinct ways, intelligence is based on these three components regardless of culture.

RELATIVE INFLUENCE OF HEREDITY AND ENVIRONMENT ON INTELLIGENCE. The impact of heredity on intelligence can be shown through genetic studies and by looking at factors such as parental IQ and studies of twins. Genetic studies have shown what are believed to be genetic markers for intelligence on three different chromosomes. Studies on parental IQ have demonstrated that biological parents have a stronger influence on IQ than adoptive parents, implying a strong genetic component. Finally, identical twins are closer in IQ than are fraternal twins, again showing the strong genetic component of intelligence, although there is also evidence that environment has a small impact on IQ of identical twins.

The environmental factors that impact intelligence are family of origin, education, economics, race, and gender. Family efforts to expand the skills and talents of a child do increase the child's IQ score, as does providing an academically enriched environment. When parents engage in more and higher-quality communication with a child, especially in the first three years of life, IQ increases. Outside of the family itself, high-quality early education opportunities can increase intelligence.

A family's economic situation correlates to IQ, as well, in part because families with a secure economic base may be more able to provide an enriched environment. Because economic status also correlates with other factors, such as education level and parental IQ, it is difficult to isolate the contribution of economic status alone. Similarly, although there are correlations between ethnicity and scores on IQ tests, the correlations are distorted by other issues, such as educational opportunities, family background, and expectations of failure. In fact, some studies have shown that after events that boost ethnic pride, people perform better on IQ tests. Finally, some cultures foster intelligences that may not be measured by standard IQ tests, such as social compatibility, narrative story telling, or physical dexterity. In addition, the very act of taking a time-based IQ test by oneself is a violation of cultures that value cooperative group work and underplaying one's unique qualities.

MEASURING INTELLIGENCE

Intelligence is typically measured as an intelligence quotient (IQ) by means of an IQ test. A score below 70 indicates an intellectual disability or an intellectual developmental disorder. A score above 130 indicates intellectual giftedness.

VARIATIONS IN INTELLECTUAL ABILITY. There is wide variation among human beings in both types of intelligences and general intelligence as measured by an IQ test. This variation ranges from very low intelligence to very high intelligence.

Intellectual disability (formerly known as mental retardation) or intellectual developmental disorder is the term currently used in the Diagnostic Statistical Manual (DSM-5). It is characterized by deficits in general mental abilities that hinder adaptive functioning in one or more domains, an onset during the developmental period, and an IQ score lower than 70 points. Generally speaking, the lower the IQ score, the greater the impairment in functioning.

On the opposite end of the spectrum, those individuals scoring above 130 on the IQ test are characterized as gifted. They have advanced ability in one or more areas. The specific qualities of gifted people vary widely but may include those shown below.

SOME EXPRESSIONS OF GIFTEDNESS

Varied interests and strong curiosity

Highly developed language skills

Strong ability to process and integrate information

Ability to recognize complex relationships

Creative problem-solving abilities

Active imagination

Inclination to question authority; nonconformity

Emotional sensitivity

There are hereditary and environmental causes for intellectual disabilities and intellectual giftedness. Familial patterns for intellectual impairment have been found, but no direct cause has been identified at this point. A gene has been identified that is thought to contribute to the thickness of the frontal cortex, which is one influence on intelligence. There are many environmental factors that can impair intelligence, especially during pregnancy or early childhood. One example is fetal alcohol syndrome, caused by the presence of alcohol in the womb environment during critical periods of fetal development.

CONSCIOUSNESS

Consciousness refers to the degree of awareness of what is taking place in the environment, both internal and external.

States of Consciousness

There are various states of consciousness, including alertness, sleep, and meditative or hypnotic states.

ALERTNESS. The individual's **alertness** or awareness of their surroundings is an ever-changing state that can be measured using the Glasgow scale or another similar measure. Alertness can also be measured biologically by measuring neural responsiveness to stimuli in the brain.

SLEEP. Sleep is a state of consciousness that is altered from waking consciousness in that there is a reduction in the perception of sensory information, a reduction of muscle tension, and a disengagement of voluntary muscle movement.

There are five stages of sleep. (See Table 6.1.) Stages 1 to 4 constitute the **non-REM** (non-Rapid Eye Movement) phase of sleep through which a person passes during the first hour of sleep. Stage 5 is the REM phase of sleep. The stages of sleep can be distinguished by brain wave measurements on an EEG machine. Stage 1 is referred to as drowsiness, in which the EEG waves move lower and the cortical brain waves become more frequent. In stage 2, or light sleep, the EEG waves continue to become slower and sleep spindles begin. Sleep spindles are random surges of brain activity that indicate the individual has fallen asleep. They last only a few seconds at a time. During stage 3, moderate to deep sleep, the amplitude of low-frequency brain waves continues to rise while there is a decrease in the frequency of sleep spindles. Stage 4 is the deepest level of sleep, in which the individual produces delta brain waves. These brain waves are low frequency and high amplitude. In stage 5, the individual enters REM sleep and the brain registers waves similar to those of a person who appears to be awake. After a short period of REM sleep, the individual returns to cycle back through stages 2–5 of sleep again. The first sleep cycle, consisting of stages 1–5, lasts between 70 and 100 minutes. Following cycles are even longer because the REM stage lasts longer with each cycle.

Table 6.1 Stages of Sleep

Stages of Sleep	Characteristics	Brain Wave Activity
Stage 1	Drowsiness	Brain waves move lower. Cortical brain waves are more frequent.
Stage 2	Light sleep	Brain waves are slower. Sleep spindles begin.
Stage 3	Moderate to deep sleep	Amplitude of low-frequency brain waves rises. Sleep spindles decrease.
Stage 4	Deepest sleep	Low-frequency, high-amplitude delta brain waves
Stage 5	REM—rapid eye movement	Brain waves resemble a state of consciousness.

Dreams generally occur during the REM stage of sleep. They can also occur during other phases of sleep but are most often remembered during REM. If someone wakes up during REM, it is likely that the person will remember any dreams clearly and vividly.

Sleep is regulated by a number of biological and natural processes that occur in approximately 24-hour cycles (**circadian rhythm**). This regulation represents the interaction between external influences, such as sunlight, and internal events, such as melatonin production. Certain aspects of modern life, including artificial light, stress, and lack of physical activity can disrupt the circadian rhythms and interfere with sleep regulation.

More than 70 million Americans suffer from insomnia, a reflection of how easily the natural sleep cycle can be disturbed. In addition to factors mentioned above, many millions of people suffer from sleep apnea, in which breathing stops momentarily, sometimes for up to a minute. The resulting oxygen deprivation wakes the sleeper.

Another common sleep disorder is narcolepsy. People with this disorder appear to fall asleep in the middle of the day without warning. Narcolepsy is related to an inadequate supply of the neurotransmitter orexin, which helps people maintain states of wakefulness and sleep. Finally, people whose muscles do not become paralyzed during REM sleep are said to have REM behavior disorder and are able to walk, hit, kick, or punch during REM sleep.

MEDITATION AND HYPNOSIS. Hypnosis is a state of consciousness characterized by a reduced perception of environmental stimuli along with a heightened focus of attention. At the same time, there is an increased susceptibility to suggestion, although hypnotized people cannot be made to perform actions that they would refuse to do in normal consciousness. Hypnosis can be either self-induced or induced by another person. Hypnosis has a number of therapeutic applications, including the reduction of pain during medical procedures and access to past memories.

Meditation is another altered state of consciousness. It typically involves being physically still and yet alert. The meditator may focus on a sound, image, or sensation or may be openly alert to internal and external stimuli. Meditation has a number of generally positive effects on physiological processes. It is used to manage stress, lower blood pressure, decrease anxiety, support substance abusers in managing the triggers to their abuse, and promote improved outcomes for cancer patients. It has been shown to lead to increased intelligence.

Drugs that Alter Consciousness

There are five common classifications of drugs that alter consciousness—stimulants, depressants, narcotics, hallucinogens, and marijuana.

Stimulants are drugs that increase energy and alertness by working on either the release or reuptake of dopamine in the brain. Stimulants include amphetamines, cocaine, Ritalin (methylphenidate), caffeine, and nicotine. Ritalin is used as a treatment for people with attention deficit hyperactivity disorder (ADHD) to help them focus their attention. Some negative consequences associated with the use of stimulants include sleeplessness, increase in blood pressure, psychosis, heart problems, behavioral changes (agitation, aggression, stealing/robbery to pay for drugs), and death.

The most common depressants are alcohol and benzodiazepines. Both of these drugs work on the nervous system by increasing the ability of GABA to attach to its receptor. GABA is a neurotransmitter that inhibits neural activity. Depressants initially provide a person with a feeling of relaxation, may reduce their inhibitions or anxiety, or act as a sleep aide. Depressants may also impair memory or judgment if taken in excess. People may quickly form a dependence upon benzodiazepines and when taken with other medications (opiates) or alcohol, an accidental overdose can easily occur.

Hallucinogens operate on the nervous system in a variety of unique ways. LSD produces hallucinations by working on serotonin receptors. People taking LSD have the experience of mood swings or intensified emotions. They may become delusional or hallucinate. The experience usually lasts 12 hours. However, they may have flashbacks afterward for a few days or up to a year. Panic attacks are not uncommon. PCP (Phencyclidine) or "angel dust" can cause hallucinations, paranoia, delusions, high anxiety, and agitation. The effect can last four to six hours and repeated use can result in dependence. PCP was developed in the 1950s as an anesthetic. It works on the nervous system by inhibiting a glutamate receptor.

MDMA, also known as Ecstasy, X, or Molly straddles two drug categories—those of hallucinogens and stimulants. It works on the brain by stimulating the neurons that release serotonin. This in turn stimulates the release of oxytocin and vasopressin, hormones that regulate social behaviors involved in love, sex, trust, and empathy.

Cannabis, or marijuana, is typically classified in a category by itself for a number of reasons. It does not have hallucinogenic or stimulant properties. Although it decreases pain, it is different from a narcotic or depressant. It activates negative feedback receptors of excitatory and inhibitory neurotransmitters. Marijuana has been found to cause distorted perceptions, impaired concentration, difficulty thinking and problem solving, and difficulty with learning and memory. In heavy users, the effects of marijuana can last for weeks after consumption. For those with a predisposition to thought disorders, marijuana can instigate or worsen a psychotic episode.

Narcotics such as morphine, heroin, and other opiates activate the endorphin synapses. When heroin reenters the body, the body converts it to morphine. The morphine is absorbed by the body's opioid receptors. These are located throughout the body and are responsible for a variety of body functions. Some receptors are located in the brainstem, which houses a number of autonomic body functions. Heroin overdoses have been known to interfere with or stop the autonomic body functioning regulated by the brainstem, such as breathing, body temperature regulation, blood pressure, arousal, and respiration.

Drugs are used and abused because they target the neurotransmitters and endorphins in the body that release pleasurable sensations. Often serotonin or dopamine is involved, and the drug produces a euphoric feeling. There is a chain of reactions in the brain (**reward pathway**) that reinforces certain behaviors (such as taking a drug) by increasing the release of dopamine. The more a drug is taken, the stronger the reinforcing power of the reward pathway.

The reward pathway is an old structure evolutionarily. Stimulation by drugs is much stronger than the natural stimulation that the reward pathway is evolutionarily designed to reinforce, such as food. Therefore, the reinforcement of drugs by the reward pathway is powerful and results in a dependence that is very difficult to overcome.

MEMORY

Memory involves the encoding and storage of information so that it can be retrieved in the future. Memory is intimately connected with the learning process. Impairments to memory, including damage and decline, may significantly impact quality of life, depending on their severity.

Encoding

Encoding is the process by which information from sensory input is converted into stored memory. The thalamus region of the brain combines related sensory inputs to form a unified experience. The hippocampus processes this information and determines whether the information will be encoded into long-term memory. Encoding can take place with varying degrees of depth. A memory that is deeply encoded is easier to recall than one that is less deeply encoded. The three primary types of information that are encoded are visual (picture), acoustic (sound), and semantic (meaning).

The more meaningful or important an experience is deemed by the individual, the easier it is to encode. The more deeply a stimulus is encoded, the easier it is to retrieve later. Culture has an impact on what people choose to encode as well. The items that reflect the values of the culture are more likely to be encoded. Emotion intensifies encoding. There is a biological basis for the intensified effect, as adrenal hormones (cortisol and epinephrine) stimulate the area of the brain responsible for memory storage.

In a list of items, the first items (the **primacy effect**) and last items (the **recency effect**) are encoded more deeply than the other items. Other factors that can contribute to enhancing memory are repetition, distinctiveness, association with moderate emotion, and words or facts that were learned early in life. Factors that impair memory include distractions, learning things later in life, or pairing with an arousing stimuli.

Storage

Memory storage includes **sensory memory**, **short-term memory**, **working memory**, and **long-term memory**. Sensory memory is a very brief but highly complex impression of a particular sense. Sensory memory may last less than a second and if not transferred to short-term memory in that time, it is lost. Iconic, echoic, and haptic sensory memory refer to visual, auditory, and tactile sensations, respectively. Sensory memory is not subject to conscious control.

Short-term memory can hold information for a matter of seconds. Through the conscious repetition of information (**rehearsal**) short-term memory can be extended by 10–20 seconds. Working memory is distinguished from short-term memory in that working memory processes and organizes information, whereas short-term memory stores information.

Long-term memory holds information for an indefinite period of time. The contents of long-term memory can be divided into **explicit** and **implicit memory**. Explicit memory involves the conscious memory of the details of one's life. Implicit memory involves memory of how to perform certain tasks, such as playing tennis or singing a song, and typically cannot be recalled consciously.

INTERFERENCE THEORY OF MEMORY. The interference theory of memory teaches that forgetting occurs because something that has been learned is interfering with memory recall. In **retroactive interference**, new information hinders the recall of old information. In contrast, **proactive interference** occurs when one has difficulty retaining new information because of existing information and/or memories.

STORAGE THEORY. Information can be viewed as existing in a **semantic network**, or a web of facts that are interrelated. Items that are more closely related are closer together in the network. The theory of **spreading activation** states that the working memory is able to retrieve information faster when the semantic networks of the brain have already been activated by providing the individual with relevant contextual information. For example, a person will be able to describe a teacher more quickly if he or she has been reminded that the teacher wears black glasses and taught Introductory Psychology.

This is an example of **priming**. Priming occurs in implicit memory storage when one stimulus is paired with another. It increases or improves memory recall through association.

TEST QUESTION

A calculus professor encourages the students in a class to work through a math problem "in their head." What type of memory do the students use to solve the math problem?

(A) Explicit memory

(B) Short-term memory

(C) Semantic memory

(D) Working memory

(D) The students must use working memory to process and organize information to solve the problem.

ENCODING STRATEGIES. Encoding strategies can be used to improve memory storage and facilitate memory retrieval. Examples of encoding strategies include mnemonics, chunking, self-reference, state-dependent learning, and encoding specificity.

Mnemonics are an organizational approach that assist in recall. An example is "**P**lease **E**xcuse **M**y **D**ear **A**unt **S**ally" (**PEMDAS**), which helps students remember the order of mathematical operations: **P**arenthesis, **E**xponents, **M**ultiplication, **D**ivision, **A**ddition, **S**ubtraction.

Chunking, in contrast, is used to group a long series of unrelated information into shorter and more meaningful chunks or bits to increase memory recall. It is easier to remember a phone number as 867 and 5309 than to remember the chain 8-6-7-5-3-0-9.

Self-reference refers to the fact that information is encoded differently and is easier to recall when it is related to the individual.

State-dependent learning refers to the individual's state of consciousness. It suggests that an individual will remember the information most easily if he or she is in the same state of consciousness as when the memory was encoded.

In contrast to state-dependent learning, **encoding specificity** suggests that emotional cues guide memory retrieval. Memories can be accessed if external emotional cues are the same as at the time the memory was stored.

Retrieval

Retrieval is the final stage of the memory process. It is the act of recovering a memory from storage.

TYPES OF RETRIEVAL. There are three distinct types of retrieval—recall, recognition, and relearning. **Recall** involves retrieving a memory with minimal help of associative clues or reminders. An example of a question that might require recall is "Name three people in your second grade class." **Recognition** involves identifying the correct response to a memory task out of a list of possible responses. An example might be "Which of these people was in your second grade class—Andy, Rosa, or Celia?" **Relearning** is the process of rehearsing or repeating information from a memory so that it becomes easier to retrieve in the future. Looking at a yearbook from second grade and matching the faces to the names would involve relearning. Relearning can also occur when the same question is repeated multiple times.

RETRIEVAL CUES. A stimulus is encoded by linking it to associations at the time of learning. These associations are called **retrieval cues**. A retrieval cue is an associated category that is imprinted with the memory that makes retrieval easier if it is offered when recall is desired. Researchers Endel Tulving and Donald M. Thomson hypothesized that the more associations formed at the time of encoding, the easier the retrieval later ("Encoding Specificity and Retrieval Processes in Episodic Memory," in *Psychological Review,* 1973, Vol. 80, No. 5). An example of the use of retrieval cues is "What was the name of that little red-haired boy who was in your second-grade class? He got sick at your birthday party." The addition of the visual cues ("little," "red-haired") and contextual cues ("boy," "got sick at party") makes use of associations that make it much easier to recall the name "Andy" than simply asking for the name of someone who was in the same second-grade class.

TEST QUESTION

An elementary school teacher begins a science lesson on weather by reminding the students of a cold and rainy day in order to activate prior knowledge in the students. He describes the thunder and lightning of a particular day in the previous month to speed up their memory retrieval of the prior knowledge. Which memory storage theory is the teacher applying to the lesson?

(A) Spreading activation

(B) Recognition

(C) Retrieval cues

(D) Rehearsal

(A) Spreading activation states that working memory is able to retrieve information more quickly when provided with contextual cues.

THE ROLE OF EMOTION IN MEMORY RETRIEVAL. When strong emotion is associated with the formation of a memory, the memory is encoded either in a way that makes it easily retrievable or in a way that prevents it from being retrieved. In the first case, a **flashbulb memory** is imprinted on the mind. A flashbulb memory is a bright, striking memory that does not fade. The death of a beloved public figure, especially if sudden, creates flashbulb memories for many people, who years later remember many details, such as where they were when they heard the news, who told them, what they were doing, and how they felt about it.

Repression is the defense mechanism employed by the mind to protect itself from a memory that is overwhelmingly painful. With repression that memory is blocked from conscious awareness. This occurs most often with traumatic events and is a symptom of post-traumatic stress disorder.

A man is in a serious car accident and is taken to the hospital. When he regains consciousness, the authorities try to question him to develop an understanding of how the crash occurred. He states that he is unable to answer their questions because he does not remember the accident. Why is he unable to remember the accident?

Solution: The man is demonstrating repression, which is a common defense mechanism employed by the brain to protect the individual from the trauma of a painful memory.

Forgetting

Several factors result in "forgetting" information. These include natural aging processes, memory dysfunctions, such as dementia, and inherent limitations in the storage and retrieval of memory.

AGING. Forgetfulness is an expected part of the **aging process**. After the age of 65, people may have more difficulty binding information in memory and making and retrieving associations. They may also have deficiencies in processing new memories. Memories that are not usually affected by aging include procedural memories (problem solving or "how to" knowledge), semantic knowledge (vocabulary), and emotionally imprinted memories.

MEMORY DYSFUNCTIONS. Memory dysfunction refers to pathological conditions that fall under the category of dementia. The clinical definition of dementia is memory loss that is severe enough to impair a patient's functioning. Two major types of dementia are **Korsakoff's syndrome** and **Alzheimer's disease**.

   Korsakoff's syndrome occurs as a result of a thiamine deficiency. Thiamine deficiencies occur infrequently and are generally the result of alcoholism, dialysis, hyperemesis gravidarum, or a post-surgery vitamin deficiency. Patients with dialysis may develop Korsakoff's syndrome because their blood is removed from their body for cleaning and the thiamine may be removed from the blood at that time. If it is not replaced by diet or a vitamin supplement, the patient is at risk. For pregnant women, hyperemesis gravidarum is a serious medical condition in which the mother is not able to keep down food or water. If this continues for an extended period of time, the mother may develop a thiamine deficiency. Finally, in some cases, patients are not able to eat after they have had surgery, and this may lead to a thiamine deficiency and Korsakoff's syndrome. With Korsakoff's syndrome, patients may show symptoms of chronic memory loss, difficulty learning new things, poor short-term memory, and gaps in long-term memory. They may appear to function well in some situations but then fail to remember what happened a few minutes ago. To compensate for this, the mind fills in the gaps with made-up information (**confabulations**). The confabulations are not lies but rather coping mechanisms of the brain, and the individual believes that the events occurred.

   Alzheimer's disease is different than Korsakoff's in etiology and symptomology. Alzheimer's disease is believed to be the result of a breakdown in the ability of the brain to transmit messages across neurons. Plaques and tangles have been indicated as causing some of the brain damage that contributes to Alzheimer's disease, although their exact role in the disease is not fully understood at this time. Plaques are deposits of beta-amyloid that accrue in the spaces among the nerve cells. Tangles are gnarled fibers made of tau protein that deposit on the inside of the nerve cell. It is suspected that plaques and tangles block communication of the nerve cells.

Individuals with Alzheimer's disease may experience many types of changes and cognitive losses that contribute to their symptomology. Personality changes are not uncommon. Some patients develop aggressive and occasionally violent behaviors after a lifetime of gentleness. Memory failure is known as the classic symptom with Alzheimer's and can have an impact on executive, short-term, or long-term memory. An individual may lose procedural memories such as the steps involved in putting on one's shoes or getting home. He or she may experience long-term memory loss, such as forgetting the name or face of a loved one.

MEMORY LIMITATIONS. There are neurological limitations to the accuracy of memory, such that forgetting or inaccurate remembering can take place through the processes of decay, interference, memory construction, and inaccurate source monitoring.

Memory decay refers to nonpathological neurological processes that result in a memory becoming less available for retrieval over time. There are two theories about why a memory may decay. The first is that unused memories are replaced by newer, more relevant or important information. The second theory suggests that as new information is added to memory, old memories are displaced. Memories that are rarely retrieved may tend to disappear.

Interference refers to the fact that old memories can interfere with the storage and retrieval of new memories, and new memories can interfere with the retrieval of old memories. Interference is most pronounced when the old and new memories have similar contexts.

Memory construction refers to the phenomenon in which the mind fills in details of a memory. The information that is filled in is typically fabricated and has little basis in reality. However, it can be difficult for an individual to distinguish between the actual memory and constructed memory.

During encoding, a memory is impacted by all of the events that the individual is currently experiencing, including mood, environment, and situation. A memory is not an exact, factual replication of what occurred and is subject to human error and personal bias. When the memory is retrieved, it is subject to the mood and environment of the current moment. Memories are influenced by a wide range of often arbitrary cognitive processes occurring at the time of encoding and time of retrieval.

Source monitoring is the process in which the mind tries to distinguish the source of information in a memory. This might include trying to determine who loaned one a certain book or whether one actually turned off the stove or simply thought about doing so. Erroneous source monitoring (a **source monitoring error**) can interfere with accurate recall.

Synaptic Connections in Memory and Learning

Neuroplasticity refers to the brain's flexibility for learning. Even into old age the brain maintains the ability to learn new information, form new memories, and learn new skills. In addition, if a previous ability is lost, neuroplasticity allows the brain to relearn the ability, using a different neural pathway.

> **PRUNING**
>
> Synaptic pruning occurs when unused neural pathways die.

Learning is essentially the storage of memory, and memory involves the creation of new neural pathways. The creation of new neural pathways involves the formation of new synaptic connections between neurons. New experiences stimulate axons to form new synaptic connections with neurons in different parts of the brain. These new pathways become stronger the more they are used, meaning that there is an increased potential for that pathway to be activated again. This is called **long-term potentiation**.

Humans have the maximum number of synapses around three years of age. They lose those that are not used through **synaptic pruning**. New synapses can become established with use.

Pruning is usually turned off around age 7. New research suggests that in some individuals with schizophrenia, the gene responsible for turning off pruning fails to function. As a result, the individual's brain continues to prune synapses, causing brain damage to the prefrontal cortex that eventually presents as schizophrenia.

LANGUAGE

Language is a highly specialized cognitive function that distinguishes human beings from other animals and generally dominates human experience. Whereas other animals have forms of communication, language is unique in its complex grammatical structure and its ability to convey an infinite range of meaning with a limited set of symbols.

> **LANGUAGE**
>
> All animals communicate, but human language is unique in its complexity. It can convey a virtually infinite range of information using a finite set of symbols.

Theories of Language Development

There are many perspectives on how language is learned. These perspectives are represented in three specific theories.

THE LEARNING PERSPECTIVE. From a general learning perspective, language is learned in much the same way that all other behaviors are learned. This includes through observation and imitation, direct instruction, and conditioning.

THE NATIVIST PERSPECTIVE. One weakness of the learning perspective is that it does not seem capable of explaining how children can acquire the highly complex grammar of a language—grammar that even adults are typically unable to explicitly explain—in the space of four or five years. Instead, the Nativist perspective argues that humans are born with the biological ability to learn language. Noam Chomsky is the main theorist associated with this perspective. The Nativist perspective proposed that all humans are born with a **language acquisition device** (LAD) that accounts for the order in which children learn structure, the mistakes they make as they learn language, and the ability to rapidly generalize grammar from a limited set of input. The biological basis of language learning is supported by the fact that children across all cultures learn language structures in much the same order, and they learn specific elements of language at the same age. The fact that children nearly universally learn language effortlessly also supports the biological basis of language and the existence of the LAD. Finally, children who have not been exposed to adult language typically invent language with virtually the same structures as other human language.

THE INTERACTIONIST THEORY. This perspective combines elements of the above two perspectives. It argues that language development is both biological and social. Language learning is influenced by the desire of children to communicate with others. The theory suggests that children are born with a brain that has the inherent ability to learn language. It then adds that children learn language socially, through conversation with older people.

The Influence of Language on Cognition

To a large extent language and cognition are inseparable. Language is the medium in which much of cognition takes place. The structures of the specific language spoken by a person influence that person's view of the world. For example, speakers of languages that do not require different pronouns for males and females might be inclined to hold less rigid views of male and female roles than speakers of a language that requires every noun and adjective to indicate gender. Speakers of languages that add grammatical elements to nouns to indicate shapes and functions might have better skills at perceiving these qualities than speakers of other languages. Some languages have distinct structures for distinguishing distant past events from more recent past events and from present and future events. Other languages do not have distinct structures for indicating these tenses. Speakers of these two distinct types of languages are likely to hold different perspectives on time.

In addition, language can be used to influence the perceptions of others. Telling someone that what he or she just said is "a bit of a fib" has a different effect from telling that person that he or she lied. Likewise, how one speaks to oneself (self-talk) influences behavior. A person whose self-talk is negative, critical, or pessimistic is likely to behave differently from someone whose self-talk is positive.

Brain Control of Language and Speech

Specific areas within the human brain specialize in processing linguistic information. The left hemisphere of the brain is mainly responsible for processing language information. Wernicke's area, located in the left temporal lobe, enables human beings to understand spoken words and produce coherent written and spoken language. Broca's area, located in the left frontal lobe, directs the patterns of muscle movement necessary for producing speech. The angular gyrus processes written language.

CONSTRUCTS OF BEHAVIOR

Behavior is determined by psychological-biological constructs, social constructs, and learning, including changes to attitude and behavior.

Psycho-Bio Constructs of Behavior

The psychological-biological constructs of behavior include biological and genetic aspects of behavior, personality, emotion, motivation, attitude, stress, and psychological disorders.

BRAIN CHEMISTRY AND MENTAL ILLNESS

Medication can be used to balance neurotransmitters in the brain to alleviate symptoms of depression, anxiety, psychosis, and attentional deficits.

BIOLOGICAL BASES OF BEHAVIOR

The biological bases of behavior include neurological processes, effects of hormones, genetic factors, and physiological developmental processes.

Influence of Neurons

In the brain, messages are transferred by electrical impulses between neurons. The myelin sheathing, a layer of fat and protein that protects nerve cells, is not fully developed until the age of 25. Myelin speeds transmission of nerve impulses, but delayed maturation of myelinated axons aids in the development of new synaptic connections. It has been shown that before the myelin sheathing is formed, individuals are more impulsive. Nutritional deficiency in omega-3 fatty acids, which contribute to the myelin sheath, has been linked to decreased synaptic and behavioral plasticity and increased anxiety in adulthood. Other forms of abnormal myelinated axon formation in brain neurons have been associated with the onset of schizophrenia in adolescence.

Influence of Neurotransmitters

Neurotransmitters are chemicals in the brain that facilitate communication between neural synapses. Insufficient amounts of neurotransmitter or blockage of neurotransmitter reception or reuptake can affect communication between neurons and in turn affect behavior. Common neurotransmitters are serotonin, dopamine, gamma aminobutyric acid, and norepinephrine. Imbalances in these neurotransmitters can result in depression, anxiety, psychosis, and deficits in attention.

Effects of the Endocrine System on Behavior

The endocrine system affects behavior through the action of hormones on the brain and other organs. The brain regulates hormone secretion through the action of the hypothalamus on the pituitary gland. Hormones in turn affect the brain and other organs through their circulation through the bloodstream. Hormones are critically important as a mechanism for responding to environmental stimuli. Hormones regulate physiological and behavioral responses to hunger, thirst, sexual attraction, and changes in body temperature. Hormones are also critically important during development. Behavioral changes associated with adolescence, childbearing, and menopause are strongly influenced by changes in hormone levels. For example, the sex hormones testosterone and estrogen both affect the limbic system and levels of the neurotransmitter serotonin, which in turn affects arousal and mood. Changes in these hormone levels during puberty can result in emotional swings and behavioral volatility characteristic of adolescence.

Behavioral Genetics

Although environment plays a large role in behavior, much of the foundation of behavior is genetic.

GENES, TEMPERAMENT, AND HEREDITY. The personality traits that help shape an individual's overall temperament are partly controlled by heredity. Temperament is defined as one's general perspective on life. It includes characteristics such as activity level, response to stress, introversion or extroversion, arousal needs, intellectual curiosity, agreeableness, and resilience.

Each person is born with genetic predispositions that guide behavior. However, research into behavioral genetics is a relatively new field, and the specific genes involved and degree of personality that can be attributed to heredity have not yet been determined. Recent discoveries, though, illustrate that heritable traits may have far more of an influence than previously thought. In 2000, psychiatrist David Reiss discovered that tendencies toward delinquency, school achievement, risk-taking, and sociability might be overwhelmingly influenced by genetic factors. Furthermore, the study found evidence that parental influence may have very little actual impact upon these and other factors that ultimately determine success.

ADAPTIVE VALUE OF TRAITS AND BEHAVIORS. Evolutionary psychologists and biologists argue that many of the behaviors and traits exhibited by humans are fundamentally adaptive and once served an important role in survival and reproduction. Social animals, including humans, must learn to interact, cooperate, and harmonize with others within their species. Consequently, the brain of social animals has developed unique complex mechanisms to facilitate social interaction. Behaviors and traits such as attachment, social recognition, collaboration, group security, altruism, and compromise improved survival chances and became encoded in the genetic makeup of humans.

Many behaviors exhibited by modern humans might once have served an important adaptive social function. Prejudice against outside groups, for example, is thought to once have been crucial to group survival. Isolation from outside groups might have protected a group from exposure to viruses or bacteria to which they could have been vulnerable.

INTERACTION BETWEEN HEREDITY AND ENVIRONMENTAL FACTORS. It is generally accepted that genetic and environmental factors are not competing forces but are instead complementary influences on human physical and social development. Individuals are born with a predetermined and unchangeable genetic configuration that predisposes them to certain personality traits, psychiatric conditions, behaviors, or tendencies. Nevertheless, environmental influences determine the manner in which these traits are expressed or whether they are expressed at all. Genetic makeup may determine how one reacts to environmental conditions, but environmental conditions dictate whether or not those behavioral reactions are acceptable.

It is possible for the environment to change heredity. Epigenetics is the study of environmental factors that result in heritable changes. Epigenetic changes are not changes in DNA sequences but rather in the expression of genes. For example, environmental stresses on a parent can result in epigenetic changes in offspring that can affect learning and memory. Epigenetic changes have been associated with the occurrence of schizophrenia, substance abuse, eating disorders, and other psychological disorders. Epigenetics is reviewed in Chapter 3, Biology.

Genetic and Environmental Factors that Affect Behavior

Behavior is obviously affected by the environmental circumstances in which people find themselves. In such cases behavior can draw on past experience, if the present situation is similar to one that the person has experienced before. Alternately, a situation may be unfamiliar, in which case the behavior is not based on the past and may be a novel response. In addition to environmental influences on behavior, genetics influences behavior in specific ways.

REGULATORY GENES AND BEHAVIOR. Genes can affect behavior through the expression of proteins that affect neural networks. Differences in behavior between individuals and species may be the result of differences in the genes that code for protein, or they may result from changes in regulatory genes that affect gene expression. For example, regulatory genes in certain species of wild mice affect whether the mice are monogamous or promiscuous. Although the coding regions of the gene are the same in both species, transfer of the regulatory region of the gene from one species to another can cause promiscuous mice to become faithful to a single mate. In honeybees, inhibition or activation of regulatory genes by hive pheromones determines the developmental switch that triggers a sedentary hive worker to become an active forager or an aggressive guard. The role of regulatory genes in human behavior is a subject of current investigation.

GENETICALLY BASED BEHAVIORAL VARIATIONS IN NATURAL POPULATIONS. Genetic variation in natural populations includes variation in behavioral genes. As a result, not only do individuals within a population show genetic behavioral differences, but populations of the same species may also differ in behavior. Populations may show variation in food preference, habitat selection, foraging times, and responses to prey or predators, as well as in courtship displays, territorial defense, and mate choice. These differences may result from subtle variations in the sequences of coding genes, or they may result from changes in regulatory regions. Many behavioral genes appear to be conserved between populations, species, and higher taxonomic groups, and observed behavioral differences are caused by the effect of regulatory genes on gene expression. Some behavioral traits have been linked to single genes, such as the *period* gene in fruit flies, which affects species-level differences in courtship behavior. However, most complex behavioral differences are likely the result of multiple coding and regulatory genes, pleiotropic effects, and epigenetic interactions between genes, behaviors, and the environment.

Human Physiological Development

The section below describes how physiological development in childhood and adolescence affects behavior. The section begins with a review of the major stages of prenatal neurological and motor development.

PRENATAL DEVELOPMENT. After fertilization of an egg, cell division begins, creating a mass of cells. The mass of cells attaches itself to the wall of the uterus within a week, becoming a **blastocyst**. The developing organism is referred to as an embryo from attachment through 8 weeks and is referred to as a fetus from 8 weeks until birth. The average pregnancy is 40 weeks.

The stages of pregnancy constitute three trimesters. The most significant period of development takes place during the first trimester. During the first month, the cells are differentiating, and the embryo is developing organs. The brain, nervous system, digestive system, and heart form. Small buds of what will become appendages start to take shape.

In the second month, the embryo develops facial features that can be recognized. Eyes, a nose, and a mouth all take shape. The organs continue to develop, becoming more complex. At this point, the embryo weighs approximately a third of an ounce and is less than one inch long.

During the third month, the embryo becomes a fetus and the appendages begin to develop. Arms and legs grow from the buds that formed in the first months. Hands and feet grow, including the nails, and hair follicles develop. Eyelids emerge over the eyes. Although still not fully developed, all of the organ systems are in place and growing. Bone growth begins to replace cartilage. The fetus begins to move.

In the second trimester the toes and fingers, which were previously webbed on each hand and foot, now separate. The fetus grows skin, hair, and fingerprints. The fetus has a heartbeat and may suck its thumbs. The fetus has stages of sleeping and waking.

In the third trimester, fetal development must proceed to the point that the child is able to survive outside of the mother's womb. Development of internal organs and the brain and nervous system continues. The skin tissue develops a layer of fatty tissue underneath it. Infants become viable between the 22nd and the 25th week of gestation, with the 24th to 25th weeks appearing to be turning points for survival. Premature infants are at high risk for health problems, mental health problems, and neurological problems through their lives.

MOTOR DEVELOPMENT. During early childhood through adolescence, one of the strongest influences on behavior is physiological development. The stages of development are predictable, although the actual timeline for the stages varies with each child. For each age group, the motor development typical for that age is described below.

Birth–3 months	Rooting/suckling instinct for feeding.
	Struggles to hold head up, slightly raises head when lying on stomach, fist clenching.
	Survival depends on liver production of surfactant.
3–6 months	Able to lift head and chest.
	Rolls/pushes body over, scoots forward, grabs and pulls objects toward self and into the mouth.
	Teething (6 months), turns toward others, recognizes sounds and familiar faces.
6–9 months	Strength and agility, sits without assistance, crawls.
	Coordinates toy transfer from one hand to the other.
	Elementary feeding, begins to make sounds.
9–12 months	Stands and walks.
	Throws things, tactile orientation, begins to feed self with hands.
	Always moving, will interact with and perform for an audience, understands and obeys simple requests, expresses opinions.
	Some children are talking.
12–24 months	Handles stairs with minimal assistance, opens doors, runs, scribbles and colors, holds own glass to feed, emerging language 3–50 words.
24–36 months	Runs, jumps, kicks, and balances.
	Tosses a ball, turns pages in a book, makes necklaces with beads, draws circles with crayons, begins trying to dress self, begins using utensils to feed self.
	Diurnal potty training is attainable for most children. Nocturnal potty training is well underway. Vocabulary exceeds 50 words.
Early Childhood	
Age 3	Walks and runs steadily, climbs stairs, beginning to dress self, feeds self with utensils, assists in bathing and cleaning routines, and goes to toilet by self.
Age 4	Good balance, very physically active. Age-appropriate magical play, dresses self, feeds independently, no toileting accidents even at night, but may need help wiping.
Age 5	Physically calmer than 3 or 4 year olds. Able to engage in more complex play activities. More focused attention. Increased social independence. Language mastery increases.
Middle–Late Childhood	
Age 6–8	Refined coordination and physical motor skills. Physical play.
Age 9–11	Continues to refine and develop motor skills. Use and control of body improves (balance, flexibility, strength).

DEVELOPMENTAL CHANGES IN ADOLESCENCE. The physiological changes of adolescence and puberty have a rapid and profound impact on behavior. The main stages of development in adolescence are shown below.

Puberty

Girls: 9–12 years	Girls take a romantic interest in boys earlier because the onset of puberty is generally 2–4 years earlier. Girls mature faster than boys. Girls often date boys who are older.
Boys: 11–14 years	Later onset.

Endocrine Glands Release Hormones

Girls	Production of estrogen and progesterone stimulates growth of breasts, nipples, pubic hair, hips, uterine and vaginal areas. Menstruation begins.
Boys	Production of testosterone stimulates voice changes and growth of testicles, scrotum, facial hair, pubic hair, and chest.
General	Teens seek to conform to their peers, engage in self-condemnation, and avoid criticism. This is often more pronounced for girls than boys.

Height and Weight Gain

Girls	Full height by approximately 16 years. Growth spurt of 2–5 inches. Girls outweigh boys during this age and may be taller than boys.
Boys	Full height by approximately 18–20 years. Growth spurt of 2–5 inches. Boys tend to be taller and heavier than girls at the end of the growth spurt.
General	Unequal growth throughout the body lends the appearance of awkwardness and can result in teasing or bullying.

Early and Late Maturation

Girls	Early maturers face higher risk for alcohol, depression, eating disorders, and earlier sexual experiences. Late developers outperform other students academically.
Boys	Early maturers are perceived as more attractive, popular, and self-assured but are at higher risk for aggression and abuse of alcohol and drugs. Late maturing boys are perceived as immature.

PERSONALITY

Personality encompasses the totality of a person's behaviors, beliefs, attitudes, and emotions. Personality can be understood from a number of perspectives. (See Table 6.2.)

> ### PERSONALITY
>
> Personality is the complex web of genetic and physiological factors, conditioning, and intelligence that determine how each person lives. Maladaptive personalities can lead to physical and emotional difficulties.

Table 6.2 Psychological Approaches to Personality: The Three Forces

First Force	Behaviorist	Ivan Pavlov	Classical conditioning
		B. F. Skinner	Operant conditioning
		Albert Bandura	Social-cognitive learning
Second Force	Psychoanalytic	Sigmund Freud	Id, ego, superego; Unconscious, preconscious, and conscious mind
Third Force	Humanistic	Carl Rogers Abraham Maslow	Freedom of choice; Innate drive toward personal growth

Theories of Personality

THE PSYCHOANALYTIC APPROACH. The psychoanalytic perspective of personality was developed by Sigmund Freud. It cannot be understood without also discussing his beliefs on the mind and consciousness. He believed that the mind consists of three components: the conscious mind, the preconscious mind, and the unconscious mind. The unconscious mind conceals thoughts, feelings, and urges that cannot be tolerated because to become aware of them would cause too much psychological distress. Those thoughts may or may not be rational. The preconscious mind holds regular memories that can be retrieved at will. The conscious mind holds those thought processes of which a person is aware. People are able to think and talk about conscious processes.

Freud defined the personality as being divided into three structures—the id, the ego, and the superego. The id is the structure that is present at birth and is the source of one's most primitive, biological, sexual, and instinctive urges and behaviors such as lust, hunger, thirst, and rage. It operates on the pleasure principle and demands immediate gratification. The id is the source of psychic energy that creates tension and anxiety between the ego and the superego. The superego is the part of the personality that possesses rules and a sense of right and wrong. It holds us to our ethical and moral standards. The ego is the part of the personality that mediates between the id and the superego, provides balance, and is responsible for decision making. The ego operates between the conscious, preconscious, and unconscious minds as it contributes to memory and decision-making processes.

THE HUMANISTIC APPROACH. The humanistic theory of personality development has been called the "third force" of psychological schools of thought, the "first force" being psychoanalysis and the "second force" being behaviorist schools of thought. Humanists believe that people are not controlled by their unconscious drives, wishes, or conflicts (as psychoanalysts believe), but rather they have freedom of choice, regardless of their environment. Humanists also believe that people have an innate drive toward personal growth and that one's subjective point of view is more important than an objective view of the world. Carl Rogers and Abraham Maslow contributed to the field of humanistic personality development. Rogers's contribution to the field was the idea that children develop a self-concept of who they are and who they want to be. By assessing the discrepancies in an individual's self-concept, a therapist decreases the stress of the client. Rogers also proposed that individuals interact with "unconditional positive regard," a concept that has since become the basis for interactions between therapists and their clients. Abraham Maslow furthered the field of humanistic psychology by focusing on how an individual can achieve full potential, thus becoming self-actualized.

THE TRAIT APPROACH. The trait theory of personality has developed based on the belief that all people have similar personality features that can be identified, measured, and placed on a continuum. These personality traits have been condensed into the "Big Five": openness, conscientiousness, extraversion, agreeableness, and neuroticism. Openness is a measure of one's readiness to experience new things, engage in thought-provoking activities, and experience the world in different ways. Conscientiousness is a person's tendency to take care of business, follow through on things, be self-disciplined, and be high achieving. An extraverted person likes being with other people and is friendly and sociable. An agreeable person is caring, sympathetic, and concerned for the well-being of others. The personality trait of neuroticism refers to a person's emotional stability and mood swings in their relationships with other people. Personality Trait Theory is objective, easy to understand, has been quantified, and can be tested through the Thematic Apperception Test. The criticism of trait theory is that it does not account for development or personality change and cannot be used to predict behavior.

THE SOCIAL COGNITIVE APPROACH. The social cognitive perspective of personality development began with Albert Bandura's Social Learning Theory, which stated that individuals can learn from observing the behavior of another person. Bandura's concept of Reciprocal Determinism states that an individual acts on the environment to influence it and then the environment acts in turn on the individual's development, behavior, and personality.

The biological approach. The biological approach to personality is primarily concerned with how brain chemistry influences personality, including the role of brain chemistry in the context of rewarding and punishing stimuli. Three researchers—Hans Eysenck, Jeffrey Gray, and C. Robert Cloninger—have posited theories relating personality to biological development of the brain. Eysenck—whose work fundamentally follows a trait approach—put forth a **three-factor model** for viewing personality. He associates two of these factors with specific areas of the brain, as shown in Table 6.3.

Table 6.3 Eysenck's Three-Factor Model

Quality	Description	Brain Region
Extraversion	Degree of being outgoing	Reticular formation
Neuroticism	Degree of emotional stability or instability	Limbic system
Psychoticism	Degree of hostility and antisocial behavior	Unspecified

Gray's reinforcement sensitivity theory suggests that the brain has three neurological systems of response to rewarding or punishing stimuli, as shown in Table 6.4.

Table 6.4 Gray's Reinforcement Sensitivity Theory

System	Emotion Mediated	Personality Trait
Fight-Flight-Freeze System	Fear, avoidance of danger	Fearful, avoidant
Behavioral Inhibition System	Anxiety, risk assessment	Anxious
Behavioral Approach System	Anticipation of pleasure	Optimistic, impulsive, pleasure oriented

Cloninger's model of personality posits three general responses to rewarding or punishing stimuli and links them to neurotransmitters in the brain (Table 6.5).

Table 6.5 Cloninger's Model of Personality

Dimension	Personality Trait	Neurotransmitter Status
Novelty seeking	Impulsivity	Low dopamine
Harm avoidance	Anxiety	High serotonin
Reward dependence	Need for approval	Low norepinephrine

THE BEHAVIORIST APPROACH. Behaviorist theory of personality development was inspired by theorists such as Pavlov, Skinner, and Bandura. Pavlov is famous for his experiments with dogs' salivary reactions, which led him to develop his theories about classical conditioning. Skinner built upon Pavlov's research with his theories of operant conditioning. Bandura's contribution to the field evaluates how personality develops in response to social-cognitive learning. He posits that thinking and reasoning must occur, not just the presence of automatic stimuli (as Skinner and Pavlov have stated) for personality development and learning to occur.

The Situational Perspective on Behavior

The situational perspective on behavior stands in contrast to the perspectives presented above. This perspective, posited by Mischel, states that behavior is influenced primarily by external circumstances, and for that reason, it is not particularly helpful to categorize people's personality traits. A situational perspective would, for example, not be overly concerned with the fact that a person tends to be timid because in the appropriate situation the person is likely to be aggressive. In general, psychologists believe that both internal and external factors influence behavior.

PSYCHOLOGICAL DISORDERS

A **psychological disorder** is defined as impairment in an individual's behavior, thinking, or mood caused by psychological symptoms that significantly impact the person's functioning in one or more areas of life, such as family, work, school, or community. There are two primary models through which psychological disorders are viewed: the biomedical model and the biopsychosocial model. The **biomedical model** looks at a psychological disorder as an illness that needs to be cured. The emphasis is placed upon the biology, physiology, and genetics that influence the illness, and the goal is to cure the illness. In the **biopsychosocial model**, a patient is evaluated in the context of the biological, psychological, and social factors that are contributing to the person's difficulties. The person's risk and resiliency factors are considered and incorporated into the treatment plan. The focus is on treating the person in the context of the environmental and social factors acting on that person, as well as the biological factors. By effecting a change to the entire system, a lasting positive treatment outcome is considered more likely.

A patient visits a doctor with complaints about sleeplessness, weight gain, irritability, lack of energy, and isolating behaviors. The doctor diagnoses the patient with depression and suggests that the patient begin exercising, attend activities at church, and undergo therapy before deciding to take antidepressant medication. What treatment model is the doctor using in formulating this treatment plan?

Solution: The doctor is using the biopsychosocial model of treatment. Exercise and diet address the biological treatment needs. Therapy addresses the patient's psychological treatment needs. Active participation in a church addresses the social needs. This holistic treatment plan may be sufficient to bring about a change in mood without the need for antidepressants. If the doctor chooses to add medication later but continues to emphasize exercise, therapy, and social engagement, this would still adhere to a biopsychosocial treatment plan. A treatment plan that prescribes antidepressants without addressing the other functional domains would be characteristic of the biomedical model.

Classifying Psychological Disorders

Diagnosis and classification of psychological disorders is done using the Diagnostic and Statistical Manual of Mental Disorders version 5 (**DSM-5**), published in May 2013 by the American Psychiatric Association. Psychiatrists, psychologists, social workers, and marriage and family therapists are all eligible to receive licenses to diagnose and treat patients with mental disorders using the DSM-5. It is important to note that only a person so licensed can make a diagnosis of a psychological disorder and that the diagnosis must meet the criteria in the DSM-5. Practitioners are not allowed to make a casual diagnosis of any psychological disorder based on their personal opinions or definitions.

The DSM classifies disorders by accumulating a cluster of symptoms and developing a biopsychosocial case formulation of the client. The manual cautions that it is not sufficient to merely check off the symptoms listed for a disorder when making a diagnosis.

Incidence of Psychological Disorders

About 27% of Americans over 18 years old suffer from a diagnosable psychological disorder in a given year. Anxiety disorders, obsessive compulsive disorder, and trauma disorder combined affect about 18% of adult Americans. Depression affects about 6.5% of the adult American population. Bipolar disorder affects about 2.5%. Schizophrenia affects about 1%. A significant number of people have more than one psychological disorder. The incidence of any particular disorder may vary with age, gender, or other factors.

Psychological Disorder Types

There are nine major categories of psychological disorders that will be discussed here, based on DSM-5—anxiety, trauma, obsessive compulsive, somatic symptom, depression, bipolar, schizophrenia, dissociative, and personality disorders. Each category comprises a number of distinct diagnoses. In addition, certain specifiers can be added to a diagnosis. A notable example of a specifier is **panic attack**. Thus, there could be two distinct diagnoses of, for example, agoraphobia without panic attack and agoraphobia with panic attack.

Many categories in the DSM-5 also include the following diagnostic options, which take into account that a set of symptoms might be caused by pharmaceuticals, by a particular medical condition, or by some other cause not covered in DSM ("medical/other" options):

Substance/medicine-induced disorder	Indicates that the symptoms for that category could have been brought on by a medication or other substance
Disorder due to another medical condition	Indicates that the symptoms of this disorder have their etiology in another medical condition
Other specified disorder	Symptoms are similar to but do not exactly match a certain disorder. Clinician must specify exactly how the symptoms correspond to or differ from the diagnostic criteria.
Unspecified disorder	Symptoms are similar to but do not exactly match a certain disorder. Clinician is not required to specify exactly how the symptoms correspond to or differ from the diagnostic criteria.

ANXIETY DISORDERS. Anxiety disorders are characterized by fear and anxiety and the behaviors that result from fear and anxiety. There are ten diagnoses under the category of anxiety disorders, the six shown below plus four medical/other diagnoses.

Separation anxiety disorder	Childhood disorder. Characterized by a developmentally inappropriate fear of separation from major attachment figures.
Selective mutism	Childhood disorder. Failure to speak in a variety of social situations such as school or in public not due to a language delay or speech impairment.
Specific phobia	Extreme anxiety or fear caused by everyday objects or stimuli (such as elevators, heights, spiders, specific animals) on a consistent basis for at least 6 months.
Social anxiety disorder	Fear of being judged by others in a social situation or being negatively assessed by others to the degree that social situations are avoided.
Agoraphobia	A feeling of extreme anxiety in a location other than the home, accompanied by a desire to escape but a sense that escape is not possible (such as schools, crowds, elevators).

Generalized anxiety disorder	Fear and anxiety that cannot be controlled. Can center around any facet of life. It is present for at least 6 months and occurs more days than not.
Panic disorder	A repeated series of panic attacks that occur without warning. The individual engages in behaviors designed to decrease occurrence of the attacks or to avoid triggers that would bring about the attacks.

The medical/other diagnoses are substance/medication-induced anxiety disorder, anxiety disorder due to another medical condition, other specified anxiety disorder, and unspecified anxiety disorder.

TRAUMA AND STRESSOR-RELATED DISORDERS. This category is new in DSM-5 and it allows for **post-traumatic stress disorder (PTSD)** to be distinguished based on its etiology—the trauma that causes its symptoms. Disorders in this category are shown below.

Adjustment disorder	An adverse reaction to a stressor that occurs within 3 months but less than 6 months of the stressor and affects the individual's ability to function in one or more domain.
Acute stress disorder	Individual experiences or witnesses a traumatic event and experiences the symptoms of post-traumatic stress disorder for 1 day to 1 month. Symptoms fall into the following categories: adverse mood, intrusive thoughts, dissociative, avoidant, and aroused symptoms.
Post-traumatic stress disorder (PTSD)	Symptoms may include but are not limited to disassociation, avoidance of reminders of the trauma, hypervigilance, and startle responses. Occurs in response to a life- or health-threatening trauma.
Reactive attachment	Childhood disorder. First symptoms occur between 9 months and 5 years. Child has suffered severe neglect and/or abuse. Child has difficulty forming adaptive attachments. The child manifests lack of responsiveness, limited positive affect, sadness, fear, irritability; appears isolated and withdrawn; believes others do not care about him/her; hard to engage socially or in tasks.

Disinhibited social engagement disorder	Childhood disorder. First symptoms occur between 9 months and 5 years. Child has suffered severe neglect and/or abuse. This child appears overly friendly, befriends and goes with strangers, lacks boundaries in social situations, does not understand that strangers can pose danger, compliments adults, curries favor and asks to come home with those he/she does not know. Seeks to bond with everyone he/she meets.

OBSESSIVE-COMPULSIVE DISORDERS. Obsessive-compulsive disorders are characterized by either an obsession or a compulsion. An obsession is defined as an intrusive or unwanted thought or urge. A compulsion is a repetitive, sometimes ritualistic or rule-driven behavior that is a response to the obsession. Diagnoses included in this category are shown below.

Obsessive-compulsive disorder	Intrusive obsessions (intrusive thoughts) or compulsions (behaviors or thoughts that are ritualistic in nature and are designed to reduce anxiety) that hinder an individual's ability to function in one or more domains.
Body dysmorphic disorder	The individual perceives a physical defect in his or her appearance that others either do not see or do not believe is significant. The patient engages in behaviors to reduce his anxiety about the defect (e.g., excessive grooming, reassurance seeking).
Hoarding disorder	Significant distress about discarding things. Strong desire to save things, regardless of value, even at the expense of safety or health.
Trichotillomania	Hair loss caused by pulling out one's own hair despite repeated attempts to stop this compulsive behavior.
Excoriation	Compulsive skin picking resulting in lesions.

In addition, there are the medical/other categories of substance/medication-induced obsessive-compulsive disorder, obsessive-compulsive and related disorders due to another medical condition, other unspecified obsessive-compulsive-related disorders, and other specified obsessive-compulsive-related disorders.

SOMATIC SYMPTOM AND RELATED DISORDERS. These diagnoses focus on a patient's somatic symptoms and the patient's response to those symptoms. Patients with somatic symptoms are more likely to present in a medical clinic than in a mental health treatment setting, so it is important that a medical clinician be aware of how to identify these diagnoses.

Somatic symptom disorder	Characterized by somatic symptoms that interfere in life functioning.
Illness anxiety disorder ("hypochondria")	Individuals continually believe they are sick in the absence of significant medical symptoms.
Conversion disorder, or functional neurological symptom disorder	Presence of symptoms of altered voluntary motor or sensory function without any physical cause, brought on by stress.
Psychological factors affecting other medical conditions	A new diagnosis that acknowledges the mind-body connection. Applies to individuals who either have a medical illness that is not improving because of psychological factors or the psychological factors are interfering with treatment.
Factitious disorder	Characterized by the patient deliberately falsifying symptoms of an illness.

Finally, the medical/other diagnoses in this category include other specified somatic symptom and related disorders and unspecified somatic symptom and related disorders.

The fact that a medical diagnosis cannot be found for a patient who reports specific symptoms should **not** be used as a basis for concluding that the patient has an underlying psychological disorder. Diagnosis of a psychological disorder must be made according to criteria in DSM-5.

DEPRESSIVE DISORDERS. The most well-known of the depressive disorders is **major depressive disorder**, with a prevalence of 7%. Major depression affects women at a much higher rate than men. Depression in children is characterized by angry outbursts, physical aggression, and irritability. For this reason, children with these symptoms are given the diagnosis of **disruptive mood dysregulation disorder**. Further, this diagnosis is designed to identify children who exhibit extreme rage but do not meet full criteria for bipolar disorder. Namely, they do not demonstrate mania on an episodic basis. Instead, they are triggered by external factors. **Persistent depressive disorder** (formerly dysthymia) is a diagnosis given to those who exhibit long-term, low-grade depression. **Premenstrual dysphoric disorder**, occurring in between approximately 2% and 6% of menstruating women, is recognized as a diagnosable condition in DSM-5. The medical/other disorders included in the category of depressive disorders are substance/medication-induced depressive disorders, depressive disorder due to another medical condition, other specified depressive disorder, and unspecified depressive disorder.

BIPOLAR AND RELATED DISORDERS. Bipolar disorders and depressive disorders were previously categorized together under mood disorders. The DSM-5 has separated them out, recognizing that the component of mania in Bipolar Disorder necessitates a different approach to

BIOPOLAR DISORDER AND SUICIDE

One out of four completed suicides is attributed to bipolar disorder. The risk of suicide is 15 times higher in an individual with bipolar disorder than in the general population.

case conceptualization, assessment, diagnosis, and treatment for these individuals. **Bipolar 1** disorder is diagnosed if there is one episode of mania during the individual's life (**hypomania**—mild form of mania—may or may not be present), and there may be a depressive episode but it is not required. The risk of suicide for individuals with bipolar disorder is 15 times higher than in the general population and is estimated to account for 25% of the completed suicides in the United States.

Bipolar 2 is distinguished from Bipolar 1 in that an individual with Bipolar 2 never progresses beyond hypomania and an episode of major depression is required. **Cyclothymia** is considered a mild, long-term form of Bipolar Disorder, diagnosed for individuals when they exhibit hypomanic and depressive symptoms (as opposed to episodes).

The medical/other disorders that fall under the bipolar classification are substance/medication-induced bipolar and related disorders, bipolar and related disorders due to another medical condition, other specified bipolar and related disorder, and unspecified bipolar and related disorder.

TEST QUESTION

A 26-year-old woman goes to the doctor with the following complaints. She has not slept in days; she is engaging in risky sex with unknown partners; she is irritable; her thoughts are "moving a million miles a minute;" she cannot concentrate; she has recently spent an exorbitant amount of money on a motorcycle. She describes feeling as if she knows secrets that nobody else knows but is unable to articulate them. She speaks very quickly as she describes her complaints. What are these symptoms characteristic of?

(A) Anxiety

(B) Mania

(C) Psychosis

(D) Depression

(B) Manic behaviors are characterized by a decreased need for sleep, pressured speech, distractibility, racing thoughts, high impulsivity with poor judgment, inflated self-esteem or grandiosity, and reckless behaviors.

SCHIZOPHRENIA SPECTRUM AND OTHER PSYCHOTIC DISORDERS. Schizophrenia and other psychotic disorders are typically characterized by symptoms of **hallucinations** and **delusions**. Hallucinations are sensory perceptions that occur without stimulation. Examples are a visual hallucination, such as seeing someone who is not present, or an auditory hallucination, such as hearing voices that are not present. Delusions are a fixed set of beliefs that the patient refuses to modify even when presented with convincing evidence to the contrary. There are six general categories of delusions: persecution, grandiosity, referential, erotic, somatic, and nihilistic. Delusions can be described as either **nonbizarre** or **bizarre**. A delusion is nonbizarre if it could actually happen. A common example is the belief that the FBI is spying on the individual. A delusion is bizarre if it is outside of the generally accepted realm of possibility, for example being abducted by people from the future.

Disorders diagnosed in this category are **delusional disorder**, **brief psychotic disorder**, **schizophreniform disorder**, **schizophrenia**, and **schizoaffective disorder**. The factors that differentiate these disorders from each other include the length of presentation of symptoms, the presence or absence of depressive symptoms with the psychotic symptoms, and the sequence in which the symptoms occurred (did the psychosis or the mood symptoms occur first). The prevalence rates of psychotic disorders are considered to be quite low, below 1% for the general population.

The medical/other disorders that fall under this category include psychotic disorder due to another medical condition, substance/medication-induced psychotic disorder, catatonia associated with another mental disorder, catatonic disorder due to another medical condition, unspecified catatonia, unspecified schizophrenia spectrum and other psychotic disorder, other specified schizophrenia spectrum, and other psychotic disorder.

DISSOCIATIVE DISORDERS. Dissociative disorders are disorders that interfere with the regular functioning of memory, identity, emotion, consciousness, perception, body, motor control, and behavior. Dissociative disorders may develop as a result of a trauma. Disorders classified in this category are shown below.

Dissociative identity disorder	The individual develops two or more discrete personality states or a possession, often the result of extreme abuse or trauma.
Dissociative amnesia	An individual suddenly forgets his or her relevant personal information. This may be brought on by an extreme trauma such as a natural disaster or war.
Depersonalization/derealization disorder	Depersonalization: the person feels separated from his or her own body. Derealization: The person has the sense that his or her surroundings are not real. The person's reality testing is solid.

The medical/other diagnoses in this category include Other Specified Dissociative Disorder and Unspecified Dissociative Disorder.

PERSONALITY DISORDERS. Personality disorders involve characteristics that are intrinsic to an individual's personality structure and that impact the individual's thoughts, emotions, interpersonal relationships, and degree of impulsivity. These characteristics may be contrary to cultural norms, cause difficulties in functioning, or represent a way of interacting and behaving over time that is inflexible. Such personality characteristics may or may not be distressing to the individual and generally begin in adolescence or early adulthood.

The disorders in this category are grouped into three clusters—A, B, and C. Cluster A disorders are generally characterized by odd or eccentric behaviors. The disorders in this cluster are shown below.

Cluster A
(typified by odd or eccentric behaviors)

Paranoid personality disorder	A universal suspiciousness (paranoia) of the motives of others that impairs relationships and functioning in a variety of settings.
Schizoid personality disorder	Disengagement from social relationships and a narrowed range of emotions in social settings. Preference to be alone.
Schizotypal personality disorder	Social and interpersonal deficits. Reduced capacity for close relationships. Cognitive or perceptual distortions. Eccentric behaviors.

Cluster B disorders are characterized by erratic, emotional, or dramatic behavior. The disorders in this cluster are shown below.

Cluster B
(typified by erratic, emotional, or dramatic behaviors or characteristics)

Antisocial personality disorder	Sociopathy or psychopathy characterized by a pervasive pattern of violating the rights of others.
Borderline personality disorder	Disequilibrium in self-image, interpersonal relationships, and affect. Significant impulsivity.
Histrionic personality disorder	Attention-seeking behavior and extreme emotionality.
Narcissistic personality disorder	Need for admiration from others, a lack of empathy, and a history of grandiosity.

People with Cluster C personality disorders suffer from fear and anxiety. The disorders in this cluster are shown below.

Cluster C
(typified by fear and anxiety)

Avoidant personality disorder	Person feels inadequate, afraid of criticism, and socially inhibited.
Dependent personality disorder	A pathological need to be taken care of in the extreme. Clinging and/or submissive behaviors. A fear of separation.
Obsessive-compulsive personality disorder	Fixation with orderliness, cleanliness, perfectionism, and control (mental and interpersonal). No space for flexibility or openness.

The medical/other categories of other personality disorders include personality change due to another medical condition, other specified personality disorder, and unspecified personality disorder.

Biological Bases of Nervous System Disorders

Biology plays a part in the development of many nervous system disorders, including disorders that are diagnosed as psychological. Specifically, schizophrenia, depression, Alzheimer's disease (see page 731), and Parkinson's disease have strong biological components.

SCHIZOPHRENIA. Much research has been conducted on the biological etiology of **schizophrenia**. Many studies of twins, adoptions, and families indicate that there is a genetic tendency toward the disease. In a study published in January 2016 in the *Journal of Nature*, researchers revealed new findings that many individuals who develop schizophrenia carry a gene that accelerates or intensifies neurosynaptic pruning and that the brain overprunes neurons in the prefrontal cortex, which is responsible for thinking and planning. This places these individuals at higher risk for schizophrenia. Further, there may be as many as 14 genes linked to schizophrenia but none have been found to be a consistent cause of the disease. It is also hypothesized that biological stressors during fetal development may impair the nervous system of the fetus, predisposing the individual to develop schizophrenia. These stressors include a maternal illness/infection during birth, maternal malnourishment, difficult pregnancy, stress or trauma during pregnancy, a difficult child birth, or extended labor with difficulties. Because development of the nervous system continues after birth, it is assumed that interruptions in development after birth can also contribute to a disposition toward schizophrenia, including exposure to toxins or parasites. Brain scans have demonstrated that a brain with schizophrenia has a different structure than a brain without schizophrenia. The prefrontal areas of the brain have a diminished number of neural connections. The hippocampus and parts of the cerebral cortex are on average slightly smaller in the brains of people with schizophrenia. It is possible, however, that brain differences in people with schizophrenia are attributable to substance abuse, rather than schizophrenia per se.

DEPRESSION. The biological basis for **depression** is found in the chemistry, rather than the structure, of the brain. Neurotransmitters such as serotonin, dopamine, and norepinephrine allow the brain to efficiently and effectively carry messages from one neuron to another. When there is an imbalance in these chemicals, clinical depression may result. Genes are also implicated in depression but at this time it is not known which genes contribute to the depressive process. Depression may be influenced by dietary nutritional factors, such as omega 3 fatty acids, folic acids, and B-12 intake. Thyroid dysfunction may lead to depression.

PARKINSON'S DISEASE. Though not strictly a psychological disorder, Parkinson's is another example of a neurological disorder with a biological basis. In Parkinson's disease, a patient exhibits a decrease in dopamine, resulting in symptoms of shaking or tremors. The decrease in dopamine occurs because of progressive deterioration of the dopamine-producing neurons in the substantia nigra section of the brain. There is evidence that there may be genetic and environmental factors for Parkinson's.

STEM CELL-BASED THERAPY FOR REGENERATING CNS NEURONS. Because damaged nerve cells do not readily regenerate, damage to neurons in the brain is difficult to heal. Potential therapy for central nervous system injury includes the use of stem cells—undifferentiated cells capable of differentiating into a variety of cell and tissue types. Stem cells naturally occur in early embryos and in some adult tissues. Embryonic stem cells have the ability to divide indefinitely and differentiate into any adult tissue type, including nervous system tissue. In addition, new techniques have shown that stem cells from adult tissues, which normally only regenerate their tissue type of origin, can be induced to differentiate into nerve cells. Stem cells could be cultured and transplanted to repair and replace damaged cells. Another possible therapy would be to induce a patient's own endogenous neural stem cells to divide and regenerate damaged tissue. Both approaches are currently undergoing active research.

TEST QUESTION

A patient who is prescribed a selective serotonin reuptake inhibitor (SSRI) is most likely being treated for what?

(A) Genetic abnormalities

(B) Vitamin B-12 deficiency

(C) Structural brain damage

(D) Depression

(D) The biological basis of depression is found in the chemistry of the neurotransmitters of the brain. Serotonin is a neurotransmitter. A medication that affects the reuptake of a neurotransmitter is likely being prescribed to focus on changing the balance of neurotransmitters in the brain.

EMOTION

Emotion is one of the most critical and complex influences on motivation, personality, temperament, and overall affect.

The Three Components of Emotion

Emotion is defined as an individual's physiological, behavioral, and cognitive response to his or her environment. Even though emotional expression varies from person to person, these three elements are universal components of emotion.

> **EMOTION**
>
> Emotion is a complex expression of the interactions between physiological, behavioral, and cognitive components.

PHYSIOLOGICAL COMPONENTS. The body exhibits several physiological changes in response to emotional experience. These may include heart rate fluctuations, dilated pupils, sweating, piloerection, digestive upset, increased respiration, and flushing of the skin.

BEHAVIORAL COMPONENTS. Behavioral responses to emotion include both expressions of emotion and changes in physical behavior. Expressions of emotion are behaviors that people generally identify with a specific emotion, such as smiling, scowling, laughing, crying, and pouting. Changes in physical behavior may include aggressiveness, isolation, change in tone or rate of speech, nervous tics, agitation, or fatigue.

COGNITIVE COMPONENTS. Although emotional experience may not primarily be a cognitive experience, cognition serves to analyze and evaluate the circumstances accompanying the emotion.

Universal Emotions

In 1872, Charles Darwin proposed that human emotions were biologically adaptive and could be universally interpreted across diverse cultures. In the 1960s, Dr. Paul Ekman elaborated upon Darwin's theory in an extensive study of emotional expression within a variety of Eastern and Western societies. Ekman concluded that there are seven human emotions that are universally expressed regardless of cultural context. The seven universal emotions are fear, anger, happiness, surprise, joy, disgust, and sadness.

Adaptive Role of Emotion

It has long been theorized that emotions serve an adaptive function for humans. In his book *The Expression of Emotions in Man and Animals* (1872), Charles Darwin proposed that the manner in which ancestral humans responded to their environment, communicated, and bonded with others was

> **UNIVERSAL EMOTIONS**
>
> The seven emotions that occur in all human populations are fear, anger, happiness, surprise, joy, disgust, and sadness.

essential to their survival as a species. Consequently, universal emotional expressions evolved through natural selection as protective, social, and motivational mechanisms in humans. Modern theory suggests that emotions evolved as a means of encouraging prosocial behavior in ancestral humans. Fear or dislike of people who were dissimilar might have been advantageous to ancestral humans who competed with other communities for scarce resources. Displays of rage toward a disruptive group member might motivate cooperation within the group, which was essential for both security and acquiring food. Finally, experiencing love toward a child or partner might motivate protectiveness, nurturance, and trust.

Theories of Emotion

The three theories described below offer distinct frameworks for understanding emotion.

JAMES-LANGE THEORY. The James-Lange theory of emotion states that individuals respond with emotion only after physical changes occur in the body in reaction to a stimulus. According to James and Lange, events or conditions in the environment cause a primary physiological reaction such as muscle tension, increased heart rate/respiration, or sweating. Any emotional response occurs as a direct result of physiological arousal and is therefore secondary.

CANON-BARD THEORY. The Canon-Bard theory of emotion, published in 1915, directly disputed the conclusions reached by James and Lange. The Canon-Bard theory states that emotion is primarily experienced in the thalamic region of the brain. Any physiologic response occurs either simultaneously or secondarily. Emotional response is not a direct result of physical response.

SCHACHTER-SINGER THEORY. The Schachter-Singer theory, also called the two-factor theory of emotion, was developed in the 1960s when scholars began to focus more attention on the role of emotion in emotional expression. The Schachter-Singer theory states that physiological stimulation does play a crucial role in emotional experience. However, it is the individuals' perception of and interpretation of their physical reaction to an event that results in an emotional response. The theory posits that an appropriate emotion is experienced only as a result of the cognitive process of identifying the cause of physical arousal. People first feel a physiological response and then assign meaning to that response and experience the corresponding emotion.

The Role of Biological Processes in Perceiving Emotion

Emotion has a strong physiological component. The roles of the limbic system, prefrontal cortex, and autonomic nervous system are reviewed below.

THE ROLE OF THE LIMBIC SYSTEM. Multiple brain regions are responsible for the generation and experience of emotion. Together, these parts form the **limbic system**, which regulates emotion and plays a key role in long-term memory formation. The limbic system includes the amygdala, the hippocampus, the hypothalamus, the basal nuclei, the orbitofrontal cortex, the cingulate gyrus, the olfactory bulbs, the insula, and parts of the cortex and midbrain. (See Figure 6.1.)

The Limbic System

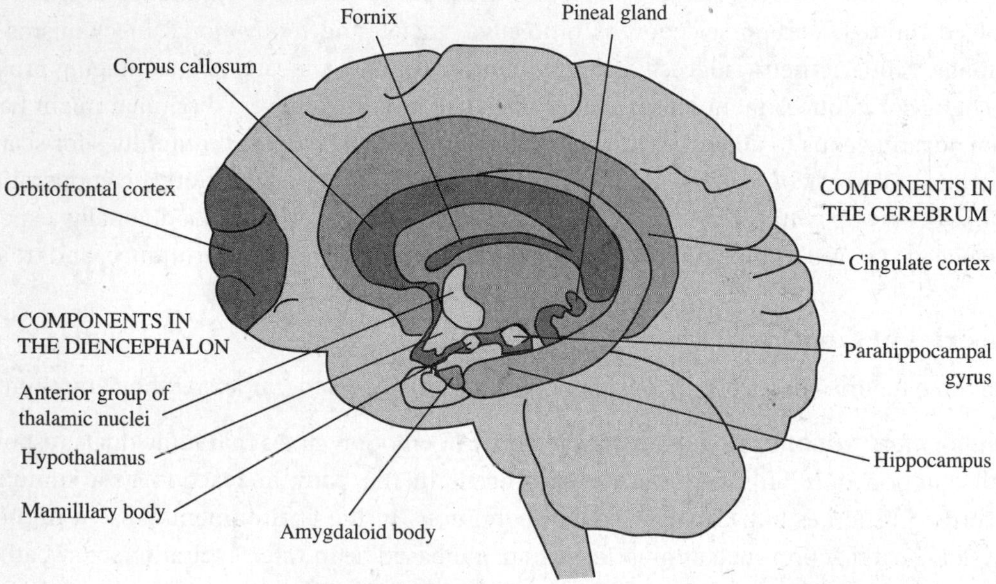

Figure 6.1. The limbic system. [Image courtesy *Blausen.com* staff (2014).]

A primary role of the limbic system is to aid in memory formation through the linkage of memory with emotional response. The association of the olfactory system with the limbic system results in the sense of smell being closely linked with memory and emotion. Strong emotions in particular generate strong memories, and similar circumstances can trigger sudden recollection of past emotion. For example, in post-traumatic stress syndrome, survivors of traumatic events are subject to continually reexperiencing emotional trauma when exposed to sounds, smells, or other circumstances that trigger memories of the event. The limbic system is also tied with the dopamine pathway (mesolimbic pathway) in the brain, particularly through the ventral tegmental area (VTA) and the nucleus accumbens (NA) of the basal nuclei. This results in the strong association between memory and motivational and pleasure centers in the brain. Activation of this pathway is involved with the pursuit of pleasurable activity and with the development of destructive addictive behaviors. Aspects of the limbic system are summarized in Table 6.6.

Table 6.6 Main Components of the Limbic System

Brain Structure	Partial List of Functions	Related Disorders
Orbitofrontal cortex	Assesses anticipated rewards, punishments, and emotional value of reinforcement; evaluates expectation vs. outcome to facilitate adaptive learning; integrates information from limbic system; used when making judgments based on intuition	Drug addiction, withdrawal, and craving; ADHD; OCD; impulse control; and perhaps Alzheimer's disease
Cingulate gyrus	Affects the relationship between behavioral outcomes and motivation; emotion; behavior; motivation; long-term memory	Individuals with schizophrenia have been found to possess a smaller cingulate gyrus than those without schizophrenia
Amygdala	Seat of social and emotional intelligence and emotional memory; conditioned learning; fear; anxiety; aggression; sexual responsiveness; face recognition	Inability to associate a stimulus with an emotional response; autism
Hippocampus	Long-term memory formation; spatial memory	Inability to form new memories
Basal nuclei	Motivation and volition; regulation of movement	Parkinson's disease; obsessive-compulsive disorder; addiction
Insula	Regulates physical homeostasis; cognitive-emotional processes (interoceptive awareness); pain and self-awareness; emotions such as happy, sad, fear, anxiety, disgust	Aphasia; Alzheimer's disease; addiction cravings

ROLE OF THE PREFRONTAL CORTEX. The limbic system is also under control of the prefrontal cortex, which regulates strategic planning and executive function. The prefrontal cortex exerts higher-level emotional control and is responsible for delayed gratification and the assessment of consequences of alternate behaviors. Direct stimulation of the hypothalamus by the amygdala results in an immediate and involuntary response from the autonomic nervous system; however, the cortex can exert slower, more deliberate, conscious control over emotional reactions to stimuli. The prefrontal cortex's ability to inhibit the fear response from the amygdala may contribute to temperamental differences between individuals in terms of innate anxiety levels and susceptibility to stress. In the other direction, emotional input from the limbic system to the prefrontal cortex can aid in and influence decision making.

PLANNING AND EXECUTIVE FUNCTION ROLES OF THE PREFRONTAL CORTEX

The prefrontal cortex is responsible for thinking and planning, impulse control, organizing emotional responses, focusing and organizing attention, filtering external distractions, and processing multiple sources of competing information simultaneously. It is the seat of personality.

EMOTION AND THE AUTONOMIC NERVOUS SYSTEM. Because of the involvement of the hypothalamus in the limbic system, generation of fear or anger by the amygdala can trigger the flight-or-fight responses of the sympathetic nervous system, including increased heart and respiration rate, pupil constriction, and the movement of blood toward the extremities. Similarly, pleasurable emotions associated with food or social interactions trigger the parasympathetic nervous system to stimulate pupil dilation, digestion, and sexual arousal. Stimuli that trigger the autonomic nervous system can in turn have a profound effect on memory. Because the hypothalamus also regulates the endocrine system, emotion is interconnected with hormone levels and endocrine function.

PHYSIOLOGICAL MARKERS OF EMOTION. A person experiencing emotion exhibits corresponding physiological changes associated with different emotions. These physiological changes, or somatic markers, include involuntary changes in heart rate, pupil dilation, posture, muscle tone, and facial expression. The perception of emotional somatic markers in others can influence an individual's own emotional state, affecting mood and decision making. For example, a smile on another person's face can arouse feelings of happiness, whereas downcast, tear-filled eyes can evoke sadness. Exposure to a grimace of rage can trigger the sympathetic nervous system and a fight-or-flight response. Similarly, emotion in the voice of another person triggers distinct spatial "signatures" in the listener's primary auditory cortex. Recognition of emotion in others and reciprocal response to somatic and auditory markers is adaptive in social animals and contributes to the development of empathy.

TEST QUESTION

Which of the following emotional responses is governed by the sympathetic nervous system?

(A) Impulsive decisions
(B) Racing thoughts
(C) Sexual arousal
(D) Racing heartbeat

(D) Racing heartbeat is governed by the sympathetic nervous system. Sexual arousal is governed by the parasympathetic nervous system. Impulsive decisions and racing thoughts are governed by the prefrontal cortex.

MOTIVATION

Motivation is the force that initiates human behavior. Motivation influences how successfully an individual achieves goals, how committed one is to a task, and how much effort one is willing to devote to reach objectives. Motivation is a complex process engaging an individual's biological, psychological, cognitive, behavioral, and social systems. Motivation results from internal drives, external influences, or a combination of both. Motivation can also be either a conscious or unconscious process. Major motivational theories of behavior have been developed in an effort to determine what specific factors influence motivation.

Factors that Influence Motivation

There are three factors that influence motivation—**instinct**, **arousal**, and **needs/drives**. Instinct refers to unconscious, innate biological behaviors that typically are genetically programmed. Arousal refers to the internal state of energy of the organism. When the energy levels are too low, an individual is motivated to act in ways that raise the energy level, such as exercising. When energy levels are too high, there is a motivation to act in ways that reduce the energy level, such as meditation or listening to quiet music.

The state of arousal influences the ability to perform an action. Increased arousal makes it easier to act, compared with lower states of arousal. However, if arousal increases beyond a certain point, it begins to interfere with performance. Excess arousal can be experienced as anxiety, nervousness, or feeling too "wired" to concentrate or perform.

Humans are also motivated by internal drives, which can be defined as the urge to reduce an uncomfortable state of arousal caused by an unmet physiological need. A drive can be biological or psychological, meaning that the need can be either physical or emotional—a need for food or a need for approval or attachment. Biological needs are regulated by a **negative feedback loop** (see Figure 6.2), in which physiological signals lead to a behavior that reduces or reverses the physiological signals. For example, when blood sugar is low because of hunger, the physiological changes that take place are eliminated or reversed when food is eaten. Eating stops the signals that urge the individual to eat.

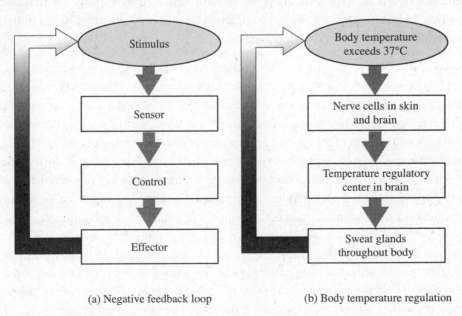

(a) Negative feedback loop   (b) Body temperature regulation

Figure 6.2. Negative feedback loops. (Image courtesy of OpenStax.)

Theories of How Motivation Affects Behavior

DRIVE REDUCTION THEORY. Also referred to as learning theory, drive reduction theory proposes that the human body is constantly striving to maintain systemic balance, or homeostasis. When the body senses an imbalance or need, an individual is biologically or psychologically motivated to eliminate discomfort to maintain equilibrium. When the individual addresses and satisfies a need through a behavior, that behavior is reinforced and the individual learns to behave similarly in the future. Drive reduction theory does not adequately account for human behaviors that seem organically irrational, such as binge eating in the absence of hunger. It furthermore fails to explain secondary reinforcers that do not satisfy a biological or psychological need, such as the motivation to work for financial compensation or attention-seeking behaviors.

INCENTIVE THEORY. Incentive theory was advanced in the 1940s by behaviorists who theorized that individuals are motivated by expectations of a real or imagined external reward. This idea contradicts earlier theories such as drive reduction theory, which contend that behavior is biologically driven.

COGNITIVE VERSUS NEED-BASED THEORIES. Need-based theories of motivation posit that individuals are motivated to satisfy their most pressing needs, which can be physiological, such as food and shelter, or higher-order needs such as esteem and love. This is considered drive reduction. Cognitive theories of motivation suggest that individuals take action based on their thoughts, beliefs, and values.

Applications of Theories of Motivation to Behavior

Biological, cognitive, and behavioral theories of motivation are instrumental in explaining behaviors and can be applied to working with compulsive behaviors such as substance abuse, eating disorders, and sexual compulsions. Researchers believe that cognitive and behavioral interventions are most influential during acquisition, the early phase of compulsion and addiction, when behavior is highly influenced by environment and expectations. Interventions based on biological theories of motivation apply during the **maintenance phase**, when an individual is compelled to practice certain behaviors due to the individual's need to maintain neurobiological homeostasis.

BIOLOGICAL FACTORS. According to recent research, compulsive behaviors all have a similar biological basis. Addictive substances, food, and sex activate the mesolimbic system, amygdala, and prefrontal cortex in the brain, which are in control of rewarding adaptive behaviors through the release of the neurotransmitter dopamine. Binge eating, sexual gratification, and addictive substances trigger the release of dopamine, which not only produces pleasure but also conditions the brain to desire these behaviors and assign them a high priority. **Adaptive** activities (those with survival value) such as sex and eating are typically rewarded with a moderate and appropriate level of dopamine. Compulsive behaviors, however, cause the brain to release an excess of dopamine. As a result, when the behavior or substance is withdrawn, dopamine levels fall below normal. Abnormally low dopamine levels cause symptoms of distress such as severe depression, angst, anger, self-hatred, and guilt. The individual becomes physiologically incapable of feeling good without the addictive behavior or substance.

The action of cocaine is representative of this phenomenon. Because of the blockage of dopamine reuptake by cocaine, dopamine remains in the synapse much longer, continuing to stimulate dopamine receptors, resulting in a longer and stronger feeling of pleasure. This can result in desensitization and tolerance. Abnormally high dopamine level in the presence of cocaine reduces the number of dopamine receptors in the post-synaptic neuron. Subsequently, in the absence of cocaine, dopamine uptake is reduced below normal, leading to cravings and the symptoms of withdrawal.

The need to stimulate dopamine production causes a person to focus exclusively on attempting to repeat the compulsive behavior that produced the original dopamine surge, even though the behavior also caused the depletion of dopamine. Essentially, the need for drugs, alcohol, sex, bingeing, or gambling becomes more important—in order to restore dopamine levels to normal—than the need for adaptive behaviors. This perspective on compulsive behaviors is consistent with both incentive theory and drive reduction theory.

A further complication is that acute physical dependence can develop with certain substances, resulting in a biological requirement for it. Alcohol, for instance, is dangerously addictive. Improper detoxification of a compulsive alcoholic may cause fatal disruptions in the neurobiological and physiological processes that depend upon alcohol. Other substances such as opiates may not induce fatal withdrawal symptoms, but abruptly quitting without medical intervention can leave an individual in physical agony for as long as a month.

> **NEUROBIOLOGY OF ADDICTION**
>
> In addiction, cravings, withdrawals, and compulsive behaviors are driven by the depletion of dopamine levels and the need to increase dopamine production.

SOCIOCULTURAL FACTORS. Compulsive behavior in an individual may originate from sociocultural factors. Social cognitive theory explains that people are motivated to acquire new behaviors in order to gain approval or avoid rejection from their peers, even if the behaviors have clearly negative consequences. In other words, the need for peer approval becomes stronger than the need for behaviors that have biological survival value.

ATTITUDE

Attitude is a favorable or unfavorable appraisal of another person, group, event, or object that is expressed through one's behavior, emotions, or beliefs. Attitudes can be either implicitly held or outwardly expressed. The three primary components of an attitude are **cognitive** (beliefs and ideas), **affective** (emotional components such as anger, fear, joy, love, sympathy, depression), and **behavioral** (actions.)

> **ATTITUDE**
>
> The components of attitude include beliefs, emotions, and actions.

Attitudes serve four functions. First, they allow people to connect with others who have similar views. Second, they help people develop a store of knowledge about their environment. Third, they provide people a way to express their beliefs to others. Fourth, attitudes are **ego-defensive** in that individuals often use them as a means of defending self-esteem. Attitudes are used as defense mechanisms—such as denial, justification, or projection—to assuage guilt and defend a sense of self-worth.

Attitude development is determined by several factors. Personal experiences such as success or failure, education level, parental influence, or cultural expectations contribute significantly to one's general perspective. Social interaction and observation are also key contributors to attitude development.

The Link Between Attitude and Behavior

Attitudes influence and lead to behaviors. If a person believes that it is good to recycle, that person will tend to save recyclable products and deliver them to a recycling location. Behavior in turn can influence attitude. If the same person is in a hurry to pick up a friend from the airport and throws a recyclable object into the garbage, the person may reframe the attitude by saying that sometimes friendships are more important than recycling. Social psychologists have concluded that people often do not act in accord with the attitudes that they claim to hold. When there is a conflict between a held attitude (recycling is good) and other pressures (need to pick up friend), the resulting mental discomfort (**cognitive dissonance**) usually results in a shift in the attitude ("sometimes a friend is more important than an object"). Once the shift has occurred, the mental discomfort disappears.

HOW ATTITUDE INFLUENCES BEHAVIOR. Although attitude is generally a poor determinant of behavior, there are certain conditions in which the influence of attitude is more pronounced. The **theory of planned behavior**, introduced by Icek Ajben and Martin Fishbein in 1977, proposes that attitude has more power in influencing behavior under three conditions. They argued that the factors that make it more likely that attitude will lead to behavior are the person's relationship to social norms and behavioral consequences, how specific an attitude is to a given situation, and the person's perception of control in a situation.

In the first case, if an individual is not overly swayed by social norms and consequences, it is more likely that, when there is a conflict between what society expects and what the person believes, the person's behavior will be consistent with the person's attitudes.

The second case has to do with how specific an attitude is toward a given situation. For example, a person who holds a belief that it is good to support local business may be only minimally motivated to attend a game of a local baseball team. However, a person who holds the specific belief that it is important to support your local baseball team at the first game of their season is highly likely to act on that belief.

Finally, people's perception of control in a situation influences their attitude about the feasibility of performing a task. The more control people perceive, the more likely they are to act according to their attitudes.

The influence of attitude on behavioral outcomes also depends on situational conditions. Attitudes that result from experience tend to be more stable, as are attitudes that are habitually accessed and exhibited. Attitude is also more consistently expressed when the individual is an expert

> **ATTITUDE, BEHAVIOR, AND CONTROL**
>
> The more control people perceive they have in a situation, the more likely they will take the attitude that a task is manageable and will work to achieve that task.

on the subject under consideration. Expectations of reward or punishment influence attitude expression, as well as situations in which an individual risks losing something valued as a consequence of the behavior.

HOW BEHAVIOR INFLUENCES ATTITUDE. People's own behaviors can cause their beliefs to change, as in the example above of the person who concludes that sometimes friends are more important than recycling. In addition, people often actively attempt to change the beliefs of others. The **foot-in-the-door** phenomenon is an effective behavioral strategy, frequently used in sales, for changing the attitudes of others. The ultimate goal is to subtly encourage others to comply with a request. The technique involves first getting another person to agree to an insubstantial proposition before introducing a more considerable one. The technique is effective due to our tendency to behave in accordance with the **theory of successive approximations**. The theory states that individuals who comply with smaller demands are more inclined to sustain a behaviorally consistent course of action, thus compelling them to agree to a more demanding plea.

> ### SHAPING BEHAVIOR
>
> The theory of successive approximations is used by parents when they reward children for engaging in a behavior that is close to the desired behavior in order to teach the children to behave in the desired manner.

Further reasoning behind the foot-in-the-door phenomenon is founded on our inherent social tendencies. Compliance with the initial, reasonable request establishes a simple relationship between the requester and requestee. The requestee justifies his or her own compliance by imagining that he or she is in a partnership with the solicitor. When a greater demand is then placed upon the requestee, he or she feels obligated to agree in order to avoid discomfort.

The **role-playing effect** also influences attitudes. In 1972, Phillip Zimbardo conducted a now classic experiment that exemplifies the degree to which role-playing behavior can dramatically affect attitude, even if only temporarily. His objective was to determine whether prison abuse resulted from the innate, anti-social personalities of guards and prisoners or from the fact that both parties changed their attitudes in order to conform to role expectations. Zimbardo constructed a mock prison in a building on the Stanford campus and recruited 24 average and emotionally stable young men to act as prisoners and guards. By the second day of the experiment, the behavior of the "guards" had degenerated to the point of psychological abuse and vicious retribution against "prisoners." They humiliated, separated, isolated, and even withheld food and clothing from their fellow students. "Prisoners" became unruly, defiant, and eventually riotous, resulting in an abrupt end to the ordeal because of ethical concerns.

The Zimbardo experiment illustrates how completely people can become absorbed by a role, even when their values, ethics, and morality are severely compromised. Zimbardo reported that some participants even experienced an identity crisis and severe disturbance as a result of completely assuming an alternate personality. As another example, conformity to gender-role expectations has been shown to affect the values of young women, causing them to downplay strength, independence, and intelligence in an effort to attract men.

COGNITIVE DISSONANCE THEORY. Cognitive dissonance theory, advanced in 1957 by Leon Festinger, is central to understanding the association between attitude and behavior. Festinger proposed that individuals feel anxious when they experience inconsistency, or dissonance, in thought or behavior. They consequently modify their attitudes in order to restore integrity. Dissonance is especially pronounced under three distinct conditions. First, dissonance is strongest when the conflicting cognition is central to one's value system, identity, and self-esteem. Second, the degree of variance between two conflicting cognitions impacts the stress that an individual experiences. Finally, individuals are especially anxious when they fail to sufficiently justify or explain the reasons for conflicting thoughts.

In order to resolve the conflict and alleviate stress, individuals employ one of three strategies for dissonance reduction. They can either change their behavior in order to align themselves with dissonant thought, justify their behavior by changing belief, or account for their behavior by adding new principles.

STRESS

Stress is a state of physiological and/or emotional tension due to a life circumstance that presents a challenge.

The Nature of Stress

The amount of stress experienced in most situations is dependent on the individual's **appraisal** of the stressful situation. Appraisals can be highly subjective. The first step of appraisal involves determining whether a challenge is negative or positive. A positive challenge involves a situation that the individual believes will result in a benefit even though it may require a significant effort. A negative challenge is one in which the individual believes the result may be harmful or painful. In the face of a negative challenge, the amount of stress experienced by the individual depends on the individual's appraisal of how harmful the situation might be and how likely the individual is to overcome the challenge.

TYPES OF STRESSORS. Stressors can be classified by the amount of stress they are perceived to evoke in an individual. The Holmes and Rahe stress scale ranks 43 major life events in order of stressfulness. Included in this list are events such as weddings, births, deaths, or moving. Crisis/catastrophes/cataclysmic events are those that are beyond the control of the individual and that have a broad negative effect, such as an earthquake or a war. Micro-stressors include the annoyances of everyday life. Ambient stressors are environmental factors that may or may not have an impact on the individual, such as crowds, noise, or bad weather.

EFFECTS OF STRESS ON PSYCHOLOGICAL FUNCTION. Stress can produce physical, emotional, and/or mental exhaustion (burnout). Stress can also produce impaired task performance, such as increased distractibility, overthinking, or freezing up on tasks. **Post-traumatic stress disorder** is a manifestation of a trauma-based mental health diagnosis that includes symptoms of flashbacks, avoidance, fears, and irritability. Finally, stress can produce or contribute to other psychological disorders such as anxiety, depression, sexual dysfunction, schizophrenia, insomnia, nightmares, poor school/work functioning, eating disorders, and/or alcohol use/dependence.

Outcomes and Responses to Stress

Individuals express and respond to stress in physical, emotional, and behavioral ways.

PHYSIOLOGICAL. The body adapts physiologically to stress through the **general adaptation syndrome (GAS)** (see Figure 6.3). There are three stages to the syndrome. In the alarm phase, the stress is recognized and the body prepares for flight or fight. In the resistance phase, the body adapts to ongoing stress, such as by shutting down certain systems to conserve energy.

In the exhaustion phase, the body loses the ability to continue fighting the stress and collapse may result.

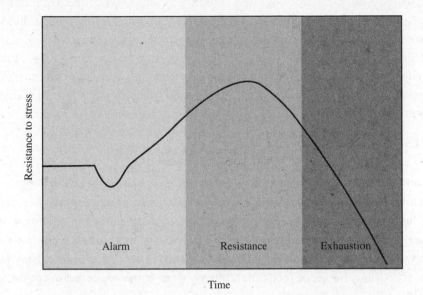

Figure 6.3. General adaptation syndrome. (Courtesy of David. G. Myers.)

EMOTIONAL. The emotional responses to stress include fear, anxiety, depression, disempowerment, loss of interest, motivation, esteem, suicidality, hopelessness, helplessness, guilt, shame, anger, rage, or ambivalence.

BEHAVIORAL. The behavioral response to stress may be withdrawal, isolation, depressive actions, anxiety, suicidal thoughts or behaviors, psychomotor agitation, irritability, aggression, hostility, violence, decompensation, increase or decrease in sleeping or eating habits, increase in substance use/abuse, and/or increase in accidents/distractibility.

Stress Management

Ongoing or repeated stress can weaken the immune system and reduce the energy available to cope with life situations. Stress can be managed in ways that are positive (lead to long term benefit) or negative (involve short-term stress reduction but long-term harm). Examples of **positive stress management** include relaxation, exercise, spiritual activities, meditation, guided imagery, changing the stressful situation, changing the way one thinks about the situation, or distracting oneself. **Negative stress management** may include activities such as cutting/superficial self-harm, addiction/dependence on drugs/food/or alcohol, or attempting suicide.

Social Constructs of Behavior

Individual behavior is affected not only by biological and genetic factors but also by social factors, specifically by the impact of the presence of others on individual behavior.

SOCIAL FACILITATION

The mere presence of other people can significantly impact an individual's performance on certain tasks. According to social facilitation theory, being observed while attempting to complete an exercise can either improve or diminish one's performance depending upon whether the task assigned is simple and familiar or complex and novel. The presence of others causes physiological arousal, often resulting in improved concentration, heightened awareness, and increased drive. When a task is familiar and uncomplicated, individuals typically improve in its execution when others are present. However, when a task is unfamiliar and complex, having others present usually results in poor task performance. This is attributed to the fact that, when engaged in a challenging task, individuals are often less confident and self-assured. Consequently, having an audience tends to elicit fear of judgment and nervousness.

TEST QUESTION

Jerry and Maria are both trying out for drill team. Jerry has been busy with homework and family obligations and therefore has been unable to practice. Maria has skipped doing her homework in order to have more time to practice for the drill team. When they arrive at the tryouts, they are surprised to find that many of their peers are present to watch the event. Jerry and Maria look at each other and express a high degree of anxiety. Using the social facilitation theory, what is the expected outcome of the tryouts?

(A) Jerry and Maria both perform poorly.

(B) Jerry performs better than expected, but Maria performs worse than expected.

(C) Jerry performs worse than expected, but Maria performs better than expected.

(D) Jerry and Maria both perform better than expected.

(C) Social facilitation theory states that the anxiety provoked by an audience improves performance for an individual who has been practicing the skill while it hinders performance for one who has not practiced.

DEINDIVIDUATION

Deindividuation is the process by which individuals relinquish their identity and norms of behavior when they immerse themselves in a group. Deindividuation theory states that when individuals become part of a group, they tend to adopt and support the identity of the group, leaving them potentially vulnerable to influence. Being a group member may cause individuals to become less self-aware and more susceptible to social pressure from other group members. Consequently, they may find themselves exhibiting behaviors that they otherwise would find reprehensible. This phenomenon can be attributed to two factors.

DEINDIVIDUATION

In deindividuation, individuals become vulnerable to the influence of others when they set aside their own identity to immerse themselves in a group identity.

Anonymity

When part of a larger group, individuals might feel less inhibited due to their apparent anonymity. Individuals in a group may become convinced that they will not be held accountable for their behavior.

Diffusion of Responsibility

Another reason that individuals in a group often feel less personal accountability for their actions is that they hold the group as a whole responsible, diminishing their personal contribution to the behavior of the group.

BYSTANDER EFFECT

The **bystander effect** is a social psychological theory that explains why individuals in a group may not feel compelled to offer assistance in an emergency situation. According to the bystander effect theory, people are less likely to offer help in an emergency situation if there are other people present witnessing the event. When there are others present, individuals tend to feel less personal responsibility to act, often believing that somebody else will intervene. Furthermore, the presence of others may increase pressure on an individual to conform to the behaviors of the group. Consequently, if no one else in the group is showing alarm, an individual may often feel pressured to exhibit ambivalence, as well.

SOCIAL LOAFING

Social loafing theory proposes that individuals tend to exert less effort when they are part of a group than when they are working alone. When an individual is working independently, he or she is solely responsible for an assignment and is typically more motivated and accountable. When working as group members, individuals often exert less effort because they tend to assume that the other members will take responsibility. Typically, larger groups experience more social loafing because individual members conclude that their participation will not significantly effect the group's overall success.

PEER PRESSURE

Peer pressure is the influence that an individual's peers exert on that individual's behavior. More specifically, peer pressure is based on an individual's perception—which may or may not be accurate—of the peers' expectations of how the individual should behave. Although the influence of a peer group can have a positive effect on identity formation, the term "peer pressure" typically refers to the negative effect when an individual feels compelled to act in a way that conflicts with his or her core values because of expectations of the peer group. Acting in this way can undermine identity and self-worth. Negative influence may result in adverse behavior, such as bullying, experimentation with drugs or alcohol, promiscuity, criminal activity, or disinterest in school.

GROUP PROCESSES

Group polarization and **groupthink** are processes that affect the behavior of individuals in a group setting.

Group Polarization

This is the process by which decision-making groups may arrive at decisions that are more ideologically extreme than the preferences of each individual group member. If the members of a group are individually inclined to take a risk, the group decision will involve a more extreme degree of risk. If the members tend to be cautious, the group decision will involve more extreme caution. Group polarization occurs in part because members of the group tend to overstate their position in order to influence others. At the same time, members want to be accepted by others in the group and may change their attitudes to match the exaggerated attitudes that they hear being expressed.

Groupthink

Groupthink is the tendency of a decision-making group to make fundamentally unsound and potentially harmful decisions as a result of emphasizing group harmony over rationality. Groupthink is especially pronounced when a group is under pressure, resulting in insufficient examination of evidence, dismissal of outside opinion, failure to devise alternate plans, and decreased concern for potential hazards.

EIGHT CONDITIONS THAT CONTRIBUTE TO GROUPTHINK

1. Illusion of invulnerability
2. Collective rationalization for decisions
3. A group belief in the inherent morality of their actions
4. Stereotyped or critical opinions of outside criticism
5. Direct pressure on dissenters within the group
6. An illusion of unity
7. Individual censorship of opinion that conflicts with group ideology
8. Self-appointed "mind guards" who conceal external censure from fellows

---

Employing certain key strategies in group processes can counteract groupthink. The group leader should remain neutral and encourage discussion of alternative viewpoints. Outside opinion should be solicited. Groups should be separated into smaller units on occasion to alleviate pressure and encourage evaluation. Finally, voting should be anonymous, allowing the individuals the freedom to express dissent without fear of reprisal.

Learning, Attitude, and Behavior

Learning is the process of acquiring new knowledge, behaviors, or attitudes. The many complex processes for learning and the theories that describe these processes are summarized for easy review below.

ASSOCIATIVE LEARNING

Associative learning is the process of learning through the development of automatic, conditioned responses in the presence of specific stimuli. Associative learning is the most straightforward manner in which humans learn novel behaviors, biases, abilities, and beliefs.

> **LEARNING**
>
> Learning occurs through conditioned (automatic, unconscious) as well as through conscious (observation, verbal instruction) processes.

Classical Conditioning

Ivan Pavlov advanced the theory now known as classical conditioning in the late nineteenth century after conducting a biological experiment that was designed to study digestion in dogs. Pavlov noticed that, over time, the dogs' physical responses to food subtly changed. The dogs typically salivated when food was placed before them, but their mouths began to water far before the food arrived. He discovered that the dogs were responding to sounds that were consistently present during feeding, such as the sound of the food cart entering the laboratory. He thus concluded that the animals had essentially been trained to associate certain sounds with food and salivated in anticipation of being fed.

The theory of classical conditioning details the process by which an individual learns to respond to a new stimulus by associating it with presence of a previously conditioned stimulus. In his experiments, Pavlov first observed and recorded the dogs' **unconditioned response (UR)**, or automatic reaction, to an **unconditioned stimulus (US)**, or a stimulus that elicits an automatic response. In this case, Pavlov noted that the dogs salivated in response to food.

He next introduced a **neutral stimulus (NS)**. Initially, a neutral stimulus does not produce a response relative to the unconditioned stimulus. Pavlov rang a bell each time the dogs received food. At first, the bell elicited no response. After a period of time, the dogs began to associate the sound of the bell with eating. Eventually, the animals began to salivate at the sound of the bell alone, a behavior that Pavlov labeled the **conditioned response (CR)**. The sound of the bell was initially a neutral stimulus but became a **conditioned stimulus (CS)**, a stimulus that through conditioning comes to elicit a response.

Pavlov recorded several phenomena that frequently occur with the process of conditioning. He first described the process of **acquisition**, or the initial stages of learning a CR. Pavlov determined that successful acquisition depended upon both the noticeability of the stimulus and the time elapsed between the introduction of the US and NS. His second finding was that a CR is vulnerable to **extinction**, becoming weaker and eventually vanishing when the CS is frequently supplied in the absence of the US. **Spontaneous recovery**, retrieval of the CR, could just as easily occur, even after a substantial amount of time has passed. Finally, Pavlov observed **stimulus generalization** and **discrimination**. Stimulus generalization occurs when the CR is induced by an unrelated stimuli that resembles the CS. Stimulus discrimination is the process by which one learns to differentiate between the CS and other stimuli that are associated with but not equivalent to the CS.

Operant Conditioning

The fundamental differences between classical conditioning and **operant conditioning** lie in the nature of the stimuli applied in order to influence behavior, when the stimuli are applied, and the type of behavior that is affected, as shown in Table 6.7.

Table 6.7 A Comparison of Classical and Operant Conditioning

	Type of Stimulus	When Applied	Type of Behavior
Classical	Neutral	Before behavior	Involuntary
Operant	Positive or negative	After behavior	Voluntary

Thus, operant conditioning attempts to increase or decrease the likelihood of a voluntary behavior by applying certain stimuli after the occurrence of a behavior. Operant conditioning is concerned with observable external behaviors rather than with the measurement of internal mental events. In operant conditioning, stimuli that increase the chances of a particular behavior involve **reinforcement**, and stimuli that decrease the likelihood of a behavior involve **punishment**.

TYPES OF REINFORCEMENT. Reinforcers are either primary or secondary. A **primary reinforcer** is a stimulus that has an inherently pleasant effect, such as food and sex. Primary reinforcers are also referred to as **unconditioned** because nearly all individuals experience them as pleasant without having to learn to do so. **A secondary reinforcer** is a stimulus that by itself is neutral but has been conditioned to be experienced as pleasant because it has been paired with another stimulus that is already pleasant. An example is the chime of a kitchen timer that is regularly used to indicate that cookies in the oven are ready to eat. Hearing the chime is enough to make the mouth begin to water.

Reinforcement can be either positive or negative. **Positive reinforcement** involves the application of a stimulus (**reinforcer**) after a behavior, such that the frequency of the behavior increases. Typically, a positive reinforcer is experienced as pleasant. An example would be giving a child ice cream after the child completes a homework assignment, with the result that the child is more likely to complete the next homework assignment.

Negative reinforcement involves the removal of an unpleasant (**aversive**) stimulus after a behavior. For example, if a student feels anxious because a homework assignment is due soon, the completion of the homework assignment results in the removal of the negative stimulus (anxiety). The removal of the anxiety is pleasant and increases the likelihood that the student will complete a homework assignment in the future.

Escape and avoidance learning are examples of negative reinforcement. **Escape** involves removing an aversive stimulus, such as washing the dishes in order to stop someone from complaining that the dishes were not washed. **Avoidance** involves preventing an aversive stimulus from occurring, such as not going home because someone there might complain that the dishes were not washed. In both cases, the likelihood of a behavior increases (washing the dishes or staying away from home) because the behavior removes or avoids an aversive stimulus.

Practice Question

An author is writing a book about psychology. Each time that her coauthor calls on the phone to talk about the project, the author's dog barks. To quiet the dog, the author picks it up. After a few months of this behavior, she picks up the dog each time she sits down to write. Describe the learning process that the author went through.

Solution: Through operant conditioning, the author learned to pick up the dog each time that she sat down to write. The barking is the negative stimulus. It was applied after she sat down and answered the phone. The author's decision to pick up the dog was voluntary.

PUNISHMENT. Punishment and negative reinforcement are often confused. Table 6.8 outlines the differences between the types of reinforcement and punishment.

Table 6.8 A Comparison of Punishment and Reinforcement

	Pleasant Stimulus	Aversive Stimulus
Punishment	Remove *(Negative punishment)*	Apply *(Positive punishment)*
Reinforcement	Apply *(Positive reinforcement)*	Remove *(Negative reinforcement)*

Note the difference between punishment and negative reinforcement. Punishment diminishes the likelihood that a behavior will occur. It is accomplished either by applying an aversive stimulus or removing a pleasant one. Negative reinforcement results in increasing the likelihood of a behavior through the removal of an aversive stimulus.

The following are examples of positive and negative punishment.

POSITIVE PUNISHMENT: A child does not complete a homework assignment and the parent spanks the child (applying an aversive stimulus—spanking).

NEGATIVE PUNISHMENT: A child does not complete a homework assignment and the parent takes away the child's electronic game (removing a positive stimulus—the game).

SHAPING AND EXTINCTION. Shaping is the process of reinforcing a complex behavior by successively reinforcing approximations of that behavior. For example, to teach a cat to jump through a flaming hoop, one might first reinforce the cat stepping over the hoop, then reinforce the cat stepping over a slightly raised hoop, then jumping through the hoop, and then jumping through the hoop while only part of the hoop is burning, and then while the entire hoop is burning.

Extinction refers to the fact that a behavior that is not reinforced tends to eventually decrease in frequency. If a child has regularly gotten ice cream after cleaning the bathroom, if the parents stop giving ice cream, the child will tend to stop cleaning the bathroom. When the parents first stop giving ice cream, the child might experience an **extinction burst**, in which the child frantically cleans the bathroom even more frequently than before, hoping that this will result in ice cream. When it does not, the extinction burst ends and the behavior of cleaning the bathroom becomes less frequent because of extinction.

> **PARTIAL REINFORCEMENT SCHEDULES**
>
> Four types:
> 1. fixed interval
> 2. variable interval
> 3. fixed ratio
> 4. variable ratio

REINFORCEMENT SCHEDULES. A reinforcement schedule is a specific plan that outlines exactly how often and under what conditions reinforcement is applied. A reinforcement schedule can be either continuous or partial. In a continuous reinforcement schedule, the targeted behavior is reinforced each time that it occurs. During phases of early learning, this type of a reinforcement schedule is important to reinforce the positive association between the desired behaviors and the rewards. After the behavior has been learned, it is more effective to switch to a partial reinforcement schedule.

Using the partial reinforcement schedule, behavior is reinforced only a portion of the time, rather than after every response. One benefit of partial reinforcement is that the response is less likely to be subject to extinction. There are four variations of partial reinforcement: fixed interval schedule, variable interval schedule, fixed ratio schedule, and a variable ratio schedule. A fixed interval schedule reinforces an individual after a set period of time, for example, giving a treat every 30 minutes. A variable interval schedule is reinforced after an unpredictable amount of time, for example, giving a treat at random time intervals.

Fixed ratio schedules reward individuals after a specified number of responses, for example, giving a treat every fourth time that a subject answers correctly. In a variable ratio schedule, a reinforcement is provided after a variable number of responses, for example, giving a treat after a random number of correct answers. With a variable ratio schedule the subject is likely to perform the rewarded action more times without a reward because he or she has learned that the reward may come at unpredictable intervals. This model is frequently used in casinos and explains why a person who has won money at a slot machine once may continue playing—and losing—for hours, hoping that the reward will come again at some unpredictable time.

TEST QUESTION

Receiving a paycheck twice a month is an example of which type of reinforcement schedule?

(A) Fixed interval schedule

(B) Variable interval schedule

(C) Fixed ratio schedule

(D) Variable ratio schedule

(A) A paycheck received twice a month is on a fixed interval.

Cognitive Processes that Affect Associative Learning

Associative learning is an intrinsic ability and therefore is usually an automatic and largely unconscious process. However, cognitive processes can either reinforce or counteract the associative learning. Consider a situation in which parents read a story to a child at bedtime only if the child has not complained when asked to go to bed. The child has learned to respond to the request "time to go to bed" by avoiding complaining. If it occurs to the child that it would be nice to hear two stories instead of one (a cognitive realization), the next time the child hears "time to go to bed" there might be a different response, such as "If I'm really good, will you read me two stories?" This is an example of a cognitive process changing the conditioned response in the direction of reinforcement.

If the child would very much like to go outside and play with friends instead of going to bed, the response to "time to go to bed" might be to sweetly beg to be allowed to go outside and play. The learned response of not complaining still applies but it has been modified to lead in a different direction—going outside instead of going to bed. This is again the result of a cognitive awareness.

There is a famous but most likely untrue story about a psychology class that decided to condition the professor—who originally spoke in a formal way from behind the podium—to eventually sit on the edge of the stage and lecture informally. This was supposedly done by the students being attentive when the professor moved forward toward the edge of the stage and talking among themselves when the professor moved back toward the podium. In some variations of the story, the professor was trained to stand on a wastebasket while lecturing. Whether the story is true or not, such associative learning depends on the fact that the subject is not consciously aware of being trained. As soon as there is a cognitive awareness, cognition takes over to either acquiesce with the process or resist it.

Biological Factors that Affect Associative Learning

Associative learning is influenced by biologically **innate** (instinctive) **behavior**, as well as by learned behaviors. Examples of innate behaviors in humans are mating, feeding, nursing their young, "nesting" instincts, protective instincts, and expressing emotions. **Learned behavior** requires practice, training, or reinforcement.

Biological preparedness is the genetically inherent tendency to form associations that will enhance survival. For example, a fear of snakes, rats, or spiders in humans is biologically adaptive and enhances survival.

HABITUATION AND DISHABITUATION

In associative learning a positive or negative reinforcement influences the likelihood of a response to a stimulus. However, even in cases in which there is neither a positive nor a negative reinforcement, behavior can be influenced by a continual exposure to a stimulus. Such learning in the absence of reinforcement is called **nonassociative learning**. In nonassociative learning, changes in behavior occur through habituation or dishabituation.

Habituation

When a person is exposed to a stimulus over a period of time, the response to the stimulus decreases, provided there is no reinforcement. This process is called **habituation**. Habituation occurs with both positive and negative responses. For example, a person who buys a new painting may have a strong feeling of pleasure when first viewing it, but with time the feeling diminishes. Similarly, a person at a new job may find the new situation highly stressful but with time the stress decreases. In each case the individual develops a physical and/or psychological tolerance to the stimulus, essentially becoming acclimated to its effects.

Habituation should be distinguished from sensory adaptation. Sensory adaptation (for example during exposure to strong light or a loud sound) is a neural response to a simple sensory input and occurs in the brain. Habituation occurs throughout the body in response to a more complex stimulus.

Dishabituation

In **dishabituation**, a response that has been diminished through habituation returns when the stimulus is removed for a period of time and then reintroduced. Alternately, dishabituation can occur when the stimulus is paired with a new stimulus that tends to evoke the initial response. If the new painting is removed for a week, the owner may feel the original excitement again on viewing it when it is returned.

OBSERVATIONAL LEARNING

Observational learning is learning by watching and repeating what someone else is doing. Observational learning is fundamentally imitation and is a characteristically human form of learning, though other animals also learn by observation. Observational learning is particularly important for children, who may rely on it to a greater degree than do adults. Gross physical activity—such as walking, running, throwing, dancing—is particularly suitable for observational learning. Subtler physical activities, such as hand motions (using a phone, turning on lights, gesturing) and facial expression, may also be learned through observation. Predominantly mental activities—reading, solving problems—may have only a very small observable component and thus are not learnable observationally. However, the aspect that is observable might be copied, such as when a child pretends to read.

In many cases the person being observed is not aware that someone is learning from them. However, a person might also consciously demonstrate (**model**) a behavior in order to teach someone else. Modeling is an important method of teaching because it is independent of verbal instruction.

There is a biological basis to the observational learning process. **Mirror neurons** are brain cells that are activated both when an individual performs an action and when an individual sees someone perform the action. In this way, observing an action becomes a mental rehearsal for performing the action, laying the foundation for observational learning. Mirror neurons explain why, when watching football on TV and seeing the quarterback get tackled, people flinch as if they feel it themselves. Mirror neurons are also responsible for the vicarious experience of emotions, such as feeling sad when observing a person who is crying.

Observational learning is important to consider in the context of explaining individual behaviors. Impressionable people might view someone who they admire in some way, such as being successful, attractive, or confident, as a model for behaviors that might prove to be antisocial or harmful. Much maladaptive teen behavior can be explained by this kind of observational learning, including cutting, drug use, and sex games. On the other hand, people can also learn positive behaviors such as kindness, generosity, or selflessness through observation.

THEORIES OF ATTITUDE AND BEHAVIOR CHANGE

There are several theoretical models for understanding changes in attitude and behavior that are involved in learning.

Elaboration Likelihood Model

The **elaboration likelihood model (ELM)** is a theory of attitude change that describes how motivation level, knowledge, and ability influence one's response to persuasive messages. According to ELM, attitude change can occur through either a **central** or **peripheral route**. Central route processing occurs when an individual is eager to hear the message and is cognitively capable of interpreting the information. Central route processing allows an individual to more thoroughly and critically appraise the persuasive message, resulting in an informed decision. Peripheral route processing occurs when there is little motivation to learn about the topic or if the topic exceeds cognitive abilities. In this case, the individual focuses on peripheral information, or information that is unrelated to the persuasive message, and tends to make more impulsive attitudinal decisions.

Social Cognitive Theory

Developed by Albert Bandura in 1977, **social cognitive theory** states that motivation is driven by both intrinsic (internal) factors and external factors, such as the observation of others and expectation of reward. According to Bandura, an individual observes the behavior of others and whether that behavior has positive or negative consequences. Based on this observation, the individual is either likely or unlikely to imitate the behavior. The external factors are the behavior of others and the consequences of that behavior. The internal factors are the evaluation of whether or not to imitate the behavior.

Factors that Affect Attitude Change

In addition to the abovementioned factors that contribute to attitude, how readily a person's attitudes change depends on many factors, such as age and personality traits. In general, children more readily change their attitudes compared to middle-aged adults, who tend to change more readily than the elderly. People with more flexible or accommodating personalities are more likely to change attitudes than people with rigid personality traits.

SELF-PERCEPTION AND INTERACTION WITH SOCIETY

The development of the personal self is the foundation for the interactions between people that form the basis of society. This section reviews the formation of self-identity, the attitudes and beliefs that influence social interactions, and behaviors and processes that underlie social interactions.

The Notion of Self and Identity Formation

This section outlines the processes involved in the formation of the notion of self and the sense of identity.

SELF-CONCEPT AND IDENTITY

This section reviews definitions of identity, the role of self-esteem and locus of control, and types of identities.

> **SELF AND SOCIETY**
>
> Just as the physical organism interfaces with the environment in which it exists, the self must interface effectively with society.

Definitions

The terms self-concept, identity, and social identity are defined below.

SELF-CONCEPT. Self-concept refers to perception of oneself as an individual and as a member of various social groups. Self-concept is an assessment of oneself based on such factors as sexuality, racial identity, socioeconomic status, and gender. These largely universal characteristics are referred to as **self-schemas**. Self-schemas are reevaluated and amended continuously throughout one's life. Consequently, self-concept becomes more complex with age and experience.

IDENTITY. Identity is each individual's unique expansion upon his or her self-concept. An individual's identity is formulated as one assesses and assigns meaning to one's self-concept. A person's identity encompasses that person's myriad values, beliefs, strengths, and weaknesses, which are all heavily influenced by environment. Consequently, one of the most significant contributors to identity development is an individual's interaction with other people and social systems. Charles Horton Cooley developed a key concept in identity formation, the idea of **the looking-glass self**, in 1902. Cooley argued that we continually evaluate others' reactions to our conduct and adjust our beliefs, values, and behavior to reflect other people's judgments. This phenomenon can result in a **self-fulfilling prophecy**. For instance, children who are told that they are capable and intelligent might begin to act as though they are capable and intelligent, ultimately confirming others' perception of them.

SOCIAL IDENTITY. Social identity is the aspect of a person's identity that includes the groups with which they associate. Individuals typically belong to various social groups, such as families, schools, clubs, or political parties. Membership in a social group, whether it is voluntary or compulsory, has a profound impact upon both one's identity formation and treatment of others. **Social identity theory**, proposed by Henri Tajfel in 1979, suggests that group membership provides one with self-esteem, belongingness, and validation. Group membership is so critical to self-regard that group members often develop contrary attitudes and behaviors toward nonmembers. This behavior, known as **in-group/out-group bias**, reflects humans' innate tendency to favor those similar to them. Bias is also an attempt by group members to elevate the prestige of their social group above "others," thereby contributing to their individual feeling of self-worth. In-group/out-group biases are the primary foundation for discrimination and prejudice.

The Role of Self-Esteem, Self-Efficacy, and Locus of Control in Self-Concept and Self-Identity

Self-esteem, self-efficacy, and locus of control play crucial roles in the development of self-concept and self-identity.

SELF-ESTEEM. This refers to individuals' perception of their overall value, purpose, and ability, and how they emotionally respond to this self-appraisal. Self-esteem is powerfully influenced by one's relationships with other people, beginning with the degree of nurturance and attention one receives as an infant. The quality of affection bestowed upon children has an indelible impact upon their perception of their intrinsic and extrinsic value. A child who experiences support, love, reasonable boundaries, encouragement, and security is more likely to develop positive coping mechanisms, healthy relationships with others, confidence, and resilience. Conversely, children exposed to neglect, abuse, irrational criticism, and unrealistic expectations often have difficulty functioning in society, manifested in symptoms such as depression, anxiety, insecurity, and unstable personal relationships.

Self-esteem is transformed during adolescence. During this period, relationships with others become more complex, and young adults begin to develop their own opinions about what is desirable and acceptable within their social world. Adolescents begin to compare their appearance, social skills, interests, athleticism, and intelligence to their peers, and ultimately judge themselves in relation to others. Acceptance or rejection by peers is especially important in self-esteem development during adolescence. Peer validation can result in confidence, increased motivation, and high self-worth. Conversely, rejection can be devastating, resulting in self-hatred, isolation, anger, and depression.

During adulthood, self-esteem becomes less dependent upon social feedback. Adults tend to evaluate their self-worth according to their own values and beliefs instead of the opinions of others. Adults base their self-esteem on such factors as their success at work, the quality of their relationships, personal integrity, and their degree of control over their environment. Even though self-esteem is well-established in adulthood, major life transitions can create a crisis. Birth, death, unemployment, and retirement are all scenarios in which one's self-esteem may be challenged and reevaluated.

SELF-EFFICACY. Self-efficacy can be defined as a person's sense that he or she has the tools and the ability to cope with life events. Individuals have an innate sense of their level of commitment, motivation, and ability when faced with a challenge or assignment. Individuals who have faith in their ability to perform a task effectively in order to achieve a goal are said to possess a high degree of self-efficacy. Self-efficacy shapes self-concept and identity by influencing an individual's approach to facing life challenges. Individuals with high self-efficacy generally are confident in their capabilities and effectiveness when working in pursuit of a goal. These people are consequently more enthusiastic, committed, driven, and less likely to give up following setbacks. Individuals with low self-efficacy have less faith in their ability to effect change and often attempt to avoid arduous tasks. They often lack motivation and perseverance and blame their own inadequacy for failures that they experience. Self-efficacy is an instrumental factor in determining an individual's response to the various trials faced in life. Self-efficacy has been proven an especially important determinant of the choices people make in regard to their physical health. High self-efficacy can mean the difference between life and death, as individuals with increased self-efficacy are more likely to alter their lifestyle (smoking, diet, exercise) and commit to change. People with low self-efficacy might instead feel as if they have no control over their body and no power to change health-related issues. They often relinquish their will, surrendering to illness or poor habits because they have no confidence in their ability to transform themselves.

LOCUS OF CONTROL. The term *locus of control* refers to individuals' perceptions of whether the events of their life are controlled by their own inner resources (**internal locus of control**) or by circumstances outside of their control (**external locus of control**). People with an internal locus of control feel as if they have a significant influence over the conditions in their environment. People with an external locus of control feel that other individuals or social systems have ultimate control. Whether one has an internal or external locus of control affects one's stress level, functioning, and overall quality of life. When one feels powerless, the emotional and physical self tend to suffer, and conditions related to poor self-esteem, such as depression, anxiety, and a fatalistic world view, may emerge. A classic example of the impact of external locus of control on identity is the decline in mental and physical health of elderly people who are transferred to nursing homes where they are not actively involved in the decision-making process. When power is relinquished, a sense of helplessness and worthlessness may set in, hastening their deterioration. On the other hand, having a strong internal locus of control can empower individuals, strengthening their self-worth and character. Elderly people who enter an assisted living situation where they are actively included in daily planning and encouraged to pursue personal interests have more positive emotional and physical outcomes.

Different Types of Identities

There are several categories of personal and social identity that individuals use to describe themselves and their connections with other people. The most commonly recognized are gender, sexual preference, nationality, race, religion, political beliefs, age, socioeconomic status, level of education, and occupation.

FORMATION OF IDENTITY

In humans, identity develops in predictable stages. The development of identity is influenced by other individuals, by groups, and by the culture as a whole, as well as by many biological and cognitive factors.

Stages of Identity Development

Identity formation is the development of an individual's unique identity and ultimate comprehension of how he or she fits into his or her social world (see Table 6.9). Identity formation, also called **individuation**, is the establishment of the characteristics that distinguish a person from other individuals and social groups. Several theories of identity formation have been advanced that attempt to outline the complex evolution of individual identity. Each theory contends that individuation occurs in stages and is influenced by a multitude of factors such as social environment, culture, biology, motivation, parental attachment, and judgment.

Table 6.9 Theories of Identity Development

Freud	Psychosexual development	Personality development is influenced by erogenous zones governed by the id. Personality development is complete in adolescence.
Erickson	Psychosocial development	Individuals must resolve developmental tasks, which are influenced by social and cultural factors. Personal growth continues throughout the lifespan.
Vygotsky	Sociocultural theory	Culture and socialization guide personality development and knowledge acquisition. Language is important in development.
Kohlberg	Theory of moral development	Moral development follows a path of fixed stages and is dependent upon cognitive abilities and social environment. Development continues throughout the lifespan.

FREUD'S THEORY OF PSYCHOSEXUAL DEVELOPMENT. Sigmund Freud advanced the foundational modern theory of identity formation in 1905. Freud theorized that an individual's personality develops in five distinct stages that focus on a particular erogenous zone in the body. Freud believed that humans are born with an inherent sexual drive, or **libido**, that guides one's progression through childhood. The libido is governed by the **id**, or the wellspring of an individual's subconscious, primal desires. Freud believed that it was crucial during the first five years of life that the individual learn to regulate the id through the development of **ego** (social norms) and **superego** (morals/values). He believed that failure to do so would result in psychological instability.

Each stage of psychosexual development features a conflict that must be resolved in order for a stable personality to develop. An individual's libidinous needs are either fulfilled, denied, or overindulged. If they are fulfilled, an individual advances unencumbered to the next stage. When needs are thwarted, tension and resentment arise. Overindulged needs result in a subconscious hesitancy to abandon the comfort of the present stage in order to progress. Overindulgence and underindulgence both create **fixation**, or the process by which the unsatisfied sexual needs from one stage cause **neurosis**, or mental dysfunction, that will govern character and behavior.

Freud's five stages of psychosexual development are:

1. **ORAL STAGE** (Birth–18 months). Erogenous zone = mouth. An infant is entirely driven by instinct, or id, and receives sustenance, comfort, and stimulation through the mouth. Infants instinctively breastfeed and explore their environment by placing objects in their mouths. If properly nurtured, infants will feel secure and will develop trust. The central conflict during the oral stage is weaning, or the discontinuation of breastfeeding and reduced reliance on the caregiver. Fixation at this stage results in a preoccupation with oral satisfaction, as exhibited through such behaviors as smoking, nail biting, or eating. Individuals fixated here may also tend to display an immature dependence upon others.

2. **ANAL STAGE** (18 months–3 years). Erogenous zone = anus. The anal stage is characterized by discipline via the development of the ego. During this stage, a child faces the task of toilet training, which involves redirecting the impulses of the id by learning to control bodily functions. A child also learns to apply this principle of self-control to its behavior, responding to parental expectations. Parental influence on toilet training significantly impacts the successful completion of the anal stage. Parents who approach their children at the appropriate time, issue reasonable requests, offer encouragement and understanding, and praise effort will foster a sense of competency and achievement in their child. Parents who are demanding and judgmental with toilet training may cause their child to develop an **anal-retentive personality**, characterized by anxiety, obsessiveness, and preoccupation with sanitation. Too much parental leniency may result in an **anal-expulsive** personality, featuring poor self-control, carelessness, and sloppy hygiene.

3. **PHALLIC STAGE** (3–6 years). Erogenous zone = genitalia. Through observation, children discern the physical difference between boys and girls. Freud believed that young boys were unconsciously sexually attracted to their mothers and girls to their fathers, creating both internal conflict and a rivalry with their same-sex parent. In young boys, the conflict known as the **Oedipus complex** is resolved when they ally themselves with their father, accepting his superiority over women. According to Freud, in girls, their **Electra complex** is rooted in **penis envy**, or the feelings of inadequacy that result from lacking a penis. When they eventually identify with the mother, resolving the conflict, they never truly overcome their sense of inferiority to men. Freud theorized that this was the source of insecurity and passivity in all women. If the central conflict of this stage is not resolved, uncontrollable or abnormal sexual compulsions may develop later in life, complicating the development of meaningful relationships.

4. **LATENCY STAGE** (6 years–puberty). Libido is inactive. During latency, sexual drive recedes for a period of time while social relationships are cultivated and interests are explored. The instinctive demands of the id are set aside in favor of ego development, or the process of learning to delay gratification. A child learns the importance of self-sacrifice and compromise in personal relationships.

5. **GENITAL STAGE** (puberty onward). Erogenous zone = genitalia. According to Freud, an interest and desire for members of the opposite sex (Freud did not address same sex

attraction in this stage) develops with the onset of sexual maturity at puberty. Individuals explore sexual relationships, identity, and accountability. Independence is featured, and ego directs behavior toward personal and mutual connections with others. Previously unresolved conflicts will create an inability to connect meaningfully with sexual partners and friends or to otherwise enjoy professional or intellectual fulfillment.

Freud's theory of psychosexual development transformed the modern approach to mental illness and personality disorders. Both were previously attributed to biological conditions such as neurological disease. Freud's theory shifted the focus to an individual's environmental conditions, social relationships, and self-perception. Freud was the first to propose that negative childhood experiences could profoundly obstruct healthy development by creating obsessiveness and insecurity. Although there were many contextual failings in Freud's theory, such as his negative view of women and homosexuality, his work has provided a firm foundation for a deeper understanding of the multiple factors that help shape an individual's identity.

ERIKSON'S STAGES OF PSYCHOSOCIAL DEVELOPMENT. Erik Erikson, a student of Freud, published his **theory of psychosocial development** in 1958. Freud's theory of psychosocial development organically influenced Erikson's theory, but Erikson proposed that human development was more heavily influenced by social interaction than by sexuality. Erikson also separated development into stages, but unlike Freud, he believed that personal growth does not end with adolescence. Instead, identity formation is a lifelong and highly interactive endeavor that only ends upon death.

Erikson embraced Freud's principle that personality is composed of the id, ego, and superego. However, Erikson argued that the ego, not the id, guided individuation. He proposed that social and cultural experiences shape the development of **ego identity**, or fundamental awareness of who we are as individuals. As people mature, the ego identity is regularly reevaluated and reconceptualized in accordance with our evolving understanding of the world. Erikson believed that individuals progress through eight distinct stages of development. In each stage, a psychosocial conflict based on environmental and social conditions is encountered. Individuals' successful resolution of this conflict determines the course of their development and affects their successful advancement through subsequent stages. If the conflict remains unresolved, the individual may struggle with related issues later in life. Erikson's eight stages follow:

> ### ERIKSON'S STAGES OF DEVELOPMENT
>
> Erikson's stages extend beyond adolescence. He believed that personal development continues throughout the lifetime.

1. **TRUST VERSUS MISTRUST** (Birth–18 months). The infant develops either basic trust or mistrust in others depending on the quality of care and nurturance received by caregivers. If the infant develops trusting relationships, it will emerge with a sense of hope.

2. **AUTONOMY VERSUS SHAME** (18 months–3 years). This stage is characterized by curiosity and experimentation. Children begin to investigate their world and attempt new behaviors. If their curiosity is safely encouraged, children develop a sense of competence and certainty. If attempts to explore are restricted or discouraged, children learn to doubt their abilities. Successful resolution of the conflict in this stage encourages the development of healthy determination.

3. **INITIATIVE VERSUS GUILT** (3–5 years). Children begin to take deliberate action to achieve goals. There is a marked effort to manipulate their environment and exert their will. For the first time, children experience guilt as they analyze the effects of their behavior and receive reward or punishment from others. If children are encouraged to take initiative,

they emerge from this stage with a sense of purpose and effectiveness. Children who encounter disapproval and discouragement experience guilt and shame.

4. **INDUSTRY VERSUS INFERIORITY** (5–12 years). School-aged children gradually become less focused on play-based learning and devote their energy to formal education. Children concentrate on both acquiring complex concepts and sharpening their abilities. Acknowledgment from parents, teachers, and peers is essential to the development of a positive self-concept. Children who receive encouragement approach adolescence with enhanced self-esteem, initiative, and a strong sense of competence. Children who are overly criticized or derided feel ashamed and inferior.

5. **IDENTITY VERSUS ROLE CONFUSION** (13–19 years). Erikson considers this stage to be the most crucial in healthy identity development. During adolescence, children experiment with individuality and determine how to function in accordance with the behavioral and social standards of their culture. According to Erikson, children undergo a pivotal yet essential **identity crisis** characterized by experimentation with authority, sexuality, boundaries, and obligations. Adolescents explore different roles, interests, and beliefs, and are heavily influenced by the opinions of their peers. Their effort to distinguish themselves as unique and independent may trigger conflict with parents and teachers. Adolescents often struggle with reconciling their childhood identity with their vision of who they hope to be as an adult. Beliefs and ideals adhered to as a child are sometimes abandoned as a more mature understanding of self emerges. Children emerge from this stage as young adults. If their healthy experimentation is fostered by adults and supported by peers, they attain **identity achievement**. Those whose attempts at individuation are rejected exhibit insecurity and might ultimately face confusion and conflict in regard to self-worth.

6. **INTIMACY VERSUS ISOLATION** (20–39 years). Ideally, adolescent experimentation recedes and individuals begin to seek fulfillment from their relationships with others. Friendships coalesce and romantic relationships deepen. If individuals are secure in their identity and willing to commit, they may find a permanent romantic partner. Those who successfully navigate relationship dynamics such as compromise and trust gain intimacy with and love for others. Individuals who retain adolescent self-doubt and confusion typically have more trouble with relationships and proceed through adulthood feeling lonely, isolated, anxious, or depressed.

7. **GENERATIVITY VERSUS STAGNATION** (40–64 years). The focus in middle adulthood is the desire to contribute in a meaningful way to society, work, and family in order to ensure stability for future generations. Love develops more complexity during parenthood, with the focus shifting away from sexual connection. Individuals strive for integrity and efficacy, longing for pride in their own achievements and in the accomplishments of their family members. Egocentric and greedy individuals fail to find deeper meaning in their lives and consequently experience stagnation.

8. **EGO INTEGRITY VERSUS DESPAIR** (65 years–death). The final stage of life is devoted to reflection upon the quality and impact of one's life. If individuals are satisfied with their personal relationships and professional achievements, ego integrity is achieved, and they feel as if their life has been meaningful. Conversely, if individuals have only failure and regret to reflect upon, they will fall into desolation and despair.

Erikson's theory of psychosocial development had a great impact on the field of psychotherapy. It emphasized the importance of early parental and social influence on children, ultimately influencing the focus of childcare and education. Erikson's theory also allows psychotherapists to identify and target any acquired behaviors, beliefs, influences, or maladaptive coping mechanisms that might have affected an individual's ability to function.

VYGOTSKY'S SOCIOCULTURAL THEORY. Lev Vygotsky developed his **theory of sociocultural development** in the early part of the twentieth century, roughly around the time that Jean Piaget's cognitive theory was published. However, the repressive political climate in Russia under Joseph Stalin prevented Vygotsky's work from becoming universally available until the 1970s. Since its publication and translation, however, the theory of sociocultural development has deepened our understanding of the role of culture and socialization in child development. Piaget theorized that children progress sequentially through a series of stages in which cognitive development necessarily precedes personality development. Vygotsky contends that sociocultural factors largely determine the direction of personality development and knowledge acquisition. Furthermore, he states that the most significant influence upon both personality and cognitive ability is a child's social interaction with parents, teachers, and other more experienced adults. Finally, Vygotsky focuses on the use and importance of language in the developmental process.

Vygotsky argues that infants are born with a universal set of **elementary mental functions** that become increasingly complex and refined through social interaction. These fundamental cognitive abilities are **attention**, **sensation**, **perception**, and **memory**. Children gradually acquire **higher mental functioning** as they interact with adults, learning cultural values and expectations. Each culture has distinct beliefs and practices concerning the most adaptive way to use one's intellectual capabilities. These **tools of intellectual adaptation** determine both the skills and values children learn and how they interpret this information. For instance, children in Western cultures are taught that reading and writing are essential to cognitive development. Children in these cultures are educated through the use of **cultural artifacts**, such as books, or through accepted practices, such as formal education. Children raised in a culture without a formal written language have no use for books or note taking. These cultures may emphasize oral traditions, such as storytelling, and use costumes or ceremonies as tools for education.

According to Vygotsky, children learn through a collaborative process in which they receive instruction (formal or informal) from a more experienced individual. The teacher, referred to as the **more knowledgeable other** (**MKO**), does not necessarily have to be an adult. An MKO must just possess more sophisticated skills and/or information than the child. Learning occurs in the **zone of proximal development**, defined as the assortment of concepts or skills that a child cannot complete on his or her own, but can accomplish with instruction and assistance from a MKO. When working collaboratively on a difficult task, a child follows the guidance of the instructor and learns to autonomously apply the acquired knowledge to future tasks, ultimately furthering cognitive development.

Another important concept in collaborative learning is **scaffolding**, or the process by which an instructor continually adapts the level of support and guidance offered to best suit the abilities of the learner and to encourage mastery of a task. When children first attempt a new skill, they need considerable support. For instance, a parent may have to physically support a baby who is learning to walk. Gradually and with practice, though, the child improves in ability, and less support is necessary. The parents adapt their level of assistance so that they are still guiding the child, but also allowing the child to rely increasingly on its own abilities. For instance, as a baby learns how to balance and move, the parent will periodically let go of the child, encouraging him or her to walk on his or her own.

Finally, Vygotsky emphasizes the importance of language in development. Children initially learn new concepts, values, and behavior through the transmission of verbal instruction using language. These lessons are then internalized by the child and become **private speech**, or the internal dialogue that all individuals use to moderate their behavior. Private speech in young children is often still verbalized, such as when a three-year-old talks aloud while attempting a puzzle. Eventually, though, private speech becomes a silent process that organizes and governs thought and action. Ultimately, individuals no longer need external guidance for certain behaviors because they have memorized appropriate skills and cultural expectations and can determine for themselves the most appropriate course of action.

KOHLBERG'S THEORY OF MORAL DEVELOPMENT. Lawrence Kohlberg was intrigued and inspired by Piaget's theory of moral development but felt that it was incomplete. He devoted his psychological career to expanding and elaborating upon Piaget's initial conclusions. Like Piaget, Kohlberg presented his subjects with a hypothetical moral dilemma and evaluated their opinions about how to appropriately resolve the issue. However, whereas Piaget focused on the moral complexity of the actual resolution provided by a subject, Kohlberg felt that the underlying moral rationale for a decision was far more crucial in understanding an individual's moral maturity. Kohlberg also theorized that moral development proceeds through fixed stages, but he believed that it does not conclude with adolescence. Instead, moral development is a lifelong and highly individual endeavor, with some reaching a higher level than others based on cognitive ability and social environment. Kohlberg proposed three levels of development, each level consisting of two stages. Kohlberg's three levels and six stages follow:

LEVEL ONE: PRECONVENTIONAL MORALITY. At this level, children judge behavior according to reward or punishment. Rules of behavior are established by parents or other authority figures.

STAGE ONE: OBEDIENCE AND PUNISHMENT ORIENTATION. If a behavior results in negative consequences, a child learns that it is "wrong" and should be avoided. The severity of a consequence determines how negatively a child judges that behavior.

STAGE TWO: NAÏVE HEDONISM. Behavior is motivated by a personal desire for reward or validation. Although another person may also inadvertently benefit, general concern for the welfare of others remains limited and secondary to one's own.

LEVEL TWO: CONVENTIONAL MORALITY. During this level, adolescents and adults behave in accordance with social norms in order to gain acceptance. The objective is to avoid blame or rejection while fostering personal relationships.

STAGE THREE: "GOOD BOY"/"GOOD GIRL" ORIENTATION. In stage three, an individual focuses on being accepted and valued by others. The primary objective is to be considered a "good" person. During stage three, the opinions of others are highly influential.

STAGE FOUR: SOCIAL-ORDER MORALITY. Moral dilemmas are resolved through strict interpretation of laws and social regulations. Rules are considered sacred and essential to the perseverance of human society. Moral exceptionalism based on need is forbidden. Many adults never progress past this stage.

LEVEL THREE: POSTCONVENTIONAL MORALITY. Individuals interpret laws and social norms from a more subjective, philosophical angle. Individuals consider human rights, personal ideals, and integrity when determining right or wrong behavior. They concede that established laws and social conventions are not always just and may need to be challenged in order to serve a higher purpose.

STAGE FIVE: SOCIAL CONTRACT ORIENTATION. Individuals adhere to laws that reflect the democratic principle of majority rule. Laws should be challenged and amended if they fail to offer universal justice or otherwise disadvantage others. Laws that are fair and universally beneficial are respected as **social contracts** that must be obeyed.

STAGE SIX: MORALITY OF INDIVIDUAL PRINCIPLES OF CONSCIENCE. The final and most idealistic stage is also virtually impossible to attain. At this level, individuals are guided exclusively by their conscience and desire for justice. Formal laws must be discarded if they are morally questionable and should be replaced with edicts that systematically take into account the needs of everyone affected.

Lawrence Kohlberg's theory of moral development was profoundly influential, ultimately giving rise to a new school of psychological thought devoted solely to moral reasoning. Nevertheless, it has faced strong criticism due to perceived cultural and gender biases embedded in Kohlberg's methodology. Culturally, it has been argued that Kohlberg's conclusions are relevant only in Western societies, which value individual rights. Critics assert that collectivist cultures that emphasize community welfare are excluded. Kohlberg's focus on the centrality of justice to moral reasoning has also come under fire. Some argue that the emphasis on justice and adherence to laws is based on an inherently masculine definition of morality. Notably, in the 1970s psychologist Carol Gillian proposed her own theory of moral development that considers a more feminized explanation of moral reasoning. She argues that women are not motivated by principles alone but are largely affected by the impact that their decisions have on those that they love. Women, therefore, are guided by values such as compassion, sensitivity to human rights, and caretaking.

The following example is often given to illustrate Kohlberg's stages.

Heinz's wife was dying from cancer. A new drug was created that could possibly save her life. Heinz went to the pharmacist to purchase the drug but was unable to afford it because the pharmacist was charging 10 times what it cost to make the drug. Heinz was unable to borrow the money from friends or family. Heinz pleaded with the pharmacist to sell him the drug, but the pharmacist declined. Should Heinz break into the pharmacy and steal the drug to save his wife's life?

Responses vary according to the stage of development:

Stage 1	Obedience and punishment	Heinz should not steal the medication for fear of the consequences. Stealing is against the law, and he will be punished.
Stage 2	Self-interest/ hedonism	Heinz should steal the medication because he will feel better, regardless of the consequences.
Stage 3	Conformity	Heinz should not steal the medication because he is a law-abiding citizen.
Stage 4	Law and order; Social order morality	Heinz should not steal the medication because it is against the law. If he does, though, he should take responsibility for the consequences of his behaviors.
Stage 5	Social contract; Human rights	Heinz should steal the medication because his wife's right to life is greater than the pharmacist's right to make a profit.
Stage 6	Universal human ethics; Individual morality	Heinz should steal the medication because the right to life supersedes the right to unrestricted commerce.

Influence of Social Factors on Identity Formation

Identity formation is influenced both by individuals and by social groups.

INFLUENCE OF INDIVIDUALS. Individuals serve as models of identity formation for children through the processes of imitation and role taking. Humans are evolutionarily hard-wired to imitate (**mimic**) the behavior of others in order to establish social connections. The frontal and prefrontal cortexes of the brain contain **mirror neurons** that enable people to emulate behavior.

Parents, friends, siblings, and even media serve as models of behavior for children as young as 6 months old. By as early as 9 months, infants are capable of **deferred imitation**, or the ability to replicate observed behavior from memory. Deferred imitation is an important cognitive milestone that indicates a child's ability to begin to think abstractly, or symbolically, about his or her environment. Imitation is crucial to healthy cognitive, social, and emotional development in that it teaches us to communicate effectively with our complex social milieu. The feedback that one receives in response to imitation ultimately guides values and conduct. When a child mimics a modeled behavior, the child receives either punishment or encouragement. Behaviors that are rewarded with praise become **incentivized**, whereas behaviors that are censured eventually become extinct.

Identity formation is also dependent on **role taking**, or social perspective taking. Social roles provide individuals with social norms and expectations of behavior within their assigned role. Roles are essentially the values, responsibilities, principles, and mannerisms that are associated with an individual's occupation, age, culture, sexuality, race, nationality, gender, occupation, or social status. In the context of identity formation, role taking allows people to imagine how others both perceive their environment and judge one's behavior or beliefs.

Sociologists Charles Cooley and George Herbert Mead both independently addressed the importance of role taking in identity development. Cooley introduced the concept of the "looking-glass self," which theorized that self-concept is developed through social interaction. People devise a fundamental appraisal of themselves—an identity—in reaction to their perception of how other people judge them.

George Herbert Mead postulated that people not only imagine how others judge them but then use these judgments to construct an individualized and ubiquitous social consciousness that he termed the **generalized other**. The generalized other is an individual's conception of the values and norms that guide the social system in which the individual lives. The generalized other is used to clarify one's position within society. Mead stated that, without the generalized other, an individual would lack social perspective and would face rejection and confusion, ultimately resulting in loneliness, dysfunction, and hopelessness.

INFLUENCE OF GROUPS. Identity is influenced by **reference groups**. A reference group is any social group that serves as a model to an individual for standards of self-esteem, goals, experiences, accomplishments, ideals, and values. Individuals use reference groups as standards by which they assess either the acceptability or deviancy of their actions and ideals.

Influence of Culture and Socialization on Identity Formation

Culture refers to the values, principles, rituals, traditions, language, dress, hierarchies, role expectations, creative expression, and social systems within a particular population. Cultural values and beliefs become an important part of a person's identity.

Cultural values are communicated symbolically through a shared language and are preserved across generations through **socialization**. Socialization is the process by which individuals learn the cultural norms of their particular social environment. Socialization occurs through social interaction and gradual cultural exposure and teaches individuals how to function within their social milieu. Through socialization, individuals are indoctrinated into a complex system of social expectations, group allegiances, codes of conduct, and political realities. Family, schools, religious institutions, media, economic systems, peers, and government are all **agents of socialization** (people and institutions that determine the predominant social conventions). Individuals absorb and internalize these core tenets from their surroundings and integrate them into their ultimate identity.

The most crucial agent of socialization is the family. Parents, caregivers, and siblings exert a powerful influence on a child's perception of relationships, boundaries, self-worth, sexuality, morality, expectations, and gender roles. Family influence is most powerful in regard to an individual's self-esteem, autonomy, political ideology, academic or occupational goals, and ethnic identity.

TEST QUESTION

In neighborhoods where they are present, gangs can function as an agent of socialization for young people. Is this statement true or false and why?

(A) True, because gangs bring much-needed income to a neighborhood.

(B) True, because gangs establish social conventions within their neighborhood.

(C) False, because the social conventions established by gangs are typically negative.

(D) False, because gangs replace missing family support.

(B) True. Gangs are established environmental institutions in the neighborhoods in which they exist and are responsible for socializing those who live in their territories, whether for good or for bad. Choice A is incorrect because bringing in income is not directly relevant to disseminating social norms. Choice C is incorrect because socialization includes both prosocial and antisocial norms. Choice D is incorrect because supplying missing family support is an example of socialization.

Attitudes and Beliefs that Affect Social Interactions

Social interactions are affected by people's perceptions of, attitudes toward, and attribution of the motives of others. Attitudes such as prejudice, bias, and stereotypes influence social interactions.

ATTRIBUTIONS AND PERCEPTIONS

Attribution Theory

Attribution theory details the process by which people attribute causes to, or explanations for, their own behavior or the behavior of others. For example, if an employee witnesses a supervisor acting rudely toward a visitor, the employee is likely to interpret the supervisor's state of mind and motivation, perhaps attributing to the supervisor an inherent meanness or, on the other hand, imagining that the supervisor may not have slept well the night before. The originator of attribution theory, Fritz Heider (1958), proposed that all people are "naïve psychologists" who are engaged in an endless quest to contextualize their experiences. Humans possess an innate need for interpreting and understanding their social environment. Although the attribution of another's motivation may be wildly incorrect, the need to find an explanation for the motivation of others is nearly universal.

Before an individual can begin the attributional process, certain criteria must be satisfied. Behaviors or events must first be directly observed and then judged to be both voluntary and intentional. Once these conditions are met, Heider determined that people develop explanations based on their perceived locus of control.

The **correspondent influence theory of attribution** explains how people interpret the behavior of others in their environment. The behaviors of other individuals are interpreted and subsequently attributed to their innate personality characteristics. These attributions are then used as predictors of the person's future behavior. Individuals base their judgment of others' behavior on three criteria. The first, degree of choice, refers to whether the action was voluntary or compulsory. Next, individuals evaluate whether or not the observed behavior had social consequences or negative repercussions for others. Finally, behavior or actions are judged for appropriateness in accordance with the prevailing social norms. Intentional, consequential, and unorthodox behaviors are more likely to be considered reflective of inherent character. They are then considered accurate indicators of the person's future behavior. In other cases, a person's behavior may be seen as caused by an environmental factor rather than by a personality trait, or as being the result of an impulse, in which case the behavior is less likely to be repeated.

FUNDAMENTAL ATTRIBUTION ERROR. People have a universal susceptibility to attributing other people's behavior to inherent personality characteristics. In doing so, people often commit a **fundamental attribution error** in judgment by discounting the influence of circumstantial factors. The end result is a human bias toward holding individuals exclusively accountable for their actions, even when there exists clear evidence of discrete situational factors. This is especially true when an individual is judging a stranger, due to a sense of detachment from the situation.

The fundamental attribution error has potentially destructive social consequences, as illustrated in the common practice of "blaming the victim" for somehow provoking the crime or abuse visited upon them. In their appraisal of certain events, outsiders often engage in **hindsight bias**, or a retrospective belief that a victim of injustice could have behaved differently or taken more precautionary measures in order to avoid mistreatment. Blaming the victim is common in cases of sexual assault, when it is suggested that the victim should have taken such preventative measures as not drinking alcohol or dressing more conservatively. It is also a significant feature in blaming the poor for their poverty or the infirm for their illness. Ironically, there is a tendency for people to attribute their own successes to internal factors while blaming failures on external influences (**self-serving bias**).

HOW CULTURE AFFECTS ATTRIBUTIONS. Cultural beliefs have a measurable impact on an individual's attributional tendencies. Individualistic and collectivistic cultures in particular exhibit fundamental differences in how behavior is explained. Individualistic cultures, such as Western Europe and the United States, appreciate autonomy and individual accomplishment. These cultures are particularly inclined toward applying the fundamental attribution error due to their almost singular emphasis on personal accountability for success or failure. Collectivist cultures, including Asian or Latin American nations, believe in the importance of interdependence, dedication to community, and group cooperation. These cultural beliefs result in a decreased propensity for holding any one individual exclusively responsible for his or her behavior. Collectivist cultures are more likely to consider the situational context of an individual's behavior before drawing conclusions.

How Self-Perceptions Shape Perceptions of Others

People perceive others (**social perceptions**) through the filter of their own self-concept, experiences and expectations, needs or motives, attitude, and personal interests. One's sense of self essentially colors the interpretation of other people's behaviors and actions and is the common cause of eight perceptual errors and distortions. The first, **selective perception**, is the tendency to attend only to information that is most personally relevant or attractive and may lead a person to ignore potentially significant information, resulting in bias. **Projection** is a tendency to evaluate other people according to one's own characteristics. When an individual projects his or her own traits onto another, the individual is predisposed to exaggerate any information that confirms their prejudgment. For instance, a thief may be inherently suspicious of most other people due to his or her own deceitfulness.

Stereotyping consists of judgments of people that are based upon group membership, such as race, nationality, sexuality, gender, or age. Individuals learn social categorization and group dynamics from their social environment and ultimately integrate generalizations about particular social groups into their self-concept. These generalizations, or stereotypes, are subsequently used to evaluate single members of that group without accounting for other factors. People also mistakenly rely on **inference** (presumption) in interpreting another person's behavior. Information gathered through inference is misleading because it is incomplete. **Impressions**, especially first impressions, of another person are also used as indicators of another person's character. However, like inference, impressions are insufficient and fragmented information that do not often accurately reflect an individual's complex personality.

The fundamental attribution error is a common distortion explained in the previous section. **The halo effect** is the tendency to draw conclusions about another person's general personality based upon a single observed characteristic. The halo effect is a logical trap resulting from the human preference for grouping similar qualities together, like generosity and kindness or stinginess and bitterness. This phenomenon is a frequent cause of misjudgment of character by assumption. The final perceptual error is to rely on one's **perceptual set** to make inferences about another person. A perceptual set consists of an individual's beliefs and information about one person that are then applied to a different individual who is similar to the first in some way.

PREJUDICE AND BIAS

Prejudice is the conscious choice to disparage an individual or social group based solely on discernable characteristics, including race, gender, age, sexuality, or religious beliefs. It is usually a deep-seated belief founded on irrational thought and is therefore not easily swayed by reasonable, logically supported arguments. Prejudice can be either positive or negative, but negative prejudice is more destructive because of its manifestation in hateful and discriminatory behaviors. In its most destructive form, prejudice can be used to subjugate or destroy an entire population.

Bias, on the other hand, is a preference for a certain standpoint instead of a deeply held belief. Bias inclines an individual toward certain behaviors or attitudes but typically results from lack of information or limited exposure to other groups. Unlike prejudice, biased beliefs can be revised when an individual is confronted with rational arguments that are based on logical evidence.

Causes of Prejudice

Prejudice can fundamentally be attributed to the intergroup dynamics that guide social structure and behavior. Prejudice is an in-group, out-group phenomenon whereby a social group seeks to elevate its status by identifying another group as inferior (as a **scapegoat**). Essentially, prejudice is borne of feelings of inadequacy, and scapegoating is an opportunity for an insecure group of people to identify and blame others for their problems. Prejudice has also been attributed to a variety of other social factors, including socialization, conformity, economic strategy, authoritarian personalities, ethnocentrism, group closure, and conflict theory.

Family is the primary influence on socialization, and attitudes and beliefs are easily transferred from one generation to the next. If a child is exposed almost exclusively to prejudiced opinions, the child will likely be conditioned through socialization to believe in the inferiority of another group. **Conformity** is another powerful social influence that guides one's beliefs and actions. Individuals have an overwhelming and intrinsic desire for the acceptance by and approval of others. Consequently, if a person is surrounded by prejudiced people, he or she will often conform to the prevailing attitude in order to avoid rejection.

EMOTIONAL AND COGNITIVE COMPONENTS OF PREJUDICE. Prejudice is fundamentally an emotional response, based on various fears about one's security. Many of the fears behind a prejudice are not conscious. Beliefs that are expressed by people who hold a prejudice are expressed in terms that may sound logical but are rationalizations for deeply held emotions. This helps explain why a person's prejudicial beliefs typically cannot be modified through logical argument.

Research on prejudice conducted over the last decade by Fiske, Cuddy, and Glick found that emotions play a role in prejudices. Specifically, the emotions of envy, pity, disgust, and pride can be used to predict an individual's negative behaviors toward a group of which the individual is not a member.

A large urban police department has 7000 police officers on the force. Of those, 354 are African American, 1986 are Hispanic, and 4460 are white. In the general population, 9% of Americans are African American, 48% are Hispanic, and 43% are white. Which of the following statements is true?

(A) These statistics represent a system of institutionalized racism in the police department.

(B) These statistics demonstrate an explicit bias on the part of the leadership of the police department.

(C) This is an example of symbolic prejudice because the minority groups clearly haven't taken advantage of the opportunities available to them in the police department.

(D) This is an example of a microaggression because the hiring practices do not limit access to employment in the police department.

(A) The police department is an established community institution. These statistics represent institutionalized racism within the police department. Proportions would be in line with the general population if there were no institutionalized racism. In that case, the police department would consist of approximately 630 Black/African American, 3360 Hispanic/Latin American, and 3010 White/Caucasian officers.

Factors that Contribute to Prejudice

Prejudice is fed by the dynamics of power, prestige, and class. Prejudice has economic advantages for certain people. The systematic disfranchisement of a population gives the more powerful group control over economic and political systems, effectively eliminating competition for resources. Prejudice is particularly pronounced during periods of economic or social unrest, when minority groups are commonly singled out and condemned as the source of the crisis.

The presence of both authoritarian personalities and ethnocentrism within a population fuels intolerance. Individuals with **authoritarian personalities** are described as easily indoctrinated, blindly loyal, convinced of their relative superiority, and fundamentally conservative in regards to religion and sex. When political or religious leaders have an authoritarian personality, extremist political or religious principles increase the potential for widespread prejudice. In this case, certain groups are identified as nonconformist and threatening and are subsequently targeted for persecution. **Ethnocentrism** refers to the judgment of another social group according to the cultural standards and beliefs of one's own culture. The perceived differences between two groups are exacerbated by ethnocentric comparison, causing individuals to disregard any similarities that may exist.

Group closure occurs when a group ideologically or physically isolates itself from other populations. The separation of two populations prevents both from becoming familiar with each other, giving rise to stereotyping and suspicion. Finally, **conflict theory** explains that powerful and entitled social groups are primarily committed to retaining their social, economic, and political advantages over others. The dominant population controls political expression, education, information, and resources by any means necessary, including violence. The subjugated group may revolt against their oppression in an effort to obtain long-denied economic and political freedoms.

Expressions of Prejudice

Prejudice can be expressed either **explicitly** or **implicitly**, also referred to as **overt** and **covert**, respectively. Individuals who deliberately display their negative and judgmental views of others practice explicit prejudice. Conversely, implicitly prejudiced people may endorse negative opinions of other groups but conceal their beliefs from others in order to avoid recrimination. Alternately, implicitly prejudiced people may not consciously be aware that they hold a prejudice even though they act in a prejudiced way. Though explicit prejudice has gradually declined over the course of the last century, social psychologists argue that implicit prejudice persists. Thus, prejudiced behavior continues to affect one's behavior despite an individual's conscious belief that prejudice is wrong. This behavior, known as **aversive prejudice**, is far more prevalent today than **dominative prejudice**, or open displays of intolerance.

Aversive prejudice manifests itself in four behaviors—symbolic, subtle, ambivalent, and benevolent prejudice.

SYMBOLIC PREJUDICE. The first, **symbolic prejudice**, occurs when an individual blames a minority group for the group's failure to take advantage of its newfound opportunities. The inability of certain groups to progress politically, economically, or socially is blamed on their perceived apathy or irresponsibility. The elimination of overt discrimination is cited as evidence that all individuals have access to equal opportunities, so failure is attributed to lack of initiative. Legitimate reasons including educational inequality or entrenched socioeconomic power are disregarded. Such principles are nevertheless supported by certain political factions and are, as such, justified and seemingly sanctioned by others.

SUBTLE PREJUDICE. The hallmarks of **subtle prejudice** include disregarding, mocking, or treating minority groups differently than other groups. Subtle racism is insidious in that it is expressed as a superficially benign action, but its effects are obvious and damaging to those who experience it. A classic example is the controversial discovery that some police officers target more African American than Caucasian people who are driving luxury cars. Such indirectly prejudiced behavior is difficult to confront because it is seemingly legal. To those who experience it, however, subtle racism is a deeply disturbing reality that undermines their self-worth and confidence.

AMBIVALENT PREJUDICE. Ambivalent prejudice is founded in cognitive dissonance theory and results from simultaneously positive and negative opinions about a minority group. Conflicted attitudes toward another group result in inconsistent behavior toward them. Because of ambivalence, an individual then experiences a sense of guilt, or dissonance. This frustration may result in misplaced resentment toward the group that is manifested in negative or discriminatory behavior.

BENEVOLENT PREJUDICE. The final category of aversive prejudice, **benevolent prejudice**, results from an individual's best intentions. Benevolent prejudice occurs when seemingly supportive and favorable opinions are expressed toward a social group. Under scrutiny, however, such comments further reinforce existing stereotypes and consequently perpetuate the marginalization of a population. Common expressions of benevolent prejudice include the statement that all members of a group are great athletes or good at art. Although apparently flattering, such expressions are ultimately indicative of belief in the separateness and inferiority of another group.

STEREOTYPES

Stereotypes—generalizations about an entire group of people—are a particular form of prejudice. Stereotypes are essentially preconceived expectations about how another person or group should behave. When people behave in accordance with a stereotype, the stereotype is confirmed. When people's behaviors do not conform to the stereotype, the behaviors are attributed to the situation or to environmental conditions, in order to protect the stereotype.

Living under the shadow of a stereotype has been shown to have profoundly negative repercussions, especially in regard to motivation for success. For instance, **stereotype threat** describes apprehension experienced by individuals who fear that their behavior or performance will confirm a negative stereotype about their social group. Stereotype threat has been blamed for the enduring racial and gender gap in academic achievement due to its detrimental effect on one's ability to perform. The pressure to transcend stereotypes causes acute anxiety and stress that ultimately undermine academic performance. Stereotype threat is also related to self-blame, depression, self-sabotage, lack of ambition, and social isolation. Stereotype threat then is a **self-fulfilling prophecy**. That is, the fear of performing poorly on a test causes people to perform poorly on the test.

Actions and Processes Underlying Social Interactions

This section reviews the main process of social interaction, including verbal and nonverbal communication, controlling the impressions one makes on others, and expressing and detecting emotions. In addition, the section reviews types of social behaviors, including both cooperative and aggressive behaviors.

SELF-PRESENTATION AND INTERACTING WITH OTHERS

Self-presentation is behavior that is intended to convey a message or image about oneself to another person. Self-presentation is also referred to as impression management, a concerted effort to create an image in the minds of others.

Impression Management

All social interactions are essentially guided by the innate human desire to leave a positive impression on other people. According to **impression management theory**, both individuals and social groups continually struggle to influence other people's perceptions about people, places, or events. They do so by tactically choosing what information to share with others in social interaction.

Self-presentation theory, derived from impression management theory, is focused specifically on how individuals attempt to construct, manipulate, or otherwise control their own image or appearance in order to gain social approval.

Self-presentation serves three essential functions for humans. The first function is to help meet needs such as food, shelter, and social acceptance. By presenting oneself in a way that is consistent with social expectations, an individual avoids social rejection or punishment.

The second function of self-presentation is to construct an identity and enhance self-esteem. An individual relies heavily on others for the recognition, acceptance, and validation of his or her self-concept and sense of self-worth. People who feel valued by others will in turn value themselves. Although self-concept is largely an internal evaluation, one's identity and feelings of self-worth are ultimately dependent upon corroboration from other people.

Self-presentation may assist in either identity creation or identity reinforcement. In the first case, an individual may experiment with different personas in public. The individual then analyzes other people's reactions before deciding on which identity to assume. This behavior is especially prevalent during adolescence and young adulthood.

The third function of self-presentation is to dictate and regulate the parameters of social interaction. Social interaction is a complex process that requires navigating differing personalities, goals, needs, preferences, temperaments, ideologies, values, genders, and cultural backgrounds. Without implicit guidelines to direct communication, human society would be virtually impossible. Social interaction is organized through the assignment of roles and the concurrent expectation that people will behave in accordance with their assumed role. Social roles help people both categorize and anticipate the behavior of others within a social setting and provide individuals with expectations of how they themselves should be treated.

THE DRAMATURGICAL APPROACH. In 1959, Erving Goffman proposed a theory that analyzed the extent to which self-presentation both directs social interaction and influences self-concept. In his theory, called the **dramaturgical approach**, Goffman argues that social interactions are no different than theatrical productions in that all individuals involved are essentially actors, who must give a convincing performance of their assumed role. Performers receive personal validation and identity security by persuading the audience of the authenticity of their "performance."

> **DRAMA**
>
> According to Goffman, interactions between people are much like roles in a play.

According to Goffman, the critical presence of the audience causes an individual to create two distinct personas, referred to as the **front-stage** and **backstage** selves. The **front-stage self** is the persona that is strategically constructed and presented to an audience. The front-stage self is dependent upon both the social setting and the intended audience. Different "selves" are required for different situations. Individuals use various, situation-dependent impression management tools in order to ensure a successful and convincing performance. These include dress, personal appearance, mannerisms, language, and nonverbal communication. Ultimately, the front-stage self is a carefully constructed, contextually appropriate, and deliberately performed persona that reveals only those personal characteristics on which an actor wishes to be judged.

Goffman considers the alternative self, the **backstage self**, to be more authentic and therefore more representative of one's true nature. Because the audience is prohibited from entering the backstage area, the actor does not feel evaluative pressure and allows himself or herself an opportunity to step out of his or her role. Backstage, the actor has an opportunity to relax, prepare for another performance, and act without fear of judgment or rejection. An individual who is backstage may also reveal certain opinions or behaviors that were deliberately withheld from the audience in order to adhere to social norms. For example, a woman who compliments a friend on her outfit may later tell another person that her friend's dress was ugly.

A woman insists on cleaning the house before company arrives. This is an example of:

(A) backstage self.

(B) front-stage self.

(C) impression management.

(D) self-presentation theory.

(B) The woman wants to put her best foot forward by showing a clean home, which is the creation of a strategically constructed image for presentation to her audience, the company.

Expression and Detection of Emotion

A critical element of social interaction is the expression of emotion and the detection and interpretation of the emotions expressed by others. Although there are certain basic universal expressions of emotion, the ways in which emotion is expressed are influenced by both gender and culture. In particular, culture and gender are particularly influential in determining guidelines regarding who is allowed to express specific feelings, when they can be expressed, and which emotions are acceptable.

HOW CULTURE AFFECTS EXPRESSION. Culture affects how emotions are displayed through the use of **display rules** and **emblems**, which dictate socially accepted norms of emotional expression. Expression is also shaped by whether a culture is collectivistic or individualistic.

Display rules are cultural beliefs regarding which emotions are acceptable to display. For instance, collectivistic cultures discourage negative emotional expression because of the value placed on interdependence. The reasoning is that the negative emotions conveyed by one individual ultimately impact the entire group. Individualistic cultures, on the other hand, value personal accountability, and individuals feel entitled to and solely responsible for their behavior. Collectivistic cultures also place a high value on emotions such as shame and regret due to the function that these emotions serve in preserving group cohesiveness. Individualistic cultures, however, emphasize the necessity of feeling proud, confident, and assertive, as these are essential to intrinsic motivation and individual achievement.

Emblems are culturally specific nonverbal gestures or expressions. For instance, the thumbs-up sign means "good job" in the United States, whereas in Saudi Arabia it is interpreted as an insult. Cultural norms determine the meaning and appropriateness of certain gestures and expressions. Eye contact, personal space, touching, and head nodding are also considered emblems that express different emotions depending upon the cultural context. In Western cultures, direct eye contact is considered emblematic of honesty, confidence, and capability. In many Eastern cultures, however, children are taught to avoid eye contact to display respect and humility, and direct eye contact is considered offensive.

HOW GENDER AFFECTS EXPRESSION. Men and women also exhibit differences in their emotional expressiveness. Generally speaking, women are expected to be more emotionally expressive, sensitive, and perceptive. Men are expected not to express emotion. According to research, women and men differ in nonverbal emotional expression in four basic areas. First, women tend to smile more than men and display warmth toward others more readily. Second, women display more frequent and animated nonverbal gestures and expressions in contrast to the reserved demeanor typical of men in the same setting. Third, women seem to be more emotionally astute in that they are more successful in reading and interpreting other people's nonverbal messages. Finally, women are more inclined to offer assistance to people who are struggling and are more effective at providing emotional support.

Verbal and Nonverbal Communication

Presenting oneself to and communicating with others takes place through both **verbal** and **nonverbal communication**. **Verbal communication** is defined as using language. Typically, this refers to spoken language, but both written language (such as a text message) and a manual/visual (sign) language might also be considered verbal. Verbal communication does not include sounds such as groans, humming, sighing, or growling, as these are not linguistic elements.

Nonverbal communication consists of nonlinguistic information that nevertheless conveys meaning. Such communication is nonlinguistic because it is not subject to rules of grammar. Typically, nonverbal communication is not conveyed through the voice but rather through gestures, actions, facial expression, eye contact, posture, tone of voice, clothing, and touch. However, voiced sounds such as a laugh or snort are examples of nonverbal communication.

Nonverbal communication is the primary indicator of characteristics such as status, health, sociability, stability, honesty, and mood. Nonverbal communication is so crucial to human existence that certain facial expressions have become intrinsic and are universally expressed regardless of cultural or social influence. Universal facial expressions of anger, fear, disgust, happiness, surprise, and sadness are even present in infants and children born without sight.

Animal Communication

All living things interact with their environment and with members of their own and other species and as such communicate. Human communication is distinct from animal communication in the complexity of concepts that can be communicated through human language. However, primates and other animals have shown the ability to understand a small amount of abstract vocabulary. Some, such as bees and ants, have complex systems for communicating location of food sources and other information critical to their existence. It is likely that communication serves a critical need in maintaining social connections in many species, as well as in communicating specific information.

SOCIAL BEHAVIOR

Social behavior is the act of communicating with members of the same species or with society at large. Human social behavior is fundamentally conflicted. On the one hand, humans have a powerful need to connect to and cooperate with others. On the other hand, much human behavior is characterized by aggression.

Aggression

Aggression, from the standpoint of psychology, is a behavior that causes or threatens to cause physical or emotional harm toward oneself, another person, or group of people. Aggressive behavior may be primarily physical, verbal, or psychological.

Aggression can be classified as either instrumental or hostile. **Instrumental aggression** is calculated behavior that is driven by the desire to fulfill a specific goal, such as acquiring new land. In addition to material goals, the goal may also be to assert dominance or to intimidate.

Hostile aggression, on the other hand, occurs in response to a perceived threat from another person or group. The aggressor's emotional reaction to the threat is anger, and the hostility is both a physical manifestation of the emotional state and a means of relieving frustration.

Aggression can also be divided into predatory versus affective aggression. **Predatory aggression** is planned, goal oriented, and under conscious control. **Affective aggression** is unplanned and uncontrolled. Affectively aggressive people are not able to control their aggressive impulses, even if they have a conscious desire to do so.

Cooperative Behavior

Unlike aggressive behavior, most social behavior is aimed at increasing harmony. Three categories of cooperative behavior are attraction, attachment, and social support.

ATTRACTION. Attraction refers to positive feelings that one person holds in relation to another person. Because enjoying such a person's presence is pleasurable, attraction typically implies a desire to spend time with that person. According to social psychologists, there are four factors that influence attraction—propinquity, reciprocity, similarity, and physical attractiveness.

Propinquity refers to proximity and exposure. People are attracted to individuals whom they encounter on a regular basis. Essentially, individuals feel more comfortable around familiar people and are therefore far more likely to develop deeper relationships with them.

The second factor, **reciprocity**, is a phenomenon by which individuals are more attracted to people who hold a positive opinion of them. Surrounding oneself with people who like them makes individuals feel validated and supported. The third factor, **similarity**, refers to the fact that people tend to prefer the company of those who share comparable beliefs, values, opinions, socioeconomic background, personality traits, interests, and life experiences. Studies have shown that relationships in which two individuals share similar views tend to be more stable and enduring.

The final factor affecting attraction is **physical attractiveness**. In his **matching hypothesis**, social psychologist Erving Goffman concludes that individuals are drawn toward people whom they rate as being similar to themselves in physical attractiveness. There are certain physical features that are considered attractive regardless of cultural background, such as large eyes, prominent cheekbones, and youth. However, there is a substantial degree of cultural variation in regard to physical beauty.

ATTACHMENT. Attachment refers to an extended, long-term bond between two individuals, in which there is a felt need for being in each other's presence and in which separation from each other results in anxiety. John Bowlby's **attachment theory** argues that an individual's expectations and beliefs about adult relationships are profoundly influenced by the type of attachment that they had as a child with their primary caregiver. In the 1970s, psychologist Mary Ainsworth proposed that children could experience five possible types of attachment with their primary caregiver. Subsequent researchers have expanded on her research by detailing precisely how each attachment type influences a child's future beliefs about and behavior toward others.

The first attachment category is **secure attachment**, which results from a caregiver who provides consistent boundaries and exhibits attentiveness, affection, support, and reasonability. Securely attached children grow into adults who are secure in themselves, independent, appropriately trusting, and optimistic. They are the most successful in navigating adult relationships.

The second category, **anxious attachment**, results from a caregiver who is on constant guard and who discourages exploration and independence. Anxiously attached children can become emotionally demanding adults who require a great deal of attention in order to feel secure.

Avoidant attachment refers to a caregiver who ignores the child's various needs, even if the child is in obvious emotional or physical pain. Emotional expression is discouraged or punished. Avoidant attachment in adulthood is characterized by emotional detachment, excessive independence, isolation, and mistrust of others.

The fourth type of attachment is **ambivalent/resistant**, which is attributed to inconsistent and even negligent care. Ambivalent/resistant caregivers often only respond to their child when he or she becomes excessively clingy. Because of the uncertainty in their lives, ambivalently attached adults often experience anxiety, depression, and fear. They may also exhibit disordered behaviors that provide a sense of control, such as obsessive-compulsive behaviors or eating disorders.

The final and most destructive attachment type is **disorganized attachment**. In this case, caregivers are cruelly abusive, terrifying, detached, and a source of pain and confusion. These caregivers are sometimes mentally ill, addicted to substances, or otherwise emotionally incapacitated. Adults who were subjected to this level of neglect as children may display hostility, self-harm, hatred, depression, and social inappropriateness. They may also develop severe personality disorders and have an extreme difficulty forming even casual relationships.

SOCIAL SUPPORT. Another aspect of cooperative social behavior is social support. Social support refers to the network of family, friends, healthcare providers, and community resources that are essential to one's physical and emotional health. There are three categories of social support. The first, **emotional support** is the level of affection, trust, warmth, and concern provided by friends and family. The second, **instrumental support**, is tangible support provided by the community or by healthcare providers. It includes financial resources, transportation, physical assistance, or any other supportive service. Finally, **appraisal support** includes the evaluative comments and opinions about oneself that are received from others. Appraisal support helps people contextualize their lives and deepen their self-awareness.

Social Behavior in Animals

Animal social behavior has similarities to, and can shed light on, human social behavior. In animals that forage together for food, foraging requires minimizing competition/aggression and maximizing cooperation. For situations in which animals compete with each other, game theory is a useful tool for understanding the results of the choices that each "player" may make in terms of cost of energy and gain of food/mate/status. For example, a young male baboon may attack a dominant male if the cost (calories, injuries) is lower than the probable gain (a dominant position, access to food, or mating privileges).

SUMMARY

This chapter began by describing perception and cognition. First sensory processing was covered. Then the foundations of cognition were reviewed, starting with attention and covering information processing, the stages of cognitive development, biological factors that affect cognition, and problem solving. Then the concepts of intelligence were reviewed, including the theory of multiple intelligences.

Next the processes of consciousness, memory, and language were covered, including states of consciousness, memory encoding, storage, retrieval, memory loss, and genetic and environmental factors of language development.

The second part of the chapter reviewed the constructs of behavior. First, the psycho-biological constructs were reviewed, including the biological bases of behavior (neuro-logical, hormonal, and genetic factors), theories of personality, psychological disorders as defined by the DSM-5 and the biological bases of the disorders, components and theories of emotion, theories of motivation, the link between attitude and behavior, and stress. Next the social constructs of behavior were reviewed, including social facilitation, deindividuation, the bystander effect, social loafing, peer pressure, and group processes. The second part of the chapter ended with a review of learning, attitude, and behavior. Topics reviewed included associative (classical and operant conditioning) and observational learning, habituation and dishabituation, and theories of attitude and behavior change.

The final part of the chapter reviewed self-perception and interaction with society. First, the notion of identity was reviewed, including self-concept and the formation of identity. Next, the chapter covered the attitudes and beliefs that affect social interactions, including attributions and perceptions, prejudice, bias, and stereotypes. Finally, the chapter reviewed the actions and process that underlie social interactions, including impression management, expression and detection of emotion, verbal and nonverbal communication, and aggressive versus cooperative behavior.

PSYCHOLOGY PRACTICE EXERCISES

> **DIRECTIONS:** This psychology passage is followed by a series of questions. Read the passage, and then for each question choose the one answer that is best. If you are not sure of an answer, eliminate the answer choices that you think are wrong and choose one of the remaining answers.

PASSAGE I

Society has become increasingly aware of mental illness in children, including mood disorders. Approximately one in seven children experiences some type of mood disorder.

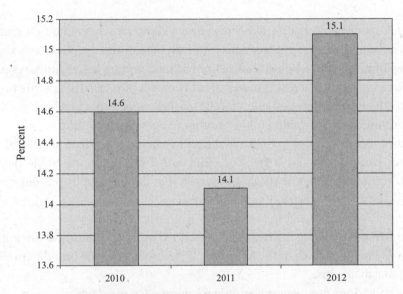

Figure 1. Percentage of all children under 15 who experienced a mood disorder in three recent years

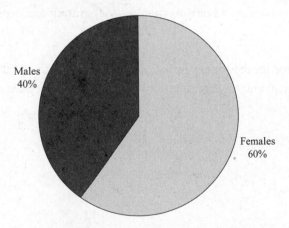

Figure 2. Percent of children under 15 suffering from a mood disorder by gender, 2010–2012

Among mood disorders, depressive disorder is one of the most common. The symptoms of a depressive disorder in a child differ from those in an adult. A child may persistently feel sad or hopeless, have low self-esteem, feel inappropriately guilty, or be hypersensitive to criticism, rejection, or failure. A child might feel like he or she wants to die, might talk about wanting to run away, or might engage in self-harming behavior such as cutting. Other symptoms of depression that can appear in a child include difficulty concentrating, a loss of interest in activities that the individual once enjoyed, disrupted sleeping patterns, decreased energy, irritability, hostility, aggression, significant weight gain or loss, difficulty making or maintaining relationships with peers or adults, and somatic symptoms.

In adults the symptoms of depression include depressed mood, a loss of interest, weight gain or loss, an increase or decrease in sleep patterns, psychomotor agitation or retardation, loss of energy, feelings of worthlessness or guilt, difficulty concentrating, or recurrent thoughts of death.

Case Study: A six-year-old male child comes into a clinic six weeks into first grade with the following symptoms: he does not share his toys with his siblings; he cries every day when his mother takes him to school; he runs away from school; and he has nightmares about being kidnapped by monsters. When his mother tries to distract him with his favorite toys or games before school, he is not interested in them. His teacher reports that he is sad all day at school and stares out the window waiting for his mother to come back for him.

The teacher, in an attempt to improve the child's behavior, rang a small bell just before snack period. Later in the day, when the child was exhibiting undesirable behaviors, the teacher would ring the bell. The teacher observed that the boy briefly relaxed when the bell was rung.

1. If a clinician were to diagnose the child described in the case study as having separation anxiety, which of the following, if true, would be the best defense for making this diagnosis.
   (A) The child does not meet the criteria for depressive disorder.
   (B) The child exhibits at least two behaviors consistent with missing his mother.
   (C) The child exhibits anxious behavior only when his mother is not present.
   (D) The child's behavior matches the criteria for separation anxiety listed in the DSM-5.

2. Based on the figures for the three years shown in Figure 1, out of 1,000 children younger than age 15, on the average approximately how many females have experienced a mood disorder?
   (A) 73
   (B) 88
   (C) 146
   (D) 600

3. According to Bowlby, the child in the case study could be best characterized as having:
   (A) a secure attachment because he views his mother as a safe base.
   (B) an avoidant attachment because his bonding pattern with his mother is inconsistent.
   (C) a disorganized attachment because he expects that his mother will not meet his needs.
   (D) an anxious/ambivalent attachment because he is distressed by separation from his mother.

4. Based on the passage, all of the following are symptoms of depression shared by adults and children EXCEPT:
   (A) a sad mood.
   (B) loss of weight.
   (C) sensitivity to rejection.
   (D) recurrent thoughts of death.

5. The child in the case study has a broken ankle and has been taking pain medication for the last six weeks. Which of the following is the best defense for NOT diagnosing the child with separation anxiety disorder?
   (A) The side effects of the medication are more consistent with attention deficit hyperactivity disorder than with separation anxiety disorder.
   (B) The child's current symptoms began several months before he broke his ankle.
   (C) Physical disorders such as a broken ankle are not covered by the DSM.
   (D) Before diagnosing a client with a psychiatric condition, a clinician must rule out medical conditions as a contributing factor.

6. The teacher's use of ringing a bell is an example of what kind of behavior modification?
   (A) Classical conditioning, because the ringing of the bell comes before the eating of the snack
   (B) Operant conditioning, because the relaxing occurs after the ringing of the bell
   (C) Operant conditioning, because the ringing of the bell is the positive reinforcement and the relaxing is the target behavior
   (D) Operant conditioning, because the ringing of the bell when there is no snack is negative punishment

7. According to Erickson's model, which of the following is the developmental task that the child in the case study should next resolve?
   (A) Industry versus inferiority, which children normally resolve between the ages of 5 and 12
   (B) Autonomy versus shame, which children normally resolve between 18 months and 3 years
   (C) Trust versus mistrust, which children normally resolve between birth to 18 months
   (D) Identity versus role confusion, which children normally resolve between 3 and 7 years of age

PASSAGE II

Case Study: A twenty-six-year-old man returned from military service in the Middle East three years ago. He recently married a twenty-eight-year-old woman who has two children from a previous marriage. He has a thirteen-year-old son from another relationship. He and his wife have a two-year-old girl together. During a severe storm, the family's car was caught by flooding waters. The family was rescued by first responders. The two-year-old girl was handed through the window first, and her family followed. The rescue of the remaining family members took some time because of difficulties caused by the water currents. During this time, the little girl was being held by a first responder while the other rescue workers focused on rescuing the remaining family members.

Present in the little girl's play are reenactments of the rescue. She began having nightmares about four nights a week shortly after the rescue. The family has brought the little girl to the doctor because since the rescue, she has begun to show distress any time she hears a siren or sees a rescue vehicle. She avoids car rides. The little girl locks doors and closes windows in the house and is afraid to leave her parents' side, even to go with close family members.

8. What is the most likely diagnosis of the little girl?
    (A) Separation anxiety disorder
    (B) Adjustment disorder
    (C) Specific phobia
    (D) Post-traumatic stress disorder

9. When the mother takes the little girl to the doctor, she asks the thirteen-year-old son to get dressed nicely for a grandparent's birthday party later that evening. When she returns, the mother finds that he has changed into torn jeans and his favorite hoodie. Based on the information in the passage, which of the following best explains his behavior?
    (A) His behavior is an age-appropriate demonstration of adolescent individuation.
    (B) He is intentionally defying his stepmother because he has not formed a secure attachment with her.
    (C) He is exhibiting symptoms of ADHD.
    (D) His behavior is an expression of the Oedipus complex as described by Freud.

10. Social learning theory would suggest that:
    (A) the little girl has learned to lock doors and windows after observing her father's behavior.
    (B) the father is the more knowledgeable other and she has learned to be hypervigilant in response to his modeling.
    (C) the rescue provided reinforcement for the child's hypervigilance.
    (D) in this scenario, reciprocal determinism suggests that the father's military service has caused his daughter's PTSD symptoms.

11. Repetitive play is an example of _____ in a child.
    (A) flashbacks or intrusive memories
    (B) mirror neurons
    (C) flashbulb memory
    (D) backstage self

12. Which of the following would suggest that the two-year-old girl may be at high risk for developing PTSD?
    (A) She is from a blended family.
    (B) She is the youngest child.
    (C) She is living in a middle-income community.
    (D) Her father may have developed PTSD during his military service.

13. Which of the following is most likely true of the child's play?
    (A) Piaget would identify it as age-appropriate magical thinking.
    (B) Erickson believed that it would contribute to the development of mastery and self-esteem.
    (C) If untreated, it could develop into a psychotic disorder.
    (D) It is an example of a symptom that can be found in the DSM.

ANSWER KEY

1. D	**3.** D	**5.** D	**7.** C	**9.** A	**11.** A	**13.** D
2. B	**4.** C	**6.** A	**8.** D	**10.** B	**12.** D

ANSWERS EXPLAINED

1. **(D)** Choice D is correct. A clinical diagnosis is not a "casual" assessment but requires that certain specific criteria are met. To diagnose separation anxiety, the criteria of the DSM must be met. Choice A is incorrect because not meeting the criteria for depressive disorder is not sufficient to prove that the criteria for separation anxiety have been met. Choices B and C are incorrect because, although they may be consistent with separation anxiety, they are not enough to establish a diagnosis. Only meeting the criteria in the DSM can do that.

2. **(B)** Choice B is correct. The average percent for the three years is 14.6. For 1,000 children, there would be 146 with mood disorders. 60% of these are female, based on Figure 2. Even without doing the math, 60% must be more than half (which is 73) but less than the whole (146) so the only answer in the correct range is 88. Choice D is 60% of the entire 1,000.

3. **(D)** Choice D is correct. Being distressed by separation from the caregiver is a defining quality of anxious/ambivalent attachment. Choice A is incorrect because, in secure attachment, the child believes the caregiver will always return. Choice B is incorrect because the reason given is actually the definition of disorganized attachment. Choice C is incorrect because the reason given is the definition of avoidant attachment.

4. **(C)** Choice C is correct because only children are described as being hypersensitive to rejection. Although an adult with depression might experience this symptom, it cannot be defended from the passage that adults experience this. Choice A is incorrect because both children and adults are listed as suffering from sadness or a depressed mood. Choice B is incorrect because both are listed as experiencing weight gain. Choice D is incorrect because the passage specifically states that this is a symptom for adults and states that children might feel like they want to die.

5. **(D)** Choice D is correct because the categories in the DSM all have an exception for when a set of symptoms is the result of a medical condition or drug. To confirm a diagnosis of separation anxiety disorder, it is necessary to rule out the diagnosis of substance/medication-induced anxiety disorder. Choice A is incorrect because, if anything, it would reinforce separation anxiety disorder as the diagnosis. Choice B is incorrect for the same reason. Choice C is incorrect because it is irrelevant. Although it is a true statement, it does not change the fact that medical conditions must be ruled out as the cause of a set of symptoms.

6. **(A)** Choice A is correct because classical conditioning applies a neutral stimulus before a behavior. Operant conditioning applies a nonneutral (reinforcing or punishing) stimulus after a behavior. The other choices are incorrect for this reason. Additionally, choice D is incorrect because the ringing of the bell is not a reinforcement. Choice D is incorrect because the ringing of the bell is neutral, not punishment.

7. **(C)** Choice C is correct because the child's symptoms indicate that he has not yet resolved this task. Choice A is incorrect because the child is not old enough to be

expected to resolve this. Choice B is incorrect because the tasks must be resolved in order and trust and mistrust must be resolved before autonomy versus shame. Choice D is incorrect because it comes after autonomy versus shame as well as trust versus mistrust, and also the child is not yet old enough to be expected to have resolved this.

8. **(D)** Choice D is correct because after the little girl experienced a traumatic event, she began demonstrating symptoms consistent with a diagnosis of post-traumatic stress disorder. Choices A and C are not correct because these diagnoses do not account for symptoms such as repetitive play or nightmares. Choice B is incorrect because adjustment disorder is used only after other disorders are ruled out and PTSD better explains the child's symptoms in the context of the trauma.

9. **(A)** Choice A is correct because choosing clothing that expresses individuation is age appropriate at thirteen years old. Choice B is incorrect because the boy's choice of clothing was not related to his attachment to his stepmother. Choice C is incorrect because ADHD symptoms do not accurately explain the boy's behavior. Choice D is incorrect because the Oedipus complex manifests at around age four and involves an unconscious sexual attraction to the mother; neither of these is the case here.

10. **(B)** Social learning theory would suggest that the child has learned to be hypervigilant by observing her father. Choice A is incorrect because social learning theory requires not just modeling but the presence of a more knowledgeable other. Choice C is incorrect because the rescue was not an example of reinforcement. Choice D is incorrect because the father's wartime traumas do not produce reciprocal determinism.

11. **(A)** Choice A is correct because repetitive play is an example of flashbacks or intrusive memories in a child. Choice B is incorrect because repetitive play is not an example of mirror neurons. Choice C is incorrect because repetitive play is not an example of encoding a flashbulb memory. Choice D is incorrect because repetitive play is not an example of the backstage self.

12. **(D)** Choice D is correct because a vulnerability to PTSD in one family member is a risk factor for other family members. Choice A is incorrect because coming from a blended family is not a risk factor for PTSD. Choice B is incorrect because birth order is not a risk factor for PTSD. Choice C is incorrect because living in a middle-income household is not a risk factor for PTSD.

13. **(D)** Choice D is correct because repetitive play is an abnormal behavior. Any abnormal behavior can be characterized as a symptom. The DSM approaches diagnosis through the use of symptoms. Choice A is incorrect because repetitive play is not an example of magical thinking as defined by Piaget. Choice B is incorrect because repetitive play is not a feature of Erickson's theory. Choice C is incorrect because repetitive play is not a prodromal symptom for a psychotic disorder.

For online practice, go to
http://barronsbooks.com/tp/mcat

Sociology

7

→ **THEORETICAL APPROACHES**

→ **CULTURE**

→ **SOCIALIZATION**

→ **SOCIAL INSTITUTIONS**

→ **ELEMENTS OF SOCIAL INTERACTION**

→ **DEMOGRAPHIC CHARACTERISTICS OF SOCIETY**

→ **SOCIAL CLASS**

→ **PREJUDICE AND DISCRIMINATION**

→ **SPATIAL INEQUALITY**

→ **HEALTH DISPARITIES**

→ **HEALTHCARE DISPARITIES**

Sociology is one of the components of the Psychological, Sociological, and Biological Foundations of Behavior section of the MCAT. About 30% of the questions in this section will be drawn from sociology. The sociology topics on the test are based on concepts taught in an introductory college-level sociology course.

INTRODUCTION

The discipline of sociology is relatively new compared to other sciences such as history, astronomy, or mathematics. It arose out of the social turmoil created by the Industrial Revolution in Western Europe in the eighteenth and nineteenth centuries. Social theories were introduced at that time to help people make sense of the rapidly changing world around them. Sociology, the study of the social processes of society, to this day attempts to understand our social world. This chapter is divided into two parts: foundational concepts of sociology and components of social stratification. A groundwork for sociology is laid in the discussion of sociology's key concepts in the first part of the chapter. The second part emphasizes an additional concept, social stratification, and concludes by considering the effects of social stratification on our health and healthcare system.

FOUNDATIONAL CONCEPTS OF SOCIOLOGY

This section of the chapter consists of the following topics: theoretical approaches, culture, socialization, social institutions, the elements of social interaction (which includes groups and organizations), and the demographic characteristics of society.

Theoretical Approaches

There are three major theoretical approaches or paradigms of sociology, along with one secondary approach, that are discussed here. Using these frameworks, sociologists build theories that attempt to make sense of our social world. Each theoretical approach is unique and offers a distinct insight into understanding society.

FUNCTIONALISM

Functionalism, also known as structural functionalism, is a conservative perspective that generally perceives society as a harmoniously functioning whole with all of its constituent parts (**structures** and institutions) working together to maintain societal equilibrium.

The early British sociologist, Herbert Spencer, a prominent structural functionalist, is famous for comparing society to a living organism, like the human body, with its various parts—structures and institutions—functioning like organs and biological systems to maintain society's existence. Functionalism, which focuses on widespread social behavioral patterns and institutions, is considered to have a macro-level view of society.

> ### STRUCTURE
>
> Sociologists define this term differently than how it is commonly understood. A structure is any pattern of behavior.

CONFLICT THEORY

Conflict theory also takes a macro-level perspective on society, seeing the big picture. This paradigm basically views society as being composed of two competing forces, those who have power and those who do not. The nineteenth-century German sociologist and founder of conflict theory, Karl Marx, focused his attention on the pronounced class conflict of his day between the bourgeois (capitalists, or owners of production) and the proletariat (workers or producers). Marx, like the conflict theorists who have followed him, demonstrated how conflict in society is generated from the fact that those who are powerful in society work to maintain their societal advantage, while the subordinate strives to acquire more power. Two manifestations of conflict theory in contemporary times are race-conflict theory (focusing on the power struggle between whites and minorities) and gender-conflict theory (focusing on the power struggle between men and women). Conflict theory differs from the other sociological paradigms in that it advocates for a sociologist's active role in bringing about social equality.

SYMBOLIC INTERACTIONISM

Of the three main sociological theoretical approaches, **symbolic interactionism** is the only one that takes a micro-level perspective. It is primarily concerned with the study of individual or small group social interactions and how these shape society. Symbolic interactionists focus on the symbols people use to communicate with others and how these symbols are interpreted. From the standpoint of symbolic interactionism, an issue such as teenage smoking is seen not merely as a result of insufficient warnings about the dangers of tobacco but as an activity that is given symbolic meaning through the interactions of teenage peers. For example, smoking may be given the symbolic value of representing rebellion against adult authority. Symbolic interactionists believe that such symbolic meaning—acted on by a group—provides the best insight into society. Whereas functionalists might look at the phenomenon of teenage smoking in a very large context that includes the agricultural aspects of tobacco growing, the economic sphere of the tobacco industry, and the attitudes of several generations, the symbolic interactionist focuses on the dynamics of the interactions of a small group of people (peers). Similarly, symbolic interactionism has a narrower focus than conflict theorists, who look at the power struggle between the wealthy tobacco industry, the government, and segments of society that are powerless to protect themselves from addictive products.

SOCIAL CONSTRUCTIONISM

Closely related to symbolic interactionism is a secondary approach called **social constructionism**. Social constructionism is a school of thought that is concerned with how knowledge is generated in everyday social interactions. A central concept of social constructionism is the **social construction of reality**, which is defined as the social reality that is created through social interactions. This is a fundamental concept of symbolic interactionism. For example, the meaning of a coin is defined by the agreement among individuals that the coin has worth, rather than by the value of the metal in the coin itself.

Two examples of how social constructionism can be applied to the field of medicine are as follows: (1) The manner in which doctors set up their offices, dress, and conduct themselves is a powerful force in the construction of reality with their patients, determining whether or not patients see a doctor as being in control and proficient. (2) Appropriate standards of health vary from one society to another or even among different segments of the same society. This difference can be explained using the social constructionist's perspective. Through interactions with those around them, individuals learn what an appropriate standard of health is.

Culture

Culture can be defined broadly as the learned behaviors shared by a people. These learned behaviors dictate how people make and use objects (material culture) as well as how they think (symbolic culture). Culture has allowed humans to adapt to their environment much in the same way that biological evolution allows organisms to adapt. However, cultural evolution occurs much more rapidly than biological evolution, providing a mechanism for rapid cultural response to environmental change even within a single generation.

Culture in turn can result in environmental changes that may then lead to biological evolution and adaptation in human groups. For example, the domestication of cattle by some groups in Europe and Africa within the last ten thousand years has resulted in convergent evolution of lactose tolerance in these populations.

MATERIAL CULTURE

Physical objects (cars, clothing, digital devices, houses) are tangible components of culture, also known as artifacts, and constitute **material culture**. Material culture can differ greatly among distinct cultural groups.

SYMBOLIC CULTURE

Symbolic culture refers to the nonmaterial elements of culture. These include symbols, language, values, beliefs, norms, and rituals.

Symbols and Language

Symbols are objects, images, sounds, or actions that are associated with a meaning. Often the relationship between the symbol and the meaning is arbitrary, such as a red light meaning "stop." For this reason most symbols must be learned, and a culture is defined in part by the set of symbols that are mutually understood among a people. An object, image, sound, or action that has symbolic meaning in one culture may not convey any meaning at all in a different culture. Alternately, it may convey a dramatically different meaning in another culture, which can result in misunderstandings and conflict. For instance, the "thumbs up" symbol meaning "Good job!" in the West is understood in Iran as an offensive act toward another person.

Language is a system of symbols that is able to convey highly complex and sophisticated meaning in a way that other types of symbols cannot. Language is so important to culture that it is seen as one of the defining characteristics of a particular culture. In fact, language is indispensable for **cultural transmission**. Cultural transmission is the passing on of a culture to succeeding generations. There are nearly 7,000 different languages in the world today. Over 300 languages are spoken in the United States alone. Many languages today are in danger of extinction, which can happen when a language with a limited number of speakers is replaced by a socially or economically more dominant one. More than 50 percent of languages worldwide are spoken by fewer than 10,000 people each.

Values and Beliefs

Values are broad standards or principles that define qualities that a culture holds to be important. All cultures have values that are shared by most members. There can be a sharp contrast between the values of one culture and those of another. One culture might value individuality and another communality. One might value hard work and another leisure. Other contrasting pairs of values include competitiveness versus cooperation, science versus spirituality, and democracy versus consolidated authority.

Whereas values are general, **beliefs** are *specific* notions that people share about what is true or false. Beliefs are shaped and guided by values. Within the framework of a cultural value that education is important, people might hold a specific belief that medical doctors can help prevent or cure illnesses, based on their education.

Norms

Norms are rules and regulations that a society uses to guide the behaviors of its members. Norms are enforced in society by sanctions that punish and reward behaviors. There are two types: mores (MORE-ayz) and folkways.

MORES. **Mores** are norms that deal with moral issues and that have strong support among society's members. The punishments for violating mores are often severe and are often formally spelled out in legal statutes or codes. Examples of mores are incest taboos, prohibitions against stealing, and prohibitions against murder.

FOLKWAYS. **Folkways** are norms that have weaker support among society's members and that carry less severe, informal punishments for their violators. An example of a folkway is what is considered a proper place setting for meals. Generally, this folkway is casually adhered to in our society, but on more formal occasions it becomes more expected. A host who puts the forks on the wrong side of the plate at a formal dinner will not be reported to authorities for his infraction but may meet with some disapproval from guests.

Paying your restaurant bill only with pennies would be a violation of this type of norm, _____, whereas knowingly paying your restaurant bill with counterfeit money would be an example of violating this type of norm, _____.

(A) values; beliefs

(B) mores; folkways

(C) beliefs; values

(D) folkways; mores

(D) The first example illustrates a norm violation that may generate surprised looks and murmurs (informal punishments) from restaurant staff and fellow patrons but will not lead to police involvement (formal punishments). The second example constitutes criminal fraud, punishable by heavy fines or imprisonment (formal punishments). Choice A is incorrect because even though values and beliefs may influence norms, they are not norms. Choice B is incorrect because it is opposite to the correct answer. Choice C is incorrect for the same reason that choice A is incorrect.

Rituals

A **ritual** is an established pattern of formal behavior that is conducted on special occasions. It can be religious or secular. The Inauguration of a President in Washington, D.C., is an example of a nonreligious ritual. Rituals serve to reinforce the sense of a common bond among members of a culture by drawing on feelings of deep common purpose and shared values.

CULTURE SHOCK AND CULTURAL LAG

Culture can sometimes be the source of personal and societal confusion. For example, first-time travelers to a developing country from a developed country (or vice versa) will often have a revelational experience of a way of life that is far different than their own. When someone initially experiences such an unfamiliar culture, they may undergo a period of disorientation known as **culture shock**.

Technological innovations in society produce new objects of material culture. These, in turn, bring about changes in society to which symbolic culture—such as norms—adapts and tries to regulate, if necessary. The longer symbolic culture takes to catch up to these societal changes, the more chance there is for confusion and conflict in society. The disturbance in society caused by symbolic culture not keeping pace with societal changes brought about by new material culture is called **cultural lag**. The transformations in society accompanying the proliferation of cell phones and smartphones over recent decades and the societal confusion created by unsolidified norms of etiquette and law for using these devices is a good example of cultural lag.

SUBCULTURES

Whereas a culture includes a set of common values shared by a group of people, within any society there are often segments that share a set of values different to some

SUBCULTURES

African-American, Hispanic-American, Asian-American, Jewish, and Muslim subcultures are examples of prominent subcultures in the United States.

extent from those of the wider society in which they live. These segments are called **subcultures**. The most significant subcultures are based on factors such as ethnicity, national origin, religion, or language—elements that are part of a person's identity. In such cases people are members of the subculture by virtue of who they are, even if being a member brings negative consequences, such as discrimination. Other subcultures are based on interests or hobbies, such as being a wine enthusiast or Star Trek fan. Membership in these subcultures is based on what a person does and is voluntary.

ASSIMILATION AND MULTICULTURALISM

A society with many cultures may hold a value that it is better for minority cultures to blend into the dominant culture (**assimilation**), or it may hold a value that maintaining diverse cultures is beneficial (**multiculturalism**).

Assimilation is the process by which members of a subculture take on the characteristics of the dominant culture in society. Assimilation can help members of a subculture avoid prejudice and discrimination but at the possible cost of losing their cultural heritage and self-esteem.

Multiculturalism is an appreciation of cultural diversity. It is in contrast to the belief that subcultures should adopt the values of the dominant culture. An appreciation of multiculturalism in a society reduces the pressure for members of subcultures to assimilate.

Socialization

Socialization refers to the process through which cultural values, beliefs, and norms are transmitted from one generation to the next. Socialization serves to guide the behavior of individuals within a society. It begins at a very early age and continues throughout life.

From the perspective of moral development, socialization moves people beyond a self-centered perspective to a perspective that accommodates others. At the same time, a well-developed moral sense may lead some people to reject certain values imparted by socialization.

AGENTS OF SOCIALIZATION

Although socialization takes place in every social interaction, there are several specific **agents of socialization** that have the most pervasive influence on members of society. These agents include family, school, peers, mass media, and the workplace.

Family

For most people, the family is the most important agent of socialization. It is in this setting that infants and toddlers are cared for by parents and other family members. Children learn skills and values almost exclusively in the family until they are old enough to go to school and, if homeschooled, even longer. In addition, a child's social identity is transmitted to them by their family. This involves both racial and class identities.

School

Most of the socialization that takes place in school is a consequence of what is called the **hidden curriculum**—the informal and unofficial, often unintended, lessons learned by students in school. For many children, the school is the first place where they are exposed to others of different races and different class backgrounds. This experience tends to strengthen their own social identities. Children tend to group with others of the same race, class, and gender. Schools also reinforce gender roles children have already developed in the family. For many children, the school is their first exposure to the rules and regulations of formal bureaucratic institutions.

Peers

In school, children often become members of a peer group. A **peer group** is composed of individuals who share common characteristics, such as age, interests, and social position. Peers become most influential in the socialization process in adolescence. This is the time of life when children often seek independence from their family and begin to establish their own identity. At this age, the peer group differs from the family and school, in that, there is, generally, less adult supervision. As a result, members of the peer group may become involved in harmful or illegal activities, such as drinking and drug abuse. Another aspect of peer groups is **anticipatory socialization**. Anticipatory socialization is the process by which individuals conform to a group's behavior primarily out of a desire to be a part of the group.

Mass Media

Mass media—including newspapers, radio, television, films, and the internet—is unique among other agents of socialization in that ideas and values of the broader society, including of the world as a whole, are conveyed to large numbers of people in a short time. The groups that control mass media have the potential to exert a disproportionate influence on values, beliefs, and norms.

Workplace

The workplace is the setting for **organizational socialization**. This socialization is the process by which new employees learn what is necessary to assume a role in an organization. Through organizational efforts like orientations and trainings, a new employee develops skills and learns about the values and procedures of an organization.

DEVIANCE AND STIGMA

Failure to follow the rules of society (**deviance**) can result in negative consequences (**stigma**) for an individual.

Deviance

Deviance refers to actions that depart from and violate cultural norms. The source of many pioneering insights into deviance, the classical French sociologist Emile Durkheim revealed that deviance is needed to affirm society's values and norms. The response to deviance can be mild to severe depending on the degree of the offense to society. For example, **crime**, a type of deviance in which a society's criminal law has been violated, is usually punished more severely than a violation of a folkway, a cultural norm that has weaker support among society's members. Whether or not punishments for violating cultural norms are formal or informal, they serve as mechanisms for **social control**. Social control is the way in which society attempts to regulate the behaviors of its members.

Theories of deviance. Since Durkheim, other sociologists have studied the theory of deviance. American sociologist Robert Merton developed the concept of **strain theory**. (See Figure 7.1.) Strain theory states that deviance is the result of society not supplying the sufficient conventional or institutionalized means (education and employment) for members to achieve society's socially approved cultural goals (the American dream and financial success).

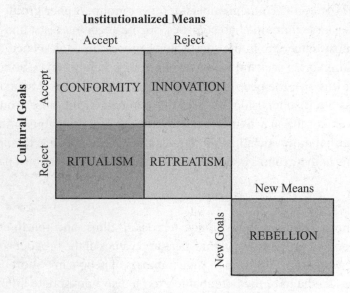

Figure 7.1. Robert Merton's typology of deviance

According to Merton, there are five responses to the strain created in this social environment. **Conformity** (the only nondeviant response) consists of using socially accepted means—hard work, talent, and education—to try to achieve the cultural goals of society. **Innovation** occurs when those with little or no conventional means, often the poor, use unconventional means (dealing drugs, stealing, other crimes) in their attempts to achieve culturally approved success. **Ritualism** is an adherence to conventional means, especially to an excessive degree, with a lost hope of ever achieving out-of-reach cultural goals. **Retreatism** is a rejection of both society's approved goals and the accepted means to reach those goals. Social dropouts—drunkards, drug addicts, and outcasts—are considered retreatists. Finally, **rebellion** is like retreatism in that it is a rejection of society's means and goals, but instead of a withdrawal, it engages society with new means and goals. Counterculturalists and political revolutionaries are examples of rebels.

Two other theories that provide insight into understanding deviance are **labeling theory** and **differential association theory**. **Labeling theory** focuses on how people react to behavior more than on the behavior itself. It points out the relativity of defining behavior as deviant. What some people consider deviant, others may not consider deviant at all. Edwin Sutherland's **differential association theory** emphasizes the role of groups in determining the likelihood of whether or not an individual will engage in deviant behavior. The theory reveals a strong correlation between the amount of time an individual spends in peer groups that encourage deviant behavior and the probability that the individual will engage in that behavior.

A hardworking factory worker who rigidly follows company policies but who believes she will never get a promotion to help her move to a better neighborhood is an example, according to Merton, of:

(A) conformity.

(B) innovation.

(C) ritualism.

(D) retreatism.

(C) Choice C is correct because this factory worker is an example of someone who adheres to the institutionalized (conventional) means of hard work and obedience but who has lost hope of even making the next step toward the American Dream. Choice A is incorrect because even though she conforms to following the institutionalized means to success (hard work and obedience), she does not conform to believing she can achieve that success. Choice B is incorrect because the factory worker is not using any unconventional means of innovation, such as drug dealing or stealing, and is no longer pursuing culturally approved success. Choice D is incorrect because even though, like retreatists, the factory worker is not pursuing society's approved goals of the American Dream and financial success, she has, unlike retreatists, not rejected society's institutionalized means. In fact, it is her strict adherence to the means of hard work and obedience that give her some consolation of self-respect.

Stigma

When deviant behavior by an individual is persistent, the individual can acquire a **stigma**. A stigma is a strongly negative label that society associates with an individual. Such a label changes the individual's self-concept and social identity. A person who has been stigmatized may internalize society's negative label and may become socially isolated.

CONFORMITY AND OBEDIENCE

The desires to conform to norms and to obey authority play a strong role in socialization.

Conformity

Conformity is the process by which an individual modifies his or her behavior in direct response to the influence of another person or group. Conformity occurs as a direct result of both **informational social influence** and **normative social influence**. With informational social influence, an individual is unsure how to act in a particular situation and relies on information gained by observing the actions of others in similar situations.

With normative social influence, an individual's behaviors, appearance, beliefs, and/or values are influenced, consciously or unconsciously, by the desire to act like others in order to be accepted and liked by them. Conformity to social norms within a group can result in a conflict between personal values and need for social validation. As a result, a person may publicly comply with predominant social norms but privately disapprove of the group's behavior. Normative influence is most pronounced when the group is important to an individual (**strength**), when the group is close in space and time at the moment of conformity (**immediacy**), or when there are a large number of people in the group (**number**).

Obedience

Informational and normative social influence play a substantial role in **obedience**, or compliance with other people's demands. Obedience is also driven by a need to please others, especially if the other in question is an authority figure. Most people have been socialized to defer to authorities, experts, or other people in positions of power in order to avoid punishment, embarrassment, or rejection. Obedience to authority is common in emergency situations. In obeying authority in such situations, people generally trust both that the authority figures know how to react and that they are acting in the best interest of the public.

Social Institutions

Social institutions are major areas of social life that meet or attempt to meet the needs of society's members. Types of social institutions include religion, the family, education, health and medicine, and government and economy.

RELIGION

The primary focus of **religion** is meeting the spiritual needs of society's members. Religion gives meaning and purpose to human existence. Religion helps separate the **sacred**, what is holy or set apart, from the **profane**, what is ordinary or mundane. In many societies there is a state-affiliated religion that has significant influence on governmental policy. Because of the emotional power of religious beliefs, religious institutions have a strong influence on the social and political values of their members.

THE FAMILY

The **family** is considered the basic unit of society. Sociologists that adhere to the functionalist approach consider the family to be the "backbone of society" because of the family's socialization and supportive functions. Because the family is the primary institution through which individuals receive their social identity, conflict theorists focus on how the family perpetuates class, race, ethnic, and gender inequality in society.

There are two main classifications of the family: the extended family and the nuclear family. The **extended family**, which includes parents, children, and kin, plays a greater role in preindustrialized societies. The **nuclear family**, which can have one or two parents and their children, plays a greater role after industrialization, a period marked by increased social mobility and migration.

> **EXTENDED FAMILY**
>
> The extended family is a great asset for preindustrial, agrarian societies. Because there are more caretakers, families can have more children, strengthening the agriculturally based economic unit of the large, extended family. Older members contribute their knowledge of farming to younger generations.

EDUCATION

Education is a social institution that transfers society's knowledge to its members. The quality of education received by society's members can be affected by factors such as class, race, ethnicity, and/or gender.

HEALTH AND MEDICINE

The social institutions of **health and medicine** serve to maintain the health and well-being of the members of society. Different societies may set different standards for acceptable physical and mental health.

Social epidemiology and holistic medicine are two areas of health and medicine that are of special interest to sociologists. **Social epidemiology** is the study of how diseases and health are spread throughout society. **Holistic medicine** is an alternative practice of medicine that places more emphasis on a person's physical and social environment than the more pervasive scientific model of medicine.

GOVERNMENT AND ECONOMY

The social institution of **government** functions to assign authority and guide society as a whole. It is closely related to the social institution of the **economy**, which serves to regulate the production, distribution, and consumption of society's goods and services. Historically, the close connection between the government and economy is evidenced by the tendency of particular forms of government to coexist with specific economic systems. Examples of this include monarchy with feudalism, democracy with capitalism, and communism with socialism.

Elements of Social Interaction

Social interaction is the exchange of actions among people in a society. To more fully understand this process, it is important to be familiar with the different elements that can affect it. These elements include status, roles, social groups, networks, and organizations.

STATUS

Status is the social position that a person holds in society. A person's status influences how that person interacts with others and how others interact with that person. One person can hold more than one status. For example, someone might have the statuses of professor, being middle-aged, a spouse, a parent, and a coach. A **status set** inlcudes all of the status positions held by a particular person.

There are two types of status: ascribed status and achieved status. **Ascribed status** includes status that is given to a person at birth or later in life through little or no effort of that person. Status that is determined by a person's age, sex, race, ethnicity, and family background is ascribed status. Becoming a parent, losing a spouse, or being disabled in an accident are examples of how ascribed status can be assumed after birth. **Achieved status** is status that is voluntarily acquired through a person's effort (or lack thereof). A person's occupation is considered an achieved status. Nobel Prize Laureate, honor-roll student, high school dropout, criminal, and city council member are all examples of achieved status.

Most achieved statuses are influenced by ascribed statuses. For example, a person who comes from a wealthy family (ascribed status) has a better chance of becoming a doctor (achieved status). Likewise, a person who was raised in poverty (ascribed status) is more likely to be unemployed, be underemployed, or have a low-wage job (achieved status).

ROLES

An individual who holds a particular status is expected to behave in a way that is appropriate for that status. The expected behavior that is attached to a status is a **role**. Most statuses are accompanied by more than one role. For instance, some common roles that mothers have are nurturer, nurse, disciplinarian, and confidant to their children. **Role set** is the term used to define the various roles of a single status.

Sometimes roles of a single status can come into conflict. For example, attorneys have a duty to the court to always tell the truth, but attorneys also have a duty to zealously advocate for their clients. Sometimes these two roles come into conflict, and this explains why criminal attorneys typically will not ask their clients if they have committed a crime in question. Conflict between roles of a single status is called **role strain**.

Sometimes a person experiences tension between roles, not of the same status, but of different statuses of their status set. This is called **role conflict**. A working parent who is pulled between the responsibilities of work and home is experiencing role conflict.

GROUPS

A **social group** consists of two or more people who interact with and feel connected to one another. A social group can be classified as either a **primary group** or a **secondary group** depending on how closely connected group members are to one another. Close personal relationships in small groups characterize primary groups, where interactions are viewed as ends in themselves and not as means to another end. The family is the most important primary group in society. A peer group of friends is also a primary group. A secondary group is a large group composed of impersonal relationships. Unlike a primary group, in which members share a number of activities together, secondary groups are centered around a focused activity. Interactions between secondary group members are generally guided towards specific goals. Students in the same school or co-workers in the same company are considered secondary groups.

A major effect that groups have on social interaction is that they promote group conformity. Experiments by Solomon Asch and Stanley Milgram have shown that members of a social group will conform to a standard group behavior even if this behavior is illogical. Additionally, Irving L. Janis coined the term **groupthink** to explain the propensity of social group members to conform to a narrow view on some issue being examined by their social group.

Practice Question

How does the proverb "blood is thicker than water" relate to primary and secondary groups?

Solution: A common understanding of this proverb is that family ties are stronger and more important than ties with those outside the family. The family is considered the most important primary group, more significant than a circle of friends (the other example of a primary group). This proverb also considers secondary groups to be bound together with much weaker impersonal relationships.

NETWORKS

Networks are loose associations of people that often comprise many people over great distances. The World Wide Web is considered the largest network. Unlike social group members, network members have no real sense of belonging. People in a network may or may not know each other, and social interactions rarely, if at all, take place between them. For job seekers and immigrants who have newly arrived, increased social interactions in networks can be extremely valuable in helping them meet their goals.

ORGANIZATIONS

Organizations or, as called by sociologists, formal organizations, are large secondary groups that are characterized by bureaucracy. **Bureaucracy** is a model of organization that emphasizes rationality, hierarchy, specialization of skills, and impersonal rules and regulations. Government agencies and conventional corporations are examples of formal organizations. Bureaucracy, in effect, streamlines social interactions with the goal of increased organizational efficiency and productivity.

Bureaucracy, however, has its downside. The classical German sociologist, Max Weber, who believed that bureaucracy was the most efficient way to organize social interactions, also realized that the highly rationalized and impersonal treatment of people in a bureaucratic organization leads to their dehumanization and alienation. He saw bureaucracy as transforming people into cogs in a machine, trapping them in an "iron cage." Another German sociologist, Robert Michels, developed a theory called the **iron law of oligarchy**. It maintains that all bureaucracies, even democratic ones, will inevitably be controlled by an elite few (an **oligarchy**). Robert Merton was the first to use the term **bureaucratic ritualism** to describe the rigid adherence to rules and regulations in a bureaucracy that undermine an organization's goals.

Demographic Characteristics of Society

Demography is the statistical study of the characteristics of human populations. By providing information and explanations of the composition and shifts of a society's population throughout time, demography helps enlighten the understanding of society and the social interactions that take place there.

DEMOGRAPHIC CATEGORIES

Demographic categories include age, gender, race and ethnicity, immigration status, and sexual orientation.

Age

Awareness of the age composition of a society can help a society prepare to meet the needs of its population. For example, demographic knowledge of the entry of "baby boomers" in the United States into their senior years is critical in helping U.S. health and medical, government, and economic institutions prepare for the needs that this will precipitate.

Sex

One important demographic variable that is used to study the composition of males to females in society is the **sex ratio**. The sex ratio is the number of males to every 100 females in society. Another important tool for analysis is the **age–sex pyramid**, which graphically illustrates the sex composition of different age **cohorts** or groups in society. A demographic analysis of the sex composition of the Russian Federation is a good illustration of how this type of study can help one understand society and social interactions. In the Russian Federation, there are a disproportionate number of females to males in the working-age cohorts. This has been explained by the high rates of male death in these cohorts caused by diseases and accidents.

RACE AND ETHNICITY

Race is determined by biological characteristics, whereas ethnicity is determined by cultural ones.

Race and Ethnicity

Race and ethnicity is another demographic category that is of interest to demographers. The information that people report as to what they consider to be their racial and/or ethnic identity is used for demographic purposes.

A **race** is a category of people with distinct biological or visible characteristics that a society deems to be important. **Ethnicity** is based on the shared cultural traits (ancestry, language, and religion) of a people. Both racial and ethnic categories are considered to be socially constructed and are only distinguished as society finds a need to do so.

TEST QUESTION

The Amharic language and Oriental Orthodox Christianity are for many Ethiopian Americans cultural characteristics that comprise their _____. Many Ethiopian immigrants to the United States, because of the color of their skin, have faced for the first time in their lives barriers to upward social mobility based on their

_____.

(A) race; ethnicity
(B) ethnicity; ancestry
(C) ethnicity; race
(D) ancestry; race

(C) The correct answer for the first blank is "ethnicity" because language and religion are both important characteristics comprising a people's ethnicity. The correct answer for the second blank is "race" because skin color is a biological characteristic often used to define race. Ancestry (line of descent) is not a correct response for the first blank. It is considered another shared cultural characteristic, like language and religion, that makes up a people's ethnicity. Ethnicity is not a correct response for the second blank, because it is the shared cultural characteristics of a people and is not based on biological or visible characteristics such as skin color.

Immigration Status

Immigrants are the foreign-born population in a society. A demographic study of immigration in the United States in the last 50 years reveals a major change in the characteristics of this segment of U.S. society. According to the U.S. Census Bureau, in 1960, 1 in 20 of the

U.S. population was an immigrant, probably from Europe, and likely settled in the Northeast and Midwest. In 2010, 1 in 8 of the U.S. population was an immigrant, probably from Latin America or Asia, and likely settled in the West and South.

Sexual Orientation

The three main categories of sexual orientation that have been studied by demographers are heterosexuality, homosexuality, and bisexuality. According to demographic findings, most people have a heterosexual orientation. In the United States, men that have a homosexual orientation are between 3 percent and 9 percent of the population and women who have a homosexual orientation are between 1 percent and 5 percent of the population. The percent of those with a bisexual orientation has been difficult to determine on account of the different definitions used to define bisexuality—sexual attraction to both sexes to a near equal degree or sexual attraction to both sexes in any degree.

Determining the demographics for sexual orientation is difficult, in part because many people who are not strictly heterosexual may not identify themselves. In addition, there is a wide gap between the number of people who claim to be exclusively gay and the number of people who report having had some feelings for a member of the same sex. In one of the largest surveys done, about 2.5 percent of both men and women reported being either gay or bisexual. However, 8 percent of men and 15 percent of women had either had a sexual experience with someone of the same sex or had been attracted to someone of the same sex.

Being transsexual (transgendered) involves one's sense of gender identity and is independent of the gender to which one is attracted.

DEMOGRAPHIC SHIFTS AND SOCIAL CHANGE

The demographic makeup of society is constantly changing. As demographics change, the values of society also change. This section reviews the forces that contribute to demographic change.

Demographic Transition

Demographic transition theory links the transitions of a society to technological changes. (See Figure 7.2.) According to this theory, preindustrialized societies' populations remain fairly constant in size because the high birth rates in these societies—encouraged by the need for labor provided by children for agricultural economies—is balanced by high death rates, which are caused by low living standards and primitive medical technology. The beginning of industrialization brings a shift according to this theory because industrialization brings higher food supplies and better medical technology, which lowers death rates. Birth rates remain high, so populations increase rapidly. Demographic transition theory states as industrialization more fully develops, birth rates fall because children in this period are more likely to reach adulthood, so parents tend to feel less pressure to have additional children. Also, because living standards are higher, children become more of an economic liability for families. Death rates continue to fall with medical advancements, but overall, the population only grows steadily. With postindustrialization, birth rates continue to fall with increased living standards and death rates remain constant. Population growth is slow in this period.

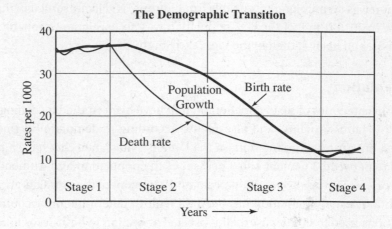

Figure 7.2. Demographic transition. Stage 1 is preindustrialized. Stage 2 is the beginning of industrialization. Stage 3 is more fully developed industrialization. Stage 4 is postindustrialization.

Fertility, Migration, and Mortality

Fertility, mortality, and migration lead to changes in a society's population size and composition. **Fertility** is the number of births in a given population. Demographers measure fertility by the variable of the crude birth rate. The **crude birth rate** is the number of annual live births for every 1,000 people in a population. **Mortality** is the number of deaths in a given population. Demographers measure mortality using two variables: the crude death rate and the infant mortality rate. The **crude death rate** is the number of annual deaths for every 1,000 people in a population. The **infant mortality rate** is the number of annual infant deaths for every 1,000 live births in a population. The term **migration** as primarily used by demographers means the immigration and emigration of a population. **Immigration** is the movement of people into a society's land. **Emigration** is the movement of people out of a society's land.

Migration can be explained by **push** and **pull factors**. Push factors are those elements in people's environment *pushing* them away, such as unemployment, war, famine, and persecution. Pull factors are those elements in another geographical area that are *pulling* or attracting those people, such as job opportunities, peace, attractive climate, and freedom.

Social Movements

A **social movement** is a collective push for social change or to maintain the status quo in society. Social movements for social change can culminate in war, bringing about significant decreases in a society's population caused by war fatalities and emigration.

Globalization

Globalization refers to the overall tendency for social processes to become increasingly more global and less territorial in scope. The main elements of society—economics, education, culture, religion, and law—have become increasingly intertwined across national borders. Nearly every facet of modern life contributes to globalization, including electronic communication, which virtually erases geographical distance as a significant factor. Globalization can only be expected to expand in the foreseeable future.

Urbanization

Urbanization is the tendency for people to move from rural areas to urban areas. The tendency for people to gather in large populations has been operating from ancient times but has accelerated in recent centuries. It is most advanced in developed countries but is a strong trend in developing countries as well. The United Nations predicts that over 64 percent of the population in developing countries will live in urban settings by 2050 and that nearly 86 percent of the population in developed countries will be urbanized. Urbanization affects both economics and environment. Economics is affected by the excess of labor in the cities and the dearth of labor in agricultural areas, among other factors. Environment is affected by the large land areas that are paved and the lack of vegetation, as well as concentrated pollution from industry and transportation.

COMPONENTS OF SOCIAL STRATIFICATION

Social stratification refers to the differences between layers of society distinguished on the basis of status, economics, power, and politics. Some important aspects of social stratification include the concepts of social class, prejudice and discrimination, spatial inequality, health disparities, and healthcare disparities.

Social Class

Social class is the foundation of social stratification.

ASPECTS OF SOCIAL STRATIFICATION

The most important aspects of social stratification include the elements of class, status, and power; cultural capital and social capital; social reproduction; privilege and prestige; and the intersections of race, gender, and age.

Class, Status, and Power

These three interrelated elements determine the extent to which people are able to maintain or improve their situation in society. **Class** typically refers to an economic division between upper, middle, and lower income people. However, people who do not meet the usual criteria for membership in a particular class may possess other characteristics that define a class, such as educational level, culture, and speech. For example, a person born into a lower-class family might develop an income considered to be upper class and yet have the speech and habits of a person from the lower class. In some societies, membership in a class is hereditary and may not be defined by wealth, as in the example of hereditary nobility.

Status, like class, indicates a person's relative standing in relation to others. Status differs from class in that it is not necessarily based on wealth but on how one is viewed by others. Status can be achieved by actions or through reputation. In some societies, status is primarily inherited.

Power refers to the ability to manipulate elements of society to one's benefit. Economic standing confers power but some people may achieve power without class standing or status through their own actions or personalities.

> **CLASS**
>
> It is common to perceive the U.S. class system as having four divisions: upper class, middle class, working class, and lower class.

Cultural Capital and Social Capital

The term **capital** refers to resources that can be used to improve one's circumstances. Cultural and social capital are noneconomic resources. **Cultural capital** refers to cultural qualities that are valuable in improving social standing. They include education, intelligence, manner of dress, and manner of speech. **Social capital** refers to the social connections established by a person, on which the person can draw to improve standing.

Social Reproduction

Social reproduction is the phenomenon in which social standing is preserved from one generation to the next. Both high standing and low standing are preserved through social reproduction. Social reproduction, then, is responsible for the perpetuation of social inequality.

Privilege and Prestige

The concept of **privilege** is that some people have access to certain societal benefits through characteristics over which they have no control, such as gender, race, and age. Privilege is granted through the values of others, rather than earned. The concept is important because people who benefit from privilege often mistakenly believe they have earned benefits through their own actions and may not understand why others, without privilege, do not do so. **Prestige** refers to the respect granted to individuals because of their status, class, or power. Prestige may or may not correlate with the individual's actions or attributes.

Intersections of Race, Gender, and Age

The dynamics that result in class, power, and status in a society do not apply in the same way to all people. Actions that would be sufficient to result in high status for one person may not have that result for people who are members of a racial minority. Similarly, a woman is likely to have a harder time achieving class, status, or power than would a man in the same circumstances. A woman who is a member of a racial minority would have an even harder time. In the case of a woman who is both older and a member of a racial minority, the disadvantage is compounded.

PATTERNS OF SOCIAL MOBILITY

Social mobility refers to the ability to move from one class or status to another. Social mobility usually applies to patterns that affect groups of people. There are typical patterns that apply to mobility. Mobility can change from one generation to the next or within a generation. In addition, mobility can be downward as well as upward. Mobility may or may not reflect a particular person's abilities and skills.

Intergenerational and Intragenerational Mobility

Intergenerational mobility refers to the changes in status that take place from one generation to the next. In a society in which people have a status that is very similar to the status of their parents, there is little intergenerational mobility. Intergenerational mobility is of most significance at the lower levels of society. It can be improved by programs that provide support for young children of lower-class families. **Intragenerational mobility** occurs within one generation. It is correlated with individual efforts and support programs aimed at adults. Changes in legislation can support intragenerational mobility by removing discriminatory laws.

Downward and Upward Mobility

Whereas most people hope that their situations improve, mobility can occur both in an upward direction (improved status) and in a downward direction (decreased status). A pervasive pattern of downward mobility for a group of people is an indication that significant negative societal forces are acting on that group.

Meritocracy

Meritocracy is the belief that people should benefit in proportion to their merits. Merits include abilities, skills, productivity, intelligence, and talent, among other qualities. Meritocracy stands in opposition to the belief that certain people are entitled to power or status by virtue of belonging to certain groups or by heredity. A belief in meritocracy favors the upward mobility of oppressed groups, although members of those groups may need additional support to develop the merits from which they can benefit because discrimination acts to prevent people from access to developing merits.

POVERTY

In some societies, there is a greater gap between the wealthy and the poor. In other societies, the gap is smaller. However, few, if any, societies can avoid having an impoverished class. Poverty is a concern because people living in poverty have a poor quality of life. In addition, the existence of a large impoverished class also affects the quality of life of middle- and upper-class people.

Relative and Absolute Poverty

Absolute poverty refers to a lack of the basic necessities of life—food, clothing, shelter, and medical care. **Relative poverty** is in reference to the average material wealth of people in a given society. People in relative poverty may have the basic necessities but are not able to live as well as others in the society.

Practice Question

When discussing poverty in the United States, what type of poverty is generally being referred to?

Solution: Although a small percentage of the U.S. poor are plagued by absolute poverty, most poverty in the United States, as in other wealthy nations, is relative poverty. In general, the U.S. poor have a much higher standard of living than the poor of developing countries. Some developing countries have over a half of their population living without the basic necessities needed to sustain life.

Social Exclusion: Segregation and Isolation

Social exclusion refers to the process by which certain groups are excluded from access to goods or services that are available to other members of society. For example, in some societies certain groups are not allowed to attend public school. Social exclusion keeps certain groups separate from mainstream society (**segregation**) and at the same time forces them into their own closed society (**isolation**). Social exclusion helps keep marginalized groups from accessing the resources that could make them upwardly mobile.

Prejudice and Discrimination

Prejudice, bias, and discrimination are powerful forces that perpetuate social stratification. Prejudice and bias are defined and described in Chapter 6, Psychology. **Discrimination** is the act of treating people in a specific way because of their membership in a particular group or their placement in a particular category. Typically, discrimination involves treating people in a way that is worse than if they did not belong to that group or category. Discrimination differs from **prejudice** in that prejudice refers to the beliefs and attitudes held by a person, whereas discrimination refers to the actions that result from those beliefs and attitudes.

INDIVIDUAL VERSUS INSTITUTIONAL DISCRIMINATION

Discrimination is often thought of as the action of individuals. However, discrimination is also built into the structure of many institutions, including governmental, economic, religious, and educational institutions. Institutional discrimination may be difficult to change, even if individuals within an institution are in favor of change, because of the relative inflexibility of institutional structures in general.

HOW POWER, PRESTIGE, AND CLASS INFLUENCE DISCRIMINATION

People in the upper classes of society who possess power and prestige have the ability to influence society to their own benefit. As a result, a powerful person can use influence to perpetuate personal prejudices. This can be done by implementing discriminatory policies in the institutions controlled by the powerful person. It can also be done through supporting discriminatory organizations, through propaganda in the mass media, and through supporting politicians who hold similar prejudices. In this way, a person with power can perpetuate discrimination that is far more damaging than the discrimination that a less powerful person can.

Spatial Inequality

Spatial inequality refers to a discriminatory pattern of access to products or services based on location. In other words, groups that are kept physically isolated by means of social exclusion may not have access in their communities to resources that people living in mainstream communities have. These resources include work, education, health services, and food, as well as other resources that could potentially increase their upward mobility.

Residential Segregation

Residential segregation refers to the phenomenon by which certain groups are restricted in the areas in which they may live. Residential segregation can be the result of laws that restrict where people can live. In the United States, residential segregation occurs primarily because of discriminatory housing practices on the part of property owners that prevent people of specific groups from buying or renting in certain neighborhoods.

Environmental Inequality

People living in neighborhoods that are segregated by ethnicity or socioeconomic status may find that they do not have the power to protect their neighborhood from industrial or environmental pollution, such as toxic chemicals or loud noise. People in more affluent neighborhoods are more successful in keeping such dangers out of their communities.

Global Inequality

Many regions of the world suffer from spatial inequality because, compared to the developed world, they are impoverished and segregated. Entire regions lack adequate access to education, employment, healthcare, and even basic necessities of life. In this way global society functions as a macrocosm of national societies.

Health Disparities

Health disparities exist based on race, gender, and socioeconomic class. Racial health disparities are primarily due to the effects of discrimination and the resulting lower socioeconomic statuses, rather than to any racial characteristics. People who do not have access to adequate prenatal or pediatric medical care may have children with health problems that will carry over into adulthood.

Significant differences have been noted among different racial groups in the incidence of obesity, diabetes, stroke, heart disease, and cancer. It is difficult to isolate the relative contribution of factors such as genetics, socioeconomic status, and dietary habits in creating and addressing these discrepancies. However, aside from clear genetic differences among groups, most differences are considered to arise from low socioeconomic status.

In general, about 16 percent of nonelderly Hispanic and African Americans indicate that they are in poor health. By comparison, only 10 percent of nonelderly Caucasian Americans state that they are in poor health.

There are also health discrepancies between males and females. Although worldwide, women statistically live longer than men by as much as an average of eight years, women and girls suffer from less access to healthcare, along with reduced access to education and to material resources. Men, on the other hand, are more likely to suffer from accidents and physical violence, including voluntary or forced participation in the military. Certain diseases by their nature are more likely to affect one gender than the other, though this is equally deleterious for men and women.

Class disparities in health are related to socioeconomic status. Upper-class people have more access to healthcare and are more likely to get care sooner. In addition, the advanced education that typically goes along with upper-class status makes people better informed about health.

> **RESIDENTIAL SEGREGATION**
>
> A notorious example of residential segregation enacted and enforced by laws is the former residential segregation of blacks, coloreds, and whites under the system of apartheid in South Africa.

Healthcare Disparities

As would be expected, the same forces that create health disparities among different racial groups and classes and between the genders also affect access to healthcare for many of the same reasons. The percent of Americans who do not have a regular source of healthcare is 30 percent for Hispanics, 20 percent for African Americans, and 16 percent for Caucasian Americans. African Americans (18 percent) and Hispanic Americans (13 percent) are more likely to rely on a hospital or clinic for healthcare than Caucasian Americans (8 percent).

A woman's access to healthcare correlates to some extent with the attitudes of the woman's family and community. Families and communities that have more restrictive views of roles for women may also have more restrictive views on access to healthcare. Women in such situations may also have fewer economic resources and less education. In general, the fact that women tend to earn less than men for the same work means that women are less able to afford healthcare.

SUMMARY

This chapter reviewed the foundations of sociology and focused on the issues of social stratification. The foundational concepts covered four theoretical approaches to sociology and then definitions of culture, including material and symbolic culture, subcultures, and assimilation and multiculturalism.

Next the concept of socialization was defined, including agents of socialization, deviance and stigma, and conformity, and obedience. The social institutions of religion, family, education, health, government, and economy were discussed. Then the elements of social interaction were defined, including status, roles, groups, networks, and organizations. The foundational concepts ended with a discussion of demographics. Demographic criteria include age, sex, race and ethnicity, immigration status, and sexual orientation. Demographic shifts include transition, fertility, migration, mortality, social movements, globalization, and urbanization.

The second part of the chapter reviewed the components of social stratification. Social class was discussed, including the various elements that contribute to stratification—class, status, power, cultural and social capital, social reproduction, privilege and prestige, and issues of race, gender, and age. The patterns of mobility that affect social class were reviewed, including intergenerational and intragenerational mobility, upward and downward mobility, and meritocracy. Then poverty was discussed in relation to social class, including relative and absolute poverty, and segregation and isolation.

The next aspect of social stratification covered in the chapter was discrimination. Individual and institutional discrimination were defined and the effects of power, prestige, and class on discrimination were discussed. Spatial inequality was the third aspect of social stratification, and the chapter reviewed residential segregation, environmental segregation, and global inequalities. The discussion of social stratification ended with a discussion of health disparities and healthcare disparities in society.

SOCIOLOGY PRACTICE EXERCISES

> **DIRECTIONS:** This sociology passage is followed by a series of questions. Read the passage, and then for each question choose the one answer that is best. If you are not sure of an answer, eliminate the answer choices that you think are wrong and choose one of the remaining answers.

PASSAGE I

Residential segregation is the separation of categories of people into different neighborhoods. In the United States, residential segregation is primarily based on factors of race and income. Although open acts of residential segregation are illegal in the United States, this type of segregation persists through more covert discriminatory housing practices and by personal choice. The three categories of people that are most negatively affected by residential segregation are African Americans, Hispanics, and the poor.

A study conducted in 1993 on two neighborhoods in a U.S. metropolitan area revealed not only the presence of residential segregation in this area but also unexpected statistics on the effects of residential segregation on segregated neighborhood members. Neighborhood A is an inner city neighborhood, and Neighborhood B is a more affluent city neighborhood. The factors that were measured included the percent of residents living below the poverty level, the percent of non-Hispanic whites, the average cost per pound for apples, and the average concentration of lead found in the blood of residents, measured in micrograms per deciliter. Concentrations above 10 are considered to be excessive. Twenty years later a follow-up study was done in the same neighborhoods. The results of the studies are shown below.

1993 Study

	Neighborhood A	Neighborhood B
% below poverty	24%	2%
% of non-Hispanic whites	24%	97%
Average cost of apples per pound	$0.85	$0.60
Average lead concentration in blood, µg/dL	40	3

2013 Study

	Neighborhood A	Neighborhood B
% below poverty	38%	2%
% of non-Hispanic whites	16%	83%
Average cost of apples per pound	$2.90	$1.50
Average lead concentration in blood, µg /dL	35	3

In 2013, a new component of research was added to this study on residential segregation to include undercover researchers who conducted housing searches with real estate agents representing property in Neighborhood A. Different pairs of researchers posing as married couples approached the agents on the same day. The results were analyzed to look for signs of racial discrimination.

1. Which of the following, if true, is a valid explanation of the discrepancy in blood lead levels between Neighborhood A and Neighborhood B that points to environmental inequality?
    - (A) The residents of Neighborhood A who asked their landlords to remove lead paint were routinely evicted.
    - (B) Some ethnic groups have a genetic susceptibility to lead absorption in the blood.
    - (C) The number of residents willing to be tested in Neighborhood A was much smaller than the number of residents tested in Neighborhood B.
    - (D) Researchers expected the residents of Neighborhood A to have higher blood levels and this expectation affected the results.

2. In the undercover research described in the last parargraph of the passage, which of the following groups would be likely to give the most reliable evidence of racial discrimination if they were to approach the real estate agents?
    - (A) A couple in which one person is African American and the other person is white
    - (B) A first couple that is white representing themselves as highly educated and a second couple that is African American representing themselves as high school dropouts
    - (C) A first couple that is Hispanic, representing themselves as highly educated and a second couple that is white, representing themselves as highly educated
    - (D) A first couple in which the man is white and the woman is Native American and a second couple in which the man is Native American and the woman is white

3. Which of the following conclusions about changes from 1993 to 2013 is best supported by the results of the two studies, as shown in the tables?
    - (A) Adjusted for inflation, the disparity in cost of produce between the two neighborhoods is the same.
    - (B) Environmental health disparity between the two neighborhoods has increased.
    - (C) Racial segregation in Neighborhood B has increased.
    - (D) Racial segregation in Neighborhood A has increased.

4. Which of the following is the most reasonable explanation for the difference in the price of apples between the two neighborhoods?
    - (A) There are few, if any, growers of apples in lower-income neighborhoods.
    - (B) Because of the limited mobility of the residents of Neighborhood A, store owners are able to charge higher prices.
    - (C) People with near poverty level incomes spend a larger percentage of their income on food.
    - (D) People in lower-income neighborhoods buy proportionally less fruit than people in more affluent neighborhoods.

5. Extrapolating from the information in the passage, which of the following is most likely to be true of an ethnically homogenous region of the world in which the average income is extremely low?

(A) There would be a high level of racial discrimination in housing.

(B) Environmental pollution would have increased in the last 20 years.

(C) The people of the region would not be able to protect themselves from environmental pollution.

(D) There is a wide disparity in the prices of different fruits and vegetables.

PASSAGE II

In an attempt to understand the social influences behind public opinion shifts in the United States, a team of sociologists conducted two nationwide surveys using random sampling methods. The surveys were conducted in 2005 and, a decade later, in 2015. Identical questionnaires were used both years. The study revealed a dramatic rise of public support for legalizing the recreational use of marijuana. In addition to asking respondents whether or not they supported legalizing the recreational use of marijuana, the survey also asked respondents to select one of three major agents of socialization that most influenced their decision—peers, including coworkers; family; and mass media. The results of the surveys concerning respondents in support of legalizing the recreational use of marijuana are below.

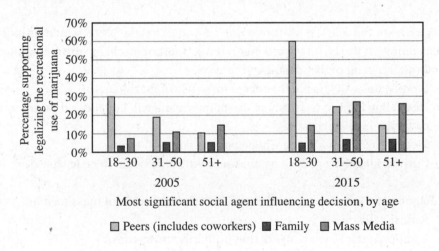

Most significant social agent influencing decision, by age

□ Peers (includes coworkers) ■ Family ▨ Mass Media

6. What is the best explanation for the stronger peer influence on the cohort of 18–30-year-olds compared with the other age cohorts?

(A) Older people do not have as many friends.

(B) Because peers are most influential in the socialization process in adolescence, the 18–30-year-olds are most influenced by peers because of the group's closer age proximity to adolescence.

(C) The 18–30-year-olds have less contact with mass media sources than the other age groups.

(D) A family's influence on 18–30-year-olds is significantly less than on the other age groups.

7. Which one of the following statements about the study's findings is best supported by the passage?
    (A) Those in the 31–50 age group are the most supportive of legalizing the recreational use of marijuana.
    (B) The number of 31–50-year-olds who support legalizing the recreational use of marijuana doubled over the 10-year study period.
    (C) People over 50 years old are the most supportive of legalizing the recreational use of marijuana.
    (D) The number of 18–30-year-olds who support legalizing the recreational use of marijuana doubled over the 10-year study period.

8. Which of the following is/are considered a primary group?

    I. a peer group of friends
    II. family
    III. coworkers

    (A) I only
    (B) II only
    (C) I and II only
    (D) I, II, and III

9. Which one of the following future events, if it were to take place, would be most consistent with the trend toward increased support of legalizing the recreational use of marijuana in all of these adult age cohorts?
    (A) More states will legalize the recreational use of marijuana.
    (B) Laws allowing the recreational use of marijuana will be repealed in states that currently have such laws.
    (C) Medical use of marijuana will be outlawed in all 50 states.
    (D) Current illegal drugs like cocaine and heroin will begin to be legalized.

10. Which one of the following is NOT considered an example of mass media?
    (A) A local newspaper
    (B) A national television network that primarily shows movies
    (C) A clergy's sermon to a local congregation
    (D) Horror movies

ANSWER KEY

1. A	3. D	5. C	7. D	9. A
2. C	4. B	6. B	8. C	10. C

ANSWERS EXPLAINED

1. **(A)** Choice A is correct because it exemplifies how people living in segregated neighborhoods lack power to keep environmental pollution out of their community. Choice B is incorrect because, even if it were the cause of the discrepancy, it is not an

example of environmental inequality. Choice C is incorrect for the same reason. Choice D is incorrect because this would invalidate the results and because it is not an example of environmental inequality.

2. **(C)** Choice C is correct because the relative qualifications of the two couples are the same (highly educated) so any difference in how they are treated by the agents would reflect the difference in ethnicity. Choice A is incorrect because there is no second couple to compare them with. If they are turned down, there is no way to know the reason. Choice B is incorrect because the two couples differ in education, so if the white couple is given a preference, it may be because of their more advanced education. Choice D is incorrect because any difference in how the two couples are treated would be due to a combination of gender and race, not just race.

3. **(D)** Choice D is correct because Neighborhood A was originally 76 percent minority (24 percent white) and in 2013 was 84 percent minority. Choice A is incorrect because in 1993 the cost of apples in Neighborhood A was nearly 50 percent higher than Neighborhood B, but in 2013 it was nearly double. Choice B is incorrect because the ratio of lead concentrations between the neighborhoods was first 40:3 and then 35:3, so the disparity decreased. Choice C is incorrect because Neighborhood B was more diverse in 2013, with a lower percentage of non-Hispanic whites.

4. **(B)** Choice B is correct because people in lower income neighborhoods constitute a "captive customer," and thus store owners can charge higher prices. Choice A is incorrect because more affluent neighborhoods in the city are equally unlikely to have fruit growers. Choice C is incorrect because, although true, this by itself does not explain why store owners can charge higher prices. Choice D is incorrect for the same reason.

5. **(C)** Choice C is correct. Such a region functions much like a segregated, lower-income neighborhood, in which a certain ethnic group is isolated. Like the people in a lower-income neighborhood, people in this region would not have the power to control their environment. Choice A is incorrect because there is only one ethnic group in the region. Choice B is incorrect because, although it might be true, it cannot be inferred from the information in the passage, in which lead content decreased slightly. Choice D is incorrect because the passage does not reflect a disparity in prices of different types of produce but rather a discrepancy between produce prices in one region versus another region.

6. **(B)** It is true that peers are most influential in the socialization process in adolescence, and the 18–30-year-olds are closest to adolescence when compared with the other age groups in this study. This is the best explanation of the stronger peer influence evidenced in this group in the study. Choice A is incorrect because no evidence supports that older people have fewer friends. Choice C is incorrect because no proof supports the claim that the 18–30-year-olds have less contact with mass media sources than other age groups. Choice D is incorrect because although the findings show that the 18–30-year-olds are least influenced by family, the difference when compared with the other age groups is not significant (only 2 percent).

7. **(D)** The 2005 survey revealed that a total of 40 percent of the respondents from the 18–30-year-olds supported legalizing the recreational use of marijuana, and the 2015 survey revealed that a total of 80 percent of the respondents from that age group supported this legalization. Choice A is incorrect because the findings of the study show that 18–30-year-

olds are the most supportive of legalizing the recreational use of marijuana. Choice B is incorrect because the 2005 survey revealed that a total of 35 percent of the respondents from the 31–50-year-olds supported legalizing the recreational use of marijuana, whereas the 2015 survey revealed that a total of 60 percent of the respondents from this same age group supported this legalization (not quite double). Choice C is incorrect because the findings of the study show that the 18–30-year-olds are the most supportive of legalizing the recreational use of marijuana.

8. **(C)** A peer group of friends and family are characterized by close personal relationships in small groups, where interactions are viewed as ends in themselves and not a means to another end. These same characteristics define a primary group. Choice D is incorrect because coworkers are considered a secondary group. Secondary groups are characterized by impersonal relationships that are centered around a focused activity (work), where interactions among members are generally guided toward specific goals.

9. **(A)** It is logical to infer that in a democratic society, increasing support for legalizing the recreational use of marijuana among the voting-age populace will result in more states legalizing recreational marijuana use. Choice B is incorrect because increasing support for legalizing the recreational use of marijuana would have the opposite effect. Instead of laws allowing the recreational use of marijuana being repealed, there would be more laws enacted to legalize the recreational use of marijuana. Choice C is incorrect because the medical use of marijuana is generally more supported in society than the recreational use of marijuana. Therefore, if support of the recreational use of marijuana continues to increase, support for the medical use of marijuana will also increase, not decrease. Choice D is incorrect because there is no evidence that an increase in support of legalizing the recreational use of marijuana has any correlation to increased support for legalizing other illegal drugs.

10. **(C)** The audience of the sermon is confined to a congregation of limited size. Mass media is characterized by its ability to convey ideas and values of the broader society to large numbers of people in a short time. Choice A is incorrect because newspapers, even if local, are a form of mass media. Choice B is incorrect because television is a form of mass media. Movies also convey ideas and values to large groups of people. Choice D is incorrect because movies meet the definition of mass media, regardless of their genre.

For online practice, go to
http://barronsbooks.com/tp/mcat

## PART 3

Critical Reasoning

Critical Analysis and Reasoning Skills

8

→ **AN OVERVIEW**

→ **TACKLING THE PASSAGE**

→ **UNDERSTANDING THE QUESTIONS**

→ **GETTING THE ANSWER**

→ **SAMPLE PASSAGE**

This chapter will help you understand the patterns that the Critical Analysis and Reasoning section is testing. You will learn strategies for organizing your time, for orienting yourself to the passage, and for getting the correct answer. A sample passage will be analyzed in depth to help you learn how to apply the strategies. Finally, you will have a chance to take a short MCAT-style Critical Analysis and Reasoning section and read the explanations.

AN OVERVIEW

The Critical Analysis and Reasoning Skills (CARS) section of the MCAT is similar to the task that is called Reading Comprehension on other tests. The long passages are drawn from the social sciences and humanities. Do not be too surprised if they seem particularly boring. There are typically nine passages. Each one has from five to seven questions. The time limit for the section is 90 minutes.

> ### SUBJECTS FOR CARS PASSAGES
>
> **Humanities:** architecture, art, dance, ethics, literature, music, philosophy, popular culture, religion, theater, studies of diverse cultures
> **Social Sciences:** anthropology, archaeology, economics, education, geography, history, linguistics, political science, population health, psychology, sociology

Is It Possible to Improve on CARS?

If CARS were just a test of how well people read, improving would probably be difficult. The good news is that CARS is very learnable. This section will go over powerful strategies for setting up the passage, for analyzing the questions, for working through the answers, and for proving which answer is indisputably correct. CARS contains hidden agendas and secret patterns, and they will be revealed in the following pages. By mastering these CARS strategies and combining them with the important timing strategies covered in the Introduction, most MCAT takers can expect to increase their scores significantly.

There is a notable difference between CARS and the physical and social science sections. On the sciences, the test taker may be missing some content or factual knowledge. On the CARS, everything needed to solve the problem is given in the passage. Another difference is that CARS has no independent questions.

Mastering Timing

Timing strategy is just as important on the CARS as it is on the sciences. To get the most out of this section, you may want to review the section on timing strategy in the Introduction.

The first step in timing strategy is to rank the passages in order of difficulty. The difficulty is subjective. What is easy for one test taker might be impossible for another. Simply glance at the passage. If the topic seems unpleasant, it probably will be. The only other factor to consider is the complexity of the language. Theoretically, a passage could be on an interesting topic but be written in a way that makes it hard to understand. The opposite is also true. A passage may be about a difficult topic but may be relatively easy to follow.

If two passages are equally difficult but one has more questions, choose the one with more questions. It offers more possible points for the same setup time. However, never choose a harder passage just because it has more questions. The more questions rule applies only to passages of equal difficulty.

After taking a timed practice section, evaluate the effectiveness of your timing strategy. To do this, you need to know how much time you spent on each question. After marking an answer, make a note on scratch paper of the time it took to the nearest half of a minute. Score the section, and then review your strategy.

STEPS FOR TIMING

1. Rank the passages in order of difficulty.
2. Set up the easiest passage.
3. Do all the questions but not necessarily in order. Give each question up to 3 or 4 minutes if necessary.
4. When 3 minutes are left, fill in cold guesses.
5. Keep working until the end.
6. If starting a new passage with only a few minutes left, don't read. Go right to a detail question.

How many questions were wrong, ignoring the questions that were blind guesses? If you chose more than one or two wrong answers, then there is room for improvement. How? Suppose you have five wrong answers. In theory, you could have skipped two of those questions and used the time to get the other three correct. Look at the questions that were wrong. How much time did you spend on them? If there are many wrong answers on which you spent only 1 or 2 minutes, you may be rushing. Compare the person who works on 30 questions and gets 12 right with the person who works on 16 questions and gets all of them right. Who has the better score?

Work on timing strategy until you are missing no more than two answers on a timed section. Check that you spent at least 3 or 4 minutes on the questions that were wrong. Do not worry right now if the score is not where it should be. Focus on accuracy. Look carefully at each wrong answer, and try to determine why you were not able to get it correct. Was something confusing? Were there two answers that were very close? The next step is to master the CARS strategies that will help to get more questions correct more quickly.

How to Practice

Most practice on the CARS—maybe 80 percent—should be done untimed. Working untimed means practicing and discovering strategies for getting the right answer no matter how long it takes. Thoroughly working on one question may take 20 or 30 minutes or even more. This is fine. If a particular question becomes frustrating, rather than giving up, set it aside, take a break, and come back to it later.

Even when practicing untimed, use a watch and write down the time spent on each question. On many questions, it may feel like you are taking too long. However, it may turn out that you solve the problem within 3 to 5 minutes. On the real test, it is OK to spend that much time on the more difficult questions. Keeping track of time helps you adjust your internal sense of what is too much time and what is acceptable. On questions that you get wrong despite your best efforts, it will also show whether you gave the question enough time.

Occasionally do a CARS section timed to evaluate timing strategy under testing conditions. Do a timed section now as you begin your studying and then again every few weeks. Before taking a timed section, think about how to apply new timing strategies. On the actual test, watches are not allowed. You must use the clock on the computer to keep track of time.

It is OK to use a watch at home as you practice. Write down the time spent on each question. Keep track of which questions you worked on and which questions were cold guesses. Every question should be either worked on thoroughly or guessed on cold. There should not be anything in between. During the last 3 minutes, put down cold guesses for questions that there is not enough time to answer. Do not take time to work these questions partially or to eliminate answers. Other than during the last 3 minutes, do not guess on any question unless you have already spent 3 to 4 minutes on it.

Many MCAT takers will get their best score by working on only four or five of the passages and guessing blindly on the remaining questions. The person who works on four passages and gets every question correct will score higher than the person who works on most of the questions but gets half of them wrong.

TACKLING THE PASSAGE

> **THE THREE SKILLS FOR MASTERING CARS**
>
> 1. Organize the passage.
> 2. Analyze and understand the questions.
> 3. Prove the correct answer, and find the flaws in the wrong ones.

UNTIMED PRACTICE

You should do 80 percent of your practicing untimed.

Untimed practice is the best way to build strategies.

It's OK to spend 20 or 30 minutes figuring out what makes a question difficult.

NO WATCHES ON THE MCAT!

Practice using the clock on the computer to keep track of time.

How to Set Up the Passage

What is the most efficient way to set up a passage? What must you remember, what must you understand, and what can you ignore? A typical CARS passage contains 20, 30, or more specific facts. However, a passage tests only three or four of those facts. The rest of the questions test what can be called big picture information. These include the main idea, the author's tone, and the function of a particular phrase. The test taker who is trying to absorb all of the facts is doing too much work. Consider using a different approach.

All questions are either big picture questions or fact questions. For a fact question, you can always go back to the passage and review that fact. This is an example of using the eyes, not the memory—a strategy that was reviewed in the Introduction. Indeed, even if you tried to remember the facts the first time through the passage, you would not be able to remember them accurately enough to answer the questions. A better, faster, and more accurate strategy is to go back and get facts as they are needed.

This means it is not necessary to memorize facts when reading the passage. Then why bother to read the passage at all? To answer a big picture question, you must first have a clear sense of the big picture—the overall structure and movement of the passage. The real purpose of the initial skimming of the passage, then, is to find the big picture.

The big picture of a passage has some predictable elements. Learning to recognize these elements makes it relatively easy to find the big picture in any CARS passage.

Most CARS passages—and perhaps all of them—are built around what can be called a dichotomy. This is a contrast or a tension between two opposing things, something "on the one hand" versus something else "on the other hand." Consider the discussion given in the strategy section of the Introduction about the two vehicles: the Toyota and the Subaru, one red and one silver, one a car and one a truck. This is a clear example of a dichotomy. Two things are compared and contrasted. There may or may not be similarities, but there must be a fundamental contrast.

The dichotomy can take the form of a problem to be solved, a dilemma, a paradox, or a contradiction as well as a simple contrast between two things.

Because the supply of petroleum is decreasing steadily, we will need increasingly more sources of energy in the future.

Until recently, scientists believed that asteroids traveled alone.

Whereas the inquisitorial system of law allows for more cooperation between all parties, the adversarial system often results in more information being brought to light.

The theory of evolution replaced earlier attempts to explain biological variations as remnants of primordial differences.

Beethoven believed that traditional standards of musical composition were not sacred, that they should be broken at the whim of the creative force, and yet today, many teachers of composition hold Beethoven's own standards up as guidelines to be rigorously learned and followed.

Identify the dichotomies in these examples. It may be helpful to use expressions such as "On the one hand, there is a red Toyota pickup. On the other hand, there is a silver Subaru wagon."

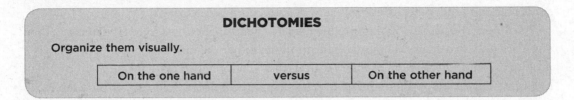

MCAT passages use certain kinds of dichotomies regularly. One of the most common is the dichotomy between an old phenomenon and a new phenomenon. The theory of evolution is a new theory replacing an old theory. Beethoven's standards were new compared with the traditional (old) standards from before his time.

Another very common type of dichotomy is a dichotomy between theories. The passage that discusses the theory of evolution is a good example. Very often, one theory is old and the other new. However, passages can also use contemporary theories that are being contrasted with each other. Because a new theory is not usually presented unless it corrects flaws in a previous theory, the author of a passage will usually find the new theory better, at least in some ways.

The big picture involves not just a dichotomy but what the passage does with the dichotomy. All of this together creates what we can call the structure of the passage. Here are examples of structures.

Structure 1

- A theory is presented.
- Facts supporting it are given.
- A fact that weakens it is given.
- The author concludes that the theory is good, despite the weakness.

Structure 2

- An attitude or belief from the past is presented.
- The current belief about the same subject is presented.
- Support for the superiority of the current belief is given.
- Additional support for the current belief is given.
- The author concludes that the current belief is superior.

Structure 3

- A dilemma is presented.
- A solution is given.
- Evidence to support the solution is given.
- The author points out a new problem that the solution would create.
- A way to overcome the new problem is given.
- The author concludes that the original solution has merits but also has drawbacks and states that further research is needed.

The passage establishes the dichotomy and then builds a structure by incorporating combinations of elements such as definitions, explanations, clarifications, and examples. From there, it goes on to present elements such as solutions, partial solutions that create new problems, support for a view, objections to or criticisms of a view, rebuttals to objections, similarities and differences between *A* and *B*, and interim conclusions.

The flow of the passage is often predictable. If a theory, belief, or solution is defended, then there are only two ways the passage can continue. Either the defense holds up, or there is a problem with it. If there is a problem with it, there are only two ways the passage can then continue. Either the problem can be overcome and the defense holds up, or the problem is fatal and the defense does not hold up.

The ending of a passage is often particularly important. A passage may introduce something new at the end or may give critical insights into the author's main point. The ending can confirm that a particular view or theory is correct or that it is correct but with some qualifications. Alternately, the passage may conclude that the view or theory is incorrect or that it is incorrect with some redeeming qualities. The passage may conclude that a further line of investigation is needed. It may propose a new synthesis that provides an alternative to either of the original two elements of the dichotomy. It may even suggest a whole new area that could be investigated as a result of the passage's line of inquiry.

TIP

ENDINGS ARE IMPORTANT!

Notice how the passage ends. Often there will be a question about it.

Finding the Big Picture (Structure)

Try skimming the passage below in order to find the big picture. Start at the beginning of the passage, and skim until you find something that could be a dichotomy.

Relationships among elements of the natural world are often more complex than we realize, so that our actions affecting one element may have unexpected, and often negative, effects on another. For example, grasslands, which, of course, are grazed by various animals in a natural setting, may be adversely affected when grazing takes place under conditions altered by people.

Many grasslands in the West have been grazed under altered conditions for well over a hundred years. Scientists have been recently studying the effects of grazing by the American bison, commonly known as the buffalo, because it has a less harmful effect on grasslands than most other domestic grazing animals. Two factors have been measured—the health of the grasses and the health of the range area in general. Health of the grasses is measured by counting the number of grass clumps per acre still alive at the end of the season. Health of the range is measured by calculating the number of different species of plants per acre and the total mass of vegetation produced per acre for the season. By comparing bison-grazed range areas with ungrazed control areas, researchers found that the more palatable, fine-textured grasses, such as Indian Rice Grass, suffered significant damage, whereas less tasty, coarse grasses, such as Sacaton, showed virtually none. Overall range health declined in areas dominated by Indian Rice Grass but not in those dominated by Sacaton.

It is still unclear whether a decrease in the health of grasses, even with the more vulnerable ones, necessarily results in a decrease in range health in the long run. Rangelands dominated by the slower-growing, fine-textured species will obviously be more susceptible to permanent damage, but the ultimate effect on a rangeland depends on four identifiable factors. Areas with these characteristics would be most adversely affected: a high ratio of fine grasses to coarse grasses; a high ratio of grasses to nongrass plants; low annual rainfall; and high average seasonal temperatures. It would be a good idea to identify range areas with a combination of these characteristics and take special restorative measures with them, because they are most susceptible to being damaged by human-directed grazing.

The first paragraph does not contain any significant dichotomies. It gives a general statement and an example. It refers to a possible problem but offers no binary choice—no choice between two distinct things.

The second paragraph starts with facts. Facts are not dichotomies. The passage does mention that the bison is different from other domestic grazing animals. This fact could be the basis for a dichotomy, but the passage does not pursue such a dichotomy. The passage goes on to mention two additional factors—the health of grasses and the health of rangeland. Whereas there are differences between these two factors, the passage does not pursue a conflict between them.

Only when the passage introduces the distinction between fine-textured grasses and coarse grasses is there a clear, black-and-white distinction. Fine grasses do not hold up to grazing. Coarse grasses do. The final paragraph does not pursue this dichotomy further but does return to the dichotomy between the health of grasses and the health of rangelands— the dichotomy that was mentioned earlier in the passage but not pursued at that time. Thus, health of grasses versus health of rangelands does turn out to be another significant dichotomy. The paragraph states that the solution to the problem is unclear. It identifies further factors that need to be considered.

> **FACTS ARE NOT DICHOTOMIES**
>
> A dichotomy must involve a conflict or contrast between two things.

The ending tells us that we can use information about the difference between fine- and coarse-textured grasses and the information about how the health of grasses influences the health of rangeland to help solve the problem of damage caused by human-directed grazing.

The big picture of the passage can be condensed to its essentials. Fine grasses are more susceptible to damage than coarse grasses in grazing conditions that have been altered by people. Damage to grasses alone does not determine whether the rangeland is damaged; other factors are needed. We can use this information to protect vulnerable areas.

Why is it important to identify dichotomies and the big picture? First, big picture questions cannot be accurately answered without a clear grasp of the big picture. Second, many of the detail questions are specifically designed to confuse the reader between the facts on opposite sides of the dichotomy. What color was the vehicle that had four-wheel drive? Often the test uses terms that sound similar to create additional confusion. For example, a passage might contrast neurolinguistic therapy with linguistic neuropathology.

Keeping dichotomies clear and separate in the memory is very difficult. A diagram on paper, on the other hand, is an almost foolproof way of keeping two sets of data distinct. Once the dichotomy is clear, put it down on paper immediately.

> **CARDINAL RULE!**
>
> Use your eyes, not your memory.
> Don't try to remember facts. Go back and check them.
> Don't organize information in your head. Put it on paper.

Diagramming the Big Picture

Theoretically, it is possible to draw a complete diagram of all of the dichotomies and facts in a passage, along with their relationships. However, this is far too time-consuming to do in the actual test. During the test, you need to write down only the main dichotomies and basic facts. Go back to the diagram of the differences between the two vehicles in the Introduction, the Toyota and the Subaru. It is a good example of a basic working diagram. Even though it is only a part of the whole setup, it is a complete diagram of that part. Such a diagram would make it nearly impossible to become confused.

In order to develop a sense of how much to diagram and how much to leave out, start by fully diagramming one or two passages. After that, try cutting back to what feels like just the essentials. If you get questions wrong because the diagram was too incomplete, try diagramming a little more. If a diagram contains information that was never needed to answer the questions, try doing less.

Diagramming is similar to making an outline of a passage. However, instead of putting headings down the side of the page, make columns across the top. The columns are usually in pairs—one side of the dichotomy versus the other side. Consider the following example.

> *Until 1959, most social scientists considered the family unit to be the only valid subject of sociological research.*

Is there a dichotomy? At first glance, this example may seem only to give facts. However, the statement "Until 1959" actually creates a dichotomy: what was true before 1959 versus what was true after 1959. This is a very common kind of dichotomy. It may be introduced with wording such as "until recently," "up to now," or "before the 4th century A.D."

> *In the 1960s, sociologists at some major universities began interviewing single adults about their work habits, social relationships, and personal goals.*

This reveals the other half of the dichotomy—what was true after 1959. The dichotomy can be diagrammed. Note that the diagrams below are formatted for easy reading. An example of how to diagram by hand is shown at the end of this section.

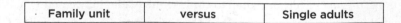

| Family unit | versus | Single adults |

Additional information about each side of the dichotomy can be added.

TIP

THE IMPORTANCE OF DICHOTOMIES

Nearly all CARS passages are based on dichotomies, even though they might not seem to be at first glance.

Family unit	versus	Single adults
< 1959		> 1959

If the passage gives more facts about the earlier studies, those facts can go under "Family unit." Facts about the later studies can go under "Single adults."

Suppose the passage's next sentence said:

> *Modern researchers are divided as to whether young single adults constitute a sociological reality distinct from single senior citizens.*

This sentence introduces a new dichotomy between younger and older, but it falls under the "Single adults" column. It is a dichotomy within one-half of an existing dichotomy. One category splits into two.

Family unit	versus	Single adults	
< 1960		> 1960	
		younger	older

> *Young singles can typically look forward to an increasing income and are more flexible in developing new friends and interests.*

This sentence gives specific information about the "younger" category. It also gives implied information about the "older" category because they are contrasted.

Family unit	versus	Single adults	
< 1960		> 1960	
		younger	older
		increasing $	fixed $
		more flexible, friends/interests	less flexible

> *However, most sociologists now believe that these differences are insignificant compared with the similarities among all ages of single people in free time and amount of social contact.*

What has happened here? The author has reconciled the dichotomy. The problem is solved, the two sides brought together and the tension removed.

Family unit	versus	Single adults	
< 1960		> 1960	
		younger	older
		increasing $	fixed $
		more flexible, friends/interests	less flexible
		⌄	

Below is an example of how to diagram big picture dichotomies by hand on your scratch paper.

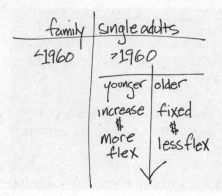

To summarize, then, there is a basic dichotomy, a new dichotomy within a branch of the original dichotomy, and the coming together (merging or bridging) of the two sides of a dichotomy. All of these were diagrammed, along with the details that go into each category.

Dichotomies are often indicated by words or phrases like "however," "on the other hand," and "in contrast." These show a switch from one side of a dichotomy to another. For example, "John is happy with his job. However, he is dissatisfied with his living situation." Words or phrases such as "similarly," "likewise," and "in the same way" show that the author is continuing to talk about the same side of the dichotomy.

Once a dichotomy has been introduced, there are usually only a few directions in which the passage could go next. It could give examples. It could explain theories. It could evaluate whether something is good or bad. It could bridge a dichotomy. It could create a dichotomy within a dichotomy. Keeping these possibilities in mind helps you recognize more quickly where the passage is going.

Identifying dichotomies is such a powerful organizing tool that it can be used to understand the structure of a passage even when the content of the passage is too difficult or complex to follow. The next passage is based on the most complex recent theories in astrophysics. For most people, the details of the passage would be so incomprehensible as to prevent understanding the big picture. To avoid being sidetracked by complex detail, try skipping the details and sticking only with the big picture. The passage has been modified below to simulate that. The actual details are replaced with simple variables, A and B.

Until 1956, people thought that stars generated their energy by A. New research, however, indicated that Theory A could not explain Observation O. Theory B was put forward to explain Observation O. Theory B was widely attacked because calculations based on it came up with a different estimate for the life span of our Sun than those based on previous observations. Professor X reviewed the previous observations and found that the observations themselves were inaccurate, and once corrected, the new calculations matched those predicted by Theory *B*. Theory *B* not only gives us a more consistent explanation of how stars produce their energy but also reassuringly gives life on Earth an extra 15 million years before our Sun dies.

Even though the topic is highly complex, the structure of the passage is easy to spot by simply sidestepping the details.

THE POWER OF THE BIG PICTURE

With the big picture, you can even understand a passage on advanced thermonuclear theory.

MCAT passages include topics drawn from the social sciences and humanities. The MCAT test writers choose topics that most people do not have much experience with. As a result, many of the topics may be difficult to understand or may simply be boring. Test takers who come across the rare interesting passage are sometimes caught off guard, getting hooked into it, and forgetting about time. Be careful to avoid this.

READ SELECTIVELY

If you are reading the whole passage, you are doing too much work and taking too much time!
Skim.
Look for the big picture.
Don't obsess over details.

How to Skim

Start skimming for the big picture at the beginning of the passage. If the first few sentences contain only facts but no dichotomies, continue until you find a dichotomy. Identify the two parts of the dichotomy clearly. You should take extra time on this step in order to be accurate.

Passages can be thought of as an analysis of an interesting something. This mnemonic contains four implied questions that help build the big picture. What is the something? What makes it interesting? In what way is it analyzed? How does the analysis end up?

In the astrophysics passage, the something being analyzed was two theories. It was the contrast and tension between them that made the topic interesting. The analysis consisted of showing problems posed by Theory *A* and a partial solution (Theory *B*) with its own problems. The analysis concluded by showing how the problems with Theory *B* had been overcome.

AN ANALYSIS OF AN INTERESTING SOMETHING

What is the something?
What makes it interesting?
How is it analyzed?
How does it end up?

Each of the four questions has certain common answers that help quickly identify the structure of the passage.

Analysis of an Interesting Something

1. What is the something that is interesting?
   Theory
   Event
   Action
   Definition
   Phenomenon (social, political, natural, and so on)
2. What is interesting about it?
   Contrast (*A* versus *B*, old versus new)
   Dilemma/problem/inadequacy/unknown
   Paradox/discrepancy/paradoxical contradiction
3. In what way is it analyzed?
   Definitions/explorations/clarifications/examples
   Solutions
   Partial solutions with additional problems
   Support for a view
   Criticisms of or objections to a view
   Similarities between *A* and *B*
   Differences between *A* and *B*
   Interim conclusions
4. How does it end up?
   A view or solution holds up.
   A view or solution holds up with qualifications.
   A view or solution does not hold up.
   A view or solution does not hold up but has some redeeming qualifications.
   Further inquiry is needed.
   A new synthesis is proposed.

UNDERSTANDING THE QUESTIONS

There are only about seven types of questions on the CARS. And all of the questions fall into just two categories—detail questions and big picture questions. Detail questions ask for facts that are specifically stated in the passage or that can be implied from information specifically stated. Big picture questions test an understanding of the overall purpose and structure of the passage. When beginning work on a question, start by orienting to the question. Identify the question type, and review the strategy for that type.

> **USE THE TWO FUNCTIONS OF YOUR BRAIN**
>
> Big picture thinking and detail thinking are two different ways in which the brain processes information.
> Can you notice when you are using one or the other?

It would be nice to think that there is just one strategy for each type. Unfortunately, it is not that simple. One main idea question, for example, may throw completely different obstacles at the test taker than another main idea question. To master strategy, you must work carefully with hundreds of questions.

The good news, though, is that all questions of a particular type have certain things in common. Learning these common elements will help you quickly and accurately get right to the heart of what the question is asking.

The CARS Tests Four Thinking Skills

1. **COMPREHENSION.** Has the reader understood the facts presented in the passage?
2. **EVALUATION.** Can the reader identify the relationships among the various elements of the passage?
3. **APPLICATION.** Can the reader apply information in the passage to other situations?
4. **EXTENSION.** Can the reader use new information presented in the question stem to evaluate information in the passage?

Notice that the last three of these skills are big picture skills. By learning to evaluate the big picture, a test taker will be better able to answer the more complex questions.

Big Picture Questions

Big picture questions test your holistic understanding of the passage as opposed to mastery of specific facts. Big picture question types include:

CARS TESTS FOUR SKILLS
Comprehension
Evaluation
Application
Extension

1. Main idea
2. Author's tone
3. Logical organization
4. Literary techniques
5. Extension

Each of these types can be asked in a variety of ways. For example, a main idea question can be worded in a simple way, such as "Which of the following is the main idea of the passage?" or in a more complex way, such as "Most likely the author would identify which of the following as most closely matching his or her primary purpose?" Complex wording often makes the question type difficult to identify.

Carefully examine the wording of each VR question. You must know what type of question it is before trying to answer it. Become familiar with all of the many variations of wording for each type.

Below are some fairly straightforward variations along with specific strategies for the particular question type.

MAIN IDEA

1. The author's main point is . . .
2. The author's major contention is . . .
3. The main idea expressed in the passage is . . .
4. The passage best answers which of the following questions?
5. Which statement below is the best title for the passage?

Strategy for Main Idea Questions

To be correct, the answer must meet two criteria. First, it must be a statement that is true and consistent with the passage. Second, it must match the structure (big picture). Beware of choosing an answer that is true or consistent but is not the main idea.

TYPES OF BIG PICTURE QUESTIONS

Main idea	Logical organization	Extension
Author's tone	Literary techniques	

TONE

1. The tone of the passage is best described as . . .
2. For what audience is the author most likely writing?
3. The attitude of the scholar mentioned in the second paragraph can best be described as . . .

Strategy for Tone Questions

Every passage has what can be called a voice. Consider the following passage.

> Most politicians try to be tactful when they are talking to the public, but not good old Congressman Harry Paxton. Harry recently told a group of constituents that they had the brains of a banana slug when it came to understanding the federal budget. He told them that one of their fellow citizens complained that the government was giving too much money to people on welfare who weren't doing anything to earn it. But the complainer was himself living on disability payments. The country would be a better place if we had more politicians like Harry.

What are the voices in this passage? Does the author have a voice? In any passage, the author either has an opinion about the information or is neutral. A neutral passage is like a newspaper article. It presents only the facts without expressing an opinion. If the author's voice is not neutral, it will be either positive, in support of the information presented, or negative, critical of the information.

On the MCAT, if the author's voice is positive, it will be either totally positive or positive with some qualifications or reservations. In the above article, the author is totally positive about Harry Paxton. No reservations are expressed. If the last line had read, "*The country would be a better place if we had more politicians like Harry, but he would be wise to tone down his approach or he may not get reelected,*" then the author's voice would be positive with qualifications. Note that the phrase "but not good old Congressman Harry Paxton" in the first sentence already indicates that the author is positive. If the author's voice is negative, it will likewise be either totally negative or negative with some positive qualifications.

MCAT tone questions ask about tone, or voice. In the above passage, there are three distinct voices. One is the author's. Whose voice is reflected in the statement "they had the brains of a banana slug when it came to understanding the federal budget"? Whose voice is reflected in the statement "the government was giving too much money to people on welfare who weren't doing anything to earn it"? The first is Harry's voice. The second is the voice of the person on disability. Be careful to identify the various voices in a passage and to keep them separate. Generally, tone questions ask about the author's voice.

In tone questions, answers are often on a continuum. For example,

(A) Bitter
(B) Unconcerned
(C) Cautiously supportive
(D) Ecstatic

Note that these answers start with a totally negative tone, move through neutral to a moderately positive tone, and then move to a fully positive tone. First identify where on the continuum the author's voice falls. If the author is positive but mentions some drawbacks, this is the qualifiedly positive position, which is answer choice C. It is not necessary to agree with the exact wording, "cautiously supportive." The correct place on the continuum takes precedence over the specific wording of the answer, even if the wording does not seem to be perfectly accurate.

TIP

START WITH THE BIG PICTURE

You can't answer a big picture question without having a good sense of the big picture. Be sure to skim the passage first for the big picture, and avoid memorizing details.

LOGICAL ORGANIZATION

1. In which way does the author develop his or her argument?
2. The relationship between the first and second paragraphs can best be described as . . .
3. The author's argument depends on the assumption . . .
4. The event described in the third paragraph is most likely based on . . .

Strategy for Logical Organization Questions

These questions require you to have a clear sense of the relationships between paragraphs. Careful skimming for the big picture is the best tool for understanding how the parts of the passage are related to each other and to the main idea.

LITERARY TECHNIQUES

1. The author uses the analogy of a balloon in order to . . .
2. The word *candid* would be best substituted for by which of the following?
3. The author mentions volcanoes in order to . . .
4. The author's statement that college graduates should be ready to "spring off the starting block" suggests which of the following about the author's view of life?

Strategy for Literary Technique Questions

These questions are similar to logical organization questions but focus more closely on a specific word or phrase and on its function in the overall presentation. The clues are often found somewhere in the five lines before and five lines after the cited expression.

EXTENSION

1. With which assertion below would the author most strongly disagree?
2. The paragraph following the passage would most likely . . .
3. The passage was most likely taken from . . .
4. If dinosaur fossils were found in Alaska, it would be most logical to conclude . . .
5. Which of the following most seriously weakens the argument presented in the passage?
6. A logical expectation for a person who agrees with the author would be . . .
7. Can these contradictory statements be reconciled by the author's argument?
8. Which of the following provides the best evidence that . . .

Strategy for Extension Questions

Extension questions give additional information—an extension of the passage—and ask which statement is consistent with the passage or which can serve as a conclusion. Some extension questions present options for a paragraph that would follow the passage. In ordinary writing, almost anything could follow a passage, even a switch to a barely related topic. On the MCAT, however, the correct answer must be consistent with, and an extension of, the original big picture.

Extension questions often require that you interpret information presented in the passage or that you take new information and relate it to the information in the passage.

DETAIL QUESTIONS

Unlike big picture questions, detail questions must be defendable by information stated in the passage.

Detail Questions

All detail questions ask for facts. These may be facts that are specifically stated in the passage (specific detail questions) or facts that follow logically from the information that is explicitly stated (implied detail questions). Correct answers typically do not depend on outside knowledge. If you choose an answer based on your own outside information, it cannot be the correct answer unless it can also be defended based on information stated in the passage. Be careful, especially on science passages, not to bring in outside knowledge.

SPECIFIC DETAIL

1. The author states that . . .
2. According to the passage . . .
3. Which of the following is NOT stated in the passage?

Strategy for Specific Detail Questions

The correct answer must be defendable by words stated in the passage. The test of a correct answer is to be able to point to the specific words in the passage that undeniably prove that the answer must be true.

IMPLIED DETAIL

1. The author suggests/implies that . . .
2. It can be inferred from the passage that . . .
3. If the author's claim about wild boars is true, which of the following is also true?
4. Which of the following is supported by the conclusion?
5. Which of the following is most defensible?
6. The author implies which relationship between the two parties?

Strategy for Implied Detail Questions

As with specific detail questions, the answer must be defendable by pointing to specific words in the passage. However, the answer is derived from facts in the passage through the application of logic. It is not specifically stated in the passage.

> *Anyone who has worked at the Anderson Coal Mine during the past*
> *20 years can participate in the upcoming class action suit. Jamie Peters*
> *began work at the mine five years ago.*

It can logically be concluded from the above two facts that Jamie Peters is eligible to participate in the suit. This fact is not stated in the passage, but it follows indisputably from the facts that are given.

Watch out for two traps with implied detail questions. First, a conclusion that goes too far beyond what is stated cannot be logically defended. In the above example, it cannot be defended that Jamie Peters suffered injuries or illness while working in the mine. That conclusion goes too far.

The other trap is to reject a conclusion because it seems to be explicitly stated in the passage rather than implied. It is highly unlikely that an MCAT question will ask you to distinguish between one answer choice that is explicitly stated and another that is derived through logic. If an implied detail answer is absolutely defendable, it must be correct, even if it appears to be a restatement of a fact in the passage. Generally, on closer inspection, it turns out that the answer is not completely a restatement. There is usually some small leap of logic that the test taker did not notice.

Some answer choices may seem too obvious or too simple to be correct. However, if they can be defended by words in the passage, they must be the correct answer. Remember that there are actually many easy-level questions on the test. Do not try to make the question more difficult than it is.

Answers to detail questions are often highly literal. If an answer choice says "Most of the people in cities suffer from allergies," you must prove by words in the passage that at least one more than half of the people in cities suffers from allergies. This is what *most* literally means—at least one more than half.

> ### TWO TYPES OF DETAIL QUESTIONS
> Specific detail   Implied detail

AAMC Question Type Categories

When you read explanations of CARS questions in AAMC materials, you will find that the AAMC refers to three broad categories that encompass the question types you have learned in this chapter.

Foundation of comprehension questions are supposed to deal with the basic information in the text. Questions in this category include assumptions, the author's viewpoint, inferences and conclusions, the main idea, explicitly or overtly stated facts, understanding the passage, and the use or meaning of a word or phrase.

Reasoning within the text questions focus on integrating information given in the passage. These questions can include assessing the author's attitude or opinion, assessing evidence that might support conclusions, considering the author's logic, drawing conclusions, and the function of elements of the passage.

Reasoning beyond the text questions involve applying information in the passage to a new situation, assessing how new information would affect the points in the passage, and interpreting a new scenario from the perspective of the passage.

GETTING THE ANSWER

As described in the Introduction, you must use strategies when answering MCAT questions in order to increase your score. This holds true for CARS questions.

Strategies for Answering Questions

The first step in getting an answer is to orient to the question or, more specifically, to the question stem. The question stem is the part of the question leading up to, but not including, the answer choices. Orienting means going beyond simply reading the stem by taking time to make sure you clearly understand the meaning or by identifying what is unclear. Orienting includes getting a sense of which part of the passage this question relates to, how the question fits in to the structure of the passage, and what might need to be done to answer it correctly. Orienting need not take more than 15 to 30 seconds, but it is a critical step. It is a big picture strategy in which you let the information in the question sink into your mind more thoroughly. Test takers commonly get questions wrong because they never clearly understood what the question meant or how it fit into the passage.

After orienting to the question stem, the steps for solving a CARS problem are the same as those outlined under "The Generic Way to Answer a Question" in the testing strategy section of the Introduction. Quite often in CARS, the second step is to go back to the passage and look for information. For example, if the question asks, "Which of the following is a form of torture prohibited by the Geneva Convention?" the first step is to scan the passage for information about forms of torture and the Geneva Convention. What if you can find nothing? Some information must be in the passage because the answer must be defendable by statements in the passage. If you cannot find any information, look again. If there is only one reference to torture and the Geneva Convention, for example "the rack is prohibited under the Geneva Convention," the answer must be based on that reference.

THE FOUR STEPS FOR GETTING AN ANSWER

(STEP 1) Orient to the question stem.

(STEP 2) Decide on a plan of attack.

(STEP 3) Make one pass through the answer choices, using elimination.

(STEP 4) Use the adversarial approach to evaluate the remaining answer choices.

Many test takers do not realize at first that in the CARS, the answers must be correct for very literal and specific reasons. Look carefully for the exact reason that one of the answers must be correct. Look for the fatal flaws in the other answers. It is almost never the case that one answer is better than another. One is right. The others are dead wrong. Usually an answer is dead wrong because it either violates what is actually stated in some subtle way or is simply not defendable by anything stated.

A wrong answer is not necessarily wrong because it contains wrong facts, although some answers are wrong for this reason. Instead, answers are often wrong because they violate logic or they contain one word that is not defendable. For example, consider a passage that states that many people in the United States do not like to eat liver. Suppose a question says, "Which of the following is consistent with the passage?" Evaluate the answer that says, "Most Americans find eating liver unpleasant." First consider the phrase "find eating liver unpleasant." The information that we have is that "many people in the United States do not like to eat liver." Is this the same as saying that people find it unpleasant? Yes. It can be defended from the dictionary definitions of these terms that they are interchangeable. The same can be said about the terms "American" and "people in the United States."

The term "most," on the other hand, is dead wrong. *Most* means at least one more than half. The passage only states that "many" people do not like to eat liver. It is impossible to defend that at least one more than half of Americans do not like to eat liver. The fatal flaw here is a logical and semantic one.

ARE EXTREME ANSWERS WRONG?

Not necessarily! If the passage makes an extreme statement, such as "All Americans hate liver," then an extreme answer will be correct. However, you should always be suspicious of extreme answers and check to see if they are defendable. Often, they are not.

There are hundreds of patterns of fatal flaws and correct answers. At first, they can be difficult to identify correctly. In order to learn the most from each question, do not stop working on the question until it is clear exactly why the right answer is right and exactly why the wrong answers are wrong.

When there are two remaining possible answers, the most powerful tool for finding the correct answer is the adversarial approach, described in the strategy section of the Introduction. Be careful to keep the defending and attacking stages completely separate. When test takers find they cannot use the adversarial approach successfully, it is usually because they are mixing the two stages.

YOUR MOST POWERFUL STRATEGY

The adversarial approach is your most powerful tool for getting tough answers.

(STEP 1) Attack the answer you like.

(STEP 2) Defend the answer you don't like.

When you attack, totally attack. When you defend, defend like your life depends on it!

BEWARE THE DEFAULT MULTIPLE-CHOICE QUESTION!

Which multiple-choice answer below do you think would be the correct one?

- (A) The moon is made of green cheese.
- (B) The Sun revolves around Earth.
- (C) Life is based on complex biological processes.
- (D) It is easier for a woman to become a doctor than for a man.

Most people would probably choose C. It is the only answer that is factually correct. Is C the correct answer? Notice that there was no question stem given. If a person chooses C, what question stem are they answering? In the absence of a question stem, most people assume what we can call the default multiple-choice question, "Which of the following is true in the real world?"

Sometimes a CARS stem does ask the default question. However, if the question is something else, there is a danger that your brain will revert to the default question. Obviously, this would result in getting a wrong answer. Go back regularly to reread the question while working through the answer choices. If the question above had been "Which of the following statements is a belief that was held in the past but is no longer widely held?" choice C would be the wrong answer. Perhaps we can say that it would be the right answer to the wrong question.

Important Tips for Better Reading

Be an active reader. Have a plan and have tools for implementing your plan. Here are some additional tools that will help you be a more effective active reader.

SHOULD I TAKE NOTES AND HIGHLIGHT?

Do this only if it helps! Some people take far too many notes and highlight too much. If you look back at a passage and find that you never needed most of your notes and highlights, cut back.

DO NOT READ THE QUESTIONS FIRST

Does it help to read all the questions first before reading the passage? People who do this may feel that they will be able to spot the answers to detail questions as they read the passage. Many detail questions, however, are so specific that unless you are focusing on the question, the answer will not be easy to find. Thus, reading all of the questions in advance may only waste time.

Sometimes it is helpful to go directly to one question instead of reading the passage. If you start a new passage with only a few minutes left in the test, it would be a waste of time to set up the passage. In this case, go directly to a detail question and then search the passage for the information needed to answer that question.

SIGNAL WORDS

As you skim the passage, look for words that show whether the author is continuing a line of thought or switching to a contrasting one.

READING MORE QUICKLY AND ACCURATELY

Many test takers find that the language in CARS passages is so complex that it is difficult to understand. Often test takers simply guess at what they think is being said. Often their interpretations are wildly wrong, albeit creative. If you are a slow reader or you find yourself struggling with understanding the complex sentences in the CARS, keep in mind these helpful strategies.

---

1. Take a friendly approach to the passage.
2. Avoid details. Look for the big picture.
3. Study and use sentence diagramming.
4. Do lots of untimed practice.

Clearly, interesting topics are easier to "get into" than boring ones. However, even with a boring or obnoxious topic, you can take a friendly attitude. Namely, pretend that you are interested. It may make your mind a little more receptive.

The purpose of skimming the passage, as has been discussed earlier, is to see the big picture. Read only enough detail to be able to follow the flow of the passage. As with the passage on the theories of how the Sun generates energy, stepping back from the complex details helps improve both reading speed and comprehension. Avoid getting bogged down in details.

Sentence diagramming is one of the most powerful tools for breaking down a highly complex sentence. Do this only if it is necessary for getting an answer, because it does take time. Diagramming a sentence means identifying the basic parts of the sentence—subject, verb, object, modifiers, and connecting words—and drawing a picture of the relationships between these parts.

Mastering diagramming will probably take more instruction than can be given here. However, the following example may help show how even an extremely complex sentence can be broken down into simple relationships. Let's start simply with the child.

What does the child do? The child eats.

What does the child eat? The child eats bread.

When does this happen? During the war, the child eats bread.

TIP

DIAGRAMMING SENTENCES

Sentence diagramming is a powerful tool that helps you break apart the grammatical structure and understand the real relationships in the sentence.

What child does this? During the war, the child who lost her family eats bread.
Which war was it? During the war between the two ethnic groups, the child who lost her family eats bread.

This process could continue and result in the following.

> *During the last war between the two ethnic groups occupying the territory in the eastern region of what was formerly known as Herzegovina, the child who lost her family on the trek from the mountains to the sea coast during the evacuation of the most vulnerable populations eats bread that she found in an abandoned cow shed as a photographer from the western press, moved by the mixture of sorrow and wisdom in her expression, quietly and surreptitiously snaps her portrait for posterity.*

Is it clear that the basic sentence is still "the child eats" and that every new bit of information tells more about an earlier bit? This sentence would be challenging to diagram. Try answering these questions.

What kind of war?
Which ethnic groups?
Which region?
What specific trek?
When did she lose her family?
Evacuation of whom?
What do we know about the bread?
What do we know about the photographer's motivation?
In what manner did the photographer snap her picture?

Formal diagramming teaches specific strategies for quickly identifying parts of sentences and their relationships. If you find many sentences too complex to follow, find a good guide to diagramming.

Diagramming should be practiced untimed. Do not worry if it is taking more time than can be spent on the actual exam. Just like the other CARS skills, diagramming skill improves by practicing slowly, carefully, and patiently. Eventually, you will be able to diagram under the actual time constraints of the test if needed.

VOCABULARY

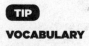

VOCABULARY

CARS is not designed to be a test of vocabulary. If you see a word you don't know, other clues will help you get the answer.

Some people find it helpful to study vocabulary words that may be on the test. For people who have limited study time, that time is probably better spent, however, on practicing other CARS strategies. An unfamiliar word in a passage should not be an obstacle. The passage almost always contains other clues to clarify what the word means. CARS is not really a vocabulary-based task. Studying even hundreds of vocabulary words may not increase your score.

READING CHALLENGING ARTICLES

Some people have reported that regularly reading challenging material, such as articles in technical or scientific journals, has helped them perform better on CARS. The test taker's first priority should be to master the strategies given here and apply them to MCAT style passages.

Keep in mind that MCAT CARS passages are designed specifically to be based on a dichotomy and to challenge the reader in certain specific ways. Other challenging material is not likely to be organized in this way but may help improve analytical skills.

SAMPLE PASSAGE

Here is the passage that was introduced earlier, along with seven questions. Try using strategies on these. Then check the explanations for an in-depth look at how to best apply strategy.

Relationships among elements of the natural world are often more complex than we realize, so that our actions affecting one element may have unexpected, and often negative, effects on another. For example, grasslands, which, of course, are grazed by various animals in a natural setting, may be adversely affected when grazing takes place under conditions altered by people.

Many grasslands in the West have been grazed under altered conditions for well over a hundred years. Scientists have recently been studying the effects of grazing the American bison, commonly known as the buffalo, because it has a less harmful effect on grasslands than most other domestic grazing animals. Two factors have been measured—the health of the grasses and the health of the range area in general. Health of the grasses is measured by counting the number of grass clumps per acre still alive at the end of the season. Health of the range is measured by calculating the number of different species of plants per acre and the total mass of vegetation produced per acre for the season. By comparing bison-grazed range areas with ungrazed control areas, researchers found that the more palatable, fine-textured grasses, such as Indian Rice Grass, suffered significant damage, whereas less tasty, coarse grasses, such as Sacaton, showed virtually none. Overall range health declined in areas dominated by Indian Rice Grass but not in those dominated by Sacaton.

It is still unclear whether a decrease in the health of grasses, even with the more vulnerable ones, necessarily results in a decrease in range health in the long run. Rangelands dominated by the slower-growing, fine-textured species will obviously be more susceptible to permanent damage, but the ultimate effect on a rangeland depends on four identifiable factors. Areas with these characteristics would be most adversely affected: a high ratio of fine grasses to coarse grasses; a high ratio of grasses to nongrass plants; low annual rainfall; and high average seasonal temperatures. It would be a good idea to identify range areas with a combination of these characteristics and take special restorative measures with them, because they are most susceptible to being damaged by human-directed grazing.

Take as much time as necessary on these questions to give yourself a chance to try new strategies. After the questions is a discussion of the answers.

1. Which of the following is the main idea of the passage?
   (A) Whereas natural relationships are complex, grazing is generally more beneficial for grazing animals than it is for plants.
   (B) Use of grasslands to raise bison has had a deleterious effect on rangelands dominated by Indian Rice Grass.
   (C) Human impact may be endangering the health of certain rangelands.
   (D) Grazing of bison can reduce the health of some grasses but probably does not affect the health of the rangeland in general.

2. According to the passage, the health of a rangeland with a significant population of grasses the health of which has been damaged by grazing may not decline if which of the following is true?
   (A) The rangeland has an above average number of trees and shrubs.
   (B) Most of the precipitation the rangeland receives comes in the summer.
   (C) The rangeland is not subject to high winds.
   (D) Coarse-textured grasses become more palatable.

3. It can be inferred from the passage that the absence of a measurable decline in the health of rangelands dominated by Sacaton supports the conclusion that grazing can reduce the health of a rangeland because
   (A) Sacaton is grazed by more types of animals than are most grasses.
   (B) Sacaton grows mostly in the control plots used in this research.
   (C) Sacaton is similar in many ways to Indian Rice Grass but is known to taste bad to bison.
   (D) Sacaton grows in areas similar to those in which Indian Rice Grass grows but is more tolerant of high temperatures.

4. It can be inferred from the passage that which of the following would be true of range areas grazed by domestic animals other than bison?
   (A) The health of some palatable grasses may have decreased even more than in areas grazed by bison.
   (B) Most of the grazing would have occurred in Sacaton plants.
   (C) The overall health of the rangeland would probably be about the same as on the rangeland grazed by bison.
   (D) They would produce a better profit per acre than rangeland grazed by bison.

5. The passage suggests that which of the following is true about rangeland health as defined?
   (A) The range's health decreases when certain species die out without being replaced by species that previously did not grow there.
   (B) The range's health decreases when the total number of plants decreases.
   (C) The range's health is probably low if it contains many fine-textured grasses.
   (D) The range's health is high if it has not been grazed under human control.

6. It can be inferred from the passage that which of the below types of rangeland would be LEAST likely to decline in health under human-directed grazing?
    (A) A rangeland with only a few species of fine-textured grasses
    (B) A rangeland with a relatively high number of nongrass species
    (C) A rangeland in a hot, dry area consisting predominantly of unpalatable grasses
    (D) A mixed shrub and grass rangeland with a large number of fine-textured grass species

7. Which of the following is most likely an assumption behind the author's suggestion in the last sentence?
    (A) If a human action harms the environment, the action should be stopped.
    (B) It is probable that human-directed grazing will continue.
    (C) Maintaining the health of rangelands pays off economically.
    (D) Repairing a damaged environment is more expensive than preventing an environment from becoming damaged in the first place.

Explanations and Strategies

QUESTION 1

"Which of the following is the main idea of the passage?"

Question 1 Answer Choices
(A) Whereas natural relationships are complex, grazing is generally more beneficial for grazing animals than it is for plants.
(B) Use of grasslands to raise bison has had a deleterious effect on rangelands dominated by Indian Rice Grass.
(C) Human impact may be endangering the health of certain rangelands.
(D) Grazing of bison can reduce the health of some grasses but probably does not affect the health of the rangeland in general.

Let's review the systematic process for answering questions. The first step is to orient to the question. This question is straightforward. The second step is to consider what approach to take. In this case, quickly review the big picture. The next step is to review all the answer choices, crossing out ones that are clearly wrong, such as those that go in the wrong direction. During this step, it is not necessary to evaluate each answer choice in depth. Spending a few minutes carefully evaluating answers A, B, and C would turn out to be wasted time if answer D is clearly and obviously correct. After this first pass through all four answer choices, if the answer is not clear, use the adversarial approach to evaluate the answers that are left.

There are really two aspects to finding a correct answer for a main idea question. The correct answer must be true according to the passage, and it must be the main idea. Just being true is not good enough. Consider choice A. Is it true according to the passage? Is it consistent with the passage? Yes, it is. However, it is not the main idea. Choice A is out.

Is choice B true or consistent? Yes. By checking the passage, it is clear that Indian Rice Grass is one of the grasses that would be overgrazed. Is this the main idea? No. Choice B is out.

Is choice C true or consistent? Yes. Is it the main idea? Possibly. Leave it in for now.

Is choice D true or consistent? That is questionable. The first part is true. However, the passage does not contain evidence that would defend the fact that it is unlikely that bison would affect the health of rangeland. In fact, it could be defended that bison grazing, when combined with some of the four factors of adversity, would affect the health of rangeland. Choice D does not pass the test of being true according to the passage or consistent with it. Three answers are out.

Double check choice C. Is it the main idea? This step may seem unnecessary to you, but it is an important safeguard against making careless errors. Verifying that this is indeed the main idea takes only seconds. However, if an error had been made and choice C were not the correct answer, the error would show up now because choice C would not hold up to the scrutiny of a double check. You would then reevaluate the other answer choices.

Here is a very common error to watch out for. You eliminate three answers but are not very happy with the remaining answer. You choose it anyway because everything else is out. Inevitably, it turns out that you had eliminated the correct answer. Avoid the temptation to go with the remaining answer. Go back and reevaluate each answer using the adversarial approach.

If this happens often, be more conservative about crossing out answers. It is better to leave an answer in during the first pass through and then evaluate more carefully during the second pass.

QUESTION 2

"According to the passage, the health of a rangeland with a significant population of grasses the health of which has been damaged by grazing may not decline if which of the following is true?"

Question 2 Answer Choices
(A) The rangeland has an above average number of trees and shrubs.
(B) Most of the precipitation the rangeland receives comes in the summer.
(C) The rangeland is not subject to high winds.
(D) Coarse-textured grasses become more palatable.

Remember the first step? Orient to the question. Does this question seem confusing? It should. Notice the complexity of the wording. You must break down the meaning before going on. First, notice that it is a fact question. It says "according to the passage." Find the grammatical subject of the sentence and the verb that goes with it. "The health . . . may not decline. . . ." This is followed by an "if" statement. Put the "if" statement first. "If one of the following is true, the health . . . may not decline." Note that the subject, health, is vague. Clarify this by asking what kind of health? "Health of a rangeland." Clarify further by asking what kind of rangeland. "Rangeland with a significant population of grasses." Clarify even further. What about these grasses? "Their health has been damaged by grazing." Does this clarify the sentence?

Step two is to consider a plan of attack. Before looking at the answer choices, go back and review the factors that cause a rangeland's health to decline. Remember that one of the dichotomies is health of grasses versus health of rangeland. These are separate. Certain things hurt health of grasses. However, they are not necessarily the same as what hurts the health of rangeland. Do not rely on memory. "Use your eyes, not your memory." There are four factors: a high ratio of fine grasses to coarse grasses; a high ratio of grasses to nongrass plants; low annual rainfall; and high average seasonal temperatures.

An answer that includes one of these factors will go in the wrong direction. It will cause the rangeland to decline. If three answers do this, the remaining answer must be the correct one. Make a first pass through the answers. If an answer does not contain one of the four factors that lead to decline, it might contain a factor that does not affect range health at all. Instead, it might contain a factor that actually improves range health. You need to realize that the correct answer does not have to improve range health.

What about choice A? Trees and shrubs are nongrasses. It goes in the direction of a lower than average ratio of grasses to nongrasses, which is the opposite of one of the four factors of decline. This could be the answer.

What about choice B? It sounds like it would help the health of the rangeland. However, the correct answer has to be defendable based on the four factors. Answer B does not relate to the four factors. Having low annual rainfall would still be possible even though that rainfall comes in the summer. On closer inspection, choice B is not defendable. Could it be the irrelevant answer that is right because the others are clearly wrong? Maybe. Leave it in.

What about choice C? There is nothing about winds in the four factors. Note that choices B and C both contain irrelevant factors. This means it is highly unlikely that the correct answer could be an irrelevant one. More likely, the correct answer will contain a factor that will strengthen the rangeland.

What about choice D? Palatability is a factor in the health of the grasses, not of the rangeland. Being clear on the dichotomy between the two helps to avoid making an error on this answer. Even though it is not one of the four factors of range decline, let's be safe and evaluate it. Grasses that previously tasted bad now taste good. They will get grazed more. The health of the rangeland will, if anything, get worse. Answer D goes in the wrong direction.

Answer A is the only one that contains a factor that would increase the health of the rangeland. On the actual test, this would be enough evidence to choose answer A. However, as an exercise, try to attack choice A, using the adversarial approach. Even on the real test, you should look briefly at choice A again to make sure there are no significant concerns. Notice that looking for reasons to justify answer A only confirms your original prejudice. It is more helpful to see if choice A can be attacked.

The only possible attack on answer A is that it does not prove that we will have a high ratio of nongrasses to grasses, only that it will be higher than average. Given the flaws in the other answer choices, this is not enough to question answer A's validity.

"It can be inferred from the passage that the absence of a measurable decline in the health of rangelands dominated by Sacaton supports the conclusion that grazing can reduce the health of a rangeland because:"

Question 3 Answer Choices
- (A) Sacaton is grazed by more types of animals than are most grasses.
- (B) Sacaton grows mostly in the control plots used in this research.
- (C) Sacaton is similar in many ways to Indian Rice Grass but is known to taste bad to bison.
- (D) Sacaton grows in areas similar to those in which Indian Rice Grass grows but is more tolerant of high temperatures.

Orient to the question. Again, the wording is complex. The basic sentence is "it can be inferred." What is *it* that can be inferred? Find just the simple subject, verb, and object. "It can be inferred that the absence supports the conclusion." What is it the absence of? "A measurable decline." Continue asking questions to get more detail.

Another way to organize a complex sentence is to work backward or outward from the middle. Start with the phrase "rangelands dominated by Sacaton." Expand this to "the health" of those rangelands. Expand that to "a decline" in that health. Remember that part of what the MCAT is testing is the test taker's ability to understand these complex sentences.

The question, then, says, "Rangeland dominated by Sacaton does not decline. How does this support the conclusion that grazing can hurt rangeland?" Notice that the question asks for an inference. This is a fact but not one that is specifically stated. It is one that can be concluded from stated facts. Also notice that the question seems paradoxical. How can an example in which the rangeland is not hurt be used to explain why grazing can hurt rangeland?

The plan of attack is to use the eyes, not the memory, to scan the passage for information about the relationship between Sacaton and the health of rangelands. Sacaton is a coarse grass, and the word *grasses* appears in two of the four factors: "a high ratio of fine grasses to coarse grasses; a high ratio of grasses to nongrass plants."

Having oriented to the question, consider choice A. In more complex questions, it is easy to forget exactly what the question is asking. If necessary, glance at the question again. Choice A seems irrelevant.

What about choice B? This also seems irrelevant.

What about choice C? Answer C is true and consistent with the passage. It also highlights the fundamental difference between coarse grasses and fine grasses. Remember the dichotomy between health of grasses and health of rangeland? Within the health of grasses there is an additional dichotomy—coarse versus fine—with coarse being unpalatable and fine being palatable. Answer C is obviously relevant in some way. However, is it the reason why the scenario in the question described supports the conclusion? Leave it for now and look at choice D.

Answer D also compares the two types of grasses but does so in terms of tolerance for high temperature as opposed to palatability. Leave choice D in for now.

Now compare choice C and D using the adversarial approach. In the adversarial approach, attack the answer choices that seem good and defend the answer choices that seem poor.

Sometimes you should also look for the defense of the answer that looks good and the attack for the answer that looks bad.

Try to attack choice D. Consider this. Answer D says that Sacaton withstands heat. The conclusion that needs to be defended has to do with how grazing can hurt rangeland. Withstanding heat is not directly related to grazing.

Compare this with choice C. Palatability is directly related to grazing. If the grass tastes better, it will be grazed more. Choice C is the answer.

QUESTION 4

"It can be inferred from the passage that which of the following would be true of range areas grazed by domestic animals other than bison?"

Question 4 Answer Choices
(A) The health of some palatable grasses may have decreased even more than in areas grazed by bison.
(B) Most of the grazing would have occurred in Sacaton plants.
(C) The overall health of the rangeland would probably be about the same as on the rangeland grazed by bison.
(D) They would produce a better profit per acre than rangeland grazed by bison.

Orient to the question. This is an inferred fact. Create a plan of attack. This question refers to a dichotomy between bison and other grazing animals. Go to the passage to find any relevant information on this dichotomy. Remember to use your eyes, not your memory. The passage says, "the American bison, commonly known as the buffalo, because it has a less harmful effect on grasslands than most other domestic grazing animals."

The passage contains only one fact. Other domestic grazing animals cause more damage than bison. The correct answer must reflect greater damage.

Answer A refers to the health of grasses rather than the health of rangeland. However, it does go in the right direction, namely that palatable grasses will be worse off. Leave it.

Look at choice B. It may be true that heavier grazers might eat more Sacaton than less heavy grazers. However, the question asks about rangeland in general. There may not be any Sacaton there. "Most" means more than half. Even if it were known that the Sacaton comprised more than half of the rangeland, it cannot be proven that more than half of the grazed plants were Sacaton. Choice B is undefendable.

Choice C contradicts the only known difference between bison and other domestic grazing animals. It is out.

Choice D is a distracter. Some people, especially if they have experience with ranching, may think bison are a poor choice economically. However, this interpretation reads in too much. Nothing in the passage would defend this view, even if it might be true in the real world. Choice D is out.

Everything is out except answer A. Double-check choice A. A possible attack on choice A is that it talks about health of grasses rather than that of rangelands, and the question asks about the effect on rangelands. Now rebut this attack. Destroying the grasses on a rangeland would lead directly to a diminishing of the health of the rangeland.

QUESTION 5

> "The passage suggests that which of the following is true about rangeland health as defined?"
>
> ### Question 5 Answer Choices
> (A) The range's health decreases when certain species die out without being replaced by species that previously did not grow there.
> (B) The range's health decreases when the total number of plants decreases.
> (C) The range's health is probably low if it contains many fine-textured grasses.
> (D) The range's health is high if it has not been grazed under human control.

Orient to the question. It is straightforward. It is a fact or, possibly, inference question. The plan of attack is to review what the passage says about rangeland health. The four factors have already been identified. Is there anything else? The second paragraph tells how to measure rangeland health. "Health of the range is measured by calculating the number of different species of plants per acre and the total mass of vegetation produced per acre for the season." Is this enough to answer the question?

Answer A introduces new information. However, it does make sense and is consistent with the passage. Remember not to eliminate an answer unless it is clearly out. Leave in choice A.

Choice B seems consistent with the passage. Leave it in.

Choice C is consistent with the passage. The word *probably* might not be defendable. However, wait until the second pass through the answer choices to analyze it more deeply.

Choice D says that as long as there is no human control, the rangeland health will be high. This implies that there are no other factors that could affect the rangeland health. Whereas this implication might be true, it is unlikely. Additionally, nothing in the passage supports it. Answer D is out.

Use the adversarial approach to compare choices A, B, and C. The original attack on answer A was that it seems to introduce new information. Try to defend choice A. To do so, it must be matched with one of the given factors that affect rangeland health. Answer A has no relationship either to the human-controlled grazing or the four factors of rangeland health.

Try fitting answer A to the factors for measuring the health of the rangeland—the number of different species of plants per acre and the total mass of vegetation produced per acre for the season. If a certain species dies out without being replaced by a species that previously did not grow there, the total number of different species of plants will be reduced on that same acreage. If this is not clear from the words, quantify the argument. Start with fifteen species of plants per acre. Three of those species die out. Twelve remain. If the plants of those twelve species spread, there are more plants but still only twelve species.

This is a strong argument for choice A. However, it will be important to quickly make sure that choices B and C do not hold up. Using the same measure of rangeland health, answer B gives us fewer plants. Does this necessarily mean that there will be either a lower number of species per acre or less mass of vegetation per acre? The fact that there are fewer plants seems like it should lead to less in general. To attack this impression, try to prove that there could be fewer plants and yet a greater number of species. The proof can be mathematical.

	Before	After
# of plants	1000	400
# of species	8	30

Compare the two scenarios. Before choice B takes place, there may have been 1000 plants but they may have all been of eight species. After choice B takes place, there are only 400 plants but there is a broader variety of species. It may seem counterintuitive, but nothing in the passage prevents this scenario. The number of plants simply does not necessarily correlate to the number of species.

The same argument will hold up for the relationship between fewer plants and total mass of vegetation.

	Before	After
# of plants	1000	1
Mass of vegetation in kg	350 kg	500 kg

In this example, an absurd situation has been used to make a point. Even if an area were reduced from 1000 plants to one, if that one plant were huge, the mass could be greater than before. There is no necessary correlation between the number of plants and the mass of vegetation, despite the commonsense, but false, assumption that fewer plants should result in less mass. Answer B is out.

Answer C implies that the presence of many fine-textured grasses correlates to poor range health. It is only the ratio of fine-textured to coarse grasses that correlates to range health. The number of fine-textured grasses alone does not tell us anything about the ratio. This can be proven by stating that there could be many fine-textured grasses and twice as many coarse ones. Note also that the term *many* is not a quantitative term. There is no way to prove that a certain number constitutes *many*. Depending on the situation, the word *many* could refer to any quantity more than one.

QUESTION 6

"It can be inferred from the passage that which of the below types of rangeland would be LEAST likely to decline in health under human-directed grazing?"

Question 6 Answer Choices
(A) A rangeland with only a few species of fine-textured grasses
(B) A rangeland with a relatively high number of nongrass species
(C) A rangeland in a hot, dry area consisting predominantly of unpalatable grasses
(D) A mixed shrub and grass rangeland with a large number of fine-textured grass species

Orient to the question. It asks for an inferred fact. The word LEAST is in capital letters because, like the words EXCEPT or NOT, the question is asking for the opposite of what the test taker might expect. It would be more natural to look for something that would cause the rangeland to decline. The question asks for the opposite.

What is the plan of attack? If it is possible to prove that three of the answers would lead to decline, then the remaining answer would be correct, even if it were irrelevant. On the other hand, the correct answer may be one that actively goes in the direction of improving rangeland. The wrong answers, then, could either contain conditions that would lead to decline or could be irrelevant.

Review the four factors that lead to decline: "a high ratio of fine grasses to coarse grasses; a high ratio of grasses to nongrass plants; low annual rainfall; and high average seasonal temperatures."

Answer A, with only a few species of fine grasses, would lead in the direction of minimal damage. Leave it in.

Choice B refers to a "relatively high number" of nongrass species. This correlates with less damage. Leave it in.

Choice C has some factors that go in the right direction and some that go in the wrong direction. It cannot be completely thrown out at this point.

Choice D also contains information that seems to go in both directions.

No answers were clearly out. Make a second pass through the answers using the adversarial approach. Start with choice A, and try to attack it. A defense of choice A would be based on claiming that a low ratio of fine grasses to coarse ones would be least likely to lead to decline. Can that claim be attacked? Look carefully at what answer A actually says, namely "only a few species" of fine grasses. Is this the same as a low ratio of fine grasses to coarse ones? Prove that it is not.

	Fine	Coarse	Ratio of Fine to Coarse
# of species	3	45	0.06
# of plants	100,000	4500	2222.20

The mathematical example above proves that the number of species does not correlate with the number of plants. The predictive rule—a high ratio of fine to coarse—is based on the number of plants.

Choice B results in a "relatively high" number of nongrass plants. In this case, the number of plants is the correct measurement. The term *relatively* means it is in relation to something else, the number of grass plants. This is an exact match for a condition that would lead to the least amount of damage.

In choice C, the "hot, dry" condition definitely goes in the wrong direction, that of damage. "Unpalatable grasses" goes in the direction of less damage. It is not possible to determine from the information given which of these factors would be strongest. Theoretically, the conditions in choice C could lead to less damage than would those in choice B. However, proving that they would is not possible. Answer C is out.

Answer D is wrong for the same reasons. It is actually even weaker than choice C. Even though the large number of fine grasses is clearly in the wrong direction, the "mixed" shrub and grassland does not definitely establish that there is a low ratio of grass to nongrass.

This question tries to confuse the test taker between two close but distinct concepts—the number of groups and the number of members of a group. If at a convention 15 groups are representing Cleveland and three groups are representing Atlanta, which city has more people at the convention?

Similarly, some questions confuse ratio and actual number. If 40 percent of the people in City *A* have BMWs and only 3 percent of the people in City *B* do, which city has more BMWs? It cannot be determined. Three percent of the people in New York City would be more than 40 percent of the people in a small town.

QUESTION 7

"Which of the following is most likely an assumption behind the author's suggestion in the last sentence?"

Question 7 Answer Choices
(A) If a human action harms the environment, the action should be stopped.
(B) It is probable that human-directed grazing will continue.
(C) Maintaining the health of rangelands pays off economically.
(D) Repairing a damaged environment is more expensive than preventing an environment from becoming damaged in the first place.

Orient to the question. It is an unusual question type and relates to logic. To answer this, you must know that an assumption is an unstated fact that is necessary to make the argument work. If the assumption is removed or negated, the argument will fall apart. For example, consider the following argument. "All white cats are deaf. Little Binky is white. Therefore, Little Binky is deaf." What is the assumption in this argument? What is the unstated but necessary fact? Could it be that "Little Binky is a cat"? Test it out by removing or negating it, namely, by saying that Little Binky is something other than a cat, such as a rhinoceros. If Little Binky is a rhinoceros, the argument does not hold up. This is proof that "Little Binky is a cat" is an assumption of the argument.

What is the plan of attack? Reread the last sentence of the passage, and orient to the argument it is trying to make.

"It would be a good idea to identify range areas with a combination of these characteristics and take special restorative measures with them, because they are most susceptible to being damaged by human-directed grazing."

What about choice A? Is this a fact that is required to make the argument work? Negate it. "If a human action harms the environment, it does not necessarily have to be stopped." Does this ruin the argument? It does not seem to. Choice A is not necessary to make the argument work.

Choice B seems too simpleminded and possibly irrelevant. However, it cannot yet be thrown out.

Try negating choice C. "Maintaining the health of the rangeland does not pay off economically." Does this weaken the argument? Possibly. There would be less incentive to maintain the rangeland. Keep it in for now.

ASSUMPTION QUESTIONS

To test an answer, negate it. If the argument falls apart, that answer was the necessary fact.

Does the author need to believe choice D for the argument to work? It does not seem likely. The author is not addressing a choice between preventing and restoring. Answer D is out.

Answers B and C are left. Choice B did not seem like a strong answer. However, at this stage, you must be careful. Because choice C is the favored answer, attack it. The defense for answer C was that lack of an economic reason for maintaining the health of rangeland might weaken the argument. However, this can be the author's assumption only if the author is concerned with economic payoff. No evidence in the passage would prove that the author's main concern is economic.

Because choice B was the least-favored answer, try to defend it. Negate answer B. "Human-directed grazing will not continue." Try to defend that this will affect the argument. If there is no more human-directed grazing, is it not true that the threat to these more-vulnerable rangelands is gone? The argument falls completely apart. It is no longer necessary to recommend protection from human-directed grazing.

Without the negation test, it was very difficult to see how choice B was anything more than a simpleminded, self-evident fact. This demonstrates the power of negation in assumption questions.

The patterns in these questions represent a handful of the hundreds of patterns on the test. Some of the patterns are quite common. Others may show up only rarely. Learn as many patterns as possible by working carefully and analytically on each practice question.

SUMMARY

This chapter covered a number of important points that you should review regularly as you practice.

You learned that there are specific strategies you can use to improve on the CARS. You learned how to control your time to increase your score. You learned several ways of practicing in order to master your CARS strategies.

This chapter showed you skimming methods for setting up the passage and for iden- tifying and diagramming its structure (Big Picture.) It discussed the two main categories of questions—Big Picture and Detail—and the specific types of questions within each of those categories. Big Picture questions include Main Idea, Tone, Logical Organization, Literary Techniques, and Extension. Detail questions include Specific Detail and Implied Detail.

This chapter taught you specific strategies for getting to the correct answer. Among the main strategies are orienting to the question, making two passes through the answer choices, and using the adversarial approach.

The chapter demonstrated many strategies and techniques for you. Review the chap- ter periodically and practice what you have learned as you work on the tests.

PASSAGE I

The creative person attempting to be true to the leanings of his or her own spirit in this all-too-concrete world that is both our home and our prison must find a way to turn the gentle energy of artistry that warms him or her into a weapon with which to fight against the nearly irresistible current of modern materialism. If the artist, musician, or poet cannot find the way to do this while young, the chance may be lost. Were he, instead of a poet, a businessman or lawyer or soldier, the young man would be trained by his eager elders, taught the weapons of his war, and sent off to make his way, proud family cheering him on. But as a poet, an artist, he stands apart from the world of logic, of money, of laws—a lone orchid in a desert of scrub and cacti.

Of all the creative souls, I believe the loneliest must be the musician. The poet has at least the language in common with his fellows. When needed, a fine letter from his pen may accomplish a practical task—arranging a trip, setting right a misunderstanding, communicating with an attorney. His art is but a higher use of a faculty which he can rehearse daily, albeit in a cruder form.

But with whom can the musician practice her art? At the mechanic's, can she sing her concerns, or play on the piano her lack of understanding of why a small replaced part costs two weeks' income? Can she present the traffic policeman with a fine new waltz to explain why her license was left at home? Walking in the street, sitting in the café, hearing the ongoing verbal give and take that distinguishes mankind from our furry cousins, it is for her but noise—perhaps a rhythm here and there, but mostly random. For her, communication means to put the noise in order, to let it resonate with the heart, the belly, and to broadcast it into the world as a way to heal chaos. Who, walking by her in the street, even hears her?

What guidance, then, can we, an older generation, offer the young musician—most isolated of all artists—so that she can find the strength to turn her plowshare into a sword? The way is simple. Set aside concerns about the outer world—that strange and foreign land—and start with what comes most naturally—the gift of making music. From trusting in this comes confidence in one's strength. If the young musician follows this path, she will sooner or later discover that she can communicate with others on her own terms. It is not necessary to communicate with everyone. That is the mistaken notion of youth, born out of loneliness. My primary advice is "Communicate only with those who can hear you." Then, in life as in music, the young musician begins to gain an appreciative audience.

I have said that the way is simple, but it is also not easy. Many are the landmines that lay hidden beneath the green fields of musical creativity. Foremost—and most particularly dangerous for the youngest and newest of musicians—is a smoldering impatience with the length of time it takes for the first few signs of appreciation from other people to appear. To avoid this fatal trap, hold close to your heart these two weapons: savor without greed even the tiniest successes; and remind yourself again and again that you work only for expressing what you must, as if you were the only human on Earth.

The true enemy of the young musician is a two-headed beast: one head Failure, breathing fire and spitting venom; the other, Success, luring her into sweet oblivion. If recognition comes too soon, before the musician has grounded herself in her own creativity, she may become addicted to the approval of others, only to find that when she is most vulnerable, the approval disappears. Having struggled so desperately to reach her goal and then losing it so quickly, she may not have the will to try again. But is this not a sign that, all along, her goal was still the approval of others? That she had still not returned to the spirit of creating for herself only?

Perhaps the ideal of creating for oneself alone sounds selfish, isolated, uncaring for the world around one. Nothing could be more untrue. How long would an oak tree survive if it sent its roots out into the air in all directions, hoping some passing wind or rain would bring nourishment? To thrive, the musician must put her roots down deeply into the source of her own creativity. Only then can she grow to her full stature, spreading her arms to shade and shelter others and sharing her songs to soothe them.

1. In the fourth paragraph, the author mentions that the young musician may eventually be able to "communicate with others on her own terms." Based on how it is used in the passage, the statement suggests that a young musician should:
   (A) stand up for what she believes in.
   (B) develop certain "weapons" for dealing with people.
   (C) shift from external to internal motivation.
   (D) use a similar but cruder form of her own art to communicate with others.

2. It can be inferred from the passage that a successful musician would find which of the following most gratifying?
   (A) Being able to communicate with her peers on her own terms
   (B) Staying in touch with her own creativity
   (C) Earning recognition in later life from those who truly can appreciate her work
   (D) Continuing to publish new work in her middle years

3. Which of the following facts about young creative people is NOT supported by the passage?
   (A) A creative talent can help them in dealing with the demands of daily life.
   (B) They have guidance to offer other artists, including musicians.
   (C) Some of them may find success as dangerous as failure.
   (D) Their families may not approve of their plans for the future.

4. If it were known to be true that nearly two-thirds of young musicians who have achieved some success eventually fail, which of the following would be the most direct cause of this failure according to information given in the passage?
   (A) They did not focus on creating for themselves only.
   (B) They became addicted to approval.
   (C) They did not savor the small successes.
   (D) They became discouraged because they did not continue to be successful.

5. What is the author's purpose in using the line "turn her plowshare into a sword" in the fourth paragraph?
   (A) It creates a parallel between the poet's pen and the musician's instrument.
   (B) It indicates the seriousness of the mistaken notion of youth referred to later in the same paragraph.
   (C) It emphasizes the difference between the situations of creative people in general, including poets, and those of musicians.
   (D) It extends an analogy previously applied to poets.

6. Which of the following is NOT an example of a recommendation that the author has for young musicians?
   (A) A young musician gives up trying to communicate with people on any terms.
   (B) A young musician throws an expensive celebration party for his friends even though a publisher has simply agreed to look over a score.
   (C) A young musician spends less time listening to the music of her favorite composers and more time creating variations on children's songs.
   (D) An otherwise timid young musician takes a course in weaponry to learn how to deal with the world more aggressively.

7. Which of the following bits of advice to young creative people by a different author most strongly conflicts with the statements in the passage?
   (A) It's not how many people you know but whom you know.
   (B) Both failure and success can make you or break you.
   (C) Work on your music as though you were the last person on Earth.
   (D) Let little things affect you in a big way.

PASSAGE II

Heliocentrism is the theory that Earth and the planets revolve around the Sun and that the Sun is stationary and is the center of the universe. There is a historic rivalry between heliocentrism and geocentrism, which theorized that Earth stood motionless at the center of the universe. Writings espousing heliocentrism are found as early as the 3rd century B.C. However, heliocentrism did not become a scientifically viable theory until the 16th century, when Nicolaus Copernicus was able to create a mathematical model of the motion of the Sun and planets. Subsequently, both Johannes Kepler and Galileo Galilei added to Copernicus's model. Galileo was able to confirm visually some of the predictions of the model using the newly invented telescope.

To the naive observer looking up into the sky, Earth seems to stand still while the celestial objects move across the sky in a daily rhythm. It is no wonder that the geocentric model had its appeal. However, consistent observation of the skies soon reveals discoveries that cannot be explained by a strict geocentric theory. Even before the heliocentric theory came to the fore, astronomers had proposed that certain planets revolved around the Sun, while the Sun itself, along with those planets, revolved around Earth.

Heliocentrism comes in conflict not just with "common sense" but also with the Church. Copernicus's ideas contradicted certain well-known verses from the King James Bible. 1 Chronicles 16:30 says, "The world also shall be stable, that it be not moved." Psalm 104:5 says, "[the Lord] Who laid the foundations of the earth, that it should not be removed for ever." Ecclesiastes 1:5 says, "The sun also ariseth, and the sun goeth down, and hasteth to his place where he arose."

While privately many learned officials of the Church described the value of Copernicus's theory, in public the Church remained opposed, holding to the geocentric model. The conflict between the two models put the Church in a difficult position. To acknowledge the new model would mean having to admit that the Bible itself was either wrong or was to be interpreted in a limited, poetic way. This was also a tacit admission that the Church had erred in its interpretation of the Bible. Unable to take this course, the public voice of the Church repudiated heliocentrism to the extreme degree that Galileo himself was tried and found guilty, spending his final years under arrest.

Technically, of course, the heliocentric system is not correct. Although Earth and the planets revolve around the Sun, the Sun is not the stationary center of the universe. During the 18th and 19th centuries, evidence mounted that the Sun was simply one of the countless stars in the sky. It was not until the 20th century that the concept of some fixed focal point in the universe was overturned by Einstein's special theory of relativity.

Despite the science, it may be that on some level human beings will never let go of the deeply intuitive feeling that we are at the center of everything. If we, our planet, cannot be at the center, then there must be some other center of the universe that we can depend on in an otherwise chaotic world. Are we ready to live in a universe with no such center?

8. According to the passage, proponents of geocentrism would most object to the claim that:
    (A) Earth moves.
    (B) the Sun moves around Earth.
    (C) the Biblical description of astronomy may not be literally true.
    (D) the heliocentric theory is not technically correct.

9. All of the following statements about Copernicus are consistent with the passage EXCEPT:
    (A) some believers in his theory were tried and found guilty.
    (B) Galileo's observations with the telescope helped Copernicus form his theory.
    (C) some officials of the Church privately expressed some support for his theory.
    (D) his ideas were in conflict with parts of the Bible.

10. Which of the following statements about heliocentrism can be inferred from the passage?
    (A) It is not completely acceptable because humans need to believe in a central focus point of the universe.
    (B) The Church consistently objected to it.
    (C) It acknowledges that the Sun does not act any differently than other stars do.
    (D) Heliocentrism existed before Christianity.

11. Which of the following is an example of a poetic interpretation of "the world also shall be stable, that it be not moved"?
    (A) Even though the crust of Earth moves, we can trust in the predictability and orderliness of the movements.
    (B) Earth itself is held in orbit by forces beyond our understanding.
    (C) We can depend on nature to provide us with food and shelter, no matter what else changes.
    (D) The infinite changes and movements of the universe are guided by an underlying intelligence.

12. Which of the following can be inferred about Einstein's special theory of relativity based on information in the passage?
    (A) It was the final proof of the heliocentric model.
    (B) It predicts that the universe is continually getting warmer.
    (C) The Church opposes it publicly while privately acknowledging its importance.
    (D) It challenges a fundamental human belief.

13. What does the author most likely mean by the phrase "common sense"?
    (A) Believing something because most other people believe it
    (B) Believing something because the senses give a certain impression
    (C) Believing something because it is supported by writings of spiritual authorities
    (D) Believing something because it is a simple, logical conclusion

PASSAGE III

Despite its complicated narrative style and the absence of the supposedly indispensable love motive, the novel *Robinson Crusoe*, by Daniel Defoe, was received well in the literary world. The book is considered one of the most widely published books in history. It has been popular since the day it was published, and continues to be highly regarded to this day.

Novelist James Joyce noted that the true symbol of the British conquest is Robinson Crusoe: "He is the true prototype of the British colonist. . . . The whole Anglo-Saxon spirit is in Crusoe: the manly independence, the unconscious cruelty, the persistence, the slow yet efficient intelligence, the sexual apathy, the calculating taciturnity."

In a sense Crusoe attempts to replicate his own society on the island. This is achieved through the application of European technology, agriculture, and even a rudimentary political hierarchy. The idealized master-servant relationship Defoe depicts between Crusoe and Friday can also be seen in terms of cultural imperialism. Crusoe represents the "enlightened" European whilst Friday is the "savage" who can only be redeemed from his supposedly barbarous way of life through assimilation into Crusoe's culture.

According to J. P. Hunter, Robinson is not a hero, but an everyman. He begins as a wanderer, aimless on a sea he does not understand, and ends as a pilgrim, crossing a final mountain to enter the promised land. The book tells the story of how Robinson becomes closer to God, not through listening to sermons in a church but through spending time alone amongst nature with only a Bible to read.

Whether colonial hero or enduring everyman, the story is one of personal triumph over hostile circumstances through the enduring goodness of providence. There is, however, a different and darker interpretation of *Robinson Crusoe*, and that interpretation is a psychological one. It sees the story as one of a man whose great failure is the inability to find and maintain a relationship of love, or indeed, even of friendship.

In sailing from his homeland, Crusoe abandons society for the company of a small group of men alone in a vast sea. In being shipwrecked, he leaves behind even that small remnant of humanity. From a psychological standpoint, his inability to love—to love friends, to love a woman—eventually drives him into complete and utter isolation.

Robinson Crusoe is in fact the ultimate workaholic. What he sees as his great triumphs, we can only see as evidence of his skewed focus. The more marvelous his accomplishments, the sadder his situation in our eyes. Though he tries to prove how much he can do on his own, by himself, we know that he is trying to prove the wrong point.

It would be gratifying to the psychologically minded reader if Robinson Crusoe would recognize the emotional gap that his workaholism is trying to fill. At least then he could begin to move slowly toward the ability to love. Being stranded would have been the perfect opportunity. We can imagine him sitting alone in the sunset saying, "You know, all that I've accomplished is really meaningless without friends." But he never does. Even his relationship with Friday is not a friendship. It is a master/servant work relationship, without equality.

Why does Defoe allow his hero to drown in workaholism without the possibility of redemption? The answer is likely that Defoe himself saw Crusoe's endless work as redeeming. Quite possibly it was Defoe who filled the void of love in his own life with the fantasy adventures of his eternally lonely hero.

Adapted from "Robinson Crusoe" in *Wikipedia, The Free Encyclopedia*
http://en.wikipedia.org/w/index.php?title=Robinson_Crusoe&oldid=358449298
(accessed April 26, 2010).

14. According to the author, all of the following would be good ways to work toward a relationship of love or friendship EXCEPT:
    (A) moving to an industrial city.
    (B) noticing an emotional gap in oneself.
    (C) showing a potential friend a difficult project that you completed.
    (D) reflecting on one's life situation.

15. Which of the following is the author's attitude about Daniel Defoe, author of *Robinson Crusoe*?
    (A) He is supportive of Defoe because Defoe used a vivid imagination to portray a situation that he never personally experienced.
    (B) He is supportive of Defoe because Defoe accurately portrayed the emotions of a man torn between survival and longing for friends.
    (C) He is critical of Defoe because Defoe built his own blind spots into his character.
    (D) He is critical of Defoe because Defoe does not have his character ultimately triumph over his environment.

16. The author suggests that which of the following may have been Crusoe's true motivation for sailing on a ship?
    (A) Crusoe hoped to start a new life in a friendlier place.
    (B) Crusoe hoped to prove his ability to take care of himself.
    (C) Crusoe thought he might enjoy becoming a sailor.
    (D) Crusoe felt a need to avoid painful situations.

17. If a lost chapter of *Robinson Crusoe* were found, which of the following events in that chapter would most weaken the author's argument?
    (A) Crusoe tells Friday to draw pictures of Crusoe's family as Crusoe describes them.
    (B) Crusoe tells Friday to take a week off for himself.
    (C) Crusoe tries to build a grain storage container, fails, and gives up.
    (D) Friday tells Crusoe he was a leader among his people and expects to be treated as an equal.

18. Which of the following characterizes James Joyce's feelings about the Anglo-Saxon spirit?
    (A) He feels positive about it because he is proud of the British Empire.
    (B) He feels ambivalent about it because, whereas it is persistent, it is too slow.
    (C) He would feel better about it if it would recognize its own cruelty.
    (D) He feels negative about it because colonialism has predominantly been hurtful to the colonized.

What is a child worth? For today's parents, the answer would undoubtedly be in terms of love, joy, and gratification. However, in earlier times, these might not have been the terms in which a parent would answer the question.

Consider the child in a primitive agricultural society. By the time the child was four or five, it would probably be expected to participate in some of the tasks required for sustaining the community. A small child might help harvest grains, carry baskets from the field to the village, or deliver items from one community member to another. By the age of 10, a child would probably be spending many hours a day helping with tasks as well as learning new skills. By the early teenage years, children were likely to function as adults, with compensation made for their still-limited strength, endurance, and skills. A child in such a society had specific economic worth. The child produced material goods required by the community.

The worth of a child had economic value not only in primitive societies. Consider the Industrial Revolution, a mere two to three hundred years ago. If anything, the Industrial Revolution made children even more of a commodity, removing them further from the emotional life of the family and from a natural and healthy environment. In many ways, the emotional value of the child was crushed. Only the economic value remained.

This seems a complete reversal of how modern parents see their children. How did the modern view, which by our standards seems the natural view, come about? A number of changes happened at the same time. In the late 1800s, reformers began campaigning for child labor regulation and for compulsory education, arguing that children should be given the opportunity to learn and to that end should be spared from exploitative work. At the same time, as industry evolved, there was less demand for child labor, making the child's economic worth less valuable. Additionally, the concept of the family united by love rather than duty began to grow. All in all, the child came to be seen as emotionally precious rather than economically valuable. In fact, the greater the gap that could be created between what was seen as the coarse economic world and the life of the child, the greater the preciousness.

At the end of the 19th century, when children were no longer seen as having an economic value, a family in Georgia sued for damages when their child was killed in an accident. The court ruled that they were due no monetary damages because the child did not contribute economically to the family. Ironically, as the new attitude toward children evolved in the 20th century, the almost otherworldly emotional value of the child came to be assigned a corresponding economic value. A couple in New York in the late 1970s was awarded $750,000 for the accidental death of their child.

By looking at this example more closely, we can see what is perhaps a unique shift in the definition of worth or value. For possibly the first time in history, it is emotional value that is dictating economic worth, rather than the other way around. A modern parent, responding to the question "What is your child worth?" might well respond, "A million dollars," not because of the child's earning potential but because we value love as highly as money.

19. Based on information in the passage, if the Industrial Revolution had not occurred, which of the following would most likely have been true?
    (A) People from primitive societies would not have moved to industrialized societies.
    (B) Children would not have had to work as many hours.
    (C) Children would have had less economic value to their parents.
    (D) Parents would have had stronger emotional connections to their children.

20. The phrase "as well as learning new skills" about children in primitive societies serves what function in the passage?
    (A) It shows that the economic value of a child in primitive societies was greater if their skills were greater.
    (B) It shows that some primitive attitudes toward children are different from our modern attitudes.
    (C) It shows that some primitive attitudes toward children are similar to our modern attitudes.
    (D) It leads into the discussion of how the attitudes toward children changed during the Industrial Revolution.

21. What is the author's purpose in citing the two cases of parents suing over the accidental death of a child?
    (A) It emphasizes that some families value the emotional worth of their child over the economic worth.
    (B) It emphasizes that modern society believes that economic worth and emotional worth are related.
    (C) It emphasizes that modern society believes that a child's economic value should not be determined by the child's emotional value.
    (D) It emphasizes that different regions of the country hold different values about a child's worth.

22. What is the meaning of the word "otherworldly" in the passage?
    (A) Children are believed to be a spiritual or religious gift.
    (B) Modern parents draw a strong distinction between the world of work and the life of the family.
    (C) A child's value is spiritual, not material.
    (D) Children are in touch with things that we as adults have lost touch with.

23. Which of the following statements would the author most likely agree with?
    (A) The change to placing an emotional value on children in the 19th century was caused in part by reformers.
    (B) The change to placing an emotional value on children in the 19th century was caused in part by parents who had stronger bonds with their children.
    (C) It is hard to know why parents in primitive societies required so much work from their children.
    (D) Many things changed in the 19th century in relation to children, but it is hard to say what was the primary cause.

PASSAGE V

The myth of the free-market economy is that prices in our current economy reflect the free interplay of the costs of production and demand and that, because of this, nothing should be done by government to interfere with any of these components. If the basic premise were true, then the system would not need any outside interference to make it work better. The premise, however, is not, in fact, true.

Consider two chicken farmers. One takes her accumulated chicken manure to the city dump and pays the dump fee. The other throws his chicken manure into the nearby river. The first farm will have a higher production cost and thus, will have to charge more for its eggs. If there is no corresponding difference in quality, this may drive the first farmer out of business.

If the government creates a law against dumping manure in the river, the second farmer may complain that they are interfering with his ability to do business. In fact, any fine for dumping manure in the river simply pays for the actual cost of cleaning up the manure. This is a bona fide cost of production from which the farmer has tried to escape.

In his book *The Ecology of Commerce*, Paul Hawken describes modern business as an environment in which companies compete in trying to escape as much actual cost of production as possible in order to keep their prices low. Industries lobby the government to protect them from having to pay costs such as the expense of processing discarded packaging, the costs of recycling old products, and medical expenses incurred when people become sick from using the industry's products or being exposed to the industry's toxic waste.

These expenses are all real. They must be paid for by someone. Under the current system, Hawken points out, the general public must pay the cost.

Suppose that a company wished to be more responsible. It would be in the position of the first chicken farmer. Its prices would be higher than its competitors. Perhaps a small number of conscientious consumers would voluntarily pay a higher price. In the long run, however, it would be unlikely to succeed. How, then, can the current system be changed if not one company at a time?

Hawken suggests a different approach. Consider the analogy of a family in which, at dinnertime, everyone grabs food as quickly as possible and those who are slow go hungry. If one family member recognized the unfairness, not to mention the unhealthiness, of having to grab and gulp food and if that family member refrained from grabbing, that person would simply get no food. If, however, that person held a meeting of all the family members and got them to agree that the system was bad for all of them, they might arrive at a healthier arrangement that they would all agree to.

If businesses were to agree to a fairer set of rules, none would actually suffer. A fairer set of rules in modern commerce would mean that businesses would be responsible for costs that are the direct result of their products. If a company produced drinks in plastic bottles that ended up in the municipal dump, they would be charged for the cost of processing those bottles. However, so would all of their competitors.

One benefit of a set of fairer rules is rather unexpected. Instead of spending all of their efforts on pushing production costs onto the public, companies could focus instead on creating better, more efficient, less toxic, and more environmentally friendly products. In fact, that would be the only way for companies to become more competitive.

24. The author would agree with all of the following statements EXCEPT:
    (A) when companies evade production costs, they create inferior products.
    (B) Hawken's approach can work only if individual companies start changing their policies.
    (C) a fair free-market economy is theoretically possible.
    (D) a business should not complain about expenses if their competitors are subject to the same expenses.

25. According to the passage, which of the following is relevant in determining whether a company should be regulated by society?
    (A) The company's products are inferior to those of its competitors.
    (B) The company charges excessively for its products because it holds a monopoly.
    (C) People who drink the company's soft drink develop diabetes at a higher rate than the general public.
    (D) The company's executives make far more money than other people in the community doing similar work.

26. According to the passage, which of the following would lead to a fairer system of allocating costs of production?

    I. All companies in an industry agree to pay full disability costs for their workers.
    II. All companies in an industry agree to provide discounts for the truly needy.
    III. All companies in an industry agree not to undercut each other's prices.

    (A) I only
    (B) I and II only
    (C) II only
    (D) II and III only

27. Paul Hawken's own company attempts to accept its costs of doing business, especially in terms of being more environmentally conservative. Why then would Hawken agree that the system cannot be changed "one company at a time"?
    (A) Few companies have the commitment that is needed.
    (B) A company that changed in this way would have to charge more than its competitors.
    (C) A single company cannot realistically calculate the costs of its environmental impact.
    (D) The actions of small groups are unlikely to change the system on a larger scale.

28. The author implies that which of the following could be a way to improve the current system without involving government regulation?
    (A) Certain conscientious companies could begin making a change on their own.
    (B) Consumer groups could advocate buying from only companies that do not evade actual production costs.
    (C) All members of an industry could agree on an industry-wide set of rules.
    (D) Industries could lobby the government to protect them from unnecessary costs.

PASSAGE VI

It is a rare thing today to hear a logical argument between two people that deserves the designation "logical." Especially in the arena of politics, there is much yelling, much shaking of fists, much assertion of questionable facts, but very little that really amounts to an exploration of the truth of an issue.

Perhaps the art of logic could be salvaged if some guidelines and definitions were set forth and then followed by those who would argue together. Let us then define what we can call a true logical discussion. A logical discussion is an exchange between two or more people in which the shared goal is to come to the truth—which the arguers both agree must exist—by employing valid logic and by avoiding certain pitfalls that result, not in logical discussion, but in a logical yelling match.

The first pitfall to consider is the emotionally laden argument. Most arguers today rely heavily on emotionally charged topics or statements. One might say that passion for a point of view is a sign of sincerity on the part of the arguer. There are two points of confusion here. The first is a confusion between the role of the arguer and the role of the audience. To have a true logical discussion, the audience must be ignored, or at least considered as secondary. It is not the goal of the logical discussion to move an audience—as is often the case in common logical argument—but rather to arrive at a truth that both arguers agree on. The arguer who uses emotion to blind the audience may end up also blinded. The second confusion is about the role of emotion. In a logical discussion, emotion is a response to the truth, not a tool for establishing truth.

A second pitfall is the use of what might be called "potential" facts. The arguer makes an assertion such as, "Everyone knows that most people want no new taxes." This assertion, if true, would bolster the argument. However, the arguer rarely bothers to document the potential fact. To have a true logical discussion requires establishing facts before using them to support an argument. Establishing a fact may require citing reliable sources or having one's opponent concede that the fact is true. Until a fact is established, using it to make a point is fundamentally no different than making an emotional argument. It is based on wishful thinking.

What makes a logical discussion effective? From the standpoints of both the arguers and the audience, it is simply that the illogical and the emotional have been avoided, the facts have been established, and the logic that has been applied is valid. An argument that is appealing just on an intuitive level is not effective. It is only persuasive. A persuasive argument may have the power to move people to action, but that action is likely to be harmful. One need only look to Hitler's Germany for examples. To become effective, an intuitively appealing argument must be held up to closer inspection.

If logical discussion were to be used by politicians, the format of political dialogue would need to change dramatically. Instead of the two-minute expositions followed by one minute of emotional backlash, each candidate would need to have time to lay out arguments and establish facts. It could require a series of such discussions over many weeks to find the pitfalls and avoid them and to begin to create an effective argument. The great question is whether the politicians, not to mention the public, are up to the task.

29. Which of the following best describes the author's purpose?
    (A) To present a consistent logical discussion
    (B) To uncover the characteristics of logical discussion
    (C) To describe a process for verifying an emotional stance
    (D) To show viable alternatives to logical discussion

30. Which of the following is an assumption made in the author's argument?
    (A) Some kinds of logical argument are more logical than others.
    (B) Arguments that avoid emotional stances are not convincing.
    (C) To understand a logical discussion as a listener, it is necessary to have experience as an arguer.
    (D) An effective argument is simply one that convinces on an intuitive level.

31. The passage offers logical support for which of the following statements?
    (A) An argument can move people to action without being effective.
    (B) An emotional stance may blind the arguer as well as the audience.
    (C) Potential facts are as important as real facts.
    (D) The reactions of the audience should not be the primary goal of the arguers.

32. The author rejects the validity of an emotional argument because:
    (A) emotionally tainted facts cannot be proven.
    (B) an emotional argument assumes that the highest truth has the strongest emotional appeal.
    (C) an emotional argument encompasses both potential feelings and documented feelings.
    (D) an emotional argument focuses on the response to truth rather than the establishment of truth.

33. Based on information in the passage, it can most accurately be inferred that logical discussion must be able to distinguish:
    (A) a potential fact from an established fact.
    (B) an emotional fact that is relevant from one that is not.
    (C) whether an audience is responding to an argument or not.
    (D) an established fact with emotional impact from one without impact.

34. A reporter attending a Congressional debate noted that, even though Congresswoman Johnson was a far more dramatic orator than Congressman Martinez, Martinez's argument brought tears to the reporter's eyes because of its dispassionate assessment of the truth. This statement supports which assertion in passage?

(A) The passion of an arguer has the power to move the audience.

(B) The emotional responses of the audience may influence the arguer.

(C) The arguer must assume that the truth exists.

(D) Emotional response should flow from the recognition of the truth, not vice versa.

35. Which statement below, if true, would weaken the author's argument about logical discussion?

(A) Arguers vary in the extent to which they express their emotions.

(B) A good argument does more than simply arouse a response.

(C) It is often hard to pinpoint the exact nature of an emotion being expressed.

(D) The primary purpose of an argument is to move people to action, regardless of which action.

PASSAGE VII

The conventional theory explaining the origins of the Milky Way, the galaxy in which our sun lies, holds that the galaxy was formed relatively quickly, over a 200-million-year period. Approximately 13 billion years ago, a cloud of gas is believed to have collapsed in on itself, forming the distinctive disk of the galaxy, surrounded by a halo. In this scenario, the stars in the galaxy would then have to be roughly the same age.

In recent years, astronomers have been able to observe certain stars that are believed to date from the beginning of the galaxy. These stars are part of globular clusters, a spherical collection of tightly bound stars in the halo of the Milky Way. Stars in a globular cluster are often at the same stage of stellar evolution, indicating that they originated at the same time. As remnants of the formation of the galaxy, globular clusters hold valuable clues to that period.

Our galaxy contains over 150 known globular clusters. While studying a number of globular clusters, astronomers have found an unexpected variation in the clusters' ages. One cluster was found to be 2 billion years older than the average cluster, and others were 2 to 5 billion years younger. These findings conflict with the suppositions of the conventional theory that the entire galaxy formed within a mere 200 million years.

Astronomers are now willing to look at alternative theories—theories that they previously had no reason to consider—in order to reconcile the conventional theory with the new facts pointing to a much slower development of the Milky Way. One such theory, proposed by Yale astronomer Richard Larson, contends that the Milky Way formed over a period of a billion years, rather than a mere 200 million. Larson theorizes that the galaxy came into being through the interaction of hundreds of smaller gas clouds, which eventually coalesced into a single system.

In considering not just the Milky Way but other galaxies as well, Larson explains that up to this point, two models have been postulated about galaxy formation. One is based on collapse and one on merger. The collapse model cannot account for the formation of a disk but does at least account for the general structure of typical elliptical galaxies. Larson states that there has been much debate about the role of mergers in galaxy formation. "There is compelling evidence that mergers do sometimes occur" and that they play a role in the formation of some elliptical galaxies and probably also in some early spiral galaxies.

According to Larson, postulating two separate models is not particularly helpful. In reality, he says, most galaxy formation is likely a complex process involving both collapse and merger. The process of galaxy building is tied to the environment in which it is taking place. In certain environments, galaxy formation may happen relatively at one time. In others, there may be an ongoing attraction of newer stars. Size is also important. Merger is unlikely to have been an important factor in smaller galaxies.

36. Which of the following, if true, would most support a hypothesis that is an alternate to the conventional theory?
    (A) The vast majority of the globular clusters in the Milky Way are nearly identical in age.
    (B) Most of the galaxies studied by astronomers were formed by the merger method.
    (C) The globular clusters that are older than 200 million years originated in other, nearby galaxies.
    (D) 130 of the known globular clusters in the Milky Way are at least a billion years older or younger than the average star in the galaxy.

37. Which of the following opinions would the author of this passage most likely agree with?
    (A) Richard Larson's theory is the best alternative to the conventional theory.
    (B) The existence of a few exceptions to the predictions of a model is cause to question that model.
    (C) Specifically identifying causes of galaxy formation is not possible.
    (D) Dwarf galaxies were not created by merger.

38. It can be inferred that Larson's theory of the origin of the Milky Way was predominantly based on:
    (A) the merger model because hundreds of clouds merged into one cloud.
    (B) the merger model because the Milky Way contains a disk.
    (C) the collapse model because hundreds of clouds collapsed into one cloud.
    (D) the collapse model because the Milky Way is a smaller galaxy.

39. Which of the following new facts, if true, would most weaken the author's argument?
    (A) Most globular clusters were not formed at the same time as the galaxy of which they are a part.
    (B) Most globular clusters in a galaxy are about the same age.
    (C) Globular clusters are nearly always formed by the same process as the galaxy of which they are a part.
    (D) Globular clusters of the smallest galaxies were formed by merger.

40. All of the following information about a newly found galaxy would help predict the forces that formed the galaxy EXCEPT:
    (A) the galaxy's size.
    (B) whether it is elliptical or spiral.
    (C) whether it contains a disk.
    (D) whether its formation was similar to that of the Milky Way.

ANSWER KEY

1. C	**6.** D	**11.** C	**16.** D	**21.** B	**26.** A	**31.** A	**36.** D
2. B	**7.** B	**12.** D	**17.** A	**22.** B	**27.** B	**32.** D	**37.** B
3. B	**8.** A	**13.** B	**18.** C	**23.** D	**28.** C	**33.** A	**38.** B
4. A	**9.** B	**14.** C	**19.** D	**24.** B	**29.** B	**34.** D	**39.** A
5. D	**10.** D	**15.** C	**20.** C	**25.** C	**30.** A	**35.** D	**40.** B

ANSWERS EXPLAINED

1. **(C)** The passage states that learning to communicate with others on one's own terms comes from confidence in one's strength, which in turn comes from setting aside the outer world and trusting the inner. Answer A is never discussed. Choice B involves weapons, which are mentioned in other parts of the passage but do not relate to the quote. Answer D is stated as a characteristic of poets.

2. **(B)** The passage clearly states that the most fundamental quality needed for success, and therefore the most gratifying quality, is to send "roots down deeply into the source of her own creativity." The other answer choices represent positive events but are all secondary to choice B.

3. **(B)** The passage cites offering guidance as something that the older, not younger, generation does. The other answer choices are all derived from specific statements in the passage.

4. **(A)** The passage cites both working only for expressing what you must and working from the source of one's creativity as the root sources of success. The passage states that becoming addicted to approval is caused by failure to create for oneself, so it is a secondary cause, as are choices C and D.

5. **(D)** The first paragraph includes the poet, along with the artist and musician, in the analogy of turning a gentle energy into a weapon. The quoted passage extends this analogy. The quote does not refer to the musician's instrument.

6. **(D)** The author does not imply that creative people should literally learn to use weapons. Answer A is an example of setting aside the concerns of the outer world. Choice B is an example of savoring without greed even the tiniest successes. Answer C is an example of being less influenced by others and being more focused on one's own creativity.

7. **(B)** The passage states that both failure and success can "break" one but never states that failure can "make" one. So this statement contradicts the passage. Answer A is consistent with the advice that a young musician does not need to communicate with everyone but should instead communicate with only those who can listen. Choice C is very close to a specific statement in the passage. Answer D refers to savoring even the tiniest successes.

8. **(A)** The passage states that one of the defining assumptions of geocentrism is that Earth is stationary.

9. **(B)** Galileo's work came after Copernicus's. The other answers are all consistent with the passage.

10. **(D)** The passage mentions references to heliocentrism from the 3rd century B.C. Choice B is incorrect because the Church privately acknowledged its benefits. Answer C is incorrect because, unlike other stars, the Sun is believed to be the center of the universe.

11. **(C)** Answers A and B are scientific interpretations, taking the word "world" literally. Answer D is poetic, but it is not an interpretation of the quote.

12. **(D)** The last paragraph explains the effect on our beliefs of eliminating the possibility of a static center of the universe.

13. **(B)** The passage refers to the sensory impression of the sky moving around the observer.

14. **(C)** Choice C, which demonstrates a pride in personal accomplishments, represents a movement away from love, based on the author's statement that "what he sees as his great triumphs" we see as evidence of his skewed values. Choice A is consistent with the author's view of moving toward love because it is a move toward other people and away from being isolated. Choices B and D are cited directly by the author as moving toward love.

15. **(C)** The blind spot is described by the author as not recognizing the inability to love and instead filling that emptiness with work.

16. **(D)** The author implies that Crusoe was escaping from social situations that made him uncomfortable. Choice B is incorrect because, whereas Crusoe may have believed this was his motivation, the author does not.

17. **(A)** This answer shows that Crusoe is thinking about his family and wants to see their faces. Choice B does not change the fact of a master/servant relationship. Answer D might change that relationship but does not necessarily lead to friendship. Choice C is only a small setback in Crusoe's workaholism.

18. **(C)** Joyce condemns "unconscious cruelty," implying that it would be better if the British colonizer at least became conscious of the cruelty. Answers A and D do not reflect the mix of positive and negative traits. Choice B is not factually correct.

19. **(D)** The passage states that the Industrial Revolution removed children further from the emotional life of the family. It does not say whether children worked more hours or made more money.

20. **(C)** The value on education and learning new skills is the same as in our modern attitudes.

21. **(B)** The passage states that emotional value is now recognized as having an economic worth and that loss of a child should be compensated economically. Answer C states the opposite of this.

22. **(B)** The quote refers to the relatively new attitude that children should be sheltered from and separated from the world of work.

23. **(D)** The author poses the question of what caused the change and answers by describing several changes that occurred at the same time. It is left unclear whether they are causes of the change or reflections of it. This is the reason for choices A and B being wrong. Answer C is wrong because the author specifies the reasons why parents in primitive societies needed the children to contribute.

24. **(B)** The passage states the opposite. All companies must agree to change at the same time.

25. **(C)** The answer choice implies that the drink causes health problems, the costs for which will then be borne by the public. In choice B, a monopoly is a manipulation of the demand side of free enterprise. However, the passage focuses on the cost of production.

26. **(A)** Choice I is an example of companies paying for costs that they have actually incurred. This leaves only answers A and B. Choice II is admirable but not an example of accepting responsibility for costs incurred. Choice III goes in the wrong direction because it is an example of price fixing.

27. **(B)** By taking on more of its actual costs, a company would have to charge more, whereas a competitor who is evading costs can charge less.

28. **(C)** The author's suggestion that all members of an industry would have to agree to a fairer set of rules implies that this could be done without government involvement. Answer A is wrong because the passage specifically states that changing one company at a time would not work.

29. **(B)** The point of the article is to describe what makes an argument a logical discussion.

30. **(A)** The author must believe that some kinds of arguments are more logical than others for the passage to proceed. If the author believed that choices B, C, and D were not true, the passage would not be affected.

31. **(A)** The passage supports answer A by giving an example of it. The other answers, though put forth as true, are not logically supported with examples, statistics, or other information.

32. **(D)** The passage states that the fundamental problem with an emotional argument is that it uses emotions to try to establish truth, whereas emotion should be the response to truth.

33. **(A)** A logical discussion, as defined, must be able to distinguish facts that are not yet documented (potential facts) from facts that have been documented. The passage does not discuss the importance of whether an emotional fact is relevant. Choice C is wrong because the passage states that the reaction of the audience is not relevant.

34. **(D)** The reporter's emotional response was a reaction to the truth, not to an emotional appeal (answer A). Choices B and C do not match the situation.

35. **(D)** Answers A, B, and C are consistent with the author's argument. Answer D directly contradicts one of the author's assertions and would thus weaken the argument.

36. **(D)** Answers A and C support the conventional theory. Choice B is irrelevant, because it does not talk specifically about the Milky Way.

37. **(B)** The author calls into question the conventional theory on the basis of three exceptions to its predictions. Answer A is wrong because the author does not state that Larson's theory is best. Choice D is wrong because the author is merely reporting Larson's findings without indicating agreement with them.

38. **(B)** Because collapse cannot account for the formation of a disk, the disk of the Milky Way must be explained by the merger model. Answers A and C are incorrect in part because the result was not one cloud but a galaxy. Choice D is incorrect because no information indicates that the Milky Way is a smaller galaxy.

39. **(A)** The argument depends on the fact that the globular clusters were formed at the same time as the galaxy itself. Choice B is wrong because the argument is based on a handful of findings that are exceptions to the conventional theory.

40. **(B)** Size would indicate collapse. A disk would indicate merger. Both collapse and merger can account for spiral galaxies. However, not enough information is provided about elliptical galaxies.

For online practice, go to
http://barronsbooks.com/tp/mcat

PART 4

Practice Tests

Get additional practice online at
http://barronsbooks.com/tp/mcat

Answer Sheet: Practice Test 1

CHEMICAL AND PHYSICAL FOUNDATIONS

1. Ⓐ Ⓑ Ⓒ Ⓓ	13. Ⓐ Ⓑ Ⓒ Ⓓ	25. Ⓐ Ⓑ Ⓒ Ⓓ	37. Ⓐ Ⓑ Ⓒ Ⓓ	49. Ⓐ Ⓑ Ⓒ Ⓓ
2. Ⓐ Ⓑ Ⓒ Ⓓ	14. Ⓐ Ⓑ Ⓒ Ⓓ	26. Ⓐ Ⓑ Ⓒ Ⓓ	38. Ⓐ Ⓑ Ⓒ Ⓓ	50. Ⓐ Ⓑ Ⓒ Ⓓ
3. Ⓐ Ⓑ Ⓒ Ⓓ	15. Ⓐ Ⓑ Ⓒ Ⓓ	27. Ⓐ Ⓑ Ⓒ Ⓓ	39. Ⓐ Ⓑ Ⓒ Ⓓ	51. Ⓐ Ⓑ Ⓒ Ⓓ
4. Ⓐ Ⓑ Ⓒ Ⓓ	16. Ⓐ Ⓑ Ⓒ Ⓓ	28. Ⓐ Ⓑ Ⓒ Ⓓ	40. Ⓐ Ⓑ Ⓒ Ⓓ	52. Ⓐ Ⓑ Ⓒ Ⓓ
5. Ⓐ Ⓑ Ⓒ Ⓓ	17. Ⓐ Ⓑ Ⓒ Ⓓ	29. Ⓐ Ⓑ Ⓒ Ⓓ	41. Ⓐ Ⓑ Ⓒ Ⓓ	53. Ⓐ Ⓑ Ⓒ Ⓓ
6. Ⓐ Ⓑ Ⓒ Ⓓ	18. Ⓐ Ⓑ Ⓒ Ⓓ	30. Ⓐ Ⓑ Ⓒ Ⓓ	42. Ⓐ Ⓑ Ⓒ Ⓓ	54. Ⓐ Ⓑ Ⓒ Ⓓ
7. Ⓐ Ⓑ Ⓒ Ⓓ	19. Ⓐ Ⓑ Ⓒ Ⓓ	31. Ⓐ Ⓑ Ⓒ Ⓓ	43. Ⓐ Ⓑ Ⓒ Ⓓ	55. Ⓐ Ⓑ Ⓒ Ⓓ
8. Ⓐ Ⓑ Ⓒ Ⓓ	20. Ⓐ Ⓑ Ⓒ Ⓓ	32. Ⓐ Ⓑ Ⓒ Ⓓ	44. Ⓐ Ⓑ Ⓒ Ⓓ	56. Ⓐ Ⓑ Ⓒ Ⓓ
9. Ⓐ Ⓑ Ⓒ Ⓓ	21. Ⓐ Ⓑ Ⓒ Ⓓ	33. Ⓐ Ⓑ Ⓒ Ⓓ	45. Ⓐ Ⓑ Ⓒ Ⓓ	57. Ⓐ Ⓑ Ⓒ Ⓓ
10. Ⓐ Ⓑ Ⓒ Ⓓ	22. Ⓐ Ⓑ Ⓒ Ⓓ	34. Ⓐ Ⓑ Ⓒ Ⓓ	46. Ⓐ Ⓑ Ⓒ Ⓓ	58. Ⓐ Ⓑ Ⓒ Ⓓ
11. Ⓐ Ⓑ Ⓒ Ⓓ	23. Ⓐ Ⓑ Ⓒ Ⓓ	35. Ⓐ Ⓑ Ⓒ Ⓓ	47. Ⓐ Ⓑ Ⓒ Ⓓ	59. Ⓐ Ⓑ Ⓒ Ⓓ
12. Ⓐ Ⓑ Ⓒ Ⓓ	24. Ⓐ Ⓑ Ⓒ Ⓓ	36. Ⓐ Ⓑ Ⓒ Ⓓ	48. Ⓐ Ⓑ Ⓒ Ⓓ	

CRITICAL ANALYSIS AND REASONING

1. Ⓐ Ⓑ Ⓒ Ⓓ	12. Ⓐ Ⓑ Ⓒ Ⓓ	23. Ⓐ Ⓑ Ⓒ Ⓓ	34. Ⓐ Ⓑ Ⓒ Ⓓ	45. Ⓐ Ⓑ Ⓒ Ⓓ
2. Ⓐ Ⓑ Ⓒ Ⓓ	13. Ⓐ Ⓑ Ⓒ Ⓓ	24. Ⓐ Ⓑ Ⓒ Ⓓ	35. Ⓐ Ⓑ Ⓒ Ⓓ	46. Ⓐ Ⓑ Ⓒ Ⓓ
3. Ⓐ Ⓑ Ⓒ Ⓓ	14. Ⓐ Ⓑ Ⓒ Ⓓ	25. Ⓐ Ⓑ Ⓒ Ⓓ	36. Ⓐ Ⓑ Ⓒ Ⓓ	47. Ⓐ Ⓑ Ⓒ Ⓓ
4. Ⓐ Ⓑ Ⓒ Ⓓ	15. Ⓐ Ⓑ Ⓒ Ⓓ	26. Ⓐ Ⓑ Ⓒ Ⓓ	37. Ⓐ Ⓑ Ⓒ Ⓓ	48. Ⓐ Ⓑ Ⓒ Ⓓ
5. Ⓐ Ⓑ Ⓒ Ⓓ	16. Ⓐ Ⓑ Ⓒ Ⓓ	27. Ⓐ Ⓑ Ⓒ Ⓓ	38. Ⓐ Ⓑ Ⓒ Ⓓ	49. Ⓐ Ⓑ Ⓒ Ⓓ
6. Ⓐ Ⓑ Ⓒ Ⓓ	17. Ⓐ Ⓑ Ⓒ Ⓓ	28. Ⓐ Ⓑ Ⓒ Ⓓ	39. Ⓐ Ⓑ Ⓒ Ⓓ	50. Ⓐ Ⓑ Ⓒ Ⓓ
7. Ⓐ Ⓑ Ⓒ Ⓓ	18. Ⓐ Ⓑ Ⓒ Ⓓ	29. Ⓐ Ⓑ Ⓒ Ⓓ	40. Ⓐ Ⓑ Ⓒ Ⓓ	51. Ⓐ Ⓑ Ⓒ Ⓓ
8. Ⓐ Ⓑ Ⓒ Ⓓ	19. Ⓐ Ⓑ Ⓒ Ⓓ	30. Ⓐ Ⓑ Ⓒ Ⓓ	41. Ⓐ Ⓑ Ⓒ Ⓓ	52. Ⓐ Ⓑ Ⓒ Ⓓ
9. Ⓐ Ⓑ Ⓒ Ⓓ	20. Ⓐ Ⓑ Ⓒ Ⓓ	31. Ⓐ Ⓑ Ⓒ Ⓓ	42. Ⓐ Ⓑ Ⓒ Ⓓ	53. Ⓐ Ⓑ Ⓒ Ⓓ
10. Ⓐ Ⓑ Ⓒ Ⓓ	21. Ⓐ Ⓑ Ⓒ Ⓓ	32. Ⓐ Ⓑ Ⓒ Ⓓ	43. Ⓐ Ⓑ Ⓒ Ⓓ	
11. Ⓐ Ⓑ Ⓒ Ⓓ	22. Ⓐ Ⓑ Ⓒ Ⓓ	33. Ⓐ Ⓑ Ⓒ Ⓓ	44. Ⓐ Ⓑ Ⓒ Ⓓ	

BIOLOGICAL AND BIOCHEMICAL FOUNDATIONS

1. Ⓐ Ⓑ Ⓒ Ⓓ	13. Ⓐ Ⓑ Ⓒ Ⓓ	25. Ⓐ Ⓑ Ⓒ Ⓓ	37. Ⓐ Ⓑ Ⓒ Ⓓ	49. Ⓐ Ⓑ Ⓒ Ⓓ
2. Ⓐ Ⓑ Ⓒ Ⓓ	14. Ⓐ Ⓑ Ⓒ Ⓓ	26. Ⓐ Ⓑ Ⓒ Ⓓ	38. Ⓐ Ⓑ Ⓒ Ⓓ	50. Ⓐ Ⓑ Ⓒ Ⓓ
3. Ⓐ Ⓑ Ⓒ Ⓓ	15. Ⓐ Ⓑ Ⓒ Ⓓ	27. Ⓐ Ⓑ Ⓒ Ⓓ	39. Ⓐ Ⓑ Ⓒ Ⓓ	51. Ⓐ Ⓑ Ⓒ Ⓓ
4. Ⓐ Ⓑ Ⓒ Ⓓ	16. Ⓐ Ⓑ Ⓒ Ⓓ	28. Ⓐ Ⓑ Ⓒ Ⓓ	40. Ⓐ Ⓑ Ⓒ Ⓓ	52. Ⓐ Ⓑ Ⓒ Ⓓ
5. Ⓐ Ⓑ Ⓒ Ⓓ	17. Ⓐ Ⓑ Ⓒ Ⓓ	29. Ⓐ Ⓑ Ⓒ Ⓓ	41. Ⓐ Ⓑ Ⓒ Ⓓ	53. Ⓐ Ⓑ Ⓒ Ⓓ
6. Ⓐ Ⓑ Ⓒ Ⓓ	18. Ⓐ Ⓑ Ⓒ Ⓓ	30. Ⓐ Ⓑ Ⓒ Ⓓ	42. Ⓐ Ⓑ Ⓒ Ⓓ	54. Ⓐ Ⓑ Ⓒ Ⓓ
7. Ⓐ Ⓑ Ⓒ Ⓓ	19. Ⓐ Ⓑ Ⓒ Ⓓ	31. Ⓐ Ⓑ Ⓒ Ⓓ	43. Ⓐ Ⓑ Ⓒ Ⓓ	55. Ⓐ Ⓑ Ⓒ Ⓓ
8. Ⓐ Ⓑ Ⓒ Ⓓ	20. Ⓐ Ⓑ Ⓒ Ⓓ	32. Ⓐ Ⓑ Ⓒ Ⓓ	44. Ⓐ Ⓑ Ⓒ Ⓓ	56. Ⓐ Ⓑ Ⓒ Ⓓ
9. Ⓐ Ⓑ Ⓒ Ⓓ	21. Ⓐ Ⓑ Ⓒ Ⓓ	33. Ⓐ Ⓑ Ⓒ Ⓓ	45. Ⓐ Ⓑ Ⓒ Ⓓ	57. Ⓐ Ⓑ Ⓒ Ⓓ
10. Ⓐ Ⓑ Ⓒ Ⓓ	22. Ⓐ Ⓑ Ⓒ Ⓓ	34. Ⓐ Ⓑ Ⓒ Ⓓ	46. Ⓐ Ⓑ Ⓒ Ⓓ	58. Ⓐ Ⓑ Ⓒ Ⓓ
11. Ⓐ Ⓑ Ⓒ Ⓓ	23. Ⓐ Ⓑ Ⓒ Ⓓ	35. Ⓐ Ⓑ Ⓒ Ⓓ	47. Ⓐ Ⓑ Ⓒ Ⓓ	59. Ⓐ Ⓑ Ⓒ Ⓓ
12. Ⓐ Ⓑ Ⓒ Ⓓ	24. Ⓐ Ⓑ Ⓒ Ⓓ	36. Ⓐ Ⓑ Ⓒ Ⓓ	48. Ⓐ Ⓑ Ⓒ Ⓓ	

PSYCHOLOGICAL, SOCIAL, AND BIOLOGICAL FOUNDATIONS

1. Ⓐ Ⓑ Ⓒ Ⓓ	13. Ⓐ Ⓑ Ⓒ Ⓓ	25. Ⓐ Ⓑ Ⓒ Ⓓ	37. Ⓐ Ⓑ Ⓒ Ⓓ	49. Ⓐ Ⓑ Ⓒ Ⓓ
2. Ⓐ Ⓑ Ⓒ Ⓓ	14. Ⓐ Ⓑ Ⓒ Ⓓ	26. Ⓐ Ⓑ Ⓒ Ⓓ	38. Ⓐ Ⓑ Ⓒ Ⓓ	50. Ⓐ Ⓑ Ⓒ Ⓓ
3. Ⓐ Ⓑ Ⓒ Ⓓ	15. Ⓐ Ⓑ Ⓒ Ⓓ	27. Ⓐ Ⓑ Ⓒ Ⓓ	39. Ⓐ Ⓑ Ⓒ Ⓓ	51. Ⓐ Ⓑ Ⓒ Ⓓ
4. Ⓐ Ⓑ Ⓒ Ⓓ	16. Ⓐ Ⓑ Ⓒ Ⓓ	28. Ⓐ Ⓑ Ⓒ Ⓓ	40. Ⓐ Ⓑ Ⓒ Ⓓ	52. Ⓐ Ⓑ Ⓒ Ⓓ
5. Ⓐ Ⓑ Ⓒ Ⓓ	17. Ⓐ Ⓑ Ⓒ Ⓓ	29. Ⓐ Ⓑ Ⓒ Ⓓ	41. Ⓐ Ⓑ Ⓒ Ⓓ	53. Ⓐ Ⓑ Ⓒ Ⓓ
6. Ⓐ Ⓑ Ⓒ Ⓓ	18. Ⓐ Ⓑ Ⓒ Ⓓ	30. Ⓐ Ⓑ Ⓒ Ⓓ	42. Ⓐ Ⓑ Ⓒ Ⓓ	54. Ⓐ Ⓑ Ⓒ Ⓓ
7. Ⓐ Ⓑ Ⓒ Ⓓ	19. Ⓐ Ⓑ Ⓒ Ⓓ	31. Ⓐ Ⓑ Ⓒ Ⓓ	43. Ⓐ Ⓑ Ⓒ Ⓓ	55. Ⓐ Ⓑ Ⓒ Ⓓ
8. Ⓐ Ⓑ Ⓒ Ⓓ	20. Ⓐ Ⓑ Ⓒ Ⓓ	32. Ⓐ Ⓑ Ⓒ Ⓓ	44. Ⓐ Ⓑ Ⓒ Ⓓ	56. Ⓐ Ⓑ Ⓒ Ⓓ
9. Ⓐ Ⓑ Ⓒ Ⓓ	21. Ⓐ Ⓑ Ⓒ Ⓓ	33. Ⓐ Ⓑ Ⓒ Ⓓ	45. Ⓐ Ⓑ Ⓒ Ⓓ	57. Ⓐ Ⓑ Ⓒ Ⓓ
10. Ⓐ Ⓑ Ⓒ Ⓓ	22. Ⓐ Ⓑ Ⓒ Ⓓ	34. Ⓐ Ⓑ Ⓒ Ⓓ	46. Ⓐ Ⓑ Ⓒ Ⓓ	58. Ⓐ Ⓑ Ⓒ Ⓓ
11. Ⓐ Ⓑ Ⓒ Ⓓ	23. Ⓐ Ⓑ Ⓒ Ⓓ	35. Ⓐ Ⓑ Ⓒ Ⓓ	47. Ⓐ Ⓑ Ⓒ Ⓓ	59. Ⓐ Ⓑ Ⓒ Ⓓ
12. Ⓐ Ⓑ Ⓒ Ⓓ	24. Ⓐ Ⓑ Ⓒ Ⓓ	36. Ⓐ Ⓑ Ⓒ Ⓓ	48. Ⓐ Ⓑ Ⓒ Ⓓ	

Periodic Table of the Elements

1 H 1.0																	2 He 4.0
3 Li 6.9	4 Be 9.0											5 B 10.8	6 C 12.0	7 N 14.0	8 O 16.0	9 F 19.0	10 Ne 20.2
11 Na 23.0	12 Mg 24.3											13 Al 27.0	14 Si 28.1	15 P 31.0	16 S 32.1	17 Cl 35.5	18 Ar 39.9
19 K 39.1	20 Ca 40.1	21 Sc 45.0	22 Ti 47.9	23 V 50.9	24 Cr 52.0	25 Mn 54.9	26 Fe 55.8	27 Co 58.8	28 Ni 58.7	29 Cu 63.5	30 Zn 65.4	31 Ga 69.7	32 Ge 72.6	33 As 74.9	34 Se 79.0	35 Br 79.9	36 Kr 83.8
37 Rb 85.5	38 Sr 87.6	39 Y 88.9	40 Zr 91.2	41 Nb 92.9	42 Mo 95.9	43 Tc (98)	44 Ru 101.1	45 Rh 102.9	46 Pd 106.4	47 Ag 107.9	48 Cd 112.4	49 In 114.8	50 Sn 118.7	51 Sb 121.8	52 Te 127.6	53 I 126.9	54 Xe 131.3
55 Cs 132.9	56 Ba 137.3	57 La 138.9	72 Hf 178.5	73 Ta 180.9	74 W 183.9	75 Re 186.2	76 Os 190.2	77 Ir 192.2	78 Pt 195.1	79 Au 197.0	80 Hg 200.6	81 Tl 204.4	82 Pb 207.2	83 Bi 209.0	84 Po (209)	85 At (210)	86 Rn (222)
87 Fr (223)	88 Ra (226)	89 Ac† (227)	104 Rf (261)	105 Db (262)	106 Sg (266)	107 Bh (264)	108 Hs (277)	109 Mt (268)	110 Ds (281)	111 Rg (280)	112 Cn (285)	113 Uut (284)	114 Fl (289)	115 Uup (288)	116 Lv (293)	117 Uus (294)	118 Uuo (294)

★	58 Ce 140.1	59 Pr 140.9	60 Nd 144.2	61 Pm (145)	62 Sm 150.4	63 Eu 152.0	64 Gd 157.3	65 Tb 158.9	66 Dy 162.5	67 Ho 164.9	68 Er 167.3	69 Tm 168.9	70 Yb 173.0	71 Lu 175.0
†	90 Th 232.0	91 Pa (231)	92 U 238.0	93 Np (237)	94 Pu (244)	95 Am (243)	96 Cm (247)	97 Bk (247)	98 Cf (251)	99 Es (252)	100 Fm (257)	101 Md (258)	102 No (259)	103 Lr (260)

Practice Test 1

CHEMICAL AND PHYSICAL FOUNDATIONS
OF BIOLOGICAL SYSTEMS

Time: 95 minutes
     59 Questions

DIRECTIONS: The majority of questions in the Chemical and Physical Foundations of Biological Systems section are organized into groups, with each group containing a descriptive passage. Read the passage, and then select the one best answer for each question. Some questions are not drawn from a passage and are also independent of the other questions. When answering questions, eliminate the choices that you are sure are incorrect and then choose the best remaining answer. When you have chosen an answer, mark it in the corresponding location on the answer sheet. A periodic table can be found on the back of your answer sheet. You may consult it as needed.

PASSAGE I

Many chemical systems have been studied as a means of understanding chemical reaction mechanisms. One of the earliest was the reaction between hydrogen and iodine gases to form gaseous hydrogen iodide. The reaction mechanism has been determined by experimental means and is shown below.

Step 1	$I_2 \leftrightarrow 2I$	(fast)
Step 2	$I + H_2 \leftrightarrow H_2I$	(fast)
Step 3	$H_2I + I \rightarrow 2HI$	(slow)

Some basic thermodynamic data for selected compounds in the reaction is shown in Table 1.

Table 1
Thermodynamic Data

Compound	ΔH°_f (kJ/mole)	ΔG°_f (kJ/mole)	S° (J/mole K)
H_2	0	0	131
I_2	0	0	261
HI	27	2	207

The value for the equilibrium constant for the synthesis of HI is on the order of 10^{-1}. For the synthesis of hydrogen chloride from its elements, the equilibrium constant is on the order of 10^{16}.

1. Given the equilibrium constants for the syntheses of hydrogen iodide and hydrogen chloride from their elements, the rate of synthesis of HCl compared to the rate of formation of HI (at the same temperature):
   (A) is 10^{17} times greater.
   (B) is 10^{17} times less.
   (C) is 17 times greater.
   (D) cannot be determined based on the information provided.

2. Which of the following is the most stable intermediate in the reaction described by steps 1–3?
   (A) H_2I
   (B) H_2
   (C) I
   (D) I_2

3. The overall entropy change for the formation of HI from hydrogen and iodine as described in the passage is:
   (A) close to zero because the products and reactants have nearly identical masses.
   (B) close to zero because the number of moles of gases does not change.
   (C) close to zero because products and reactants have similar thermodynamic stability.
   (D) positive because hydrogen iodide is a more acidic compound than either hydrogen or iodine.

4. The figure below shows the energy diagram for the reaction.

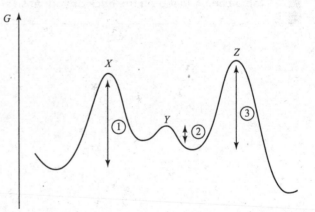

   Which arrow corresponds to the fastest step?
   (A) 1
   (B) 2
   (C) 3
   (D) It cannot be determined based on the information in the graph.

5. Compared to aqueous HCl, aqueous HI is a:
   (A) stronger acid because I⁻ ions are larger than Cl⁻ ions, making HI bonds weaker than HCl bonds.
   (B) weaker acid because I⁻ ions are larger than Cl⁻ ions, making HI bonds weaker than HCl bonds.
   (C) stronger acid because I⁻ ions are larger than Cl⁻ ions, making HI bonds stronger than HCl bonds.
   (D) weaker acid because I⁻ ions are larger than Cl⁻ ions, making HI bonds stronger than HCl bonds.

6. Hydrogen iodide is a:
   (A) polar compound because electrons are shared evenly between the hydrogen and the iodine atoms.
   (B) polar compound because electrons are shared unevenly between the hydrogen and iodine atoms.
   (C) nonpolar compound because electrons are shared evenly between the hydrogen and the iodine atoms.
   (D) nonpolar compound because electrons are shared unevenly between the hydrogen and the iodine atoms.

PASSAGE II

A balanced diet consists of a healthy mixture of fats, carbohydrates, and proteins. Each of these nutritional categories is further divided into subcategories with specific and unique functions in metabolism and other cellular processes. Proteins, for example, are composed of unique blends of amino acids that give them diverse functionality. Table 1 below lists the major categories of amino acids and an example of each.

Table 1 Amino Acid Categories

Category	Example	Side Chain	pK_R
Nonpolar	Phenylalanine		—
Branched Chain	Valine		—
Uncharged Polar	Tyrosine		10.46
(+) Charge	Arginine		12.48
(−) Charge	Glutamate		4.07

Foods such as eggs and quinoa are composed of mixtures of proteins that contain all essential amino acids: arginine, histidine, isoleucine, leucine, lysine, methionine, phenyl-alanine, threonine, tryptophan, and valine. This combination of amino acids with varying acidity, hydrophobicity, and reactivity ensure the completion of biological processes necessary for survival. In an experiment to test the protein content of an unknown cut of fish, the fish was ground, and protein was extracted. Purified proteins were loaded onto an electrophoresis gel, which separates proteins based on their isoelectric point (pI), and compared to crude egg and quinoa protein samples to determine protein similarities. The results are shown in Figure 1.

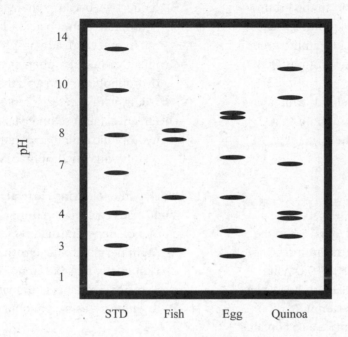

Figure 1. Proteins present in unknown fish sample compared to standard protein sample, egg protein, and quinoa protein

7. Which of the following properties of an amino acid is responsible for its amphiphilic character?
   (A) The positively charged amino group (NH_3^+) that can lose a hydrogen to form NH_2 and participate in acid–base reactions
   (B) The variation in R-groups among different amino acids that produces variable reactivity
   (C) The combination of a basic amino group (NH_2) and acidic carboxyl group (COOH)
   (D) The combination of an acidic amino group (NH_2) and a basic carboxyl group (COOH)

8. Of the amino acids listed in Table 1, which have the ability to be used as a fluorophore?
   (A) Phenylalanine and tyrosine
   (B) Phenylalanine only
   (C) Arginine and glutamate
   (D) Glutamate only

9. In Figure 1, the protein found at pH 5.3 in the egg sample contains six essential amino acids and has a molecular weight of 35 kDa. What information does this suggest about the protein at pH 5.3 in the unknown fish sample?
   (A) The protein in the fish sample also contains six essential amino acids.
   (B) The pI of the protein in the fish sample is 5.3.
   (C) The protein in the fish sample contains at least six essential amino acids.
   (D) The protein in the fish sample is 35 kDa.

10. Phenylketouria (PKU) is a disorder characterized by impaired phenylalanine catabolism, presented phenotypically by mental retardation. Would IV drug administration (water solubility required) be effective or ineffective in treating PKU?
    (A) Ineffective, because phenylalanine is a hydrophylic amino acid that would be unreactive with a hydrophobic IV drug
    (B) Ineffective, because phenylalanine is a hydrophobic amino acid that would likely not interact with a hydrophilic IV drug
    (C) Effective, because phenylalanine is a hydrophobic amino acid that would react readily with a water-soluble IV drug
    (D) Effective, because phenylalanine is a hydrophilic amino acid that would react readily with a hydrophilic IV drug

11. Which of the following correctly ranks the amino acids tyrosine, arginine, and glutamate in order of increasing acidity?
    (A) Arginine, glutamate, tyrosine
    (B) Glutamate, tyrosine, arginine
    (C) Tyrosine, arginine, glutamate
    (D) Arginine, tyrosine, glutamate

12. Arginine is capable of being synthesized by the body but is quickly broken down into urea. Would this classify arginine as an essential or nonessential amino acid?
    (A) Essential, because urea is a necessary metabolic intermediate
    (B) Essential, because even though the body produces arginine, it is confined to the urea cycle
    (C) Nonessential, because the body can synthesize arginine
    (D) Nonessential, because urea can be produced from other sources aside from arginine

PASSAGE III

Experiment 1

A group of students is interested in studying the reactions between solid metals and solutions containing ions of those metals. They react five metals in combination with 0.10 M solutions of the nitrate ions of those metals and record their observations, which are summarized in Table 1.

Table 1 Reactions Between Metals and Metal-Nitrate Solutions

Metal	$AgNO_3$	$Cu(NO_3)_2$	$Mg(NO_3)_2$	$Pb(NO_3)_2$	$Zn(NO_3)_2$
$Ag_{(s)}$	X	NVR	NVR	NVR	NVR
$Cu_{(s)}$	Gray ppt	X	NVR	NVR	NVR
$Mg_{(s)}$	Gray ppt	Red-brown ppt	X	Gray ppt	Gray ppt
$Pb_{(s)}$	Gray ppt	Brown ppt	NVR	X	NVR
$Zn_{(s)}$	Gray ppt	Brown ppt	NVR	Gray ppt	X

NVR = no visible reaction; ppt = precipitate; X = reaction not performed

Experiment 2

In a separate experiment, each of the metals is placed in a 1.0 M solution of sulfuric acid, H_2SO_4, and the results are recorded in Table 2.

Table 2 Reaction Between Metals and Sulfuric Acid

Metal	Reaction with H_2SO_4	Reaction with HCl
Ag	NVR	NVR
Cu	NVR	NVR
Mg	Bubbling, solution becomes hot	Bubbling, solution becomes hot
Pb	Bubbling	NVR
Zn	Bubbling, solution becomes warm	Bubbling, solution becomes hot

NVR = no visible reaction

13. Based on the data in Table 1, what is the order of these metals from most to least active?
    - (A) $Ag > Cu > Pb > Zn > Mg$
    - (B) $Mg > Zn > Pb > Cu > Ag$
    - (C) $Mg > Cu > Ag > Zn > Pb$
    - (D) $Mg > Zn > Cu > Pb > Ag$

14. What was the identity of the gas formed when magnesium reacted with the sulfuric acid?
    - (A) SO_2
    - (B) SO_3
    - (C) H_2
    - (D) O_2

15. When an aqueous solution of silver nitrate reacts with an aqueous solution of sodium chloride, a white precipitate forms. What is the formula of this precipitate?
    - (A) $AgCl_2$
    - (B) $NaNO_3$
    - (C) $AgCl$
    - (D) $Na(NO_3)_2$

16. When the boiling points of the silver nitrate and lead nitrate solutions are compared, what results are obtained? (Both solutions are 0.1 M.)
    - (A) Lead nitrate is higher because it is more soluble.
    - (B) Lead nitrate is higher because it dissociates into more ions.
    - (C) Lead nitrate is higher because it has a higher molar mass.
    - (D) Silver nitrate is higher because it is better able to dissolve at the higher temperatures.

17. When the piece of magnesium metal is placed in a solution of copper(II) nitrate, which of the following occurs?
    - (A) Mg metal is oxidized and Cu^{+2} ions are reduced.
    - (B) Mg metal is reduced and Cu^{+2} ions are oxidized.
    - (C) Mg metal is oxidized and Cu metal is reduced.
    - (D) Mg metal is reduced and Cu metal is oxidized.

18. When lead reacts with sulfuric acid, what is the most likely product?
    - (A) PbS
    - (B) $PbSO_4$
    - (C) $Pb(SO_4)_2$
    - (D) Pb_2SO_4

The following questions do not refer to a descriptive passage and are not related to each other.

19. The figure below shows the phase diagram of carbon dioxide.

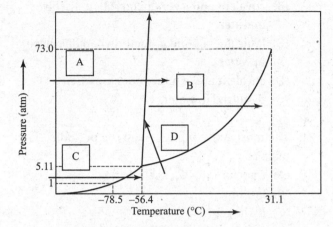

Which arrow above represents the process of sublimation?
(A) Arrow A
(B) Arrow B
(C) Arrow C
(D) Arrow D

20. Static electricity can cause charge to build up on an object:
(A) only if the object is a good conductor.
(B) only if the object is a good insulator.
(C) only if the object has a current path to ground.
(D) only if the object is not grounded.

21. Copper electrical wiring in a circuit is found to have too much resistance in a particular section of the circuit that operates at high temperature. Which of the following will NOT decrease the resistance?
(A) Replacing the wiring with a material of lower resistivity
(B) Replacing the wiring with the same type of material that has smaller cross-sectional area
(C) Replacing the wiring with the same type of material with shorter length
(D) Lowering the temperature in the environment of the circuit

22. What is the electron configuration of the most stable ion of magnesium?
(A) $1s^2 2s^2 2p^6 3s^2$
(B) $1s^2 2s^2 2p^6 3s^2 3p^2$
(C) $1s^2 2s^2 2p^6$
(D) $1s^2 2s^2 2p^6 3s^1$

PASSAGE IV

Chemical bonds involve the transfer and/or sharing of valence electrons. The main determinant of the type of bond two atoms will form is the electronegativity difference between the atoms. Ionic compounds typically involve a metal and a nonmetal, forming positive and negative ions that electrically attract each other. Ionic compounds are hard, brittle solids at room temperature. They have high melting points and often dissolve in water. Their solutions (and molten forms) conduct electricity, whereas the solids act as insulators. Covalent compounds involve electron sharing. The smaller the electronegativity difference between the atoms, the more nonpolar the bond. Covalent compounds are often liquids or gases at room temperature, and their solutions do not conduct electricity. Figure 1 shows the electronegativities of representative elements.

H 2.2								He
Li 0.98	Be 1.57		B 2.04	C 2.55	N 3.04	O 3.44	F 3.98	Ne
Na 0.93	Mg 1.31		Al 1.61	Si 1.90	P 2.19	S 2.58	Cl 3.16	Ar
K 0.82	Ca 1.00		Ga 1.81	Ge 2.01	As 2.18	Se 2.55	Br 2.96	Kr 2.9
Rb 0.82	Sr 0.95		In 1.78	Sn 1.96	Sb 2.05	Te 2.1	I 2.66	Xe 2.6
Cs 0.79	Ba 0.89		Tl 2.04	Pb 2.33	Bi 2.02	Po 2.0	At 2.2	Rn

Figure 1. Electronegativities of representative elements

Typically, bonds in which the two atoms have electronegativities of greater than 1.7 are considered ionic, whereas those with electronegativity differences of 0.4–1.7 are considered polar covalent.

23. Carbon disulfide, CS_2, is a widely used industrial solvent. It is a liquid at room temperature and is:
    (A) ionic and a conductor when dissolved in water.
    (B) covalent and a conductor when dissolved in water.
    (C) ionic and a nonconductor when dissolved in water.
    (D) covalent and a nonconductor when dissolved in water.

24. The most active nonmetal on the periodic table is:
    (A) francium.
    (B) lithium.
    (C) hydrogen.
    (D) fluorine.

25. The bond between carbon and hydrogen can be described as:
    (A) polar covalent because of uneven electron sharing.
    (B) nonpolar covalent because of even electron sharing.
    (C) nonpolar covalent because of uneven electron sharing.
    (D) ionic because of the gain and loss of electrons.

26. Which of the following pure substances would most likely have the highest boiling point?
    (A) NaCl
    (B) CaO
    (C) NH_3
    (D) OF_2

27. Which of the following pairs of compounds consists of an ionic compound followed by a covalent compound?
    (A) KCl, $CaCl_2$
    (B) CH_4, Li_2O
    (C) PCl_3, IBr_3
    (D) NaBr, CCl_4

PASSAGE V

A model that is helpful in understanding the motion of individual atoms, the specific heat, and the absorption spectra for a solid is that the solid is composed of atoms that are in an ordered structure and that vibrate about an equilibrium position. A one-dimensional model in which the vibrating atoms repel one another can be modeled as a spring. The atoms effectively elongate one spring and compress the other as they vibrate. This mechanical model is shown below in Figure 1.

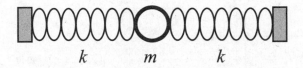

k m k

Figure 1. A mechanical spring model

In a normal Hooke's law spring, the restoring force is kx, but in the situation in which one spring pushes while the other pulls, the restoring force is $2kx$. In any oscillating system such as this, the energy goes back and forth between potential energy stored in the springs and kinetic energy due to the velocity. The total energy of the vibrating atom is (1) $mv^2_{max}/2$, where the maximum velocity is the velocity when the atom passes through equilibrium, or (2) kA^2, where A is the amplitude of the oscillations.

There are 6.0×10^{23} (Avogadro's number) molecules per mole. It is not unusual for a metal to have a heat capacity of 6 cal/mole. So a convenient energy for the single atom in this simple model would be 10^{-23} cal/atom/C°. The calorie to joule relation is roughly 4 J = 1 cal. The atomic spacing in metals is around 2×10^{-10} m. The amu is approximately 2×10^{-27} kg.

28. In analysis of the motion of the atom, what quantity is conserved?
    (A) Charge
    (B) Angular momentum
    (C) Energy
    (D) Linear momentum

29. Using the energy of 10^{-23} cal/atom/C° and taking the amplitude of the motion as 10% of the atomic spacing, what is the effective k of the model?
    (A) 0.1 N/m
    (B) 12 N/m
    (C) 0.03 N/m
    (D) 140 N/m

30. How can this model be adapted to a gas?
    (A) The model cannot be applied to a gas.
    (B) The model can be applied to a gas by lowering the spring constant.
    (C) The model can be applied to a gas by adding additional dimensions and keeping similar spring constant values.
    (D) The model can be applied as is because gas atoms arrange themselves in linear strings.

31. Using energy analysis, find the maximum velocity of a 24 amu atom.
    (A) 0.4 m/s
    (B) 1.3×10^{13} m/s
    (C) 300 m/s
    (D) 40 m/s

32. What is the approximate side of a cube of one mole of a metal?
    (A) ~1.6 cm
    (B) ~1.0 m
    (C) ~0.06 cm
    (D) ~20 m

PASSAGE VI

Experiment 1

A chemist investigated the solubilities of dimethyl sulfoxide (DMSO) and methyl-t-butyl ether (MTBE) in different solvents. The structures of the two solutes are shown in Figures 1 and 2.

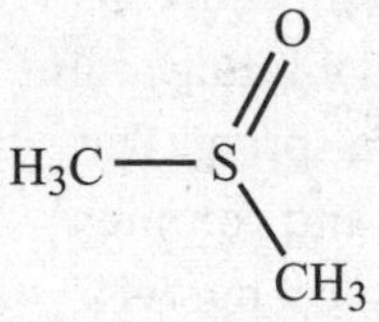

Figure 1. Dimethyl sulfoxide

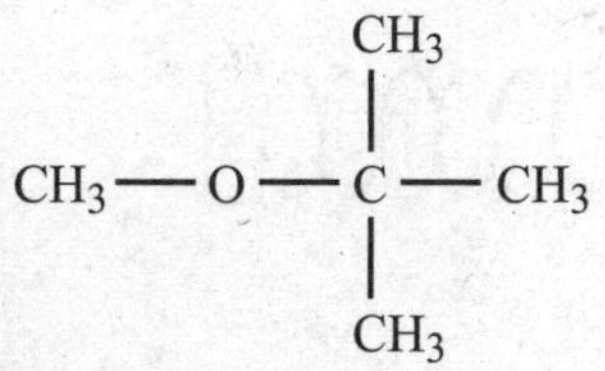

Figure 2. Methyl-t-butyl ether

The results are summarized in Table 1.

Table 1 Solubility of DMSO and MTBE in Various Solutes

Solute	Solubility in Water	Solubility in Hexane (C_6H_{14})	Solubility in Toluene ($C_{10}H_8$)
DMSO	Highly soluble	Insoluble	Insoluble
MTBE	Slightly soluble	Highly soluble	Highly soluble

Experiment 2

In a second experiment, the chemist investigated the solubility of four organic acids in water. The results are summarized in Table 2.

Table 2 Solubility of Organic Acids in Water

Organic Acid	Formula	Solubility in Water (g/100g H_2O) at 25°C
Formic acid	HCOOH	Completely miscible
Acetic acid	CH_3COOH	Completely miscible
Pentanoic acid	$CH_3CH_2CH_2CH_2COOH$	5.0
Decanoic acid	$CH_3(CH_2)_8COOH$	Insoluble

33. Based on the information in the passage, which of the following is most likely to be true about the solubility of MTBE?
    (A) MTBE is highly soluble in polar solvents because it is a polar substance.
    (B) MTBE is slightly soluble in polar solvents because it is a nonpolar substance.
    (C) MTBE is highly soluble in nonpolar solvents because it is a polar substance.
    (D) MTBE is highly soluble in nonpolar solvents because it is a nonpolar substance.

34. What prediction can be made about the miscibility of hexane and toluene?
    (A) Hexane and toluene will be miscible in each other because each can form hydrogen bonds.
    (B) Hexane and toluene will be immiscible in each other because they have dissimilar polarities.
    (C) Hexane and toluene will be miscible in each other because they can interact via London dispersion forces.
    (D) Hexane and toluene will be immiscible in each other because hexane can form dipole interactions while toluene cannot.

35. Which of the following best explains the pattern in the solubility of organic acids shown in Table 2?
    (A) As the molar mass increases, the compounds become less soluble because it is harder for water molecules to solvate them.
    (B) As the molar mass increases, the compounds become less soluble because the nonpolar hydrocarbon portion of the molecule becomes a larger fraction of the molecular structure.
    (C) As the molar mass increases, the compounds become less soluble because the compounds have less ability to generate London dispersion forces.
    (D) As the molar mass increases, the compounds become more soluble because the amount of dipole interaction between the molecules decreases.

36. What is the orbital hybridization on the carbon atoms in DMSO?
    (A) sp
    (B) sp^2
    (C) sp^3
    (D) dsp^3

37. What shape do the bonds around the sulfur atom have in DMSO?
    (A) Linear
    (B) Trigonal planar
    (C) Tetrahedral
    (D) Trigonal pyramidal

38. Sulfur atoms sometimes can form compounds with more than four pairs of bonding electrons. Which orbitals are responsible for allowing sulfur atoms to do this?
    (A) 2p
    (B) 2d
    (C) 3d
    (D) 3p

The following questions do not refer to a descriptive passage and are not related to each other.

39. How do the rates of diffusion of Ar (molar mass = 40) and Br_2 (molar mass = 160) compare assuming both gases are at the same temperature and pressure?
    (A) Ar diffuses 4 times as fast as Br_2.
    (B) Ar diffuses 2 times as fast as Br_2.
    (C) Br_2 diffuses 4 times as fast as Ar.
    (D) Br_2 diffuses 2 times as fast as Ar.

40. Methanol, CH_3OH, is manufactured commercially from the exothermic reaction of hydrogen gas and carbon monoxide.

    $$CO_{(g)} + 2H_{2(g)} \leftrightarrow CH_3OH_{(g)}$$

    Which of the following will lead to an increase in the amount of methanol produced?
    (A) Increase the temperature and increase the pressure.
    (B) Increase the temperature and decrease the pressure.
    (C) Decrease the temperature and increase the pressure.
    (D) Maintain constant temperature and pressure and add a catalyst.

41. A car is traveling at a constant speed of 30 km/hr in a circle of radius 200 m. Which of the following is true about the acceleration of the car?
    (A) It is zero since the speed is constant.
    (B) It is zero since the velocity is constant.
    (C) There is acceleration due to changing velocity.
    (D) The acceleration is negligible due to the radius of the circle.

PASSAGE VII

Human hair is made up of a series of coiling keratin alpha helices held together by cross linkages of disulfide bonds. The alpha helix is a right-hand twisted polypeptide structure, and two keratin alpha helices are coiled together to form a left-hand coiled coil. These coils are further twisted into protofilaments and protofibrils. Approximately four protofibrils are intertwined to form an intermediate filament of hair. Alpha-keratin is rich in hydrophobic amino acid residues such as alanine, valine, leucine, isoleucine, methionine, and phenyl-alanine. Ammonium thioglycolate and hydrogen peroxide are chemicals often used in the cosmetic industry to manipulate hair into forming unnatural curls (Figure 1).

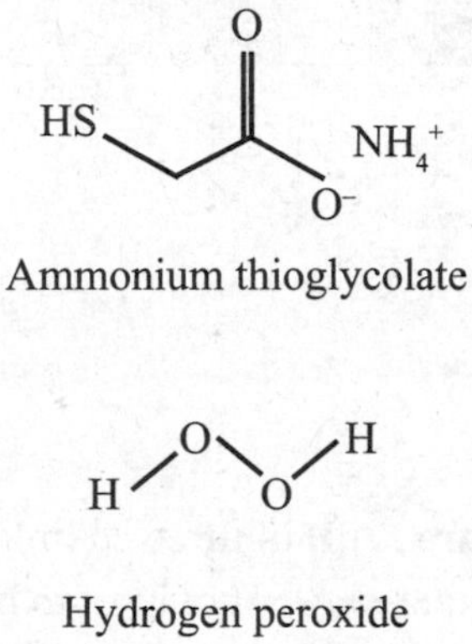

Ammonium thioglycolate

Hydrogen peroxide

Figure 1. Structures for ammonium thioglycolate and hydrogen peroxide

In order for hair to be permanently waved, ammonium thioglycolate is applied with heat after the hair has been wrapped around a coil. The heat breaks hydrogen bonds within the alpha helical structure so that the polypeptide chain uncoils, and the ammonium thiogly-colate breaks disulfide bonds, leaving amino acid residues exposed. After some time, the ammonium thioglycolate is removed, and hydrogen peroxide is added to establish new disulfide bonds to create hair coiled in a desirable way.

One concern many people have with the use of chemicals on hair is associated with the effect of pH on the hair follicle. An experiment was conducted to compare the pH levels of chemicals used in different types of hair treatments and measure the severity of hair damage and breakage caused by each chemical (Figure 2 and Table 1).

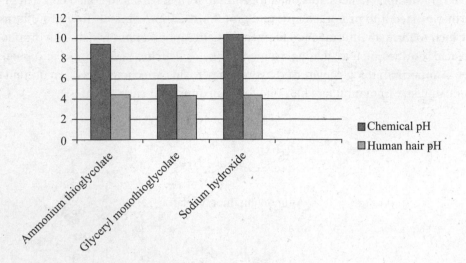

Figure 2. pH of three chemicals compared to pH of human hair

Table 1 Severity of Damage

Common Name	Chemical Formula	Severity of Damage (1–5)
Ammonium thioglycolate	$HSCH_2CO_2NH_4$	2
Glyceryl monothioglycolate	$C_5H_{10}O_4S$	1
Sodium hydroxide	NaOH	3

42. Which of the following is the purpose of ammonium thioglycolate in permanent waving?
    (A) It functions as an oxidizing agent to cleave disulfide bonds.
    (B) It functions as a reducing agent to cleave disulfide bonds.
    (C) It cleaves hydrogen bonds to uncoil the polypeptide helix.
    (D) It establishes new hydrogen bonds to coil the hair.

43. An experiment is conducted in which different proteins are sequenced. Which of the following peptide fragments would most likely belong to a keratin alpha helix?
    (A) Gly – Ala – Pro – Gly – Pro – Hyp
    (B) Gly – Ser – Gly – Ala – Gly – Ala
    (C) Ala – Val – Arg – Gln – Met – Leu
    (D) Ala – Val – Cys – Met – Leu – Cys

44. Keratin is sometimes used to coat the outside of pills to allow uptake of medicine in a desired location. Based on information in the passage, where are keratin-coated pills designed to dissolve?
    (A) Intestine
    (B) Stomach
    (C) Bloodstream
    (D) Mouth

45. A cosmetic chemist is trying to develop a safer liquid shampoo for use on fine, brittle hair. The hydroxide ion concentration of various formulas has been measured in mol/L at 25°C.

Formula M	Formula N	Formula O
6.8×10^{-5}	8.0×10^{-5}	8.7×10^{-3}

Formula P	Formula R
6.3×10^{-7}	4.0×10^{-7}

Based on this experiment and information in the passage, which of the following can be concluded?
    (A) Formula R will cause the least amount of hair damage because it is the most acidic.
    (B) Formula R will cause the most amount of hair damage because it is the most acidic.
    (C) Formula O will cause the least amount of hair damage because it is the most acidic.
    (D) Formula O will cause the least amount of hair damage because it is the most basic.

46. Globular proteins containing multiple disulfide bonds must be heated at higher temperatures for a longer amount of time than those without disulfide bonds in order to achieve denaturation. Which of the following properties explains this characteristic?
    (A) Disulfide bonds are ionic bonds.
    (B) The bond between two cysteine residues is a double bond.
    (C) Disulfide bonds are covalent bonds.
    (D) Noncovalent interactions stabilize globular proteins.

The following questions do not refer to a descriptive passage and are not related to each other.

47. The figure below shows the phase diagram of carbon dioxide.

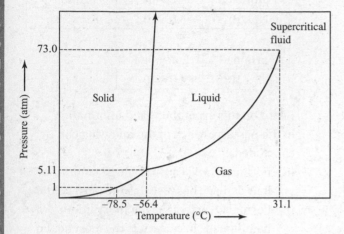

Which of the following would be most likely to change carbon dioxide at 30°C and 10 atm of pressure from a gas to a liquid?
(A) Lower the pressure.
(B) Raise the temperature.
(C) Lower the pressure and lower the temperature.
(D) Raise the pressure and lower the temperature.

48. A flash of lightning is seen and the sound is heard about 6 seconds later. The distance to the lightning is approximately:
(A) 100 m
(B) 500 m
(C) 2 km
(D) 10 km

49. A spring exerting no restoring force has a length of 80 cm. When stretched to 100 cm, the restoring force is 2N. When stretched to 150 cm, the restoring force will be:
(A) 9 N
(B) 7 N
(C) 5 N
(D) 3 N

50. Which of the following will be least effective at increasing the voltage from an electrochemical cell from the reduction of zinc ions to metallic zinc?
(A) Adding zinc nitrate to the zinc ion solution
(B) Increasing the molar concentration of the zinc ion solution
(C) Increasing the volume of the solution of zinc ions
(D) Increasing the surface areas of both the anode and the cathode

51. An ideal gas is compressed at constant temperature so that the pressure is doubled. Which of the following statements must be true?
(A) The average velocity of a molecule hitting the walls of the container is higher.
(B) The frequency of collisions of the molecules with the container walls is higher.
(C) Both the velocity and frequency of collisions is higher.
(D) Neither the velocity nor frequency of collisions is higher.

52. When transmitting electrical power over long distances, it is best to use:
(A) high current and therefore lower voltage.
(B) high voltage and therefore lower current.
(C) both high current and high voltage.
(D) Power transmission is independent of both voltage and current.

PASSAGE VIII

Skatole (3-methylindole) and 1,3-dimethylindole (Compounds **1** and **2**—see Figure 1) are appropriate models for more complex 3-alkylindoles, which are metabolites of various biological synthesis pathways. Researchers doing bromination studies of alkylindoles decided to synthesize the brominated derivatives of Compounds **1** and **2**. These molecules were to be used as synthetic intermediates and reference compounds.

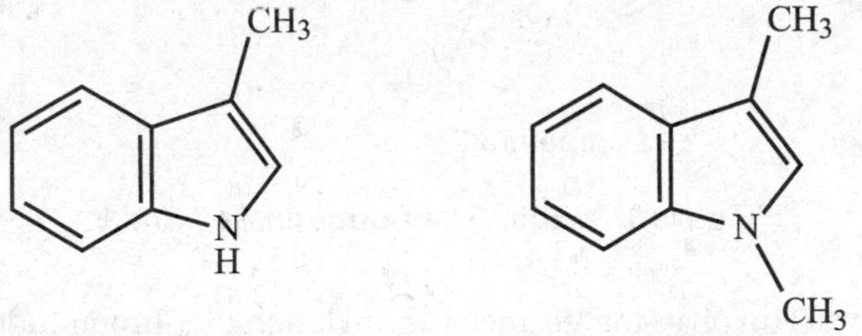

Compound 1   **Compound 2**

Figure 1. 3-methylindole and 1,3-dimethylindole

The desired brominated derivatives, Compounds **5** and **6**, were synthesized starting with commercially available 5-bromoindole (Compound **3**). The multistep process is shown in Figure 2.

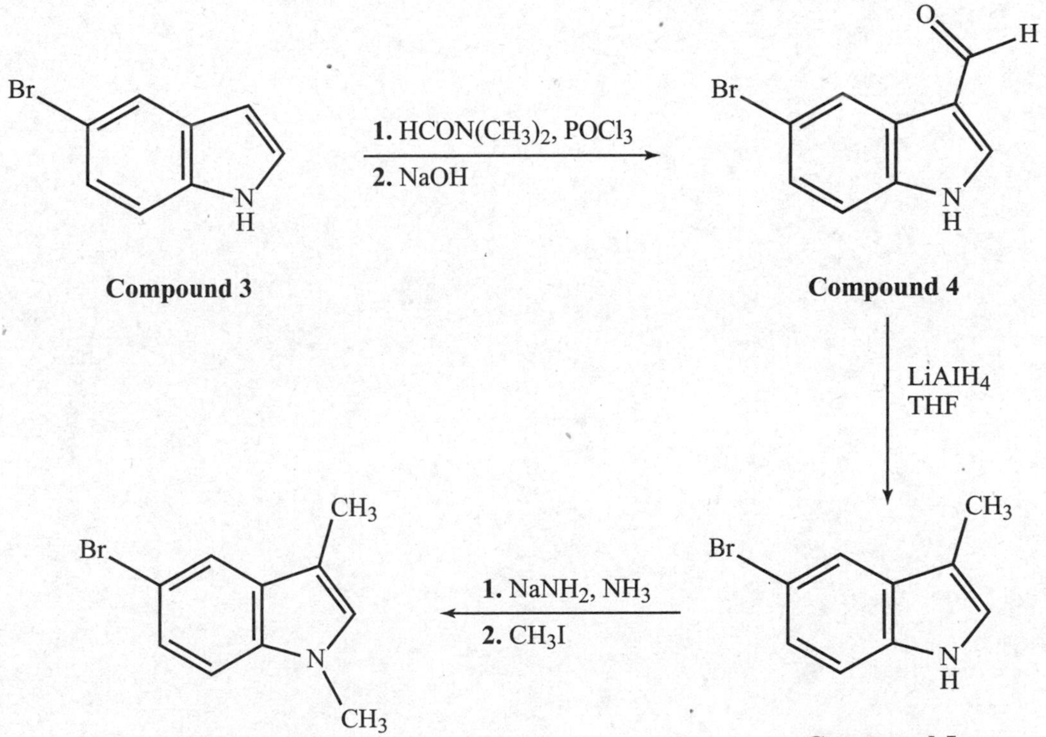

Compound 3   **Compound 4**

Compound 6   **Compound 5**

Figure 2. Synthesis of Compounds **5** and **6**

It was decided that the carboxylate derivative (Compound **8**) of Compound **6** would also be a valuable reference compound, so it was prepared according to Figure 3 shown below.

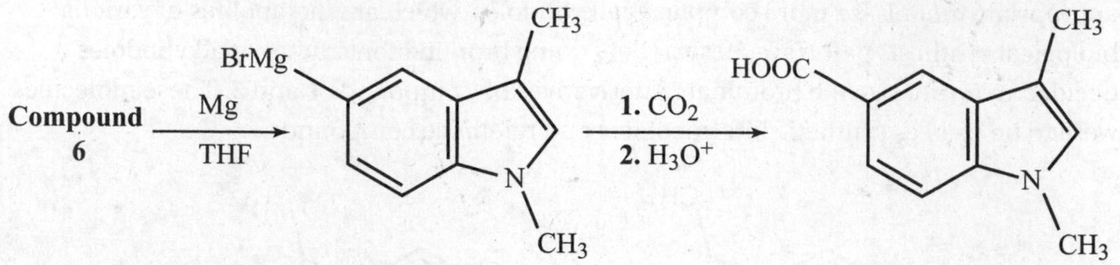

Compound 7 **Compound 8**

Figure 3. Synthesis of Compounds **7** and **8**

Step one in Figure 2 involves the Vilsmeier formylation of 5-bromoindole in the 3 position producing an aldehyde, Compound **4**. In the second step the formyl group is transformed to a methyl group by treatment with lithium aluminum hydride in the solvent tetrahydrofuran to give Compound **5**. In the last step, N-methylation of Compound **5** produced the desired 5-bromo-1,3-dimethylindole (Compound **6**). Compound **6** was then converted to a carboxylic acid (Figure 3) by forming the Grignard reagent and then carboxylating it with carbon dioxide gas. Reaction of the carboxylate anion with aqueous acid yielded Compound **8**.

53. Which of the following is *not* true about the reaction solvent used to prepare the Grignard reagent (Compound **7**)?
   (A) It contains an ether functional group.
   (B) It is a hydrogen bond donor.
   (C) It helps solvate the Grignard reagent as it forms.
   (D) It is a cyclic compound.

54. Reaction of CO_2 with Compound **7** involves:
   (A) an elimination reaction.
   (B) a rearrangement reaction.
   (C) an addition reaction.
   (D) a substitution reaction.

55. In Figure 2 if the formal group (–C=OH) of Compound **4** were reacted with CrO_3 in acidic solution the result would be:
   (A) an alcohol.
   (B) a ketone.
   (C) a carboxylic acid.
   (D) a methyl ester.

56. How many stereoisomers of Compound **6** are possible?
   (A) None
   (B) 2
   (C) 3
   (D) 4

57. The geometry of the bonds attached to the nitrogen in Compound **2** would be expected to be:
   (A) trigonal planar.
   (B) trigonal pyramidal.
   (C) tetrahedral.
   (D) square planar.

The following questions do not refer to a descriptive passage and are not related to each other.

58. The Ksp value for silver iodide, AgI, is 4×10^{-16}. What is the molar solubility of silver iodide?
   (A) 2×10^{-8}
   (B) 2×10^{-16}
   (C) 8×10^{-16}
   (D) 8×10^{-32}

59. If a sample of gas is heated from 10°C to 20°C, the volume of the gas will:
   (A) increase slightly from the original volume.
   (B) be double the original volume.
   (C) decrease slightly from the original volume.
   (D) be half of the original volume.

CRITICAL ANALYSIS AND REASONING SKILLS

Time: 90 minutes
  53 Questions

DIRECTIONS: The Critical Analysis and Reasoning section contains a number of passages. Each passage is followed by a series of questions. Read the passage and then choose the one best answer for each question. When answering questions, eliminate the choices that you are sure are incorrect, and choose the best remaining answer. When you have chosen an answer, mark it in the corresponding location on the answer sheet.

PASSAGE I

Unlike traditional evaluations of the development of young artists, the sociological approach views the development of artistic skills, particularly among young people in a major urban setting, as a community-based phenomenon that takes place only because of the mutual support provided by artists of varying degrees of accomplishment. Namely, the sociological approach identifies an intricate support system that is almost essential if young artists are to develop artistically as well as to learn how to market their creations. These support systems, which nourish and train the aspiring artist, constitute grassroots institutions, those that are intimately intertwined with the artist's daily life. They are based on informal personal relationships and mutual goals and concerns. They create a stepping stone on which the otherwise isolated artist can gain access to the more impersonal and formal institutions in the artistic world. These grassroots institutions encompass artistic peers, mentors, family, and colleagues in other artistic fields.

One main purpose of artistic support systems is artistic training. It is clear to most researchers that young artists in a major urban setting have received much of their training from their own peers and local mentors. Many young artists spend long hours working with each other or a more experienced friend, involving a mutual sacrifice of time and effort and itself an expression of a community-level support system. If one person is making a particularly strong effort, others may pitch in with artistic or financial help, not expecting any personal reward but rather as an expression of mutual support. It is not necessarily because particular young artists cannot afford more formal training that they turn to the support system. They may simply not trust that a more impersonal institution can respond to their individual needs or they may fear that they will lose their individuality in the process.

Within the urban artistic community, certain business support groups have helped artists learn the marketing skills needed to succeed financially. These groups consist of a carefully balanced blend of neophytes, more experienced artists, and members of the community who are familiar with the operations of institutions, galleries, or funding organizations. According to one researcher, nearly half of the sculptors active in Boston in the first half of the 20th century got full-time work through the help of support groups. Among young artists today, however, business support groups have become less active. Some artists, such as the potters in New York City, have developed other ways of increasing their marketing skills. In the 1950s, New York's potters began establishing internships for young artists with older firms. This gave the young artists an opportunity to learn new skills, earn a modest living, and gain exposure for their work in the hopes of attracting more lucrative employment. Painters in San Francisco in the 1960s established one-on-one mentorships between aspiring artists and well-established ones. This allowed the neophyte a highly personalized training as well as an introduction into the formal institutions of the field. Similarly, other artistic groups developed ways of working their way into the artistic upper echelons.

1. It can be inferred from the passage that which of the following would be LEAST likely to be involved in an artist's grassroots support system?
   (A) A friend involved in a different field of art
   (B) The artist's sister
   (C) An art teacher of the artist
   (D) The director of a top museum in the artists' field

2. Which of the following is an example of a grassroots support system as described in the passage?
   (A) An adult education program run through the public schools offers free art classes, taught by local accomplished artists, that are open to the public.
   (B) The mayor's office in a large city provides money for a summer program employing young artists to teach artistically gifted children.
   (C) A group of sculptors living in a San Francisco neighborhood arranges individual mentorships for themselves with well-known sculptors.
   (D) A well-known school of the arts offers scholarships to aspiring young artists who meet certain criteria.

3. Based on the passage, what can be inferred about business support groups?
   (A) Young sculptors today are more likely to find employment through a business support group than through internships or mentorships.
   (B) Younger artists are less likely to use them.
   (C) They were originated by sculptors in Boston.
   (D) They contributed to the employment of a significant number of sculptors working in Boston between 1900 and 1950.

4. Which of the following can be best concluded based on the passage?
   (A) An aspiring artist in an urban area who received no training from local mentors would not be able to succeed.
   (B) Grassroots support systems have been most active in helping young artists since 1950.
   (C) Aspiring urban artists have created a number of alternatives to the standard ways of getting artistic and business training.
   (D) The business support systems developed by various types of artists have mostly been successful because of their carefully designed formal structure.

5. Which statement below best describes the organization of the second paragraph?
   (A) The author describes a situation and then presents the historical setting from which it evolved.
   (B) The author makes an assertion and then presents a number of examples that support it.
   (C) The author outlines an argument and then presents a counter argument.
   (D) The author gives an example of a particular phenomenon and from it draws a general conclusion.

6. According to the passage, support systems provide which of the following to aspiring urban artists?
   (A) Advice on making grassroots contacts in the artistic communities of nearby major urban areas
   (B) A supportive environment that is relatively free of competitive pressure
   (C) Strategies for encouraging a formal training institution to respond to their individual needs
   (D) Contacts with people in their community who understand the workings of formal art institutions

7. Based on the passage, it can be inferred that it would be LEAST likely for a traditional evaluation of the development of young urban artists to do which of the following?

(A) Evaluate the social setting in which the artists live and work

(B) Analyze present day examples of aspiring artists as opposed to historical trends

(C) Focus on the experiences that individual aspiring artists have had in common

(D) Evaluate how artists maintain successful businesses as opposed to how they get established in successful businesses

Since the 1980s, the percentage of people falling within the definition of "middle class" in the United States has dropped dramatically. As a result, the gap between the wealthy and the poor has widened. The percentage of the nation's wealth controlled by a small number of super-wealthy has increased. The percentage of the population living in poverty has increased.

Many economists see this trend leading to disaster. They predict that the rate of loss of the middle class will snowball and that as the growing population of poor becomes increasingly demanding, uneducated, and violent, the only option for the wealthy will be to dispense with the pretense of democracy completely and establish a government of the wealthy, by the wealthy, and for the wealthy.

I wonder, however, if this view does not miss the mark. Most people would probably agree that people who have the skills to be successful in their personal and business lives also have the skills to guide the nation. There may be occasional examples of an uneducated person rising to political power, but even in those cases, this person must have had some outstanding skills—possibly charisma, leadership, eloquence—despite the lack of a formal education.

The activities of those with leadership ability, whether they be in business or government, are complex responses to complex situations. Such people must understand the forces that act on communities and nations and respond to those forces in a way that maintains the stability and prosperity of the state. To the uneducated, the poor of mind, these activities are probably incomprehensible. How could such people be expected to make electoral decisions that affect the nation's well-being?

The defining difference between the nation's business and government leaders and the great mass of the unsuccessful can be defined simply as intelligence. When the intelligent encounter an economic or political problem, they embrace it. The unintelligent rant against it or take up some violent but ineffective response. The intelligent study, research, and analyze the problem. The unintelligent are incapable of understanding that the problem has any depth to it. The intelligent, as they understand the problem, develop a new and creative response to it. This response is nearly guaranteed to be effective. The unintelligent react in the same predictable way again and again, guaranteeing that they will simply dig themselves more deeply into despair.

It is regrettable that some would paint the successful as greedy destroyers of freedom. True, greed may be the motivator that raises a superior person above the masses in the first place. However, it has been true throughout history that those who are capable of guiding the rest of humanity have risen to positions in which they could do so. For the most part they have done so not in the context of democracy but as benevolent leaders directing from above.

To bemoan the loss of the middle class and the rise of the most capable is to miss the fact that those of the middle class who were capable of excellence have risen to that role. Those who were not have taken their natural place in the lower rankings of society. To fight against the rise of intelligence in our society is, by definition, unintelligence itself.

8. In the passage, the author asserts which of the following about the middle class?

 I. The gap between the middle class and the poor in the United States has widened since the 1980's.
 II. Members of the middle class who are capable of doing so have risen to excellence.
 III. Loss of the middle class will lead to disaster.

(A) II only
(B) III only
(C) I and II only
(D) I, II, and III

9. What is the main thesis of the passage?
(A) A strong middle class is necessary for a healthy democracy.
(B) Creative problem solving is helpful in both business and government.
(C) It is natural for the economically most successful to make political decisions.
(D) Economic disaster is unavoidable.

10. If female members of a certain animal community were found to have better problem-solving skills than the male members, which of the following would the author most likely believe?
(A) The females will make the important decisions for the group.
(B) The gap between the number of females and males will likely increase.
(C) It is possible that the animals could become a threat to humans.
(D) The gap between the number of females and males will ultimately lead to disaster for the group.

11. The author's attitude toward the increasing gap between rich and poor is best described by saying that the gap:
(A) is likely to even out with time.
(B) needs to be reversed.
(C) has nothing to do with unintelligence.
(D) is not something to be concerned about.

12. If the author were to present a talk at a conference on Third World economic development, which of the following topics would be most likely for the author to discuss?
(A) The importance of an equitable distribution of wealth
(B) The importance of businesses that can help the poor increase their income
(C) The role of the wealthy in forging a plan for the future
(D) Why wealth is not important to a traditional culture

13. All of the following are examples that the author might cite to support his definition of intelligence EXCEPT:
(A) becoming fluent in a difficult language.
(B) designing a successful ad campaign to convince voters to vote for a wealthy candidate.
(C) developing an economic support plan for Congress to implement in order to prevent a recession.
(D) building a more cost-effective carburetor.

PASSAGE III

. . . As I jot this paragraph, I am out just after sunrise, and down towards the creek. The lights, perfumes, melodies—the blue birds, grass birds and robins, in every direction—the noisy, vocal, natural concert. For undertones, a neighboring wood-pecker tapping his tree, and the distant clarion of chanticleer. Then the fresh-earth smells—the colors, the delicate drabs and thin blues of the perspective. The bright green of the grass has receiv'd an added tinge from the last two days' mildness and moisture. How the sun silently mounts in the broad clear sky, on his day's journey! How the warm beams bathe all, and come streaming kissingly and almost hot on my face. . . .

Later.—Nature marches in procession, in sections, like the corps of an army. All have done much for me, and still do. But for the last two days it has been the great wild bee, the humble-bee, or "bumble," as the children call him. As I walk, or hobble, from the farm-house down to the creek, I traverse the before-mention'd lane, fenced by old rails, with many splits, splinters, breaks, holes, &c., the choice habitat of those crooning, hairy insects. Up and down and by and between these rails, they swarm and dart and fly in countless myriads. As I wend slowly along, I am often accompanied with a moving cloud of them. They play a leading part in my morning, midday, or sunset rambles, and often dominate the landscape in a way I never before thought of—fill the long lane, not by scores or hundreds only, but by thousands. Large and vivacious and swift, with wonderful momentum and a loud swelling, perpetual hum, varied now and then by something almost like a shriek, they dart to and fro, in rapid flashes, chasing each other, and (little things as they are) conveying to me a new and pronounc'd sense of strength, beauty, vitality, and movement. . . .

As I write, I am seated under a big wild-cherry tree—the warm day temper'd by partial clouds and a fresh breeze, neither too heavy nor light—and here I sit long and long, envelop'd in the deep musical drone of these bees, flitting, balancing, darting to and fro about me by hundreds—big fellows with light yellow jackets, great glistening swelling bodies, stumpy heads and gauzy wings—humming their perpetual rich mellow boom. . . . How it all nourishes, lulls me, in the way most needed; the open air, the rye-fields, the apple orchards. The last two days have been faultless in sun, breeze, temperature and everything; never two more perfect days, and I have enjoy'd them wonderfully. . . .

. . . Down in the apple-trees and in a neighboring cedar were three or four russet-back'd thrushes, each singing his best, and roulading in ways I never heard surpass'd. Two hours I abandon myself to hearing them, and indolently absorbing the scene. Almost every bird I notice has a special time in the year—sometimes limited to a few days—when it sings its best; and now is the period of these russet-backs. Meanwhile, up and down the lane, the darting, droning, musical bumble-bees. A great swarm again for my entourage as I return home, moving along with me as before.

As I write this, two or three weeks later, I am sitting near the brook under a tulip tree, 70 feet high, thick with the fresh verdure of its young maturity—a beautiful object—every branch, every leaf perfect. From top to bottom, seeking the sweet juice in the blossoms, it swarms with myriads of these wild bees, whose loud and steady humming makes an undertone to the whole, and to my mood and the hour. . . .

From Walt Whitman, *Complete Prose Works, Specimen Days and Collect, November Boughs and Goodbye My Fancy* (*http://www.gutenberg.org/dirs/etext05/7cmpr10.txt*, accessed May 2010).

14. The author is most concerned with:
    (A) a study of nature from the standpoint of a biologist.
    (B) the interrelationships of life forms as studied in ecology.
    (C) an interaction with living things from the standpoint of a poet.
    (D) an analysis of a problem concerning bees.

15. From the author's perspective, what is the significance of the bees?
    (A) They are examples of the ferocity caused by intense competition for food.
    (B) They represent the symbiosis between nature and humans, in that they pollinate our food crops and provide us with honey.
    (C) They are able to communicate complex information among thousands of individual bees.
    (D) They inspire qualities of wildness, vigor, musicality, and grace.

16. The author uses the word "wild" to describe both the bees and the cherry tree. What does the author most likely mean by the word "wild" in relation to the tree?
    (A) The tree has large, widely sweeping branches in all directions.
    (B) The spirit of the tree, like that of the bees, is not something logical or linear.
    (C) The word refers to a species of cherry tree.
    (D) The fruits of the tree are scattered all over in random fashion.

17. Which of the following is an assumption that the author makes?
    (A) Things that can cause pain can also elicit pleasure.
    (B) The countryside offers greater pleasures than the city.
    (C) In nature, beauty is in inverse proportion to size.
    (D) That which is most beautiful is most fleeting.

18. Which of the following is most likely the author's meaning for the phrase, "All have done much for me"?
    (A) The author is grateful for the people who have helped him in his life.
    (B) Nature has protected him from harm.
    (C) The author is grateful to the children for their creativity, including the names they give to creatures.
    (D) The author has enjoyed various aspects of Nature.

PASSAGE IV

Private equity in the 1980s was a controversial topic, commonly associated with corporate raids, hostile takeovers, asset stripping, layoffs, plant closings, and outsized profits to investors. As private equity reemerged in the 1990s, it began to earn a new degree of legitimacy and respectability. Although in the 1980s, many of the acquisitions made were unsolicited and unwelcome, private equity firms in the 1990s focused on making buyouts attractive propositions for management and shareholders. According to *The Economist*, "[B]ig companies that would once have turned up their noses at an approach from a private-equity firm are now pleased to do business with them."

Additionally, private equity investors became increasingly focused on the long-term development of companies they acquired, using less leverage in the acquisition. In the 1980s, leverage would routinely represent 85% to 95% of the purchase price of a company compared with average debt levels between 20% and 40% in leveraged buyouts in the 1990s and the first decade of the 21st century. KKR's 1986 acquisition of Safeway, for example, was completed with 97% leverage and 3% equity contributed by KKR, whereas KKR's acquisition of TXU in 2007 was completed with approximately 19% equity contributed.

The Thomas H. Lee Partners' acquisition of Snapple Beverages, in 1992, is often described as the deal that marked the resurrection of the leveraged buyout after several dormant years. Only two years after the original acquisition, Lee sold the company to Quaker Oats for $1.7 billion. Lee was estimated to have made $900 million for himself and his investors from the sale. Quaker Oats would subsequently sell the company, which performed poorly under new management, three years later for only $300 million.

In 1993, David Bonderman and James Coulter completed a buyout of Continental Airlines. They were virtually alone in their conviction that there was an investment opportunity with the airline. The plan included bringing in a new management team, improving aircraft utilization, and focusing on lucrative routes. By 1998, the men had generated an annual internal rate of return of 55% on their investment. Unlike Carl Icahn, who executed a hostile takeover of TWA in 1985, Bonderman and Coulter were widely hailed as saviors of the airline, marking the change in tone from the 1980s.

As the market for private equity matured, so too did its investor base. The Institutional Limited Partner Association was initially founded as an informal networking group for limited partner investors in private equity funds in the early 1990s. However the organization would evolve into an advocacy organization for private equity investors with more than 200 member organizations from 10 countries. As of the end of 2007, ILPA members had total assets under management in excess of $5 trillion, with more than $850 billion of capital commitments to private equity investments.

Adapted from "History of Private Equity and Venture Capital," on Wikipedia, *http://en.wikipedia.org/wiki/History_of_private_equity_and_venture_capital* (accessed May 2010).

19. The author is primarily concerned with:
   (A) describing the ways in which the power of private equity has been misused.
   (B) outlining the history of private equity.
   (C) contrasting an earlier quality of private equity investing with a later quality.
   (D) documenting that private equity investing can be beneficial to all parties.

20. Which of the following statements, if true, would most seriously weaken the author's contention about private equity firms in the 1990's?
   (A) Acquisitions by private equity firms often resulted in consumers having fewer and lower-quality choices.
   (B) The average percentage of leverage for acquisitions in the 1990s was only marginally greater than the corresponding percentage for the 1980s.
   (C) More than half of the businesses bought by private equity firms and then sold for a profit were later sold at a loss by the next owner.
   (D) In most of the acquisitions made by private equity firms in the 1990s, the shareholders earned less profit than what they would have without the acquisition.

21. What does the author mean by the phrase, "using less leverage in the acquisition" [paragraph 2]?
   (A) Allowing the managers and shareholders of the company being purchased to have more input on the terms of acquisition
   (B) Agreeing to avoid the most aggressive procedures, including hostile takeover, asset stripping, and plant closures
   (C) Agreeing to pay a higher percentage of equity in the purchase
   (D) Agreeing to pay most of the purchase price up front

22. Which of the following most likely represents the author's attitude about the acquisition of Snapple Beverages in 1992?
   (A) Ambivalence
   (B) Optimism
   (C) Censure
   (D) Enthusiasm

23. According to the author, all of the following would be positive results for a private equity investor who follows the principles that emerged in the 1990s EXCEPT:
   (A) higher profits.
   (B) happier management.
   (C) respectability.
   (D) praise.

24. If it were true that only the 1990s model of investing could lead to respectability and also that outsized profits prevent using the 1990s model, which of the following would also have to be true?
   (A) Anyone who avoids giving outsized profits to investors will gain respectability.
   (B) Those who do not follow the 1990s model will give outsized profits to investors.
   (C) If there are respectable private equity investors, they do not give outsized profits to investors.
   (D) There are some who follow the 1990s model but are not respectable.

PASSAGE V

Neanderthals, according to Paul Jordan (Jordan, P. *Neanderthal: Neanderthal Man and the Story of Human Origins.* The History Press, 2001), appear to have had psychological traits that worked well in their early history but finally placed them at a long-term disadvantage with respect to modern humans. Jordan is of the opinion that the Neanderthal mind was sufficiently different from that of Homo sapiens to have been "alien" in the sense of thinking differently from that of modern humans, despite the obvious fact that Neanderthals were highly intelligent, with a brain as large as or larger than our own. This theory is supported by what Neanderthals possessed and, just as importantly, by what they lacked, in cultural attributes and manufactured artifacts. Essentially, the Neanderthals lost out because their behaviors and tools eventually became second-rate.

There once was a time when both human types shared essentially the same Mousterian tool kit and neither human type had a definite competitive advantage, as evidenced by the shifting Homo sapiens/Neanderthal borderland in the Middle East. But finally Homo sapiens started to attain behavioral or cultural adaptations that allowed "moderns" an advantage. There are early glimmers of this from Zaire, where, in the area of Katanda, bone harpoon points have been found of fine workmanship, dating to perhaps 80,000 years ago. These featured backward-pointing barbs and lateral grooves so they could be easily installed on a wooden shaft, used to harpoon local fish. These appear to have been made by modern humans and make for a more sophisticated spear than any that Neanderthals are known to have made. Jordan admits that some of these innovations were "flash in the pan" local affairs that faded away for awhile, but there does not seem to be much doubt that Homo sapiens in Africa were taking steps toward better tools and a more complex social life, while the Neanderthal ways and technology remained the same. It is noted that fishing was never much of a Neanderthal accomplishment (they did eat fish on occasion) but is more a behavior of modern human types. There is an example of a barbed point made from bone, evidently made by a Neanderthal, but such finds are very rare. Per Jordan, the Nean-

derthals made wooden and stone artifacts, but bone and ivory ones were not common, implying that the Neanderthal mind tended to be rather resistant to learning new methods or materials.

Neanderthal people mastered complex tasks such as the making of fire, shelters with post holes, and stone tools. In their later career, Neanderthals appear to have sometimes buried their dead, and their placement of Cave Bear bones in order shows some sort of reverence or perhaps religion toward this animal. Yet there were many Cro-Magnon tools and behaviors that the Neanderthals seem to have never developed: organized fishing, using fish hooks and fish nets, headgear or hats, shoes, sewn clothing, needle-and-thread, and long-distance trade. It is still debated whether Neanderthals had significant art or music.

Jordan states that the Chatelperronian tool tradition suggests Neanderthals were making some attempts at advancement, as Chatelperronian tools are only associated with Neanderthal remains. It appears this tradition was connected to some sort of social contact with Cro-Magnons. There were some items of personal decoration found at these sites, but these are inferior to contemporary Cro-Magnon items of personal decoration and arguably were made more by imitation than by a spirit of original creativity. At the same time, Neanderthal stone tools were sometimes finished well enough to show some aesthetic sense. As Jordan notes, "A natural sympathy for the underdog and the disadvantaged lends a sad poignancy to the fate of the Neanderthal folk, however it came about."

Adapted from "Neanderthal," on Wikipedia, *http://en.wikipedia.org/wiki/Neanderthal* (accessed May 2010).

25. According to information in the passage, which of the following could be concluded about the period 80,000 years ago?
    (A) Neanderthals were beginning to lose cultural tools that had previously helped them survive.
    (B) There were some early humans in Africa who could be considered modern.
    (C) The Neanderthals in the Middle East were coexisting with Homo sapiens.
    (D) This was the final stage of Homo sapiens achieving cultural adaptations that gave them an advantage over Neanderthals.

26. What is the author's purpose in saying that Neanderthals "mastered complex tasks"?
    (A) To demonstrate that with larger brains than modern humans, Neanderthals excelled in certain areas
    (B) To show that when they were able to observe modern humans, Neanderthals could master new skills they might not have learned on their own
    (C) To document that there is a difference between advanced cultural skills and flexibility to learn new skills
    (D) To suggest that Neanderthals may have been just as artistic and musical as we are

27. Assuming that Cro-Magnon people were similar to us in their thoughts and emotions, based on the information in the passage, how would they have most likely felt about Neanderthal people that they observed?
    (A) Respectful of the Neanderthals' more ancient ways
    (B) Puzzled by the Neanderthals' lack of shoes
    (C) Confused by the Neanderthals' greater strength but ignorance of stone tools
    (D) Sympathetic of the Neanderthals' impending extinction

28. Recent DNA analysis strongly supports the theory that early modern humans and Neanderthals did not interbreed. Which of the following would the author most likely agree is the explanation?
    (A) The shifting boundaries of their territories kept the populations geographically separated.
    (B) The populations occupied the same geographical area but had no cultural contact with each other.
    (C) The Neanderthal mind and body were too "alien" to attract a modern human mate.
    (D) The two populations were sometimes in close proximity but were of separate species.

29. What is the author's purpose in citing the final quote from Jordan?
    (A) To highlight that no one knows how the Neanderthals met their final end
    (B) To show the author's personal emotions about an object of academic study
    (C) To provide an example of the subtle emotional faculties of modern humans
    (D) To document a truth in anthropology that the underdog seldom meets a good end

PASSAGE VI

Social Security is a social insurance program officially called "Old-Age, Survivors, and Disability Insurance" (OASDI), in reference to its three components. It is funded primarily through a dedicated payroll tax.

Reform proposals continue to circulate with some urgency, due to a long-term funding challenge faced by the program. Starting in 2016, program expenses begin to exceed revenues. This is due to the aging of the baby-boom generation (resulting in a lower ratio of paying workers to retirees), expected continuing low birth rate (compared to the baby-boom period), and increasing life expectancy.

Advocates of major change in the system generally argue that drastic action is necessary because Social Security is facing a crisis. In his 2005 State of the Union speech, President Bush indicated that Social Security was facing "bankruptcy." In his 2006 State of the Union speech, he described entitlement reform (including Social Security) as a "national challenge" that, if not addressed in a timely manner, would "present future Congresses with impossible choices—staggering tax increases, immense deficits, or deep cuts in every category of spending."

A liberal think tank, the Center for Economic and Policy Research, says that "Social Security is more financially sound today than it has been throughout most of its 69-year history" and that Bush's statement should have no credibility.

Nobel Laureate economist Paul Krugman, deriding what he called "the hype about a Social Security crisis," wrote: "[T]here is a long-run financing problem. But it's a problem of modest size. The [CBO] report finds that extending the life of the trust fund into the 22nd century, with no change in benefits, would require additional revenues equal to only 0.54 percent of G.D.P. That's less than 3 percent of federal spending—less than we're currently spending in Iraq. . . . Given these numbers, it's not at all hard to come up with fiscal packages that would secure the retirement program, with no major changes, for generations to come."

The claims of the probability of future difficulty with the current Social Security system are largely based on the annual analysis made of the system and its prospects and reported by the governors of the Social Security system. Although such analysis can never be 100% accurate, it can at least be made using different probable future scenarios and be based on rational assumptions and reach rational conclusions, with the conclusions being no better (in terms of predicting the future) than the assumptions on which the predictions are based. With these predictions in hand, it is possible to make at least some prediction of what the future retirement security of Americans who will rely on Social Security might be.

Proponents of the current system argue that if and when the trust fund runs out, there will still be the choice of raising taxes or cutting benefits, or both. They say that demographic and revenue projections might turn out to be too pessimistic, and that the current health of the economy exceeds the assumptions used by the Social Security Administration.

These Social Security proponents argue that the correct plan is to fix Medicare, which is the largest underfunded entitlement, repeal the 2001–2004 revenue reductions, and balance the budget. They believe a growth trend will emerge from these steps, and the government can alter the Social Security mix of taxes, benefits, benefit adjustments, and retirement age to avoid future deficits. The age at which one begins to receive Social Security benefits has been raised several times since the program's inception.

Adapted from Wikipedia, "Social Security Debate (United States)," on Wikipedia, *http://en.wikipedia.org/wiki/Social_Security_debate_%28United_States%29* (accessed May 2010).

30. All of the following are strategies that the author uses to support the position that Social Security is not in need of drastic action EXCEPT:
    (A) citing an authority who is acknowledged as an expert in an appropriate discipline.
    (B) questioning the motives of government officials who claim drastic action is needed.
    (C) providing specific examples of solutions for the problems faced by Social Security.
    (D) quoting opinions of political liberals.

31. Which of the following is most likely the reason for the argument that "the correct plan is to fix Medicare"?
    (A) It will be much easier to fix Medicare because it is a smaller program than Social Security.
    (B) Fixing Medicare alone will result in a growth trend.
    (C) Social Security is not the largest under-funded entitlement program.
    (D) Social Security probably cannot be fixed, so the next most reasonable program to fix is Medicare.

32. If a conservative approach is defined in contrast to a liberal approach as a desire to avoid changes to economic structures, which of the following would characterize the views of Paul Krugman?
    (A) They are liberal because he wants to radically change the system.
    (B) They are liberal because he wants to dramatically increase government spending on Social Security.
    (C) They are conservative because they are based on the report of an independent board.
    (D) They are conservative because his multi-generational plan does not call for major change.

33. Which of the following best describes the author's probable reason for the last line of the passage?
    (A) It supports the premise that Social Security has been in serious trouble before.
    (B) It is an informational point to help readers of the article understand how Social Security will affect them.
    (C) It shows that a certain adjustment that could keep Social Security from running out of money could be easily done.
    (D) It is a counterargument to a specific claim of those who say that Social Security requires dramatic change.

34. Which of the following scenarios would be most analogous to the relationship in the passage between those who claim Social Security requires dramatic change and those who claim it does not?
    (A) Several internationally recognized ecologists present research on global climate change and urge dramatic action, whereas an opposing group loudly proclaims there is no need for worry.
    (B) A teacher presents her principal with several years of data showing that her students are scoring very close to their targets, but the principal states that the teacher must make dramatic changes in her curriculum for the school to avoid censure.
    (C) A noted audiologist claims that listening to loud rock music will permanently damage hearing, whereas a group of professional rock musicians claim it is everyone's right to decide what they enjoy listening to.
    (D) A Nobel prize-winning economist demonstrates with well-researched data that certain radical but effective policy changes will eliminate the national debt in one generation, but politicians present researched evidence that voters will not elect a politician who follows those policies.

PASSAGE VII

Most people would say that they would like to be happy. In fact, many would say that being happy is one of their primary goals in life. At the same time, would not most people claim that being happy usually has to take second place to other responsibilities in their lives—work, family, social obligations? The pursuit of happiness is something, they would claim, that gets squeezed in here and there—at a movie, a quick walk around the block, in front of the television, a visit with a friend.

I would challenge this view that we only pursue happiness on rare occasions. Take as an example the person waking up groggy in the morning who would love to get another hour of sleep but needs to show up at work on time. Is this person abandoning happiness in favor of obligation? I say no. The person has, subconsciously perhaps, weighed all possible options for action at that moment and chosen the one that will result in the greatest possible happiness.

A critic might object to my point, saying that the sleepy subject of our experiment was, in fact, torn between pleasing himself or herself and pleasing the boss. This critic could say the same for all of our obligations. At one moment we postpone pleasing ourselves so that we can please our spouse. At the next moment our happiness is put aside to please a neighbor, or a child, or a client. But again I say the critic has the wrong view, a view that pits happiness against unhappiness. Suppose it is possible to do away with unhappiness altogether. Then this conflict disappears and only happiness remains.

If our sleepy subject thinks that she would rather be sleeping than getting to work to keep the boss happy, she will definitely be unhappy. However, the problem lies not in the situation but in the fact that she has not thought the situation through carefully. If, instead, she were to tell herself that all the possibilities were open and that it was only for her to decide what would make her happiest, she could then consider all the options and make a decision. Perhaps the decision would be to sleep in. Perhaps it would be to go to work. In either case, it would be the action that, after careful consideration, she felt would bring her the most happiness.

Suppose wealthy Aunt Bertha calls to say she will be spending three weeks with you. If you think in terms of your once-a-year golf vacation versus alienating Aunt Bertha, you will have no choice but unhappiness. If you ask yourself what course of action would bring you the greatest happiness, then, no matter what you choose to do after careful and patient consideration, you will be as happy as possible at that moment.

This kind of careful and patient and comprehensive thinking takes more energy than our usual reactions. It is perhaps easier to grumble one's way out of bed. It takes an active and flexible mind to consider all the possibilities for happiness. The great irony of happiness, then, may be that we choose to be unhappy because it takes less work.

35. The author responds to the critic's argument by:
    - (A) questioning the critic's credentials.
    - (B) showing that the critic's logic leads to an illogical conclusion.
    - (C) undermining an assumption of the critic's argument.
    - (D) showing that the critic has incorrectly generalized from a narrow example.

36. If it were proven that some people derive happiness from pleasing others, how would this affect the author's argument?
    - (A) It would not affect the argument.
    - (B) It would weaken the argument because such people still have to choose between pleasing themselves or others.
    - (C) It would support the author's contention that it is easier to please people than to work against them.
    - (D) It would weaken the author's contention that we choose to be unhappy because it takes less work.

37. All of the following beliefs about happiness are consistent with the passage EXCEPT:
    (A) we can be as happy as possible in every situation.
    (B) there is always a way to please others and still be able to please oneself.
    (C) unhappiness is a result of lack of effort.
    (D) there is a difference between being happy and being as happy as possible.

38. Why does the author use the word "irony" in the last sentence?
    (A) People claim that they are unhappy much of the time, and it turns out that, in fact, they are.
    (B) Even though the author has tried to prove that people are happy, it turns out that they are not.
    (C) The critics claim that people are torn between happiness and unhappiness, and it turns out they are correct.
    (D) People claim they are unhappy because of other people, but it turns out they are unhappy because of their own actions.

39. In the second paragraph, how successful is the author in challenging the idea that we pursue happiness only on rare occasions?
    (A) The author is unsuccessful because the example given is not a rare occasion.
    (B) The author is unsuccessful because the person in the example will not be happy whether he or she sleeps in or goes to work.
    (C) The author is successful because the person made the decision that resulted in the greatest happiness.
    (D) The author is successful because the author demonstrates how a common example of unhappiness is, on closer inspection, an example of happiness.

40. If a man took a female friend to a movie instead of to a play that she would have preferred, which of the following would represent the author's probable evaluation of the situation?
    (A) The man was as happy as possible in the situation because he was doing what he wanted.
    (B) The woman was as happy as possible in the situation because she avoided a conflict.
    (C) The man would be as happy as possible in the situation only if he carefully considered all of the options.
    (D) The woman would not be as happy as possible in the situation if the man did not carefully consider all of the options.

The history of human growth and development is at the same time the history of the terrible struggle of every new idea heralding the approach of a brighter dawn. In its tenacious hold on tradition, the Old has never hesitated to make use of the foulest and cruelest means to stay the advent of the New, in whatever form or period the latter may have asserted itself. Nor need we retrace our steps into the distant past to realize the enormity of opposition, difficulties, and hardships placed in the path of every progressive idea. The rack, the thumbscrew, and the knout are still with us; so are the convict's garb and the social wrath, all conspiring against the spirit that is serenely marching on.

Anarchism could not hope to escape the fate of all other ideas of innovation. Indeed, as the most revolutionary and uncompromising innovator, Anarchism must needs meet with the combined ignorance and venom of the world it aims to reconstruct.

To deal even remotely with all that is being said and done against Anarchism would necessitate the writing of a whole volume. I shall therefore meet only two of the principal objections. In so doing, I shall attempt to elucidate what Anarchism really stands for.

The strange phenomenon of the opposition to Anarchism is that it brings to light the relation between so-called intelligence and ignorance. And yet this is not so very strange when we consider the relativity of all things. The ignorant mass has in its favor that it makes no pretense of knowledge or tolerance. Acting, as it always does, by mere impulse, its reasons are like those of a child. "Why?" "Because." Yet the opposition of the uneducated to Anarchism deserves the same consideration as that of the intelligent man.

What, then, are the objections? First, Anarchism is impractical, though a beautiful ideal. Second, Anarchism stands for violence and destruction; hence, it must be repudiated as vile and dangerous. Both the intelligent man and the ignorant mass judge not from a thorough knowledge of the subject but either from hearsay or false interpretation.

A practical scheme, says Oscar Wilde, is either one already in existence or a scheme that could be carried out under the existing conditions; but it is exactly the existing conditions that one objects to, and any scheme that could accept these conditions is wrong and foolish. The true criterion of the practical, therefore, is not whether the latter can keep intact the wrong or foolish; rather, it is whether the scheme has vitality enough to leave the stagnant waters of the old, and build, as well as sustain, new life. In the light of this conception, Anarchism is indeed practical. More than any other idea, it is helping to do away with the wrong and foolish; more than any other idea, it is building and sustaining new life.

The emotions of the ignorant man are continuously kept at a pitch by the most blood-curdling stories about Anarchism. Not a thing is too outrageous to be employed against this philosophy and its exponents. Therefore, Anarchism represents to the unthinking what the proverbial bad man does to the child—a black monster bent on swallowing everything; in short, destruction and violence.

Destruction and violence! How is the ordinary man to know that the most violent element in society is ignorance; that its power of destruction is the very thing Anarchism is combating? Nor is he aware that Anarchism, whose roots, as it were, are part of nature's forces, destroys, not healthful tissue but parasitic growths that feed on the life's essence of society. It is merely clearing the soil from weeds and sagebrush that it may eventually bear healthy fruit.

Someone has said that it requires less mental effort to condemn than to think. The widespread mental indolence, so prevalent in society, proves this to be only too true. Rather than to go to the bottom of any given idea, to examine its origin and meaning, most people will either condemn it altogether or rely on some superficial or prejudicial definition of non-essentials.

Anarchism urges man to think, to investigate, to analyze every proposition; this is indeed the essence of the New. Because it distinguishes clearly the weeds of society from that which is fruitful, Anarchism is eternally New. By its nature it cannot become the Old.

Adapted from *Anarchism and Other Essays* by Emma Goldman, *www.gutenberg.org/files/2162/2162-h/2162-h.htm* (accessed May 2010).

41. The passage implies that negative attitudes about Anarchism:
    (A) are influenced by the same factors that influence racist attitudes.
    (B) can easily be overcome through intelligent discussion.
    (C) are grounded in the inherent wisdom of tradition.
    (D) fail to distinguish between two different types of destruction.

42. The passage suggests that thinking, as promoted by Anarchism, requires:
    (A) an appreciation of what can be carried out under existing conditions.
    (B) intelligence that values both knowledge and tolerance.
    (C) a certain amount of hard work.
    (D) a thorough knowledge of information in the national media.

43. Suppose that critics of Anarchism pointed to an Anarchist society that confiscated a well-run but monopolistic automobile industry, resulting in massive job loss. Which one of the following would the author most likely say in response?
    (A) The Old must be destroyed before the New can arise.
    (B) The practical must be destroyed before the ideal can arise.
    (C) The New has the power to cleanse and heal, even if some people get hurt.
    (D) The unhealthy must be destroyed for the truly practical to arise.

44. Which of the following, if true, would most strengthen the author's conclusion that Anarchism, by its nature, cannot become the Old?
    (A) Tradition commonly maintains itself at the expense of society.
    (B) Ignorance has the potential to turn into intelligence when nurtured.
    (C) It takes less effort to think than to act.
    (D) Anarchism requires not just thinking but also an emotional intensity.

45. Which of the following statements by an opponent of Anarchism, if true, would most weaken the author's argument?
    (A) The lesson of history is that what appears wrong or foolish to one generation often proves to be wise and healthy to another.
    (B) Those of us who oppose Anarchism are just as intelligent as those who support it.
    (C) People who analyze every situation may have some understanding of the mind but can never understand the heart.
    (D) The fatal flaw of Anarchism is that a true Anarchist must reject even Anarchism.

46. Based on the passage, which of the following does the author claim is true of Anarchism?

    I. It represents destruction and violence.
    II. It is rooted in the forces of nature.
    III. It does not destroy but rather builds the New.

    (A) I only
    (B) I and III only
    (C) II only
    (D) II and III only

PASSAGE IX

It is always easier to follow a beaten path than to break one's way through untrodden forests. It is easier to walk after we "learn how," and learning how is simply doing it over and over until the legs and feet have acquired habits of motion and accommodation to distances and to what is underfoot. It is easy to do anything after we have done it again and again, so that it has become second nature, and "second nature" is habit. The wise man early forms certain habits of personal care, of eating, sleeping, exercising; of study; of meeting the usual occurrences of life. The first day he spent at anything new was a hard one. Nothing was done naturally. Active attention had to be keenly held to each detail. He had to learn where things belonged, how to do this and that for the first time, how to work with his associates.

Do you remember the first hospital bed you ever made, the first bed bath you gave, the first massage? You had to be taught bit by bit, detail by detail. You did not look upon the finished whole but gave almost painful attention to each step that led to the made bed, the completed bath, or the given massage. Your fingers were probably all thumbs unless you had experience in such things before you came to the hospital. Your mind was tired from the strain of trying to remember each suggestion of your instructor. The second time, or certainly the third or fourth time, it went better. After a week of daily experience, you gave the bath or massage or made the bed with much less effort. A month later the work was practically automatic and accomplished in a fraction of the time you spent on it that first day. Now you can do it quickly and well with little conscious thought; and at the same time carry on a brisk conversation with your patient or think out your work for the day. Your mind is free for other thoughts while you perform the task easily and perfectly. Your method of doing the work has finally become a habit that saves the effort of conscious attention. The details of your routine work are directed by the subconscious. The habit will be energy and time saving in proportion to the accuracy of your first conscious efforts spent on the new undertaking. Thus, useful habit is the result of active effort.

We can acquire habits of thinking and habits of feeling as well as habits of doing.

But the other habits, the bad ones, are not acquired with effort. We fall into them. Hazy thinking is easier than clear thinking. Suppose you are by nature rather oversanguine or overdespondent, and you make no genuine attempt to evolve that nature into poise. Directing will to do what desire opposes is too difficult, and you go the way of least resistance. So easily are the bad habits formed; but only with tremendous effort of will and persistence in refusing their insistent demands can they be broken or replaced by helpful ones.

But habits can be learned; and bad habits can be broken when an overpowering emotion is aroused against them, possesses the mind, and controls the will; or when reason weighs them in the balance and judgment finds them wanting, and volition directs the mind to displace them by others.

The nurse meets in her patients numberless habits which retard recovery of body and make for an unwholesome mental attitude. Some patients have the complaint habit, some the irritation habit, some the self-protection habit, some the habit of impatience, some of reckless expression of despair, some of loss of control, some of incessant self-attention. The nurse who can arouse an incentive to habits of cheer expression when the least cause of cheer appears, who can by reason, or if that is not possible, by suggestion—by holding out incentives, or by making some privilege depend upon control—this nurse can help her patient to displace habits of an illness-accepting mind with habits of a health-accepting one. Above all, let her beware of opening the way to habits of invalidism. Some people acquire the "hospital habit" because it is easier to give way to ill-feeling, however slight, and to be cared for with comfort, than to encourage themselves to build up endurance by giving little attention to minor ailments.

Adapted from *Applied Psychology for Nurses* by Mary F. Porter, A.B., *http://www.gutenberg.org/files/18843/18843-h/18843-h.htm* (accessed May 2010).

47. Which of the following would the author most likely argue is a benefit of habit?
    (A) An habitual action takes less energy than the actions we fall into.
    (B) An action that is done many times is more likely to become a "good" habit than a "bad" habit.
    (C) One habit can displace another habit.
    (D) Habits can be helpful in dealing with completely new situations.

48. Which of the following is an assumption on which the author's logic depends?
    (A) It is not necessary to pay active attention to a task in order to do it well.
    (B) A nurse must address a patient's illness-accepting habits in order for the patient to become healthy.
    (C) A tremendous effort of will overcomes negative habits of thinking.
    (D) People who have gone through the hard work to become a nurse will empathize with the hard work a patient must do to change unhealthy attitudes to healthy ones.

49. According to the passage, which of the following should be done by nurses who find that their habitual reaction to patients exhibiting invalidism is negative?
    (A) Pay little attention to the patient's minor ailments.
    (B) Pay keen attention to the details of the patient's situation.
    (C) Do not give in when overpowering emotion is aroused.
    (D) Apply tremendous will power to resist their usual reaction.

50. Which of the following would help determine whether a patient has an unwholesome mental attitude?
    (A) The patient requests aspirin every hour.
    (B) The patient requests aspirin only when in discomfort.
    (C) The patient requests aspirin after trying breathing exercises for pain control.
    (D) The patient cannot remember ordering aspirin or other medications.

51. The author suggests that caring for a patient with comfort
    (A) can reinforce a patient's bad habits.
    (B) encourages the patient to fight old habits.
    (C) is not possible the first time a nurse tries it.
    (D) can cause a nurse to fall into invalidism.

52. All of the following are given by the author as examples of a task that a nurse may have initially struggled with but eventually learned to do naturally EXCEPT:
    (A) learning where things belong
    (B) making a bed
    (C) exercising
    (D) thinking out the work for the day

53. Based on the passage, which of the following does the author claim is NOT a positive thing for nurses to do?
    (A) Be cheerful when there is little cause for cheer
    (B) Converse with patients while trying to perform complex tasks
    (C) Encourage patients to report minor complaints
    (D) Withhold privileges from a patient who fails to display health-building attitudes

BIOLOGICAL AND BIOCHEMICAL FOUNDATIONS OF LIVING SYSTEMS

Time: 95 minutes
59 Questions

> **DIRECTIONS:** The majority of questions in this section are organized into groups, with each group containing a descriptive passage. Review the passage, and then select the one best answer for each question. Some questions are not drawn from a passage and are also independent of the other questions. When answering questions, eliminate the choices that you are sure are incorrect and then choose the best remaining answer. When you have chosen an answer, mark it in the corresponding location on the answer sheet. A periodic table can be found on the back of your answer sheet. You may consult it as needed.

PASSAGE I

Bovine spongiform encephalopathy (BSE) is a fatal neurological disorder commonly referred to as mad cow disease. BSE and related diseases such as scrapie are collectively known as transmissible spongiform encephalopathies (TSE) because the brain becomes riddled with holes. This deterioration of the brain leads to severe neurological symptoms including impaired movement, loss of cognitive function, strange behavior, and, ultimately, death. Although the exact nature of these diseases is not completely understood, a misfolded brain protein seems to be the causative agent. Misfolding of a normal cellular prion (proteinaceous infectious particle) protein, PrP^C, into an abnormal scrapie form, PrP^{Sc} creates a domino effect in the brain because when PrP^{Sc} interacts with PrP^C, the normal protein is converted into the abnormal form, and the number of infectious proteins exponentially increases.

PrP^C and PrP^{Sc} are chemically similar, but they can be distinguished by conformational differences and resistance to proteinase K. The misfolding of the protein is believed to be associated with molecular chaperone family Hsp70. Hsp70 proteins bind to unfolded proteins to facilitate correct folding pathways.

A group of students was asked to explore the minor differences between BSE and scrapie in hamsters, as well as the structural differences between PrP^C and PrP^{Sc}.

Experiment 1 was conducted to measure the amount of Hsp70 and PrP in normal, scrapie-infected, and BSE-infected hamsters. Students isolated Hsp70, normal and infectious PrP, and actin in a Western blot to visualize the relative amount of each protein in each hamster tissue sample (see Figure 1).

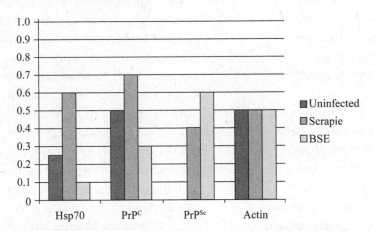

Figure 1. Relative protein values derived from a Western blot

Experiment 2 was conducted to investigate the structural differences between cellular PrP^C and infectious PrP^{Sc}. Previous literature revealed that a specific section of PrP^{Sc} from amino acid residue 27 to amino acid residue 53 contained most of the structural changes, and students were able to cleave the protein at these residues (see Table 1).

Table 1 Percentage of Secondary Structures

Prion	α-helix %	β-sheet %
PrP^C	45	15
PrP^{Sc}	21	39
PrP^{Sc} 27-53	7	76

1. Which of the following identifies a way in which PrP^Sc is distinct from other infectious agents such as viruses and bacteria?
   (A) It is unable to multiply on its own without the use of the host.
   (B) It does not contain nucleic acid.
   (C) It does not contain any amino acids.
   (D) It is able to multiply on its own without the use of the host.

2. Assuming that the students' results were accurate, which of the following is the most probable sequence of events after a cow is infected with BSE?
   (A) Chaperone proteins are up-regulated creating an influx of PrP^C. This rapid folding leads to more mistakes by Hsp70, creating infectious prions. The infectious prions convert normal protein prions and grow at an exponential rate to destroy neuronal tissue, leaving holes in the brain.
   (B) Chaperone proteins are destroyed, preventing correct folding of the prion protein, and the protein is misfolded with more β-sheets. The infectious prions convert normal proteins to prions and grow at an exponential rate to destroy neuronal tissue, leaving holes in the brain.
   (C) Hsp70 proteins are destroyed by the virus preventing correct folding of the α-helices. The prions containing excess β-sheets are unable to function correctly and cause damage to neuronal tissue. The infectious prions convert normal protein prions and grow at an exponential rate to destroy neuronal tissue, leaving holes in the brain.
   (D) Hsp70 is up-regulated creating an overproduction of PrP^C. This rapid influx leads to misfolded prions due to resistance to proteinase K. The misfolded prions convert normal protein prions and grow at an exponential rate to destroy neuronal tissue, leaving holes in the brain.

3. Which of the following can be inferred about actin from its use in Experiment 1?
   (A) Actin is a protein present in all eukaryotic cells and is unaffected by TSEs.
   (B) Actin is a protein up-regulated by Hsp70.
   (C) Actin is a type of microfilament that is present only in the cerebral spinal fluid of hamsters.
   (D) Actin is resistant to proteinase K.

4. Based on information from Experiment 1, which factor must be kept constant by the students in all samples while measuring the relative amount of protein?
   (A) The amount of proteinase K used to digest protein
   (B) The amount of agarose used in the Western blot
   (C) The amount of actin in each tissue sample
   (D) The amount of time PrP^Sc is allowed to incubate in tissue samples

5. Genetically engineering PrP-deficient farm animals has become of practical interest to researchers because the only way to guarantee protection against prion infections is the absence of PrP. However, the normal physiological function of PrP in animals remains unknown. Currently, genetic testing with knockout mice has been inconclusive. Which of the following is a probable alternative way to deactivate or avoid PrP^Sc without interfering with the normal role of cellular PrP?
   (A) Design an enzyme that targets proteins with exceptionally high α-helix content, rendering the infectious PrP nonfunctional.
   (B) Model a peptide fragment that binds to cellular PrP to stabilize its conformation and prevent misfolding.
   (C) Create an agent that degrades Hsp70 proteins but leaves PrP unaltered.
   (D) Model a peptide fragment that binds amino acid residues 27-53 of PrP^Sc to stabilize those residues in the β-sheet conformation.

The following questions do not refer to a descriptive passage and are not related to each other.

6. What would be the strongest expected intermolecular interaction between sodium acetate (the solute) and water (the solvent) in a solution?
   (A) Hydrogen bonding
   (B) Dipole–dipole interaction
   (C) Ion–dipole interaction
   (D) Dispersion forces

7. What would be an unlikely physical property of a monosaccharide?
   (A) Soluble in organic solvents
   (B) High melting point
   (C) Sweet taste
   (D) Hydrogen bond

8. What is the A+T/G+C ratio in a given species if adenine makes up 30% of bases?
   (A) 3:1
   (B) 3:2
   (C) 2:3
   (D) 1:3

9. A spirometer is used to measure a lung vital capacity of 4800 ml. Total lung capacity is estimated at 6000 ml. The difference between the two measurements reflects:
   (A) tidal volume.
   (B) expiratory reserve volume.
   (C) inspiratory reserve volume.
   (D) residual volume.

PASSAGE II

Obesity continues to increase in the United States as well as in other developed countries, contributing to several life-threatening diseases such as heart disease, hypertension, and type II diabetes. According to the Centers for Disease Control and Prevention (CDC), more than 80 percent of people with type II diabetes are obese or overweight. The pathology of diabetes includes renal failure, blindness, amputation of the extremities, heart disease, and neuropathy due to the tissues becoming insensitive to insulin. As the number of cases of type II diabetes associated with obesity continues to rise, it is important for medical science to understand the pathology and biochemistry behind the disease.

Although the inability to create insulin by type I diabetics is an autoimmune disease, the insulin resistance seen in type II diabetes is often a consequence of excess intake of lipids that the body is unable to store in adipose tissue and is instead stored in the liver and muscle tissue. Studies show that diet, exercise, and medication can help type II diabetics by aiding the liver in fatty acid metabolism, shifting metabolism toward fatty acid oxidation instead of synthesis and stimulating insulin production by the pancreas. Several hormones and enzymes play a role in energy homeostasis and metabolism and can be heavily influenced by diet and exercise. For example, when exercising, the body produces more AMP to be used by adenosine monophosphate-activated protein kinase (AMPK) for oxidation of fatty acids. When eating, the body produces more ATP, shifting metabolism toward the synthesis of fatty acids. Medications can also be used to manipulate metabolism by acting on these hormones and enzymes, as shown in Table 1.

Table 1 Various Treatments for Type II Diabetes

Prevention/ Treatment	Cellular Target	Desired Effect	Side Effects
Healthy Diet	Triacylglycerides	Restores lipid capacity in adipose tissue and restores insulin sensitivity	None
Exercise	AMPK	Aids weight loss through inhibition of fatty acid synthesis	None
Glucophage	AMPK	Increases glucose uptake in muscle and decreases glucose uptake in liver	Bloating, gas, upset stomach, and diarrhea
Amaryl	Pancreatic β cells	Stimulates insulin secretion	Low blood glucose levels, rash, and upset stomach
Avandia	PPARγ	Controls and activates expression of genes to increase action of insulin in liver and increases glucose uptake, decreasing glucose synthesis in liver	Increased risk of congestive heart failure, cold symptoms, frequent vomiting, and shortness of breath
Actos	PPARγ	Same as for Avandia above	Swelling, fluid retention, and nausea

10. An overweight 17-year-old patient with a family history of diabetes presents with symptoms such as lightheadedness, sweating and shaking, fatigue, and frequent urination. Which of the following would best determine whether this patient has type I or type II diabetes?

(A) A glucose tolerance test would determine whether blood glucose levels are abnormal.

(B) The patient's age is sufficient to determine that the patient has type I diabetes.

(C) The patient's weight is sufficient to determine that the patient has type II diabetes.

(D) An autoantibody test would determine the patient's autoimmunity.

11. Which of the following statements accurately describes AMPK?

(A) It is an enzyme activated by increased levels of AMP, and it is able to shift metabolism of fats toward oxidation.

(B) It is an enzyme activated by increased levels of AMP, and it is able to shift metabolism of fats toward synthesis.

(C) It is an enzyme activated by increased levels of ATP, and it is able to shift metabolism of fats toward oxidation.

(D) It is an enzyme activated by increased levels of ATP, and it is able to shift metabolism of fats toward synthesis.

12. Based on the information in Table 1, PPARγ is:

(A) protease.

(B) a transcription factor.

(C) kinase.

(D) G-protein.

13. A mouse gene that plays a role in appetite regulation has been discovered. This gene is labeled *DB* for diabetic because when a mouse has two defective copies (*db/db*), the mouse will be obese and diabetic. The *DB* gene codes for a leptin receptor in the brain that receives a signal to reduce fuel intake and increase energy usage. Which of the following is most likely leptin's role in a normal mouse?

(A) A gene that codes for triacylglycerides, increasing the amount of adipose tissue

(B) A hormone that controls appetite, maintaining insulin sensitivity and adipose capacity

(C) A hormone that controls appetite, decreasing insulin sensitivity and adipose capacity

(D) An enzyme that inhibits fatty acid oxidation

14. The figure below shows insulin levels in relation to the time a normal person consumes food. Assuming that meals are eaten at 8:30 A.M., 11:30 A.M., and 4:30 P.M., which of the following charts most accurately depicts the insulin levels of a type II diabetic?

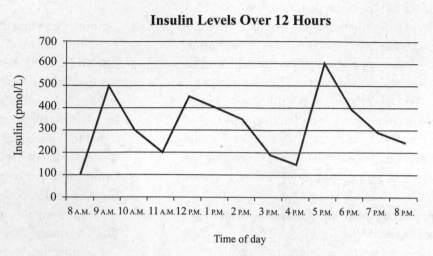

Insulin levels of a person without diabetes

(A)

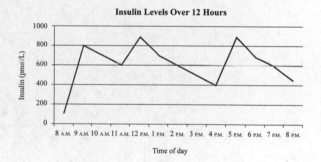

(B)

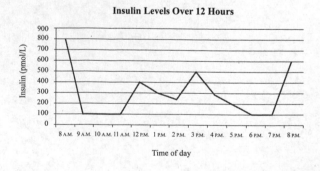

(C)

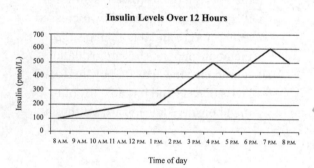

(D) None of the above; someone with type II diabetes is unable to produce insulin.

PASSAGE III

Pancreatitis is a gastrointestinal disorder characterized by extensive pain in the abdominal area surrounding the pancreas. In pancreatitis, the pancreas becomes inflamed and may cease normal functioning. Abdominal tenderness and vomiting frequently accompany pancreatitis. Dehydration may result from extensive vomiting. The heart rate and breathing rate are elevated in patients with pancreatitis. A high rate of mortality is associated with untreated acute pancreatitis.

Although there are several causes of pancreatitis, two causative factors are predominant: alcoholism and blockage by gallstones. Alcohol usage is associated with chronic pancreatitis. Gallstone blockage results in acute pancreatitis. The blood serum enzymes (serum amylase and lipase) are often elevated in pancreatitis.

Treatment of pancreatitis is designed to alleviate the severe pain and to minimize inflammation of the pancreas. Narcotic pain relievers are provided and oral ingestion of food is limited. For blockages due to gallstones, resection (removal) of the pancreas may be necessary should the blockage not resolve after a few days.

Recent evidence suggests that in some cases the hydrolytic enzymes secreted by the pancreas are activated prior to release into the duodenum. It has been hypothesized that the resulting tissue destruction can lead to bacterial infection (abscesses) characteristic of acute pancreatitis.

15. In a patient with a gallstone blockage, digestion of which nutrient would be LEAST affected?
    (A) Starches
    (B) Proteins
    (C) Lipids
    (D) Monosaccharides

16. In the pancreatic abscess cited in the last paragraph, all of the following would be expected to be found EXCEPT:
    (A) macrophages.
    (B) viruses.
    (C) bacteria.
    (D) antigens on the surface of bacterial cell walls.

17. Acute pancreatitis would be expected to most affect the blood levels of which of the following?
    (A) Albumin
    (B) Sodium
    (C) Chloride
    (D) Glucose

18. If the hypothesis about the early activation of hydrolytic enzymes mentioned in the last paragraph is correct, then which of the following can be concluded about a person experiencing this early activation?
    (A) They do not have mutations in the DNA exons coding for the hydrolytic enzymes.
    (B) Pancreatic lipase will be found in the blood.
    (C) Treatment for acute pancreatitis for the person should not be delayed.
    (D) In a laboratory setting, the hydrolytic enzymes isolated from the pancreatic duct of the person show a higher ratio than normal of pancreatic enzymes to zymogens.

19. Suppose a form of pancreatitis was determined by the presence of recessive alleles on two autosomal genes in a simple Mendelian manner. For a family affected by the disorder, which of the following could NOT be true?
    (A) Two normal parents have children who are affected.
    (B) Two affected parents have normal children.
    (C) The two genes are not linked.
    (D) Individuals who are heterozygous on both genes are not affected by the disorder.

PASSAGE IV

Vitamin D is known to stimulate the absorption of calcium from ingested food. A research study was carried out to determine the effect on blood calcium levels when different quantities of vitamin D were present in a subject's diet. Although several methods exist to measure the amount of calcium in blood, it was decided to remove aliquots of blood for laboratory analysis of the calcium concentration.

Patients were selected at random from a sample of convenience: male and female patients from an urban clinic. The patients ranged in age from 18 years to 65 years. No patient was selected who had a known condition that would prevent absorption of calcium or the action of vitamin D. The subjects were asked to save a sample of the food they consumed so it could be analyzed for vitamin D and calcium content. Blood samples were taken every other day for two weeks.

Bioavailability is defined as the ratio of a chemical's concentration in blood to its concentration in food. Chemicals with high bioavailability are readily absorbed into systemic circulation. Low bioavailability may limit the effectiveness of a pharmaceutical.

The researchers determined the amounts of calcium and vitamin D in the food using standard food chemistry protocols. The blood samples were analyzed for calcium content and the bioavailability was computed for each patient when a blood sample was taken. Representative results for two patients are shown in Figure 1 and Figure 2 below. The researchers concluded that an increase in vitamin D in the diet led to a higher bioavailability of calcium.

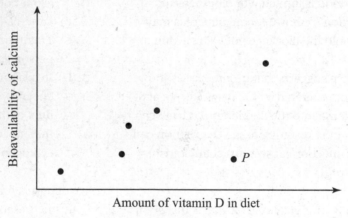

Figure 1.

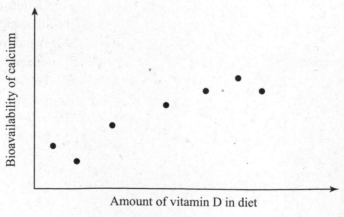

Figure 2.

20. The most probable reason for the outlier data point *P* in Figure 1 is that:
    (A) the patient took a supplement of vitamin D and did not provide a sample of the supplement.
    (B) the measured concentration of calcium in the patient's food was higher than the true value.
    (C) the patient has a disease that increases calcium uptake.
    (D) the patient has a chronic, ongoing hypocalcemia disorder, a disease in which calcium uptake is altered independently of vitamin D levels in the diet.

21. During the patient evaluation process, several patients reported chronic constipation. Evaluation of these patients' data showed lower bioavailability values for calcium compared to other patients. A hypothesis was proposed that the constipation results in lowered gut motility and less calcium ingested. Which of the following, if true, would best support the hypothesis?
    (A) The patients experiencing constipation ate less food.
    (B) The patients experiencing constipation had higher than normal levels of vitamin D in their food.
    (C) A few patients who did not report constipation also showed lower bioavailability of calcium.
    (D) A few patients who did not report constipation were on a low calorie diet.

22. A reviewer pointed out that the researchers did not screen the subjects for osteoporosis, or weakening of the bones. A patient with osteoporosis would be expected to have which of the following?
    (A) High osteoclast activity and high osteoblast activity
    (B) High osteoclast activity and low osteoblast activity
    (C) Low osteoclast activity and high osteoblast activity
    (D) Low osteoclast activity and low osteoblast activity

23. An underlying assumption the researchers made in interpreting the results of the study was:
    (A) the patients had low levels of calcitonin.
    (B) the patients had high levels of calcitonin.
    (C) the vitamin D level in the blood was the same for each individual.
    (D) the calcium level in blood was only due to dietary calcium.

24. In the experimental design, any of the following could have been a controlled variable EXCEPT:
    (A) The vitamin D content of the participants' food
    (B) The calcium content of the participants' food
    (C) The ratio of calcium in the blood to calcium in the food intake
    (D) The age of the participants

PASSAGE V

The first major reaction pathway that occurs during aerobic and anaerobic respiration is glycolysis. The purpose of glycolysis is to extract the energy from a molecule of glucose by releasing free energy in the form of ATP and NADH, and the result of this extraction is the formation of two molecules of pyruvate. The energy provided from aerobic respiration is vital to many of the cellular processes in the body, but after a period of fasting or strenuous exercise, the body needs to synthesize more glucose through a process called gluconeogenesis.

Gluconeogenesis and glycolysis share many of the same steps, but they are not the same reactions running in opposite directions. Seven of the steps in gluconeogenesis are simply the reverse of the reaction steps in glycolysis, but three of the steps are catalyzed by different enzymes because those reactions are irreversible and are highly exergonic.

The conversion of fructose-6-phosphate (F6P) to fructose 1,6-bisphosphate (F16BP) is the commitment step in glycolysis and is shown in reaction (1). The enzyme that catalyzes this step is phosphofructokinase-1 (PFK-1). The step that opposes reaction (1) in gluconeogenesis is catalyzed by fructose 1,6-bisphosphatase-1 (FBP-1) and is shown in reaction (2).

$$\text{Fructose 6-phosphate} \xrightarrow[\text{}]{\text{ATP} \quad \text{PFK-1} \quad \text{ADP}} \text{Fructose 1,6-bisphosphate} \quad (1)$$

$$\text{Fructose 1,6-bisphosphate} \xrightarrow[\text{}]{\text{ADP} \quad \text{FBP-1} \quad \text{ATP}} \text{Fructose 6-phosphate} \quad (2)$$

Regulation of glycolysis and gluconeogenesis requires several different enzymes, but reactions (1) and (2) are specifically regulated by fructose 2,6-bisphosphate (F26BP). F26BP stimulates PFK-1 in favor of glycolysis and inhibits FBP-1 to prevent gluconeogenesis.

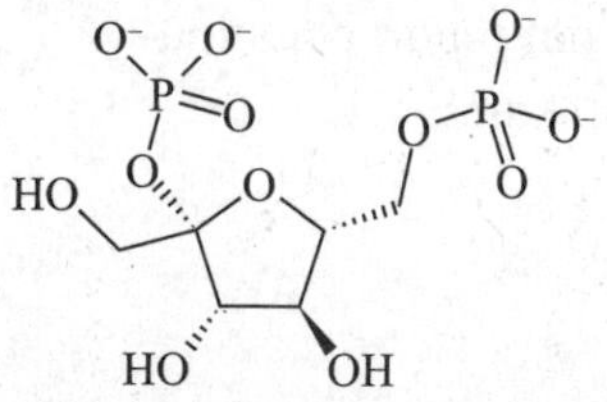

Figure 1. Chemical structure of fructose 2,6-bisphosphate

F26BP binds to PFK-1 allosterically to increase the enzyme's affinity for its substrate. On the other hand, when F26BP binds to FBP-1, it changes conformation to significantly reduce affinity for its substrate. Cellular concentration of F26BP is influenced by the hormones insulin and glucagon.

25. PFK-1 does which of the following?
    (A) Adds a phosphate group to fructose 6-phosphate
    (B) Removes a phosphate group from fructose 6-phosphate
    (C) Adds a phosphate group to fructose 1,6-bisphosphate
    (D) Removes a phosphate group from fructose 1,6-bisphosphate

26. Which of the following free-energy change values most likely corresponds to reaction (1)?
    (A) 22 kJ/mol because the reaction is spontaneous and energy is absorbed
    (B) 22 kJ/mol because the reaction is spontaneous and energy is released
    (C) –22 kJ/mol because the reaction is spontaneous and energy is released
    (D) –22 kJ/mol because the reaction is nonspontaneous and energy is released

27. Which of the following best describes the mechanism by which allosteric inhibition inhibits the function of an enzyme?
    (A) It binds to the substrate and induces the substrate's inactive conformation by changing the shape of the substrate.
    (B) It binds to the substrate on an area other than the active site to prevent the enzyme from binding.
    (C) It binds to the active site of the enzyme to prevent the substrate from binding.
    (D) It binds to the enzyme and induces the enzyme's inactive conformation by changing the shape of the enzyme.

28. Which of the following is the structure of fructose 6-phosphate?

(A)
$CH_2OPO_3^{-2}$
|
$C = O$
|
$HO - C - H$
|
$H - C - OH$
|
$H - C - OH$
|
$CH_2OPO_3^{-2}$

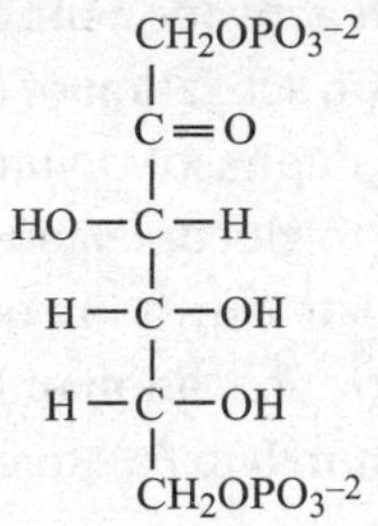

(B) 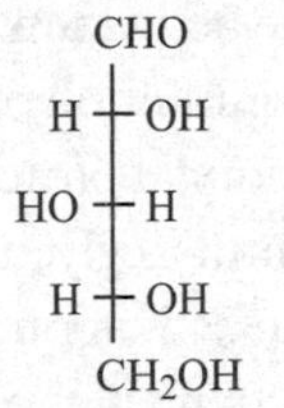
CHO
H — OH
HO — H
H — OH
CH_2OH

(C)
H   O
H — OH
HO — H
H — OH
H — OH
CH_2OH

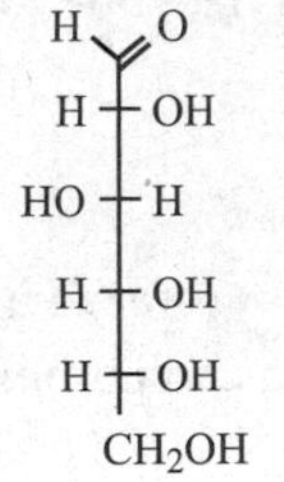

(D)
CH_2OH
|
$C = O$
|
$HO - C - H$
|
$H - C - OH$
|
$H - C - OH$
|
$CH_2OPO_3^{-2}$

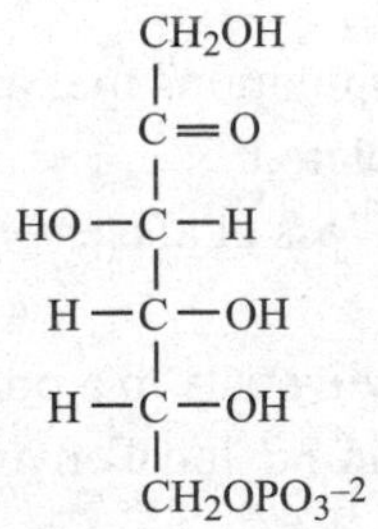

29. If insulin is increased, how will glycolysis/gluconeogenesis regulation be affected?
    (A) Insulin will inhibit activation of F26BP, leading to allosteric activation of FBP-1, which will dephosphorylate F16BP to commit to gluconeogenesis.
    (B) Insulin will stimulate activation of F26BP, leading to allosteric activation of PFK-1, which will phosphorylate F6P to commit to glycolysis.
    (C) Insulin will stimulate activation of F26BP, leading to allosteric inhibition of PFK-1, which will phosphorylate fructose 6-phosphate to commit to glycolysis.
    (D) Insulin will stimulate activation of F26BP, leading to allosteric activation of PFK-1, which will phosphorylate F6P to commit to gluconeogenesis.

The following questions do not refer to a descriptive passage and are not related to each other.

30. Genetic drift:
    (A) occurs in large populations that are geographically isolated.
    (B) results in random loss of alleles between generations.
    (C) increases genetic diversity in a population.
    (D) results in adaptation to local environments.

31. In human infants, gradual seasonal changes in environmental temperature trigger the hypothalamus to release thyrotropin-releasing hormone, which, in turn, stimulates the anterior pituitary to release thyroid-stimulating hormone (TSH). TSH acts on the thyroid to induce production of thyroid hormone. The physiological response to this hormone cascade is to:
    (A) increase metabolic rate.
    (B) dilate cutaneous blood vessels.
    (C) stimulate the parasympathetic nervous system.
    (D) decrease body temperature.

32. Benzoic acid was treated successively with the following reagents: 1. $SOCl_2$, 2. $(CH_3CH_2CH_2)_2CuLi$, 3. $LiAlH_4$, and 4. H_2O. The final product of this process would most likely be:

    (A)

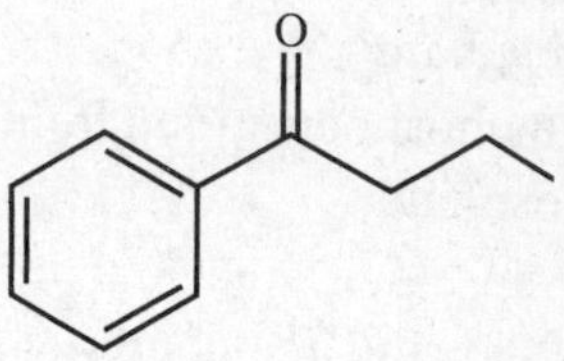

    (B)

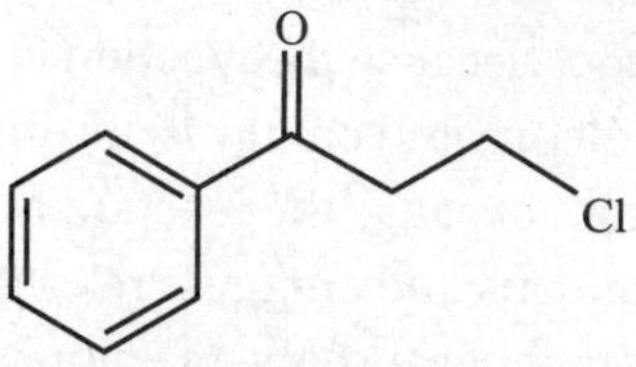

    (C)

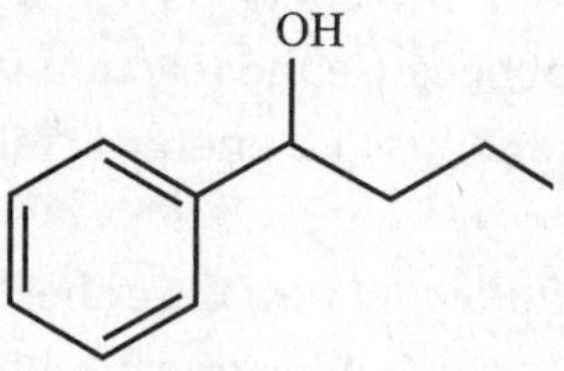

    (D)

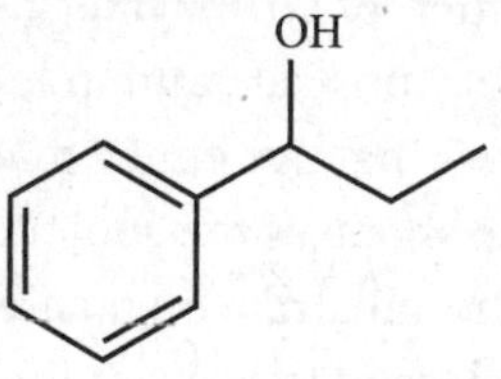

33. Which agent cannot be used to denature a protein?
    (A) Urea, a hydrogen bond disruptor
    (B) Ethanethiol, to break disulfide bonds
    (C) 0.005% sodium chloride, to break the peptide bond
    (D) Detergents, to disrupt the nonpolar core of a protein

PASSAGE VI

Glutamate is a nonessential amino acid that also acts as one of the primary excitatory neurotransmitters in the central nervous system, functioning in learning and memory storage.

Glutamate released by exocytosis from vesicles in presynaptic neuron terminals crosses the synaptic cleft and binds to postsynaptic receptors. One class of glutamate receptor, the NMDA receptor, is a nonspecific ligand-gated ion channel which, when activated by glutamate, allows influx of Ca^{2+} ions. If enough receptors are activated, changes in the electrochemical gradient will initiate an action potential in the postsynaptic neuron.

Termination of the excitatory signal occurs when extracellular glutamate is cleared from the synaptic cleft by transmembrane transport proteins found in both neurons and glial cells. Rapid uptake of glutamate by the glutamate transport protein EEAT2 is dependent on maintenance of the electrochemical gradient by the ATP dependent Na^+-K^+ pump.

If extracellular glutamate persists in the synaptic cleft, it can act as a neurotoxin. Brain injury such as stroke can result in excitotoxicity. Reductions in oxygen and glucose concentrations cause glutamate transporters to reverse direction, leading to postsynaptic mitochondrial damage and programmed cell death.

Glutamate excitotoxicity is thought to contribute to degenerative neurological disorders such as Alzheimer's disease and amyotrophic lateral sclerosis (ALS). Compound **A** is an experimental drug that is being tested for use in treating these disorders. Compound **A** deactivates NMDA receptors by acting as an antagonist, a drug that blocks the binding of a ligand to a receptor (see Figures 1 and 2).

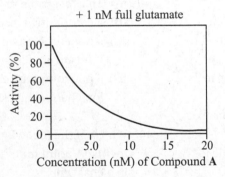

Figure 1. Effect of Compound **A** on activity of NMDA receptors

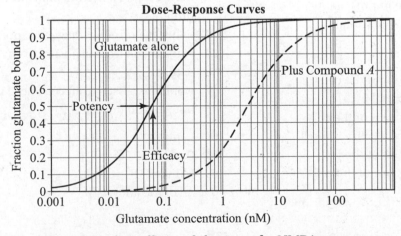

Figure 2. Binding affinity of glutamate for NMDA receptors in the presence and absence of Compound **A**

34. For glutamate to trigger an action potential, it must cause:
    (A) depolarization of the NMDA receptor.
    (B) depolarization of the postsynaptic neuron.
    (C) hyperpolarization of the postsynaptic neuron.
    (D) a threshold response in presynaptic resting potential.

35. An increase in extracellular glutamate concentration would:
    (A) increase learning and memory at low doses, and decrease learning and memory at high doses.
    (B) decrease learning and memory at low doses, and increase learning and memory at high doses.
    (C) show a steady increase in learning and memory with increasing concentration of glutamate.
    (D) show a steady decrease in learning and memory with increasing concentration of glutamate.

36. The result of oxygen and glucose deprivation to the brain is:
    (A) apoptosis of presynaptic neurons due to high levels of Na^+.
    (B) apoptosis of postsynaptic neurons due to high levels of Ca^{2+}.
    (C) mitochondrial damage in postsynaptic neurons due to high intracellular glutamate.
    (D) mitochondrial damage in presynaptic neurons due to high extracellular glutamate.

37. The electrochemical gradient of the cell is maintained at resting potential by:
    (A) simple diffusion of Na^+ out of the cell.
    (B) facilitated diffusion of Ca^{2+} into the cell.
    (C) active transport of K^+ out of the cell.
    (D) active transport of Na^+ out of the cell.

38. If Compound **A** is given to a patient suffering from stroke, the risk of damage due to glutamate excitotoxicity will:
    (A) increase, because both oxygen deprivation and Compound **A** will increase extracellular glutamate concentration.
    (B) decrease, because Compound **A** lowers the concentration of extracellular glutamate caused by oxygen deprivation.
    (C) decrease, because Compound **A** blocks the ability of glutamate to initiate a postsynaptic action potential.
    (D) neither increase nor decrease, since extracellular glutamate is taken up by glutamate transporters such as EEAT2.

39. As Compound **A** concentration increases, activity of NMDA receptors decreases. However, the effectiveness of Compound **A** was reduced by increasing extracellular glutamate concentration. This behavior suggests that Compound **A** acts on the NMDA receptor as:
    (A) an irreversible receptor antagonist.
    (B) a competitive receptor antagonist.
    (C) a noncompetitive receptor antagonist that binds to an allosteric site.
    (D) a noncompetitive antagonist that acts as an ion channel blocker.

40. Which of the following would be true statements? A point mutation of the EEAT2 gene in a glial cell:

    I. may result in a dysfunctional transport protein.
    II. may have no effect on gene expression.
    III. could result from exposure to environmental toxins.
    IV. would be passed from cell to cell via mitosis and meiosis.

    (A) I and III
    (B) II only
    (C) I, II, and III
    (D) All of the above

PASSAGE VII

Biofilms are layers (colonies) of unicellular organisms surrounding a surface. Biofilms are observed in many diverse areas such as marine environments and cooling water supplies for buildings. The presence of biofilms in food-processing equipment has serious implications for food safety.

The growth of biofilms has been investigated recently in an effort to develop effective countermeasures for use in food-processing environments. Scientists carried out the following three experiments to understand the growth and development properties of biofilms.

Experiment 1

Biofilms of bacterial species Q and bacterial species R were grown separately on a glass surface. A square portion of each was carefully excised and the two films were placed adjacent to each other with a 10 mm space between them. Upon observation for 72 hours, no growth was observed in the space between the two squares. The scientists concluded that bacterial species Q and R could not coexist in a biofilm. It was hypothesized that bacteria Q and/or R secreted a substance that inhibited the growth and adhesion of the other species.

Experiment 2

Bacterial species Q and R were homogenized using a blender. The scientists attempted to grow a biofilm from the mixed culture. The scientists measured the adhesion properties of the biofilm to a glass surface. The biofilm produced by using the mixture of species Q and R showed poor adhesion properties to the glass surface. The scientists were easily able to completely remove all bacteria on the surface.

Experiment 3

Bacterial species Q, R, and T were homogenized using a blender. The scientists attempted to grow a biofilm of the three species. The scientists measured the adhesion properties of the biofilm to a glass surface and found that the biofilm adhered as strongly to the surface as biofilms containing Q and R separately.

Figure 1 depicts a fourth experiment in which small cultures of Q, R, and T were placed separately on a culturing medium and allowed to grow. The results are shown at 15 minute intervals.

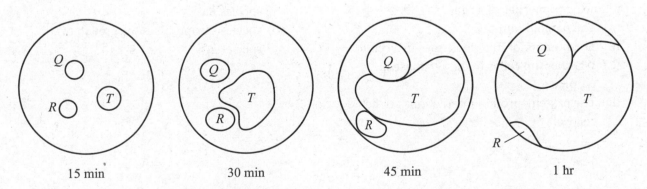

Figure 1. Experiment 4

41. The results of Experiment 2 could be explained using which of the following hypotheses?
    (A) Individually, species Q and R are unable to adhere to a glass surface.
    (B) Individually, species Q and R are non-colony-forming bacteria.
    (C) Either species Q or R secretes a substance that blocks prophase I in the other species.
    (D) Both Q and R secrete substances that block transcription of adhesion proteins in the other.

42. Which of the following inferences can be made solely from the results of Experiment 3?
    (A) Bacterial species T must suppress the growth of bacterial species Q and R.
    (B) Bacterial species T must affect the cell-cell communication pathways of species Q and/or R.
    (C) Bacterial species T has some properties that are different from the properties of bacteria Q and/or R.
    (D) Bacterial species Q and R must signal species T to increase its growth rate.

43. Which could NOT be a molecule or class of molecule secreted by bacterial species Q?
    (A) Ribonucleic acids
    (B) Deoxyribonucleic acids
    (C) Histones
    (D) β-Lactams

44. The ability of a biofilm to form on a surface most strongly depends on which of the following properties of a cell?
    (A) The haploid number
    (B) The number of free ribosomes in a cell
    (C) Whether the cell is in the G0 phase or G1 phase
    (D) The protein–protein interactions on the cell wall

45. Some bacteria are small enough to live within a host cell, such as an epithelial cell in the small intestine. Suppose some bacteria were able to infect the cells in the endoderm of an embryo. Which tissue or organ, in a newborn infant, would most likely be least damaged?
    (A) Eyes
    (B) Brain
    (C) Small intestinal epithelial cells
    (D) Hair follicles

46. In a food-processing plant, a biofilm of thickness 1.8 cm was discovered on the bottom of a food storage tank that was open to air. The bacteria living at the bottom of the biofilm were observed to be quite different biochemically from the bacteria living in the upper 0.2 cm of the biofilm. How can this fact be explained?
    (A) The bacteria on the upper 0.2 cm of the biofilm are facultative anaerobes.
    (B) The bacteria on the upper 0.2 cm of the biofilm are anaerobes.
    (C) The bacteria at the bottom of the biofilm are aerobes.
    (D) The bacteria at the bottom of the biofilm do not undergo glycolysis.

47. Based upon the results of Experiment 4, all of the following can be concluded EXCEPT:
    (A) species T grows at a faster rate than species Q and R.
    (B) species Q grows at a faster rate than species R.
    (C) species T influences the growth of species R.
    (D) species Q suppresses the growth of species T.

The following questions do not refer to a descriptive passage and are not related to each other.

48. Bile produced by the liver:
    (A) is secreted into the stomach to begin the breakdown of polypeptides.
    (B) is secreted with pancreatic enzymes to digest polysaccharides in the large intestine.
    (C) emulsifies triglycerides in the duodenum.
    (D) lowers the pH of the small intestine to aid in absorption of carbohydrates.

49. In gastropod mollusks, a midgut gland situated on top of the stomach functions in secretion of digestive enzymes and in detoxification, absorption, and excretion of the products of digestion and metabolism. These functions are performed by which of the following analogous organs in mammals?
    (A) Spleen and kidneys
    (B) Liver and pancreas
    (C) Bile duct and sweat glands
    (D) Stomach and small intestine

50. A dihybrid cross is a cross between two parents, each of which is heterozygous for two traits. In a dihybrid cross, what proportion of offspring are predicted to be heterozygous in one or both of the two traits?
    (A) All
    (B) $\frac{7}{8}$
    (C) $\frac{3}{4}$
    (D) $\frac{9}{16}$

51. Glycogen stored in animal muscles is the result of polymerization of which monomer?
    (A) Amino acids
    (B) Starch
    (C) Glucose
    (D) Nucleic acids

52. A developmental biologist is studying the M and m alleles of a particular gene in *D. melanogaster*. The scientist measures the frequency of the M allele (the dominant allele) in several generations. The results are shown below.

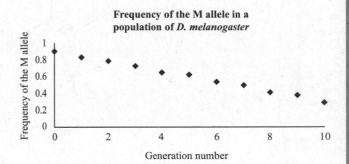

Frequency of the M allele in a population of *D. melanogaster*

All of the statements below are consistent with data presented above EXCEPT:
    (A) The frequency of heterozygotes in this study is greater than 0.1.
    (B) The M allele provides a higher fitness for *D. melanogaster* than does the m allele.
    (C) The M allele provides a lower fitness for *D. melanogaster* than does the m allele.
    (D) Neither MM nor Mm are embryo lethal.

PASSAGE VIII

It has been known for decades that a specific compound, 3-pentadecylcatechol (Structure **I**), found in the oil of poison ivy plants is largely responsible for the dermatitis-producing effect on human skin. Catechols (a general class of compounds where a benzene ring has two *ortho* substituted hydroxyl groups) are highly susceptible to oxidation, resulting in *ortho*-quinones. It is believed that the oxidation product of **I** is the active compound in a skin protein binding reaction that leads to antigen formation followed by an allergic response (see Scheme **I**).

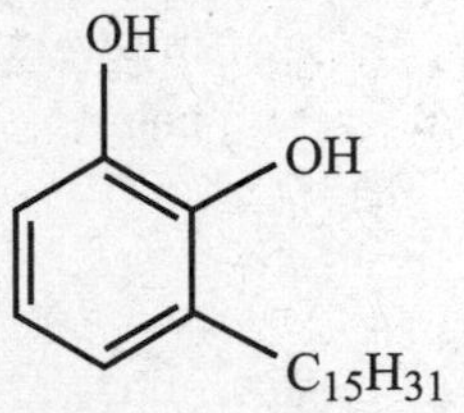

I

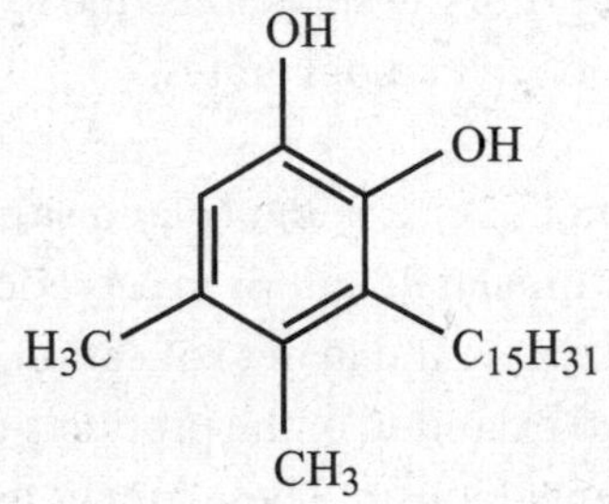

II

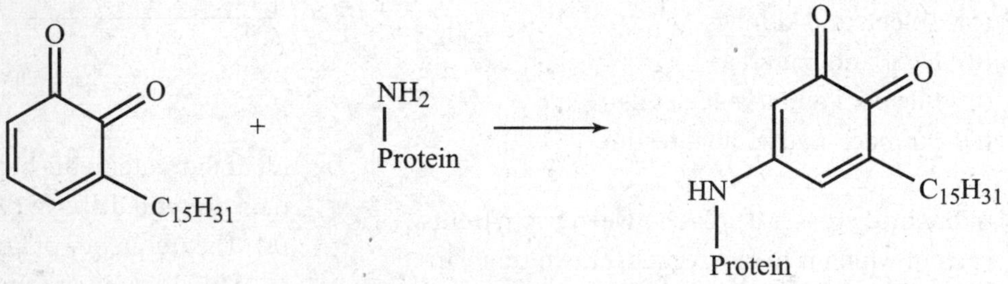

Scheme I

In an attempt to verify the allergic response mechanism, scientists synthesized an analog of **I** in which the proposed protein binding sites on the benzene ring were blocked by methyl groups (see Structure **II**). If the hypothesis concerning the compound's protein binding ability is correct, the analog, **II**, of Compound **I** should show a marked reduction in allergenic activity. Compound **II** was synthesized according to Scheme **II**, starting with 4,5-dimethylbenzene-1,2-diol (Compound **III**).

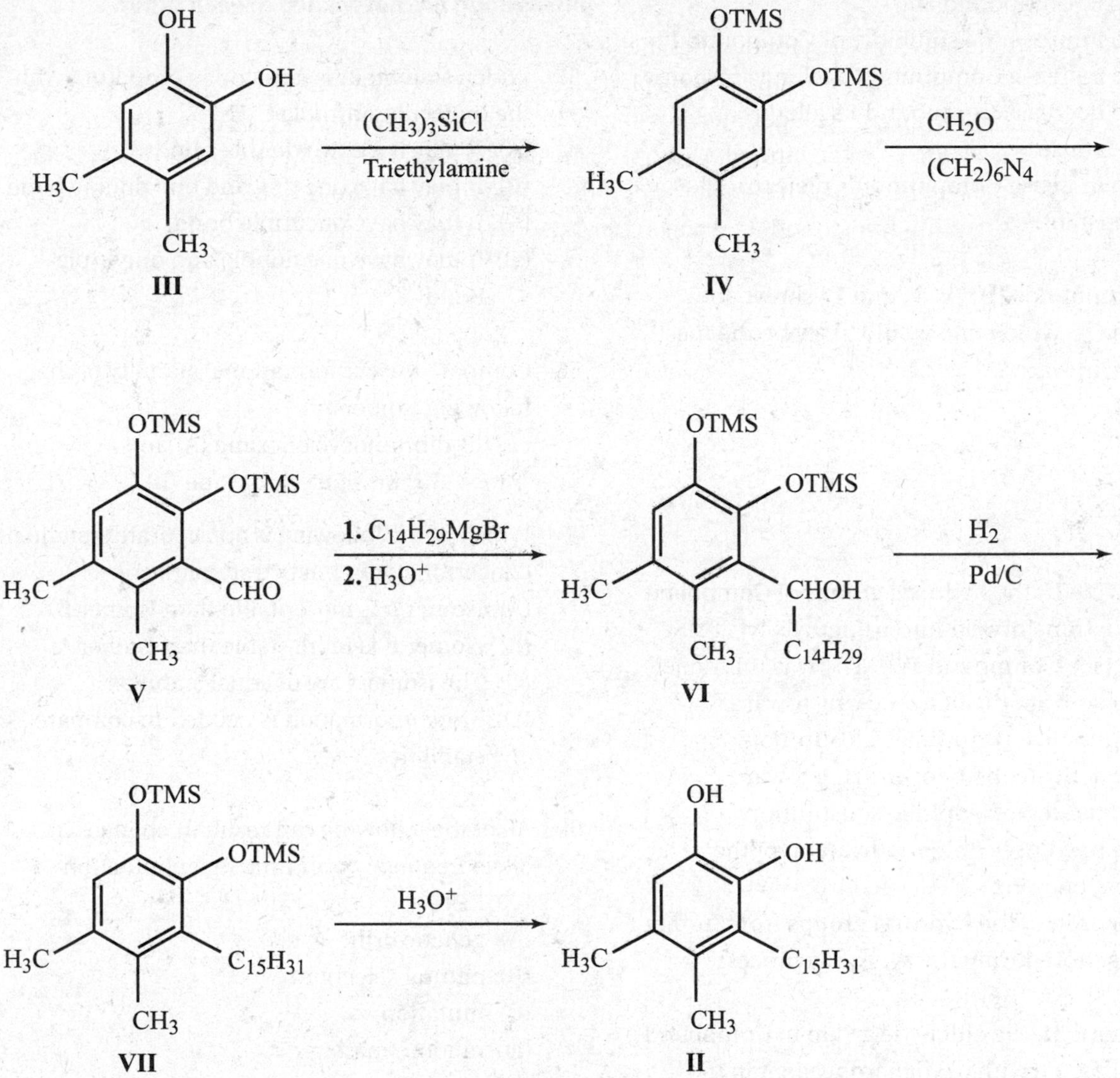

Scheme II

53. What is the proposed function of the methyl groups in Compound **II**?
    (A) To improve the solubility of Compound **I**
    (B) To increase Compound **I**'s allergic response
    (C) To decrease Compound **I**'s allergic response
    (D) To increase Compound **I**'s dielectric constant

54. Of Compounds **III**, **IV**, **V**, and **VI** shown in Scheme **II**, which one would likely be the most soluble in water?
    (A) **III**
    (B) **IV**
    (C) **V**
    (D) **VI**

55. In Scheme **II**, the hydroxyl groups of Compound **III** were transformed into trimethylsilyl (TMS) ethers (see Compound **IV**). Why was this done?
    (A) To activate the benzene ring toward aromatic electrophilic substitution
    (B) To activate the benzene ring toward aromatic nucleophilic substitution
    (C) To prevent further methylation of the benzene ring
    (D) To protect the hydroxyl groups from further reaction during the synthesis process

56. In Scheme **II**, the aldehyde group in Compound **V** was reacted with a Grignard reagent in the first step and then treated with aqueous acid (second step) to yield an alcohol. An appropriate solvent for step one of this process would be:
    (A) diethyl ether.
    (B) water.
    (C) ethanol.
    (D) acetone.

The following questions do not refer to a descriptive passage and are not related to each other.

57. Which statement is false for a compound with the molecular formula C_3H_4?
    (A) It may have two double bonds.
    (B) It may have one ring and one double bond.
    (C) It may have one triple bond.
    (D) It may have one double and one triple bond.

58. Compare the conformational stability of the following isomers:
    cis-1,3-dibromocyclohexane (A) and
    trans-1,3-dibromocyclohexane (B)

    Which of the following is an accurate statement concerning their relative stabilities?
    (A) Isomer A is more stable than isomer B.
    (B) Isomer B is more stable than isomer A.
    (C) The isomers are of equal stability.
    (D) More information is needed to compare stabilities.

59. All of the following can result in changes in allele frequency over time in a population EXCEPT:
    (A) genetic drift.
    (B) natural selection.
    (C) mutation.
    (D) random mating.

PSYCHOLOGICAL, SOCIAL, AND BIOLOGICAL FOUNDATIONS OF BEHAVIOR

Time: 95 minutes
    59 Questions

> **DIRECTIONS:** The majority of questions in this section are organized into groups, with each group containing a descriptive passage. Read the passage, and then select the one best answer for each question. Some questions are not drawn from a passage and are also independent of the other questions. When answering questions, eliminate the choices that you are sure are incorrect and then choose the best remaining answer. When you have chosen an answer, mark it in the corresponding location on the answer sheet.

PASSAGE I

A psychologist is conducting experiments on various aspects of perception. The experiments test individual subjects, one at a time.

Experiment 1

A subject is seated in a dark, soundproof room for 15 minutes. Then, a dot of red light of a single frequency is shown on the wall in front of the subject, starting faintly and then becoming increasingly brighter. The subject is asked to indicate the exact moment when the light first becomes visible. At that point the red light is turned off and an overhead 60-watt white light is turned on in the room. Every 30 seconds a buzzer sounds and a dot of bright red light is either flashed or not shown at all on the wall in front of the subject, who must report whether or not the red dot was shown. At the first buzzer, the subject reported seeing the red dot but in fact no red dot had been shown.

Experiment 2

A subject enters a dark, soundproof room and puts on a set of headphones. A tone of a single frequency is played through the headphones, starting faintly and increasing in volume. The subject is asked to indicate the exact moment when the sound first becomes audible. At that point the tone is played continuously at the same volume for three minutes. After three minutes the subject is told that at some point the volume will increase and is asked to indicate the exact moment at which the volume noticeably increases. The volume is increased by 0.5 percent every five seconds. After 35 seconds the subject reports that the volume has just noticeably increased.

At that point the volume is doubled and the sound is played at that volume for three minutes. After three minutes the subject is told that the volume will again increase at some point and is asked to report the exact moment at which the increase is noticeable. The volume is again increased by 0.5 percent every 5 seconds. In this trial, the subject does not report an increase of volume until 65 seconds.

1. In Experiment 1, using signal detection theory, what was the noise and what was the target stimulus in the experiment design?
   - (A) Target = faint red dot, noise = dark room
   - (B) Target = 60-watt light, noise = faint red dot and 30-second buzzer
   - (C) Target = bright red dot, noise = faint red dot
   - (D) Target = bright red dot, noise = 60-watt light and 30-second buzzer

2. Which of the following indicates a difference between Experiments 1 and 2 that makes the results of Experiment 2 less valid?
   - (A) Experiment 1 tests the perception of light in a dark room.
   - (B) Experiment 2 involves only sound, whereas Experiment 1 involves both light and sound.
   - (C) Experiment 2 allows the subject to begin the experiment immediately upon entering the room.
   - (D) In the second part of Experiment 1, the strength of the red light is not increased at a steady rate.

3. Which of the following best explains why it took the subject in Experiment 2 65 seconds to identify a volume increase in the second part of the experiment but only 35 seconds in the first part?
   - (A) The time required to identify a change in a stimulus varies directly with the frequency of the stimulus.
   - (B) The time required to identify a change in a stimulus varies directly with the strength of the stimulus.
   - (C) The ability to distinguish a change in a stimulus decreases during a long experiment.
   - (D) If a subject is told that a stimulus will increase, the subject is more likely to report an increase in the stimulus.

4. Which of the following is an aspect of perception theory that is incorporated in Experiment 2 but not in Experiment 1?
   - (A) Adaptation
   - (B) Perception threshold
   - (C) Difference threshold
   - (D) Top-down processing

5. In Experiment 1, the subject reported seeing the red dot when it had not been shown. This is an example of which of the following responses according to signal detection theory?
   - (A) Correct rejection
   - (B) Miss
   - (C) Hit
   - (D) False alarm

PASSAGE II

A male patient who had recently been involved in a serious automobile accident is being interviewed by a physician. The physician introduces herself as Dr. Montoya. The patient turns away to sit down as the physician puts on a lab coat and a pair of glasses and takes a seat behind her desk. The patient looks up and asks where Dr. Montoya is. The physician assures the patient that she is Dr. Montoya.

The physician places a glass of water on the desk and offers it to the patient, who reaches toward the glass but knocks it over. The patient apologizes, commenting that he did not think the glass was that close.

The physician asks the patient to report anything unusual that he has experienced since the accident. The patient reports having been sitting in his car stopped at a light and suddenly having the feeling that his car was moving backward on its own. When asked to explain, the patient reports that the car to his right was actually moving forward and that the only way he knew that it was the other car, and not his, that was moving was that his body did not feel like it was moving.

At the end of the interview Dr. Montoya points out that compared to before the accident, the patient's visual processing is worse and that the patient is exhibiting symptoms of post-traumatic stress. The patient responds by saying that the accident must have caused some damage.

6. Based on the patient's experience that his car was moving backward on its own, which of the following can be concluded?
    (A) His vestibular system was probably damaged in his recent accident.
    (B) His ability to distinguish background visual information from foreground information is impaired.
    (C) His vestibular system functioned normally during the incident.
    (D) Either his visual processing or his vestibular system did not function normally during the incident.

7. Which of the following strategies, if applied as he was reaching toward the glass of water, would be most likely to have helped the patient avoid knocking over the glass?
    (A) Looking first with one eye and then with the other
    (B) Using his left hand instead of his right
    (C) Blinking rapidly
    (D) Asking Dr. Montoya if he was getting close to the glass

8. If the patient also reported that he periodically felt dizzy and lost his balance, this would be most consistent with damage to the functioning of:
    (A) the kinesthetic sense.
    (B) the vestibular system.
    (C) perception of motion.
    (D) perception of depth.

9. Which one of the following conclusions is most supported by information in the passage?
    (A) The patient may have lost the sight in one eye.
    (B) The patient may have an impairment in long-term memory.
    (C) The patient may have an impairment in his vestibular system.
    (D) The patient may be nearsighted.

10. The patient's comment at the end of the passage is an example of which of the following?
    (A) Perceptual constancy
    (B) Bottom-up processing
    (C) Top-down processing
    (D) Applying a generalization to a specific incidence

11. The patient's failure to recognize Dr. Montoya after she put on her jacket and glasses is an example of which of the following?
    (A) Inability to use parallel processing
    (B) Charles Bonnet syndrome
    (C) Faulty binocular vision
    (D) Failure of perceptual constancy

The following questions do not refer to a descriptive passage and are not related to each other.

12. The idea that deviant behavior upholds society's norms and that the response to deviance actually brings people together in society illustrates what theoretical approach?
    (A) Functionalism
    (B) Conflict theory
    (C) Symbolic interactionism
    (D) Social constructionism

13. According to the information processing model, human beings use their senses to register data in the environment. The brain processes, interprets, and stores these perceptions, sometimes resulting in a verbal or nonverbal response called the:
    (A) yield.
    (B) opinion.
    (C) output.
    (D) feedback.

14. The alarm phase, the resistance phase, and the exhaustion phase describe how the body adapts physiologically to stress. These three stages comprise:
    (A) post-traumatic stress disorder.
    (B) the general adaptation syndrome.
    (C) generalized anxiety disorder.
    (D) the fight or flight response.

15. In isolation from the normal level of sensory input, the brain may compensate for the absence of stimuli by creating realistic hallucinatory images. This phenomenon is referred to as:
    (A) parallel processing.
    (B) accommodation.
    (C) sensory adaptation.
    (D) Charles Bonnet syndrome.

16. The act of not returning an appropriate greeting in an everyday situation is an example of:
    (A) violating mores.
    (B) a ritual.
    (C) assimilation.
    (D) violating a folkway.

PASSAGE III

A sociologist has published the results of a field study on two isolated tribes, X and Y.

Tribe X

Similar to many modernized societies, Tribe X relies on a male-dominated culture to create order and provide stability in society. Tribe X's androcentric culture places men into the role of providing for the material needs of the tribe. Men are considered to have exclusive moral responsibility for the acquisition of supplies through hunting. In addition, men are responsible for protection of the entire tribe and manual labor such as building homes. In contrast, the women serve as the caregivers and historians of society. Tasks such as childrearing and storytelling are the domain of the women. The study concludes that Tribe X society mirrors a preindustrial America and that because of its traditional view of gender roles, Tribe X society establishes an unequal balance of power in favor of the men.

Tribe Y

In contrast to Tribe X, Tribe Y has a more egalitarian assignment of roles as its norm. Tribe Y actively supports nontraditional gender roles by allowing both men and women to provide for society based on their ability rather than gender. Men who excel at childcare remain at home while women with strong hunting ability scout for game. Tribe Y typically has an overabundance of caregivers and a dearth of hunters, which leads to ongoing food shortages.

17. By valuing equal opportunity, Tribe Y causes which of the following?
    (A) Inequalities in task management
    (B) A power struggle for leadership
    (C) A society free from gender roles
    (D) Higher levels of efficiency than Tribe X

18. Based on the passage, which of the following is an example of a violation of Tribe X mores?
    (A) A father teaching his son how to hunt
    (B) The elderly chief telling stories during a festival
    (C) A women hunting to provide for her family
    (D) A child forgetting to fetch water

19. Which of the following conclusions is most supported by information in the passage?
    (A) Tribe Y lacks the ability to properly socialize their children.
    (B) Tribes Y and X have no gender roles in common.
    (C) Tribe X lacks a strong leadership.
    (D) Tribe X society has similarities to early American society.

20. If caregiving is considered a traditionally female role and hunting a traditionally male role, which of the following is probably true about Tribe Y?
    (A) More men than women are willing to take nontraditional roles.
    (B) The women who hunt are not particularly effective hunters.
    (C) The men do not like to hunt with a group of hunters consisting mostly of women.
    (D) When there is a food shortage, men and women who had been providing childcare change to hunting.

21. A study was conducted among both Tribe X and Tribe Y women who had never used any hunting weapons. The women were given a bow and arrows and asked to shoot at a target. Women from Tribe Y shot more accurately than women from Tribe X. Which of the following best explains these results?

(A) Women from Tribe X frequently watch the men shoot arrows.

(B) The women from Tribe Y knew women who shot arrows.

(C) The skills for shooting an arrow are similar to the skills for throwing a hunting spear.

(D) Women in Tribe X are more confident of their storytelling skills than are women of Tribe Y.

22. What is a disadvantage of Tribe X role allocation?

(A) Prescribed roles based on gender ignore individual strengths.

(B) It gives members an exact description of their role in society.

(C) Men who excel at childcare are not as nurturing as women who excel at childcare.

(D) An overabundance of hunters would lead to a shortage of childcare providers.

The following questions do not refer to a descriptive passage and are not related to each other.

23. According to the DSM-5, one of the central criteria for diagnosis of an intellectual developmental disorder is an IQ score lower than:

(A) 45.

(B) 70.

(C) 90.

(D) 100.

24. Sanctions that reward or punish behavior are mechanisms for:

(A) anticipatory socialization.

(B) stigmatizing.

(C) normative social influence.

(D) social control.

25. A patient who has been on dialysis for six months has recently had trouble remembering recent events, has trouble recognizing family members, and has started crafting elaborate lies. The doctor suspects that the dialysis has caused a thiamine deficiency in the patient, resulting in which of the following?

(A) Korsakoff's syndrome

(B) Alzheimer's disease

(C) Schizophrenia

(D) Generalized anxiety disorder

PASSAGE IV

One cause of memory loss is Korsakoff's disease, which is brought on by a lack of thiamine in the brain. The lack of thiamine is often associated with extreme malnutrition or alcoholism. A person with Korsakoff's typically suffers permanent brain damage due to the structural effects of the thiamine deficiencies. Individuals with Korsakoff's often have large gaps in their memory and create untrue memories to fill in those gaps to help maintain an identity in the absence of memory. Another cause of memory loss is Parkinson's disease, although this symptom is not as well known as the inevitable tremors that characterize the disease. Parkinson's disease is associated with the death of brain cells responsible for producing dopamine.

An 86-year-old female goes to the doctor with her daughter. The daughter reports that her mother has the following symptoms: decrease in appetite, indigestion, sleeping all the time, a loss of interest in family activities that she used to enjoy, and chronic forgetfulness. The mother's husband died suddenly of a stroke six months ago. However, the mother's symptoms have progressed gradually over the last three years. The daughter explains that her mother sometimes has difficulty finding the right words and then stops talking in the middle of a sentence. The mother's walking is normal and her hands are steady, but she often does not know what day or time it is. The mother sometimes does not remember how to dress herself. The daughter reports that her mother has a history of heavy drinking but has been sober for ten years.

The doctor orders a series of blood tests, an EKG, and a PET scan. The blood tests reveal moderately high blood sugar and moderately low levels of thiamine. The EKG results are normal. The PET scan shows amyloid plaque build up in the brain.

26. Based on the passage, which of the following is the most likely diagnosis of the mother's condition?
    - (A) Parkinson's disease
    - (B) Korsakoff's syndrome
    - (C) Amnesia
    - (D) Alzheimer's

27. Forgetting how to dress herself properly is an example of deficits in what kind of memory?
    - (A) Semantic memory
    - (B) Short-term memory
    - (C) Heptatic memory
    - (D) Procedural memory

28. The doctor tests the mother's memory by asking what she had to eat on the day that she played Bingo last week. What strategy is the doctor using in order to help the mother remember?
    - (A) Spreading activation theory, because it is easier to remember food than more abstract events
    - (B) Spreading activation theory, because he is referring to a memory associated with the target memory
    - (C) Primacy, because she ate before she played Bingo
    - (D) Primacy, because eating is a primary reinforcement

29. What comorbid mental health conditions should the doctor in the passage consider?
    - (A) Alcohol use disorder
    - (B) Bereavement
    - (C) Parkinson's
    - (D) Separation anxiety disorder

30. A supervisor has just dictated a list of five items that an employee is to purchase at a store, at which point the fire alarm goes off in the building. After a few minutes, an announcement indicates that the alarm was a false one. At the store, the employee remembers the first, second, and last items from the list but cannot remember the others. Which of the following statements accurately describes a psychological theory explaining the employee's behavior?

(A) The employee suffered a disruption in semantic knowledge in response to a traumatic event.

(B) The employee's memory failure occurred because information was not encoded and stored in memory.

(C) The recency effect prevented the employee from remembering earlier items in the list.

(D) The flashbulb memory formed when the alarm sounded, inhibiting the later retrieval of memories.

31. The doctor in the passage asked the mother what she did on her last vacation and the mother said that she took a vacation to the Fiji Islands. The daughter stated that no such trip took place. The mother's response is an example of:

(A) confabulation, a fabricated memory without intent of personal gain.

(B) hallucination, false sense impressions that can occur with dementia.

(C) manipulation, a falsehood told to achieve a particular end or goal.

(D) persuasion, a true or false statement made to change another person's attitude.

PASSAGE V

A researcher examines the relationship between the "Big Five" personality traits and individuals with generalized anxiety disorder. The Big Five personality traits are openness, conscientiousness, extraversion, agreeableness, and neuroticism. The researcher surveys two groups—a group of randomly selected people without generalized anxiety disorder and a group selected randomly from a pool of people with generalized anxiety disorder. Members of each group received an explanation of each of the Big Five personality traits and were asked to determine which one trait was most dominant in their personality. The results are shown below.

Table 1 Control Group Primary Traits

Control Group, $n = 500$	
Openness	20%
Conscientiousness	20%
Extraversion	25%
Agreeableness	25%
Neuroticism	10%

Table 2 Experimental Group Primary Traits

Experimental Group, $n = 100$	
Openness	20%
Conscientiousness	25%
Extraversion	5%
Agreeableness	15%
Neuroticism	35%

32. In MRI studies, the personality trait of extraversion was positively correlated with increased size of the medial orbitofrontal cortex. This region of the brain processes information about rewards for behavior. Based on this and Tables 1 and 2, which of the following conclusions can be made?
    - (A) Increased size of the medial orbitofrontal cortex is a cause of generalized anxiety disorder.
    - (B) Compared to the general public, people with generalized anxiety disorder have an enlarged medial orbitofrontal cortex.
    - (C) People with generalized anxiety disorder are more likely to act impulsively than the general public.
    - (D) People with generalized anxiety disorder respond differently to positive reinforcement than does the general public.

33. Which of the following predictions about the behavior of people with generalized anxiety disorder in comparison with the general public is best supported by the passage?
    - (A) They are better organized and more dependable.
    - (B) They have better impulse control.
    - (C) They are less curious about new ideas or experiences.
    - (D) They are less suspicious and antagonistic.

34. Which of the following pairs of traits, if they were both correlated with a particular gene, would most indicate a genetic component of generalized anxiety disorder?
    - (A) A positive correlation with openness and a negative correlation with extraversion
    - (B) A positive correlation with conscientiousness and a positive correlation with agreeableness
    - (C) A positive correlation with conscientiousness and a negative correlation with agreeableness
    - (D) A positive correlation with neuroticism and a negative correlation with conscientiousness

35. If 3 percent of the adult population has generalized anxiety disorder, approximately how many people out of 1000 randomly chosen adults would report that their primary personality trait was neuroticism?

(A) 97

(B) 100

(C) 107

(D) 350

36. Anxiety disorders may have roots in the developmental stages of personality formation. Which of the following statements about personality formation is consistent with Erikson's theory?

(A) Human behavior is primarily a response to circumstances, and the attempt to analyze a person in terms of personality traits is too narrow.

(B) Personality develops in unique ways for each person.

(C) Personality develops in stages that occur in a specific order that should be completed by young adulthood.

(D) Personality develops in stages that occur in a specific order, and development continues throughout life.

37. Which of the following can be concluded about generalized anxiety disorder from the information in the passage?

(A) Extraversion prevents general anxiety disorder.

(B) Generalized anxiety disorder causes a reduction of extraversion.

(C) There is a correlation between generalized anxiety disorder and extraversion.

(D) There is a correlation between generalized anxiety disorder and openness.

PASSAGE VI

To study the effects of gender discrimination in the medical field, 100 patients were offered the help of two doctors—one male and one female. The patients were allowed to pick which doctor they preferred to have examine them during a routine physical. Prior to choosing their doctor, a brief medical and educational history of the doctors was disclosed to the patients. The following paragraphs describe the credentials that the patients were shown for each doctor.

Doctor #1 (Female Doctor)
The credentials of this doctor were excellent in all areas. Graduating at the top of her class from a high-ranking medical school, this doctor went on to train under a well-respected mentor in the medical community. After five years of employment under her mentor, the doctor opened a private practice and has effectively treated her patients for ten years while maintaining high reviews.

Doctor #2 (Male Doctor)
The credentials of this doctor were slightly less impressive than those of the female doctor. Graduating with a 3.5 GPA from a middle-ranking medical school, this doctor immediately joined his father's local practice. After two years of employment, the doctor opened his own private practice and has been treating his patients for five years with no formal complaints on his record.

Questionnaire
At the beginning of the study, patients were shown the credentials for each doctor but without any reference to the doctors' gender. All patients were then asked to answer the following questions:

1. Which doctor would you choose?
2. Which doctor has the most impressive credentials?

They were then informed of the genders of each doctor and asked this follow-up question:

3. Knowing this information, which doctor would you choose?

Results
Upon completion of the questionnaire, the following results were gathered. Based on questions 1 and 2, Doctor #1 was the unequivocal favorite, garnering 100 percent of the votes. In contrast, Doctor #2 received 75 percent of the votes in question 3.

38. Based on the results of this experiment, which of the following can be concluded?
    (A) Gender is the most important consideration when patients choose a doctor.
    (B) Male doctors receive better training than female doctors.
    (C) Patients choose the most experienced doctor.
    (D) Most people have a gender bias when choosing a doctor.

39. Which of the following would have made the results of the study more reliable?
    (A) If the male doctor had better credentials than the female doctor
    (B) If the patients had been given a questionnaire after they received their physical to reevaluate the skills of their doctor
    (C) If the number of years of experience for both doctors was the same
    (D) If patients had been allowed to interview the doctors before choosing one

40. Upon review of the experiment, it was discovered that 65 of the participants were male. Which of the following best explains how this information serves as an extraneous variable?
    (A) Men may be uncomfortable with a woman performing their physical.
    (B) A majority male sample creates bias for questionnaire responses 1 and 2.
    (C) Males would tend to conform to how other males expect them to vote.
    (D) Men are as likely as women to believe that a female doctor is not as effective as a male doctor.

41. Which of the following exemplifies institutional discrimination?
    (A) Most of the male doctors at a hospital would prefer to go to a male doctor for their own physical exams.
    (B) A hospital has a strict policy requiring all female doctors under the age of 50 to be tested for pregnancy every three months.
    (C) The hospital committee responsible for evaluating and hiring potential new physicians is predominantly male.
    (D) All the male physicians at a hospital received their medical degrees from the same institution.

42. If the same experiment were repeated but with a female and male nurse, instead of doctor, how might this change the decision that the patients had to make?
    (A) Patients would be torn between apparent credentials and perceived medical ability.
    (B) Patients would be torn between perceived medical ability and caregiving ability.
    (C) Patients would choose the male practitioner regardless of credentials.
    (D) Patients would choose the female practitioner regardless of credentials.

43. Nutritional deficiencies can severely disrupt cognitive development in children. For instance, iodine deficiency during development can result in the loss of up to:
    (A) 5–10 IQ points.
    (B) 10–15 IQ points.
    (C) 20–25 IQ points.
    (D) 35–40 IQ points.

44. Which of the following is a characteristic NOT held in common by people with severe hearing loss and people with severe visual impairment?
    (A) Their disability is not readily apparent to many people.
    (B) They are able to communicate well within their subculture.
    (C) They may miss environmental cues that would protect people without these disabilities from danger.
    (D) Their interactions with people without disabilities are limited by their disability.

45. A child who is especially sensitive, curious, headstrong, and imaginative may be exhibiting signs of:
    (A) alertness.
    (B) attention deficit hyperactivity disorder.
    (C) separation anxiety disorder.
    (D) giftedness.

PASSAGE VII

Oppositional defiant disorder is a common diagnosis seen in many pediatric patients. The clinical presentation of the disorder includes the following: temper tantrums, disobeying parents or other caregivers, arguing, and speaking out of turn in class. In the clinical setting, these behaviors can cost physicians a great amount of time and prolong appointments because an uncooperative child hinders the physician from being able to conduct a thorough and careful physical examination. In addition, these uncooperative behaviors can be dangerous for the patient. For instance, a child who needs routine vaccinations and who will not sit still due to a temper tantrum may potentially get injured by the needle. As a result, many psychologists have looked into mechanisms to curb oppositional or defiant behaviors during medical appointments. One mechanism is to use a token rewards system, which involves giving positive praise to children periodically throughout appointments for being cooperative and reinforcing behavior with small prizes like stickers. Children can accumulate stickers and then trade in these stickers at the end of the appointment for larger prizes. Other researchers use a combination of this token rewards system plus having children observe role models (children their own age who are cooperative during appointments). The figure below illustrates outcomes using these techniques. Note that most researchers begin with an initial assessment of the frequency of oppositional or defiant behaviors exhibited during first appointment and then track frequency of oppositional or defiant behaviors across subsequent appointments.

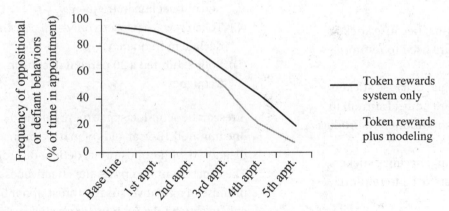

Figure 1. Change in oppositional or defiant behavior

46. What is the best explanation for adding a baseline assessment of disruptive behaviors before beginning the intervention?
    (A) It improves accuracy of intervention effectiveness by serving as a confounding variable to which treatment outcomes can be compared.
    (B) It improves accuracy of intervention effectiveness by serving as an additional dependent variable to which treatment outcomes can be compared.
    (C) It improves accuracy of intervention effectiveness by serving as an additional independent variable to which treatment outcomes can be compared.
    (D) It does not improve accuracy of the intervention effectiveness but does yield greater statistical power.

47. The token rewards system can be classified as which type of associative learning?
    (A) Classical conditioning, because stickers, praise, and prizes are neutral stimuli to which the child is conditioned to produce a reflexive behavior
    (B) Classical conditioning, because stickers, praise, and prizes are used to reinforce good behavior
    (C) Operant conditioning, because stickers, praise, and prizes are neutral stimuli to which the child is conditioned to produce a reflexive behavior
    (D) Operant conditioning, because stickers, praise, and prizes are used to reinforce good behavior

48. Which of the following best explains why both lines in Figure 1 drop rapidly after the first appointment?
    (A) Children begin to associate bad behavior with negative reinforcement.
    (B) Children begin to associate good behavior with positive reinforcement.
    (C) Children begin to associate bad behavior with negative punishment.
    (D) Children notice that other children who behave well receive rewards.

49. Which of the following is an example of negative punishment that would likely decrease the incidence of undesirable behavior in the situation described in the passage?
    (A) When the subject child exhibits undesirable behavior, the child is scolded verbally.
    (B) When the subject child exhibits desirable behavior, the researcher stops scolding the child.
    (C) The researcher rings a bell just before each instance of the subject child's undesirable behavior.
    (D) The researcher stops praising the subject child when the child exhibits undesirable behavior.

50. Which of the following treatment modalities exhibited the greatest decline in the frequency of disruptive behaviors from the second appointment to the third appointment, and what was the approximate rate of the modality?
    (A) Token rewards system only—30 percent decline in frequency.
    (B) Token rewards system and modeling—10 percent decline in frequency.
    (C) Token rewards system only—20 percent decline in frequency.
    (D) Both exhibited a 20 percent decline in frequency.

51. A researcher conducts an experiment with one hundred 12-year-olds who have been diagnosed with oppositional defiant disorder. The experiment compares the effectiveness of a promise of a treat versus the threat of not being able to watch television in convincing each child to receive an immunization shot. Which of the following could be a confounding factor in this experiment?
    (A) Children are assigned randomly to one of the two experimental groups.
    (B) Some of the children have a history of responding more positively to promises than to threats.
    (C) A child's parents have not been consistent in following up with promises and threats.
    (D) One hundred subjects is too small a number to give a significant result.

PASSAGE VIII

Researchers conduct the following psychological experiments.

Experiment 1

A 4-year-old male child and his parents are asked to complete the following tasks. The mother is asked to provide the child with instructions/prompts/commands to have the child independently change from his pajamas to his clothing in the least possible amount of time with the least possible number of prompts. Only one set of clothing is available. A period of outdoor playtime is provided with both parents. Then the father must accomplish the same task in reverse, providing the child with instructions/prompts/commands to have the child independently change from his clothing to his pajamas in the least amount of time with the least possible number of prompts. The result of the experiment was that the child completed the tasks with fewer prompts and less time for his mother than for his father.

Experiment 2

The same 4-year-old male child and his father are asked to play in a playroom while researchers observe them through a window. The father wears an earpiece so that he can hear requests from the researchers and follow their directives. The father and son are first directed to play together for three minutes. Then the father is instructed to narrate the child's play but not participate in it for three minutes. Then the father is instructed to sit in the room and not narrate the child's play but to respond to the child only if the child engages with the father for the next three minutes. Then the father is instructed to not respond to the child for three minutes. At the end, the father reengages with the child. Then the mother repeats the same pattern with the child. Researchers measure the differences in the child's responses. Finally the same pattern is repeated with both parents in the room.

The result of the experiment was that the child became irritable when the father stopped playing and narrating. He became aggressive toward his toys when his father stopped interacting altogether. However, when his mother became silent, he crawled into her lap and played with the toys until she reengaged with him, never becoming aggressive with the toys.

On the drive home after the experiments, the boy was highly upset. As the family's car approached a red traffic light, the father urged the mother, who was driving, to go through the light because their son needed to get home, where he would feel comfortable. The mother refused, stating that it was against the law to drive through a red light.

52. Which of the following is an interpretation of the two experiments that is consistent with Freud's theories?

   (A) The boy has a rivalry with his father because he is romantically attracted to his mother.

   (B) The boy has penis envy, which will be resolved when he aligns with his father and forgoes his rivalry.

   (C) The boy is in the latency stage and driven by the impulses of his id.

   (D) The boy has an anal-expulsive personality due to unresolved conflicts in the anal stage of life and is now exhibiting poor self-control, impulsivity, and aggression.

53. According to Vygotsky's theories, which of the following would be the best way for the boy to better learn how to play independently?

   (A) The boy should be left alone for increasing periods of time so that he learns to play independently.

   (B) The parents should reward the boy with positive attention whenever he plays independently.

   (C) The parents should play together with the boy but at times move away and the mother and father each play alone.

   (D) The boy's behavior cannot be expected to improve until he is older.

54. Which of the following is an explanation of the disagreement between the father and mother in the last paragraph that is most consistent with a feminist view of morality?

   (A) Women base morality on a balance of principles and the needs of the people in their lives, whereas men base morality on principles alone.

   (B) In a specific situation, some people may consider the needs of the people in their lives to be important in making a moral decision, and other people may believe that principles are more important than the needs of the people in their lives.

   (C) Two people, even if married, may have a different evaluation of the relative importance of a certain person in their lives, even if that person is their child.

   (D) Even though women are generally not as concerned with morals as men, sometimes men are more concerned with the people in their lives than with morals.

55. Which of the following is an interpretation of the two experiments that is consistent with Erikson's theories?

   (A) The boy is regressed in his relationship with his father.

   (B) The boy's mother offers him less encouragement than does his father.

   (C) The boy's father offers him less encouragement than does his mother.

   (D) The boy is regressed in his relationship with his mother.

56. An educator proposed that an important goal of elementary school education should be to help students to be able to work independently. Which of the following conclusions about this proposal can most logically be drawn?
    (A) The proposal is valid because independence is a universally appreciated value.
    (B) The proposal is valid because most people in the educator's community appreciate independence.
    (C) The proposal is invalid because many cultures do not value independence.
    (D) The proposal is invalid because children in elementary school are too young to develop independence.

57. Which of the following is an interpretation of the two experiments that is consistent with Kohlberg's theories?
    (A) The boy's behavior is motivated by his desire for praise from his father.
    (B) The boy is seeking to benefit only himself by manipulating his parents.
    (C) The boy is responding to social norms established through observation of others.
    (D) The boy is responding to the parent he expects to discipline him more severely—the mother.

The following questions do not refer to a descriptive passage and are not related to each other.

58. Two different types of memories contribute to one's overall long-term memory. The first type consists of conscious memories of the specific details of one's life. The second type stores the memory of certain physical movements, thoughts, tasks, and abilities that one has learned. These two types of memory are referred to as:
    (A) working memory and sensory memory.
    (B) recall and recognition.
    (C) explicit and implicit memory.
    (D) memory construction and flashbulb memory.

59. In which way(s) do(es) the specific language that one learns influence his or her cognitive abilities and view of the world?

    I. Speakers of a language that does not contain separate pronouns for males and females may hold less rigid views of male and female roles.
    II. Speakers of a language that has different structures for distinguishing past events from recent/present events may have a different concept of time than others.
    III. Speakers of a language that add grammatical elements to nouns in order to indicate shapes and functions may be better skilled at perceiving these qualities.

    (A) I only
    (B) I and II only
    (C) II and III only
    (D) I, II, and III

ANSWER KEY
Practice Test 1

CHEMICAL AND PHYSICAL FOUNDATIONS

1. D	13. B	25. B	37. D	49. B
2. A	14. C	26. B	38. C	50. D
3. B	15. C	27. D	39. B	51. B
4. B	16. B	28. C	40. C	52. B
5. A	17. A	29. C	41. C	53. B
6. B	18. B	30. A	42. B	54. C
7. C	19. C	31. D	43. D	55. C
8. A	20. D	32. A	44. A	56. A
9. B	21. B	33. D	45. A	57. A
10. B	22. C	34. C	46. C	58. A
11. D	23. D	35. B	47. D	59. A
12. B	24. D	36. C	48. C	

CRITICAL ANALYSIS AND REASONING

1. D	12. C	23. A	34. B	45. A
2. C	13. A	24. C	35. C	46. C
3. D	14. C	25. B	36. A	47. C
4. C	15. D	26. C	37. B	48. A
5. B	16. C	27. B	38. D	49. D
6. B	17. A	28. D	39. D	50. C
7. A	18. D	29. B	40. C	51. A
8. A	19. C	30. B	41. D	52. D
9. C	20. D	31. C	42. C	53. C
10. A	21. C	32. D	43. D	
11. D	22. A	33. C	44. A	

ANSWER KEY
Practice Test 1

BIOLOGICAL AND BIOCHEMICAL FOUNDATIONS

1. B	13. B	25. A	37. D	49. B
2. B	14. A	26. C	38. C	50. C
3. A	15. D	27. D	39. B	51. C
4. D	16. B	28. D	40. C	52. B
5. B	17. D	29. B	41. D	53. C
6. C	18. D	30. B	42. C	54. A
7. A	19. B	31. A	43. C	55. D
8. B	20. B	32. C	44. D	56. A
9. D	21. A	33. C	45. C	57. D
10. D	22. B	34. B	46. A	58. A
11. A	23. D	35. A	47. B	59. D
12. B	24. C	36. B	48. C	

PSYCHOLOGICAL, SOCIAL, AND BIOLOGICAL FOUNDATIONS

1. D	13. C	25. A	37. C	49. D
2. C	14. B	26. D	38. D	50. D
3. B	15. D	27. D	39. C	51. C
4. C	16. D	28. B	40. A	52. A
5. D	17. A	29. B	41. C	53. C
6. C	18. C	30. C	42. B	54. B
7. D	19. D	31. A	43. B	55. B
8. B	20. A	32. D	44. A	56. C
9. A	21. B	33. A	45. D	57. D
10. B	22. A	34. C	46. B	58. C
11. D	23. B	35. C	47. D	59. D
12. A	24. D	36. D	48. B	

Chemical and Physical Foundations

1. **(D)** Reaction rates cannot be determined from equilibrium constants or other thermodynamic data.

2. **(A)** Because the activation energy for step 3 is the highest (it is the slowest step), the H_2I must be the most stable of the intermediates.

3. **(B)** There are two moles of gas on both the reactants and products sides of the reaction. Calculating the change in entropy for the reaction gives a value very close to zero.

4. **(B)** The smallest activation energy corresponds to the fastest step.

5. **(A)** Because iodine atoms are larger than chlorine atoms, the bond in HI is a longer and weaker bond than the bond in HCl, making it easier to break. This means that HI is more readily dissociated into ions than HCl.

6. **(B)** The bond in HI is polar. The electrons are shared unevenly because of the higher electronegativity of iodine compared to hydrogen.

7. **(C)** Choice C is correct because amphiphilic is described as having the ability to react as both an acid and a base. The amino group of an amino acid reacts as a base, whereas the carboxyl group reacts as an acid. Choice A is incorrect because the removal of a hydrogen from NH_3^+ is an acid–base reaction in itself, but it classifies the amino group as basic, not amphiphilic. Choice B is incorrect because even though the addition of basic and acidic R-groups (carbon-based side chains) may increase the acidity or basicity of an amino acid, they are not essential for its inherently amphiphilic character. Choice D is incorrect because it incorrectly describes the amino group as acidic and the carboxyl group as basic.

8. **(A)** Choice A is correct because the benzylic rings present in phenylalanine and tyrosine allow them to act as a fluorophore. Choice B is incorrect because it does not include tyrosine. Choices C and D are incorrect because though arginine and glutamate are charged, this does not give them the ability to emit UV light as fluorophores.

9. **(B)** Choice B is correct because an electrophoresis gel separates proteins based on isoelectric point, the pH at which the protein has a neutral charge. The protein stops migrating in the gel after losing its charge, so the point at which the protein is found is pI. Choice A is incorrect because though it is possible that both proteins contain the same six essential amino acids, it is not required in order for them to have the same pI. Choice C is incorrect because the classification of amino acids as essential or nonessential is not dependent on pI. Choice D is incorrect because the molecular weight of the protein in kDa does not directly affect pI.

10. **(B)** Choice B is correct because phenylalanine is listed in the table as a nonpolar amino acid, making it hydrophobic, or insoluble in water. The hydrophilic requirement of IV drugs would prevent the solubility of phenylalanine with the drug. Choice A is incorrect because it incorrectly states that water-soluble IV drugs are hydrophobic. Choices C and D are incorrect because they wrongly state the IV drug would be effective, because of an incorrect assumption that hydrophobic and hydrophilic substances are miscible and that phenylalanine is a hydrophilic amino acid, respectively.

11. **(D)** Choice D is correct because it correctly orders the amino acids in order of decreasing pK_R, the pH at which the side chain will release a hydrogen atom. A low pK_a correlates to a higher acidity. Choices A, B, and C are incorrect because they do not correctly order the amino acids.

12. **(B)** Choice B is correct because essential amino acids must come from food while nonessential amino acids can be synthesized in the body. Though arginine is synthesized, it cannot be used in necessary metabolic functions, making it an essential amino acid. Choice A is incorrect because the importance of urea as a metabolic intermediate does not affect arginine's classification as an essential amino acid. Choice C is incorrect because of the reasons stated in the explanation of choice B. Choice D is incorrect because the production of urea from sources other than arginine does not affect arginine's reactivity once being synthesized by the body.

13. **(B)** In Table 1, magnesium reacted with four of the solutions, zinc with three, lead with two, copper with one, and silver with none. In Table 2, it is shown that Pb reacts more energetically than Cu.

14. **(C)** Sulfuric acid reacts with magnesium metal to produce hydrogen gas: $Mg_{(s)} + H_2SO_{4(aq)} \rightarrow MgSO_{4(aq)} + H_{2(g)}$. Sulfuric acid is a non-oxidizing acid (compared to nitric acid, which often produces nitrogen oxides as gaseous products).

15. **(C)** The precipitate is silver chloride, AgCl. Silver forms ions with a +1 charge.

16. **(B)** Boiling point elevation depends on the number of moles of dissolved particles. Because the comparison is between equimolar solutions of lead nitrate and silver nitrate and because lead nitrate produces 3 ions/mole and silver nitrate produces 2 ions/mole, lead nitrate will have a higher boiling point.

17. **(A)** Because magnesium is more active than copper, the magnesium metal will be oxidized to magnesium ion and the copper ion reduced to copper metal.

18. **(B)** The lead has an oxidation number of +2 in these compounds, and sulfate ions have a charge of –2, making $PbSO_4$ the correct answer.

19. **(C)** Sublimation is the physical change from a solid to a gas.

20. **(D)** Both insulators and conductors can have static electricity on them, but they must not be grounded or the charge dissipates.

21. **(B)** A smaller cross-sectional area leads to higher resistance.

22. **(C)** The most stable ion of magnesium is +2, so two electrons would be lost from the configuration $[Ne]3s^2$.

23. **(D)** Because carbon disulfide has bonds between carbon (electronegativity = 2.55) and sulfur (electronegativity = 2.58), the bond type is covalent. Covalent compounds tend to be nonconductors if they dissolve in water.

24. **(D)** The most active nonmetal (strongest oxidizing agent) is fluorine.

25. **(B)** The electrons are shared evenly (electronegativity difference = 0.35) between carbon and hydrogen, making the bond nonpolar covalent.

26. **(B)** The highest boiling point would belong to one of the ionic compounds, either NaCl or CaO. Since the ions in sodium chloride have +1 and –1 charges and those in calcium oxide have +2 and –2 charges, the electrical attraction between ions is greater in calcium oxide.

27. **(D)** Typically, binary ionic compounds involve a metal and a nonmetal, whereas covalent compounds involve two nonmetals.

28. **(C)** Notice in the passage the statement, "energy goes back and forth between potential energy stored in the spring and kinetic energy due to the velocity." This statement means that energy is conserved.

29. **(C)** The total energy is 1 cal or 4 J per atom. The amplitude is (10% of the atomic spacing). Use $E = kA^2$.

30. **(A)** The model cannot be adapted because in gases the molecules of the gas behave as independent particles.

31. **(D)** Set $mv^2_{max}/2 = E$ $v^2_{max} = (8 \times 10^{23} \text{ J})(24 \times 2 \times 10^{-27} \text{ kg})$ $v_{max} = 40 \text{ m/s}$

32. **(A)** If there are 6.0×10^{23} atoms in the mole, then a cube would have the cube root of this number of atoms along each edge. Estimate the cube root of 6.0×10^{23} as a little over 8.0×10^7. With atomic spacing roughly 2.0×10^{-10} m, the cube must have a side of roughly 1.6 cm.

33. **(D)** Because MTBE is highly soluble in nonpolar solvents, it is a nonpolar substance, as dictated by the principle "like dissolves like."

34. **(C)** Both hexane and toluene are nonpolar. Hydrogen bonding is not a phenomenon of nonpolar substances, but London dispersions forces allow nonpolar substances to interact with each other.

35. **(B)** The compounds become less soluble as the fraction of the molecule composed of nonpolar hydrocarbon increases. Because "like dissolves like," the greater the polar portion of the molecule, the greater the solubility in a polar solvent such as water.

36. **(C)** Each carbon atom has four electron pairs around it, leading to an sp^3 orbital hybridization and a tetrahedral shape.

37. **(D)** The three bonds and one lone pair around the S atom have a trigonal pyramidal shape. There are two single bonds to the methyl groups and a double bond between the S and the O. There is an additional lone pair on the sulfur atom.

38. **(C)** Expanded octets involve d orbitals. The second energy level has no d orbitals, so it cannot be correct.

39. **(B)** According to Graham's law, the rates of diffusion of gases are inversely proportional to the square roots of their molar masses. Therefore, because bromine has a molar mass four times that of argon, argon will diffuse twice as fast.

40. **(C)** This is an application of Le Châtelier's principle. Higher pressure favors the side with fewer moles of gas, in this case the products. Since the reaction is exothermic, heat can be treated as a product, and lowering the temperature will shift the system to the right.

41. **(C)** The direction of motion is changing, so the velocity is changing. Acceleration is the change in velocity over time.

42. **(B)** Choice B is correct. The passage indicates that ammonium thioglycolate cleaves disulfide bonds, leaving amino acid residues behind. In order to break the S–S bond, ammonium thioglycolate donates electrons to leave two thiol (–SH) groups. When an agent donates electrons, it is a reducing agent. Choice A is incorrect because ammonium thioglycolate is not an oxidizing agent. Choice C is incorrect because the passage states that heat is used to uncoil the polypeptide helix. Choice D is incorrect because the hair returns to a helical shape after removal of heat.

43. **(D)** The passage states that alpha keratin contains hydrophobic amino acids such as alanine, valine, leucine, isoleucine, methionine, and phenylalanine. This eliminates choices A and B. This problem requires the knowledge that disulfide bonds are formed between two cysteine amino acid residues. This eliminates choice C and leaves choice D as the correct answer.

44. **(A)** The information in Figures 1 and 2 shows that the greatest amount of damage to keratin occurs under alkaline conditions, or higher pH. This indicates that the keratin-coated pill will dissolve under alkaline conditions. The pH of the stomach is normally around 2, and the pH inside the mouth is around 5.5. This eliminates choices B and D. The pH of blood is 7.4, but the medication needs to dissolve in order to get into the bloodstream, not dissolve in the blood. This eliminates choice C and leaves choice A as the only possible correct answer.

45. **(A)** This problem requires knowledge of hydroxide ion concentration, pH, and pOH. The most acidic formula will cause the least amount of damage to hair. The formula with the lowest hydroxide concentration $[OH^-]$ is the safest formula because it has the lowest pH and the greatest acidity. The correct answer is choice A because it correctly indicates that Formula R is the most acidic.

46. **(C)** This problem asks why globular proteins with disulfide bonds are more stable than those without disulfide bonds. This requires knowledge of the stability of different types of bonds as well as knowledge about disulfide bonds. Choice A is incorrect because the disulfide bond is not an ionic bond. Choice B is tempting because disulfide bonds occur between cysteine residues, but it is incorrect because it is not a double bond. Although most globular proteins are held together by noncovalent bonds, this does not account for increased stability to withstand higher temperatures. Choice C is the correct answer because disulfide bonds are covalent bonds. The bond occurs between two identical atoms, and covalent bonds are extremely stable bonds.

47. **(D)** The graph shows that lowering the temperature and raising the pressure can both liquefy a gas.

48. **(C)** Multiply the speed of sound at about 330 m/s by 6 s.

49. **(B)** Get the spring constant from 100 cm – 80 cm = 20 cm. So 2 N/20 cm or 0.1 N/cm. Then when the spring is stretched (150 cm – 80 cm = 70 cm) this gives a 7 N force.

50. **(D)** Surface area of either the anode or cathode has no effect on cell voltage. Cell voltage is affected by ion concentration and the identity of the anode and cathode.

51. **(B)** The velocity of the molecules depends only on temperature.

52. **(B)** The equation $P = I^2R$ is relevant for power transmission. High current results in more power loss than high voltage.

53. **(B)** The acid chloride will react with the second reagent—$(CH_3CH_2CH_2)_2CuLi$, which will add a three-carbon branch to the carbonyl group—to yield a *ketone*.

54. **(C)** The reaction proceeds via *nucleophilic addition*. The nucleophilic Grignard reagent carbon adds to the electrophilic carbon of the carbon dioxide; this process is referred to as *carboxylation*.

55. **(C)** The described reaction conditions are highly oxidizing, so the formal group (an aldehyde) will be oxidized to a carboxylic acid group.

56. **(A)** Compound **6** has no carbon chirality centers (no sp^3 hybridized carbons are present). The nitrogen center in the molecule is theoretically chiral, but at room temperature it interconverts too quickly for a pair of enantiomers to exist.

57. **(A)** The nitrogen atom's lone pair is part of the aromatic ring system's delocalized electrons. The entire ring system is aromatic and geometrically flat. The bonds around the nitrogen will have approximately 120° angles.

58. **(A)** Because the concentrations of silver and iodide ions are equal, the expression to be solved is $4 \times 10^{-16} = x^2$ and $x = 2 \times 10^{-8}$.

59. **(A)** In order to qualitatively determine the effects of temperature on a gas, the temperature must be in kelvin, so the change in temperature is from 283 K to 293 K, or about 3%.

Critical Analysis and Reasoning

1. **(D)** The criteria given by the passage for members of a grassroots support system include mentors, family, and colleagues in other fields. Answer choices A, B, and C fit in these categories. The antithesis of the support system is someone from an impersonal institution, thus the answer is D.

2. **(C)** The other answer choices all involve impersonal institutions, no matter how well intentioned.

3. **(D)** The passage states that business support groups were in favor in the first half of the 20th century but not since then. Choices A and C go beyond what the passage states. Choice B is wrong because there is no evidence that today younger artists are more likely to reject business support groups than are older artists.

4. **(C)** Choice A goes too far. Choice B is incorrect because it is the alternatives to business support groups that began around 1950. Choice D is incorrect because the support systems have been informal.

5. **(B)** The paragraph's assertion is "One main purpose of artistic support systems is artistic training." The rest of the paragraph gives examples of this. A careful examination of the other answer choices shows that they do not match the structure of the paragraph.

6. **(B)** Choices C and D are wrong because they deal with formal institutions, which are not the focus of support groups. Choice A is wrong because the passage does not talk about support groups providing contacts for neighboring cities.

7. **(A)** The traditional evaluation is discussed only at the beginning of the first paragraph. The author establishes that the new approach is a community-based one, so the correct answer must include the community, or social setting.

8. **(A)** Choice A is correct because Roman numeral II is stated in the last paragraph. Roman numeral I is not valid, as the author asserts that the gap is between the wealthy and the poor, not the middle class and the poor. Roman numeral III is not valid because it is "many economists" who state this, not the author, who questions it.

9. **(C)** Choices A and D are part of the argument that the author is rebutting. Choice B is consistent with the author's argument but is not the main point.

10. **(A)** The author equates problem-solving ability with the ability to lead.

11. **(D)** The author believes this widening gap is natural and will lead toward better leadership. Choice A could be true, but it is not stated in the passage. Choice C is wrong because the author believes that the gap has to do with relative intelligence and unintelligence among people.

12. **(C)** The author clearly believes that the wealthy should control the political and economic planning.

13. **(A)** The author defines intelligence as the ability to solve economic or political problems. Answer A is the only one that does not involve solving an economic or political problem.

14. **(C)** The other answer choices focus on a scientific approach, whereas the author is writing poetically.

15. **(D)** Each of the qualities in answer choice D is exemplified by statements in the passage. Choices A, B, and C are not defendable by the passage and do not represent the author's primary attitude of appreciation of the qualities in choice D.

16. **(C)** The hyphenation indicates that "wild-cherry" may be a type of cherry tree. This also indicates that it is not the tree that is wild (choices A, B). Choice D implies that the cherries are wild, which is not logical.

17. **(A)** The author greatly appreciates the bees at the same time that they pose the threat of stinging him. The author never compares the country with the city (choice B). Choice C is false because the author finds the trees beautiful. This also negates choice D, as trees are not fleeting.

18. **(D)** The phrase refers to Nature, not to people or children. The author gives no examples of Nature protecting him. Describing Nature as marching like an army is a distractor.

19. **(C)** The article sets up at its beginning a contrast between the negative and positive aspects of private equity investing. Choices A and D focus on only one of these aspects. Choice B ignores the contrast.

20. **(D)** The author contends that in contrast to the negative activities of the 1980s, private equity firms in the 1990s wanted to make their transactions attractive to management and shareholders. Answer D makes the transaction unattractive to shareholders.

21. **(C)** The example of KKR makes it clear that a purchase consists of leverage and equity. If there is less leverage, there must be more equity.

22. **(A)** The author hails the acquisition as marking a return of leveraged buyouts—a positive—but describes the subsequent inflated sale price, demise of the company, and ultimate loss to the new parent company as negatives.

23. **(A)** The author describes the 1990s approach as one that seeks respectability (choice C) and offers a better deal to management (choice B). In the Continental Airlines example of this approach, the investors earned praise (choice D). There is no evidence that this approach will inherently result in higher profits.

24. **(C)** To be respectable requires following the 1990s model. Following that model requires not giving outsized profits. Choice A is incorrect because those avoiding outsized profits could still use either model. Choice B is wrong because those who do not use the 1990s model can choose to give or not give outsized profits. Choice D could be true—and is likely true—but it does not have to be true based on the given information. It could be that all who follow the 1990s model are respectable.

25. **(B)** The people in Zaire are given as an example of modern humans. The passage then refers to these people as being in Africa. Choice A is wrong because the Neanderthals did not lose tools but fell behind the advanced tools of Homo sapiens. Choice C is wrong because the passage does not defend that the two groups coexisted. Choice D is incorrect because the period is cited as "early" evidence.

26. **(C)** The point of the paragraph is to show that despite having certain skills that were exceptional, the Neanderthals did not have the flexibility to develop other skills that modern humans mastered.

27. **(B)** The passage states that, unlike Cro-Magnon, the Neanderthals never made shoes. Given the obvious utility of footwear, this would seem puzzling to Cro-Magnon observers. The Neanderthal ways may have been more ancient but they were also more primitive (choice A). The Neanderthals had stone tools (choice C). It is unlikely that impending extinction could have been observed or comprehended by Cro-Magnon, and nothing in the passage supports that it would (choice D).

28. **(D)** The final paragraph implies that the two groups were in close enough proximity for Neanderthals to learn some Cro-Magnon technology. This eliminates choices A and B. Choice C is incorrect because it is not necessary to attract a mate in order to breed. In answer D, separate species by definition cannot interbreed.

29. **(B)** The quote is an emotional expression, not a statement of facts or theories (choices A and D). By saying, "As Jordan notes," the author is concurring with the statement.

30. **(B)** The passage discusses the views of the president but not his motives.

31. **(C)** The passage describes Medicare as the largest underfunded entitlement program, implying that saving Medicare will free money for other programs, such as Social Security.

32. **(D)** Krugman specifically says that Social Security can be made workable for many generations without major changes. This meets the definition given of *conservative*. Choice

B is wrong because the only definition given for liberal is, by inference, wanting to make major changes. Choice A is wrong because Krugman does not propose this.

33. **(C)** The last paragraph mentions several factors that could easily be adjusted to avoid deficits, among them, changing the age for qualifying for benefits. The last sentence documents that this has already been done in the past. Choice D is incorrect because, even though it is part of an argument against those who call for dramatic change, there is no specific claim that it is rebutting.

34. **(B)** The key elements of the passage are a documented argument against the need for radical change versus an undocumented opinion for radical change. Whereas choice D deals with a parallel situation—the national debt—it does not match these elements. In Answer A, the informed sources are in favor of radical change.

35. **(C)** The author undermines the assumption that happiness and unhappiness must stand in opposition by questioning whether unhappiness needs to exist at all.

36. **(A)** It is irrelevant to the author whether people please themselves or others. The author's argument is concerned with whether the decision to act is carefully thought out or not.

37. **(B)** The author's approach does not promise that one can please oneself and others at the same time. The person who consciously decides to sleep in has done what makes him or her as happy as possible but may make the boss angry. Choices A and D are implied by the author's discussion. Choice C is stated explicitly.

38. **(D)** The passage starts with the assertion that people do not have much time for happiness because of their obligations to others. The author concludes that unhappiness is a result of people's own lack of energy to think carefully.

39. **(D)** The author is successful in proving that situations for happiness are not rare by taking a common situation that would not normally be considered an opportunity for happiness and showing that it is.

40. **(C)** The author's criterion for being as happy as possible does not depend on pleasing oneself or others but in carefully considering all the options. Choice D is incorrect because the woman's happiness, from the author's standpoint, does not depend on what the man does.

41. **(D)** The passage states that Anarchism destroys not healthy tissue, as opponents suggest, but parasitic growths. Although the author might find parallels between racism and anti-Anarchist feelings, the passage mentions nothing about racism. Choices B and C go in the wrong direction.

42. **(C)** The passage states that it takes "less mental effort to condemn than to think." This implies that thinking requires some effort. Choices A and B draw on statements from the passage but not correctly. Choice D confuses the need for thorough knowledge of a subject with the possibility of hearsay, which the media might represent.

43. **(D)** The passage clearly states that it is only the unhealthy that needs to be destroyed. The question involves the destruction of livelihood resulting from a change. Choice A defends the change by saying that the Old must be destroyed. Though not incorrect, it misses the point that it is the unhealthy aspects of the old that must be destroyed. Choice

B makes the practical into a negative, whereas the author defines the practical as a positive. Choice C is incorrect because in the passage the author does not defend hurting people for the sake of progress.

44. **(A)** In saying that Anarchism cannot become the Old, the author is defining the two as opposites. Tradition is an element of the Old. "Maintaining itself at the expense of society" is a definition of parasitism. Anarchism by definition destroys the parasitical. Answer A strengthens the argument that Anarchism is the opposite of the parasitical (Old). The other answers would not strengthen this argument. Choice D is a distractor that tries to insert some emotional interest into the question.

45. **(A)** The author defines Anarchism as being practical and defines practical as eliminating the wrong and foolish. Answer A establishes that it is not possible to accurately know what is wrong or foolish and thus destroys the ability for Anarchism to act practically. Choice B does not weaken the argument because the author has already admitted that there are intelligent people among the opponents of Anarchism. Choice C points to a missing emotional element in Anarchism, but the author does not base her argument on the need for an emotional element. If choice D were true, it would pose some logical concerns about how to define Anarchism, but it does not weaken the arguments that the author makes.

46. **(C)** Choice C is correct because Roman numeral II is stated in the eighth paragraph. Roman numeral I is not valid because it represents the view of the ignorant toward Anarchism. Roman numeral III is not valid because the author states that Anarchism destroys "parasitic growths."

47. **(C)** The author states that a good habit has the ability to displace a bad habit. Choice A is wrong because actions we fall into do not take any energy. The passage does not contain information that would defend choice B. Choice D violates the author's definition of habit.

48. **(A)** The author says that once a habit is established, work is directed by the subconscious, whereas a new task requires "active attention." If the author did not assume that work could be done well subconsciously, there would be no benefit to habit. The other answers are all possible but are not necessary to the author's argument.

49. **(D)** The question mixes two situations—nurses recognizing a bad habit in themselves and the injunction to help patients avoid negative attitudes. Answer D is the advice given in the passage to people facing a bad habit in themselves. Choice A confuses the advice that patients should pay little attention to minor ailments. Choices B and C confuse other information in the passage.

50. **(C)** The main criterion given in the passage for determining whether a patient has a good or bad attitude is giving way to ill-feeling versus encouraging him or her to build endurance. Choices A, B, and D do not indicate whether the patient is trying to build endurance or not. Answer C shows that the patient is trying to build endurance and therefore would allow the determination that the patient does not have a bad attitude.

51. **(A)** Choice A is correct. The last paragraph says that habits of invalidism involve wanting to be "cared for with comfort," so a nurse doing so can reinforce the bad habit of invalidism. Choice B is incorrect because caring with comfort can reinforce bad habits, not encourage new ones. Choice C is incorrect because the passage does not state that

any activities are impossible the first time they are tried. Choice D is incorrect because it is not the nurse but the patient who can fall into invalidism.

52. **(D)** Choice D is correct because making a bed is mentioned in the passage not as a task that a nurse must learn but as something that the nurse is able to do while doing a task that has become automatic. The other answer choices are all examples of tasks that people in general learn to do (in the first paragraph) or that a nurse in particular learns to do (in the second paragraph.)

53. **(C)** Choice C is correct because encouraging patients to report minor complaints is an example of something that might reinforce invalidism. Choice A is incorrect because the author encourages nurses to be cheerful when there is little cause for cheer. Choice B is incorrect because the author states that conversing with patients is something nurses do naturally when performing a task has become automatic. Choice D is incorrect because the author claims that withholding privileges under specific circumstances is an approach that a nurse can use to help patients build good habits.

Biological and Biochemical Foundations

1. **(B)** Viruses and bacteria contain nucleic acid, and prions are unique because they are infectious proteins. Choice A is incorrect because viruses and prions are unable to multiply without hijacking the host, and choice D is incorrect because bacteria are able to multiply on their own, but viruses and prions are not. Choice C is incorrect because all proteins are made up of amino acids, so prions must contain amino acids.

2. **(B)** Choice B is correct because it is the only option that correctly describes the results that the students found for tissue samples infected with BSE. Choice A is incorrect because it describes the results found for tissue samples infected with scrapie, not BSE. Choice C is incorrect because it says that a virus destroys Hsp70. Prions are infectious proteins, and they are classified separately from viruses. Choice D is incorrect because it not only describes the partial events of tissues infected with scrapie, but it also suggests that these events happen because of resistance to proteinase K, and that is not the case.

3. **(A)** Choice A is correct. Because actin remains constant in all tissue samples under all conditions, it can be inferred that it is a control that is unaffected by TSE. Actin is commonly used as a control in Western blots because it is a microfilament present in all eukaryotic cells and provides a standard for the variables in a Western blot. None of the other choices can be inferred from the information given in the passage.

4. **(D)** The passage reveals that PrP^{Sc} grows at an exponential rate once it has infected a mammal. Tissue samples must be inoculated with PrP^{Sc} at the same time in order for experimental results to be reliable. If PrP^{Sc} were allowed to infect a certain tissue sample longer than the others, the results would be dramatically skewed, and this means choice D is the correct answer. Choice A is incorrect because the amount of proteinase K used to digest proteins is not important unless the resistance to proteinase K is being measured, and in Experiment 1 it is not. Choice B is incorrect because although the amount of agarose used should be kept consistent, the precise amount of agarose used would not dramatically affect the results. Choice C is incorrect because although actin is used as a standard, the amount of actin present in each tissue sample cannot be controlled by the students.

5. **(B)** Choice B is correct because this suggestion is the only option that protects the naturally occurring PrP^C and its function. Misfolding is the cause of infectious prion diseases, so prevention of misfolding is ideal. Choice A is incorrect because it suggests that the infectious PrP^{Sc} is composed of exceptionally high α-helix secondary structure, but referring to Experiment 2 in the passage reveals that PrP^{Sc} is composed of exceptional β-sheet structure. Choice C is tempting because it seemingly bypasses the cellular PrP, but it is incorrect because degradation of the chaperone Hsp70 protein would result in more misfolded prion proteins. Choice D is incorrect because maintaining β-sheet conformation in PrP^{Sc}, the infectious prion protein, will only stabilize the infectious protein.

6. **(C)** The solute, sodium acetate, is the salt of acetic acid, and being ionic would completely ionize when dissolved in water (the solvent). The sodium and acetate ions would be surrounded and separated by polarized water molecules; thus, the interactions between the solute and solvent species are ion–dipole.

7. **(A)** Saccharides (commonly referred to as sugars) have many hydroxyl functional groups attached to their carbon backbones. This makes them highly polar compounds and would preclude them from dissolving to any reasonable extent in nonpolar organic solvents.

8. **(B)** If $A = 30\%$, then $T = 30\%$, and $A + T = 60\%$; $G + C = 40\%$. $(A + T)/(G + C) = 60/40 = 3:2$.

9. **(D)** Vital capacity is the maximum volume of air that can be moved into and out of the lungs. Residual volume refers to the amount of air left in the lungs after maximum exhalation. Total lung capacity is the vital capacity plus the residual volume.

10. **(D)** The distinguishing factor between type I and type II diabetes is that type I is an autoimmune disease that destroys β cells, whereas type II is a desensitizing of tissues to insulin. Choice D is correct because it determines the presence of autoimmune disease. Choice A is incorrect because both type I and type II diabetics display elevated levels of blood glucose. Choice B is incorrect because although a young age often points to type I diabetes, this is not enough to definitively distinguish between the two types. Choice C is incorrect because although being overweight often points to type II diabetes, this is not enough to definitively distinguish between the two types.

11. **(A)** The passage explicitly states that AMPK acts on AMP to shift metabolism toward fatty acid oxidation, so choice A is correct. The other options are incorrect because fatty acid synthesis promotes weight gain, whereas AMPK promotes weight loss, and ATP is produced during rest and eating to store fat.

12. **(B)** Choice B is correct because Table 1 describes the actions of Avandia and Actos as acting on PPARγ, activating expression of genes to increase action of insulin in the liver. Transcription factors are factors that activate genes. Choice A is incorrect because proteases are enzymes that cleave bonds. Choice C is incorrect because kinases are enzymes that phosphorylate targets. Choice D is incorrect because a G-protein is not able to activate gene expression.

13. **(B)** Choice B is correct. It can be inferred that leptin is a hormone because of the way it is transmitted as a signal to the leptin receptor in the brain. Leptin must also be a hormone that promotes weight loss and therefore maintains insulin sensitivity and adipose capacity in which fat can be appropriately stored. Choice A is incorrect because increasing

triacyglycerides is not characteristic of a mouse without diabetes. Choice C is incorrect because decreasing insulin sensitivity and adipose capacity are characteristic of a mouse that has diabetes and that is missing the leptin receptor. Choice D is incorrect because leptin is not an enzyme, and it encourages fatty acid oxidation.

14. **(A)** In type II diabetes, the person is insensitive to insulin and must produce much more than the average person after eating a meal. The only chart that matches this description is the first one, and choice A is correct. Choices B and C are incorrect because they do not accurately show insulin increases after meal times. Choice D is incorrect because although type I diabetics do not produce insulin and must have injections, type II diabetics do produce their own insulin.

15. **(D)** The pancreas secretes enzymes that digest protein, starches, and fats. This secretion is blocked by a gallstone, so no hydrolytic enzymes would be released. Monosaccharides are not hydrolyzed by enzymes in the small intestine, so their digestion is not affected.

16. **(B)** An abscess results from tissue dying and becoming infected with bacteria. The macrophages of the immune system recognize the antigens on the bacteria cell wall and trigger endocytosis of the bacteria. Viruses need a living cell as a host and are not found in an abscess.

17. **(D)** The pancreas secretes insulin into the blood. Insulin reduces blood glucose levels. A lack of insulin will strongly affect the blood glucose level.

18. **(D)** Answer D is correct because zymogens are the inactive form of enzymes. Choice A is incorrect because not all mutations result in nonfunctional enzymes. Choice B is incorrect because the pancreas secretes pancreatic lipase into the small intestine, not into the blood. Choice C is incorrect because the passage implies that whereas the early activation of enzymes will result in tissue damage, the damage does not necessarily result in infection.

19. **(B)** Answer B is correct because if both parents are homozygous recessive at both loci, they can only pass on recessive genes to their offspring, all of whom would be affected. Choice A could be true if both parents are heterozygotes at the two loci. For choice C, if two genes are on different chromosomes, they are not linked. In choice D, heterozygotes will not have the disorder because the presence of one dominant gene will prevent expression of the disorder.

20. **(B)** The measured calcium level is too high in the food, so the bioavailability is too low. For choice A, taking a vitamin D supplement would cause an increase in the bioavailability of the calcium, which is inconsistent with the outlier's low bioavailability. For choice C, if the patient has a disease that increases the calcium uptake, then the bioavailability should be higher than expected. For choice D, if there was a hypocalcemia disorder that is independent of vitamin D level, then all data points would show lower than normal bioavailability.

21. **(A)** To support the hypothesis, there must be evidence for lowered amounts of calcium ingested. If the constipated patients ate less food, they would have lower amounts of calcium ingested.

22. **(B)** Osteoblast cells deposit new bone, whereas osteoclast cells resorb (destroy) bone. Thus in osteoporosis, osteoblast activity is lower than osteoclast activity.

23. **(D)** The authors did not take into consideration any effect on blood calcium levels due to factors other than diet. For instance, the effect of bone resorption on bioavailability of calcium was not addressed.

24. **(C)** By definition, the results of an experiment—in this case, the ratio of blood calcium to dietary calcium intake—are not controlled. The quantities used to determine the result are controlled.

25. **(A)** This question requires the ability to read the chemical reaction that shows the action of PFK-1. Reaction (1) shows that PFK-1 takes a phosphate group from adenosine triphosphate (ATP) to fructose 6-phosphate to create fructose 1,6-bisphosphate. Knowing that kinases always phosphorylate their substrates also reveals that choice A is correct. Choice B is incorrect because removing a phosphate from fructose 6-phosphate would result in fructose. Choice C is incorrect because the enzyme acts on fructose 6-phosphate, not fructose 1,6-bisphosphate. Choice D incorrectly describes both the enzymatic activity and the substrate of PFK-1.

26. **(C)** The passage states that glycolysis is a highly exergonic series of reactions, and reaction (1) is a commitment step of glycolysis. Exergonic reactions have negative free-energy values (ΔG), and they release energy and are spontaneous. Because reaction (1) is a commitment step, these characteristics of the reaction make sense because a large amount of energy would need to be put into the reaction to make it go in the other direction. Choice C is the only choice that correctly describes all of these characteristics in reaction (1). Choices A and B are incorrect because the free-energy change value for reaction (1) is negative. Choice D is incorrect because a negative free-energy value represents a spontaneous reaction.

27. **(D)** The passage states that F26BP allosterically reacts with PFK-1 or FBP-1 and changes conformation to significantly reduce affinity for its substrate. Choice D is the only choice that correctly states this. Choice A incorrectly states that the conformation of the substrate is changed, whereas it is the enzyme whose conformation is altered. Choice B is incorrect because it states that the inhibitor binds to the substrate's active site. The active site is located on the enzyme. Choice C is also incorrect because it describes competitive inhibition instead of allosteric inhibition.

28. **(D)** The name "fructose 6-phosphate" indicates that there is one phosphate group on the sixth carbon. The correct structure is shown in choice D. Choice A is incorrect because the structure shown contains two phosphate groups. Choices B and C show structures without any phosphate groups. Figure 1 shows the cyclic conformation of fructose 2,6-bisphosphate, and using this as a reference may help elucidate the structure of fructose 6-phosphate.

29. **(B)** Insulin is increased after eating a meal, and it causes cells in the liver to absorb glucose. If glucose is readily available, it will be converted to energy through the process of glycolysis. This eliminates choices A and D because gluconeogenesis is not needed when there is an abundance of glucose. Choice C is almost correct, but it suggests that the deactivation of PFK-1 leads to glycolysis, whereas it is actually the activation of PFK-1 that leads to glycolysis.

30. **(B)** Genetic drift is the random loss of alleles in small, geographically isolated populations, resulting in reduced genetic diversity.

31. **(A)** Thyroid hormone acts to increase metabolic rate and body temperature, and it acts as a vasoconstrictor.

32. **(C)** The first reagent, $SOCl_2$, in the sequence will produce an *acid chloride* from the carboxylic acid group of benzoic acid. The acid chloride will react with the second reagent (($CH_3CH_2CH_2)_2CuLi$, which will add three carbon branches to the carbonyl group) to yield a *ketone*. Reaction of the ketone with $LiAlH_4$, followed by treatment with water (steps 3 and 4), will transform the ketone into an *alcohol*.

33. **(C)** Dilute (0.005%) sodium chloride cannot denature a protein and cannot cleave the peptide bond.

34. **(B)** The neurotransmitter triggers depolarization of the postsynaptic neuron.

35. **(A)** Given the S-shape of the curve showing response of NMDA receptors to glutamate, glutamate is increasingly effective at increasing doses up to 50% of maximum response, after which the effectiveness decreases with increasing concentration. Also, at normal physiologic concentrations, glutamate is responsible for learning and memory, but at high concentrations it acts as a neurotoxin.

36. **(B)** Oxygen deprivation results in disruption of the electrochemical gradient of the cell because of failure of the sodium potassium pump. Glutamate transporters reverse direction, resulting in high extracellular glutamate and triggering prolonged release of calcium ions into the post-synaptic neuron, leading to mitochondrial damage and apoptosis.

37. **(D)** The sodium-potassium pump requires ATP to pump Na^+ out of the cell and K^+ into the cell.

38. **(C)** According to the passage, oxygen deprivation causes glutamate transporters to reverse direction, increasing the concentration of extracellular glutamate in the synapse. However, Compound **A** deactivates NMDA receptors that respond to glutamate. So even in the presence of high levels of glutamate, postsynaptic neurons are not overstimulated, and the risk of excitotoxicity is reduced.

39. **(B)** Compound **A** binds to NMDA receptors and blocks glutamate from binding, decreasing the activity of the receptors and causing the dose-response curve for glutamate to shift to the right. Because increasing the concentration of glutamate decreases the effect of Compound **A**, these two substances must be competing for binding sites. The substance that is in higher concentration will reversibly bind to more receptors.

40. **(C)** Point mutations have a wide range of effects depending on the location and type of mutation. They may be caused by exposure to environmental factors over a person's lifetime and may be passed from cell to cell via mitosis. Glial cells undergo mitosis but not meiosis.

41. **(D)** Adhesion proteins would be involved in the adhesion of biofilm. Blocking transcription of these proteins would prevent adhesion. Choices A and B are factually incorrect. Choice C is incorrect because prophase I is part of meiosis, which bacteria do not undergo.

42. **(C)** Clearly species *T* must have some properties that are different from *Q* and *R*, or else the combination of the three would have behaved as did the combination of just *Q* and *R*.

The other answers could possibly be true, but there is no evidence from the experiment that would defend them.

43. **(C)** It is not possible for bacterial species Q to secrete histones. Histones are eukaryotic proteins that wrap the DNA into a chromosome. For answer choices A and B, it could be true that DNA or RNA is secreted from bacterial species Q as the passage does not provide further detail.

44. **(D)** The ability of a biofilm to form is a direct result of protein–protein interactions of cell-wall proteins with proteins of another cell. For answer choices A and C, the haploid number and stage of the cell cycle is not relevant for bacteria.

45. **(C)** This question tests knowledge of which embryonic tissue layer gives rise to which tissue in an infant. The ectoderm of an embryo will develop into the eyes, brain (nervous system), and hair follicles. The endoderm develops into the digestive tract, including the small intestinal epithelial cells.

46. **(A)** The bacteria in the upper part of the biofilm are more likely to be exposed to oxygen than bacteria in the lower part of the biofilm. Thus the bacteria in the upper 0.2 cm of the biofilm are most likely facultative anaerobes.

47. **(B)** After 1 hour, R has grown significantly less than Q; however, the most probable cause is not growth rate but the suppressive effect of T on R. Choice D can be concluded because at 1 hour, Q has occupied some of the area previously occupied by T.

48. **(C)** Bile is released into the duodenum. Bile contains bile salts that emulsify lipids to aid in breakdown by pancreatic enzymes.

49. **(B)** The liver is responsible for detoxification of metabolic byproducts, glycogen storage, breakdown of red blood cells, and secretion of bile. The pancreas secretes digestive enzymes.

50. **(C)** Write out the Punnett square for the cross: AaBb × AaBb.

1/16 AABB	2/16 AABb	1/16 AAbb
2/16 AaBB	4/16 AaBb	2/16 Aabb
1/16 aaBB	2/16 aaBb	1/16 aabb

The genotypes heterozygous for one or both traits are AaBB, AABb, AaBb, aaBb, and Aabb. The probability of any progeny with one of these genotypes is $\frac{12}{16} = \frac{3}{4}$.

51. **(C)** Glycogen stored in muscles and the liver is the result of polymerization of glucose.

52. **(B)** Choice B is an exception, and therefore the correct answer. Choice B cannot be true because the frequency of the M allele declined steadily throughout the study. If M provided higher fitness, its frequency would be expected to increase. Choice A is true, and not an exception, because the lowest frequency of heterozygotes, from the graph and Hardy Weinberg, is $2 \text{ pq} - 2(.9)(.1) = .18$. Choice C is true, and not an exception, as reduced fitness for the M allele would result in a decline in the frequency of the allele. Choice D is true, and not an exception, because if MM and Mm were embryo lethal, then the M allele would drop to zero frequency in the second generation.

53. **(C)** The purpose of the methyl groups is to prevent protein binding and thus reduce the compound's allergenic properties.

54. **(A)** Compound **III** has two hydroxyl groups, both of which can hydrogen bond with water and increase its solubility. None of the other compounds has this property.

55. **(D)** TMS is a common protecting group for alcohols. Silyl ethers are inert to many common organic reaction reagents; however, they can later be hydrolyzed with acid to regenerate the alcohol functional group.

56. **(A)** Diethyl ether is the only solvent choice that will not react with the Grignard reagent used in step one of the transformation of the aldehyde group to an alcohol.

57. **(D)** According to the general chemical formula for an alkane (C_NH_{2N+2}), the formula C_3H_4 is missing 4 hydrogen atoms. This indicates the compound has *two degrees of unsaturation*. Answer D would require *three*.

58. **(A)** Isomer A is more stable (has lower energy) because both bromine substituents can be placed in equatorial positions. This is not possible for isomer B.

59. **(D)** Random mating is one of the Hardy–Weinberg conditions required for the maintenance of stable allele frequencies in a population. Nonrandom mating, such as inbreeding, leads to changes in gene frequencies, as do genetic drift, natural selection, gene flow, and mutation.

Psychological, Social, and Biological Foundations

1. **(D)** The target in a signal detection experiment is the stimulus that the subject has to identify as present or not present. In this case, it is the bright red dot. The noise consists of any other sensory input that is present, which makes detecting the target more difficult. In this case, both the 60-watt light and the buzzer are present. Only choice D matches this information.

2. **(C)** Choice C is correct because in Experiment 1 the subject is allowed time to adapt to the testing surroundings (sensory adaptation), which contributes to all subjects having a similar baseline for their just-noticeable threshold when tested. Choice A is incorrect because it does not affect the validity of Experiment 1. Choice B is incorrect because testing both light and sound does not make an experiment more valid. Choice D is incorrect because the experimental design does not require that the strength be increased, and, if anything, choice D would point out a flaw in Experiment 1, not Experiment 2.

3. **(B)** Choice B is correct because, as predicted by Webber's law, the strength of the just-noticeable difference varies in direct proportion to the baseline. The baseline is higher in the second part of the experiment and so the time needed to notice the change is longer. Choice A is incorrect because the just-noticeable difference does not vary by frequency of the stimulus. Choice C is incorrect because the experiment was not long enough to produce this kind of fatigue. Choice D is incorrect because the subject was told to expect an increase in both trials, so this does not explain the difference.

4. **(C)** Choice C is correct because the difference threshold measures the subject's ability to detect a change in a signal, rather than the presence of a signal. Only Experiment 2 tests this. Choice A is incorrect because adaptation—a physiological change in response

to being exposed to a stimulus or to the absence of a stimulus for a period of time—is present in both experiments. Choice B is incorrect because the perception threshold measures the ability to detect the presence of a stimulus and is tested in both experiments. Choice D is incorrect because top-down processing—applying overall knowledge to specific details—is not measured in either experiment.

5. **(D)** Choice D is correct because a false alarm is defined as reporting that the stimulus is present when it is not. Choice A is incorrect because correct rejection is defined as correctly identifying when the stimulus is not present. Choice B is incorrect because a miss is defined as not reporting when the stimulus is actually present. Choice C is incorrect because a hit is defined as correctly reporting when the stimulus is present.

6. **(C)** Choice C is correct because the patient's body did not feel like it was moving, which is a sign that the vestibular system was functioning correctly. Choice A is incorrect for this reason. Choices B and D are incorrect because the illusion that the patient experienced is not a sign of pathology and occurs in unexceptional people.

7. **(D)** Choice D is correct because the patient's actions demonstrate a failure of depth perception and asking for external input would compensate. Choices A and C are incorrect because if one of his eyes is unable to see, these strategies would not improve his depth perception. Choice B is incorrect because the problem was due to depth perception, not hand coordination.

8. **(B)** Choice B is correct because the vestibular system is responsible for balance. Choices C and D are incorrect because they are related to vision. Choice A is incorrect because it is related to the positioning of the body in the world and would not on its own produce a sense of dizziness.

9. **(A)** Choice A is correct because the passage provides the most evidence for the patient having lost binocular vision (depth perception). Choice B is incorrect because there is no impairment in his long-term memory, but rather his short-term memory or his perceptual constancy. Choice C is incorrect because his vestibular was functioning correctly when he experienced a common optical illusion. Choice D is incorrect because near-sightedness is not a consideration with depth perception.

10. **(B)** Choice B is correct because the patient is responding to the pieces of information provided by Dr. Montoya to construct a theory of what must have occurred, the definition of bottom-up processing. Choice A is incorrect because this is not an example of perceptual constancy. Choice C is incorrect because this is an example of bottom-up, not top-down processing. Choice D is incorrect because it describes top-down processing.

11. **(D)** Choice D is correct because the patient's inability to recognize the doctor once her appearance had changed slightly is the definition of a failure of perceptual constancy. Choice A is incorrect because the example does not pertain to parallel processing. Choice B is incorrect because the patient is not experiencing quick blindness and sensory deprivation followed by a hallucination as is common with Charles Bonnet syndrome. Choice C is incorrect because the faulty binocular vision was pertinent to the client knocking the glass over in his lack of depth perception, but not his failure to recognize the doctor.

12. **(A)** Choice A is correct because the structure of deviance is being described as supporting society. The concept of society's structures and institutions working together

to maintain societal equilibrium is a functionalist one. Choice B is incorrect because conflict theorists focus on how those in power in society label who and what is deviant to their own advantage. Choice C is incorrect because symbolic interactionists focus on how micro-level interactions in small groups affect how people define or label deviance. Choice D is incorrect because social constructionists focus on how definitions of deviance are constructed in interactions that take place in small groups.

13. **(C)** Choice C is correct because output can be defined as the response that results from the registration of environmental information. Choice A is incorrect because the word "yield" is not used in information processing to mean the output. Choice B is incorrect because the output is not necessarily an expression of opinion. Choice D is incorrect because feedback in an information system refers to output that is then used as a further input to elicit another response.

14. **(B)** Choice B is correct because the process by which the body adapts physiologically to stress occurs in these three stages. Choice A is incorrect because post-traumatic stress disorder is a mental health diagnosis often brought on by extreme stress. Choice C is incorrect because generalized anxiety disorder is a mental health diagnosis in which an individual remains consistently fearful or anxious for a period of at least six months. Choice D is incorrect because the fight or flight response is only the first stage of the general adaptation syndrome.

15. **(D)** Choice D is correct because this is the definition of Charles Bonnet syndrome. Choice A refers to the processing of multiple inputs at the same time. Choice B refers to the modification of thoughts or behaviors in response to new information. Choice C refers to the neurological changes that accompany ongoing exposure to a sensory input.

16. **(D)** Choice D is correct because this example illustrates the failure to comply with a societal norm that does not involve a moral component or have strong societal support, as do mores. Choice A is incorrect for the same reason. Choice B is incorrect because rituals are conducted on special occasions involving patterned behavior. Choice C is incorrect because assimilation is the process by which minorities take on the characteristics of the dominant culture, and this example does not mention minorities or indicate any type of conformity.

17. **(A)** Choice A is correct because by allowing all members of Tribe Y to choose their role in society, the opportunity for certain roles to be ignored or marginalized is greater. Choice B is incorrect because nothing in the passage defends that there is a power struggle among leaders. Choice C is incorrect because even though Tribe Y allows both men and women to enact opposite gender roles, it does not eliminate their presence in society. Choice D is incorrect because the food shortages and inequalities in task management present in Tribe Y display inefficiency.

18. **(C)** Choice C is correct because it violates the strict societal roles in which men have the exclusive responsibility for hunting. Choice A is incorrect because, as a male in Tribe X, it is a son's duty to learn how to hunt and provide for the tribe. Choice B is incorrect because there is nothing in the passage that indicates that an elderly chief could not do this. Choice D is incorrect because it displays a folkway violation. It may be a child's duty to fetch water, but there are no rules present to demand such a task.

19. **(D)** Choice D is correct because Tribe X's androcentric society matches pre-industrial U.S. society that consistently values the efforts of men above women. Choice A is incorrect because Tribe Y's overabundance of caregivers supplies its children with more than the necessary quantity of agents of socialization. Choice B is incorrect because although Tribe X and Y reflect opposite systems of role allocation, Tribe Y's equal opportunity allows members to enact gender roles much like those of Tribe X. Choice C is incorrect because Tribe X grooms its men from birth to adopt leadership roles, thus providing them with the ability to be a strong leader.

20. **(A)** Choice A is correct because the passage states that there are too many childcare providers and not enough hunters. Given a male:female ratio of about 50:50, this means there are more men who chose childcare than women who chose hunting. Choice B is incorrect because the food shortage is not due to inefficient hunting. Choice C is incorrect because there is nothing in the passage to defend that hunting groups are mostly women. Choice D is incorrect because then there would be no ongoing food shortage.

21. **(B)** Choice B is correct because the expectation that one's gender is able to accomplish a task can enhance performance, and expectation that one's gender cannot perform a task, which would be the case for the women from Tribe X, can diminish performance. Choice A is incorrect because, if anything, it would lead to better skills. Choice C is incorrect because neither group of women had used a hunting weapon. Choice D is incorrect because it is irrelevant to shooting an arrow and if anything, greater confidence in general does not explain why the women from Tribe X performed worse with the bow.

22. **(A)** Choice A is correct because by predetermining roles for men and women, Tribe X passes over its members' individual strengths. A woman who excels at hunting and could be an asset as a hunter is required to be a mother and caretaker. Choice B is incorrect because having an exact description of one's role can have the advantage of eliminating doubt in one's place and use in society. Choice C is incorrect because it would only pertain to Tribe Y. Choice D is incorrect because unlike in Tribe Y, in Tribe X the balance of hunters and childcare providers is tied to the balance of men and women, and it is unlikely that the proportion of women would become too low.

23. **(B)** Choice B is correct. Choice A is much too low for a threshold of intellectual developmental disorder. Choices C and D are in the normal range.

24. **(D)** Choice D is correct because social control is defined as the way in which society tries to regulate the behaviors of its members, and sanctions are a significant way that society does this. Choice A is incorrect because anticipatory socialization involves the desires of an individual to be a part of a group, which could include rewards but does not directly involve punishments. Choice B is incorrect because stigmatizing involves placing a negative label on an individual (punishment) but does not involve a reward. Choice C is incorrect because, like anticipatory socialization, normative social influence concerns a person's desires to be accepted by a group (rewards) but does not directly involve punishments.

25. **(A)** Choice A is correct because Korsakoff's syndrome is caused by thiamine deficiency and results in the symptoms described. Choices B, C, and D are incorrect because Alzheimer's would not be consistent with an onset due to thiamine deficiency.

26. **(D)** Choice D is correct because the amyloid plaque in the brain is a characteristic of Alzheimer's. In addition, all of the other answer choices can be eliminated. Choice A is incorrect because the mother does not experience any tremors or difficulty walking. Choice B is incorrect because the mother stopped drinking ten years earlier, and any alcohol-induced thiamine deficiency would have resulted in symptoms at that time. Choice C is incorrect because most of the mother's symptoms are not related to forgetting information.

27. **(D)** Choice D is correct because procedural memory involves knowing how to perform physical tasks. Choice A is incorrect because semantic memory involves remembering vocabulary. Choice B is incorrect because knowing how to dress requires long-term, not short-term, memory. Choice C is incorrect because heptatic memory involves remembering shapes, sizes, and grip of objects. Although heptatic memory may be involved in holding and manipulating items of clothing, forgetting how to put clothes on or in what order to put them on goes beyond heptatic memory.

28. **(B)** Choice B is correct because spreading activation theory involves accessing a memory by activating memories associated with the target memory. Choice A is incorrect because spreading activation theory is as described for choice B. Choices C and D are incorrect because primacy refers to remembering the first item in a list.

29. **(B)** Choice B is correct because the loss of the mother's husband could be expected to cause bereavement. Choice A is incorrect because the mother stopped using alcohol ten years ago. Choice C is incorrect because the absence of tremors rules out Parkinson's. Choice D is incorrect because separation anxiety disorder is a disorder of children.

30. **(C)** Choice C is correct because the recency effect makes it more likely that the last item on a list (the item most recently reviewed) is remembered accurately, while earlier items tend to be forgotten. The first item, and possibly the second, was remembered because of the primacy effect. Choice A is incorrect because semantic knowledge involves vocabulary. Choice B is incorrect because the fact that several of the items were remembered proves that the information was stored. Choice D is incorrect because a flashbulb memory refers to a memory that is vivid and intense because of a trauma or shock that occurred when the memory was formed.

31. **(A)** Choice A is correct because there is no evidence that the mother's response was intended to achieve any personal gain or change the doctor's attitude. Choice B is incorrect because the mother's response is not an example of false sensory impressions. Choice C is incorrect because there is no evidence that the mother was trying to achieve a personal end. Choice D is incorrect because there is no evidence that the mother was trying to influence the doctor's attitude.

32. **(D)** Choice D is correct because significantly fewer people with generalized anxiety disorder have extraversion. As a result, they would have on the average smaller medial orbitofrontal cortex and less ability to process information about rewards for behavior, on which positive reinforcement depends. Choices A and B are incorrect because generalized anxiety disorder is correlated with smaller orbitofrontal cortex. Choice C is incorrect because the medial orbitofrontal cortex is not necessarily involved with impulsivity.

33. **(A)** Choice A is correct because people with generalized anxiety disorder ranked themselves higher in conscientiousness, which is associated with organizational skills and

dependability. Choice B is incorrect because impulsivity is associated with lower conscientiousness. Choice C is incorrect because curiosity correlates with openness and the incidence of openness is the same in both groups. Choice D is incorrect because lower suspicion is associated with higher agreeableness, but the generalized anxiety group had lower agreeableness.

34. **(C)** Choice C is correct because, to indicate a genetic component, the gene would have to be correlated with differences between the general population and people with generalized anxiety disorder. In choice C, the presence of the gene correlates with more conscientiousness and less agreeability, which is consistent with the findings in the study. Choice A is incorrect because it would result in more openness and less extraversion. The study shows that openness does not differ between the groups, so choice A is not as strong as choice C. Choice B is incorrect because it would result in more conscientiousness (which is consistent with the study) and more agreeableness (which is not consistent). Choice D is incorrect because it would result in more neuroticism (consistent) and less conscientiousness (not consistent).

35. **(C)** Choice C is correct. Out of 1000 people, 970 would not have the disorder and 30 would. Of the 970 (97), 10 percent would have neuroticism as their main trait. Of the remaining 30 (10.5), 35% would have neuroticism as their main trait. The total is 107.5.

36. **(D)** Choice D is correct because Erikson postulates that personality is developed in predictable stages that must be gone through in order. This contradicts choice B. In contrast to Freud, Erikson believes that personality continues to develop throughout life. This contradicts choice C. Choice A reflects the situational approach to behavior.

37. **(C)** Choice C is correct because there is a clear relationship between the two but that is not enough to defend that there is a causal relationship, as implied in choices A and B. Choice D is incorrect because openness was ranked the same for both groups.

38. **(D)** Choice D is correct because the dramatic change in doctor preference once gender was identified shows that a bias was operating. Choice A is incorrect because although a large majority of respondents changed their vote during question 3, 25 percent still believed that the female doctor was more qualified. Choice B is incorrect because the study itself does not provide any evidence to support this, even if people believe it. Choice C is incorrect because the results clearly show that when gender is involved, some participants ignore the doctors' experience.

39. **(C)** Choice C is correct because it would eliminate one possible extraneous variable, namely that some people preferred a doctor who was more recently out of medical school. Choice A is incorrect because it would have masked the fact that patients were choosing the male because of gender. Choice B is incorrect because it would be irrelevant. The point of the study was to evaluate preferences based on gender and credentials only. Choice D is incorrect for the same reason.

40. **(A)** Choice A is correct because feeling uncomfortable with the opposite gender performing a physical confuses the issue of which doctor the patients feel is more competent. Choice B is incorrect because without knowing the gender prior to responses 1 and 2, there can be no sexually discriminate bias. Choice C is incorrect because each participant is not only unaware of his or her fellow participant's answers, but each is not informed of their answers to the questionnaire. Choice D is incorrect because if men

and women have equal bias, then the fact that there are more men does not distort the results.

41. **(C)** Choice C is correct because if the hiring committee is dominated by men, this constitutes discrimination at an institutional level. Choice A is incorrect because this does not affect institutional policy. Choice B is incorrect because this does not represent discrimination. It may be that it is important for female doctors to know if they are pregnant for their own safety and health. Choice D is incorrect because this does not necessarily lead to any discrimination. The word "institution" is a distractor.

42. **(B)** Choice B is correct because, although patients predominantly value medical skill in a doctor—for which they have a preference for males—they may also value caregiving skills in a nurse, and this would cause a conflict between the two values. Choice A is incorrect because it is the same conflict that existed in the original experiment. Choice C is incorrect because patients may prefer female qualities in a nurse. Choice D is incorrect because patients may still prefer a male.

43. **(B)** Choice B is the correct range. The other choices are too low or too high.

44. **(A)** Choice A is correct because people with a severe hearing loss do not necessarily look different or move differently compared to people without a disability. A hearing loss is typically only apparent when trying to communicate verbally. By contrast, the movements of a person with a visual impairment are typically readily visible. Choice B is incorrect because hearing-impaired people can communicate fluently with other people who share their nonverbal mode of communication. People with visual impairment are not impaired in verbal communication. Choice C is incorrect because people with hearing impairments may miss sounds such as police sirens, oncoming traffic, and falling objects. People with visual impairments may miss visual cues. Choice D is incorrect because people with hearing impairments are limited in verbal communication, and people with visual impairments are limited by mobility.

45. **(D)** Choice D is correct because gifted children typically exhibit all of the traits mentioned. Choice A is incorrect because alertness refers to awareness and would not include being headstrong. Choice B is incorrect because attention deficit hyperactivity disorder is characterized by the inability to focus attention. Choice C is incorrect because separation anxiety disorder refers to children who exhibit anxiety when separated from an attachment figure.

46. **(B)** Choice B is correct because the frequency of disruptive behaviors is a dependent variable, and accuracy of the experimental outcomes is improved by getting an initial frequency of disruptive behaviors before beginning treatment. Choice A is incorrect because a confounding variable is something that influences outcomes and may not yield a truly accurate depiction of behavior. Choice C is incorrect because the frequency of disruptive behaviors is a dependent variable. Choice D is incorrect because statistical power increases with adding more measurements/subjects, and this also helps improve accuracy.

47. **(D)** Choice D is correct because operant conditioning applies a reinforcer that is non-neutral (either pleasant or aversive) after a behavior. Choice A is incorrect because classical conditioning applies a neutral stimulus before a reflexive behavior. Choice B is

incorrect for the same reason. Choice C is incorrect because stickers, praise, and prizes are not neutral.

48. **(B)** Choice B is correct because over time, children receiving either tokens alone or tokens plus modeling begin associating good behavior with rewards. Choice A is incorrect because negative reinforcement means removing an undesired stimulus, and in this case, there are no stimuli being removed. Choice C is incorrect because negative punishment would mean taking something desirable away for bad behavior, and in the token reward system, no stickers are taken away. Choice D is incorrect because it applies only to the tokens plus modeling group.

49. **(D)** Choice D is correct because negative punishment is the removal of a desired stimulus after an undesirable behavior. Choice A is incorrect because it involves the application of a negative stimulus, rather than the removal of a positive one. Choice B is incorrect because it involves reinforcing a behavior and is an example of a negative reinforcer. Choice C is incorrect because applying a stimulus before a behavior is an example of classical, not operant, conditioning and does not affect the incidence of the behavior.

50. **(D)** Choice D is correct because both treatment modalities do exhibit a 20 percent decline in the frequency of oppositional or defiant behaviors from the second appointment to the third appointment. For the token reward system only modality, the frequency of oppositional or defiant behavior from the second to the third appointment were approximately 80 percent and 60 percent, respectively, whereas the frequency of oppositional or defiant behavior from the second to the third appointment for the token reward system plus modeling modality was approximately 70 percent and 50 percent, respectively. Choice A is incorrect because the token reward system only exhibited a 20 percent decrease in oppositional or defiant behavior frequency, not 30 percent. Choice B is incorrect because the token reward system plus modeling modality exhibited a 20 percent decrease in the frequency of oppositional or defiant behaviors, not 10 percent. Choice C is incorrect because even though the token reward system only modality did exhibit a 20 percent decrease in the frequency of oppositional or defiant behavior, so did the token reward system plus modeling modality.

51. **(C)** Each child's personal history with his or her parents' promises and threats is a confounding variable that can skew the results of the experiment. Choice A is incorrect because a valid experiment requires a random assignment. Choice B is incorrect because the children's preferred responses to reward and punishment are the dependent variables being tested. Choice D is incorrect because 100 subjects is a significant sample size.

52. **(A)** A Freudian would interpret the results as evidence of an Oedipus complex, involving an attraction to the mother and rivalry with the father. Choice B is incorrect because, according to Freud, girls, not boys, experience penis envy. Choice C is incorrect because in Freudian theory the latency stage does not begin until the age of 6 and involves ego impulses, not id. Choice D is incorrect because there is no evidence of an anal-expulsive personality. Aggression is not in and of itself such evidence.

53. **(C)** Vygotsky believed that children learn through interaction with others, especially more knowledgeable others. In choice C the child learns through observing his parents play independently. Choice A is incorrect because it does not put the child in contact with others. Choice B is incorrect because, although it might be successful for other

reasons, it does not conform to Vygotsky's principles. Choice D is incorrect because the child is old enough to learn some independent behavior.

54. **(B)** Choice B captures the essence of the feminist argument that some people are guided by principle alone and others take into account the lives of those around them. Choice A is incorrect because, in this case, it is the mother who bases her morality on principles alone. Choice C is incorrect because it is not the case that the mother valued the child less than did the father. Rather, she felt that the principle was more important than her value of the child. Choice D is incorrect because feminist theory does not believe that women are not moral but that they base their morality on factors that differ from those on which men base their morality.

55. **(B)** Choice B is correct because the boy is in the stage of Initiative versus Guilt. That he exerts his own will when with his father is a sign that he feels greater comfort with his father, which in turn is a sign that he receives more encouragement from his father than his mother. Choice A is incorrect because there is no evidence suggesting regression. Choice C is incorrect for the same reasons that choice B is correct. Choice D is incorrect because there is no evidence to support it.

56. **(C)** Choice C is correct because collectivist cultures value interdependence and cooperation rather than independence, so the educator's proposal would be considered harmful by people from such cultures whose children attend such a school. Choice A is incorrect because it is not true. Choice B is incorrect because even if true, the policy would be harmful for people with collectivist values. Choice D is incorrect because it is not true.

57. **(D)** Choice D is correct because in the preconventional stage, children respond to the expectation of punishment. Choice A is incorrect because the boy behaves worse with his father. Choice B is incorrect because Kohlberg does not address these dynamics. Choice C is incorrect because the boy has not developed past the preconventional stage.

58. **(C)** Choice C is correct because of the definitions of explicit and implicit memory. Choice A is incorrect because working memory organizes information, and sensory memory is a brief impression of a sensory experience. Choice B is incorrect because recall refers to the ability to retrieve a memory with little effort, and recognition refers to identifying a correct answer on a memory task. Choice D is incorrect because memory construction occurs when the mind fills in missing information, and flashbulb memory is a memory that is easily retrieved because it is associated with a strong emotion.

59. **(D)** Choice D is correct because I, II, and III all describe the effects of specific languages on cognition and/or view of the world.

Answer Sheet: Practice Test 2

CHEMICAL AND PHYSICAL FOUNDATIONS

1. Ⓐ Ⓑ Ⓒ Ⓓ 13. Ⓐ Ⓑ Ⓒ Ⓓ 25. Ⓐ Ⓑ Ⓒ Ⓓ 37. Ⓐ Ⓑ Ⓒ Ⓓ 49. Ⓐ Ⓑ Ⓒ Ⓓ
2. Ⓐ Ⓑ Ⓒ Ⓓ 14. Ⓐ Ⓑ Ⓒ Ⓓ 26. Ⓐ Ⓑ Ⓒ Ⓓ 38. Ⓐ Ⓑ Ⓒ Ⓓ 50. Ⓐ Ⓑ Ⓒ Ⓓ
3. Ⓐ Ⓑ Ⓒ Ⓓ 15. Ⓐ Ⓑ Ⓒ Ⓓ 27. Ⓐ Ⓑ Ⓒ Ⓓ 39. Ⓐ Ⓑ Ⓒ Ⓓ 51. Ⓐ Ⓑ Ⓒ Ⓓ
4. Ⓐ Ⓑ Ⓒ Ⓓ 16. Ⓐ Ⓑ Ⓒ Ⓓ 28. Ⓐ Ⓑ Ⓒ Ⓓ 40. Ⓐ Ⓑ Ⓒ Ⓓ 52. Ⓐ Ⓑ Ⓒ Ⓓ
5. Ⓐ Ⓑ Ⓒ Ⓓ 17. Ⓐ Ⓑ Ⓒ Ⓓ 29. Ⓐ Ⓑ Ⓒ Ⓓ 41. Ⓐ Ⓑ Ⓒ Ⓓ 53. Ⓐ Ⓑ Ⓒ Ⓓ
6. Ⓐ Ⓑ Ⓒ Ⓓ 18. Ⓐ Ⓑ Ⓒ Ⓓ 30. Ⓐ Ⓑ Ⓒ Ⓓ 42. Ⓐ Ⓑ Ⓒ Ⓓ 54. Ⓐ Ⓑ Ⓒ Ⓓ
7. Ⓐ Ⓑ Ⓒ Ⓓ 19. Ⓐ Ⓑ Ⓒ Ⓓ 31. Ⓐ Ⓑ Ⓒ Ⓓ 43. Ⓐ Ⓑ Ⓒ Ⓓ 55. Ⓐ Ⓑ Ⓒ Ⓓ
8. Ⓐ Ⓑ Ⓒ Ⓓ 20. Ⓐ Ⓑ Ⓒ Ⓓ 32. Ⓐ Ⓑ Ⓒ Ⓓ 44. Ⓐ Ⓑ Ⓒ Ⓓ 56. Ⓐ Ⓑ Ⓒ Ⓓ
9. Ⓐ Ⓑ Ⓒ Ⓓ 21. Ⓐ Ⓑ Ⓒ Ⓓ 33. Ⓐ Ⓑ Ⓒ Ⓓ 45. Ⓐ Ⓑ Ⓒ Ⓓ 57. Ⓐ Ⓑ Ⓒ Ⓓ
10. Ⓐ Ⓑ Ⓒ Ⓓ 22. Ⓐ Ⓑ Ⓒ Ⓓ 34. Ⓐ Ⓑ Ⓒ Ⓓ 46. Ⓐ Ⓑ Ⓒ Ⓓ 58. Ⓐ Ⓑ Ⓒ Ⓓ
11. Ⓐ Ⓑ Ⓒ Ⓓ 23. Ⓐ Ⓑ Ⓒ Ⓓ 35. Ⓐ Ⓑ Ⓒ Ⓓ 47. Ⓐ Ⓑ Ⓒ Ⓓ 59. Ⓐ Ⓑ Ⓒ Ⓓ
12. Ⓐ Ⓑ Ⓒ Ⓓ 24. Ⓐ Ⓑ Ⓒ Ⓓ 36. Ⓐ Ⓑ Ⓒ Ⓓ 48. Ⓐ Ⓑ Ⓒ Ⓓ

CRITICAL ANALYSIS AND REASONING

1. Ⓐ Ⓑ Ⓒ Ⓓ 12. Ⓐ Ⓑ Ⓒ Ⓓ 23. Ⓐ Ⓑ Ⓒ Ⓓ 34. Ⓐ Ⓑ Ⓒ Ⓓ 45. Ⓐ Ⓑ Ⓒ Ⓓ
2. Ⓐ Ⓑ Ⓒ Ⓓ 13. Ⓐ Ⓑ Ⓒ Ⓓ 24. Ⓐ Ⓑ Ⓒ Ⓓ 35. Ⓐ Ⓑ Ⓒ Ⓓ 46. Ⓐ Ⓑ Ⓒ Ⓓ
3. Ⓐ Ⓑ Ⓒ Ⓓ 14. Ⓐ Ⓑ Ⓒ Ⓓ 25. Ⓐ Ⓑ Ⓒ Ⓓ 36. Ⓐ Ⓑ Ⓒ Ⓓ 47. Ⓐ Ⓑ Ⓒ Ⓓ
4. Ⓐ Ⓑ Ⓒ Ⓓ 15. Ⓐ Ⓑ Ⓒ Ⓓ 26. Ⓐ Ⓑ Ⓒ Ⓓ 37. Ⓐ Ⓑ Ⓒ Ⓓ 48. Ⓐ Ⓑ Ⓒ Ⓓ
5. Ⓐ Ⓑ Ⓒ Ⓓ 16. Ⓐ Ⓑ Ⓒ Ⓓ 27. Ⓐ Ⓑ Ⓒ Ⓓ 38. Ⓐ Ⓑ Ⓒ Ⓓ 49. Ⓐ Ⓑ Ⓒ Ⓓ
6. Ⓐ Ⓑ Ⓒ Ⓓ 17. Ⓐ Ⓑ Ⓒ Ⓓ 28. Ⓐ Ⓑ Ⓒ Ⓓ 39. Ⓐ Ⓑ Ⓒ Ⓓ 50. Ⓐ Ⓑ Ⓒ Ⓓ
7. Ⓐ Ⓑ Ⓒ Ⓓ 18. Ⓐ Ⓑ Ⓒ Ⓓ 29. Ⓐ Ⓑ Ⓒ Ⓓ 40. Ⓐ Ⓑ Ⓒ Ⓓ 51. Ⓐ Ⓑ Ⓒ Ⓓ
8. Ⓐ Ⓑ Ⓒ Ⓓ 19. Ⓐ Ⓑ Ⓒ Ⓓ 30. Ⓐ Ⓑ Ⓒ Ⓓ 41. Ⓐ Ⓑ Ⓒ Ⓓ 52. Ⓐ Ⓑ Ⓒ Ⓓ
9. Ⓐ Ⓑ Ⓒ Ⓓ 20. Ⓐ Ⓑ Ⓒ Ⓓ 31. Ⓐ Ⓑ Ⓒ Ⓓ 42. Ⓐ Ⓑ Ⓒ Ⓓ 53. Ⓐ Ⓑ Ⓒ Ⓓ
10. Ⓐ Ⓑ Ⓒ Ⓓ 21. Ⓐ Ⓑ Ⓒ Ⓓ 32. Ⓐ Ⓑ Ⓒ Ⓓ 43. Ⓐ Ⓑ Ⓒ Ⓓ
11. Ⓐ Ⓑ Ⓒ Ⓓ 22. Ⓐ Ⓑ Ⓒ Ⓓ 33. Ⓐ Ⓑ Ⓒ Ⓓ 44. Ⓐ Ⓑ Ⓒ Ⓓ

BIOLOGICAL AND BIOCHEMICAL FOUNDATIONS

1. Ⓐ Ⓑ Ⓒ Ⓓ 13. Ⓐ Ⓑ Ⓒ Ⓓ 25. Ⓐ Ⓑ Ⓒ Ⓓ 37. Ⓐ Ⓑ Ⓒ Ⓓ 49. Ⓐ Ⓑ Ⓒ Ⓓ
2. Ⓐ Ⓑ Ⓒ Ⓓ 14. Ⓐ Ⓑ Ⓒ Ⓓ 26. Ⓐ Ⓑ Ⓒ Ⓓ 38. Ⓐ Ⓑ Ⓒ Ⓓ 50. Ⓐ Ⓑ Ⓒ Ⓓ
3. Ⓐ Ⓑ Ⓒ Ⓓ 15. Ⓐ Ⓑ Ⓒ Ⓓ 27. Ⓐ Ⓑ Ⓒ Ⓓ 39. Ⓐ Ⓑ Ⓒ Ⓓ 51. Ⓐ Ⓑ Ⓒ Ⓓ
4. Ⓐ Ⓑ Ⓒ Ⓓ 16. Ⓐ Ⓑ Ⓒ Ⓓ 28. Ⓐ Ⓑ Ⓒ Ⓓ 40. Ⓐ Ⓑ Ⓒ Ⓓ 52. Ⓐ Ⓑ Ⓒ Ⓓ
5. Ⓐ Ⓑ Ⓒ Ⓓ 17. Ⓐ Ⓑ Ⓒ Ⓓ 29. Ⓐ Ⓑ Ⓒ Ⓓ 41. Ⓐ Ⓑ Ⓒ Ⓓ 53. Ⓐ Ⓑ Ⓒ Ⓓ
6. Ⓐ Ⓑ Ⓒ Ⓓ 18. Ⓐ Ⓑ Ⓒ Ⓓ 30. Ⓐ Ⓑ Ⓒ Ⓓ 42. Ⓐ Ⓑ Ⓒ Ⓓ 54. Ⓐ Ⓑ Ⓒ Ⓓ
7. Ⓐ Ⓑ Ⓒ Ⓓ 19. Ⓐ Ⓑ Ⓒ Ⓓ 31. Ⓐ Ⓑ Ⓒ Ⓓ 43. Ⓐ Ⓑ Ⓒ Ⓓ 55. Ⓐ Ⓑ Ⓒ Ⓓ
8. Ⓐ Ⓑ Ⓒ Ⓓ 20. Ⓐ Ⓑ Ⓒ Ⓓ 32. Ⓐ Ⓑ Ⓒ Ⓓ 44. Ⓐ Ⓑ Ⓒ Ⓓ 56. Ⓐ Ⓑ Ⓒ Ⓓ
9. Ⓐ Ⓑ Ⓒ Ⓓ 21. Ⓐ Ⓑ Ⓒ Ⓓ 33. Ⓐ Ⓑ Ⓒ Ⓓ 45. Ⓐ Ⓑ Ⓒ Ⓓ 57. Ⓐ Ⓑ Ⓒ Ⓓ
10. Ⓐ Ⓑ Ⓒ Ⓓ 22. Ⓐ Ⓑ Ⓒ Ⓓ 34. Ⓐ Ⓑ Ⓒ Ⓓ 46. Ⓐ Ⓑ Ⓒ Ⓓ 58. Ⓐ Ⓑ Ⓒ Ⓓ
11. Ⓐ Ⓑ Ⓒ Ⓓ 23. Ⓐ Ⓑ Ⓒ Ⓓ 35. Ⓐ Ⓑ Ⓒ Ⓓ 47. Ⓐ Ⓑ Ⓒ Ⓓ 59. Ⓐ Ⓑ Ⓒ Ⓓ
12. Ⓐ Ⓑ Ⓒ Ⓓ 24. Ⓐ Ⓑ Ⓒ Ⓓ 36. Ⓐ Ⓑ Ⓒ Ⓓ 48. Ⓐ Ⓑ Ⓒ Ⓓ

PSYCHOLOGICAL, SOCIAL, AND BIOLOGICAL FOUNDATIONS

1. Ⓐ Ⓑ Ⓒ Ⓓ 13. Ⓐ Ⓑ Ⓒ Ⓓ 25. Ⓐ Ⓑ Ⓒ Ⓓ 37. Ⓐ Ⓑ Ⓒ Ⓓ 49. Ⓐ Ⓑ Ⓒ Ⓓ
2. Ⓐ Ⓑ Ⓒ Ⓓ 14. Ⓐ Ⓑ Ⓒ Ⓓ 26. Ⓐ Ⓑ Ⓒ Ⓓ 38. Ⓐ Ⓑ Ⓒ Ⓓ 50. Ⓐ Ⓑ Ⓒ Ⓓ
3. Ⓐ Ⓑ Ⓒ Ⓓ 15. Ⓐ Ⓑ Ⓒ Ⓓ 27. Ⓐ Ⓑ Ⓒ Ⓓ 39. Ⓐ Ⓑ Ⓒ Ⓓ 51. Ⓐ Ⓑ Ⓒ Ⓓ
4. Ⓐ Ⓑ Ⓒ Ⓓ 16. Ⓐ Ⓑ Ⓒ Ⓓ 28. Ⓐ Ⓑ Ⓒ Ⓓ 40. Ⓐ Ⓑ Ⓒ Ⓓ 52. Ⓐ Ⓑ Ⓒ Ⓓ
5. Ⓐ Ⓑ Ⓒ Ⓓ 17. Ⓐ Ⓑ Ⓒ Ⓓ 29. Ⓐ Ⓑ Ⓒ Ⓓ 41. Ⓐ Ⓑ Ⓒ Ⓓ 53. Ⓐ Ⓑ Ⓒ Ⓓ
6. Ⓐ Ⓑ Ⓒ Ⓓ 18. Ⓐ Ⓑ Ⓒ Ⓓ 30. Ⓐ Ⓑ Ⓒ Ⓓ 42. Ⓐ Ⓑ Ⓒ Ⓓ 54. Ⓐ Ⓑ Ⓒ Ⓓ
7. Ⓐ Ⓑ Ⓒ Ⓓ 19. Ⓐ Ⓑ Ⓒ Ⓓ 31. Ⓐ Ⓑ Ⓒ Ⓓ 43. Ⓐ Ⓑ Ⓒ Ⓓ 55. Ⓐ Ⓑ Ⓒ Ⓓ
8. Ⓐ Ⓑ Ⓒ Ⓓ 20. Ⓐ Ⓑ Ⓒ Ⓓ 32. Ⓐ Ⓑ Ⓒ Ⓓ 44. Ⓐ Ⓑ Ⓒ Ⓓ 56. Ⓐ Ⓑ Ⓒ Ⓓ
9. Ⓐ Ⓑ Ⓒ Ⓓ 21. Ⓐ Ⓑ Ⓒ Ⓓ 33. Ⓐ Ⓑ Ⓒ Ⓓ 45. Ⓐ Ⓑ Ⓒ Ⓓ 57. Ⓐ Ⓑ Ⓒ Ⓓ
10. Ⓐ Ⓑ Ⓒ Ⓓ 22. Ⓐ Ⓑ Ⓒ Ⓓ 34. Ⓐ Ⓑ Ⓒ Ⓓ 46. Ⓐ Ⓑ Ⓒ Ⓓ 58. Ⓐ Ⓑ Ⓒ Ⓓ
11. Ⓐ Ⓑ Ⓒ Ⓓ 23. Ⓐ Ⓑ Ⓒ Ⓓ 35. Ⓐ Ⓑ Ⓒ Ⓓ 47. Ⓐ Ⓑ Ⓒ Ⓓ 59. Ⓐ Ⓑ Ⓒ Ⓓ
12. Ⓐ Ⓑ Ⓒ Ⓓ 24. Ⓐ Ⓑ Ⓒ Ⓓ 36. Ⓐ Ⓑ Ⓒ Ⓓ 48. Ⓐ Ⓑ Ⓒ Ⓓ

Periodic Table of the Elements

1	2	3	4	5	6	7	8	9	10	11	12	13	14	15	16	17	18
1 **H** 1.0																	2 **He** 4.0
3 **Li** 6.9	4 **Be** 9.0											5 **B** 10.8	6 **C** 12.0	7 **N** 14.0	8 **O** 16.0	9 **F** 19.0	10 **Ne** 20.2
11 **Na** 23.0	12 **Mg** 24.3											13 **Al** 27.0	14 **Si** 28.1	15 **P** 31.0	16 **S** 32.1	17 **Cl** 35.5	18 **Ar** 39.9
19 **K** 39.1	20 **Ca** 40.1	21 **Sc** 45.0	22 **Ti** 47.9	23 **V** 50.9	24 **Cr** 52.0	25 **Mn** 54.9	26 **Fe** 55.8	27 **Co** 58.8	28 **Ni** 58.7	29 **Cu** 63.5	30 **Zn** 65.4	31 **Ga** 69.7	32 **Ge** 72.6	33 **As** 74.9	34 **Se** 79.0	35 **Br** 79.9	36 **Kr** 83.8
37 **Rb** 85.5	38 **Sr** 87.6	39 **Y** 88.9	40 **Zr** 91.2	41 **Nb** 92.9	42 **Mo** 95.9	43 **Tc** (98)	44 **Ru** 101.1	45 **Rh** 102.9	46 **Pd** 106.4	47 **Ag** 107.9	48 **Cd** 112.4	49 **In** 114.8	50 **Sn** 118.7	51 **Sb** 121.8	52 **Te** 127.6	53 **I** 126.9	54 **Xe** 131.3
55 **Cs** 132.9	56 **Ba** 137.3	57 **La** 138.9	72 **Hf** 178.5	73 **Ta** 180.9	74 **W** 183.9	75 **Re** 186.2	76 **Os** 190.2	77 **Ir** 192.2	78 **Pt** 195.1	79 **Au** 197.0	80 **Hg** 200.6	81 **Tl** 204.4	82 **Pb** 207.2	83 **Bi** 209.0	84 **Po** (209)	85 **At** (210)	86 **Rn** (222)
87 **Fr** (223)	88 **Ra** (226)	89 **Ac†** (227)	104 **Rf** (261)	105 **Db** (262)	106 **Sg** (266)	107 **Bh** (264)	108 **Hs** (277)	109 **Mt** (268)	110 **Ds** (281)	111 **Rg** (280)	112 **Cn** (285)	113 **Uut** (284)	114 **Fl** (289)	115 **Uup** (288)	116 **Lv** (293)	117 **Uus** (294)	118 **Uuo** (294)

★ Lanthanides

58 **Ce** 140.1	59 **Pr** 140.9	60 **Nd** 144.2	61 **Pm** (145)	62 **Sm** 150.4	63 **Eu** 152.0	64 **Gd** 157.3	65 **Tb** 158.9	66 **Dy** 162.5	67 **Ho** 164.9	68 **Er** 167.3	69 **Tm** 168.9	70 **Yb** 173.0	71 **Lu** 175.0
90 **Th** 232.0	91 **Pa** (231)	92 **U** 238.0	93 **Np** (237)	94 **Pu** (244)	95 **Am** (243)	96 **Cm** (247)	97 **Bk** (247)	98 **Cf** (251)	99 **Es** (252)	100 **Fm** (257)	101 **Md** (258)	102 **No** (259)	103 **Lr** (260)

† Actinides

Practice Test 2

CHEMICAL AND PHYSICAL FOUNDATIONS OF BIOLOGICAL SYSTEMS

Time: 95 minutes
59 Questions

DIRECTIONS: The majority of questions in the Chemical and Physical Foundations of Biological Systems section are organized into groups, with each group containing a descriptive passage. Read the passage, and then select the one best answer for each question. Some questions are not drawn from a passage and are also independent of the other questions. When answering questions, eliminate the choices that you are sure are incorrect and then choose the best remaining answer. When you have chosen an answer, mark it in the corresponding location on the answer sheet. A periodic table can be found on the back of your answer sheet. You may consult it as needed.

PASSAGE I

Bromate ion and bromide ion react via a redox reaction in acidic medium according to Equation 1.

$$BrO_3^-{}_{(aq)} + 5Br^-{}_{(aq)} + 6H^+{}_{(aq)} \leftrightarrow 3Br_{2(l)} + 3H_2O_{(l)}$$
Equation 1

Because bromine is a reddish brown liquid, one way to follow the rate of the reaction is by monitoring the concentration of Br_2 based on its absorption of light. The rate of the reaction can be described as the number of moles of bromine produced per second, as shown in Equation 2.

$$\text{Rate} = \Delta[Br_2]/\Delta t$$
Equation 2

The rate law can be determined by a series of experiments summarized in Table 1.

Table 1. Determination of the Rate Law

Trial #	$[BrO_3^-]$ (Mole/L)	$[Br^-]$ (Mole/L)	$[H^+]$ (Mole/L)	Reaction rate (Moles/ L sec)
1	0.10	0.10	0.10	0.8
2	0.20	0.10	0.10	1.6
3	0.20	0.20	0.10	3.2
4	0.10	0.10	0.20	3.2

The rate is determined by monitoring the intensity of light at a wavelength of 400 nm that is absorbed by the reddish-brown bromine that is formed in the reaction.

$$A = \varepsilon \ell c$$
Equation 3

In Equation 3, A is absorbance, ε is the molar extinction coefficient, ℓ is the path or cell length, and c is the molar concentration. Beer's law, shown in Equation 3, states that the absorbance of the solution is linear with respect to concentration and cell path length. The cell length is kept constant at 1.0 cm. The molar extinction coefficient, ε, is a constant at any given wavelength, and for bromine at 400 nm is 300 $M^{-1}cm^{-1}$.

1. Compared to light with a wavelength of 400 nm, light of wavelength 600 nm would have:
   - (A) a greater frequency and a greater energy.
   - (B) a greater frequency and a lower energy.
   - (C) a lower frequency and a greater energy.
   - (D) a lower frequency and a lower energy.

2. After 10 seconds, the absorbance of the solution in trial 1 is 0.900. What is the Br_2 concentration at that time?
   - (A) 2.7 M
   - (B) 0.90 M
   - (C) 0.03 M
   - (D) 0.003 M

3. Based on the data, what is the order of the reaction with respect to BrO_3^-?
   - (A) 0
   - (B) $\frac{1}{2}$
   - (C) 1
   - (D) 2

4. Pure bromine has a density of 3.2 g/cm^3 at room temperature. What is the molarity of pure bromine?
   - (A) 20.0 M
   - (B) 10.0 M
   - (C) 5.0 M
   - (D) 2.0 M

5. The overall reaction is found to follow a fourth-order rate law. What are the units of k, the rate constant?
   - (A) s^{-1}
   - (B) $M^{-1}s^{-1}$
   - (C) $M^{-2}s^{-1}$
   - (D) $M^{-3}s^{-1}$

Kinetic evaluation of enzymes is important when determining an enzyme's potential pharmaceutical use. Drugs usually react with other enzymes in the body either to activate or inhibit the enzyme. Reversible inhibitors are often structural analogs of substrates or products, and they are often used as drugs to slow down a specific enzyme. There are several ways a drug can inhibit an enzyme, and these can be represented by different Lineweaver–Burk plots. Lineweaver–Burk plots show the double reciprocal of the Michaelis–Menten equation. Competitive inhibitors bind to the active site of the enzyme, competing with the substrate to react. The maximum velocity (V_{max}) is unchanged by a competitive inhibitor, and the concentration of substrate at which the reaction takes place at one half its maximum rate (K_m) is increased as more substrate is needed to displace the inhibitor. K_m is a measure of affinity. Uncompetitive inhibition binds at a site other than the active site and binds only to the enzyme-substrate complex to decrease V_{max} and K_m. Noncompetitive inhibition can bind equally well to the enzyme or the enzyme-substrate complex to alter V_{max} but hold K_m constant. In mixed inhibition, the inhibitor does not bind to the active site, but it can bind to the enzyme or the enzyme-substrate complex. Mixed inhibition alters both the V_{max} and K_m. A series of experiments was conducted to measure the activity of two variations of a drug with the enzyme carbonic anhydrase. Carbonic anhydrase is found in red blood cells where it catalyzes the reaction

$$CO_2 + H_2O \xleftarrow{CA} H_2CO_3 \leftrightarrow H^+ + HCO_3^- \qquad (1)$$

to enable CO_2 transfer from tissues to lungs. This enzyme has a significant effect on pH and fluid levels in other areas of the human body as well.

Experiment 1 was conducted to measure the normal enzymatic activity of carbonic anhydrase on normal substrate H_2CO_3 *in vitro*. Data was plotted on a Michaelis–Menten graph (Figure 1).

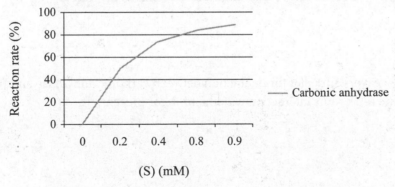

Figure 1. Change of reaction rate of carbonic anhydrase with increasing substrate concentration

Experiment 2 was conducted to more accurately measure V_{max} of carbonic anhydrase in the presence of H_2CO_3 *in vitro* by plotting the information on a Lineweaver–Burk plot. The V_{max} of carbonic anhydrase in the presence of Drug X (Figure 2) and in the presence of Drug Y was also measured *in vitro* (Figure 3).

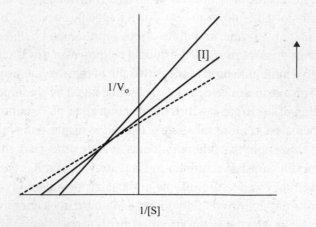

Figure 2. Lineweaver–Burk plot for interaction between carbonic anhydrase and Drug X (The dotted line represents interaction with no inhibitor present.)

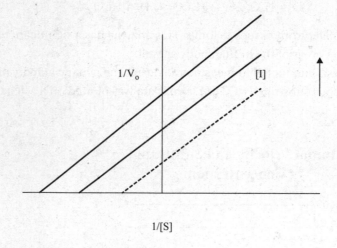

Figure 3. Lineweaver–Burk plot for interaction between carbonic anhydrase and Drug Y (The dotted line represents interaction with no inhibitor present.)

6. What is the Michaelis constant, K_m, of carbonic anhydrase in the presence of H_2CO_3?
   (A) 0.2
   (B) 0.4
   (C) 0.6
   (D) 0.8

7. What type of inhibition does Drug X exhibit on carbonic anhydrase?
   (A) Irreversible
   (B) Competitive
   (C) Noncompetitive
   (D) Mixed

8. Which of the following correctly describes the action of Drug Y on carbonic anhydrase?
   (A) Drug Y binds to the carbonic anhydrase-H_2CO_3 complex to decrease V_{max} and hold affinity constant.
   (B) Drug Y binds to the active site of carbonic anhydrase to decrease V_{max} and hold affinity constant.
   (C) Drug Y binds to the carbonic anhydrase-H_2CO_3 complex to decrease V_{max} and affinity.
   (D) Drug Y binds to carbonic anhydrase to decrease V_{max} and hold affinity constant.

9. The rate equation describing mixed inhibition is:

$$V_0 = \frac{V_{max}[S]}{(\alpha K_m + \alpha'[S])}$$

Which of the following statements describes α of carbonic anhydrase in the presence of Drug X?
   (A) α decreases as the concentration of Drug X increases, lowering the initial velocity of the reaction.
   (B) α increases as the concentration of Drug X decreases, lowering the initial velocity of the reaction.
   (C) α increases as the concentration of Drug X increases, lowering the initial velocity of the reaction.
   (D) α increases as the concentration of Drug X increases, raising the initial velocity of the reaction.

10. The three-dimensional structure of an enzyme is an important characteristic in catalysis. The enzyme must be able to lower the activation energy of a reaction by forming chemical bonds but also be able to leave the reaction without undergoing a permanent change. Taking this statement into consideration, how does carbonic anhydrase achieve lower activation energy?
   (A) Carbonic anhydrase is complementary to the substrate of the reaction and forms covalent bonds with the substrate.
   (B) Carbonic anhydrase is complementary to the transition state of the reaction and forms covalent bonds with the transition state.
   (C) Carbonic anhydrase is complementary to the substrate of the reaction and forms ionic and hydrogen bonds with the substrate.
   (D) Carbonic anhydrase is complementary to the transition state of the reaction and forms ionic and hydrogen bonds with the transition state.

11. How could a competitive carbonic anhydrase inhibitor be used to treat glaucoma?

(A) The inhibitor would bind to the active site of the enzyme to decrease affinity for its substrate, inhibiting production of H_2O. This would increase the intraocular pressure in the eye by increasing production of aqueous humor.

(B) The inhibitor would bind to the active site of the enzyme to decrease affinity for its substrate, inhibiting production of HCO_3^-. This would reduce the intraocular pressure in the eye by reducing production of aqueous humor.

(C) The inhibitor would bind to the enzyme-substrate complex to decrease affinity for its substrate, inhibiting production of HCO_3^-. This would reduce the intraocular pressure in the eye by reducing production of aqueous humor.

(D) The inhibitor would bind to the active site of the substrate to decrease affinity for its enzyme, inhibiting production of H_2O. This would reduce the intraocular pressure in the eye by reducing production of aqueous humor.

12. Consider the following reaction:

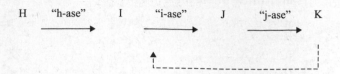

Assuming the dotted line represents feedback inhibition, what will happen to the products in this reaction if there is an abundance of K?

(A) H levels will remain the same, but I, J, and K levels will decrease.

(B) H and I levels will remain the same, but the production of J and K will decrease.

(C) All reactant levels will decrease.

(D) K levels will continue to increase, and all other product levels will decrease.

There are a number of synthetic routes that have been developed to synthesize *trans*-β-carotene (Compound **1**), a dietary source of vitamin A and a yellow food-coloring agent. Most approaches use a form of the Wittig reaction. This reaction is used to form carbon–carbon double bonds and thus prepare more complex molecules by coupling two less functionalized ones.

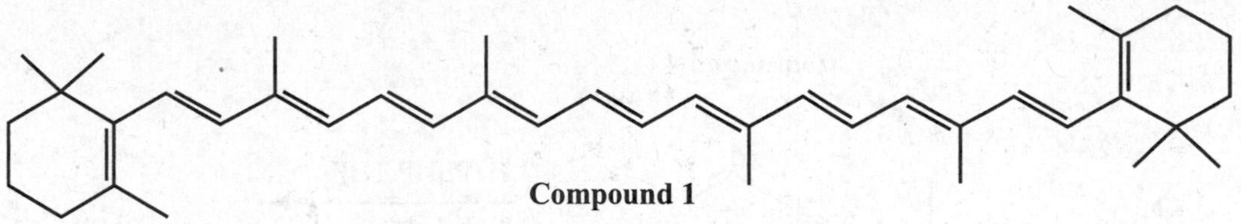

Compound 1

Preparation of Wittig "reagents" (shown in Figure 1) involves the reaction of a primary alkyl halide (sometimes secondary ones can be used) with triphenylphosphine (Compound **2**) to form an alkyltriphenylphosphonium salt. The salt is then treated with a strong base (often butyllithium, BuLi) to produce a phosphorus *ylide* (Compound **3**). The ylide reagent is then reacted with an aldehyde or ketone compound to form an alkene.

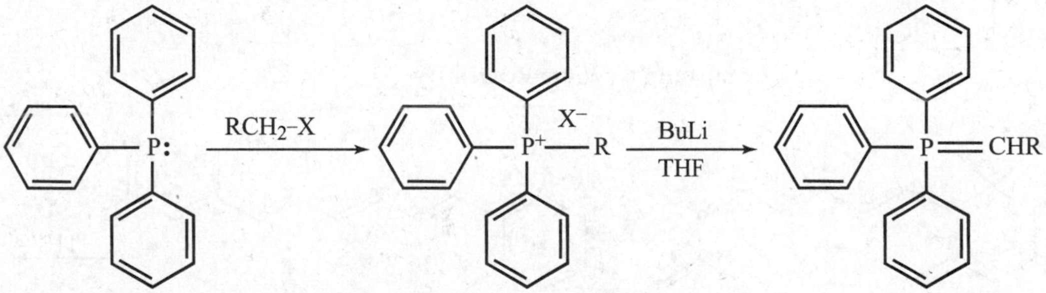

Compound 2   **Compound 3**

Figure 1. Preparation of Wittig "reagents"

Figure 2 shows a synthetic process using the Wittig reaction to prepare *trans*-β-carotene starting with a commonly available industrial intermediate used to make vitamin A, Compound **4**.

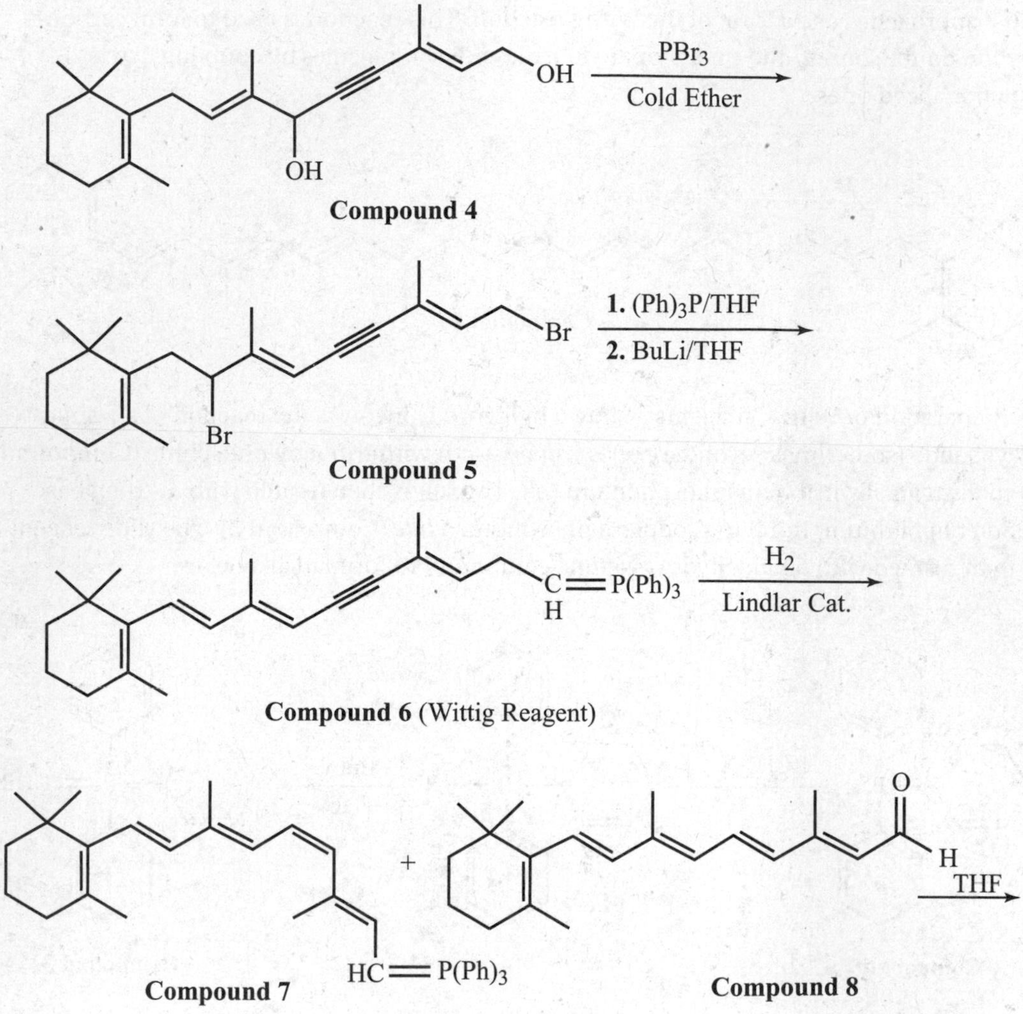

Compound 4

Compound 5

Compound 6 (Wittig Reagent)

Compound 7   +   **Compound 8**

11-*cis*-β-carotene $\xrightarrow{\text{1. Heating in Heptane}}$ *trans*-β-carotene (**Compound 1**)
2. Recrystallization from
Methylene Chloride

Figure 2. A synthetic process of preparing *trans*-β-carotene using the Wittig reaction

In the above scheme, Compound **4** is converted to the dibromide (Compound **5**) by treatment with PBr_3. The dibromide is then converted to a Wittig reagent (Compound **6**). Note that the secondary bromide group did not form an ylide and instead dehydrobromination occurred to form a double bond. Reduction of Compound **6** with H_2 using Lindlar catalyst produces the *cis* alkene Wittig reagent; Compound **7**, which is reacted with Compound **8** to give 11-*cis*-β-carotene. This intermediate is isomerized by heating and purified by recrystallization to give *trans*-β-carotene (Compound **1**).

13. By what mechanism is the formation of an alkyltriphenylphosphonium salt most likely to occur (see Figure 1)?
    (A) $E1$
    (B) $E2$
    (C) S_N1
    (D) S_N2

14. In Figure 2 why was 11-*cis*-β-carotene transformed to *trans*-β-carotene when it was heated?
    (A) The trans form is thermodynamically more stable.
    (B) The trans form is more highly substituted.
    (C) The isomerization is nonspontaneous.
    (D) ΔG for the reaction is positive.

15. When Compound **6** is reacted with hydrogen gas and Lindlar catalyst, Compound **7** is produced. If the triple carbon–carbon bond in Compound **6** were reacted with Na metal dissolved in liquid ammonia the result would be:
    (A) a ketone and aldehyde.
    (B) a cis double bond.
    (C) a carboxylic acid.
    (D) a trans double bond.

16. If the Wittig reagent, $(Ph)_3P=CH-C(CH_3)_3$, were reacted with cyclohexanone the product would be:

(A)

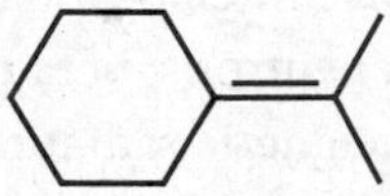

(B)

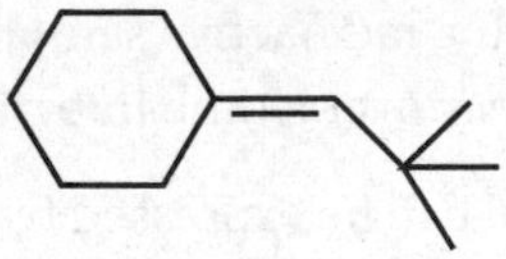

(C)

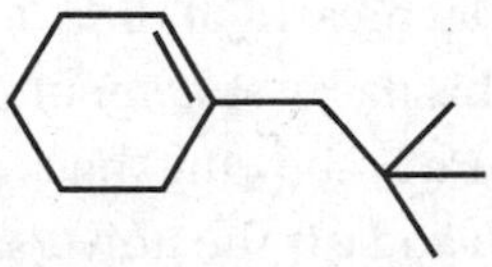

(D)

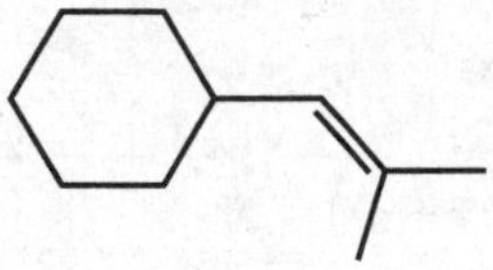

PASSAGE IV

Radioactive elements spontaneously disintegrate. Three kinds of radiation are emitted by radioactive nuclei: alpha particles that are basically helium nuclei consisting of two protons and two neutrons; beta rays that are either electrons or positrons; and gamma radiation, electromagnetic radiation of high energy photons. Positrons are the anti-particle to the electron. They have very short lifetimes.

If a radioactive sample contains N radioactive nuclei, then the number of nuclei that decay over a time interval is proportional to N. The number per time is the rate of decay and can be expressed by the equation $R = \dfrac{\Delta N}{\Delta t} = -\lambda N$, where N is the number of radioactive nuclei present at time, t, and λ is the decay constant for a given substance. The solution to this decay statement is an exponential decay described by the formula accompanying Figure 1, showing the exponential decay of N versus time. N_0 is the number present at time zero and e is the universal constant and base of natural logarithms 2.7.

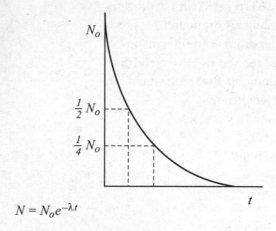

$$N = N_o e^{-\lambda t}$$

Figure 1. The exponential decay of N vs. time

An expression relating the half-life to the decay constant is $T_{1/2} = \dfrac{0.7}{\lambda}$.

Radon is a radioactive, colorless, odorless, tasteless gas, occurring naturally as part of the normal radioactive decay chain of uranium. Radon gas from natural sources can accumulate in buildings, especially in confined areas such as attics and basements. Breathing high concentrations of radon can cause lung cancer. There are two units of activity, the curie (Ci), equal to 3.7×10^{10} decays per second, and the becquerel (Bq), equal to 1 decay per second. Naturally occurring radium decays at approximately 1 Ci per gram of material.

17. The amount of radioactive radon gas goes from 12 g to 3 g in 7.6 days. What is the half-life of radon?
    (A) 3.8 days
    (B) 7.6 days
    (C) 15.2 days
    (D) 30.4 days

18. What is the activity of 10^{28} radioactive radium nuclei if $\lambda = 1.4 \times 10^{-11}$ per second?
    (A) 2.6×10^{-3} Ci
    (B) 3.8×10^6 Ci
    (C) 1026 Ci
    (D) 1.4×10^{13} Ci

19. Which of the following gives the relative order of the masses of the different kinds of radiation from high mass to low mass?
    (A) Beta, gamma, alpha
    (B) Gamma, alpha, beta
    (C) Alpha, gamma, beta
    (D) Alpha, beta, gamma

20. If the decay constant multiplied by a certain time factor is equal to 2, then the amount of radon remaining is
    (A) $N_0/2$
    (B) $N_0/2.7$
    (C) $N_0/4$
    (D) $N_0/7.3$

21. Which of the following statements about radon is false?
    (A) It is dangerous partly because it is odorless and tasteless.
    (B) Radon is often found near uranium mines.
    (C) The half-life of radon is proportional to the original amount present.
    (D) The rate of decay is proportional to the decay constant.

The following questions do not refer to a descriptive passage and are not related to each other.

22. How many protons, neutrons, and electrons would be found in the chemical species $^{44}Ca^{+2}$?
    - (A) 20 protons, 24 neutrons, 20 electrons
    - (B) 20 protons, 22 neutrons, 20 electrons
    - (C) 20 protons, 24 neutrons, 22 electrons
    - (D) 20 protons, 24 neutrons, 18 electrons

23. Reduction potentials for some common metals are shown in the table below:

Reaction	E^0
$Zn^{+2} + 2e^- \rightarrow Zn$	–0.76 V
$Cu^{+2} + 2e^- \rightarrow Cu$	+0.52 V
$Pt^{+2} + 2e^- \rightarrow Pt$	+1.21 V
$Sn^{+2} + 2e^- \rightarrow Sn$	–0.14 V

    Which of the following metals can spontaneously reduce tin ions to produce metallic tin?
    - (A) Zinc only
    - (B) Copper only
    - (C) Copper and zinc only
    - (D) Copper, zinc, and platinum

24. If the frequency of a sinusoidal wave is halved, then the:
    - (A) speed is halved.
    - (B) speed is doubled.
    - (C) period is halved.
    - (D) period is doubled.

25. The gravitational force on Mars is a little more than one-third of that on Earth. If a basketball player were to jump vertically with the same initial velocity on Mars as she does on Earth, then the amount of time taken to reach maximum height would be:
    - (A) 3 times less.
    - (B) 3 times more.
    - (C) 3^2 times less.
    - (D) 3^2 times more.

The inverse square law is popularly associated with force laws involving charges and masses. The force law of attraction (like charges) or repulsion (unlike charges) between charges is proportional to the product of the charges divided by the distance squared. In a similar way, the gravitational force of attraction of two masses is the product of the masses divided by the square of the distance between their centers. The inverse square law is also applicable in more familiar areas such as nuclear radiation, sound, and light.

Nuclear radiation is usually detected by a counter, and that counter has a specific size or opening so that as the detector is moved away from the radiation source, the number of counts decreases. The detectors typically integrate the counts over a time interval and give the radiation rate as so many counts per unit of time or equivalent. The radiation occurs spontaneously from atoms within the source and there is no preferred direction, so the source can be viewed as spherically symmetric even though in a laboratory setting the bulk of the radiation is absorbed by a surrounding container with a relatively small solid angle of radiation available for study. The number of counts follows an inverse square law of the form $N = N_0/r^2$, where N is the number of counts, N_0 is the number of counts at the source, and r is the distance from the source. Table 1 gives typical data for a radiation experiment.

Table 1. Radiation Experiment

Counts	Distance
100	10 cm
25	20 cm
11	30 cm

Sound intensity also follows an inverse square law. Sound from a spherically symmetric source radiates in all directions. The total power of the source is the intensity in W/m^2 times the surface area of a sphere of radius equal to the distance from the source (see Figure 1). Keep in mind that power is in watts and intensity is in watts per square meter.

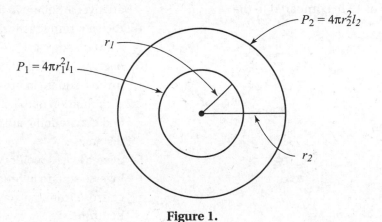

Figure 1.

The total power is the same, so the intensity ratios are found by setting these two expressions for power equal.

$$r_1^2 I_1 = r_2^2 I_2 \quad \text{or} \quad \frac{I_1}{I_2} = \left(\frac{r_2}{r_1}\right)^2$$

26. A Geiger counter with a known cross-sectional area placed at a distance from a radioactive source is able to accurately estimate the activity level of the source because:
    (A) the source radiation is spherically symmetric.
    (B) the source radiation is typically in the gamma ray region of the spectrum.
    (C) the source radiation is typically particles and not electromagnetic waves.
    (D) the counter is able to monitor the typical changes in radioactive decay rate.

27. Using the data given in the table, find the activity of a radioactive source when the counter is placed at a distance of 5 cm.
    (A) 6 counts
    (B) 400 counts
    (C) 200 counts
    (D) 50 counts

28. For a 5.0 W spherical sound source, calculate the approximate sound intensity at 10 m.
    (A) ~500 W/m^2
    (B) 60 W/m^2
    (C) (5/1200) W/m^2
    (D) (1/100) W/m^2

29. For a sound source, what is the ratio of the intensities (I_{12}/I_4) at 12 m compared to the intensity at 4 m?
    (A) 1/9
    (B) 2
    (C) 1/3
    (D) 1/6

30. The gravitational force for an object at 9 km from the surface of Earth versus 1 km from the surface of Earth is:
    (A) about 1/3, in accordance with the inverse square law.
    (B) about 3 times as much, in accordance with the inverse square law.
    (C) about the same because the distance from the center of Earth has not changed significantly.
    (D) about the same because gravity does not follow the inverse square law.

31. Human perception of loudness is that a 10-fold increase in intensity is perceived as a doubling of loudness. What approximate decrease in distance from the source produces this 10-fold increase in intensity?
    (A) ~10
    (B) ~14
    (C) ~6.4
    (D) ~3.2

32. Protons in an atomic nucleus are bound together by the strong nuclear force.
    The strong force must:
    (A) also follow the inverse square law because all fundamental forces of nature do.
    (B) decrease more rapidly with distance than an inverse square in order to overwhelm the electromagnetic repulsion only at very short distances.
    (C) decrease less rapidly with distance than an inverse square in order to overwhelm the combination of the electromagnetic force and gravitational attraction only at larger distances.
    (D) decrease less rapidly with distance than an inverse square in order to prevent nuclear collapse from the gravitational attraction of neutrons.

The following questions do not refer to a descriptive passage and are not related to each other.

33. The equation below is unbalanced.

$$ClO_3^- + Mn^{+2} \rightarrow Cl_2 + MnO_4^{-1}$$

What happens to the chlorine atoms in the process described by the equation?
(A) Chlorine atoms are reduced and each chlorine atom gains 5 electrons.
(B) Chlorine atoms are reduced and each chlorine atom loses 5 electrons.
(C) Chlorine atoms are oxidized and each chlorine atom gains 5 electrons.
(D) Chlorine atoms are oxidized and each chlorine atom loses 5 electrons.

34. Consider the following reaction:

$$2KHCO_{3(s)} + H_2SO_{4(aq)} \rightarrow$$
$$2H_2O_{(l)} + 2CO_{2(g)} + K_2SO_{4(aq)}$$

What volume of 4.0 M sulfuric acid is needed to produce 44.8 L of carbon dioxide gas at STP?
(A) 125 ml
(B) 250 ml
(C) 500 ml
(D) 1000 ml

35. A radio station broadcasts at a frequency of 90.5 MHz. Given that the speed of the radio waves is 3×10^8 m/s, what is the distance between adjacent crests of the radio waves?
(A) 3300 m
(B) 3.3 m
(C) 0.30 m
(D) 0.003 m

36. A person whirls a ball on the end of a string in a circular path above the person's head. The diameter of the circle is 0.8 m. The ball has a period of rotation of 0.25 seconds. How many meters along the circular path does the ball travel each second?
(A) 3.2π m
(B) 2.4π m
(C) 0.8π m
(D) 0.4π m

PASSAGE VI

One of the oldest chemical reactions used by humans is saponification, or the making of soap. Most saponification reactions involve the reaction of fatty acids with sodium or potassium hydroxides, although other alkali metal hydroxides can also be used. Soaps made with sodium hydroxide tend to be harder than those made with potassium hydroxide. The reaction below (Figure 1) shows the process by which tristearin, an animal fat, reacts with sodium hydroxide to make a soap and a molecule of glycerol.

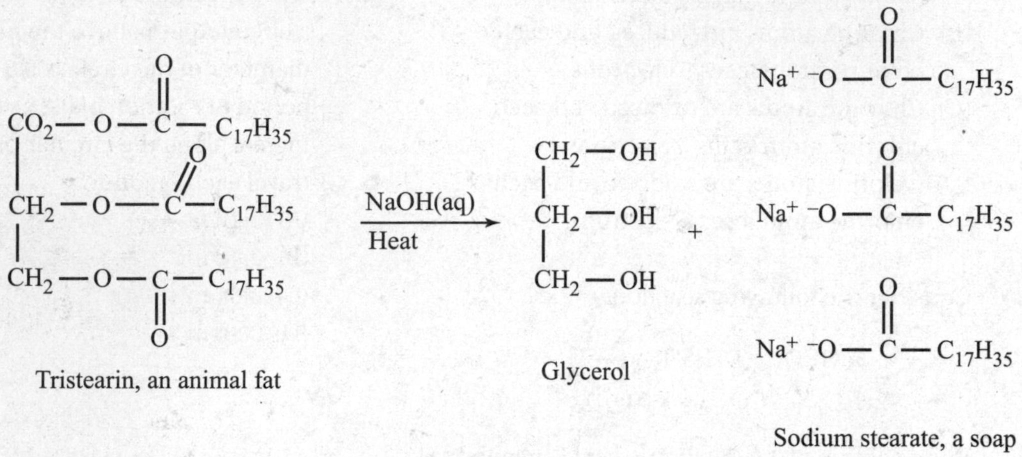

Figure 1. The reaction of tristearin with sodium hydroxide

The molecules of the soap have nonpolar and polar regions, allowing the soap to interact with both nonpolar materials and with water.

Historically, soap was made by mixing animal fat with burned bones or ashes. This produced a harsh soap that dissolved fats and oils but also was caustic to tissue. Modern soap has the unreacted base neutralized, making the soap less irritating to skin but not affecting its cleaning properties.

In the modern industrial process, beef tallow or vegetable oil is reacted with concentrated solutions of sodium hydroxide, and the salt is precipitated by the addition of sodium chloride solution. Vegetable oils tend to produce softer soaps than animal fats. The aqueous layer is removed and the glycerol formed as a byproduct is collected for other industrial uses.

One drawback of soaps is that they react with calcium or magnesium ions and produce soap scum. Detergents, on the other hand, have the ability to act as surfactants, disrupting hydrogen bonds and lowering surface tension.

37. Soft soaps, hard soaps, and detergents are all regularly used as cleaning agents. Which of the following would be used to produce a soft soap?
    (A) Sodium hydroxide and tallow
    (B) Sodium hydroxide and vegetable oil
    (C) Potassium hydroxide and vegetable oil
    (D) Glycerol and potassium hydroxide

38. The heat of combustion of tristearin (molar mass = 926) is 37,000 kJ/mole. By how many degrees Celsius could 1000 grams of water be heated using the heat produced by the combustion of one gram of tristearin? The specific heat capacity of water is 4.18J/g°C.
    (A) 0.9°C
    (B) 3.6°C
    (C) 9.0°C
    (D) 36.0°C

39. How does the boiling point of glycerol (molar mass = 93) compare to that of pentanol, $C_5H_{11}OH$ (molar mass = 88)?
    (A) Glycerol has a higher boiling point due to London dispersion forces, which increase with molar mass.
    (B) Pentanol has a higher boiling point because the OH group allows it to form hydrogen bonds.
    (C) Glycerol has a higher boiling point because it can form more hydrogen bonds than pentanol.
    (D) Pentanol has a higher boiling point because the nonpolar region of the molecule allows it to have more London dispersion forces.

40. What would be true about the boiling and freezing points of a solution made by dissolving 50 grams of glycerol in 100 grams of water compared to the freezing and boiling points of pure water?
    (A) The boiling point will be higher and the freezing point will be higher.
    (B) The boiling point will be higher and the freezing point will be lower.
    (C) The boiling point will be lower and the freezing point will be higher.
    (D) The boiling point will be lower and the freezing point will be lower.

41. Why are soaps more soluble in water than fats?
    (A) Soaps have higher molar masses than fats.
    (B) Soaps can undergo hydrogen bonding with water molecules.
    (C) Soaps can form ion–dipole interactions with water molecules.
    (D) Soaps can have strong London dispersion forces due to their high molar masses.

PASSAGE VII

Arsenic has been known and used since the middle ages as a poison, a coloring agent, and a medicine. Most arsenic is obtained by the roasting of arsenopyrite, FeAsS, in an oxygenated environment as shown in Equation 1.

$$2FeAsS_{(s)} + 3O_{2(g)} \rightarrow As_2O_{3(g)} + Fe_2O_{3(s)} + S_{2(g)}$$
Equation 1

The arsenic can then be purified by decomposing the arsenic(III) oxide as shown in Equation 2.

$$2As_2O_{3(s)} \rightarrow As_{4(s)} + 3O_{2(g)}$$
Equation 2

Arsenic compounds have been widely used as insecticides, although their toxicity to humans has led to their replacement in recent years.

Gallium arsenide is widely used to manufacture faster computer chips. Gallium arsenide is made by the process shown in Equation 3.

$$2Ga_{(s)} + 2AsCl_{3(l)} \rightarrow 2GaAs_{(s)} + 3Cl_{2(g)}$$
Equation 3

42. For a ground state arsenic atom, which answer represents the correct electron configuration?
(A) [Ar] $4s^23d^74p^6$
(B) [Ar] $4s^23d^{10}4p^65s^25p^3$
(C) [Ar] $4s^23d^54p^8$
(D) [Ar] $4s^23d^{10}4p^3$

43. Gallium arsenide has a melting point of 1240°C and is hard and brittle. Its molten form is an insulator. What type of solid is gallium arsenide?
(A) Ionic
(B) Covalent network
(C) Molecular
(D) Nonpolar

44. If a computer chip manufacturer wanted to avoid the use of arsenic compounds, which of the following would be the best candidate to test as an alternative?
(A) Ga
(B) Ge
(C) Se
(D) Sb

45. The compound arsenic trichloride obeys the octet rule. Which of the following is correct about phosphorus trichloride?
(A) It is trigonal planar in shape and is nonpolar.
(B) It is trigonal pyramidal in shape and is nonpolar.
(C) It is trigonal pyramidal in shape and is polar.
(D) It is tetrahedral in shape and is polar.

46. Arsenic(III) oxide is produced by the reaction shown in Equation 1. What is the oxidation number of the arsenic in As_2O_3?
(A) +2
(B) +3
(C) −3
(D) +5

47. Based on information in the passage, it can be assumed that arsenic compounds are no longer used as widely as they were in the past, in part because:
(A) arsenopyrite has become increasingly scarce.
(B) the cost of purification through roasting significantly exceeds the cost of electrolytic purification.
(C) manufacturers of purified arsenic are concerned for the health of their workers.
(D) due to its toxicity, arsenic no longer has any medicinal value.

The following questions do not refer to a descriptive passage and are not related to each other.

48. If a conducting ball hanging by an insulated string is attracted by a positively charged rod, which of the following statements can be true?

    I. The conducting ball was originally negatively charged.
    II. The conducting ball was originally positively charged.
    III. The conducting ball was originally neutral.

    (A) I only
    (B) II only
    (C) I and III
    (D) II and III

49. Saturated fatty acids are converted to energy by successively breaking off two carbon chunks, which are then injected into the citric acid cycle in the form of acetyl CoA. This process is referred to as:
    (A) Omega oxidation
    (B) Pentose phosphate pathway
    (C) Beta oxidation
    (D) Ketolysis

50. Which of the following pairs of 0.1 M solutions will produce a precipitate?
    (A) Silver nitrate and lead(II) chloride
    (B) Lead(II) nitrate and nitric acid
    (C) Sodium bromide and calcium chloride
    (D) Potassium nitrate and mercury(II) acetate

51. Oxidation of fats in the diet results in about twice the energy as a carbohydrate on an ATP/gram basis. The principal reason for this difference is:
    (A) during glycolysis, the organism must first invest energy by breaking ATP.
    (B) the harvesting of energy is more efficient when oxidizing fat.
    (C) the relative amount of oxygen in the two different macromolecules differs considerably.
    (D) fat can be converted to ketones.

PASSAGE VIII

Acetic acid is a widely used chemical in industry and is found in most homes. Solutions of household vinegar are 4% to 6% acetic acid in water. Industrially, acetic acid is used in the manufacturing of acetates for films and other polymers. Historically, acetic acid was made from the oxidation of ethyl alcohol, the same reaction that can turn a bottle of wine into vinegar. The reaction for this process is:

$$CH_3CH_2OH_{(l)} + O_{2(g)} \rightarrow CH_3COOH_{(aq)} + H_2O_{(l)}$$

Equation 1

Basic thermodynamic data at 25°C for the chemicals involved in equation 1 are summarized in Table 1.

Table 1

Thermodynamic Data for Equation 1

Compound	ΔH_f° (kJ/mole)	S° (J/mol K)	ΔG_f° (kJ/mole)
$CH_3CH_2OH_{(l)}$	−278	161	−175
$O_{2(g)}$	0	205	0
$CH_3COOH_{(aq)}$	−484	158	−390
$H_2O_{(l)}$	−286	70	−237

Acetic acid is a weak acid, with a K_a value of 1.8×10^{-5}. When in an aqueous solution, acetic acid dissociates according to the reaction:

$$CH_3COOH_{(aq)} + H_2O_{(l)} \leftrightarrow CH_3COO^-_{(aq)} + H_3O^+_{(aq)}$$

Equation 2

Acetic acid is used as a precursor for the manufacturing of vinyl acetate, which is used to make polyvinyl acetate (PVA), a compound found in almost all latex paints and common glues.

52. In Equation 2, water is acting as a:
    (A) Brønsted–Lowry acid because it accepts a proton.
    (B) Brønsted–Lowry acid because it donates a proton.
    (C) Brønsted–Lowry base because it accepts a proton.
    (D) Brønsted–Lowry base because it donates a proton.

53. When one mole of ethanol is oxidized in Equation 1, what mass of acetic acid is produced?
    (A) 30 g
    (B) 46 g
    (C) 60 g
    (D) 78 g

54. The molecular geometry around the oxygen atom in the hydronium ion of Equation 2 is:
    (A) linear.
    (B) trigonal planar.
    (C) trigonal pyramidal.
    (D) tetrahedral.

55. What is the change in enthalpy for the reaction $2\,H_{2(g)} + O_{2(g)} \rightarrow 2\,H_2O_{(l)}$?
    (A) −286 kJ
    (B) +286 kJ
    (C) +572 kJ
    (D) −572 kJ

56. The formation of acetic acid from the oxidation in Equation 1 is:
    (A) nonspontaneous because $\Delta G°_{rxn}$ is positive.
    (B) spontaneous because $\Delta G°_{rxn}$ is negative.
    (C) spontaneous because $\Delta S°_{rxn}$ is positive.
    (D) spontaneous because $\Delta G°_{rxn}$ is positive.

57. The entropy change in Equation 1 is:
    (A) positive because the number of moles of gaseous products is greater than the number of moles of gaseous reactants.
    (B) positive because the number of moles of gaseous products is less than the number of moles of gaseous reactants.
    (C) negative because the number of moles of gaseous products is greater than the number of moles of gaseous reactants.
    (D) negative because the number of moles of gaseous products is less than the number of moles of gaseous reactants.

The following questions do not refer to a descriptive passage and are not related to each other.

58. A farsighted man is able to focus only on objects that are at least 150 cm from his eyes. He wants to wear eyeglasses that will help him read a computer screen at 50 cm from his eyes. What must be the approximate focal length of the lenses in his eyeglasses?
    (A) −75 cm
    (B) +75 cm
    (C) −100 cm
    (D) +100 cm

59. Charges of +Q1 and +Q2 are held stationary at a distance of 3 cm. The magnitude of Q1 is double that of Q2. An electron is between the two charges at a distance of 2 cm from Q1 and at a distance of 1 cm from Q2. If the force from charge Q2 is 1 N, what is the net force on the electron?
    (A) 0 N
    (B) 0.5 N
    (C) 1 N
    (D) 2 N

Time: 90 minutes
53 Questions

DIRECTIONS: The Critical Analysis and Reasoning section contains a number of passages. Each passage is followed by a series of questions. Read the passage and then choose the one best answer for each question. When answering questions, eliminate the choices that you are sure are incorrect, and choose the best remaining answer. When you have chosen an answer, mark it in the corresponding location on the answer sheet.

PASSAGE I

The history of the sociopolitical changes of the 1960s can be reevaluated in terms of the economic factors involved in the evolution of food cooperatives, a central institution in activist university communities of the '60s. There are four tenets that are fundamental to this reevaluation.

The first tenet is that cooperative food buying already existed on a small but significant scale among suburban families in the 1950s. Establishing larger food-buying clubs and, later, coop stores, was in some ways a natural outgrowth of this. Though the heads of these '50s families had little economic incentive to organize more formal buying associations, their children going away to college in the '60s found that the financial benefits outweighed the time and effort needed to do so.

The second tenet is that contrary to the general impression of college students of the time, there were many economical and sociological differences among university communities in the '60s.

The third tenet maintains that there were two quite distinct groups involved in the creation of food coops. The first group consisted of children of less affluent families who often had no choice but to do anything possible to save money on necessities. The second group consisted of more affluent students who opted to save food money that could then be used for relative luxuries, such as clothing or entertainment. Whereas the more affluent students could afford to quit a cooperative at any time, they actually exerted a strong influence on cooperative policies and operations because, even though they were less likely to contribute their labor, their greater spending power and willingness to go elsewhere if necessary forced the coop to respond to their needs. At the beginning of the coop era, these more affluent students left the running of the coop to their less affluent comrades. However, by 1968 it became financially lucrative for the often more business-savvy affluent students to hold management positions, which they generally did to the exclusion of less affluent students.

Finally, the fourth tenet is that the entire campus food coop movement was not really a departure at all from mainstream economics. Coops operated in conjunction with the mainstream economy. However, to claim that food cooperatives represented no more than a slight variation of the same old theme ignores the dramatic social and political contributions of the coop movement, as well as the economic contributions. The food coops of the '60s certainly never achieved the economic sophistication of mainstream food stores. But what about the thousand-member coops of the major Eastern universities that created day care centers, published newsletters, and served as social hubs of the community? Perhaps some might claim that these privileged, liberal university communities were exceptions. However, the ideas and practices coming out of these communities exerted a major influence on almost all university communities throughout the country, no matter how traditional or conservative.

While this economic analysis applies to the actions of many of the less affluent coop members at dozens of campuses, we need to go one step further and relate it to the sociopolitical changes of the time. The growing disparity between the needs of the less affluent but more numerous workers and more affluent managers eventually led to a rank-and-file emphasis on a truly cooperative style of management by consensus and a commitment to the needs of the less fortunate. This attitude certainly spilled over into the political activism of the time.

1. According to the passage, which of the following statements about coop members in the '60s is most true?
   (A) More came from less affluent families than came from more affluent families.
   (B) Coop members from less affluent families were able to keep their living expenses lower than could the average university student on their campus.
   (C) Coop members were able to save more money on food than their parents had in the '50s.
   (D) By 1968, coop members from more affluent families found certain coop jobs more attractive.

2. According to the last paragraph, it is helpful to:
   (A) explain the connection between the mainstream economy and the food cooperatives.
   (B) relate the lives and attitudes of less affluent coop members to the political and sociological changes of the '60s.
   (C) make use of sociological research available on the actions of coop members from more affluent families.
   (D) differentiate the values of university students from diverse ethnic backgrounds.

3. The author uses the phrase "same old theme" [paragraph 5] to convey:
   (A) that coops were slight variations on time-tested, reliable principles.
   (B) that coops did not escape a division between the affluent and less affluent.
   (C) that coops were more than a minor change from previous economic models.
   (D) that coops addressed sociopolitical issues as well as economic ones.

4. Based on the passage, which of the following statements about food coops in the '60s is true?
   (A) Economic sophistication of the coops in the major Eastern universities never equaled that of mainstream food stores.
   (B) The sociological and artistic achievements of the major Eastern university coops have gone unacknowledged.
   (C) Coops simply borrowed the fundamental aspects of mainstream food stores and did not contribute anything unique.
   (D) Coops in conservative university towns were not significantly influenced by the privileged, liberal coops of the East.

5. According to the passage, which of the following is true of students going to college in the 1960s?
   (A) Most of them gravitated toward unskilled work rather than management.
   (B) Their economic prospects were better at college than at home.
   (C) They differed from their parents in that they were interested in cooperating with others to save money.
   (D) They found that the effort of organizing more formal buying associations paid off financially.

6. The main point of the passage is to
   (A) contrast several views of the changes of the '60s.
   (B) discuss certain economic analyses of the coops of the '60s and relate them to a more accurate understanding of the events of that era.
   (C) establish the main tenets of the mainstream sociopolitical view of the '60s.
   (D) present a reinterpretation of the history of the '60s from a sociopolitical perspective.

7. It can be inferred from the passage that college students of the '60s believed that:
   (A) many college students were ultimately not able to support themselves financially.
   (B) more students joined coops to buy necessities or to make social change than to save money for relative luxuries.
   (C) university communities across the country were very similar economically and sociologically.
   (D) many college students did not maintain strong economic connections with their parents.

8. Which of the following best represents the author's attitude toward the sociopolitical changes of the '60s?
   (A) They played a major role in the creation of new economic models such as coops.
   (B) They were slight variations on changes already taking place in the '50s.
   (C) Certain economic changes that took place due to necessity fueled sociopolitical changes.
   (D) They exacerbated the gulf between the politically liberal and conservative.

The lone hunter or gatherer, whether in pursuit of food or merely strolling through the world in reverie, has a direct and simple relationship to nature and to himself or herself. Bring even one other human being into this setting and the relationship is no longer simple. There is suddenly a fork in the road, a decision to make. Do we take the path of cooperation or the path of competition?

This choice represents the two fundamental options for human beings living together in society. In prehistory the choice was probably simple. Members of a tribe or family group predominantly needed to cooperate with each other to survive. Certainly at times there must have been rivalries within the group, but it was most likely in relation to foreign groups that competition was the driving relationship. Within the tribe, the urge to compete may have been channeled into formal games and exercises.

As human communities became larger and economically more effective, it became easier for some individuals to secure their economic position to such an extent that they did not need the cooperation of others to survive. Their relationship with others became one of competition—competing for the resources of potential customers, competing for power on the town council, competing for mates and friends.

In some societies—notably in the East—cooperation continues to be highly valued. The individual is expected to defer to the needs of society. In some totalitarian societies this is taken to an extreme, with a complete loss of individual freedom for the supposed good of the state. In the West, competition has become dominant, and nowhere more than in the United States. Some would say that competition has also gone to the extreme there.

Perhaps the balance between competition and cooperation can be seen as depending on the extent to which particular individuals believe they can meet all of their own needs without having to cooperate. In America, with streets paved with gold, with unlimited fertile farmland for the taking, with vast natural resources just a shovel's depth below the surface, it is no wonder that competition became the norm.

But the myth of independence is just that. It is a fundamental attitude, lodged somewhere in the mind, that I can take care of myself no matter what. From that perspective, others are either a nuisance or a resource to be mined. On closer inspection, this attitude does not match reality. Who is there that may not become sick or injured? Perhaps a few lucky individuals. Who is there that will not become old and lose the strength of their youth? Who is there that may not become lonely for human company in some quiet moment?

And yet in our political lives, Americans say loudly and clearly to their government, "Leave me alone. I don't want to pitch in to help others." We are resistant to giving our tax dollars for even the most worthwhile cause because, fundamentally, that represents cooperation.

Perhaps Daniel Boone was truly independent. For today's American, however, it is folly to claim independence. One cannot get in a car, walk on a sidewalk, buy groceries, collect unemployment, mail a letter, go to the doctor, without deeply participating in the cooperative efforts of society. A strong case can be made that, in today's society, cooperation is more and more important, and yet we have inherited a personal attitude toward others that finds that fact literally impossible to believe.

9. Which of the following is true about the author's assertion that in some societies, cooperation is still valued?
   (A) It is supported with evidence.
   (B) It is expanded on with further explanation.
   (C) It is contradicted by information that modern society is becoming more competitive.
   (D) It is proven to be a false generalization.

10. Which of the following statements, if true, would most weaken the author's argument about Americans?
    (A) Most Americans have voted for a political candidate who supports projects for the public good.
    (B) A large percentage of Americans have received unemployment, disability, Medicare, or Social Security payments at some time.
    (C) Many Americans would be willing to pay taxes toward a publicly funded project as long as they would personally benefit from it.
    (D) Many Americans come from countries that are less competitive than the United States.

11. Based on the passage, which of the following would be the response of a person with a fundamentally competitive attitude when faced with the argument that he or she might get sick some day?
    (A) I'm not going to get sick.
    (B) If I do, I'll never accept welfare.
    (C) If I do, I can deal with it myself somehow.
    (D) If I do, I'll find some way to make money off it.

12. If a competitive person received an offer to be involved in a cooperative project, the competitive person would most likely:
    (A) turn it down to focus on his or her own projects.
    (B) try to find out how much money each person would make.
    (C) try to find out who the leaders of the project were.
    (D) try to find out how to minimize his or her input and maximize the return.

13. The author sees competitiveness as:
    I. preventing tax money from going to worthwhile causes.
    II. a valuable part of the American spirit.
    III. unrealistic.

    (A) I only
    (B) I and II
    (C) I and III
    (D) III only

14. How might the author respond to a movement to create a new political party to represent competitive-minded people?
    (A) It is unnecessary because one of the existing parties already represents them.
    (B) It is unrealistic because there are not enough people interested in forming a third party.
    (C) It is ironic because to do so would require cooperation.
    (D) It is a good idea because competitiveness has its place and should be represented.

Colony Collapse Disorder (CCD) is a phenomenon in which worker bees from a beehive abruptly disappear. Although such disappearances have occurred throughout the history of apiculture, the term Colony Collapse Disorder was first applied to a drastic rise in the number of disappearances of Western honey bee colonies in North America in late 2006. Colony collapse is economically significant because many agricultural crops worldwide are pollinated by bees.

The exact mechanisms of CCD are still unknown. One report indicates a possible association between the syndrome and the presence of the Israel acute paralysis virus (IAPV). In 2007, the journal *Science* published research by a team of U.S. scientists and researchers that found a significant connection between IAPV and CCD in honeybees. Other factors may also be involved, however, and several have been proposed as causative agents: malnutrition, pesticides, pathogens, immunodeficiencies aggravated by environmental stresses, mites, fungus, beekeeping practices (such as the use of antibiotics, or long-distance transportation of beehives), and electromagnetic radiation. More speculative possibilities have included both cell phone radiation and genetically modified (GM) crops with pest control characteristics, though no evidence exists for either assertion.

At present, the primary source of information, and the presumed "lead" group investigating the phenomenon, is the Colony Collapse Disorder Working Group, based primarily at Penn State University. Some researchers have commented that the pathway of propagation functions in the manner of a contagious disease; however, there is some sentiment that the disorder may involve an immunosuppressive mechanism, potentially linked to stress leading to a weakened immune system. Specifically, according to researchers at Penn State: "The magnitude of detected infectious agents in the adult bees suggests some type of immunosuppression."

When a colony is dying, for whatever cause, and there are other healthy colonies nearby, those healthy colonies often enter the dying colony and rob its provisions for their own use. If the dying colony's provisions were contaminated, the resulting pattern of healthy colonies becoming sick when in proximity to a dying colony might suggest that a contagious disease is involved. However, it is typical in CCD cases that provisions of dying colonies are not being robbed, suggesting that at least this particular mechanism is not involved in CCD.

Additional evidence that CCD might be an infectious disease came from the following observation: The hives of colonies that had died from CCD could be reused with a healthy colony only if they were first treated with DNA-destroying radiation.

A few scientists have suggested that climate change can make bee hives more vulnerable to CCD, although it is not implicated as a direct cause of the disorder. "We see plants blooming at different times of the year," says amateur beekeeper Wayne Esaias, a researcher at the NASA Goddard Space Flight Center, "and that's why the nectar flows are so much earlier now. I need to underscore that I have no evidence that global warming is a key player in colony collapse disorder. But it might be a contributor, and changes like this might be upping the stress level of our bee populations."

Adapted from "Colony Collapse Disorder," on Wikipedia, *http://en.wikipedia.org/wiki/ Colony_collapse_disorder* (accessed May 2011).

15. The passage implies that Colony Collapse Disorder:
    (A) may have economic consequences outside the United States.
    (B) is difficult to identify without laboratory research techniques.
    (C) is probably caused by IAPV.
    (D) is caused by a disease that may be transmitted from bees to mites.

16. The scientists in the Colony Collapse Disorder Working Group would most likely suggest which of the following courses of action to those seeking to reduce the impact of CCD?
    (A) Temporarily stop the use of honeybees in American agriculture to allow the disease organisms to die out.
    (B) Treat infections in the bees while eliminating stresses that may lead to underlying immunodeficiencies.
    (C) Administer antibiotics to kill the microorganisms responsible for creating immunodeficiencies.
    (D) Set hives up as far as possible from cell phone towers.

17. Which of the following is NOT supported by the passage?
    (A) Global warming could lead to multiple infectious agents in some bees.
    (B) A hive affected by CCD that has not been treated with radiation cannot be safely used by a healthy colony of bees.
    (C) The provisions of dying colonies are not contaminated with disease.
    (D) CCD may cause an infestation with IAPV.

18. If an episode of CCD were traced to the kind of genetically modified crops described in the passage, what would best describe the mechanism?
    (A) The nectar and pollen from the crops were inferior in their nutritional value to bees, thus starving them.
    (B) The crops had residual radioactivity that caused genetic damage to the bees.
    (C) The crops produced genetic mutations in successive generations of bees.
    (D) The crops produced a substance that harmed or killed bees.

19. Which of the following, if true, would NOT support a theory that cell phone radiation could affect bees?
    (A) Bees use electromagnetic radiation to navigate.
    (B) Exposure to high frequency sound for long periods damages bees' immune systems.
    (C) Bees typically avoid areas around radio towers, even if the areas are rich in food.
    (D) Bees living under high voltage electric transmission lines start food collection earlier in the spring than other bees.

In many ways, the 20th century was an era in which two ideologies regarding the role and purpose of government vied and, literally, clashed. Ironically, from an historical standpoint, these two views were both relatively new. Until the advent of democracy, government was basically the rule of the powerful—sometimes with the interest of the less powerful in mind but more often at the expense of the less powerful. Democracy, an experiment first and foremost attempted in the United States, held in theory that each citizen had an equal vote in the election of government officials.

The second ideology, emerging from the work of Karl Marx and fueled by the injustices experienced in Europe, was communism—a belief that the role of government was to provide for the needs of even the lowest in society. A corollary to this was that in order to accomplish this ideal, the wealth of the country was spread among the many, leaving none destitute but none very well off. It is not primarily the political aspect of these two ideologies that has resulted in conflict but rather the economic aspect.

Even as the battle between these two ideologies raged, on the sidelines the distinctions between the two begin to blur. In many Western democracies, the governments took on an active role in providing for the economic welfare of its citizens, giving rise to social programs that included education, healthcare, and old-age support. Some communist governments let go of control of some economic activities, allowing private citizens to own and manage economic enterprises.

With the collapse of the Soviet Union at the end of the 20th century, many countries were forced to make a rapid and painful transition from an economy controlled by the state to a private one. Interestingly, some of the more socialistic Western democracies had gone that same route, albeit in a more gradual way. The United Kingdom is a clear example. In 1979, state-owned industries were losing more than 3 billion pounds annually. The government initiated a policy of selling these businesses to private owners. As a result, more than 34 billion pounds were raised from the sales, and ongoing income comes into the Treasury from the profits of the now privately run companies.

Not only has privatization of industry stopped the downward spiral of losses but it also seems to have increased productivity. Employees at British Airways and British Gas showed a 20% increase in productivity. At British Telecom, before privatization, there was always a long waiting list to have phone service installed. Afterward, there was no waiting list. At Associated British Ports, strikes and labor disputes were frequent before privatization and absent after.

One of the explanations given for the increase in productivity is that workers have been given the option to buy shares in the company. As "owners" of the company, workers suddenly had a very personal interest in its well-being. In some cases, workers have actually requested a lowering of wages in order to increase a company's overall health.

Ironically, this shift of ownership of business from government to private citizens, while anathema to the communist ideology, actually accomplished one of the primary goals of communism—a sense of ownership of the means of production by the workers. Although it can be argued that the workers will never have the control—or the profits—that the majority shareholders of the company enjoy, the sense of being partial owners—comrades, if you will—seems to have added to the lives of working people an enjoyment and a sense of importance that was not there under government ownership.

20. Which statement below is NOT consistent with the information presented by the author?
   (A) People who support democracy do not necessarily believe that the government should take care of the needs of the lowest in society.
   (B) Some non-communist countries in the 20th century have had government-run industries.
   (C) Many governments that previously owned industries have had to privatize them quickly.
   (D) The principles of democratic and communist ideologies are mutually exclusive.

21. Which of the following statements would the author most likely support?
   (A) The workers in industry are better off if the industry is privately owned and operated.
   (B) Democratic societies have a moral responsibility to take care of their citizens who have few resources.
   (C) It is important that work provide people with a sense of ownership of the means of production in a democratic as well as a communist society.
   (D) Workers can never own enough shares in a capitalistic business to make any difference.

22. Which of the following policies would most likely be supported by an advocate of communism as described in the passage?

   I. government-funded, guaranteed pensions for the elderly
   II. government ownership of industry on behalf of the workers
   III. incentives for private business to establish healthcare plans for their workers

   (A) I only
   (B) I and II
   (C) I and III
   (D) II and III

23. Which of the following can be inferred from the passage?
   (A) The United States has the lowest level of government-owned industry among democracies.
   (B) Labor disputes can significantly disrupt worker productivity.
   (C) When workers own a share of their company, their primary concern is for their level of wages.
   (D) In a democracy everyone has an equal vote.

24. Which of the following would best represent a blend of democratic and communist ideologies in a society?
   (A) No citizen is wealthy and no citizen is poor.
   (B) The means of production are owned by the workers.
   (C) The lowest of citizens has a vote equal to the richest.
   (D) The citizens of a democratic society have access to government grants for higher education.

25. What is the author's purpose in putting the word "owners" [paragraph 6] in quotes?
   (A) Just because workers own shares does not mean they make decisions about the business.
   (B) Lower-class workers can never really be considered to be equals to the ruling class, even if they own shares of the business.
   (C) The workers do not really own anything tangible because the shares of stock could easily decline in value or become worthless.
   (D) It is unlikely that owning shares made any real difference in the lives of the workers.

26. All of the following are results of privatization that are given in the passage EXCEPT:
   (A) worker ownership of the means of production.
   (B) the right for every citizen to own a business.
   (C) faster access to utilities.
   (D) a painful transition.

PASSAGE V

Some commentators on modern American society cite the long work hours required by today's employers as evidence of a loss of meaningful values, an abandonment of recreation, with its attendant pleasure and relaxation, a turning aside from nature, from family, from peace and quiet. In short, extended work hours are seen by some as a descent into dry and lifeless workaholism.

Extending the metaphor of work as addiction, some would say that modern workers are helpless victims of the ever-increasing demand to produce. The monkey on the back of workers is the system itself, out of anyone's control, requiring more and more feeding and giving back only the dry ashes of money.

I would disagree with this assessment. To look at a worker spending 50 or 60 hours a week at the office and to see a person who is missing out on life is to overlook a critical and fundamental truth. For many workers, the work done at the office is not an inferior substitute for life. It is life itself. For them, work is passion. Work is fulfillment. Work is intricate relationships with coworkers. Work is the commitment to something larger and more lasting than oneself. Work is the pain of bringing something into being, the bitter sorrow of failure, and the elation of success, all shared with one's tribe.

For most people, there is a gap, a separation between their work life and their family life. Their work life is the life described above. Their family life consists of spouse, children, and other family members comfortably centered around the home. Family life also includes extended community—people with shared recreational interests or religious interests. Family life is what we associate with fun, love, relaxation—in short, living. It is no wonder, then, that some people may come to think of work as the opposite. In reality, work is not the opposite. It is the alternate way of living.

The root of the problem is the perception that work is an unpleasant means to an end. The end is money, or financial security. Consider the state of mind of a person with this attitude. While making phone calls, the person is thinking how much more pleasant it would be to be fishing but to go fishing would get the person fired. This makes the person unhappy. Work, though, does not have to be seen as a means to an end. It can be seen as an end in itself. From this perspective, the phone call is part of a bigger picture. It is teamwork, a challenge, an opportunity to build skills, to overcome hurdles, to bring home a hunting prize to the tribe.

Even if these more dramatic elements are not part of the phone call, it is still an opportunity for art. By art, I mean an outward, creative expression of the energy of being alive, an expression that is not just internal but is shared with others. It is creative in that it is spontaneous, an activity that is not the routine or usual. Because art starts with experience, the phone call may start with listening closely to the other person. Then, because art is spontaneous, the normal ways of responding may give way to something new—a creative suggestion, a shared anecdote, an inspired question, an insight. And because art inspires others to live, the person on the other end might respond with an unexpected enthusiasm. This is what the critics of work fail to see.

27. Which of the following is the author's primary message?
    (A) Work is an important aspect of our modern lives.
    (B) Work is not the means to an end.
    (C) Creating art can be as unpleasant as working at a job.
    (D) Family life is often sacrificed in order to earn a living.

28. Which of the following is the probable reason that the author uses the word "tribe"?
    (A) The author is trying to make the tone of the article more informal.
    (B) The author is referring to not just the immediate family but also to the extended family and friends who act as extended family.
    (C) The author is indicating that the workplace consists of a close-knit group of people with common goals who have to cooperate to achieve those goals.
    (D) Many companies predominantly hire people of the same ethnic or religious background.

29. Which of the following is most likely the author's purpose in describing work as an addiction?
    (A) To clarify a premise of an argument in order to refute the argument
    (B) To use an analogy to weaken a previous argument
    (C) To attack an argument by showing that it uses a word in two contradictory ways
    (D) To establish that a particular behavior is the antecedent cause of a later behavior

30. Which of the following facts, if shown to be true, would most weaken the author's argument about work?
    (A) Most people bring work home from the office to do over the weekend.
    (B) Most people who work overtime do not do so voluntarily.
    (C) Most people see their work activities as routine and isolated.
    (D) Most people would be unhappy if their work were not a means of earning money.

31. Which of the following arguments would be most parallel to the author's argument?
    (A) Some say that caring for the environment is too much of a strain on the economy, but I say that caring for the environment is the only way to save the economy.
    (B) Some say that religion is the opiate of the people, but I say religion is an expression of passion and a source of community.
    (C) Some say that family responsibilities prevent individual expression, but I say a good family is one in which individuals can express themselves.
    (D) Some say that work is good for the soul, but I say that too much work detracts from the joy of family life.

PASSAGE VI

The study of the nervous system dates back to ancient Egypt. Evidence of trepanation, the surgical practice of either drilling or scraping a hole into the skull with the aim of curing headaches or mental disorders or relieving cranial pressure, being performed on patients dates back to Neolithic times and has been found in various cultures throughout the world. Manuscripts dating back to 1700 BCE indicated that the Egyptians had some knowledge about symptoms of brain damage.

Early views on the function of the brain regarded it as a "cranial stuffing" of sorts. In Egypt, from the late Middle Kingdom onward, the brain was regularly removed in preparation for mummification. It was believed at the time that the heart was the seat of intelligence.

The view that the heart was the source of consciousness was not challenged until the time of Hippocrates. He believed that the brain was not only involved with sensation, since most specialized organs (e.g., eyes, ears, tongue) are located in the head near the brain, but was also the seat of intelligence. Aristotle, however, believed that the heart was the center of intelligence and that the brain served to cool the blood. This view was generally accepted until the Roman physician Galen, a follower of Hippocrates and physician to Roman gladiators, observed that his patients lost their mental faculties when they had sustained damage to their brains.

In al-Andalus, Abulcasis, the father of modern surgery, developed material and technical designs that are still used in neurosurgery. Averroes suggested the existence of Parkinson's disease and attributed photoreceptor properties to the retina. Avenzoar described meningitis, intracranial thrombophlebitis, and mediastinal tumors, and made contributions to modern neuropharmacology. Maimonides wrote about neuropsychiatric disorders and described rabies and belladonna intoxication. Elsewhere in medieval Europe, Vesalius (1514–1564) and René Descartes (1596–1650) also made several contributions to neuroscience.

Studies of the brain became more sophisticated after the invention of the microscope and the development of a staining procedure by Camillo Golgi during the late 1890s that used a silver chromate salt to reveal the intricate structures of single neurons. The hypotheses of the neuron doctrine were supported by experiments following Galvani's pioneering work in the electrical excitability of muscles and neurons. In the late 19th century, DuBois-Reymond, Müller, and von Helmholtz showed that neurons were electrically excitable and that their activity predictably affected the electrical state of adjacent neurons.

In parallel with this research, work with brain-damaged patients by Paul Broca suggested that certain regions of the brain were responsible for certain functions. At the time, Broca's findings were seen as a confirmation of Franz Joseph Gall's theory that language was localized and certain psychological functions were localized in the cerebral cortex. The localization of function hypothesis was supported by observations of epileptic patients conducted by John Hughlings Jackson, who correctly inferred the organization of motor cortex by watching the progression of seizures through the body. Wernicke further developed the theory of the specialization of specific brain structures in language comprehension and production.

Adapted from "Neuroscience," in Wikipedia, *http://en.wikipedia.org/wiki/Neuroscience* (accessed May 2011).

32. Which of the following might Hippocrates and Aristotle have agreed on?
    (A) The eyes and ears are involved in intelligence.
    (B) Intelligence requires not only knowledge but also compassion.
    (C) Cool blood may be necessary for intelligence.
    (D) The heart not only circulates the blood but is also the seat of intelligence.

33. Some people have brain-based disorders that cause them to act impulsively and inappropriately toward others. If an observer were to say that such a person were acting from the heart rather than the brain, the observer's attitude would be closest to:
    (A) Hippocrates, because the brain is the center for the specialized senses such as sight and hearing.
    (B) Aristotle, because the person's brain is not functioning intelligently.
    (C) Maimonides, because a neurological disorder is causing an emotional disorder.
    (D) Wernicke, because appropriate language function is centered in the brain.

34. Based on information in the passage, where and when did Abulcasis live?
    (A) In North Africa or the Middle East, around the time of the Roman gladiators
    (B) In Europe, around the time of the Roman gladiators
    (C) In North Africa or the Middle East, in the middle ages
    (D) In medieval Europe

35. Broca's discoveries about the brain were most likely the result of what scientific method?
    (A) The principle that a correlation between physiological processes and symptoms implies a causal relationship
    (B) Experimental evidence in which electrically excited neurons are observed to affect neighboring neurons
    (C) A hypothesis that specific functions must correlate to specific parts of the brain
    (D) A statistical analysis that shows that what is true in a small number of cases holds to be true when observed in a large population

PASSAGE VII

Playing music, like the performance of most arts, is at its heart a creative expression. Just as a young child spontaneously takes finger paints and creates a completely novel work of art, so that child might also sing a made-up song. However, in both art and music, a young person cannot long pursue the creative interest without soon having to learn technique.

To coax creative expression out of an instrument requires mastering technology. The young student must first learn the basic skills for producing sound and forming individual notes. Then the more subtle techniques must be learned for moving quickly between notes, forming combinations of notes, and producing certain patterns of sound. All of this requires mastering not just the technology of the instrument but also the technology of the hands, the mouth, the breath, and so on, depending on the specific instrument.

But it can be argued that technology is the enemy of creativity. Technology is the engagement of that part of the brain that may be clever but is not original, that may be precise but is not creative, that may be dependable but is not spontaneous. Technology is the spirit that masters itself at the expense of losing contact with the world of sensual experience; and without drawing its inspiration from the world of sensual experience, technology brings forth only dead ghosts, imitations of life.

Musicians sometimes report that the more they practice technique, the less creativity comes through. Abandoning the instrument for a period of time—something that the technologically minded instructor considers a cardinal sin—often results in a burst of creativity when the musician does begin playing again. We are left with the paradox that in order to be able to play an instrument well, the student of music must study technique but in studying technique, the creativity at the heart of performance is destroyed. This paradox raises two questions: Is there a way to preserve creativity in the face of technical practice? and Why is it that the power of technique seems stronger than the power of creativity?

Consider the second question. Why does technology win out over creativity? This does not only happen in the study of music or art. It also is a pattern in our lives. Children are more spontaneous, more creative, more intuitive than adults. The younger the child, the less it knows and the more it creates. Perhaps it is a neurological fact that as the brain accumulates knowledge, it becomes less able to create spontaneously. This may have survival value evolutionarily. Those who better remembered "how to do things" survived better than those who lost themselves in creativity.

Does this mean that there is no hope? The clue lies in the experience of musicians who "forget" to practice for a while. Creativity comes surging back, only to recede again as they continue to practice. The secret may be to periodically forget everything one knows about music, to abandon the accumulated knowledge, to let it wither and compost and return, if but briefly, to the raw spontaneity of the child.

36. Which of the following would be the opposite of "dead ghosts," as used by the author?
    (A) Lively imagination
    (B) Technical brilliance
    (C) Tactile richness
    (D) Poignant memory

37. Which of the following best characterizes what the author is trying to convey in using the word "paradox" [paragraph 4]?
    (A) Creativity will usually be diminished by technology.
    (B) Technology is a necessary tool for expressing creativity.
    (C) Ironically, art and music face the same problem.
    (D) In order to express creativity, one ends up losing it.

38. Which of the following, if found to be true about learning to play an instrument, would most conflict with the author's theories?
    (A) Practicing an instrument involves continually creating new sequences of fingering and sound.
    (B) The advanced technology of many instruments required intense creativity to invent and develop.
    (C) Only the most creative musicians stick with the process of learning technique.
    (D) Practicing technique helps create skills that are not easily lost.

39. Which of the following most accurately represents the author's attitude toward art and music?
    (A) They are different in that music involves more technologically advanced instruments.
    (B) They are different in that art can be maintained indefinitely as a purely creative endeavor, whereas music soon loses its creativity.
    (C) Art and music parallel the difference between creativity and technology.
    (D) Art and music are similar in that they are both creative endeavors subject to the effect of technology.

40. If a musician wants to be able to express creativity with increased technological competence, the author would suggest that the musician:
    (A) first master creative expression and then study technology.
    (B) avoid technology and focus solely on creative expression.
    (C) study technology and then temporarily forget it.
    (D) study creative expression with someone who has mastered it.

PASSAGE VIII

Geologists have long noted certain unusual patterns of melting in the glacial areas of Iceland. For many years this phenomenon has been explained by a theory known as the mantle plume model. A group of geologists has recently raised the question of whether plumes even exist, and if they do, whether they occur regularly in the planet's mantle or are, instead, rare local phenomena.

Publishing a report of nearly a thousand pages, this group has presented a compelling case against the theory that plumes are the cause of the unusual melting patterns. This flies in the face of those who for years have held the mantle of the plume model as established truth. It is gratifying to see that there are still those scientists with enough independence of spirit to follow their instincts upstream of that which is "known" and to apply rigorous scientific inquiry to change the course of human knowledge.

What, then, is actually wrong with the plume model? The hypothesis predicts the existence of certain characteristics at the plume site, including buoyancy fluxes, time-progressive volcanic chains, a large volume of heat flow, swells, unusual volcanic activity, and a high ratio of 3He to 4He. Many of the sites actually examined lack most or all of these signs. To make the plume model work despite this lack would require radically changing some of its basic assumptions. The problem with such changes to the model is that the theory would become virtually untestable and, therefore, useless.

As an alternative to the plume model, the report offers a number of models based on plate tectonics. A plate tectonic model would explain certain phenomena that have been found in the vicinity of the unusual melting patterns—phenomena that were not explained by the plume model. These include membrane stresses, reheated slabs, leaky transform faults, propagation of cracks, decompression melting of mantle, and reactivated plate boundaries. The high number of possible plate tectonic theories that could explain the observed phenomena indicates that phenomena similar to the Icelandic one could result from differing causes.

Unfortunately, even though many novel theories have been proposed in this report, there is virtually no defense of the plume model. True, it may turn out that it becomes discarded, but given the previous vigorous belief in the plume model, it is difficult to believe that there is not something salvageable in it and that someone in the group of geologists would not have come forward in its defense.

As the results of this report spread throughout the community of geologists, one thing is clear. It will be very difficult for anyone to assert the plume model again with the certainty that it once commanded. No matter which theory wins out in the end, this report has shown the power of the scientific process to fundamentally change even firmly accepted paradigms. For that we owe it, regardless of our theoretical allegiance, a debt of gratitude.

41. At the Icelandic sites of unusual melting, which of the following observations would be most relevant in determining whether a plume model or a plate tectonic model would best explain the melting?
    (A) The propagation of cracks is observed.
    (B) The sites are ones which the group of scientists writing the above mentioned report specifically studied.
    (C) A high ratio of 3He to 4He is observed but no buoyancy fluxes are observed.
    (D) There is a large volume of heat flow but there are no reheated slabs observed.

42. What is the author's purpose in using the word "useless" at the end of the third paragraph?
    (A) It indicates that the mantle plume model has outlived its value as an explanation of unusual melting.
    (B) It calls into question the value of a model that can neither be proven nor disproven.
    (C) It questions the value of a theory whose predictions are rarely found in actual circumstances.
    (D) It indicates that a theory that has been radically changed should not be considered to be the same theory.

43. Which of the following best describes the author's attitude toward the group of scientists mentioned in the passage?
    (A) The scientists' work was exemplary.
    (B) The scientists should have been more respectful of their more experienced colleagues who previously created the plume model.
    (C) The scientists' work was valuable for two reasons and yet contains a flaw.
    (D) The scientists successfully defended the mantle plume theory but neglected to salvage useful parts of the plate tectonic theory.

44. If it were determined that one unusual melting spot in Iceland exhibited membrane stresses and another nearby one exhibited propagation of cracks, which of the following could be logically concluded?
    (A) Both melting spots have the same cause because they both exhibited signs of plate tectonic involvement.
    (B) The melting spots have different causes because one exhibited signs of mantle plumes and the other exhibited signs of plate tectonic involvement.
    (C) The melting spots have different causes because they exhibited two different signs of plate tectonic involvement.
    (D) It is unclear whether the melting spots have the same or different causes.

45. The word "upstream" [paragraph 2] most likely refers to the fact that:
    (A) volcanically heated water will move against gravity.
    (B) a new generation of scientists is more likely to make new discoveries than an older generation.
    (C) a new generation of scientists is more likely to challenge accepted theories than an older generation.
    (D) it is more difficult to challenge an accepted theory than to support it.

46. Which of the following, if true, would provide the strongest defense for the plate tectonic model?
    (A) A survey of most known unusual melting sites yields no instances of buoyancy fluxes, large volumes of heat flow, swells, or a high ratio of 3He to 4He.
    (B) Plumes are proven to be rare local phenomena.
    (C) Membrane stresses and propagation of cracks are found at nearly all unusual melting sites.
    (D) Most of the geology community comes to believe that the plate tectonic model is correct.

47. Which of the following is an assumption held by the author?
    (A) It is possible to appreciate a scientific theory even without believing it is true.
    (B) It is possible to appreciate a scientific endeavor even without believing the theory it proposes.
    (C) It is possible to question an accepted theory even if one believes the theory to be true.
    (D) It is possible to salvage a theory even if it has been seriously attacked.

The annual Local Talent concert has traditionally brought into the public eye—or more accurately the public ear—previously unknown and yet talented local musicians. This year's concert was no exception. Perhaps the most striking from among the wide range of ages and styles was a young woman named Francesca, who introduced her music with a single word, "Primitive."

Francesca performed on the piano. Her first piece did indeed evoke a sense of the primitive. The rhythms were earthy, fundamental, simple, and yet powerful. And yet it is ironic that the instrument itself from which this primitive music emanated is anything but primitive. The piano is a highly technical instrument, the result of hundreds of years of mechanical perfection. It has a technical precision that requires ongoing maintenance by highly trained piano "engineers."

Had Francesca performed with gourds, with handmade pipes or reeds, by pounding on hollowed stumps or by squeezing sound from inflated bladders, had she simply wailed, daubed, perhaps, in mud, the feeling of primitiveness would have been enhanced. And yet there is no doubt that, playing the piano, she moved that which is primordial in the audience.

It would have added to the effect of the performance if it had been the case that Francesca had learned her skills self-taught by following the irresistible pull of her own primitive intuitions. Deepening the irony further is the truth—that she holds a doctorate in music from one of the top conservatories in the country. Can this highly technical, highly trained music be called primitive?

When asked what primitive means to her, Francesca reports that it has taken her years of study to perfect a technique that she feels is truly primitive. Surely, we asked, were not her first untrained attempts at music as a child by definition primitive? No, she responds. They were stiff, uncreative, mechanical acts of necessity, performed to please adults or to gain attention. Primitiveness, she explains, does not lie in lack of knowledge or absence of technical training, nor does it lie in the medium through which it is expressed. Lack of knowledge is simply ignorance. Lack of technical skill is simply clumsiness.

Primitiveness, according to Francesca, is direct experience. It is the language of the skin, the bones, the nose, and the eye. It is deeper even than the language of the heart, for the heart cannot help but want to change the world to its own end, whereas primitiveness goes directly with what is, no matter where it leads.

To express primitiveness requires being in touch with it, Francesca explains. But being in touch is not enough. Primitiveness itself must learn how to touch the keys just so, how to weave the sounds in order to say what it will. Primitiveness must become master of the technique. To her, there is no contradiction between the primitive and the technically sophisticated.

As true as her argument may ring, another event comes to mind that raises doubts about her view. Five elders sat in a semi-circle on the ground under a ponderosa pine. Four had flutes that looked handmade. One had a drum of animal skin stretched over a roughly carved, hollowed log. The music itself was simple, not complicated, sometimes slightly dissonant. The rhythm of the drum was straightforward, hardly varying during the entire session. And yet those who listened lost themselves in the sound and felt that they had truly experienced the primitive.

48. It can be inferred from the passage that Francesca's artistic abilities were the result of:
    (A) beginning to experiment with music as a child.
    (B) interpreting music through her heart rather than through her technical knowledge.
    (C) studying music with people from primitive cultures.
    (D) mastering the technical aspects of instruments and performance.

49. Which of the following best describes the author's intent in putting the word "engineers" in quotes in the second paragraph?
    (A) The author wants to indicate that piano tuners are more than just technicians.
    (B) The author wants to emphasize the contrast between a piano technician and the primitive.
    (C) The author is calling into question whether primitive people have the capacity to master engineering.
    (D) The author is indicating that although piano tuners are not technically engineers, their training is equivalent to that of a degreed engineer.

50. Which of the following, if true, would most contradict Francesca's implication that her approach to music as a child had no relation to her later musical interest in primitiveness?
    (A) As a child, she got the most positive response from adults when she concentrated on how the music felt in her body.
    (B) The more she practiced as a child, the more she was able to please the people listening to her.
    (C) She developed unusually good keyboard skills as a child.
    (D) As a child, adults often told her that her music was primitive.

51. Based on the last paragraph, the author believes which of the following about primitive music?
    (A) There is no contradiction between primitiveness and technical sophistication.
    (B) A flute is more primitive than a piano.
    (C) Primitiveness sometimes lies in the medium through which it is expressed.
    (D) Given equal levels of musical sophistication, less sophisticated instruments will produce a more primitive effect.

52. The word "primordial" [paragraph 3] is used in a way that is most similar to which of the following phrases:
    (A) language of the heart
    (B) simply ignorance
    (C) absence of technical training
    (D) lost themselves in the sound

53. Which of the following is NOT a belief that Francesca holds about primitive music?
    (A) Music that is in touch with direct experience will be primitive.
    (B) Music that is not in touch with direct experience cannot be primitive.
    (C) Primitiveness may be expressed if there is mastery of technique.
    (D) Without mastery of technique, primitiveness might not be expressed.

BIOLOGICAL AND BIOCHEMICAL FOUNDATIONS OF LIVING SYSTEMS

Time: 95 minutes
   59 Questions

DIRECTIONS: The majority of questions in this section are organized into groups, with each group containing a descriptive passage. Review the passage, and then select the one best answer for each question. Some questions are not drawn from a passage and are also independent of the other questions. When answering questions, eliminate the choices that you are sure are incorrect and then choose the best remaining answer. When you have chosen an answer, mark it in the corresponding location on the answer sheet. A periodic table can be found on the back of your answer sheet. You may consult it as needed.

The body's immune system is designed to recognize antigens and mount a commensurate response to them. The immune system must be able to distinguish the body's own tissue and proteins from foreign tissues and proteins. Viruses, parasitic worms, tumors, and bacteria make up the majority of antigens that the immune system must respond to. The intensity of the immune response and the triggers of the immune response must be tightly regulated to avoid allergic or autoimmune reactions. The major components of the immune system are the innate and the adaptive immune systems.

The innate immune system is the first layer that a pathogen will encounter in the human body. The innate immune system consists of macrophages, mast cells, leukocytes, and other cell types. These cells provide an immediate, but generally nonspecific, response to a pathogen. As such, there is no immunological memory of a pathogen the body was previously exposed to.

The adaptive immune system provides a more specific response to a pathogen. Due to the necessary alteration in gene expression, the adaptive immune response results in a time delay between pathogen exposure and maximal immune response. The adaptive immune system provides an immunological memory for pathogens to which the body was previously exposed. This immunological memory has been hypothesized to be a cause of sensitization in exposure to allergens.

Nuts are considered complete foods because they provide protein, fat, and carbohydrates. The tree nut allergy and the peanut allergy are two common food allergies. In the tree nut allergy, proteins present in the fruits (nuts) of trees such as the Brazil nut, chestnut, hazelnut, and walnut can cause a severe allergic response in people who have this allergy. Management of the tree nut allergy involves abstaining from the offending nut types. In case of accidental exposure, the standard treatment protocol is injection with epinephrine.

The effects of these foods can be understood through consideration of the Type I hypersensitivity pathway that mediates both mild allergic symptoms as well as the more severe form known as anaphylaxis. During the initial phase of sensitization, E class antibody is produced in response to allergen exposures through a process involving several cell types. These IgE antibodies are then released into the blood, where they will ultimately bind to high affinity Fc receptors on mast cells and basophils. This very sensitive receptor-IgE complex arms these cells so that subsequent contact with the antigen or any other stimulus capable of cross linking adjacent antibody-receptor complexes results in aggregation of the Fc receptors and degranulation. This results in release of histamine and heparin but also the release of a number of other important products of arachidonic acid metabolism including prostaglandins and leukotrienes. These messengers mediate a number of responses, including widespread vasodilation, increases in capillary permeability, and severe bronchoconstriction. This severity of reaction appears to be under genetic control and ranges from mild allergic disease such as occasional hay fever through asthma to the full blown anaphylactic responses. In many cases, after sensitization, subsequent exposures trigger a worsening of symptoms; paradoxically, though, it seems at least in some cases, allergic patients can be desensitized to the offending antigen through repeated contact with very small doses which are then gradually increased until acceptable levels of tolerance are reached.

1. Which of the following physiological responses would be expected to occur in a patient with peanut allergy?

   I. Vasodilation
   II. Reddening of the skin and increased skin temperature
   III. Increased glomerular filtration

   (A) I only
   (B) II only
   (C) I and II only
   (D) I, II, and III

2. Which of the following might explain why patients with a peanut allergy have less severe symptoms when eating baked peanut cookies compared to eating raw peanuts?
   (A) The heat denatures the fats in the peanuts.
   (B) The heat denatures the antigens in the peanuts.
   (C) The heat denatures the antibodies in the peanuts.
   (D) The heat denatures the carbohydrates in the peanuts.

3. New treatments being developed for the treatment of severe asthma and nut allergies are immunologically based and consist of monoclonal anti-IgE antibodies. These attack and neutralize only free IgE or that bound to the low affinity Fc receptor, such as those on cells destined to become plasma cells and not IgE bound to the high affinity Fc receptor. The need for this selectivity derives from which of the following properties?
   (A) That this would cripple the immune system by blocking needed protective antibodies on a variety of cell types
   (B) That such drugs could disrupt signal transduction in B lymphocytes resulting in immune-incompetence
   (C) That such drugs might actually cause anaphylaxis through their binding of IgE-Fc receptor complexes
   (D) That such drugs would lead to an up-regulation of Fc receptors, making basophils and mast cells even more sensitive to the antigen

4. A biotechnology company has recently proposed using ribozymes in the treatment of peanut flour to render the food edible to people who have a peanut allergy. Ribozymes are molecules that consist only of ribonucleic acid and function as catalysts. Ribozymes and most enzymes differ in which of the following?
   (A) Enzymes do not display substrate selectivity, whereas ribozymes do.
   (B) Enzymes are built from amino acids, whereas ribozymes are built from nucleic acids.
   (C) Enzymes are held together with hydrogen bonds, whereas ribozymes cannot be held together with hydrogen bonds.
   (D) Enzymes do not have a secondary structure, whereas ribozymes do have a secondary structure.

5. The passage states that severe allergic reactions have occurred even after the patient has remained stable for 2–6 hours. Which of the following statements best explains this?
   (A) The innate immune system is responsible because it remembers the peanut antigen and mounts a delayed response.
   (B) The innate immune system is responsible because it produces antibodies specifically against the peanut antigen.
   (C) The adaptive immune system is responsible because it denatures the antigen and renders the antigen more potent.
   (D) The adaptive immune system is responsible because it contains a memory for the antigen.

6. The stimulus for degranulation is found to be associated with a rapid increase in calcium and the involvement of membrane phospholipids. Which second messenger system is likely responsible for degranulation?
   (A) Voltage gated Ca^{+2} channels opening in response to closure of a K^+ channel
   (B) Phosphatitidl inositol and derivatives operating through protein kinase C and diacylglycerol
   (C) Transcription factors activated through the MAPK cascade
   (D) Through a G protein, which subsequently causes an increase in cAMP, which activates protein kinase C

The most common ring systems found in natural organic compounds are cyclohexanes. These six-membered carbon rings can assume low energy conformations that almost completely eliminate ring strain. This is unusual because most small and medium-size carbon ring structures are strained. The lowest energy conformer that cyclohexane can assume is called the *chair* conformation. Hydrogens and other substituents attached to cyclohexane rings in the chair conformation occur in two relative positions, *axial* and *equatorial* (see Figure 1, in which unsubstituted cyclohexane is shown in the chair conformation).

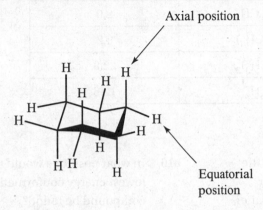

Figure 1. Unsubstituted cyclohexane in the chair conformation

Because the cyclohexane ring is conformationally mobile at room temperature, the chair conformation rapidly interconverts between left and right forms. This process is called ring flipping. It is illustrated in Figure 2. The energies of these two conformers are identical.

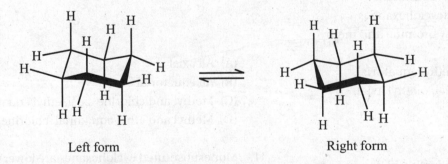

Left form ⇌ Right form

Figure 2. Ring flipping

Careful study of Figure 2 shows that as the cyclohexane ring "flips," the axial and equatorial positions interconvert. After much study, it has been found that substituents larger than hydrogen occupy *equatorial* positions in the lowest energy conformations of cyclohexane compounds. The more bulky the substituent, the more the cyclohexane compound is stabilized by assuming a conformation where the group is equatorial. Rings with multiple substituents assume low energy conformations where the larger groups are equatorial and the smaller ones are axial. Table 1 shows the normalized (relative to the –F substituent) sizes of some substituents commonly bonded to cyclohexane rings.

Table 1 Relative Sizes of Common Cyclohexane Substituents

Substituent	Size
–F	1.0
–Cl	2.0
–Br	2.0
–OH	4.2
–CH$_3$	7.6
–CH$_2$CH$_3$	8.0
–CH(CH$_3$)$_2$	9.2
–C(CH$_3$)$_3$	22.8
–C$_6$H$_5$	12.6

7. At room temperature, what would be the relative ratio of the left and right chair conformers (respectively) of cylcohexane?

    (A) 90:10
    (B) 10:90
    (C) 50:50
    (D) More information is needed to make an estimate.

8. If the lowest energy conformation of *cis*-1-bromo-4-methylcyclohexane is "ring flipped," the new bromine and methyl positions will be:

    (A) bromine axial, methyl equatorial.
    (B) bromine equatorial, methyl axial.
    (C) both equatorial.
    (D) both axial.

9. Cyclopentane is considerably higher in energy than cyclohexane. Why?

    (A) Increased ring strain
    (B) Increased torsional strain
    (C) Increased steric strain
    (D) Both A and B are true.

10. In what positions would the substituents of the lowest energy conformation of the following compound be found?

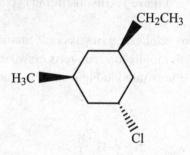

    (A) All axial
    (B) All equatorial
    (C) Methyl and chlorine axial, ethyl equatorial
    (D) Methyl and ethyl equatorial, chlorine axial

11. Monosubstituted cyclohexanes are lower in energy when the substituent is in the equatorial position. Why?

    (A) Less steric strain
    (B) More steric strain
    (C) Less torsional strain
    (D) Less ring strain

PASSAGE III

Hydrogen cyanide (HCN), a compound used commercially in the production of plastics and pesticides, is a fast-acting metabolic poison that causes serious physical damage or death when inhaled, ingested, or absorbed through the skin or eyes. HCN prevents the transfer of electrons to oxygen and the reduction of oxygen to water, inhibiting cellular respiration. The mechanism for this is generally considered to be the binding of the cyanide ion (CN^-) to a receptor on cytochrome c oxidase in the electron transport chain.

When HCN enters the human system, it is distributed to virtually every part of the body, causing widespread cell death and loss of organ function. It inflicts the most profound damage on those organs that have the highest oxygen requirements, such as the brain and heart. In acute cases, death can occur within minutes as a result of cellular asphyxiation.

Mild chronic exposure may result in damage to the central nervous system, optic nerve, and thyroid gland. Resulting symptoms can include general weakness, unusual sleepiness, dizziness, headache, confusion, strange behavior, coma, shortness of breath, and seizures. There is no evidence that cyanide has mutagenic or carcinogenic effects.

One approach to the treatment of cyanide poisoning is to administer nitrites, which convert hemoglobin to methemoglobin. Methemoglobin contains iron in the ferric state (+3) instead of the usual ferrous state (+2) and binds avidly to cyanide, thus displacing it from the ferric heme moiety of cytochrome C oxidase. The product, cyanmethemoglobin, is relatively nontoxic. Methemoglobinemia, however, is a type of poisoning in its own right. The ferric heme group enhances cooperativity among the other three heme groups of the hemoglobin molecule such that affinity for oxygen becomes too great for significant transfer to occur at the tissues, which results in tissue hypoxia. This must be carefully monitored and subsequently treated with methylene blue, which converts methemoglobin back to hemoglobin. The hope in such a treatment is to trade the very lethal form of histotoxic hypoxia that is cyanide poisoning for a potentially less dangerous and more easily managed oxygen delivery disorder.

12. Testing of tissues of people exposed to HCN can reveal elevated levels of lactate. All of the following explanations for elevated lactate are correct EXCEPT:
    (A) pyruvate cannot be converted to Acetyl-CoA.
    (B) the Krebs Cycle cannot function without NAD+ and FADH+ from the electron transport chain.
    (C) oxidative phosphorylation is disrupted.
    (D) cells shift from anaerobic to aerobic metabolism.

13. Exposure of brain cells to HCN may result in reduced decision-making ability in humans because the inactivation of cytochrome c oxidase results in:
    (A) hyperpolarization of sensory neurons.
    (B) lowered oxygen levels in blood supply to the brain.
    (C) inability of brain tissue to utilize oxygen.
    (D) disruption of signals passing between brain hemispheres through the corpus collosum.

14. Referring to the differences in cooperativity between hemoglobin and methemoglobin, what is the effect of nitrites on the shape of the plot of Hb-O2 versus oxygen pressure curve?
    (A) The relationship goes from hyperbolic to sigmoidal.
    (B) The relationship remains sigmoidal, only steeper before displaying saturation effects.
    (C) The relationship goes from sigmoidal to hyperbolic.
    (D) The relationship remains sigmoidal, only less steep before displaying saturation effects.

15. Cyanide exposure can damage the myelin sheath that insulates nerve axons. Damage to myelin can cause:
    (A) polarization of the axon.
    (B) depolarization of the axon.
    (C) hyperpolarization of the axon.
    (D) a decrease in the propagation rate of action potentials

16. The treatment of cyanide poisoning can be best summarized as:
    (A) a form of chelation therapy using the patient's own blood as the chelating agent, which involves significant risk.
    (B) a series of redox reactions that serve to remove the competitive inhibition of cyanide on cytochrome c but that also simultaneously interferes with oxygen transport.
    (C) a series of reactions that improves oxygen carrying capacity to offset the invariably more dangerous effects of histotoxic hypoxia.
    (D) the use of methylene blue to neutralize the effects of cyanide.

17. In blocking the electron transport chain, cyanide also blocks the transport of H^+ ions across the inner mitochondrial membrane. This blocking results in:
    (A) increased ATP synthesis.
    (B) decreased ATP synthesis.
    (C) increased availability of NAD^+.
    (D) denaturation of ATP synthase.

The following questions do not refer to a descriptive passage and are not related to each other.

18. The products of the complete combustion of a hydrocarbon are primarily:
    (A) carbon black and water.
    (B) hydrogen gas and water.
    (C) carbon black and carbon dioxide.
    (D) carbon dioxide and water.

19. Mass spectrometry involves the production and detection of:
    (A) positively charged species.
    (B) negatively charged species.
    (C) neutral species.
    (D) positively and negatively charged species.

PASSAGE IV

The somatic nervous system of the body provides the fine-motor skills necessary to use the fingers and hands. The sensory or afferent nervous system provides the sensory inputs necessary for agile use of the extremities. Normal function of the hand and fingers relies on efficient nerve conduction to and from the extremities. The ulnar nerve in the forearm runs parallel to the radius and ulna bones. The ulnar nerve bends at the elbow and is located in the cubital tunnel in the upper arm. The ulnar nerve is a sensory neuron responsible for sensation in the small and ring fingers. The median nerve runs parallel to the ulnar nerve and serves as a conduit for sensation in the thumb, index, and middle fingers, and half of the ring finger. The radial nerve is responsible for sensation in the back of the hand and part of the thumb.

Compression or pinching of the ulnar nerve at the elbow results in loss of sensation in the small and ring fingers. Compression of the nerve is common when sleeping with the elbow bent. The tingling sensation usually resolves within a few minutes. Patients whose symptoms are mild are advised to wrap a bath towel around their elbow to prevent bending of the elbow while sleeping. In more severe cases, surgery may be necessary to move the ulnar nerve to minimize pinching.

Although elbow bending is a major source of ulnar nerve compression, other sources of nerve compression may occur. The following sources have been documented in the medical literature: elbow and arm fractures, infections, tumors, and artery aneurysms. Aneurysms are blood-filled bulges of arterial walls. Each of these sources puts pressure on the nerve and inhibits neural conduction. This results in the loss of sensation.

20. A patient experiences loss of sensation only in the middle and index fingers. Which of the following could best account for this clinical observation?
    (A) Compression of the ulnar nerve
    (B) Compression of the median nerve
    (C) Compression of the radial and ulnar nerves
    (D) Compression of the radial and median nerves

21. An aneurysm adjacent to a nerve would be expected to cause which of the following changes in physiology?
    (A) An increase in saltatory conduction along the neuron
    (B) An increase in the frequency of depolarization and hyperpolarization of the neurons
    (C) A decrease in the frequency of depolarization and hyperpolarization of the neurons
    (D) An increase in the frequency of opening of voltage gated potassium channels

22. Which of the following molecules would be present in the greatest amount in the synapse of a motor neuron and a muscle cell? Assume the neuron has just experienced an action potential.
    (A) Acetylcholinesterase
    (B) Acetylcholine
    (C) Choline
    (D) Serotonin

23. Although rare, exposure of the fetus to teratogens results in compromised neuronal development and may lead to premature neuron death. This premature death often triggers paralysis of muscles. In which layer(s) of the embryo must the teratogen act for this to occur?
    (A) Endoderm
    (B) Mesoderm
    (C) Ectoderm
    (D) Ectoderm and mesoderm

24. Surgical treatment to move the ulnar nerve to reduce pinching must involve cutting which structure(s)?
    (A) Epiphysis of the ulna bone
    (B) Smooth muscle of the forearm
    (C) Tendon and smooth muscle of the forearm
    (D) Fibrous connective tissue

PASSAGE V

The use of secondary or tertiary alkyl halide substrates, polar protic solvents, and mildly basic nucleophiles leads to reaction mechanisms in which primarily S_N1 and $E1$ products are produced. The first and rate-determining step of these mechanisms is the formation of a carbocation intermediate that then, in the second step, either undergoes an addition (attack by a nucleophile) or elimination (deprotonation by a base) process to give the product(s). Many factors can affect the composition of the final product mixture.

Chemists studied the rates of three alkyl bromides toward S_N1 reaction with ethanol (see Figure 1) to produce ethers. In these reactions the ethanol served as both the nucleophile and the solvent.

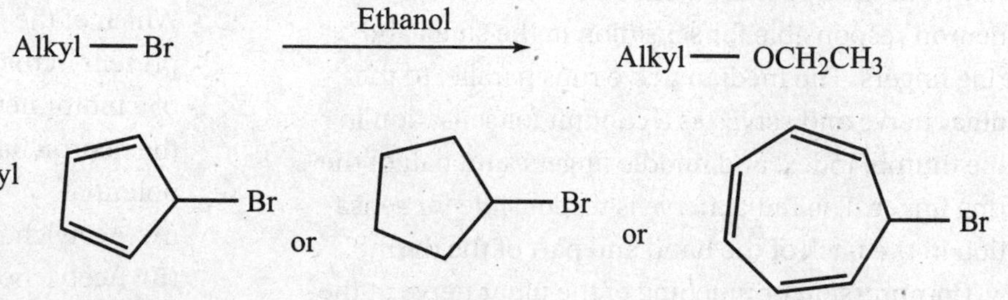

Where the alkyl bromide is:

Compound 1 **Compound 2** **Compound 3**

Figure 1. The rates of three alkyl bromides toward S_N1 reaction with ethanol

A comparison of the reaction rates of Compounds **1**, **2**, and **3** showed Compound **3** to be the most reactive and Compound **1** the least. Compound **2** was in between.

25. Compound **3** is the most reactive because:
    - (A) the ether product formed from it is the most thermodynamically stable.
    - (B) the activation energy needed to form a carbocation from it is the lowest.
    - (C) it is the least sterically hindered to nucleophilic attack by ethanol.
    - (D) the ether product formed from it is more soluble in ethanol.

26. The carbocation formed from Compound **1** can be classified as:
    - (A) nonaromatic.
    - (B) aromatic.
    - (C) antiaromatic.
    - (D) tertiary.

27. The carbocation formed from Compound **3** can be classified as:
    - (A) nonaromatic.
    - (B) aromatic.
    - (C) antiaromatic.
    - (D) primary.

28. The reaction kinetics associated with the processes shown in Figure 1 would be:
    - (A) zero order.
    - (B) first order.
    - (C) second order.
    - (D) third order.

29. If the reactant used with Compound **2** in Figure 1 had been sodium ethoxide instead of ethanol, which of the following would be true?
    - (A) The alkene product would predominate.
    - (B) The ether product would predominate.
    - (C) Approximately a 1:1 alkene/ether product mixture would be formed.
    - (D) No reaction would occur.

The following questions do not refer to a descriptive passage and are not related to each other.

30. Smooth muscle fibers may be found in all of the following EXCEPT the:
    (A) uterus.
    (B) blood vessels.
    (C) urinary bladder.
    (D) heart.

31. Conn's syndrome is characterized by excessive levels of aldosterone, which normally stimulates Na^+ reabsorption from the proximal convoluted tubules of the kidneys. Which of the following changes may be seen in Conn's syndrome?
    (A) Decreased blood volume and pressure
    (B) Decreased blood volume and increased pressure
    (C) Increased blood volume and pressure
    (D) Increased blood volume and decreased pressure

32. How many isoprene units make up the structure of the terpene compound caryophyllene, shown below?

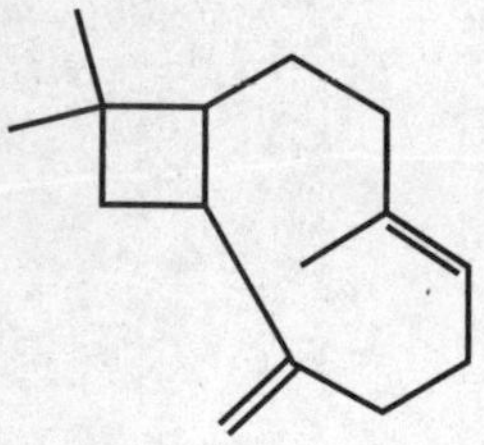

    (A) 1
    (B) 2
    (C) 3
    (D) 4

33. The cell membrane is composed of a phospholipid bilayer. Which of the following correctly represents the components of one phospholipid molecule?
    (A) Hydrophilic head only
    (B) Hydrophilic head and 1 hydrophobic tail
    (C) Hydrophilic head and 2 hydrophobic tails
    (D) 1 hydrophobic tail only

34. Cellular repolarization in neurons is most correctly described by which of the following statements?
    (A) Sodium ions move out of the cell.
    (B) Sodium ions move into the cell.
    (C) Potassium ions move out of the cell.
    (D) Potassium ions move into the cell.

PASSAGE VI

The HIV virus that causes AIDS is a lentivirus and is part of the retrovirus family of viruses. This means that it carries its own copy of reverse transcriptase, an enzyme that converts the virus's native RNA genome into a DNA genome, which then integrates with the host (or infected cell's) DNA. The cell then reproduces normally, in the process also replicating the viral DNA and translating viral proteins, which are then assembled in the cytoplasm to create new viruses.

After infection, HIV attaches to host cells by either of two pathways. The first is by recognizing CXCR 4, a chemokine receptor, on host cells, and binding to it, and the second is by attaching to CCR5, another chemokine receptor. Once the virus is firmly attached to the cell, its glycoprotein envelope fuses with the host cell's plasma membrane, and in this way the virus is internalized into the cell.

HIV mainly targets CD_4^+ T lymphocytes, the so-called T helper cells of the immune system, and kills them. In doing so, it slowly reduces their number and concentration. As their concentrations decline, so does the effectiveness of the immune system in fending off pathogens, and so a number of infections and cancers may be seen in patients. Their frequency and severity increases as the CD_4^+ cell concentration decreases.

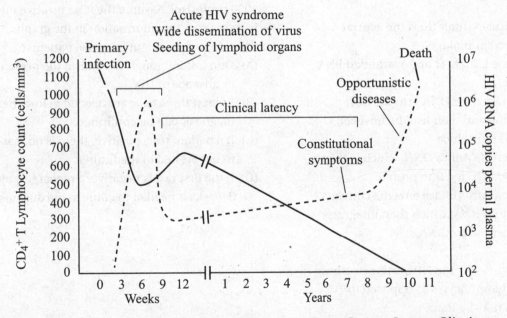

Figure 1. The frequency and severity of cancer in HIV patients. Source: Jurema Oliveira, on Wikipedia, *http://en.wikipedia.org/wiki/File:Hiv-timecourse.png* (accessed May 2011).

35. Which of the following best explains the trends depicted in the graph?
   (A) Once the number of HIV RNA copies exceeds 10^5 copies per ml, opportunistic diseases will occur.
   (B) There is a clinical latency of at least several years before constitutional symptoms and opportunistic infections develop.
   (C) CD_4^+ counts initially increase after infection is acquired, then decrease steadily.
   (D) HIV RNA copies increase steadily after infection is acquired.

36. A retrovirus is an:
   (A) RNA virus that carries the reverse transcriptase enzyme.
   (B) RNA or DNA virus that integrates its genome into the host cell.
   (C) enveloped RNA virus.
   (D) enveloped DNA virus.

37. How do retroviruses differ from the central dogma of molecular biology?
   (A) They can use either (+) or (–) stranded RNA to replicate.
   (B) They integrate their DNA into the host cell's genome and then use the host cell's elements to reproduce.
   (C) They convert RNA into DNA, which is then eventually converted into protein.
   (D) The reverse transcriptase enzyme converts their DNA into RNA, which then integrates with the host cell's mRNA.

38. One of the reasons why the HIV virus selectively attacks CD_4^+ T lymphocytes as opposed to other cell types may be that:
   (A) when CD_4^+ cells try to attack and kill the HIV virus, their defenses are weakened and it is easier for the HIV virus to enter them.
   (B) The HIV virus has a tropism for MHC II antigens on CD_4^+ lymphocytes.
   (C) CD_4^+ lymphocytes are the most common type of cells in the human body.
   (D) The HIV virus displays the CCR5 receptor necessary for HIV to enter the cell.

39. If a scientist conducting AIDS research were to encounter a population of subjects who were resistant to infection with the HIV virus, which of the following might be a plausible reason explaining this resistance?
   (A) The population has a unique type of immune system cell not found in other human populations.
   (B) The population carries a CCR5 or CXCR 4 mutation.
   (C) The population has secondary immunity from prior infection.
   (D) The population has a normal CD_4^+ count nearly 300 cells per mm^3 higher than the average for humans.

40. Suppose that a scientist were to develop a new diagnostic test for HIV that measured the amount of RNA copies per ml in plasma. The lowest detectable concentration of the test is 1000 copies/ml. Assume the false positive rate is zero. From the information in the graph, what should the scientist advise patients?
   (A) One test is enough to confirm the presence or absence of HIV.
   (B) At least three tests are needed before the diagnosis can be confirmed.
   (C) If a patient tests positive, there is no reason to be retested in the future.
   (D) If the first test is negative, a repeat test after 3 weeks is needed to confirm the diagnosis.

PASSAGE VII

Mitochondria can be considered one of the most essential membrane-bound organelles of the eukaryotic cell. Catabolic metabolism is carried out in the mitochondria. The Kreb's cycle and the coupled oxidative phosphorylation pathway provide the cell with ATP for homeostasis. In addition, the intermediates of the Kreb's cycle may be used as biochemical building blocks in the synthesis of biomolecules.

Mitochondria possess a circular DNA chromosome that codes for mitochondria-specific proteins. The other proteins needed by the mitochondria are synthesized by the host cell. Mitochondria replicate independently of the host cell, and growth is stimulated by increased energy demands of the cell. Mitochondria are maternally inherited insomuch as the sperm does not contribute any mitochondria to the zygote.

Mitochondria are small compared to the size of the host cell, which is consistent with the notion that the mitochondrial-host relationship resulted from incomplete phagocytosis. The number of mitochondria in a cell may be determined experimentally by cell fractionation studies using differential gradient centrifugation. Fluorescence techniques were used to determine the relative number of mitochondria in a normal mammalian cell over the course of several days. One aspect of fluorescence techniques is fluorescent bleaching. Fluorescence bleaching is the loss of fluorescence as a result of chemical degradation of the fluorescent dye. The results are shown in Figure 1.

Relative Number of Mitochondria in a Mammalian Cell as Determined through Fluorescence Assay

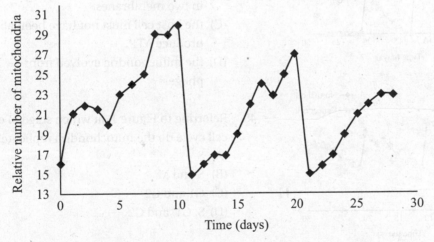

Figure 1. Relative number of mitochondria in a mammalian cell as determined through fluorescent assay.

41. The researchers determined the relative number of mitochondria in a cancer cell using the same experimental protocol as for the data presented in Figure 1. Which of the following graphs could represent the cancer cell data if plotted with the normal cell's data?

(A)

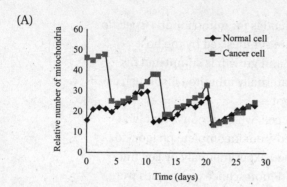

(B)

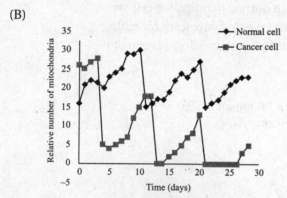

(C)

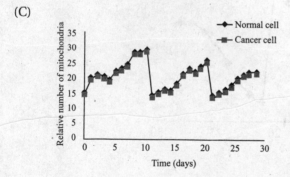

(D)

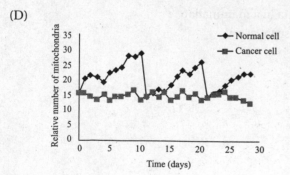

42. The large drop in number of mitochondria at day 11 and day 21 can be attributed to which cellular or chemical process?
   (A) Mitosis
   (B) Meiosis
   (C) Apoptosis
   (D) Fluorescence bleaching

43. A father has a disease that is attributable to a defect in a mitochondrial protein. What is the probability that at least one of his three children will have this disorder?
   (A) 100%
   (B) 75%
   (C) 33%
   (D) 0%

44. The reference to "incomplete phagocytosis" in paragraph 3 suggests that:
   (A) the mitochondria were originally involved in a parasitic relationship with their host.
   (B) the mitochondria should be encapsulated in two membranes.
   (C) the host cell must not have been able to produce ATP.
   (D) the mitochondria evolved from a phage.

45. Referring to Figure 1, at which stage(s) of the cell cycle do the mitochondria replicate?
   (A) S
   (B) S and M
   (C) G1 and G2
   (D) S, G1, and G2

46. Which of the following best describes the cellular metabolic reactions that occur in the mitochondria?
    (A) Glucose → Glycogen
    (B) Glucose → Pyruvate
    (C) Pyruvate → NADH, $FADH_2$, CO_2, and Acetyl CoA
    (D) Acetyl CoA → Fatty Acids

47. Radioactive glucose will be absorbed the most by which of the following cell types?
    (A) An epithelial cell
    (B) A muscle fiber
    (C) A cell of the pancreas
    (D) A Schwann cell

The following questions do not refer to a descriptive passage and are not related to each other.

48. Which of the following correctly describes the functions of the smooth and rough endoplasmic reticulum, respectively?
    (A) Protein production and lipid production
    (B) Lipid production and protein production
    (C) Post-translational modification of proteins and of lipids
    (D) Post-translational modification of lipids and of proteins

49. What is the site of the electron transport chain within the eukaryotic cell?
    (A) Inner mitochondrial membrane
    (B) Outer mitochondrial membrane
    (C) Mitochondrial cytoplasm
    (D) Intermembrane mitochondrial space

50. Which of the following is correct about the human female reproductive cycle?
    (A) On day 14 of the menstrual cycle, an FSH surge occurs.
    (B) The number of primary oocytes does not change after birth.
    (C) Oogonia start dividing only after birth to create oocytes.
    (D) Oocytes start dividing immediately after birth to create oogonia.

51. Which of the following correctly describes the phases of mitosis?
    (A) Prophase, metaphase, anaphase, telophase
    (B) Metaphase, telophase, anaphase, prophase
    (C) Anaphase, metaphase, telophase, prophase
    (D) Anaphase, telophase, metaphase, prophase

52. Which of the following is an example of the skin's role in the immune system?
    (A) Erector pili muscles controlling hair
    (B) Sensory nerve cells at various levels
    (C) Stored fat cells
    (D) Langerhans cells

PASSAGE VIII

Glomerular filtration rate (GFR) is a standard measure of kidney function. A low GFR signifies a low rate of filtration resulting from advanced renal dysfunction. The measurement of GFR is accomplished by determination of the rate of filtration of a substance from the blood into the urine relative to its concentration in blood plasma.

A common approximation of GFR is a test for **creatinine clearance** (CrCl). Creatinine is a normal product of the breakdown of creatine phosphate in muscle tissue. Production rate of creatinine is fairly constant and depends on muscle mass, which is affected by age, sex, and race. Creatinine production can also be affected by the amount of protein in the diet. Creatinine is removed from the bloodstream by glomerular filtration and is not reabsorbed by the tubules. The excretion rate is therefore proportional to glomerular filtration rate. A small amount of creatinine actively secreted in renal tubules can affect estimates of CrCl. The drug cimetidine inhibits tubular secretion and can result in a more accurate detection of CrCl.

CrCl can be measured directly, by urine sample over 24-hour period, or indirectly, through estimation, which is referred to as eCrCl, based on blood serum levels. The Cockcroft–Gault formula estimates eCrCl from blood plasma and corrects for variance due to age, sex, and body mass.

$$eCrCl = \frac{(140 - Age) \times Mass\ (kg) \times [0.85,\ if\ Female]}{72 \times Serum\ Creatinine\ (mg/dL)}$$

53. GFR measures the rate of filtrate passing from capillaries into the:
    - (A) nephric duct.
    - (B) Bowman's capsule.
    - (C) proximal convoluted tubule.
    - (D) ureter.

54. Assuming constant body mass and serum creatinine, what would be the ratio of the GFR of an 80-year-old man to that of a 20-year-old man, as approximated by eCrCl?
    - (A) 1:4
    - (B) 1:2
    - (C) 3:4
    - (D) 2:1

55. Which of the following would NOT be a consequence of a low GFR?
    - (A) Electrolyte imbalance
    - (B) Changes in extracellular fluid volume
    - (C) High levels of urea in urine
    - (D) High blood creatinine

56. Active secretion of creatinine from peritubular capillaries into the kidney tubules would cause approximations of GFR to be:
    - (A) overestimated, due to decreased serum creatinine levels.
    - (B) underestimated, due to increased serum creatinine levels.
    - (C) unaffected, because alterations in serum creatinine affect eCrCl but not GFR.
    - (D) unaffected, because neither eCrCl nor GFR are affected by tubular secretion.

The following questions do not refer to a descriptive passage and are not related to each other.

57. In general terms, which of the following phrases best defines fermentation?
    (A) Production of alcohol and carbon dioxide from the breakdown of sugar or other nutrients
    (B) Production of any gas as a result of oxidation of sugar or other nutrients
    (C) The partial breakdown of sugars and other nutrients using an electron acceptor other than oxygen
    (D) A redox reaction pair that reduces one reactant while oxidizing another

58. Sugar polymers consist of sugars attached to one another by either alpha or beta glycosidic linkages. Glycogen, amylopectin, amylose, maltose, and sucrose are easily digested by the human body, whereas cellulose, cellobiose, and lactulose are not. The digestible carbohydrates contain alpha glycosidic linkages whereas the indigestible ones do not. Many bacteria can subsist on beta glycosidically linked carbohydrates. Ruminants must use bacteria in the digestion of cellulose.

    From this information it can be concluded that:
    (A) humans and ruminants lack enzymes needed to break down the beta glycosidic linkages.
    (B) bacteria lack the enzymes needed for breaking down alpha glycosidic linkages.
    (C) ruminants lack enzymes for alpha glycosidic linkages.
    (D) humans lack enzymes for alpha glycosidic linkages.

59. Enzymes are responsible for accelerating virtually every chemical reaction on which an organism depends. Which of the following statements best characterizes the general mechanism by which all enzymes operate?
    (A) They increase the speed of the desired direction of the reaction while reducing the speed of the back reaction by coupling an exergonic reaction to the process.
    (B) They increase the speed of the forward reaction only through a reduction in the energy of activation.
    (C) They increase the speed of both forward and reverse reactions by lowering the energy of activation.
    (D) They increase the speed of the desired reaction of the reaction while reducing the speed of the back reaction by both a reduction in the energy of activation and the coupling of an exergonic reaction to the overall process.

PSYCHOLOGICAL, SOCIAL, AND BIOLOGICAL FOUNDATIONS OF BEHAVIOR

Time: 95 minutes
59 Questions

DIRECTIONS: The majority of questions in this section are organized into groups, with each group containing a descriptive passage. Read the passage, and then select the one best answer for each question. Some questions are not drawn from a passage and are also independent of the other questions. When answering questions, eliminate the choices that you are sure are incorrect and then choose the best remaining answer. When you have chosen an answer, mark it in the corresponding location on the answer sheet.

PASSAGE I

A 54-year-old male presents to his primary care physician with a chief complaint of increasing pain in the back of his head. The patient's past medical history includes color-blindness with perception of only blue, yellow, and shades of gray colors. The patient states that his vision is getting worse and that he particularly has problems seeing things on the right side of his field of view. He states that he does not wear corrective lenses. The rest of the history is otherwise unremarkable. The physician suspects that a lesion in the brain impinging on the optic nerve may be causing the patient's increasing pain and loss of vision in the right field of view. MRI study confirms that a mass is present in the posterior aspect of the patient's brain.

1. Which of the following structures is responsible for the perception of color?
   (A) Rods
   (B) Cones
   (C) Cornea
   (D) Retina

2. Based on the patient's past medical history, what classification of color blindness does he have?
   (A) Blue color blindness
   (B) Monochrome color blindness
   (C) Red-blue color blindness
   (D) Red-green color blindness

3. Which of the following is the most probable location of a lesion that affects vision?
   (A) Frontal lobe
   (B) Occipital lobe
   (C) Medulla oblongata
   (D) Pituitary

4. The perception of objects that are on the right side of the field of vision is processed in which area(s) of the brain?
   (A) Both the left and right sides of the brain
   (B) Right side of the brain only
   (C) Left side of the brain only
   (D) Anterior cortex and right side of the brain

5. Which of the following statements best fits the criteria for the opponent process theory of visual perception?
   (A) There are four cones associated with the perception of color, and they cannot be simultaneously stimulated.
   (B) There are four cones associated with the perception of color, grouped into pairs of red-green and blue-yellow. Only one group can be stimulated at a given time, and both cones in the stimulated group are active simultaneously.
   (C) There are four cones associated with the perception of color, grouped into pairs of red-green and blue-yellow. Only one group can be stimulated at a given time, and only one cone in the stimulated group will be active.
   (D) There are four cones associated with the perception of color, grouped into pairs of red-green and blue-yellow. Each group can be stimulated simultaneously, but only one cone from each group can be activated at a given time.

6. A person who goes from a bright room to a dark room would exhibit which of the following to adapt to the new environment?
   (A) Increased sensitivity of both rods and cones
   (B) Increased sensitivity of rods and decreased sensitivity of cones
   (C) Reduction of pupil size
   (D) Visual constancy

PASSAGE II

A medical sociologist examining the effects of societal factors on healthcare attainment conducts a study using data from a sample of 1000 patients suffering from post-traumatic stress disorder (PTSD). The sample had the following racial breakdown: 250 Caucasian, 250 African American, 250 Hispanic, and 250 Native American. In this study, the medical sociologist set out to determine whether there existed a correlation between patient recovery and socioeconomic status.

All participants were asked to volunteer personal information regarding their annual incomes. In addition to income reports, the medical sociologist received information regarding the amount of income allocated for treatment purposes. From these two sets of data, the percentage of income spent on treatment was calculated. The results from the study are shown in Table 1.

Table 1

Participant Racial Group	Average Annual Income	Average % of Income Spent on Treatment	Average % of PTSD Patients Who Recovered
Caucasian	$95,375	12.4	55
African American	$62,468	8.7	53
Hispanic	$54,945	5.5	29
Native American	$46,720	4.1	25

7. According to the results of the study, what correlation can be viewed between Average Annual Income and Average % of Income Spent on Treatment?
    (A) Racial groups with lower annual incomes spent a greater percentage of their income on treatment.
    (B) Racial groups with higher annual incomes spent a greater percentage of their income on treatment.
    (C) Racial groups with higher and lower annual incomes spent an equal percentage of their income on treatment.
    (D) There is no correlation present between Average Annual Income and Average % of Income Spent on Treatment.

8. The majority of the Caucasian patient's were upper middle class. Which of the following can be concluded from the results of the study?
    (A) Upper-middle-class people have more access to healthcare services.
    (B) Upper-middle-class people are likely to spend less on treatment.
    (C) Upper-middle-class people tend to care more about their health than do lower-class people.
    (D) Upper-middle-class people are better informed about their health and are more likely to seek treatment.

9. What sociological concept accounts for the lower socioeconomic status of some racial groups?
    (A) Reverse discrimination
    (B) Functionalism
    (C) Discrimination
    (D) Sexism

10. Despite the large income gap between Caucasian and African American samples, there is only a 2 percent differential in recovery rate. Which of the following, if true, would best explain this phenomenon?
    (A) Caucasian families are less likely to refer a family member for treatment for PTSD.
    (B) The incidence of PTSD is higher among African Americans than among Caucasians.
    (C) African American families spend 13 percent of their annual income on medical expenses in general.
    (D) African American families provide a strong support system that facilitates healing.

11. All of the following are possible solutions to the issue of healthcare disparities based on socioeconomic status presented in this study EXCEPT:
    (A) nationwide access to affordable healthcare based for people at all income levels.
    (B) information centers to educate lower-income families about treating health concerns.
    (C) policy change that addresses healthcare discrimination against upper-middle-class racial minorities.
    (D) more clinics in low-income neighborhoods.

The following questions do not refer to a descriptive passage and are not related to each other.

12. At 6–9 months of age, a child is first capable of:
    (A) lifting the head and chest, rolling over or pushing up, and recognizing familiar faces.
    (B) sitting without assistance, crawling, making purposeful sounds, or attempting self-feeding.
    (C) standing and walking, interacting or performing for others, or throwing objects.
    (D) opening doors, holding a glass, and self-feeding, or scribbling and coloring.

13. In which of the following pairs is the first concept defined by biological factors and the second concept defined by cultural factors?
    (A) Ethnicity; race
    (B) Race; ethnicity
    (C) Ethnicity; immigration status
    (D) Race; immigration status

14. Proponents of the humanistic approach to development argue that personality is determined by:
    (A) the "Big Five" personality traits that are universal and easily identified, measured, and placed on a continuum.
    (B) the unconscious drives, wishes, or conflicts of each individual.
    (C) freedom of choice and an innate drive toward personal growth.
    (D) one's social environment, including learning from the behaviors of others.

A pediatric psychologist studying attention designs and conducts an experiment based on the classic Stroop task to observe how well children in different age groups can hone in on one stimulus when presented with multiple interfering stimuli. The children were grouped in the following age categories: 5–8 years, 9–12 years, and 13–16 years. Thirty participants were placed in each of the age categories for a total of 90 participants. Each participant was presented with a paper on which were printed 20 words, each of which was the name of a color. Each word representing a color was printed in colored ink, but the color of the ink did not necessarily match the color named by the word. For example, the first word—green— was printed in red ink.

The list consisted of the following elements:

Word	Ink color	Word	Ink color
GREEN	Red	YELLOW	Red
RED	Light blue	RED	Yellow
BLUE	Green	ORANGE	Green
YELLOW	Dark blue	YELLOW	Green
ORANGE	Green	RED	Purple
PURPLE	Yellow	GREEN	Red
GREEN	Red	BLUE	Green
GREEN	Green	BLUE	Red
GREEN	Gray	GREEN	Green
BLUE	Green	PURPLE	Green

The participants were individually asked to say only the *color* of each word aloud and *not* the word itself from left to right in the order presented. The participants were then given a score based on how many colors were named correctly out of 20. The results were then averaged for each group and converted to a percent. Table 1 shows the results from the experiment.

Table 1

Participant Age Group	Average Number of Correctly Named Colors (out of 20)	Average % of Correctly Named Colors
5–8 years ($n = 30$)	11.7	58.5
9–12 years ($n = 30$)	12.1	60.5
13–16 years ($n = 30$)	16.4	82.0

15. Which of the following conclusions is most consistent with the results of the experiment?
    (A) Older children were more distracted by multiple stimuli than were younger children.
    (B) Younger children were more distracted by multiple stimuli than were older children.
    (C) 16-year-olds were less distracted by multiple stimuli than were 13-year-olds.
    (D) The top performers in the 5- to 8-year-old group performed as well as the lowest performers in the 9- to 12-year-old group.

16. Which of the following would most strengthen the results of the experiment?
    (A) Decreasing the number of participants in each age category and adding another age category for 17–18-year-olds
    (B) Recruiting a separate set of participants for each age category and testing their ability to read and the ability to correctly identify colors
    (C) Testing the same participants in each category for the ability to read and the ability to correctly identify colors
    (D) Having a control group that performs the same task that the subjects in the experiment performed

17. Which of the following is NOT part of the clinical presentation in pediatric patients with ADHD?
    (A) Developmental deficits in the frontal cortex and its circuitry
    (B) Increased attention to many tasks at once
    (C) Inability to focus on one given task
    (D) Overproduction of catecholamines

18. Which of the following is the dependent variable in this study?
    (A) Age categories
    (B) Twenty words with different colors
    (C) Percent of words that matched their colors
    (D) Percent of words correctly identified

19. Which of the following, if it occurred, would be an extraneous variable in the study?
    (A) Randomly drawing a sample of participants from public schools
    (B) Allowing the parents of the subjects to watch through a one-way mirror as their children perform
    (C) Only selecting subjects who are not color-blind
    (D) Finding that several of the subjects had the same first name

20. In this study, what is the distracting stimulus?
    (A) Color of the words
    (B) Age category of the participant
    (C) Words alone
    (D) Number of words

PASSAGE IV

A psychologist studying social anxiety disorder in young adults wants to see whether or not fear of social situations involves a greater cognitive element or a greater behavioral element in his patients' clinical presentations. To do this, the psychologist recruits patients with a confirmed diagnosis of social anxiety disorder and randomly assigns them to one of four treatment groups: a control group that receives no therapy, a cognitive therapy group only, a behavioral therapy group only, and a combined cognitive-behavioral therapy group. Before the start of treatment, each participant is administered the Liebowitz social anxiety scale to assess baseline level of social anxiety. The patients are asked to repeat this assessment after each therapy session until the cessation of therapy to compare start to finish level of social anxiety. The scores across participants were averaged for each of the four treatment modality categories at baseline, 3 months, 6 months, 9 months, and 12 months. The Liebowitz score ranges from 0 to 124: the higher the score is, the greater the level of social anxiety symptoms in the patient. Note that a score of 95 or more on the Liebowitz scale indicates very severe social anxiety. A score of less than 30 is considered average. The results from the study are depicted in Figure 1.

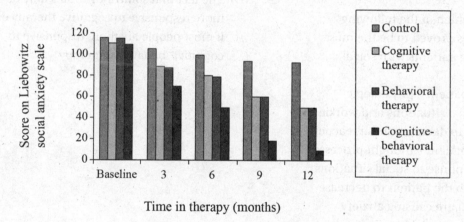

Figure 1. Results of the study

21. Based on data in Figure 1, which modality of treatment is the best for treating social anxiety disorder?
    - (A) No treatment/control group
    - (B) Cognitive therapy
    - (C) Behavioral therapy
    - (D) Cognitive-behavioral therapy

22. Which of the following theories of emotions postulates that in a potentially threatening environment a stimulus first results in a physiological response and then the brain interprets that response as an emotion such as fear?
    - (A) James-Lange theory
    - (B) Cannon-Bard theory
    - (C) Schachter's theory
    - (D) Lazarus's theory

23. Based on Figure 1, which of the following therapeutic strategies proved to be the most successful in treating patients with social anxiety?
    - (A) Addressing the patient's physiologic responses to social situations and working with the patient to decrease these reactions
    - (B) Addressing the patient's thought processes that occur in response to social situations and working with the patient to decrease the thoughts that are causing anxiety
    - (C) Addressing the patient's thoughts and physiologic responses to social situations and working with the patient to decrease maladaptive physiology and thoughts that are causing the anxiety
    - (D) Addressing how the patient's previous encounters in social situations and experiences may be affecting behavior and how the patient's personality may be playing a role in the patient's fear of social situations

24. Which structure in the brain is thought to play a significant role in the fear response and may decrease fear almost entirely upon removal?
    - (A) Amygdala
    - (B) Pituitary
    - (C) Hypothalamus
    - (D) Pineal gland

25. For the group with the least reduction of anxiety over the course of the study, which of the following most likely accounts for the measured reduction in anxiety?
    - (A) The placebo effect of receiving any therapy at all
    - (B) The effect of being in the study and taking the anxiety test
    - (C) Being around peers whose anxiety is diminishing significantly
    - (D) The fact that some individuals may be more responsive to cognitive therapy even if most people are more responsive to cognitive-behavioral therapy

The following questions do not refer to a descriptive passage and are not related to each other.

26. Which of the following explains why a Native American woman in her early fifties might be more disadvantaged in regard to achieving a higher class, status, or power than a Native American woman in her thirties and a Native American man in his early fifties?

I. Age discrimination
II. Racial inequality
III. Reverse discrimination

(A) I only
(B) II only
(C) I and II only
(D) I and III only

27. The incidence of Americans who suffer from a diagnosable psychological disorder during any given year is approximately:

(A) 9 percent.
(B) 18 percent.
(C) 27 percent.
(D) 32 percent.

28. According to the DSM-5, fear and anxiety that cannot be controlled and are present most days for a minimum of six months is referred to as:

(A) agoraphobia.
(B) panic disorder.
(C) separation anxiety disorder.
(D) generalized anxiety disorder.

PASSAGE V

The ability to satisfy both physical and psychosocial needs is at the heart of motivation. Motivation helps shape behavior by propelling individuals to act in order to meet the needs of the person. Countless needs can be identified in humans, especially the need to satisfy thirst, hunger, and even social aspects like the need to feel accepted by others. Motivation has a very strong tie to the biology of the organism, especially for hunger. For instance, when the stomach is empty and the body requires additional nutrients, the stomach secretes a peptide hormone called ghrelin that goes to the arcuate nucleus of the hypothalamus and causes the activation of neurons called NPY and AgRP, which then stimulate cells in the paraventricular nucleus that ultimately leads to the sensation of hunger. Leptin is another hormone involved in the process of hunger by inducing satiation when it is secreted by adipocytes. However, the lack of leptin secretion by adipocytes leads to hunger. Similarly, the hormone insulin that regulates blood sugar levels after a meal by causing uptake of glucose into cells can travel to the arcuate nucleus of the hypothalamus and activate POMC and α-MSH neurons that will ultimately lead to satiation.

Disruption of the normal physiology can lead to maladaptive behavior. Nowhere is this more evident than in obesity, in which individuals intake more nutrients than utilized and thus have an excess that is stored as adipose. Individuals afflicted by this condition constantly feel hunger, despite having an excess of calories.

29. According to the drive-reduction theory, what type of drive is hunger?
    (A) A primary drive
    (B) A secondary drive
    (C) A tertiary drive
    (D) A quaternary drive

30. Which of the following may lead to an increased drive to eat?
    (A) Increased insulin
    (B) Lack of ghrelin
    (C) Lack of leptin
    (D) Lack of glucagon

31. Which of the following may occur in someone suffering from anorexia nervosa?
    (A) Decreased drive due to low levels of ghrelin and leptin
    (B) Increased drive due to high ghrelin, low leptin, and high glucagon
    (C) Decreased drive due to high levels of ghrelin and leptin
    (D) Increased drive due to high levels of ghrelin, high leptin, and low glucagon

32. What structure in the brain is important in regulating temperature, thirst, and hunger homeostasis?
    (A) The pituitary gland
    (B) The pineal gland
    (C) The hypothalamus
    (D) The amygdala

33. According to Maslow's hierarchy of needs, which of the following may be true of individuals suffering from anorexia nervosa?
    (A) They have achieved a sense of self-actualization.
    (B) Self-esteem and confidence will not be reached until the physiologic needs of the individual are met.
    (C) The need to maintain homeostasis is not as important as the drive to seek nourishment.
    (D) They have a strong desire to seek safety in their environment.

34. Patients with type 1 diabetes mellitus are unable to produce sufficient insulin levels. Which of the following may be true of diabetic patients who do not undergo treatment?
    (A) They will have a higher drive due to increased activation of NPY and AgRP neurons.
    (B) They will have a higher drive due to increased secretion of leptin.
    (C) They will have a lower drive due to increased production of ghrelin.
    (D) They will have a lower drive due to increased activation of POMC and α-MSH neurons.

PASSAGE VI

In American society, the pursuit of equality is at the forefront of social issues. In recent decades, the debate on accepting same-sex couples into the institution of marriage has been a hot topic issue with media sources portraying adequate supporters for each side.

With the aforementioned debate in mind, a team of sociologists set out to examine a newer, younger generations' perspective on the topic. Through use of random sampling, 3250 college students ranging in age from 18 to 25, both men and women, and with equal representation of ethnicities, were asked the question of whether they supported same-sex marriage or not. To monitor the effects of socialization on the study's sample, the students were also asked how they believe their parents, peers, and the general American public would answer the same question. By asking for the source of each student's answer, the team of sociologists hoped to prove that socialization evolves over time and replaces past norms, in this case, the traditional stance that same-sex marriage is a deviation from commonplace societal practices.

In addition to asking college students, the team of sociologists chose to expand the experiment by asking the same question of an older generation, adults aged 40 to 60. They hoped the comparison of both younger and older generations would allow a further look into the evolution of socialization over time.

Table 1 displays the results of asking the sample of 3250 college students the study's key, two-part question.

Table 1

(18–25)	Self	Parents	Peers	General American Public
# of Yes Responses	2624	2050	2864	1937
# of No Responses	626	1200	386	1313

Table 2 displays the results of asking the sample of 3250 adults ages 40–60 the study's key, two-part question.

Table 2

(40–60)	Self	Parents	Peers	General American Public
# of Yes Responses	1865	478	1677	1812
# of No Responses	1385	2772	1573	1438

35. Based on the data in Tables 1 and 2, which of the following statements best describes the results of the experiment?
    (A) The majority of subjects display negative views of same-sex marriage.
    (B) Table 2 subjects exhibit higher levels of acceptance than Table 1 subjects.
    (C) The older generations' personal responses are significantly influenced by how they perceive their parents' beliefs.
    (D) Younger generations exhibit a higher level of perceived acceptance in relation to all variables.

36. What is the purpose of sampling a diverse population in a socialization experiment?
    (A) The topic of same-sex marriage is important to most people.
    (B) Socialization affects each gender, age, and ethnicity in distinct ways.
    (C) The experiment highlights the differences of opinion based on gender.
    (D) Diverse populations provide a wider range of results in all cases.

37. Based on the data presented, what is the most likely outcome of polling a sample of people from age 70 to 80?
    (A) Levels of acceptance equivalent to Table 2 subjects
    (B) Increased levels of dissent toward same-sex marriage
    (C) Levels of dissent equal to the data presented in the "Parents" section of Table 2
    (D) There is not enough data to predict the outcome.

38. Based on Table 1, which agent of socialization appears to have the greatest influence on personal perspective?
    (A) Parents
    (B) The general American public
    (C) Media
    (D) Peers

39. The experiment observes norm deviance in society. Which of the following is a likely mechanism for explaining how a behavior once considered deviant becomes accepted?
    (A) Definitions of deviance are the learned perceptions of each generation.
    (B) Over time, prior definitions of deviance become inapplicable to modern society.
    (C) Only through legislative action can past deviant behavior be accepted by society.
    (D) A deviant behavior must go through restructuring to transform it into an accepted norm.

40. Which of the following best explains why Table 1 shows a majority of "yes" answers?
    (A) Subjects know that their parents, their peers, and the general American public all agree with them.
    (B) Subjects believe that their perspective is largely shared in society.
    (C) On being polled, the subjects' parents and peers agreed with the subject.
    (D) Subjects support same-sex marriage.

41. The generation and experience of emotion is directed by the amygdala, hippocampus, hypothalamus, basal nuclei in the basal forebrain, olfactory bulbs, and parts of the cortex and midbrain, all of which make up the:
    (A) endocrine system.
    (B) lymphatic system.
    (C) limbic system.
    (D) circulatory system.

42. The biological need for homeostasis motivates individuals to behave in a manner that will eliminate any psychological or physical discomfort/imbalance. When a behavior satisfies a need and restores equilibrium, the behavior is reinforced and an individual learns to behave similarly in the future. This theory of motivation is known as:
    (A) incentive theory.
    (B) drive-reduction theory.
    (C) cognitive dissonance theory.
    (D) attribution theory.

43. Which of the following pairs of words represents a negative belief and attitude about a category of people and the actions that result from that belief and attitude, respectively?
    (A) Discrimination; prejudice
    (B) Individual discrimination; institutional discrimination
    (C) Prejudice; discrimination
    (D) Institutional discrimination; individual discrimination

44. Which of the following represents the correct order of Freud's five stages of psychosocial development?
    (A) Oral, anal, phallic, latency, genital
    (B) Genital, anal, phallic, latency, oral
    (C) Latency, oral, anal, phallic, genital
    (D) Anal, oral, latency, phallic, genital

45. A county government first attempted to place a landfill site in the vicinity of a predominantly upper-class community but was met with strong resistance. Subsequently, it was decided that the landfill site would be placed near a predominately poor community, which did not have the resources to challenge the county government's decision. This is an example of:
    (A) global inequality.
    (B) environmental inequality.
    (C) prejudice.
    (D) residential segregation.

PASSAGE VII

Habituation, which is defined as the dampening of response to an ongoing or repeated stimulus in the environment, has a very strong tie with the biological basis of neurotransmission. Neurons "adapt" to a stimulus by suppressing the number of action potentials released in response to that stimulus and ultimately the signal may go out of notice consciously. The treatment of many anxiety disorders is linked to habituation. The habituation curve in Figure 1 graphs level of anxiety as a function of exposure or habituation.

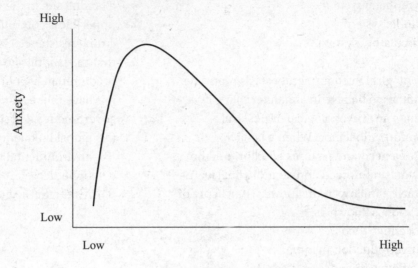

Figure 1. Habituation curve

46. After undergoing neurosurgery to remove certain tissues, a patient reports having very little anxiety and little fear in response to stimuli that were frightening before the surgery. Based on this information, which of the following did this patient have removed?
    (A) Amygdala
    (B) Pituitary gland
    (C) Hypothalamus
    (D) Pineal gland

47. Which of the following statements best summarizes Figure 1?
    (A) Over time, chronic exposure to a stimulus leads to exacerbation of anxiety.
    (B) Over time, chronic exposure to a stimulus leads to relapse of anxiety.
    (C) Over time, chronic exposure to a stimulus leads to remission of anxiety.
    (D) Initial exposure to a stimulus leads to remission of anxiety.

48. Which of the following would be consistent with dishabituation in a patient with social anxiety disorder?
    (A) Ongoing exposure leads to attenuation of anxiety symptoms.
    (B) Ongoing exposure leads to heightened anxiety symptoms.
    (C) Social rejection leads to remission of anxiety symptoms.
    (D) Social rejection leads to a relapse of anxiety symptoms.

49. How might the release of adrenaline (epinephrine) lead to an exacerbation of a patient's anxiety?
    (A) Adrenaline participates in a negative feedback loop that increases anxiety symptoms such as shaking, sweating, and arousal.
    (B) Adrenaline participates in a positive feed forward loop that increases anxiety symptoms such as shaking, sweating, and arousal.
    (C) Adrenaline participates in a negative feedback loop that decreases anxiety symptoms such as shaking, sweating, and arousal.
    (D) Adrenaline participates in a positive feed forward loop that decreases anxiety symptoms such as shaking, sweating, and arousal.

50. How does facilitation of neurons contribute to the high anxiety paired with low exposure in Figure 1?
    (A) Threshold potential of neurons is increased, making the neurons more excitable to a lower stimulus.
    (B) Threshold potential of neurons is decreased, making the neurons more excitable to a lower stimulus.
    (C) Resting potential of neurons is decreased, making the neurons more excitable to a lower stimulus.
    (D) Resting potential of neurons is increased, making the neurons more excitable to a lower stimulus.

51. Which of the following physiological events occurring in neurons leads to a remission of anxiety symptoms with long-term exposure, as depicted in Figure 1?
    (A) Threshold potential of neurons is elevated to make them less excitable.
    (B) Threshold potential of neurons is decreased to make them less excitable.
    (C) Stimulus that is facilitating neurons is removed, making them less excitable.
    (D) Neurons are facilitated to make them less excitable.

PASSAGE VIII

A sociologist selected 100 subjects, 50 male and 50 female, to participate in a simple observational test. Before beginning the test, all subjects were briefed as a group. The sociologist told them that in previous runs of this test male participants had scored much higher than the female participants. The sociologist deliberately made the false claim that the reason behind the gender achievement disparity was that men have more reliable short-term memory than do women due to biological factors. Subjects were called into the experiment room one at a time. While one participant was taking the test, the remaining 99 participants were left to talk among themselves in the briefing room. As expected, the male and female participants argued about the sociologist's false claim of male superiority.

During the test, each subject entered a room that contained a desk on which were 20 assorted objects. The objects were easily identifiable and found commonly in everyday life. Upon exiting the test room after the allotted five minutes, each subject was asked to list from memory as many objects as possible that they had seen.

Table 1 shows the results for all 100 subjects during the five-minute test. The numbers across the top represent the number of correctly remembered items. The row marked *F* shows how many female subjects correctly identified a specific number of items. For example, exactly two women correctly identified five items. The row marked *M* similarly shows the results for the male subjects.

Table 1.

	1	2	3	4	5	6	7	8	9	10	11	12	13	14	15	16	17	18	19	20
F					2		3	20	6	5		3	4	5						2
M			1		2			3		4		5			15	5		10	3	2

52. Which theoretical approach to sociology is best represented by the participants' debates?
   (A) Conflict theory, because the debates emphasized class conflict
   (B) Functionalism, because the debates reflected unharmonious structures
   (C) Conflict theory, because the debates emphasized gender conflict
   (D) Symbolic interactionism, because of shared meanings of agreements

53. Of the following statements, which best exemplifies the theory of social constructionism in the passage?
   (A) The participants' acceptance of the sociologist's false claims based on his occupation
   (B) The shared understanding that men outperform women on the test
   (C) The self-fulfilling prophecy of male success rates
   (D) The debates brought on by the sociologist's false claims

54. Which of the following is the dependent variable in this study?
   (A) The sociologist's false claims
   (B) Quality of short-term memory
   (C) Number of objects identified
   (D) Number of subjects tested

55. Based on the data in Table 1, which of the following can be concluded?
   (A) Women are better than men at observational tests.
   (B) Men are inherently better at memorization than women.
   (C) Debates amongst subjects were the sole contributor to displayed results.
   (D) Expected success by subjects can influence actual results.

56. What is the primary importance of the briefing before beginning the test?
   (A) It informs the subjects of the five-minute time limit.
   (B) It creates a shared meaning of gender bias in achievement.
   (C) It creates doubt in all subjects' abilities to succeed.
   (D) It allows subjects to voice their disagreement with the sociologist's false claims.

The following questions do not refer to a descriptive passage and are not related to each other.

57. A Centers for Disease Control report states that in 2010 64.5 percent of people between the ages of 50 and 75 were up-to-date on their colorectal cancer screening. The report also states that rates of screening increased with household income. The greater likelihood of someone with a higher household income having an up-to-date colorectal cancer screening compared to someone with a lower household income is an example of:

   (A) healthcare disparities.
   (B) gender inequality.
   (C) health disparities.
   (D) age discrimination.

58. According to Vygotsky's sociocultural theory, children learn through a collaborative process in which they receive formal or informal instruction from a more experienced individual known as:

   (A) the generalized other.
   (B) the more knowledgeable other (MKO).
   (C) the superego.
   (D) the looking-glass self.

59. One of the foundations of prejudice against others is explained by social identity theory, which argues that human beings have an innate tendency to favor those similar to them and reject those who are different. This tendency is known as:

   (A) in-group/out-group bias.
   (B) social identity.
   (C) individuation.
   (D) habituation/dishabituation.

ANSWER KEY
Practice Test 2

CHEMICAL AND PHYSICAL FOUNDATIONS

1. D	**13.** D	**25.** B	**37.** C	**49.** C
2. D	**14.** A	**26.** A	**38.** C	**50.** A
3. C	**15.** D	**27.** B	**39.** C	**51.** C
4. A	**16.** B	**28.** C	**40.** B	**52.** C
5. D	**17.** A	**29.** A	**41.** C	**53.** C
6. A	**18.** B	**30.** C	**42.** D	**54.** C
7. D	**19.** D	**31.** D	**43.** B	**55.** D
8. A	**20.** D	**32.** B	**44.** D	**56.** B
9. C	**21.** C	**33.** A	**45.** C	**57.** D
10. D	**22.** D	**34.** B	**46.** B	**58.** B
11. B	**23.** A	**35.** B	**47.** C	**59.** B
12. B	**24.** D	**36.** A	**48.** C	

CRITICAL ANALYSIS AND REASONING

1. D	**12.** D	**23.** B	**34.** D	**45.** D
2. B	**13.** C	**24.** D	**35.** A	**46.** A
3. C	**14.** C	**25.** A	**36.** C	**47.** B
4. A	**15.** A	**26.** B	**37.** D	**48.** D
5. D	**16.** B	**27.** B	**38.** A	**49.** B
6. B	**17.** C	**28.** C	**39.** D	**50.** A
7. C	**18.** D	**29.** A	**40.** C	**51.** C
8. C	**19.** B	**30.** C	**41.** D	**52.** D
9. B	**20.** D	**31.** B	**42.** B	**53.** B
10. C	**21.** C	**32.** C	**43.** C	
11. C	**22.** B	**33.** C	**44.** D	

ANSWER KEY
Practice Test 2

BIOLOGICAL AND BIOCHEMICAL FOUNDATIONS

1. C	13. C	25. B	37. C	49. A
2. B	14. B	26. C	38. D	50. B
3. C	15. D	27. B	39. B	51. A
4. B	16. B	28. B	40. D	52. D
5. D	17. B	29. A	41. A	53. B
6. B	18. D	30. D	42. A	54. B
7. C	19. A	31. C	43. D	55. C
8. B	20. B	32. C	44. B	56. A
9. D	21. C	33. C	45. D	57. C
10. D	22. B	34. C	46. C	58. A
11. A	23. C	35. B	47. B	59. C
12. D	24. D	36. A	48. B	

PSYCHOLOGICAL, SOCIAL, AND BIOLOGICAL FOUNDATIONS

1. B	13. B	25. B	37. B	49. B
2. D	14. C	26. A	38. D	50. D
3. B	15. B	27. C	39. A	51. C
4. C	16. C	28. D	40. B	52. C
5. D	17. D	29. A	41. C	53. A
6. A	18. D	30. C	42. B	54. C
7. B	19. A	31. B	43. C	55. D
8. A	20. C	32. C	44. A	56. B
9. C	21. D	33. B	45. B	57. A
10. D	22. A	34. A	46. A	58. B
11. C	23. C	35. D	47. C	59. A
12. B	24. A	36. B	48. D	

ANSWERS EXPLAINED

Chemical and Physical Foundations

1. **(D)** Wavelength and frequency are inversely related, and frequency and energy are directly related.

2. **(D)** This answer can be obtained by substituting into the Beer's law equation provided: $0.900 = (300\ M^{-1}cm^{-1})(c)(1\ cm)$. Solving for c gives the answer.

3. **(C)** Comparing trials 1 and 2, in which only the BrO_3^- ion changes concentration, shows that as the concentration of bromated ion doubles, so does the reaction rate, making the order 1.

4. **(A)** One liter of liquid bromine would have a mass of 3200 grams. Dividing that by the molar mass of 160 g/mole gives 20.0 moles/L.

5. **(D)** This can be obtained by solving $Ms^{-1} = kM^4$.

6. **(A)** This question requires knowing how to read a Michaelis–Menten graph. Figure 1 shows the reaction rate on the y-axis. On a Michaelis–Menten graph, K_m is the x-value that corresponds to the y-value at $\frac{1}{2}V_{max}$, 50% of the reaction rate. Information in the passage also reveals this relationship. Choice A is correct because the x-value that corresponds to 50% of the reaction rate is 0.2 mM. The other choices are incorrect because they do not correspond to $\frac{1}{2}V_{max}$ on Figure 1.

7. **(D)** This question requires knowing how to read a Lineweaver–Burk plot because it is a double-reciprocal graph. The correct answer is D because Figure 2 shows the pattern observed for mixed inhibition. The passage also describes that mixed inhibition alters both the V_{max} and K_m, and this is also shown on the graph by the fact that the lines cross both the x- and y-axes at different points. Choice C is incorrect because the pattern observed for uncompetitive inhibitors is not displayed in Figure 2, as noncompetitive inhibitors do not alter K_m. Choice B is incorrect because a competitive inhibitor's Lineweaver-Burk plot has lines crossing the same point on the y-axis, but not the x-axis. Choice A is incorrect because an irreversible inhibitor cannot be displaced by a substrate, and this is not reflected in the graph.

8. **(A)** Uncompetitive inhibition, also known as anticompetitive inhibition, takes place when an enzyme inhibitor binds only to the complex formed between the enzyme and the substrate (the E-S complex). Choice A is correct because Drug Y is an uncompetitive inhibitor, and this choice describes the correct action on V_{max} and K_m and the correct binding site. Choice B is incorrect because uncompetitive inhibitors do not bind in the active site, and they decrease both V_{max} and K_m. Choice C is incorrect because it does not have the correct binding site. Choice D is also incorrect because it does not correctly describe the binding site or the effect of uncompetitive inhibition on V_{max} and K_m.

9. **(C)** This question requires the understanding of how variables in an equation alter the product. α is simply the factor by which the K_m is altered. Because α is in the denominator of the reaction, if it is increased with the increase in inhibitor, then the initial velocity, V_0, will be lowered. α must be directly proportional to the amount of inhibitor because it is a factor of how much the K_m is being altered. This leaves choice C as the correct answer. The other answer choices incorrectly describe the proportionality relationship between α, K_m, and V_0.

10. **(D)** This question requires knowledge about the strength of different types of bonds. The order of bond strength is covalent > ionic > hydrogen. Enzymes are complementary to the transition state of a reaction, not the substrate. If enzymes fit in a rigid lock-and-key fashion to the substrate, the enzyme would have great difficulty reacting and moving on to another reaction. The enzyme-substrate complex follows an induced fit model instead of a lock-and-key method. Choice D is correct because it correctly states that enzymes bind to the transition state with relatively weak bonds: ionic and hydrogen. Choice A is incorrect because of transition-state theory, and if the enzyme formed covalent bonds with a reactant, it would not be able to easily leave the reaction, and it would likely be permanently altered. Choices B and C are incorrect for the same reasons.

11. **(B)** Although this knowledge is not required to correctly answer this question, it is the production of HCO_3^- that draws Na^+ into the eye causing water to follow by osmosis to form the aqueous humor in the eye. In glaucoma, there is too much aqueous humor in the eye, and this excess causes increased pressure. Choice B is correct because it states that the competitive inhibitor binds to the active site of the enzyme, inhibits production of HCO_3^-, and decreases production of aqueous humor in the eye. Choice A is incorrect because the inhibitor would not inhibit production of H_2O, and even if it did, increasing pressure in the eye would not help treat glaucoma. Choice C is incorrect because it incorrectly describes how a competitive inhibitor binds. A competitive inhibitor binds to the active site on the enzyme, not the enzyme-substrate complex. Choice D is incorrect because the inhibitor does not bind to the active site of the substrate because substrates do not have active sites.

12. **(B)** Feedback inhibition is a process in which a downstream product of a reaction series inhibits an enzyme upstream in the series to inhibit production of the product. The body uses this to maintain normal levels of the product. The correct answer is choice B because the product K is shown to inhibit enzyme "i-ase" which will inhibit production of anything after that enzyme in the reaction series. In other words, the enzyme will no longer be able to convert reactant I into J. Choice A is incorrect. The levels of I will remain the same because I occurs before the enzyme affected by the inhibitor, K. Choice C is incorrect because the inhibitor will not cause all of the reactant to decrease. Choice D is incorrect because the point of feedback inhibition is to bring the final product, K, down to normal levels.

13. **(D)** The salt is prepared by bimolecular nucleophilic substitution. Triphenylphosphine acts as a nucleophile attacking the electrophilic alkyl halide. As the phosphorus–carbon bond *forms*, the halide–carbon bond *breaks*.

14. **(A)** Trans-alkenes are thermodynamically more stable than cis-alkenes.

15. **(D)** Liquid ammonia/metal reductions of alkynes produce primarily trans-alkenes.

16. **(B)** The Wittig reagent contains an alkane, –CH, which is terminated by a *t*-butyl group. Combining the reagent with a cyclic ketone (cyclohexanone) produces Compound **B**, an alkene.

17. **(A)** When the amount goes from 12 g to 6 g, then the time is 1 half-life. When the amount goes from 6 g to 3 g, this is another half-life. So the half-life is 7.6/2 = 3.8 days.

18. **(B)** Use $R = \lambda N$. This gives a value in Bq. Then convert to Ci.

19. **(D)** Alpha particles are heavier than electrons and gamma is electromagnetic radiation, so it has 0 mass.

20. **(D)** $N = N_0 e^{-2}$ or $N_0/7.3$.

21. **(C)** Half-life is proportional to decay constant.

22. **(D)** All calcium atoms have 20 protons, and the isotope with mass number 44 has 24 neutrons. Positive ions are formed by the loss of electrons, so this ion has lost two electrons, for a total of 18.

23. **(A)** Only zinc metal will reduce tin and produce a spontaneous reaction.

24. **(D)** The period is 1/frequency.

25. **(B)** $V_{final} = V_{initial} + at$.

26. **(A)** The spherical symmetry means that if the cross-sectional area is known, you have an accurate sample of the activity level.

27. **(B)** The data from 10 cm to 20 cm shows a decrease by a factor of 4, as expected in an inverse square law. Going from 10 cm to 5 cm is halving the distance, so the number of counts should increase by a factor of 4, giving 400 counts at 5 cm.

28. **(C)** Use $P = 4\pi r^2 I$ so $I = (5.0 \text{ W})/(4\pi \cdot 100 \text{ m}^2) \approx 5/1200 \text{ W/m}^2$.

29. **(A)** $4\pi(12)^2 I_{12} = 4\pi(4)^2 I_4$, so $I_{12}/I_4 = (4/12)^2 = (1/3)^2 = 1/9$

30. **(C)** Gravity does follow the inverse square law, but it is based on the distance from the center of Earth.

31. **(D)** Because of the inverse square relationship, decreasing the distance from the source by one-third produces an approximate 10-fold increase in intensity, or doubling of the perceived loudness.

32. **(B)** The strong nuclear force is stronger than the electromagnetic force at very short distances, which is why protons do not repel each other. At larger distances protons do repel, so the strong nuclear force must be decreasing more rapidly with distance.

33. **(A)** The oxidation number of the chlorine atoms is +5 in ClO_3^- and is 0 in Cl_2. Thus chlorine is reduced and each Cl atom gains 5 electrons.

34. **(B)** 44.8 L of gas is two moles at STP. Based on the stoichiometric ratio from the coefficients, there will be one mole of sulfuric acid for every two moles of carbon dioxide. One mole of sulfuric acid would be 0.25 L of 4 M solution, since M = moles /L.

35. **(B)** Wavelength = speed/frequency

36. **(A)** The circumference is $2\pi \times 0.4$ m (the radius). There are 4 rotations in a second, so 0.8π m $\times 4 = 3.2\pi$ m.

37. **(C)** The passage states that KOH produces soft soaps and that vegetable oils produce softer soaps than animal fats.

38. **(C)** This can be solved with estimation. The heat of combustion is 37,000 kJ/mole and the molar mass can be estimated as 1000. So, 1 gram is 1/1000 of a mole, and the amount of heat produced would be 37 kJ, or 37,000 J. The temperature change of the water can be

found using $\Delta H = mCp\Delta T$. 37,000 J = (1000 g)(4.18 J/g°C)(ΔT). This gives 37,000/(4000) = a bit more than 9 degrees, for the temperature change.

39. **(C)** Glycerol has three OH groups and has the potential for multiple hydrogen bonds.

40. **(B)** Dissolving a solute in a liquid always raises the boiling point and lowers the freezing point.

41. **(C)** Soaps have an ionic (COO^-Na^+) end that can form an ion–dipole interaction with polar water molecules.

42. **(D)** Arsenic atoms have 33 electrons. Following the filling diagram on an Aufbau diagram gives the correct configuration.

43. **(B)** Being brittle, having a very high melting point, and having poor conductive properties are characteristics of covalent network compounds.

44. **(D)** Arsenic will have chemical properties most similar to another element in the same group, which means the two elements have five valence electrons.

45. **(C)** Arsenic trichloride has three bonds and one lone pair around the central arsenic atom. The trigonal pyramidal shape has a lone pair at one end, resulting in a polar molecule.

46. **(B)** The sum of the oxidation numbers in a stable compound is zero. In a compound or ion, the oxidation number of oxygen is negative two, making the arsenic atoms positive three.

47. **(C)** The passage states that arsenic is toxic and, as a result, there could be valid concerns that workers exposed to it might be harmed. Choices A and B are not defendable by the passage. Choice D is incorrect because there may be medicinal uses despite the toxicity, such as in treatment of cancer.

48. **(C)** Unlike charges attract. Electrostatic induction could also cause an attraction by pushing electrons to the opposite side of the hanging sphere and attracting the resulting positive side.

49. **(C)** Choice C is correct because beta oxidation refers to the process described. Choice A is incorrect because omega oxidation describes another oxidative pathway for fats that occurs in the ER and involves attack on the omega carbon. The PPP does not involve fats. Choice D is incorrect because ketolysis refers to the breakdown of ketones.

50. **(A)** All of the reactions are double displacements. Silver chloride is an insoluble solid.

51. **(C)** Choice C is correct because in the breakdown of foods for energy, carbon and hydrogen are oxidized to form carbon dioxide and water. The smaller the percentage of oxygen, the more energy on a per gram basis of substrate. Choices A and B are true, but they do not account for the large difference due to the higher percentage of oxygen which itself cannot be "burned." Choice D involves ketone bodies, which are produced for export to other tissues by the liver and do not alter the overall metabolism of fat.

52. **(C)** Brønsted–Lowry bases are proton acceptors. In this example, the water is accepting a proton from the acetic acid.

53. **(C)** One mole of ethanol is oxidized to one mole of acetic acid, which has a molar mass of 60.

54. **(C)** In a hydronium atom, there are three bonds and one lone pair around the central oxygen atom. This leads to a trigonal pyramidal shape.

55. **(D)** The change in enthalpy is equal to the enthalpy of the products (–286 kJ/mole × 2 moles) minus the enthalpy of the reactants, which in this case is zero, because the enthalpy of formation of any pure element in its natural state is zero.

56. **(B)** The definition of a spontaneous reaction is one with a negative free energy change.

57. **(D)** The reactants have one mole of gas and the products have none, so there is a negative change in ion entropy as the reaction proceeds.

58. **(B)** Use the lens maker's formula: $\frac{1}{o} + \frac{1}{i} = \frac{1}{f}$. If the image is on the same side of the lens as the object, the image distance will be negative. The object is the computer screen, and the image is where the eye can focus, at 150 cm. The eyeglasses are only about 1–2 cm from the man's eyes, so the approximate calculation can neglect this.

$$\frac{1}{50} - \frac{1}{150} = \frac{1}{f}$$
$$\frac{3}{150} - \frac{1}{150} = \frac{2}{150} = \frac{1}{f}$$
$$f = +75 \text{ cm}$$

59. **(B)** Recall that according to Coulomb's law, the force is directly proportional to the charge and inversely proportional to the square of the distance. Since Q2 is double the charge but double the distance, this means that the force from Q2 ends up being half the force from Q1. The forces are both attractive. So we subtract one force from the other to get the magnitude of the net force. The net force is half of the force from Q1, or 0.5 N.

Critical Analysis and Reasoning

1. **(D)** Answer D is based on the fact that affluent students took management positions. Choices A, B, and C, while they may have been true, cannot be defended by information in the passage.

2. **(B)** Choice A is discussed, but not in the last paragraph. Choices C and D are relevant issues but are not discussed in the passage.

3. **(C)** The phrase has a negative connotation. The author cites the dramatic changes facilitated by coops.

4. **(A)** The passage states that the coops in the 1960s never achieved the economic sophistication of mainstream food stores. Choices B, C, and D violate information stated in the passage.

5. **(D)** Both students and parents were interested in cooperating with others to save money. Because of the students' lower income level, the effort to do so was more worthwhile.

6. **(B)** Choice A does not match the structure of the passage. Choices C and D are incorrect because they focus on a sociopolitical view. The passage focuses on an economic view.

7. **(C)** The passage states that "contrary to the general impression of college students of the time," there were major sociological and economic differences between universities.

8. **(C)** Coops were an example of economic change due to necessity and they led to socio-political change, as stated in the last paragraph. Choice A reverses the cause and effect. Choice D is not defendable by information in the passage.

9. **(B)** The statement is not supported with evidence but it is expanded on.

10. **(C)** Even though answer C has the requirement that the taxpayer benefit from the project, this is still an example of a cooperative effort, in which many people contribute together and benefit. Choices A and B do not negate the possibility that the person is fundamentally competitive. Choice D is wrong because by itself it does not guarantee that the person is cooperative.

11. **(C)** The passage states that the fundamental attitude of the competitive is that they can take care of themselves no matter what. A competitive person does not necessarily avoid the benefits of cooperative programs such as welfare (choice B) nor does the person always try to make money in every situation (choice D).

12. **(D)** Minimizing input and maximizing return makes the project less cooperative and more competitive. Choice C only hints at possible competitive motives. Choice A is based on a false assumption that competitive people do not engage in projects with others. Choice B is wrong because no matter how high the return, if everyone contributes the same and takes out the same, it is cooperative.

13. **(C)** The author clearly finds competitiveness to be negative. Roman numeral I is defendable because the author says that competitive people sometimes vote against using tax dollars even for worthwhile causes.

14. **(C)** The effort to form a party for competitive people exemplifies the competitive person's blindness to the real need for cooperation to meet his or her needs. The other answer choices could be true statements but they are not supported by anything the author says in the passage.

15. **(A)** The first paragraph states that CCD has economic significance worldwide.

16. **(B)** The Working Group reports finding a range of infectious agents and that this indicates an underlying immune deficiency. Choice A is not viable because agriculture depends on bees. Choice C has the relationship reversed.

17. **(C)** The passage states only that healthy bees do not rob the provisions of dying hives. It does not defend that those provisions are not contaminated. Choice A can be concluded because global warming is given as an environmental stress, stresses are linked to immunodeficiencies, and immunodeficiencies are linked to multiple infectious agents. Choice D is defendable because the research shows only an "association" between the two. If there is a causal relationship, it could go in either direction.

18. **(D)** The passage refers to crops that have been genetically modified with pest control characteristics. This means characteristics that would protect them from insects, possibly including the production of substances that would harm insects.

19. **(B)** Answer B confuses high-frequency sound waves with electromagnetic radiation. All the other answer choices establish a correlation between electromagnetic radiation and an effect on the bees.

20. **(D)** The passage discusses in the second paragraph how the distinctions between the two blurred.

21. **(C)** The author states that a sense of ownership leads to greater enjoyment in the lives of workers and that ownership is a characteristic shared by both ideologies. Choice A is incorrect because in the examples in which workers were better off, it was the ownership of shares that was the cause, not privatization per se. Choice D is incorrect because the author states that ownership does make a difference, even if it is unlikely for the workers to own a majority of the shares.

22. **(B)** Choice III is incorrect because under communism, as described in the passage, it is the role of government to provide services such as healthcare.

23. **(B)** In the paragraph about increased productivity, the absence of labor disputes is cited as an example, implying that the presence of labor disputes reduces productivity. Choice C is incorrect because of the example of worker/owners voting against wage increases. Choice D is incorrect because there can be qualifications, such as citizenship, gender, or age, on who can vote in a democracy.

24. **(D)** Choice A is a characteristic of a communist society. Choice C is a characteristic of a democratic society. Choice B could be either but is not a blend. Answer D blends democracy with a government-sponsored social program.

25. **(A)** In the following paragraph, the author distinguishes the workers, who do not have control or profit, from the majority stockholders, who are the real owners.

26. **(B)** Answer B is not stated or implied in the passage as a result of privatization. The other answer choices are all specifically stated as results.

27. **(B)** The author states that the root of the problem of seeing work as negative lies in seeing work as the means to an end. The author continues by saying that on the contrary, work is an end in itself. Choice A is not specific enough. Choices C and D are inconsistent with the passage.

28. **(C)** The author uses the term to describe the workplace, not the family (choice B).

29. **(A)** In discussing addiction, the author is explaining the argument that critics of long work hours would make. The author then goes on to refute the argument. Choice B is incorrect because the analogy to an addiction is not used to weaken an argument. It is part of the argument that the author later attacks.

30. **(C)** Answer C attacks the author's two definitions of work as an end in itself—being part of a bigger picture and being creative, which is defined as the opposite of routine. Choice B is incorrect because the fact that a worker is required to work overtime does not preclude the possibility that that person will enjoy the work. Choice D also does not preclude this.

31. **(B)** The essence of the passage is one argument that claims something is addictive (work) and another that claims it (work) is a creative expression of life. Answer B best matches this.

32. **(C)** This answer links the brain to intelligence while still acknowledging Aristotle's view. The other answers do not create this link.

33. **(C)** The disorder described is a neuropsychiatric one and these were observed by Maimonides. Choice D is incorrect because the impulsive actions are not necessarily verbal. Hippocrates could be the correct answer, not because of the specialized senses but rather because the brain is the seat of intelligence.

34. **(D)** After describing Abulcasis, the passage says "elsewhere in medieval Europe," implying that that was the time period and location of Abulcasis. Although the name al-Anda-luz is Arabic, it cannot be inferred that the location was the Middle East or North Africa. It refers to Andalucia, in Spain, but the passage does not provide that information.

35. **(A)** The passage states that Broca observed people with brain damage and observed how the damage affected their behavior. He then hypothesized that this correlation showed that damage to a certain part of the brain affected certain behavior. Choice C is incorrect because it is the very hypothesis he is trying to prove.

36. **(C)** The author contrasts dead ghosts with sensual experience. Only answer C is based in sensual experience.

37. **(D)** This is the only answer that expresses a paradox, a statement that is true but seemingly contradictory.

38. **(A)** Because creating new sequences is part of the definition of creativity, this answer shows that technology can lead to creativity, undermining the author's argument. The fact that creativity went into the design of an instrument (choice B) does not affect the argument. Skills not easily lost are in the realm of technique, not creativity (choice D).

39. **(D)** The author does not draw significant distinctions between art and music.

40. **(C)** The author says that technique cannot be avoided (choices B and D) but that the musician can take periodic breaks from it, temporarily forgetting what was learned. Choice A is incorrect because the author says that technology will overpower creativity.

41. **(D)** Answer D includes factors that support the plume model and attack the plate model. The other answer choices address only one model.

42. **(B)** The passage indicates that it is the untestability of the model that makes it useless, whether it has predictive value or not.

43. **(C)** The author indicates that the work was valuable because it both brought forward a better theory and exemplified the scientific process. At the same time, the author criticizes the scientists for failing to salvage what they could from the plume model. Choice D has the facts backward.

44. **(D)** The passage states only that the various signs of plate tectonic involvement could indicate different causes. Choices A and C are wrong because the causes cannot be determined from the facts given. Choice B is incorrect.

45. **(D)** The passage defines *upstream* as going against the established view.

46. **(A)** The passage states that the absence of most of the signs predicted by the plume model would require such a complete reworking of the theory that it would become useless. The other answer choices support the plate tectonic model without correspondingly weakening the other model.

47. **(B)** The author states that regardless of theoretical allegiance, we can appreciate the fact that the report shows the power of the scientific method. Although the other answer choices could be true, they are not assumptions necessary to the author's argument.

48. **(D)** In the passage, Francesca describes successful performance as a result of mastering technique. Choice B is wrong because the heart is described as being in opposition to the primitive.

49. **(B)** The second paragraph establishes a dichotomy between the primitive and the technical. Using the word *engineer* for a piano tuner exaggerates that dichotomy.

50. **(A)** Feeling music in the body is an example of primitiveness. Because Francesca was motivated by getting a positive response from adults, this concept was reinforced. Even though this was inadvertent, it led her to tune into primitiveness.

51. **(C)** The author creates a dichotomy between the event in the last paragraph and Francesca's performance. The primary difference is that the flute event uses less sophisticated instruments and less sophisticated technique and yet conveys primitiveness. Because the technique was not as good, the result must be due to the more primitive instruments. Choice D cannot be concluded because the contrast does not involve equal musical sophistication. Choice A is wrong because it was the handmade quality of the flute that made it primitive, not the fact that it was a flute.

52. **(D)** The author uses the word *primordial* as a synonym for primitive. The phrase in the last paragraph, *lost themselves in the sound*, is also meant to convey the primitive.

53. **(B)** Music that is in touch with direct experience may or may not be primitive, but lack of being in touch with direct experience guarantees that the music cannot be primitive.

Biological and Biochemical Foundations

1. **(C)** Lowering of blood pressure implies vasodilation, which results in more blood flow to the skin and an increased skin temperature. Lower blood pressure would reduce blood supply to all vital organs, including the kidneys, so III is wrong.

2. **(B)** The antigens in the peanuts are proteins that bind to the human antibodies, which results in an allergic reaction. Heating a protein denatures it and renders it inactive. Thus, cooking the peanut denatures the antigen and generates a lower grade immune response.

3. **(C)** Choice C is correct, as the most dangerous possible reaction would be to cause anaphylaxis through the binding of the antibody to the trigger like antibody-high affinity Fc complex. This is likely prevented by choosing epitomes during the development that are normally masked by the high affinity Fc receptor. Choice A is incorrect because, although such a process with other receptors, it does not apply to degranulation. Choice B is incorrect as interaction with B cells with the low affinity receptor are deliberately targeted. Antibodies themselves are highly specific, so that the drug would affect only those cells that are destined to produce more of the offending antibody. Choice D is incorrect as any encounter with the IgE-Fc complex would most likely cause degranulation.

4. **(B)** Enzymes are constructed from amino acids, whereas ribozymes are constructed from ribonucleic acids. For choice A, the question presents no information about ribozyme selectivity. For choice C, it can be inferred that ribozymes are held together

via hydrogen bonds because nucleic acids are held together via hydrogen bonds. For choice D, both ribozymes and enzymes have hydrogen bonds, so both have a secondary structure.

5. **(D)** The delayed physiological (immune) response is due to time required for the memory of the adaptive immune system to produce enough antibodies specific to the peanut antigen. It is the adaptive immune system that can remember prior antigens.

6. **(B)** Choice B is correct because the degranulation of mast cells is thought to be linked to pathways specifically mentioned in choice B, as well as microtubule metabolism. Choice A is incorrect, although other processes such as insulin secretion are associated with such a mechanism. Choice C is incorrect as transcription pathways imply a slower process than degranulation, which is immediate. Choice D is also incorrect because it describes a classic hormone mediated pathway that does not involve lipid mobilization.

7. **(C)** The left and right forms of the cyclohexane chair conformation are identical in energy, so at room temperature they will quickly equilibrate into equal amounts.

8. **(B)** In the lowest energy conformation of the compound, the methyl will be equatorial and the bromine axial. When the conformation is ring flipped, the positions are reversed. (Note that this new conformation will be a little higher in energy.)

9. **(D)** Both ring and torsional strain make cyclopentane less stable than cyclohexane.

10. **(D)** The positions of the chlorine, methyl, and ethyl groups for the lowest energy conformation of the compound can be seen in the structure below. (When this type of question is encountered on the MCAT, it is best to draw the chair form of the compound to do the analysis.)

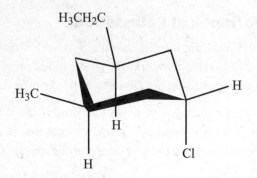

11. **(A)** Equatorial cyclohexane substituents are considerably less crowded than axial ones. This reduces steric strain.

12. **(D)** Lactate is a byproduct of anaerobic, not aerobic, metabolism. The other answer choices describe aspects of anaerobic metabolism that result in the production of lactate.

13. **(C)** Because cytochrome c oxidase is the last link in the electron chain, its inactivation by HCN prevents oxidative phosphorylation from taking place. Choice B is incorrect; oxygen levels in the blood supply to the brain are actually higher than normal because the oxygen is not being reduced.

14. **(B)** Choice B is correct because the effect of nitrites is to oxidize the heme iron. This increases cooperativity between the remaining three heme groups for oxygen molecules. Increasing cooperativity is reflected as an increase in the slope in the upstroke of the sig-

moid curve. Choice A is incorrect as hemoglobin has cooperative binding to start with and so displays the characteristic sigmoidicity of a positively cooperating protein substrate relationship. Choice C is almost correct. The kinetics may appear hyperbolic if the resolution of the curve is low, but choice B is the best response. The actual effect will be to retain a sigmoid-shaped curve, only with a steeper transition phase to the saturation plateau as concentrations. Choice D is incorrect. This would happen if the oxidation of the heme had a negative effect on cooperativity (reduction in the Hill coefficient).

15. **(D)** Myelin creates an insulating layer at the nodes of nerve cells. Insulation allows the nerve signal to propagate rapidly by saltatory conduction. Depolarization and hyperpolarization are normal events in nerve transmission, not symptoms of damage.

16. **(B)** Choice B is correct and best captures the overall sequence of interventions that employ redox reactions to transform hemoglobin so that it can capture the cyanide and then reverses this process with methylene blue. Choice A involves chelation, which scavenges metals from the body and which is incorrect. Choice C is partially correct in that methemoglobinemia is less dangerous than cyanide poisoning but actually interferes with oxygen transport. Choice D leaves out too many steps. Methylene is an antidote for methemoglobinemia but this does not address why methemoglobin was deliberately induced to form in the first place.

17. **(B)** The synthesis of ATP from ADP is driven by the energy provided by the proton (H^+) gradient created by the electron transport chain. Hence, blocking transport of H^+ ions across the membrane would decrease ATP synthesis. Choice C is incorrect because the electron carrier NADH gives up its electrons ultimately to oxygen, and the absence of oxygen would result in decreased availability of the oxidized form, NAD^+. Choice D is incorrect because no denaturation of the enzyme has occurred. If H^+ ions were able to cross the membrane, ATP synthase would continue to function.

18. **(D)** The major products of the complete combustion of any hydrocarbon are always carbon dioxide and water.

19. **(A)** Mass spectrometry uses high energy to break the covalent bonds in molecular compounds. The MS instrument detects only the positively charged species resulting from this fragmentation process.

20. **(B)** The median nerve is directly responsible for sensation in the middle and index fingers.

21. **(C)** The aneurysm will press on the nerve and inhibit nerve conduction. Nerve conduction consists of sequential depolarization and hyperpolarization cycles. Thus the frequency of these cycles will decrease. For answer choice A, the rate of saltatory conduction is decreased because conduction is inhibited. For answer choice D, the voltage-gated potassium channels open during the firing of the neuron. If conduction is inhibited, then the channels will open at a lower frequency.

22. **(B)** The neuromuscular transmitter is acetylcholine. After acetylcholine is released into the synapse, acetylcholinesterase breaks down the acetylcholine into acetate and choline. Thus the molecules with the highest concentration will be acetylcholine.

23. **(C)** Neuronal development occurs in the ectoderm. The ectoderm must be affected by the teratogen.

24. **(D)** To reach the ulnar nerve, fibrous connective tissue must be cut. Fibrous connective tissue holds the ulnar nerve in place. For answer choice A, the epiphysis of bones (or growth plate) would not be cut. For choices B and C, smooth muscle would be cut only if an artery needed to be cut.

25. **(B)** The lower a reaction step's activation energy, the faster its rate will be. Under the conditions indicated in Figure 1, the rate of formation of an intermediate carbocation from Compound **3** is highest. The positive charge can be delocalized over the entire ring.

26. **(C)** The structure of Compound **1** contains 4π electrons, which according to the $4n\pi$ electron rule makes it antiaromatic.

27. **(B)** The ion formed from Compound **3** contains 6π electrons, which according to the $4n + 2\pi$ electron rule makes it aromatic.

28. **(B)** Reactions that occur by an S_N1 mechanism exhibit first-order kinetics. Their rates depend primarily on the departure of a leaving group from the substrate to form a carbocation.

29. **(A)** Sodium ethoxide is a very strong base and would deprotonate the alkyl halide to give an alkene product.

30. **(D)** The heart contains cardiac muscle, which is an involuntary striated muscle fiber. Smooth muscles are involuntary non-striated muscles, which are generally under autonomic (and not voluntary) control.

31. **(C)** Excessive aldosterone levels will cause high Na^+ levels, which will increase blood volume and blood pressure by its osmotic effect.

32. **(C)** All terpene compounds are composed of different numbers of isoprene molecules (units). Each isoprene molecule contains 5 carbons. The compound shown is composed of 3 isoprene units because it contains 15 carbons.

33. **(C)** The hydrophilic heads face the outside, whereas the hydrophobic tails face inward.

34. **(C)** Depolarization results from sodium ions moving into cells, and repolarization from potassium moving out of the cell.

35. **(B)** This can be seen clearly on the graph's x-axis (time). Choice A is wrong because in the 6- to 9-week period the number is that high but there is no opportunistic disease. Choice C is wrong, as the graph shows them to decrease, increase, and then decrease again. Choice D is wrong for similar reasons.

36. **(A)** The passage mentions this definition. Although choice B may be correct about some viruses, not all viruses that incorporate their genome into host cells are retroviruses. The presence of an envelope has nothing to do with the retrovirus terminology.

37. **(C)** The central dogma is that DNA is converted to RNA, which is converted into protein. Retroviruses are so named because they "reverse" the dogma, as they are composed of RNA, which is reverse transcribed (by reverse transcriptase) to DNA, which then leads to protein production. The fact that this DNA has to integrate into the host cell's genome does not figure into the dogma, which simply states the flow of genetic information between the nucleic acids.

38. **(D)** Answer choice D is mentioned in the passage as necessary for the HIV virus to enter cells and cause infection. There is no support in the passage for the other choices.

39. **(B)** The passage mentions that either of these two receptors is necessary for HIV infection to occur. If they are mutated, then HIV cannot enter cells and cannot cause infection. Choice A is incorrect because it provides no evidence that the new immune cells could kill HIV. Choice C is incorrect because the population never was infected in the first place. Choice D is incorrect because the additional CD_4^+ count is not sufficiently higher than normal to counter the effect of HIV in ultimately destroying the CD_4^+ cells.

40. **(D)** The graph initially shows a window period of at least 3 weeks between primary infection and detection of the virus by the test at 1000 copies/ml. Therefore, if someone is tested during this time, and the test is negative, a second test at least 3 weeks later would be required to detect the HIV virions. In this way, only two tests are needed, not three (choice B), but one test is not enough (choice A). Choice C is incorrect because there may be clinical reasons to be retested in order to check HIV levels in the future.

41. **(A)** A cancer cell has a higher metabolic rate than a normal cell, so it is expected to have a higher number of mitochondria to supply its energy. The cancer cell also shows a decreased time for its cell cycle as it reproduces faster.

42. **(A)** From inspection of the graph, the number of mitochondria halves at days 11 and 21. This halving is consistent with mitotic division of the cell and the segregation of half the mitochondria to each daughter cell. Fluorescence bleaching is not responsible for the sudden drop in fluorescence but is responsible for the overall decrease in fluorescence.

43. **(D)** A father does not contribute his mitochondria to the zygote; therefore, the mitochondrial disease cannot be transferred to his progeny.

44. **(B)** If the "incomplete phagocytosis" hypothesis was correct, then mitochondria would be surrounded by two membranes: one from the phagocytotic vesicle and the other from the membrane of the mitochondria-precursor cell.

45. **(D)** The graph shows that the number of mitochondria fluctuates during the course of the cell cycle. The number of mitochondria increases during the S, G1, and G2 phases of the cell cycle. In the M phase, the number of mitochondria decreases sharply.

46. **(C)** The reaction Pyruvate $\rightarrow$ NADH, $FADH_2$, CO_2, and Acetyl CoA is the precursor reaction to the Krebs cycle and occurs in the mitochondria. Choice A occurs in the liver and muscles as a way to store glucose. Choice B is the overall reaction for glycolysis, which occurs in the cytoplasm. Choice D is an anabolic reaction that also occurs in the cytoplasm.

47. **(B)** A sarcomere is a cell of the skeletal muscle system; it needs large amounts of glucose for proper contraction. Thus, the sarcomere absorbs the most radioactive glucose.

48. **(B)** Ribosomes carry out protein translation and are part of the rough endoplasmic reticulum (the designation *rough* comes from the fact that the ribosomes appear as tiny dots on microscopy of the reticula). Smooth endoplasmic reticulum carries out lipid production, and Golgi apparatus carries out sorting and modification (post-translational modification) of proteins.

49. **(A)** Complexes I to IV, along with cytochrome c, are located here. Protons are pumped into the intermembrane space.

50. **(B)** Oocytogenesis is the process by which primordial follicles develop into oogonia, which then divide between fertilization and birth to create primary oocytes. These begin mitosis but remain halted in prophase 1, in which phase they may stay for up to 50 years, or the reproductive age of the individual female. The process restarts at menarche, when a few of the oocytes continue development. On day 14, an LH surge occurs, not FSH.

51. **(A)** The mitosis (or M phase in the cell cycle) may be further broken down into these stages. The other phases of the cell cycles include resting G_0, G_1, S, and G_2 (collectively termed *interphase*).

52. **(D)** Langerhans cells are involved in processing microbial antigens.

53. **(B)** Water and solutes pass from the capillaries of the glomerulus into Bowman's capsule.

54. **(B)** $(140 - 80) = 60$; $(140 - 20 = 120)$; $60/120 = \frac{1}{2}$. All other variables are constant.

55. **(C)** Low filtration rate would result in lower levels of urea in the urine, not higher. Low GFR results in high blood urea nitrogen.

56. **(A)** The additional creatinine in the urine from tubular secretion would cause an over-estimate of the glomerular filtration rate. Additional excretion of creatine from the blood via the tubules decreases serum creatinine levels, resulting in a higher value of eCrCl.

57. **(C)** Fermentation is an anaerobic process by which a fuel source is partly oxidized and uses an electron acceptor other than oxygen, but it does not involve a change in the over-all redox potential. $NAD^+/NADH$ levels remain constant as NAD^+ is regenerated. Choice A is a specific type of fermentation. Choices B and D are incomplete and/or inaccurate. Gas formation is common but occurs in many processes.

58. **(A)** Only this choice is implied by the material in the passage. Ruminants make use of bacteria to split the beta [1–4] bonds for which they lack the enzyme.

59. **(C)** Enzymes have no effect on the equilibrium of a reaction. They accelerate the reaction in both directions such that equilibrium is attained much faster no matter from which direction it comes; on occasion they are coupled to a highly exorgonic pair of reactions such as $ATP \rightarrow AMP + 2\,Pi$ to either overcome an unfavorable free-energy change or drive a reaction far to the right, but the reaction rates in both directions are accelerated.

Psychological, Social, and Biological Foundations

1. **(B)** Choice B is correct. The cones are structures found in the retina that are responsible for the perception of color. Choice A is incorrect because rods are responsible for perception of light intensity. Choice C is incorrect because the cornea does not have fibers that perceive light. However, the cornea may help bend light waves to focus it for better perception. Choice D is incorrect because it is only the cones in the retina that are responsible for color vision.

2. **(D)** Choice D is correct. In red-green colorblindness, either the red or green cones are not functioning properly, so people perceive the world in blue, yellow, and shades of gray.

Choice A is incorrect because the patient is able to perceive the color blue. In blue color blindness, the blue cones do not function, and the patient sees the world in red, green, and shades of gray. Choice B is incorrect because in monochrome color blindness, either all the cones are not functioning properly, or the cones are absent altogether. These patients see the world in gray colors. Choice C is incorrect because the patient can see blue color.

3. **(B)** Choice B is correct. The visual processing center is found within the occipital lobe of the brain. Choice A is incorrect because the frontal lobe of the brain is responsible for higher cognitive processes. Choice C is incorrect because the medulla oblongata is where the respiratory center of the brain is located. It has no role in vision. Choice D is incorrect because the pituitary gland is responsible for secreting numerous neurohormones involved in growth, metabolism, and development.

4. **(C)** Choice C is correct. The optic nerve crosses at a point called the optic chiasm. At this point, the optic nerve from both the left and right eyes divides so that fibers sensing objects on the left side of both eyes are processed on the right side of the brain, and fibers sensing objects on the right side of both eyes are processed on the left side of the brain. Thus, objects in the right field of view are processed on the left side of the brain. Choice A is thus incorrect because perception is unilateral. Choice B is incorrect because objects perceived on the right side of the brain would be located physically in the left field of view. Choice D is incorrect because it refers to the front-most (anterior) part of the brain, which encompasses both the left and right sides of the brain. Also, the right side of the brain is incorrect.

5. **(D)** Choice D is correct. According to the opponent-process theory, the four cones are grouped into two pairs: red with green and blue with yellow. Whereas each group can be stimulated, only one cone within each group can be active at a given time. Choice A is incorrect because two cones (one from each pairing of red with green and blue with yellow) can be stimulated simultaneously. Choice B is also incorrect because each group can be stimulated, though only one cone from each group can be active at a given time. Choice C is incorrect because two groups can be simultaneously active. The latter part of the statement is true, however.

6. **(A)** Choice A is correct. Even though rods become more useful than cones in dark adaptation, both the rods and cones contain light-sensitive chemicals, the concentrations of which become greater in darker environments. Choice B is incorrect because it contradicts this. Choice C is incorrect because pupils will dilate when going from a bright to dark room. Choice D is incorrect because visual constancy refers to the process of identifying an object as constant when its physical characteristics change. The change from a bright room to a darker room does not involve visual constancy.

7. **(B)** Choice B is correct because the data shows that the higher a group's annual income, the more likely they are to spend that income on treatment of their health concern. Choice A is incorrect because the lower a racial group's annual income, the more likely they are to conserve what little money they have. This leads to less being spent on treatment purposes. Choice C is incorrect because the data clearly shows that each racial group spent a different percentage of their annual income on treating their PTSD. Choice D is incorrect because there is a direct correlation between the two variables being examined in this study.

8. **(A)** Choice A is correct because class disparities play a key role in determining access to healthcare services. The higher one's class, the more likely one is to pursue and be able to attain healthcare. Choice B is incorrect because the data shows that they spent a higher percentage of their income. Choice C is incorrect because the measurement of concern for one's individual health is not examined in this study. Therefore, there is no evidence to back this statement. Choice D is incorrect because it cannot be defended by the information in the study.

9. **(C)** Choice C is correct because discrimination of certain racial groups leads to lower socioeconomic status. Choice A is incorrect because reverse discrimination is discrimination against the dominant group. Choice B is incorrect because functionalism is a theoretical approach to sociology in which the parts of society are seen to function as a whole. Choice D is incorrect because bias against women does not account for a lower socioeconomic status of minority men.

10. **(D)** Choice D is correct because a strong support system can be just as beneficial to curing medical conditions as is medical treatment. Choice A is incorrect because the number of people referred is irrelevant. The study is only concerned with those people who are receiving treatment. Choice B is incorrect for a similar reason. The incidence of PTSD in a population is not relevant to the study. Choice C is incorrect because it does not change the fact that the percentage spent on PTSD treatment was lower than for Caucasians.

11. **(C)** Choice C is correct because healthcare disparities are associated primarily with socioeconomic status. Thus, a member of a racial minority who is in the upper middle class is much less likely to experience a healthcare disparity than is a member of the same minority who is in the lower class. Choice A is incorrect because assisted healthcare being provided to low-income households would lessen the effects of socioeconomic status on an individual's ability to receive healthcare. Choice B is incorrect because teaching families how to properly treat their medical conditions would allow them to better allocate money toward quality, effective healthcare. Choice D is incorrect because one factor in healthcare disparity is an absence of medical facilities in low-income neighborhoods.

12. **(B)** Choice B is correct because all of these behaviors typically emerge between 6 and 9 months of age. Choice A is incorrect because these behaviors occur between 3 and 6 months of age. Choice C is incorrect because these behaviors occur between 9 and 12 months of age. Choice D is incorrect because these behaviors occur between 12 and 24 months of age.

13. **(B)** Choice B is correct because a society determines race by distinguishable biological or visible traits in people, and society classifies ethnicity based on cultural characteristics (ancestry, language, and religion). Choice A is incorrect for the same reason. Choice B is incorrect because it is race, not ethnicity, that is defined by biological factors, and immigration status is defined by factual information, not cultural characteristics. Choice D is incorrect because, even though the first part of the question concerning race is correct, the last part of the question is incorrect, as described above.

14. **(C)** Choice C is correct because it accurately describes the underlying philosophy of the humanistic approach. Choice A is incorrect because it describes the traits approach.

Choice B is incorrect because it describes the psychoanalytic approach. Answer D is incorrect because it describes the social cognitive approach.

15. **(B)** Choice B is the correct answer. One or more external stimuli (the words in our example) may reduce the ability of an individual to hone in on the desired stimulus (the color of the words in our example). The younger children performed more poorly because they were more distracted by the words. Choice A is incorrect because it is the opposite of choice B. Choice C is incorrect because, even though there appears to be a correlation between age and performance, the experiment does not support conclusions about the difference in performance among members of one group. Choice D is incorrect for a similar reason. Though it is possible that it is true, it is not defendably true by the results.

16. **(C)** Choice C is correct because it allows the experimenter to control for extraneous variables, including reading ability and the ability to name colors. Choice A is incorrect because even though adding another age category may or may not yield additional, compelling results, decreasing the number of participants in each age category would decrease statistical power of the results. Choice B is incorrect because recruiting a separate group of individuals does not provide information about the reading skills or ability to identify colors for the experimental participants. Choice D is incorrect because the experiment does not require a control group.

17. **(D)** Choice D is correct because catecholamines are directly proportional to the ability to pay attention. Thus, an overproduction of catecholamines would not lead to decreased ability to pay attention. In ADHD patients, it has been shown that underproduction of catecholamines can lead to poor attention. Choice A is incorrect because the frontal cortex exhibits deficits ranging from underdevelopment to improper circuitry functioning in ADHD patients. Choice B is incorrect because ADHD patients do exhibit divided attention, or focusing on multiple tasks simultaneously that leads to poor attention on the desired task. Choice C is incorrect because the hallmark of ADHD is not being able to focus on individual tasks for long periods of time.

18. **(D)** Choice D is correct because the percent of correctly identified colors is the variable being studied in different age categories and is thus the dependent variable. Choice A is incorrect because the age groups are actually the independent variables of the study. Choice B is incorrect because the 20 words with different colors are the experimental treatment given to each participant to examine attention among the age categories. Choice C is incorrect because this is not a relevant factor. Nearly all of the words did not match their colors.

19. **(A)** Choice A is correct because an extraneous variable is a factor that can distort the relationships being studied. Selecting children from the public school system only might not result in a sample that is representative of the whole population. Choice B is incorrect because it would not influence the results of the study. Choice C is incorrect because it is important for accuracy of the study to ensure that the participants are not color-blind. Choice D is incorrect because it would be irrelevant to the result. An extraneous variable is not the same as an irrelevant one.

20. **(C)** Choice C is correct because the experiment focuses on the color of ink for a word. The word itself is the distractor, as it usually represents a color different from the correct response. Choice A is incorrect because the font color of the words is what the par-

ticipants are asked to pay attention to. Choice B is incorrect because the age categories are the independent variables in the study and are not directly causing attention to be divided. Choice D is incorrect because the number of words presented to each participant is irrelevant to their ability to pay attention to the color of each word.

21. **(D)** Choice D is correct. As depicted in the figure, the combined cognitive-behavioral therapy modality had a reduction in the Liebowitz social anxiety score from approximately 110 to less than 20. This decrease was greater than all the other modalities on average over a 12-month period of treatment. Choice A is incorrect because the score remained relatively stable with hardly any decrease over 12 months. Choices B and C are incorrect because even though both exhibited a similar decline in the Liebowitz score over 12 months, the magnitude of this change was not as great as the combined cognitive-behavioral therapy modality.

22. **(A)** Choice A is the correct answer. The James-Lange theory of emotion asserts that fear arises based on our physiological response to a stimulus that may or may not be perceived as threatening. Choice B is incorrect because the Cannon-Bard theory of emotion postulates that fear and the behaviors associated with it occur at the same time and do not happen in a sequential pattern as in James-Lange. Choice C is incorrect because the Schachter theory of emotion postulates that in a threatening situation, the brain cognitively labels a physiologic change (increased heart rate, sweating, etc.) based on cues in the environment. This all happens at the same time. In contrast to the other two theories, this theory postulates that the cognitive labeling of emotion occurs based on environmental cues, not based on the physiology alone. Choice D is incorrect because the theory states that, in the presence of a threatening stimulus, the brain first assesses the environment and labels the stimulus as either threatening or not.

23. **(C)** Choice C is the correct answer. As depicted in the figure, a combined cognitive-behavioral therapy modality was the best in reducing social anxiety symptoms in patients. Thus, addressing both the patient's physiologic behaviors and thought processes to a social situation and working to correct these maladaptive behaviors is the best mechanism to treat social anxiety. Choice A is incorrect because this is addressing behavior only. Choice B is incorrect because this is addressing only the patient's cognitive processes. Choice D is incorrect because this is traditional psychoanalytic theory and is not addressing directly the thoughts and behaviors the patient has in social situations.

24. **(A)** Choice A is correct. The amygdala is a structure found in the temporal lobes of the brain bilaterally that is thought to play a large role in emotion and memories associated with emotional responses, especially fear. Several studies have demonstrated that removal of the amygdala causes decreased fear in rats and people. Choice B is incorrect because the pituitary gland is not directly involved in the fear response. Choice C is incorrect because the hypothalamus modulates and causes the pituitary gland to secrete a variety of hormones to affect metabolism, differentiation, and growth. Choice D is incorrect because the pineal gland is mainly involved in regulating internal biological rhythms, such as the sleep-wake cycle.

25. **(B)** Choice B is correct because the fact of knowing that one is in a study and of taking a test could serve as a placebo, resulting in some drop in anxiety. In addition, it is possible that there is a small decrease in measured anxiety among people who take the measure multiple times. Choice A is incorrect because the passage states that the control group

did not receive therapy. Choice C is incorrect because there is no evidence that the control group associated with other subjects. Choice D is incorrect because the control group did not receive cognitive therapy.

26. **(A)** Roman numeral I must be included because the first woman is subject to more discrimination than another woman of her ethnic background who is younger. Roman numeral II cannot be included because all three people are of the same ethnic background. Roman numeral III cannot be included because reverse discrimination is discrimination against the dominant ethnic group. The correct answer can contain Roman numeral I only, as in choice A.

27. **(C)** Choice C is correct because it is the most accurate documented percentage.

28. **(D)** Choice D is correct because it accurately describes the symptoms associated with generalized anxiety disorder. Choice A is incorrect because agoraphobia is characterized by a fear of being in public places or away from home. Choice B is incorrect because panic disorder is characterized by frequent panic attacks. Choice C is incorrect because separation anxiety disorder is a childhood disorder characterized by an inappropriate fear of separation from major attachment figures.

29. **(A)** Choice A is correct because, according to the drive-reduction theory, drives are psychological stimuli that motivate individuals to act in order to reduce that drive. Drives are categorized into primary and secondary drives. Primary drives are biological needs, such as hunger. Choice B is incorrect because secondary drives are acquired or learned over time. Choices C and D are incorrect because the drive-reduction theory does not categorize into tertiary or quaternary drives.

30. **(C)** Choice C is correct because a low level of leptin secretion by adipocytes allows NPY and AgRP neurons in the hypothalamus to be active. Both of these neurons are responsible for the sensation of hunger. Choice A is incorrect because increased insulin follows after a meal and stimulates POMC and MSH neurons that are responsible for the sensation of satiety. Choice B is incorrect because ghrelin normally stimulates NPY and AgRP neurons, which again are responsible for the sensation of hunger. Therefore, a lack of ghrelin leads to a sensation of satiety. Choice D is incorrect because a lack of glucagon indicates that the individual recently ate a meal and nourishment is not required.

31. **(B)** Choice B is correct because anorexia nervosa is a psychological condition in which individuals intentionally starve themselves in order to lose weight. Thus, an individual with this condition experiences increased hunger due to high ghrelin secretion by the stomach, low leptin production by adipocytes, and high glucagon levels. Choice A is incorrect because the drive (hunger) is increased, not decreased, and ghrelin levels are high. Choice C is incorrect because the drive increases. Additionally, leptin levels are low in a starving person. Choice D is incorrect because leptin levels are low and glucagon levels are high in a starving person.

32. **(C)** Choice C is correct because the hypothalamus is the structure in the brain responsible for regulating a variety of homeostatic mechanisms, including hunger, thirst, sex, and body temperature. Choice A is incorrect because the pituitary gland is not directly involved in the sensation of hunger and satiety. Choice B is incorrect because the pineal gland mainly regulates biological clocks, such as the sleep-wake cycle. Choice D is incorrect because the amygdala regulates emotions and memories associated with them.

33. **(B)** Choice B is correct because based on Maslow's hierarchy of needs, biological drives such as hunger, thirst, and body temperature are classified at the bottom of the hierarchy and need to be fulfilled before drives higher up on the pyramid can be fulfilled. Because confidence and self-esteem are placed higher up the pyramid in Maslow's theory, someone who is chronically starved may not have self-confidence and self-esteem, and this need is not as important to them as having their hunger reduced. Choice A is incorrect because self-actualization is at the tip of the pyramid of needs and will not be achieved until everything below it, such as the biological needs, is fulfilled. Choice C is incorrect because maintaining homeostasis is a biological process and would be on the same level as hunger and other biological needs. Hunger is another drive to maintain nutrient homeostasis. Choice D is incorrect because biological needs are more important to the individual than achieving safety, which is higher up on Maslow's hierarchy.

34. **(A)** Choice A is correct because individuals with type 1 diabetes mellitus have beta cells in the pancreas that are unable to produce sufficient levels of insulin, which normally would cause satiety by acting on MSH and POMC neurons in the hypothalamus. Because insulin levels are low, these neurons will not be stimulated, and individuals may feel a sense of hunger or need for nourishment. Choice B is incorrect because increased leptin secretion causes a lower drive and promotes satiety. Choice C is incorrect because ghrelin actually leads to an increased drive to eat. Choice D is incorrect because POMC and MSH neurons in the hypothalamus would not be active due to low insulin levels in diabetic patients.

35. **(D)** Choice D is correct because the younger subjects in Table 1 had a majority of "yes" answers in all four categories of the question model. The "yes" answers show approval of same-sex marriage in all categories according to the younger subjects. Choice A is incorrect because Table 1 clearly shows that all four categories express a positive viewpoint in relation to the question. Choice B is incorrect because the exact opposite is shown in Tables 1 and 2. Choice C is incorrect because the "Parents" category of Table 2 shows markedly lower acceptance rates compared to the "Self" category. Being socialized into acceptance of same-sex marriage would rarely come from an overwhelming negative response as is shown in Table 2's "Parents" category.

36. **(B)** Choice B is correct because the process of socialization affects each gender, age group, and ethnicity in varying ways due to each experiencing different perspectives on life and society. This varied viewpoint gives a wider range of data to examine. Choice A is incorrect because, in this case, the importance of the topic is irrelevant to who is being sampled. Choice C is incorrect because the mention of gender only informs the reader that the experiment has equal representation, not that it is a key factor in the study. Choice D is also incorrect because it is not necessarily true that a diverse population provides a wider range of results.

37. **(B)** Choice B is correct because the "parents" category of Table 2 shows high levels of dissent toward same-sex marriage. This category is indicative of the hypothesized 70–80 sample. Choice A is incorrect because the level of acceptance between the Table 2 "Self" category and "Parent" category varies greatly. At nearly a 5:1 ratio, it is far from equivalent. Choice C is incorrect because expecting perceived answers to match actual answers exactly is highly unlikely. Despite being indicative of the 70–80 sample, Table 2's "Parents" category is simply the educated guess of the subjects. Choice D is incorrect only

because it assumes that a hypothesis cannot be made with the provided information. Because the parents of the 40–60 sample would most likely fall into the 70–80 sample, it is within reason to use that data as the grounds for a hypothesis.

38. **(D)** Choice D is correct because the subjects perceive that more of their peers than any other agent of socialization would agree with their personal perspective. Choice A is incorrect because the perceived ratio of parents who agree with the subject is much lower than that of their peers. Choice B is incorrect for the same reason as Choice A, but in relation to the general American public. Choice C is incorrect because Table 1 and the experiment do not include the effects of media on personal perspective.

39. **(A)** Choice A is correct because if the definition of what is deviant is learned, then each generation has the potential to change whether it is acceptable or not. Choice B is incorrect because it implies that all deviant behaviors will become acceptable after enough time. Choice C is incorrect because legislation does not necessarily change how members of society view a behavior. Choice D is incorrect because it assumes that the only way to accept deviant behavior is to change them to mirror societal norms.

40. **(B)** Choice B is correct because the results of each agent of socialization category is the perceived view of the subject. Choice A is incorrect because, although the subject may know the exact perspective of a small population such as their parents, it is impossible to know the exact feelings of a large population such as the general American public. Choice C is incorrect because it is inaccurate. If the subjects' parents and peers agreed with the subjects, then "yes" answers would have been equivalent in all three groups. Choice D is incorrect because it only takes into account a majority of "yes" answers in the "Self" category.

41. **(C)** Choice C is correct because all of the structures listed are components of the limbic system and help direct emotional experiences. Choice A is incorrect because the endocrine system is responsible for hormonal production and regulation. Choice B is incorrect because the lymphatic system is a key component of immunity. Choice D is incorrect because the circulatory system is responsible for distributing nutrients and oxygen throughout the body while eliminating waste.

42. **(B)** Choice B is correct because it is the definition of drive-reduction theory. Choice A is incorrect because incentive theory argues that people are motivated by the expectation of reward. Choice C is incorrect because cognitive dissonance theory explains the association between attitude and behavior. Choice D is incorrect because it describes the process by which people explain their own and other people's behavior.

43. **(C)** Choice C is the correct answer because prejudice is the unfair belief and attitude about a category of people, and discrimination is the unjust actions that result from that belief and attitude. Choice A is incorrect for that same reason. Choice B is incorrect primarily because individual discrimination is an unjust action of one person, not a belief or attitude. Choice D is incorrect primarily because institutional discrimination consists of the unjust actions of an institution and is not a belief or attitude.

44. **(A)** Choice A is correct because it outlines Freud's five stages of psychosocial development in the correct order.

45. **(B)** Choice B is correct because environmental inequality is concerned with the unequal ability of communities to protect themselves from environmental pollution. In this situation, the predominately upper-class community was able to protect itself from the risk of landfill pollution, but the predominately poor community was not. Choice A is incorrect because no international comparisons are being made in this situation. Choice C is incorrect because prejudice deals with beliefs and attitudes, and this situation is concerned with the act of placing a landfill site. Choice D is incorrect because, although it can be argued that the predominately upper-class and predominately poor communities are residentially segregated, this answer does not explain their unequal ability to protect themselves from environmental pollution.

46. **(A)** Choice A is correct because the amygdala is a bilateral structure known to have a strong influence on anxiety and fear, as well as memories associated with fearful stimuli. Choice B is incorrect because the pituitary gland mainly controls the release of hormones from the thyroid, adrenal glands, and gonads that ultimately contribute to metabolism, growth, and development. Choice C is incorrect because the hypothalamus mainly plays a role in regulating thirst, hunger, sex, and regulation of the pituitary gland. Choice D is incorrect because the pineal gland is mainly involved in regulating cycles in the body, such as the sleep-wake cycle.

47. **(C)** Choice C is correct because, as the figure depicts, continued exposure to an anxiety-provoking stimulus leads to a decline in the anxiety symptoms, which is equivalent to remission of symptoms. Choice A is incorrect because symptoms are not heightened with prolonged exposure. Choice B is incorrect because the figure does not indicate that symptoms are being heightened with chronic exposure following initial treatment of anxiety. Choice D is incorrect because initial exposure to a stimulus leads to heightened anxiety and not an attenuation of symptoms.

48. **(D)** Choice D is correct because dishabituation is a return to heightened anxiety after a period of habituation. A prolonged stimulus results in habituation but if the stimulus is then removed, sensitivity to the stimulus returns (dishabituation). Choice A is incorrect because this is characteristic of habituation. Choice B is incorrect because ongoing exposure leads to a decrease, not an increase, in response. Choice C is incorrect because if ongoing exposure to social rejection did lead to remission of anxiety, this would be an example of habituation.

49. **(B)** Choice B is correct because adrenaline induces symptoms such as shaking, arousal, and sweating that may be interpreted by an individual as anxiety, which further increases symptoms in a positive feed forward loop. Choice A is incorrect because adrenaline works via a positive feed forward loop in anxiety, not a negative feedback loop. Choice C is incorrect for the same reason in that adrenaline release and increase in anxiety is through a positive feed forward loop. Choice D is incorrect because a positive feed forward loop would lead to an exacerbation of anxiety symptoms, not a decline of symptoms.

50. **(D)** Choice D is correct because neurons that are facilitated have resting membrane potentials that are elevated closer to threshold so that a lower stimulus will rapidly lead to depolarization of a neuron above threshold and excite that neuron. Choices A and B are both incorrect because the threshold level of the neuron itself is not altered. Choice C is incorrect because the resting membrane potential of facilitated neurons is elevated, not decreased.

51. **(C)** Choice C is correct because facilitation of neurons means elevating their resting membrane potential so that they are held closer to threshold and are more easily excitable with lower stimuli. Therefore, removing the trigger that is facilitating neurons lowers the resting membrane potential and makes the neurons less excitable to low levels of stimulus. Choices A and B are incorrect because threshold potential is not changed in neurons. Choice D is incorrect because neurons are not facilitated when a greater stimulus is needed to evoke a response.

52. **(C)** Choice C is correct because the debates represent a struggle of power between the two opposing forces of gender. Choice A is incorrect because the experiment does not focus on opposing classes, but on the conflict between men and women. Choice B is incorrect because functionalism is concerned with harmonious, not unharmonious, structures. Choice D is incorrect because the male and female subjects do not have a shared meaning in this debate due to opposing beliefs and therefore lack any sense of agreement.

53. **(A)** Choice A is correct because due to the sociologist's occupation alone, the subjects are willing to believe false information. Society places the occupation of scientist as an authority that is perceived to have tested the information they spread as truth. Choice B is incorrect because shared meanings of superiority fall under the theoretical approach of symbolic interactionism. Choice C is incorrect because, again, the concept of the self-fulfilling prophecy creates a shared meaning of superiority, which is better explained by symbolic interactionism. Choice D is incorrect because the debates symbolize a struggle for power between men and women. This struggle relates directly to conflict theory.

54. **(C)** Choice C is correct because the number of objects identified is the only result of the experiment listed. Choice A is incorrect because the sociologist's false claims serve as a catalyst for change in subject performance. Choice B is incorrect because the quality of the subjects' short-term memory is an independent variable that affects their ability to remember and recite what they observed during the test. Choice D is incorrect because the number of subjects tested only serves to affect the amount of data that can be reviewed after the test.

55. **(D)** Choice D is correct because the male subjects' belief that they would succeed is reflected in their higher scores as shown in Table 1. Choice A is incorrect because the results clearly show that the male subjects consistently identified more objects than the female subjects. Choice B is incorrect because of the word "inherent." No section of the passage hints at any form of natural or inherent memorization skill in men. Choice C is incorrect because the debates are only one of the variables that affected the results of the test, not the sole variable.

56. **(B)** Choice B is correct because the briefing supplied the subjects with the notion that men are better suited for the test and that previous results support this claim. Choice A is incorrect because the passage does not state that the briefing involved any information regarding the test procedure. Even if it had, the primary importance of the briefing is to create sense of gender difference. Choice C is incorrect because only female subjects experienced doubt. Choice D is incorrect because the briefing itself did not include an opportunity to voice dissent.

57. **(A)** Choice A is correct because healthcare disparities involve differences among categories of people in their ability to access healthcare. In this circumstance, colorectal cancer screening is the healthcare that lower socioeconomic categories of people have a more difficult time accessing. Choice B is incorrect because the inequality that is shown is one that involves class, not gender. Choice C is incorrect because health disparities involve the differences in health among categories of people, and this situation is specifically discussing differences in access to healthcare. Choice D is incorrect because, if any discrimination is at play in these healthcare disparities, it involves class, not age.

58. **(B)** Choice B is correct because Vygotsky coined the term MKO and described the role of such an individual in his theory. Choice A is incorrect because the generalized other is associated with symbolic interactionism and describes the general norms of behavior to which a culture expects an individual to adhere. Choice C is incorrect because it is a personality component described by Freud in his theory of psychosocial development. Choice D is incorrect because it is also used in symbolic interactionism and describes the process by which an individual develops self-concept based on how the individual believes other people view and judge him or her.

59. **(A)** Choice A is correct because in-group/out-group bias explains the intrinsic basis of prejudice in humans. Choice B is incorrect because social identity is the aspect of a person's identity that includes the groups with which they associate. Choice C is incorrect because individuation is the process of establishing characteristics that distinguish one individual from others. Choice D is incorrect because habituation/dishabituation describes a process of learning new behavior through either increased or decreased exposure to stimuli.

Index

A

Abasic sites, 409
Absolute poverty, 823
Absolute pressure, 237
Absorption spectroscopy, 552–563
Absorption spectrum, 42
Acceleration, 190–193, 205, 259–260
Accommodation, 449, 717
Accommodation reflex, 462
Acetic acid, 143
Acetyl CoA, 352–353
Acetylcholine, 449–450, 493
Acetylcholinesterase, 493
Achieved status, 815–816
Acid halides, 629–631
Acid strength, 156–157
Acid–base chemistry, 149–165
Acid–base indicators, 164–165
Acidic protons, 606
Acidity, 613
Acquired immunodeficiency syndrome, 474
Actin filaments, 335, 488, 490
Action potential, 445–446
Activated complex, 125
Activation energy, 125–126, 339
Active reading, 854
Active transport, 323, 326–328
Acute stress disorder, 745
Adaptation, 425, 717
Adaptive immune response, 469
Adaptive radiation, 428
Adenine, 370
Adenosine, 451
Adenosine diphosphate, 346
Adenosine triphosphate, 338, 346–347, 451, 496, 699
Adherens junctions, 430
Adjustment disorder, 745
Adolescence, 739, 774
Adrenal glands, 439–440
Adrenal virilism, 440

Adrenocorticoids, 434
Adrenocorticotropin, 438, 457
Aerobes, 363
Aerobic respiration, 331, 346, 352–355
Affective aggression, 794
Age–sex pyramid, 818
Aggression, 793–794
Aging, 516
Agonist, 489
Agoraphobia, 744
AIDS, 474
Albumin, 477
Alcohol fermentation, 356
Alcohols, 610–616
Aldehydes, 616–623
Aldose, 670
Aldosterone, 440
Alertness, 725
Alkali metals, 51
Alkaline earth metals, 51
Alkaline metals, 55
Alkanes, 588–599
Alkene, 549
Alkoxide, 612
Alkyl bromides, 616
Alkyl chlorides, 616
Allantois, 510
Alleles, 413
All-or-none response, 493
All-or-none threshold response, 447
Allosteric enzymes, 343
Alu sequence, 383
Aluminum, 54
Alveolar ventilation rate, 499
Alzheimer's disease, 731–732
Ambivalent prejudice, 789
Ambivalent/resistant attachment, 795
Amides, 634–636
Amines, 636–643
Amino acids, 357, 659–664
Aminoacyl-tRNA, 387

Aminoacyl-tRNA synthetases, 387
Ammonia, 693–694
Amphipathic, 322
AMPK, 701
Amplitude, 246
Amylase, 475
Amylopectin, 676
Amylose, 676
Anabolic pathways, 357
Anabolism
definition of, 683
of fats, 690
Anaerobes, 363
Anaerobic glycolysis, 494
Anaerobic respiration, 355
Anal stage, 777
Analogous traits, 429
Anal-retentive personality, 777
Analytical chromatography, 581
Anaphase, 401
Anatomical dead space, 499
Anatomy, 429–516
Anchoring and adjustment heuristic, 421
Aneuploidy, 411
Angiotensin II, 484
Angle of incline, 201
Angle strain, 595
Angstrom, 186
Angular acceleration, 230–231
Angular frequency, 258
Angular methyl groups, 678
Angular momentum, 43, 223, 230–231
Angular systems, 225
Angular velocity, 230–231
Anhydrides, 631–632
Animals
communication in, 793
social behavior in, 795
viruses that affect, 367
Anions, 58, 328
Anode, 166

Antagonist, 489
Anterior pituitary gland, 452
Antibiotic resistance, 362
Antibodies, 469, 471–472
Anticipatory socialization, 811
Anticodon, 386
Antidiuretic hormone, 437–438, 483
Antigen-presenting cells, 474
Antigens, 471
Antinodes, 248
Antiparallel strands, 370
Antisocial personality disorder, 750
Anxiety disorders, 744–745
Anxious attachment, 795
Aorta, 465
Aortic valve, 464
Apoenzyme, 341
Apoproteins, 691
Apoptosis, 334, 402
Apparent weight, 208–212
Appendicular skeleton, 486
Appraisal support, 795
Aquaporins, 326
Archimedes's principle, 234
Aromatic azo compounds, 643
Arrhenius equation, 126
Arrhenius theory, 149
Arteries, 465
Ascribed status, 815–816
Assimilation, 810
Associative learning, 766–771
Atom(s)
hydrogen, 300–301
scale of, 300
structure of, 37–40
Atomic number, 302
Atomic radius, 53
ATP synthase, 345, 355
ATP-ADP translocase, 355
Atrioventricular valve, 464
Attachment, 794–795
Attachment theory, 794
Attention, 716

Attitude, 759–762, 772–773
Attitudes, 785
Attraction, 794
Attribution theory, 784–786
Attributions, 784–786
Atwood's machine, 198–199
Aufbau diagram, 46–47
Auricle, 457
Autocrine signaling, 329
Autoimmune disorders, 474
Autoimmunity, 474
Autonomic nervous system, 454
Autonomy versus shame, 778
Autosomes, 404
Availability heuristic, 420
Average atomic mass, 39–40
Aversive prejudice, 789
Avogadro's hypothesis, 79
Avogadro's number, 94, 303
Avoidant attachment, 795
Avoidant personality disorder, 750
Axial bonds, 598
Axon hillock, 441
Axon terminals, 441
Axoneme, 335, 506
Azimuthal quantum number, 43, 45

B

B lymphocytes, 469–470
Bacillus, 359
Backcross, 419
Backstage self, 791
Bacteria, 359
Bacteriophages, 364, 365–367
Balmer Series, 42
Basal body, 335
Basal nuclei, 452
Base excision repair, 377
Basement membrane, 336, 431
Bases, 638
Basilar membrane, 459
Basophils, 470
Batteries, 271–272, 274–275
Beat, 252
Beat frequency, 252
Becquerel, 304
Beer's law, 563
Behavior, 734–773
    attitude and, 760–761
    biological bases of, 734–735
    cooperative, 794–795
    genetic and environmental
        factors that affect, 736–737
    motivation and, 758–759
    social, 793–795

social constructs of, 763–766
theories of change in, 772–773
Behavioral genetics, 735–736
Belief perseverance, 721
Beliefs, 785, 808
Benevolent prejudice, 789–790
Benzodiazepines, 726
Benzoic acid, 625
Bernoulli equation, 244–245
Beta oxidation, 357
Between-population genetic variation, 421
Bias, 721, 774, 787
Bidirectional replication, 373
Bile, 477
Binary fission, 362
Binding energy, 303
Bioenergetics, 681–683
Biofilms, 361
Biological preparedness, 771
Biological species concept, 427
Biomolecular nucleophilic substitution, 613
Biopsychosocial model, 742–743
Biotechnology, 393–398
Bipolar disorder, 747–748
Birefringence, 289
Blaming the victim, 785
Blastocyst, 511–512, 737
Blastomeres, 511
Blastulation, 511
Block problems, 201–203
Blood, 466, 478, 500
Blood pressure, 483–484
Blood-brain barrier, 337
Body dysmorphic disorder, 746
Body mass, 701–702
Bohr, Niels, 40–41
Bohr effect, 501
Bohr model, 40, 300–301
Boiling point, 88, 91, 578
Bomb calorimeter, 114–115
Bond(s)
    covalent, 59
    ionic, 57–59
Bond energy, 112–113
Bonding, 63
Bone, 485–486
Borderline personality disorder, 750
Bovine spongiform encephalopathy, 367
Bowlby, John, 794
Bowman's capsule, 482
Boyle's law, 75–76

Brain, 452–453
Brainstem, 453
Brewster's angle, 289
Brewster's law, 289
Brønsted–Lowry, 638
Brønsted–Lowry acids and bases, 149–150
Bromine, 52
Bronchioles, 497
Bronchoconstriction, 497
Brown adipose tissue, 699
Buffers, 159–160
Bulk transport, 327
Buoyancy, 234–236
Bureaucracy, 817
Bureaucratic ritualism, 817
Bursae, 488
Bystander effect, 765

C

Caffeine, 451
Cahn-Ingold-Prelog protocol, 545
Calcitonin, 438, 486
Calmodulin, 495
Calorimeter, 113–114
Calorimetry, 113–115
Cancer, 402–403
Cannabis, 727
Canon-Bard theory, 753
Capacitance, 278–281
Capacitation, 509
Capacitors, 278–281
CAP–cAMP complex, 390
Capsomeres, 364
Carbohydrates, 669–677
Carbon, 63
Carbon-13, 39
Carbon dioxide, 501
Carboxylic acids, 143, 623–629
Carcinogens, 402
Cardiac muscle, 429, 489, 495
Carnot cycle, 121–122
Carrier proteins, 326
Cartesian coordinate system, 186
Cartilage, 432, 485
Cartilaginous joints, 486
Catabolism, 683
Catalyst, 124, 130–131, 135
Catecholamines, 440
Cathode, 166
Cations, 58, 328
CD4 cells, 474
CD8 cells, 474
cDNA, 395
Cell(s)
    biology of, 319–338

communication between, 328–329
extracellular components of, 336–337
intercellular junctions, 336–337
metabolism of, 339–358
Cell cycle, 398
Cell theory, 319
Cell voltage, 171–172
Cell-mediated immunity, 469, 474
Cell-to-cell communication, 516
Cellular adhesion molecules, 431
Cellular respiration, 346
Cellular response, 329
Cellular senescence, 516
Cellulose, 336, 677
Center of gravity, 224
Center of mass, 223–224
Central dogma, 378
Central maximum, 292
Central nervous system, 452–453
Centration, 718
Centrioles, 336
Centromere, 331, 376
Centrosome, 336
Cerebellum, 453
Cerebral cortex, 452
Cerebral hemispheres, 452
Cerebrospinal fluid, 452
Cerebrum, 452–453
Cervix, 506
Channel proteins, 325–326
Chargaff's rules, 371
Charge transfer, 262–263
Charles's law, 76
Chemical change, 97
Chemical equations, 97–104
Chemical equilibrium, 131–137
Chemical reactions, 112–113
Chemical shift, 568–569
Chemically gated channels, 326
Chemiosmosis, 355
Chiasma, 406
Chirality center, 544
Cholecystokinin, 439, 480
Cholesterol, 322, 361, 478, 544, 679, 690–693
Chorionic villi, 510, 512
Chromatin, 331, 390, 401
Chromatography, 580–585
Chromosomal inversion, 409

Chromosomal translocation, 409
Chromosomes
    description of, 331, 399, 404
    mutations, 408–410
Churning, 475
Chylomicrons, 478
Chyme, 476
Chymotrypsinogen, 477
Cilia, 335
Circadian rhythm, 726
Circle, 186
Circulatory system, 463–467
Cisternae, 333
Citric acid cycle, 352–354
Class, 821
Class disparities, 825
Classical conditioning, 767
Classification, 718
Cleavage, 511
Closed manometer, 74
Coagulation, 466
Coccus, 359
Cochlea, 459
Cochlear nerve, 460
Codominance, 414
Coelom, 514
Coenzymes, 341
Cofactors, 341
Cognition, 711–734
Cognitive development,
    717–719
Cognitive dissonance theory,
    760–762
Collaborative learning, 780
Collagen, 336, 431
Collectivistic cultures, 792
Colligative properties, 90–93
Collision theory, 123
Colloids, 93, 148
Combination reaction, 98
Combined gas law, 77
Combustion reaction, 99
Commensalism, 363
Common ion effect, 146–147
Communication, 793
Competitive inhibitors, 343
Complex ion, 148
Compressions, 250
Concave spherical mirror,
    294–295
Conduction, 120, 270
Cones, 462
Confabulations, 731
Configuration
    definition of, 47
    electron, 46
Conflict theory, 788, 806

Conformational analysis, 595
Conformers, 543
Conformity, 787, 812, 813–814
Conjugate acid–base pairs,
    149–150
Conjugation, 362, 561
Connective tissue, 431–432
Connexons, 449
Conn's syndrome, 440
Consciousness, 725–727
Conservation, 718
Conservation of energy, 109,
    217
Conservative force, 215
Constitutive DNA, 331
Constructive interference, 290
Continuation words, 855
Continuity equation, 240
Contrast words, 855
Convection, 120
Convergent evolution, 428–429
Converging lenses, 296–300
Conversion disorder, 747
Convex spherical mirror,
    295–296
Cooperative binding, 467
Cooperativity, 344, 499
Coordinate covalent bond, 67
Coordinates, 194
Corona radiata, 509
Corpus luteum, 508
Correspondent influence
    theory of attribution, 785
Corticosteroids, 438
Corticotropin-releasing
    hormone, 437
Cortisol, 440, 700
Coulomb force constant, 263
Coulomb's law, 58, 263–264
Covalent bonds, 57, 59,
    533–552
Covalent modification, 344
Cranial nerves, 453
Creatine phosphate, 494
Crenate, 325
Crests, 246
Creutzfeldt-Jakob disease, 367
Crime, 811
Cristae, 332
Critical analysis and reasoning
    skills section
    AAMC question type
        categories, 851–852
    answering strategies for
        questions, 852–857
    big picture questions,
        847–850
    detail questions, 850–851

diagramming the big picture,
    842–845
dichotomies, 838–839
extension questions, 850
finding the big picture,
    840–842
implied detail questions,
    850–851
improvements in, 835–836
literary techniques
    questions, 849
logical organization
    questions, 849
main idea questions, 848
mastering of, 837
overview of, 835
passages, 837–846
practice on, 837, 869–884
questions, 846–852
reading, 854–857
skimming for the big picture,
    845–846
specific detail questions,
    850
thinking skills, 847
timing strategy for, 836–837
tone questions, 848–849
Critical angle, 287
Cross-bridges, 491
Crossing-over, 406
Crude birth rate, 820
Crude death rate, 820
Cubic curve, 186
Cultural artifacts, 780
Cultural capital, 822
Cultural lag, 809
Cultural transmission, 808
Culture
    assimilation in, 810
    attributions affected by, 786
    definition of, 807
    expression of emotions
        affected by, 792
    identity formation affected
        by, 783–784
    material, 807
    socialization, 783–784, 787,
        810–814
    subcultures, 809–810
    symbolic, 807–809
Culture shock, 809
Curie, 304
Current, 270–271
Current density, 271
Cushing's syndrome, 440
Cyanohydrins, 620
Cyclic AMP, 390
Cyclohexanamine, 637

Cyclopentanecarboxylic acid,
    624
Cyclothymia, 748
Cytochrome proteins, 355
Cytochrome P-450s, 693
Cytokines, 474
Cytokinesis, 401
Cytoplasm, 320
Cytoplasmic inheritance, 333
Cytoplasmic organelles,
    330–334
Cytoplasmic streaming, 335
Cytosine, 370
Cytoskeleton, 335–336
Cytosol, 320
Cytotoxic cells, 474
Cytotrophoblast, 512

D

d orbitals, 44
Dalton's law of partial
    pressures, 80
Damping, 260
DC, 270
Deamination, 357
Decanoic acid, 143
Decay, radioactive, 304–306
Decision making, 720–721
Decomposition reaction, 98–99
Deferred imitation, 783
Degree of unsaturation, 560
Deindividuation, 764
Deletion mutation, 409
Demographic transition theory,
    819–820
Demography, 817–819
Denaturing protein, 667–668
Dendritic cells, 470
Density, 96–97, 234
Deoxynucleoside
    triphosphates, 374
Deoxyribonucleic acid. *See*
    DNA
Deoxyribonucleotides, 369
Deoxyribose, 369
Dependent personality
    disorder, 750
Depersonalization/
    derealization disorder,
    749
Dephosphorylation, 346
Depolarization, 445
Depressive disorders, 747, 751
Depth, 238–239
Depth perception, 716
Dermis, 503
Desmosomes, 337, 430
Destructive interference, 290

Developmental biology, 511–516
Deviance, 811–812
Dextrorotatory, 547
Diagramming
  for big picture, 842–845
  sentence, 855
Diamagnetic atoms, 48
Diaphragm, 497
Diastereomers, 544
Diastole, 464
Diatomic elements, 98
Diels–Alder reaction, 605
Diencephalon, 452
Differential association theory, 812
Differentiation, 515
Diffraction, 285, 290–292
Diffusion, 81
Digestive system, 474–480
Dihedral angle, 597
Dihybrid cross, 417
Dihydroxyacetone phosphate, 349
Dilution, 145
Diploid somatic cells, 404
Dipole interactions, 84
Dipole/dipole moment, 68
Directional selection, 425
Disaccharides, 670, 675–676
Discrimination, 824
Disequilibrium, 717
Dishabituation, 771
Disinhibited social engagement disorder, 746
Disorganized attachment, 795
Dispersion, 287–288
Displacement, 189, 250
Displacement reactions, 99–100
Display rules, 792
Disproportionation reaction, 104
Disruptive selection, 426
Dissociative disorders, 749
Distal convoluted tubule, 483
Distillation, 577–580
Divergent evolution, 428–429
Diverging lenses, 296–300
Divided attention, 716
DNA
  complementary base-pairing system of, 371–372
  description of, 320, 368
  function of, 372
  mutations, 377
  nitrogenous bases of, 368
  recombinant, 393

replication of, 372–378
structure of, 370–371
DNA fingerprinting, 383
DNA gyrase, 373
DNA helicase, 373
DNA hybridization, 372, 396–397
DNA libraries, 394–395
DNA ligase, 374
DNA methylation, 391
DNA polymerase III, 373
DNA polymerases, 376
DNA primase, 373
DNA sequencing, 396
DNA supercoils, 331
DNA technology, 397–398
Dominance, 413–414
Dominative prejudice, 789
Dopamine, 437, 450, 727
Doppler effect, 255–257
Dorsal rami, 453
Double displacement reaction, 99
Double gene cross, 417–419
Double helix, 370
Double inclined planes, 200
Double-slit interference, 290–291
Down-regulation, 389
Dramaturgical approach, 791
Drift, 270
Drift velocity, 270
Drive reduction theory, 758
Duodenum, 478
Dynamic equilibrium, 87, 132

E

Ear, 457–460
Ecological niches, 428
Ectopic pregnancy, 507
Effective collision, 123
Effective nuclear charge, 48
Effusion, 81
Ego, 776
Ego identity, 778
Ego integrity versus despair, 779
Egocentrism, 718
Eicosanoids, 698
Elaboration likelihood model, 772
Elastin, 431
Electra complex, 777
Electric field, 264–266
Electric potential, 268–269
Electrical potential, 169
Electrochemical cell, 165
Electrochemistry, 165–173, 682

Electrolytes, 141, 272
Electrolytic cells, 165–166, 172
Electromagnetism, 281–285
Electromotive force, 169–173, 274–275
Electron(s)
  configuration of, 46
  number of, in energy levels, 46
  structure of, 37–38
  valence, 48, 52, 54
Electron affinity, 55
Electron transport chain, 354
Electronegativity, 55–56, 271
Electron-volt, 268
Electrophoresis, 669
Electrostatic induction, 263
Electrostatics
  charge transfer, 262–263
  definition of, 262
  electric field, 264–266
  Gauss's law, 266–267
  induction, 263
Elemental analysis, 564
Elements
  chemical properties of, 52–57
  main group, 49
  rare earth, 49
  representative, 49
Ellipse, 186
Emblems, 792
Embryogenesis, 511–515
emf, 169–173, 274–275
Emigration, 820
Emission spectrum, 42
Emotion
  adaptive role of, 753
  biological processes' role in perceiving of, 754–756
  components of, 752
  expression of, 792–793
  physiological markers of, 756
  theories of, 753–754
  universal, 753
Emotional support, 795
Empirical formula, 95–96
Empirical gas laws, 75
Emulsion, 93
Enantiomers, 544, 546–548
Encoding, 728
End replication problem, 375
Endergonic, 338
Endochondral ossification, 485
Endocrine signaling, 329
Endocrine system, 432–441, 735
Endocytosis, 327

Endolymph, 459
Endometrium, 506
Endoplasmic reticulum, 333
Endorphins, 450–451
Endoskeleton, 486
Endospore, 363
Endosymbiotic hypothesis, 332
Endothermic reaction, 108–109
Endotoxins, 360
Energy, 215–216
  law of conservation of, 109
  rotational, 233
  wavelength and, 41
Energy diagram, 126
Enhancer, 392
Enolates, 621
Enolization, 621
Enteric endocrine system, 479
Enteric nervous system, 479
Enteroendocrine cells, 476
Enthalpy, 110, 112
Entropy, 115–116
Enzymatic cascade, 686
Enzyme(s)
  activity of, 342
  allosteric, 343
  as catalysts, 339–345
  classification of, 345
  description of, 131
  in DNA replication, 374
  inhibitors of, 343–344
Enzyme elasticity coefficient, 687
Enzyme-substrate complex, 340
Eosinophils, 470
Epidermis, 502
Epididymis, 505
Epigenetic inheritance, 391
Epimers, 672
Epinephrine, 440, 450
Epithelial tissue, 430
Equatorial bonds, 598
Equilibrium
  chemical, 131–137
  definition of, 122–123
Equilibrium constant, 133–134, 136, 145, 150
Equivalence point, 162
Equivalent weight, 154
Erikson, Erik, 776, 778–780
Escherichia coli, 368
Esterification, 627–628
Esters, 633–634
Estradiol, 507
Estrogen, 441
Ethnicity, 818
Ethnocentrism, 788

Ethylene glycol, 343
Euchromatin, 331
Eukaryotic cells
    description of, 320, 331
    DNA replication in, 375–378
    replication of, 398–403
Eustachian tube, 458
Evolution, 421–429
Excitatory postsynaptic
    potential, 448
Excoriation, 746
Exhaustive methylation, 641
Exocytosis, 327–328
Exogenous DNA, 393
Exons, 383
Exonucleases, 382
Exothermic reaction, 108–109
Expanded octet, 60
Expiratory reserve volume, 498
Explicit memory, 728
Expression of emotion,
    792–793
Expressivity, 415
Extended family, 814
External locus of control, 775
Extinction, 769
Extracellular matrix, 336, 431
Extraction, 575–577
Extranuclear inheritance, 411
Eye, 460–463

F

Facilitated diffusion, 325
Factitious disorder, 747
Facultative anaerobes, 363
Facultative DNA, 331
FAD, 683
Falling bodies, 194–197
Fallopian tubes, 506
Family, 810, 814
Farad, 278
Faraday's laws, 167, 284–285
Fats, anabolism of, 690
Fatty acids
    description of, 357
    free, 688
    metabolism of, 688–693
    oxidation of, 688–689
Feces, 479
Feedback inhibition, 344
Female reproductive system,
    506–508
Fermentation, 356
Fertility, 820
Fertilization, 509
Fibronectin, 336, 431
Fibrous joints, 486
Filling diagram, 46

Fimbriae, 361
Fingerprint region, 556
First ionization energy, 53–54
First law of thermodynamics,
    119
First-order reaction, 129
Fischer esterification, 628
Fischer projections, 671
Fission reaction, 303
Fixation, 777
Flagella, 335, 361
Flagellin, 361
Flashbulb memory, 730
Flat bones, 485
Fluid(s), 234–235
Fluid mosaic model, 323
Flux, 267
Flux control coefficient, 687
FMN, 683
Folkways, 808
Follicle-stimulating hormone,
    438
Foot-in-the-door
    phenomenon, 761
Force(s), 198–207
    frictional, 203–206
    magnetic, 282
    writing of, 223
Forebrain, 452
Forgetting, 731
Form constancy, 716
Formal charge, 61–62
Formal charge calculations,
    539
Formic acid, 143
Fovea centralis, 462
Fractional abundance, 39
Fractional distillation, 579–580
Frameshift, 386
Frameshift mutation, 409
Francium, 56
Fraternal twins, 509
Free body diagram, 200
Free energy, 136
Free fatty acids, 679–680, 688
Freezing point depression, 91
Frequency, 41, 246
Freud, Sigmund, 740, 776–778
Friction, 219
Frictional forces, 203–206
Friedel–Crafts alkylation, 608
Front to back inversion, 293
Front-stage self, 791
Fructose 1,6-bisphosphatase,
    685
Fructose 1,6-bisphosphate, 349
Fructose-6-phosphate, 349
Fuel metabolism, 700

Functional group, 554–555
Functionalism, 806
Fundamental attribution error,
    785
Fundamental harmonic, 248
Furanoses, 672
Fusion reaction, 303
Futile cycle, 695

G

GABA, 450
Gabriel synthesis, 639–640
Galileo, 194
Galvanic cells, 165, 167–169,
    172
Gametes, 404, 407
Ganglia, 452
Gap junctions, 337
Gardner, Howard, 723
Gas exchange, 499–501
Gas pressure, 74
Gases, 71–83
    density of, 97
    dissolving, 143
    solubility of, 142–143
    spectra of, 301
Gas–liquid chromatography,
    583
Gastric inhibitory polypeptide,
    480
Gastrin, 480
Gastrula, 513
Gastrulation, 513
Gate control theory of pain, 715
Gated channels, 326
Gauge pressure, 237
Gauss, 281, 566
Gauss's law, 266–267
Gay-Lussac's law, 77
GC content, 372
Gel electrophoresis, 395–396
Gender, 792–793, 822
Gender-conflict theory, 806
Gene(s), 372, 378, 396, 412, 735
Gene cloning, 394
Gene deletion, 409
Gene duplication, 409
Gene expression, 372, 378,
    389–393, 396
Gene flow, 423
Gene pool, 421
Gene repression, 390
General adaptation syndrome,
    762–763
Generalized anxiety disorder,
    745
Generativity versus stagnation,
    779

Genetic drift, 423
Genetic engineering, 385
Genetically modified
    organisms, 393
Genetics, 412–420
Genital stage, 777–778
Genome, 372
Genophore, 331
Genotype, 412–413
Germ cells, 503
Ghrelin, 480, 702
Gibbs free energy, 117, 338
Giftedness, 724
Gigawatts, 186
Gillian, Carol, 782
Glial cells, 430, 443
Globalization, 820
Globular proteins, 666
Glucagon, 439, 480
Gluconeogenesis, 357, 477,
    684–685, 694–696
Glucose, 477
Glucose-6-phosphate, 348,
    684–685
Glutamate, 450
Glyceraldehyde, 670
Glyceraldehyde 3-phosphate,
    350
Glyceraldehyde 3-phosphate
    dehydrogenase, 350
Glycocalyx, 323, 361
Glycogen metabolism, 686–687
Glycogen synthase, 687
Glycogenesis, 477
Glycogenolysis, 477, 686
Glycolipids, 322, 328, 361
Glycolysis, 347–352, 684–685,
    700
Glycoproteins, 323, 328, 367
Glycosaminoglycans, 336, 431
Glycosylation, 334
Goffman, Erving, 794
Going across a group, 53
Going down a group, 53
Golgi body, 334
Golgi tendon organs, 456
Gonadotropin-releasing
    hormone, 437
Gonads, 404, 440–441
G-protein coupled membrane
    receptors, 329
Graded potential, 445
Graham's law, 81–82
Gram-negative bacteria, 360
Gram-positive bacteria, 360
Granzymes, 474
Graphing, 186–188
Gravitation, 207

Gravity, 194, 207, 224
Group closure, 788
Group polarization, 765–766
Group processes, 765–766
Groups, 816
Groupthink, 766, 816
Growth factors, 434
Growth hormone, 438
Growth hormone–releasing
    hormone, 437
Guanine, 370

H
Habituation, 771
Hair, 503
Hair follicle receptors, 456
Half-cells, 167
Half-life of first-order
    reaction, 129
Half-reactions, 103
Hallucinations, 748
Hallucinogens, 727
Halo effect, 786
Haloform reaction, 623
Halogenation, 599
Halogens, 51
Haploid daughter cells, 407
Haptens, 471
Hardy–Weinberg principle,
    420–421
Haworth projections, 673
Health disparities, 825
Healthcare disparities, 826
Hearing, 714
Heart, 463–465
Heat, 107
Heat capacity, 113–114
Heat of combustion, 114
Heat of fusion, 121
Heat of reaction, 110–112
Heat of vaporization, 121
Heat transfer, 120
Heating curve, 89–90
Heisenberg Uncertainty
    Principle, 42
Hell–Volhard–Zelinskii
    reaction, 628
Helper cells, 474
Hematocrit, 466
Hemiacetal, 620, 672
Hemolyze, 325
Henderson–Hasselbalch
    equation, 160
Henry's law, 500
Heredity, 736
Hess's law of heat summation,
    112
Heterochromatin, 331, 376

Heterocyclic amines, 638
Heterogeneous, 137
Heuristic, 420
Hexanoic acid, 143
Hexokinase, 348, 684–685
Hexoses, 672
Hidden curriculum, 810
High performance liquid
    chromatography, 585
Higher power curves, 186
Hindsight bias, 785
Histone acetylation, 391
Histones, 331
Histrionic personality
    disorder, 750
Hoarding disorder, 746
Hofmann elimination,
    641–642
Hofmann rearrangement, 635
Holoenzyme, 341
Homeostasis, 319, 467,
    683–684
Homogeneous, 137
Homologous chromosomes,
    400
Homologous pairs, 404
Homologous traits, 429
Hooke's law, 218, 220
Horizontal gene transfer, 362,
    367
Hormones, 432–434, 437–438
Hostile aggression, 794
Hückel's rule, 588
Human anatomy, 429–516
Human chorionic
    gonadotropin, 510
Humoral immunity, 469
Hund's rule, 47–48
Hybrid orbitals, 65–66
Hybridization, 396–397
Hydration, 140
Hydration number, 140
Hydration shell, 140
Hydraulics, 237–238
Hydrocarbon chemical
    reactions, 599–610
Hydrogen atom, 300–301
Hydrogen bonding, 83–84,
    612
Hydrogen bonds, 88
Hydrogen cyanide, 61
Hydrolysis, 157–159
Hydronium ion, 142, 151
Hydrophilic, 322
Hydrophobic, 322
Hydrostatic pressure, 465
Hyperadrenalism syndromes,
    440

Hyperbola, 186
Hyperpolarization, 445
Hypertonic solution, 324–325
Hypnosis, 726
Hypochondria, 747
Hypodermis, 503
Hypomania, 748
Hypophyseal portal system,
    437
Hypothalamus, 436–437, 452
Hypotonic solution, 324–325

I
Id, 776
Ideal gas law, 78–79
    deviations from, 82
Ideal gases, 75–83
Identical twins, 509
Identity
    cultural influences on,
        783–784
    definition of, 773
    description of, 774
    formation of, 776–784
    moral development theory
        of, 776, 781–782
    psychosexual development
        theory of, 776–778
    psychosocial development
        theory of, 776, 778–780
    social, 774
    social factors that affect,
        783
    socialization influences on,
        783–784
    sociocultural theory of, 776,
        780–781
    types of, 775–776
Identity achievement, 779
Identity crisis, 779
Identity versus role confusion,
    779
Ileum, 479
Illness anxiety disorder, 747
Imines, 620, 636
Immigration, 820
Immigration status, 818–819
Immiscible, 143, 576
Immune system, 468–474
Immunoglobulins, 471–472
Implicit memory, 728
Impression management, 790
Impressions, 786
Inborn errors of metabolism,
    411
Inbreeding, 423
Incentive theory, 758
Inclined planes, 199–201

Incomplete dominance, 414
Incus, 458
Independent assortment
    principle, 407
Individuation, 776
Induced fit, 340
Induction, 263, 516
Industry versus inferiority,
    779
Infant mortality rate, 820
Inference, 786
Information-processing
    model, 717
Infrasound, 254
In-group/out-group bias, 774
Inhibin, 506
Inhibitory postsynaptic
    potential, 448
Initiation factors, 388
Initiative versus guilt, 778–779
Innate immune response,
    468–469
Inner ear, 458
Inner transition metals, 51
Insertion mutation, 409
Insomnia, 726
Inspiratory reserve volume,
    498
Instantaneous power, 222–223
Instrumental support, 795
Insulin, 394, 439, 480
Integral membrane proteins,
    323
Integrins, 336, 431
Integumentary system,
    501–504
Intellectual disability, 724
Intelligence, 722–724
Intensity, 255
Intercalated disks, 495
Intercellular junctions, 337
Interference, 732
Interferons, 474
Intergenerational mobility,
    822
Interleukins, 474
Intermediate filaments, 335
Internal locus of control, 775
International Union of Pure
    and Applied Chemistry,
    552
Interneurons, 451
Interphase, 398–400
Interspersed elements, 384
Intestine, 478–479
Intimacy versus isolation, 779
Intracellular receptors, 435
Intrafusal fibers, 456

Intragenerational mobility, 822–823
Intramembranous ossification, 485
Intrapulmonary pressure, 498
Introns, 383
Inverse square law, 58, 255
Ion channels, 326, 443–444
Ionic bonds, 57–59
Ionic compounds, 59
Ions, 58–59, 138–140, 262
IQ, 723–724
Iris, 462
Iron law of oligarchy, 817
Irregular bones, 485
Irreversibility, 718
Islets of Langerhans, 477
Isoelectric point, 665
Isoelectronic, 59
Isolation, 824
Isometric contraction, 494
Isopropanamine, 637
Isotonic contraction, 494
Isotonic solution, 324
Isotopes, 39–40, 302
IUPAC. *See* International Union of Pure and Applied Chemistry

J

Jacob–Monod model, 389
James-Lange theory, 753
Jejunum, 479
Joint kinesthetic receptors, 456
Joints, 486–488, 488
Joule, 213
Juxtacrine signaling, 329

K

Karyotype, 404
Kelvin scale, 72–73
K_{eq} 133–134, 147
Keratin, 502
Keratinocytes, 502
Ketoacidosis, 477
Ketone bodies, 477, 689
Ketones, 616–623
Ketose, 670
Kidneys, 480–483
Kinases, 345
Kinematic equations, 190
Kinetic energy, 215
Kinetic energy of rotation, 233
Kinetic-molecular theory, 71–75
Kinetics, 122–131, 137
Kinetochore, 399

Kohlberg, Lawrence, 776, 781–782
Korsakoff's syndrome, 731
Krebs cycle, 352–354
K_{sp}, 146
K_{w}, 150

L

Labeling theory, 812
Labor, 510
Lac operon, 389
Lactation, 510
Lacteals, 467
Lactic acid fermentation, 356, 494
Lagging strand, 374
Laminar flow, 243
Langerhan's cells, 502
Language, 733–734, 780–781, 808
Large intestine, 479
Latency stage, 777
Lateral gene transfer, 367
Lateral inversion, 293
Lattice energy, 58
Law of conservation of energy, 109
Law of mass action, 133
Le Châtelier's principle, 134–136, 146, 164, 501, 633
Leading strand, 374
Leakage, genetic, 423
Learning
    associative, 766–771
    collaborative, 780
    nonassociative, 771
    observational, 772
Lens maker's formula, 294
Lenses, 296–300
Lenz's law, 285, 307
Leptin, 701
Leukocytes, 466, 469
Lever arm, 225
Levorotatory, 547
Lewis acid, 67, 150
Lewis acid–base theory, 150
Lewis base, 67
Lewis dot structures, 60–67, 533–537
Leydig cells, 505
Libido, 776
Ligaments, 488
Ligand gated channels, 326, 443, 492
Ligands, 148, 326–327
Limbic system, 754
Limiting reagent, 106–107

Lindlar's catalyst, 607
Linear momentum, 223
Linear motion, 188–193
Lipase, 475
Lipids, 677–681
Lipogenesis, 477
Lipopolysaccharides, 360
Lipoproteins, 478, 692
Liquids, 83–86, 88
Literary techniques, 849
Lithium, 39
Litmus, 164
Liver, 476–477
Locus of control, 774–775
Log–linear graphing, 187–188
Log–log graphing, 188
London dispersion forces, 85
Lone pairs, 63
Long bones, 485
Longitudinal waves, 245, 249–252
Long-term memory, 719, 728, 732
Long-term potentiation, 732
Looking-glass self, 774
Loop of Henle, 483
Lumen, 333
Luteinizing hormone, 438
Lyman Series, 42
Lymph, 467–468
Lymphatic system, 467–468
Lymphocytes, 469–470
Lyses, 365
Lysogenic conversion, 367
Lysogenic cycle, 366
Lysosomes, 327, 334
Lytic cycle, 365

M

Macroevolution, 421
Macrophages, 470
Mad cow disease, 367
Magnetic field, 281–282
Magnetic quantum number, 44–45
Magnetism, 281
Magnitude of K_{eq}, 133
Main group elements, 49
Major depressive disorder, 747
Major histocompatibility complex, 471
Male reproductive system, 504–506
Malleus, 458
Manometer, 74–75, 238–240
Marijuana, 727
Markovnikov's rule, 603

Mass, 207–212, 220
Mass media, 811
Mass number, 38–39, 302
Mass percent, 94–95, 145
Mass spectrometer/ spectrometry, 283–284, 563–565
Mass–spring system, 258–259
Mass-to-charge ratio, 564
Mastication, 475
Matching hypothesis, 794
Material culture, 807
Matrix, 332
Maxwell–Boltzmann distribution, 73
MDMA, 727
Mead, George Herbert, 783
Mean free speed, 270
Mechanical energy, 221
Mechanical waves, 245–257
Meditation, 726
Medulla oblongata, 453, 497
Megahertz, 186
Meiosis, 404–412
Meissner's corpuscle, 456, 504
Melanin, 502
Melanocytes, 502
Membrane permeability, 323
Membrane potential, 328
Membrane proteins, 323
Membrane receptors, 323
Memory
    aging effects on, 731
    emotion and, 730
    encoding of, 728
    explicit, 728
    implicit, 728
    limitations of, 732
    long-term, 719, 728, 732
    retrieval of, 729–730
    short-term, 719, 728, 732
    synaptic connections in, 732–733
    types of, 719, 728, 732
Memory cells, 473
Memory construction, 732
Memory decay, 732
Memory storage, 728
Menisci, 488
Menstrual cycle, 508
Menstruation, 506
Mercury manometer, 238–240
Meritocracy, 823
Merkel's cells, 502
Merton, Robert, 811
Meso compound, 549
Messenger RNA, 379
Metabolic cascade, 329

Metabolic control analysis, 687
Metabolism
    fatty acids, 688–693
    fuel, 700
    glycogen, 686–687
    hormonal regulation of, 697–702
    principles of regulation, 683–687
    proteins, 693–694
    tissue-specific, 699–700
Metallic solids, 86
Metalloids, 50–51
Metals, 57
    alkali, 51
    description of, 50–51
    valence electrons, 54
Metaphase, 400
Metric prefixes, 185
Metric units, 186
Michaelis–Menten constant, 341
Michaelis–Menten curve, 342
Microarrays, 396
Microbiology
    prokaryotic cells, 320, 359–363
    viruses, 363–367
Microevolution, 421
Microfilaments, 335
MicroRNAs, 392
Microtubule organizing centers, 336
Microtubules, 335
Migration, 820
Mirror neurons, 772, 783
Mirrors, 293–296
Miscibility, 576
Miscible, 143
Mismatch repair, 377
Missense codons, 386
Mitochondria, 332–333
Mitochondrial DNA, 333
Mitosis, 400–401
Mitotic spindle, 399–400
Mixed anhydrides, 631
Mixed inhibition, 343
Molality, 91, 144
Molar mass, 94
Molar volume of gas and gas density, 79
Molarity, 144
Mole, 94
Mole fraction, 144–145
Molecular chaperones, 668
Molecular dipole moment, 70

Molecular formula, 95–96
Molecular geometry, 62
Molecular orbital theory, 561
Molecular weight, 93–94
Mole–mole ratios, 104
Moments of inertia, 231–233
Momentum, 223
Monoatomic ions, 138–139
Monocytes, 470
Monohybrid cross, 417
Monosaccharides, 670–675
Monosynaptic reflex, 454
Moral development theory, 776, 781–782
Morality, 781
Mores, 808
Mortality, 820
Motion, 716
Motivation, 757–759
Motor development, 738
Mucous cells, 476
Multicellular, 320
Multiculturalism, 810
Multiple bonds, 537
Multiple intelligences, 722–723
Muscle spindles, 456
Muscle tissue, 429–430, 489–496
Muscle tone, 496
Muscular system, 488–496
Mutagens, 402, 408
Mutarotation, 673
Mutations, 422–423
    chromosomal, 408–410
    DNA, 377
Mutualistic, 363
Myelin sheath, 443
Myofibrils, 488
Myosin filaments, 488, 490

N

$n + 1$ splitting rule, 570
Nails, 503
Nanometer, 186, 561
Narcissistic personality disorder, 750
Narcolepsy, 726
Narcotics, 727
Natural killer T cells, 474
Natural selection, 427–428
Negative chemotaxis, 361
Negative cooperativity, 344
Negative feedback, 435
Negative punishment, 769
Negative reinforcement, 768
Nephron, 481–484
Nervous system, 441–463

Nervous system disorders, 751–752
Nervous tissue, 430
Net ionic equations, 100
Networks, 817
Neuromuscular junction, 492
Neurons, 430, 441–449, 735
Neuroplasticity, 732
Neurosecretory cells, 437
Neurosis, 777
Neurotransmitters, 449–451, 735
Neurulation, 513–514
Neutralization reactions, 100, 161
Neutrons, 38, 302
Neutrophils, 470
Newman projections, 596
Nichrome, 273
9 + 2 arrangement, 335
Nitric oxide, 451
Nitrobenzene, 608
Nitrogenous base, 368
Noble gas core notation, 48–49
Noble gases, 51
Nodes, 248
Nodes of Ranvier, 447
Nonassociative learning, 771
Nonchromosomal inheritance, 411
Noncoding sequences, 372
Noncompetitive inhibition, 343
Nonmetals, 50–51, 57
Nonpolar bonds, 68
Non-REM sleep, 725
Nonself recognition, 471
Nonsense codon, 386
Nonverbal communication, 793
Norepinephrine, 440, 450
Normality, 154
Norms, 808
Nuclear family, 814
Nuclear forces, 303–304
Nuclear lamina, 331
Nuclear membrane, 331
Nuclei, 302–303
Nucleic acids, 368
Nucleoid region, 361–362
Nucleolus, 331
Nucleophilic addition, 619
Nucleoplasm, 331
Nucleosome, 331
Nucleotide excision repair, 378
Nucleotides, 368–369

Nucleus, 38, 302–303, 331
Nuclide symbols, 38

O

Obedience, 813–814
Obesity, 701–702
Obligate anaerobes, 363
Observational learning, 772
Obsessive-compulsive disorders, 746
Obsessive-compulsive personality disorder, 750
Octanoic acid, 624
Octet rule, 57, 538
Oedipus complex, 777
Ohm, 272, 275
Okazaki fragments, 374, 376
Olfaction, 456–457
Oligarchy, 817
Oligosaccharides, 670, 676–677
Oncogenes, 402
Oncotic pressure, 465
1:2:1 genotypic ratio, 414
Oogenesis, 504, 507
Operant conditioning, 767–770
Operator, 389
Operon, 389
Opsin, 462
Optic chiasma, 463
Optic tracts, 463
Oral stage, 777
Orbital hybridization, 534–535
Orbitals, 43–44, 46–48, 65–66, 533–535
Organ of Corti, 459
Organic acids, 155
Organismal senescence, 516
Organizational socialization, 811
Organizations, 817
Organogenesis, 513–514
Origin of replication, 373
Osmolality, 467
Osmolarity, 436
Osmoregulation, 504
Osmosis, 324–325
Osmotic pressure, 92–93, 324
Ossicles, 458
Osteoblasts, 485
Osteoclasts, 484–485
Osteocyte, 485
Osteogenesis, 485
Osteoid, 485
Osteolysis, 485
Otitis media, 458
Outbreeding, 423

Oval window, 458
Ovarian cycle, 507
Ovaries, 441
Oxaloacetic acid, 685
Oxidation, 102, 166
Oxidation numbers, 100–101
Oxidative phosphorylation, 354
Oxygen capacity, 500
Oxygen group, 52
Oxytocin, 437–438

P
p53, 403
p orbitals, 43–44
Pacinian corpuscle, 456, 504
Pain, 715
Pancreas, 432, 439, 477
Panic disorder, 745
Paper chromatography, 583
Parabola, 186
Paracrine signaling, 329
Parallel
    capacitors in, 279–280
    resistors in, 276–277
Parallel evolution, 428
Paramagnetic atoms, 48
Paranoid personality disorder, 750
Parasitic, 363
Parasympathetic nervous system, 455
Parathyroid glands, 439
Parathyroid hormone, 439, 486
Parietal cells, 476
Parkinson's disease, 751
Parvocellular neurosecretory cells, 437
Pascal, 236
Pascal's principle, 237
Passive transport, 324–326
Patella, 488
Path difference, 290
Pauli Exclusion Principle, 45
Pauling scale, 55
Peak power, 222
Pedigree analysis, 517
Peer group, 811, 816
Peer pressure, 765
Peers, 774, 811
Penetrance, 415
Penis, 504–505
Penis envy, 777
Pentose phosphate pathway, 696–697
Pepsin, 344–345
Pepsinogen, 476

Peptide hormones, 433
Peptides, 665–666
Peptidoglycan, 360
Percent composition, 94–95
Percent yield, 107
Perception, 711–734, 786
Perceptual constancy, 716
Perceptual set, 786
Perforins, 474
Perilymph, 459
Periodic table
    chemical characteristics of, 49–52
    groups of, 51–52
    organization of, 49–52
Periods, 49
Peripheral circulation, 496
Peripheral nervous system, 451, 453–456
Peripheral proteins, 323
Periplasm, 360
Peristalsis, 475
Permeability, 323
Peroxisome proliferator-activated receptors, 702
Peroxisomes, 334
Persistent depressive disorder, 747
Personality
    behaviorist theory of, 742
    definition of, 739
    humanistic theory of, 740
    psychoanalytic theory of, 740
    social cognitive approach to, 741–742
    theories of, 740–742
    trait theory of, 741
Personality disorders, 749–751
pH, 164–165
pH meter, 164
pH scale, 150–152
Phagocytosis, 327
Phallic stage, 777
Pharming, 397
Pharyngotympanic tube, 458
Phase, 246
Phase diagrams, 88–89
Phase shift, 260
Phenols, 611–616
Phenotype, 412
Phenylketonuria, 411
Pheromones, 434
Phosphate group, 368
Phosphodiester bond, 370
Phosphoenolpyruvate, 351
Phosphofructokinase, 349
Phosphofructokinase-1, 685

Phospholipids, 322, 680–681
Phosphorylase A phosphatase, 687
Phosphorylation, 329, 346
Photons, 41
Phrenic nerve, 497
Physical change, 97
Physiological development, 737–739
Pi bond, 64–65, 535
Piaget, Jean, 717–718
Pinocytosis, 327
Pituitary gland, 437–438
Piwi-interacting RNA, 392
Placebo, 715
Placenta, 507, 510
Planck, Max, 40
Planck constant, 301
Planetary model, 40
Plasma, 466
Plasma cells, 473
Plasma membrane, 320, 322, 361
Plasmids, 362, 373
Plasmolyze, 325
Platelets, 466
Pluripotent, 397, 515
PO_2, 467
pOH, 150–152
Poiseuille's law, 242
Polar bonds, 68
Polarization, 285, 288–289
Polaroids, 288
Polyadenylation signal, 381
Polyatomic ions, 139–140
Polymerase chain reaction, 396
Polymers, 335
Polymorphism, 426
Polypeptides, 389
Polyploidy, 411
Polyprotic acids, 154, 165
Polyribosomes, 389
Polysaccharides, 670, 676–677
Polysynaptic reflex, 454
Pons, 453
Population, 420–421
Porins, 332
Positive chemotaxis, 361
Positive cooperativity, 344
Positive feedback, 435
Positive punishment, 769
Positive reinforcement, 768
Posttranscriptional modification, 334, 387
Post-traumatic stress disorder, 745, 762
Potential energy, 215

Potentials, 169
Poverty, 823
Power, 222–223, 275, 821
Predatory aggression, 794
Prefrontal cortex, 755–756
Prejudice, 787–790, 824
Premenstrual dysphoric disorder, 747
Prenatal development, 737
Pressure, 236–237
Prestige, 822
Primacy effect, 728
Primary group, 816
Primary reinforcer, 768
Primes, 676
Principal quantum number, 42
Principle of independent assortment, 407
Prions, 367–368
Private speech, 781
Privilege, 822
Problem solving, 720–721
Problem space theory, 722
Progesterone, 440
Projectile motion, 197–198
Projection, 786
Prokaryotic cells
    description of, 320, 359–363
    DNA replication in, 372–374
Prolactin, 438
Promoter, 389
Prophage, 366
Prophase, 400
Propinquity, 794
Proprioceptors, 456
Prostaglandins, 434
Prosthetic groups, 341
Protein kinase enzymes, 329, 346
Proteins
    description of, 379–393, 659, 665–669
    metabolism of, 693–694
Proteoglycans, 336, 431
Proton motive force, 361
Proton nuclear magnetic spectroscopy, 566–575
Proton-motive force, 355
Protons, 38, 302
Protooncogenes, 402
Proximal convoluted tubule, 483
Psychoanalytic theory, 740
Psychological disorders
    anxiety disorders, 744–745
    biomedical model of, 742

bipolar disorder, 747–748
classification of, 743
definition of, 742
depressive disorders, 747
dissociative disorders, 749
incidence of, 743
obsessive-compulsive
    disorders, 746
personality disorders,
    749–751
schizophrenia, 748–749,
    751
somatic symptom
    disorders, 747
stressor-related disorders,
    745–746
trauma disorders, 745–746
types of, 743–751
Psychosexual development
    theory, 776–778
Psychosocial development
    theory, 776, 778–780
Pull factors, 820
Pulmonary valve, 464
Punctuated equilibrium,
    428
Punishment, 769
Punnett square, 415–416, 419
Pupillary reflex, 462
Purines, 370
Push factors, 820
PV diagrams, 121–122
Pyranoses, 672
Pyrimidines, 370
Pyruvate, 352
Pyruvate dehydrogenase, 358
Pyruvate kinase, 685

Q
Q, 134, 147
Quanta, 40
Quantum mechanics, 37
Quantum numbers, 42–46,
    302
Quantum theory, 37

R
Race, 818, 822
Race-conflict theory, 806
Racemic mixture, 548
Radiation, 120
Radioactive decay, 304–306
Raoult's law, 90–91
Rare earth elements, 49
Rarefractions, 250
Rate law, 126–129
Rate-determining step, 130
Rate-limiting step, 130

Reaction mechanism, 130
Reactions
    chemical reactions,
        112–113
    thermodynamic control of,
        137
Reactive attachment, 745
Reading, 854–857
Real image, 293
Recall, 729
Recency effect, 728
Receptor-mediated
    endocytosis, 327
Reciprocal regulation, 695
Reciprocity, 794
Recognition, 729
Recombinant DNA, 393
Recrystallization, 585–588
Rectum, 479
Redox equations, 100–104
Redox titration, 165
Reducing agents, 626
Reduction, 102, 166
Reduction potential, 169
Reference groups, 783
Reflection, 285–287
Reflex arc, 454
Reflexes, 454, 462
Refraction, 285–286
Regulatory cells, 474
Reinforcement, 768–769
Relative fitness, 427
Relative poverty, 823
Relearning, 730
Religion, 814
Remodeling, bone, 485
Renal corpuscle, 482
Renin-angiotensin system,
    484
Replacement reaction, 99
Replication forks, 373
Repolarization, 445–446
Representative elements, 49
Representative heuristic, 421
Repression, 730
Reproductive system, 504–510
Residential segregation,
    824–825
Residual volume, 498
Resistance, 272–273
Resistivity, 273–274
Resistors, 275–278
Resonance structures, 66–67
Respiratory system, 496–501
Resting membrane potential,
    328
Resting potential, 444
Restriction enzymes, 393

Retina, 462
Retreatism, 812
Retrieval, memory, 729–730
Retrieval cues, 730
Retroviruses, 365, 379
Reverse transcriptase, 365,
    395
Reverse transcription, 365
Rhodopsin, 462
Ribonucleotides, 369
Ribose, 369
Ribosomal RNA, 330, 380
Ribosomes, 321, 387–388
Ribozymes, 330, 380
Right to left inversion, 293
Rigor mortis, 491
Ring strain, 595
Ritualism, 812
Rituals, 809
RNA, 368, 379–381
RNA polymerase, 380
RNA polymerase II, 380
RNA primer, 374
RNA splicing, 383
Rods, 462
Role conflict, 816
Role set, 816
Role strain, 816
Role taking, 783
Role-playing effect, 761
Roles, 816
Root mean square speed of
    gas, 81–82
Rotational energy, 233
Rough endoplasmic
    reticulum, 333
Rugae, 476
Rutherford, Ernest, 40
Rydberg equation, 41

S
Salt bridge, 167
Saltatory conduction, 447
Salts, 157–159
Sandmeyer reaction, 642
Saponification, 634, 680
Sarcolemma, 488
Sarcoplasm, 488
Satellite DNA, 376
Saturation kinetics, 341
Scaffolding, 780
Scala media, 459
Scala vestibuli, 459
Scalars, 189
Scapegoat, 787
Schachter-Singer theory,
    753–754
Schema, 717

Schizoid personality disorder,
    750
Schizophrenia, 748–749, 751
Schizotypal personality
    disorder, 750
School, 810–811
Sclera, 462
Scrotum, 505
Sebaceous glands, 503
Sebum, 503
Second law of
    thermodynamics,
    119–120
Second messengers, 329,
    434
Second order kinetics, 614
Second substrates, 341
Secondary group, 816
Secondary reinforcer, 768
Secretin, 480
Secure attachment, 795
Segregation, 407, 824
Selection, 425–426
Selective attention, 716
Selective mutism, 744
Selective perception, 786
Self-concept, 773–774
Self-efficacy, 775
Self-esteem, 774–775
Self-fulfilling prophecy, 774
Self-perceptions, 786
Self-presentation, 790–791
Self-recognition, 471
Self-schemas, 773
Self-serving bias, 785
Semen, 505
Semicircular canals, 459
Semidiscontinuous
    replication, 374
Semilunar valve, 464
Seminiferous tubules, 505
Semipermeable membrane,
    323
Senescence, 516
Sensory adaptation, 713, 771
Sensory organs, 456–463,
    711–715
Sensory processing, 711
Sensory threshold, 712
Sentence diagramming, 855
Separation anxiety disorder,
    744
Serial analysis of gene
    expression, 396
Seriation, 718
Series
    capacitors in, 280–281
    resistors in, 275–276

Series-parallel combination resistors, 277–278
Serotonin, 450
Sertoli cells, 505–506
Sesamoid bones, 485
Sex chromosomes, 404
Sex determination, 419
Sex hormones, 434
Sex linkage, 419–420
Sex pili, 361
Sex ratio, 817
Sexual dimorphism, 426
Sexual orientation, 819
Sexual selection, 426
Shaping, 769
Shivering reflex, 496
Short bones, 485
Short-term memory, 719, 728, 732
SI Units, 185
Sigma bond, 64–65, 535
Sigma factor, 381
Signal detection theory, 713
Signal sequence, 333
Signal transduction, 329
Signal transduction cascade, 329
Signal words, 854–855
Significant figures, 184
Silent mutation, 409
Similarity, 794
Simple diffusion, 324
Simple harmonic motion, 258, 260–262
Single displacement reaction, 99
Single gene cross, 415–417
Single nucleotide polymorphisms, 377
Single-slit diffraction, 291–292
Sister chromatids, 332, 399
Skeletal muscle, 429, 489–495
Skeletal system, 484–488
Skin, 501–504
Sleep, 725–726
Sliding filament model, 491
Small interfering RNAs, 392
Small intestine, 478–479
Small nuclear ribonucleoproteins, 383
Smooth endoplasmic reticulum, 334
Smooth muscle, 430, 515–516
SO_2, 467
Social anxiety disorder, 744
Social behavior, 793–795
Social capital, 822
Social class, 821

Social construction of reality, 807
Social constructionism, 807
Social control, 811
Social exclusion, 824
Social facilitation, 763–764
Social group, 816
Social identity, 774
Social identity theory, 774
Social institutions, 814–815
Social interactions
    actions and processes that underlie, 790–795
    attitudes and beliefs that affect, 784–790
    elements of, 815–817
Social learning theory, 741
Social loafing, 765
Social mobility, 822–823
Social movement, 820
Social perceptions, 786
Social reproduction, 822
Social stratification, 821–826
Social support, 795
Socialization, 783–784, 787, 810–814
Sociocultural theory, 776, 780–781
Sociology
    foundational concepts of, 805–821
    theoretical approaches, 806–807
Sodium bicarbonate, 477
Sodium-potassium pump, 326–327, 444
Solenoid, 283–284
Solids, 83–87, 142–143
Solubility, 140, 142
Solubility curve, 137–138
Solubility product constant, 145–147
Solute, 137, 324
Solution, 137, 324
Solution concentration, 144–145
Solution formation, 140
Solvation, 140–141
Solvent, 137
Somatic symptom disorders, 747
Somatosensory system, 715
Somatostatin, 437, 439, 480
Somites, 514
Sound transmission, 253–254, 459–460
Source monitoring, 732
Southern blot, 395–396

Spatial inequality, 824–825
Spatial summation, 448
Speciation, 427–429
Specific gravity, 234
Specific phobia, 744
Spectator ions, 100
Sperm, 506
Spermatids, 506
Spermatogenesis, 504, 505–506
Spermatogonia, 505
Spermatozoa, 506
Sphingolipids, 328
Sphingomyelins, 681
Spin quantum number, 45
Spina bifida, 514
Spinal cord, 453
Spirillus, 359
Spliceosome, 383
Spontaneity, 172
Spontaneous generation, 319
Spontaneous processes, 118
Spontaneous reactions, 117, 339
Stabilizing selection, 426
Standard deviation, 183–184
Standard temperature and pressure, 75
Standing wave, 247–249
Stapes, 458
Starch, 676
Starling forces, 465
Start codon, 384
State function, 109
States of matter
    gases. See Gases
    liquids, 83–86, 88
    phase changes, 87–90
    solids, 83–87, 142–143
Static electricity, 262
Stationary wave, 247–249
Status, 815–816, 821
Stem cells, 397, 751–752
Stereoisomers, 543–552
Stereotype threat, 790
Stereotypes, 790
Stereotyping, 786
Steric strain, 595
Sternberg, Robert, 723
Steroids, 678–679
Sticky ends, 393
Stigma, 813
Stimulants, 726
Stoichiometry, 93–107
Stomach, 475–476
Stop codon, 384
Straight line, 186
Strain theory, 811

Stress, 762–763
Stressor-related disorders, 745–746
Stretch reflex, 456
Strong acid, 153–154, 163
Strong base, 153–154, 162
Strong electrolytes, 141
Strontium-90, 305
Structural isomers, 543–544
Subcultures, 809–810
Substitution mutation, 409
Substitution reactions, 613
Substrate, 339
Substrate-level phosphorylation, 350
Subtle prejudice, 789
Sudoriferous glands, 503
Summation, 448, 493
Superego, 776
Surface tension, 243
Surfactant, 498
Surroundings, 108
Suspensions, 148
Sweat glands, 503
Symbolic culture, 807–809
Symbolic interactionism, 806–807
Symbolic prejudice, 789
Symbols, 808
Symmetric anhydrides, 631
Sympathetic nervous system, 454
Synapse, 447–449
Synapse fatigue, 449
Synapsis, 406
Synaptic cleft, 447
Synaptic knobs, 447
Synaptic pruning, 732
Syncytioblast, 512
Synovial fluid, 488
Synovial joints, 486, 488
Synthesis reaction, 98
System, 108
Systole, 464

T

T_3. See Triiodothyronine
T_4. See Thyroxine
T lymphocytes, 469–470
Targeting peptide, 333
Taste, 456–457
TATA box, 381
Tautomers, 621
Telomerase, 375
Telomeres, 375
Telophase, 401
Temperate phages, 366
Temperature, 73, 107, 117

Template strand, 380
Temporal summation, 448, 493
Tendons, 488
Terpenes, 679
Tesla, 281, 566
Testcross, 419
Testes, 440
Testosterone, 440
Tetanus, 493
Tetrads, 406
Tetramethylsilane, 567
Theory of planned behavior, 760
Theory of successive approximations, 761
Thermochemistry, 107–117
Thermodynamics, 118–122
Thermoregulation, 496, 503–504
Thin-layer chromatography, 581
Third law of thermodynamics, 120
3′-5′ exonuclease, 377
3:1 phenotypic ratio, 414
3-4-5 right triangle, 183
Three-factor model, 741
Thurstone, L. L., 723
Thymine, 370
Thyroid gland, 438
Thyroid-stimulating hormone, 438
Thyrotropin-releasing hormone, 436
Thyroxine, 438
Tidal volume, 498
Tight junctions, 337, 430
Titration, 106, 161–165
TLC plate, 581–582
Tonicity, 324
Torque, 223, 226–233
Torsional strain, 595
Total dead space, 499
Total internal reflection, 287
Total lung capacity, 499
Totipotent, 397, 515
Touch, 456
Transcription, 378–379, 380–382, 389
Transcription factors, 391

Transduction, 362, 367, 393
Transesterification, 633
Transfection, 394
Transfer RNA, 380, 386–387
Transformation, 362, 393
Transition metals, 49, 51
Transition state, 125
Translation, 378–379, 384–389, 389
Translation initiation complex, 388
Transmembrane proteins, 323
Transport proteins, 323
Transport vesicles, 327
Transposons, 362, 383, 408
Transpulmonary pressure, 498
Transuranic elements, 303
Transverse mutation, 409
Transverse waves, 245–247
Trauma disorders, 745–746
Triacylglycerols, 679–680
Triarchic theory of intelligence, 723
Tricarboxylic acid cycle, 352
Trichotillomania, 746
Tricuspid valve, 464
Triiodothyronine, 438
Triose isomerase, 349
Triplet codons, 384
Tropomyosin, 491
Troponin, 491
Troughs, 246
Trust versus mistrust, 778
Trypsin, 345
Trypsinogen, 477
Tumor-suppressor genes, 402
Turgor pressure, 325
Twins, 509
Tympanic membrane, 458
Tyndall effect, 93, 148

U

Ultrasound, 254
Uncompetitive inhibition, 343
Unicellular, 320
Unimolecular nucleophilic substitution, 614
Unit cell, 86
Units, 184–186
Universal emotions, 753

Unsaturated hydrocarbon chemical reactions, 601–610
Unsaturated hydrocarbons, 591
Up-regulation, 389
Uracil, 370
Urbanization, 821
Urinary system, 480–484
Urine, 483
Uterus, 506
UV/VIS absorption spectroscopy, 560–563

V

Vaccines, 473
Vacuoles, 334
Vacuum distillation, 579
Valence bond theory, 64
Valence electrons, 48, 52, 54
Valence shell electron pair repulsions theory, 62, 541–543
Values, 808
van der Waals equation, 82–83
van Leeuwenhoek, Anton, 319
Vapor pressure, 87–88, 90–91
Vasoconstriction, 467
Vasodilation, 467
Vectors, 189
Veins, 465
Velocity, 189, 216, 247, 259
Ventral body cavity, 514
Ventral rami, 453
Verbal communication, 793
Vestibular membrane, 459
Vestibular system, 715
Vestibulocochlear nerve, 460
Vibrational spectroscopy, 553
Virion, 364
Viroids, 367–368
Virtual image, 293
Viruses, 363–367
Viscosity, 241–242
Vision, 713–714
Visual processing, 463
Vital capacity, 498
Vitamin D, 504
Vocabulary, 856
Volt, 169, 268

Voltage gated channels, 327, 444, 492
Voltaic cells, 167–169
Voltmeter, 273
Volume flow rate, 241
Vulva, 506
Vygotsky, Lev, 719, 776, 780–781

W

Water-soluble vitamins, 341
Watson-Crick model, 370
Watts, 275
Wave summation, 493
Wavelength, 41, 246
Weak acids, 155–157, 162
Weak bases, 155–157, 163
Weak electrolytes, 141
Webber's law, 712
Weber, 281
Weight, 207–212
White adipose tissue, 699
White blood cells, 469
White matter, 451
Within-population variation, 421
Wittig reaction, 620
Wobble pairing, 386
Wolff–Kishner reaction, 620
Work, 121, 213–215, 274–275
Work–energy, 216–221

X

Xeroderma pigmentosum, 378
X-linked genes, 420

Z

Z lines, 490
Zeroth law of thermodynamics, 118
Zinc, 170
Zona fasciculata, 440
Zona glomerulosa, 440
Zona pellucida, 509
Zona reticularis, 440
Zone of proximal development, 780
Zwitterions, 663
Zygote, 509
Zymogen, 344